The 5 Minute Toxicology Consult

ASSOCIATE EDITORS

KATHERINE M. HURLBUT, M.D.

FACULTY
ROCKY MOUNTAIN POISON AND DRUG CENTER
DEPARTMENT OF EMERGENCY MEDICINE
DENVER HEALTH MEDICAL CENTER
DENVER, COLORADO

EDWIN K. KUFFNER, M.D.

FACULTY
ROCKY MOUNTAIN POISON AND DRUG CENTER
DENVER HEALTH MEDICAL CENTER
DENVER, COLORADO

LUKE YIP, M.D.

ATTENDING FACULTY
ROCKY MOUNTAIN POISON AND DRUG CENTER
ATTENDING PHYSICIAN
DEPARTMENT OF MEDICINE, SECTION OF CLINICAL TOXICOLOGY
DENVER HEALTH MEDICAL CENTER
CLINICAL ASSISTANT PROFESSOR
DEPARTMENT OF PHARMACEUTICAL SCIENCES
SCHOOL OF PHARMACY
UNIVERSITY OF COLORADO HEALTH SCIENCES CENTER
DENVER, COLORADO

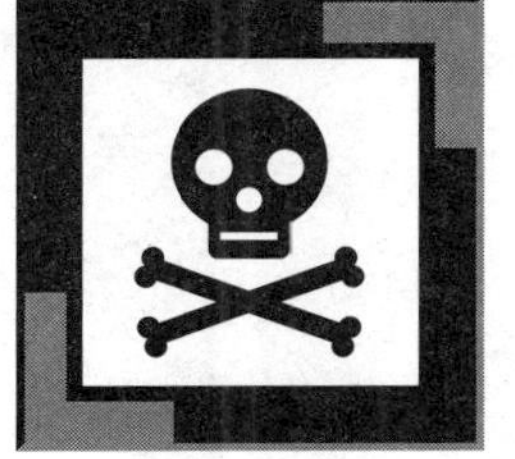
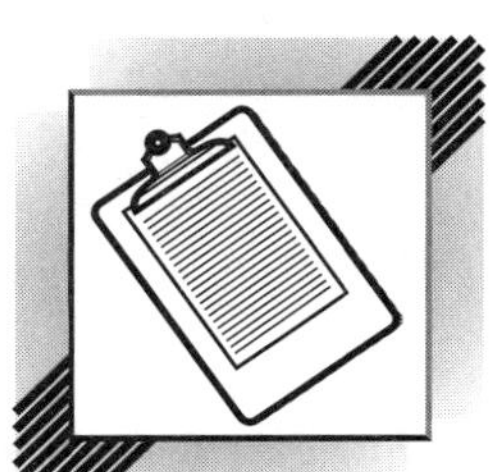
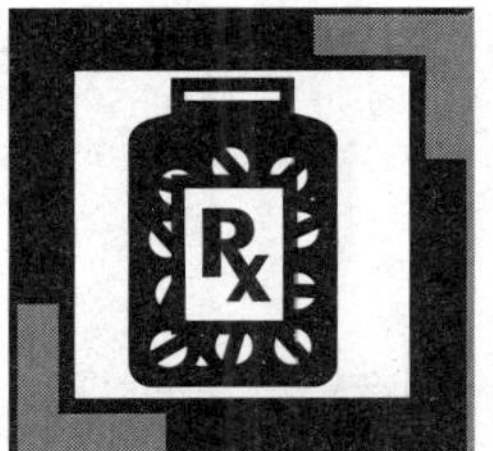
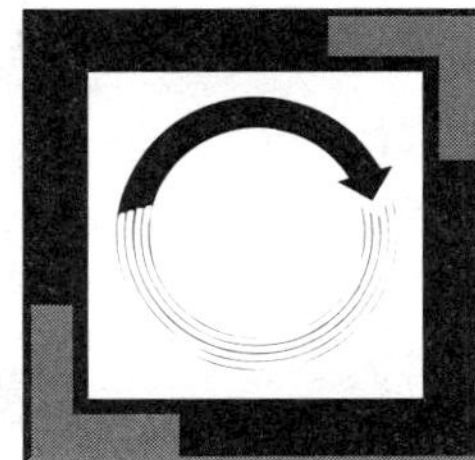
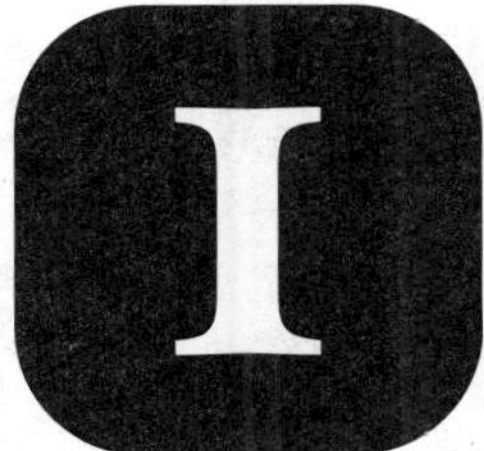
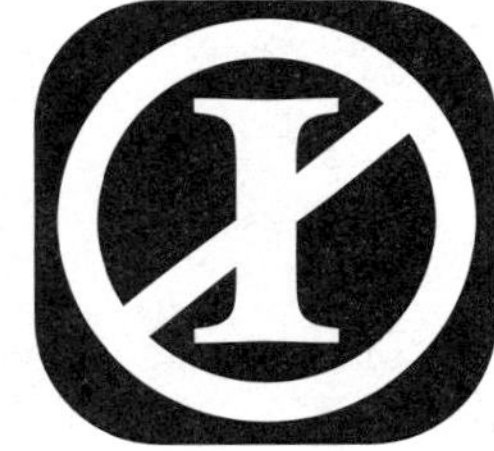
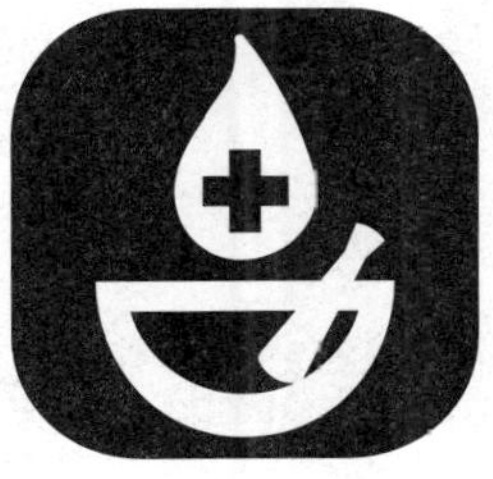
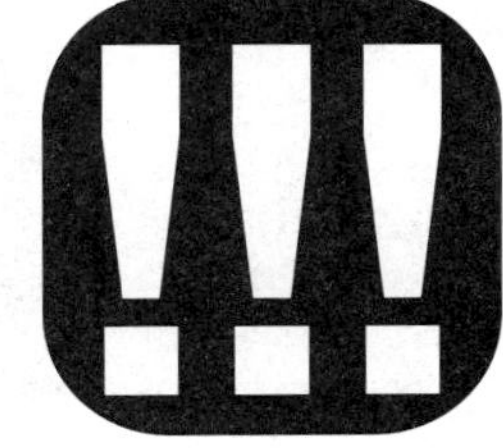

The 5 Minute Toxicology Consult

EDITOR

RICHARD C. DART, M.D., PH.D.

DIRECTOR, ROCKY MOUNTAIN POISON AND DRUG CENTER

DENVER HEALTH AND HOSPITAL AUTHORITY

ASSOCIATE PROFESSOR OF SURGERY AND MEDICINE

UNIVERSITY OF COLORADO HEALTH SCIENCES CENTER

DENVER, COLORADO

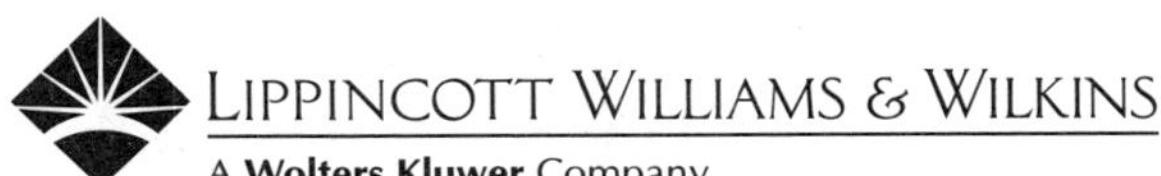

Philadelphia • Baltimore • New York • London
Buenos Aires • Hong Kong • Sydney • Tokyo

Acquisitions Editor: Elizabeth Greenspan
Managing Editor: Susan Rhyner
Supervising Editor: Mary Ann McLaughlin
Production Service: Colophon
Manufacturing Manager: Tim Reynolds
Compositor: PRD Group, Inc.
Printer: RR Donnelley/Crawfordsville

227 East Washington Square
Philadelphia, PA 19106-3780 USA
LWW.com

Printed in the USA

Library of Congress Cataloging-in-Publication Data

The 5 minute toxicology consult / editor, Richard C. Dart.
p. ; cm.
Includes bibliographical references and index.
ISBN 0-683-30202-7 (alk. paper)
1. Toxicology—Handbooks, manuals, etc. 2. Antidotes—Handbooks, manuals, etc. 3. Poisoning—Handbooks, manuals, etc. I. Title: Five minute toxicology consult. II. Dart, Richard C.
[DNLM: 1. Poisoning—Handbooks. 2. Antidotes—Handbooks. 3. Hazardous Substances—poisoning—Handbooks. QV 607 Z999 2000]
RA1215 .A14 2000
615.9—dc21 99-046468

10 9 8 7 6 5 4 3 2 1

To the patients and health care providers who have trusted the Rocky Mountain Poison and Drug Center since 1956.

To each of our callers. Their stimulating questions provided the impetus and focus to produce a practical tool for health care providers.

To the staff of the Rocky Mountain Poison and Drug Center whose dedication and commitment enable our poison center to provide high-quality care to patients throughout the United States.

To each toxicology fellow and toxicologist who trained or volunteered at the Rocky Mountain Poison and Drug Center. Their knowledge, research, and thoughtful critiques are reflected throughout this book.

Richard C. Dart, M.D., Ph.D.
Katherine M. Hurlbut, M.D.
Edwin K. Kuffner, M.D.
Luke Yip, M.D.

To NSL, LGS, KML, ASL, CRF, KAK, RC, SJI.

In Memorial: Brian and Paddy, Eddie, and Teresa.

Luke Yip, M.D.

Preface

Toxicology is an enigma to many health care providers. It involves a diverse group of medications, chemicals, natural compounds, and their interactions. Often the conditions under which toxicity develops seem arcane to the practitioner who, if faced with a diverse group of patients, find that nearly all of them are not poisoned!

The goal of this book is to simplify the life of the health care provider faced with a poisoned patient. We designed an easy-to-use tool that will provide accurate, current, and reliable information focusing on practical patient care.

To make *The 5 Minute Toxicology Consult* easy to use, standard categories are presented in each chapter so that you know precisely where to find the information you need. For example, recommendations regarding admission and discharge criteria are addressed at the same place in every chapter. Within the categories you can expect to find clinically relevant issues. Reliability and consistency have been addressed by the active involvement in every chapter of at least two experienced, board-certified, practicing emergency physicians and toxicologists.

An entire section of the book addresses the evaluation of patients who present without an identified poisoning, but in whom a poisoning is suspected. For example, what should the health care provider consider when a patient presents with pulmonary edema of possible toxicological cause?

This book was designed to be a practical and easy-to-access resource for basic care of the poisoned patient. We hope you find it useful and we encourage your comments to Lippincott Williams & Wilkins so that we can make subsequent editions even more user friendly.

Contributing Authors

MICHAEL ANDERSON
PAUL BENDER
GREGORY M. BOGDAN
ALVIN C. BRONSTEIN
THOMAS G. BURKE
CHARLES B. CAIRNS
BENJAMIN CAMP
EDWARD W. CETARUK
RICHARD CHEN
FRANK F.S. DALY
RICHARD C. DART
JOU-FANG DENG
CHRISTOPHER R. DeWITT
CHRIS FLEMING
MARTHA M. FOLEY
MARK C. GOODMAN
KATHLEEN GRAHAM
WYATT J. HALL
KENNON HEARD
KAREN BRIGID-ITA HOLOWINSKI
RIVKA S. HOROWITZ
KATHERINE M. HURLBUT
MICHAEL D. JANKOVIAK
HEATH JOLLIFF
WEI-FONG KAO
LADA KOKAN
EDWIN K. KUFFNER
CHRISTOPHER LAYTON
KEVIN M. LIER
GAYLE E. LONG
DAVID MAGILNER
JOHN P. MARSHALL
ROBIN MILLIN
JAY MULLEN
DAVID NYMAN
GERALD F. O'MALLEY
ROBERT ORMAN
JEFFREY S. PETERSON
SCOTT D. PHILLIPS
NETTI RIGGS
JEFFREY ROGERS
MELISSA J. RUYLE
JULIE SEAMAN
STEVEN A. SEIFERT
BILL SEVCIK
MICHAEL STACKPOOL
DAN STILLMAN
JANA VANDER LEEST
ROBERT E. VANDER LEEST
TIMOTHY VanDUZER
NIRMAL K. VEERAMACHANENI
MELANIE A. WELLS
BRIAN T. WILLIAMS
KATHLEEN M. WRUK
LUKE YIP

Contents

SECTION IV. CHEMICAL AND BIOLOGICAL AGENTS

SECTION I

General Approach

Nontoxic Ingestion

Basics

DESCRIPTION

A patient presentation that involves an exposure to a substance thought to be nontoxic. A compound should be considered nontoxic only if the following conditions are met:

- The product has been unequivocally identified.
- Only one product is involved.
- The label does not contain a warning from the Consumer Product Safety Commission, and the product in the bottle appears to be the original product (i.e., no substitution has occurred).
- The amount of product ingested can be accurately estimated.
- The route of exposure can be accurately determined.
- The patient is free of signs or symptoms of drug effect, both subjectively and objectively.
- Follow-up must be both available and reliable (e.g., parent or guardian).

If any of these conditions are not met or are questionable, the patient should be managed as an unknown ingestion. As Paracelsus said, "All substances are poisons; there is none that is not a poison, the right dose differentiates a poison and a remedy."

PATHOPHYSIOLOGY

By definition, a nontoxic ingestion should not produce any adverse health effects. Massive ingestions may produce some mild effects such as GI discomfort or obstruct the airway.

DRUG INTERACTIONS

Nontoxic compounds may interact with medications that are being taken therapeutically.

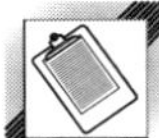

Diagnosis

DIFFERENTIAL DIAGNOSIS

Following is an alphabetical list of items generally considered to be nontoxic.

Household Items

- Ashes
- baby products
- ballpoint pen ink
- body conditioner
- bubble bath
- candles
- caps for toy guns
- caulk
- chalk produced in the United States
- charcoal
- clay
- cosmetics
- crayons produced in the United States
- deodorant
- erasers
- fabric softener
- felt-tip pens
- hand lotions
- highlighting markers
- household bleach
- indelible markers
- kitty litter
- latex paint
- laundry detergent (liquid)
- lipstick
- magic markers
- newspapers produced in the United States
- pencil lead (actually graphite)
- petroleum jelly
- pet foods or chew toys (not including pet medications)
- photographs
- plastics
- playing cards
- Play-doh
- rubber cement
- shampoos
- shaving cream
- shoe polish
- silica gel
- Silly Putty
- soaps
- spackle
- starch
- sunscreens
- sweeteners
- teething ring contents
- thermometer mercury
- toilet water
- toothpaste
- water color paints
- white glue

Medications

- Antacids
- calamine lotion
- birth control pills (if single ingestion)
- corticosteroids (if single ingestion)
- mineral oil (unless aspirated)
- oral antibiotics (some exceptions)
- water-soluble vitamins (excluding iron)
- zinc oxide
- zirconium oxide

Plants

Many plants are nontoxic. Due to regional variations in names, a poison center should be contacted if a substantial amount of any plant is ingested. A partial list of nontoxic plants is as follows:

- African violet
- aralia
- baby tears
- bird's nest fern
- bridal veil
- Coleus X hydrus
- corn plant
- creeping Jenny
- Dracaena indivisa
- dwarf schefflera
- emerald ripple
- fiddle-leaf fig
- gardenia
- grape ivy
- jade plant
- wandering Jew
- parlor palm
- peacock plant
- piggyback begonia
- piggyback plant
- prayer plant
- rubber tree
- snake plant
- spider plant
- string of hearts
- swedish ivy
- velvet plant
- wax plant
- zebra plant

Miscellaneous

Dehumidifying packets (silica or charcoal), grease and motor oils (unless aspirated), magnesium silicate, paint (indoor or latex), titanium oxide

SIGNS AND SYMPTOMS

History is a crucial element in determining a nontoxic ingestion.

- What substances did the patient have access to?
- What medications were prescribed to the patient or other family members?
- When was the last time the patient was seen?
- Were there initial symptoms that have resolved?
- Were substances at the scene brought to the emergency department for possible identification and/or analysis?
- There should be no signs or symptoms at presentation. If they do develop, the patient should be managed as an unknown ingestion.
- Refer to the specific drug chapter when particular findings suggest that drug as a possible source of toxicity. For example, rapid heart rate is covered in the Tachycardia chapter in SECTION II.

LABORATORY TESTS

If history confirms a nontoxic exposure, no testing is required. Suicidal ingestions should be managed as unknown ingestions, even if the patient claims that only nontoxic materials were ingested.

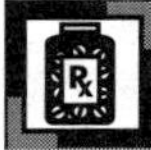

Treatment

DIRECTING PATIENT COURSE

Dosage and timing should be determined for all substances that could be involved. It is important to evaluate the need for consultation with a poison center or other specialists in order to confirm the lack of toxicity of the ingestion.

DECONTAMINATION

Do not induce emesis or other decontamination procedures for a nontoxic ingestion.

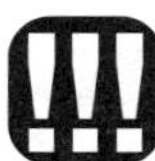

Pitfalls

Failure to accurately identify substance(s) ingested and confirm their lack of toxicity.

See also: SECTION II, Unknown Ingestion chapter.

RECOMMENDED READING

Ellenhorn MJ. Plants-mycotoxins-mushrooms. In: Ellenhorn's medical toxicology: diagnosis and treatment of human poisoning, 2nd ed. Baltimore: Williams & Wilkins, 1997.

Mofenson HC, Greensher J, Caraccio TR. Ingestions considered nontoxic. Clin Lab Med 1984;4:587–602.

POISINDEX Editorial Staff: Nontoxic ingestion. In: Rumack BH, Sayre NK, Gelman CR, eds. POISINDEX System. Englewood, CO: MICROMEDEX, Inc., November 30, 1997.

Weisman RS. Nontoxic ingestion. In: Goldfrank LR, et al., eds. Goldfrank's toxicologic emergencies, 6th ed. Norwalk, CT: Appleton & Lange, 1998.

Authors: Gregory M. Bogdan and Gerald F. O'Malley

Reviewer: Luke Yip

Elimination Enhancement

Basics

This chapter provides a description of the mechanism, indications, contraindications, and pitfalls for each of the following elimination procedures: cardiopulmonary bypass, exchange transfusion, hemodialysis, hemoperfusion, hemofiltration, multiple-dose activated charcoal, peritoneal dialysis, urinary alkalinization, urinary acidification

CARDIOPULMONARY BYPASS

Mechanism of Action

Cardiopulmonary bypass (CPB) provides hemodynamic support, allowing **endogenous** hepatic or renal clearance of the poison. It essentially "buys time" until patients can detoxify themselves.

Drug Interactions

CPB allows continued clearance of therapeutic drugs, as well.

Indications

CPB is generally performed in cases of severe overdose with hemodynamic instability from a toxicant that is normally cleared by the liver. The two drugs it has been most successful in eliminating are lidocaine and flecainide.

Contraindications and Adverse Effects

The attendant risks associated with central venous access and anticoagulation.

Pitfalls

It is important to anticipate the need for this procedure and obtain consultation early because:

- CPB requires the involvement of other specialists to initiate.
- CPB is not useful if the patient has hepatic failure.

EXCHANGE TRANSFUSION

Mechanism of Action

Serial phlebotomy and transfusion such that the patient's blood is gradually replaced with banked blood.

Drug Interactions

This procedure eliminates substantial amounts of most therapeutic drugs.

Indications

Exchange transfusion is generally performed in cases of:

- severe methemoglobinemia where the patient is unresponsive to methylene blue therapy.
- severe intoxication of an infant or neonate in whom other methods (e.g., hemodialysis and hemoperfusion) cannot be used.
- toxicant-induced massive hemolysis.

Contraindications and Adverse Effects

- The patient may experience transfusion reaction, hypothermia, hypotension, or hypocalcemia or may acquire a blood-borne infection (e.g., hepatitis).
- Thrombocytopenia and coagulopathy can develop if components other than red blood cells are not replaced appropriately.

Pitfalls

Exchange transfusion eliminates only those substances whose distribution is limited primarily to the blood volume.

HEMODIALYSIS

Mechanism of Action

Toxicants diffuse through a semipermeable membrane down a concentration gradient from blood to dialysate.

Drug Interactions

This procedure eliminates those poisons with low molecular weight, limited protein binding, and small volume of distribution.

Indications

Hemodialysis is generally performed in cases of:

- severe intoxication with water-soluble substances of molecular weight less than 500 daltons, limited plasma protein binding, and low volume of distribution (less than 1 L/kg). Some of these substances include alcohols, bromides, chloral hydrate, ethylene glycol, lithium, methanol, potassium, procainamide, quinidine, salicylate, and theophylline, among others.
- severe acidosis where the patient is unresponsive to therapy.
- severe intoxication with a substance normally eliminated by the kidney in the setting of renal failure (e.g., potassium).

Although elimination of poisons such as ethanol, isopropanol, phenobarbital, acetaminophen, and many others is increased, hemodialysis is rarely needed for these substances.

Contraindications and Adverse Effects

Hypotension, fluid and electrolyte disturbance, seizure, and the attendant risks associated with central venous access and systemic heparinization.

Pitfalls

- It is important to anticipate the need for this procedure and obtain consultation early because the initiation of hemodialysis requires the involvement of other specialists.
- Ethanol and fomepizole, used as antidotes, are also eliminated by hemodialysis. Additional doses should be administered as indicated in the Ethanol and Fomepizole chapters.
- Blood levels of toxicants may rebound after termination of dialysis. Repeated dialysis sessions may be required.
- Hemodialysis cannot be performed in severely hypotensive patients and should be initiated before intoxication becomes life threatening.

HEMOPERFUSION

Mechanism of Action

Blood perfuses across an activated charcoal cartridge, which adsorbs the poison.

Drug Interactions

This procedure also eliminates therapeutic drugs with a low volume of distribution and which are adsorbed by charcoal.

Indications

Hemoperfusion is generally performed in cases of severe intoxication of drugs with a low volume of distribution (less than 1 L/kg), low endogenous clearance, and which are adsorbed by activated charcoal. It is most commonly used for theophylline, carbamazepine, phenobarbital, and procainamide.

Contraindications and Adverse Effects

- The attendant risks associated with central venous access and systemic anticoagulation.
- Thrombocytopenia often limits the duration of hemoperfusion.

Pitfalls

- It is important to anticipate the need for this procedure and obtain consultation early because the initiation of hemoperfusion requires the involvement of other specialists.
- In most facilities, hemodialysis can be initiated much more rapidly and is usually preferred (even if hemoperfusion attains higher clearance rates under ideal conditions).
- Hemoperfusion does not correct acidemia or electrolyte abnormalities.
- Blood levels of toxicants may rebound after termination of hemoperfusion. Repeated sessions may be required.
- Hemoperfusion cannot be performed in severely hypotensive patients, and it should be initiated before intoxication becomes life threatening.

HEMOFILTRATION

Mechanism of Action

- Blood is pumped through numerous hollow fiber filters with semipermeable membranes. The toxicants are then slowly filtered out along with water, electrolytes, urea, and creatinine.
- The patient's blood pressure can be used as the pump, and hemofiltration can be performed continuously, minimizing rebound as the toxicant redistributes from peripheral tissues.

Drug Interactions

This procedure also will eliminate many therapeutic drugs.

Indications

Hemofiltration is generally performed in cases of:

• serious intoxication with compounds having a low volume of distribution (less than 1 L/kg), low endogenous clearance, and a molecular weight of less than 10,000 or 40,000 daltons (depending on the hemofilter).
• lithium and aminoglycosides intoxication, but only occasionally.

Contraindications and Adverse Effects

• The attendant risks associated with central venous access and systemic anticoagulation. However, some hemofilters do not require anticoagulation.
• Elimination rates are much lower than with hemodialysis or hemoperfusion.
• Fluid and electrolyte disturbances can develop.

Pitfalls

• Hemofiltration is a relatively new technique; its utility is not well established.
• It is important to anticipate the need and obtain consultation early because initiation of hemofiltration requires the involvement of other specialists.
• Hemofiltration cannot be performed in severely hypotensive patients, and it should be initiated before intoxication becomes life threatening.

MULTIPLE-DOSE ACTIVATED CHARCOAL

Mechanism of Action

• Repeated administration of activated charcoal may enhance elimination of the toxicant by adsorbing either the drug or the metabolite that is secreted in bile (interrupting enterohepatic recirculation).
• Alternatively, toxicant may diffuse across the intestinal wall down the concentration gradient from mesenteric vasculature into the gastrointestinal lumen, where it can be adsorbed by activated charcoal (gastrointestinal dialysis).
• Most effective for drugs that undergo substantial enterohepatic recirculation or those that have small volumes of distribution, low protein binding, and are highly adsorbed by activated charcoal.

Drug Interactions

May increase elimination of other drugs with same characteristics.

Indications

Multiple-dose activated charcoal has been used in cases of:

• Theophylline intoxication.
• Increasing elimination of phenobarbital, phenytoin, carbamazepine, quinine, dapsone, cardiac glycosides, valproate, and meprobamate intoxications. However, it has not been shown to affect the outcome for any of these poisonings.

Contraindications and Adverse Effects

• Ileus, bowel obstruction, or perforation
• Bowel obstruction or impaction, pulmonary aspiration, and fluid and electrolyte disturbances from multiple doses of cathartic

Pitfalls

• The risk of aspiration, obstruction, impaction, and fluid and electrolyte imbalance often outweigh the potential benefit.
• Never administer multiple doses of cathartics, especially to children, because fatal fluid and electrolyte disturbances may occur.

PERITONEAL DIALYSIS

Mechanism of Action

Aqueous dialysate is instilled into the peritoneal cavity. The toxicant then diffuses down the concentration gradient from blood to dialysate across the peritoneum.

Drug Interactions

This procedure eliminates therapeutic drugs that are water soluble and have a low volume of distribution, molecular weights of less than 500 daltons, and low protein binding.

Indications

Peritoneal dialysis is generally performed in cases of:

• severe intoxication with water-soluble toxicants that have a low volume of distribution (less than 1 L/kg), a molecular weight less than 500 daltons, and low protein binding. However, in most cases, hemodialysis is the preferred procedure.
• severe intoxication of an infant or neonate in whom other methods (e.g., hemodialysis and hemoperfusion) cannot be used.
• patients being transferred to a facility where hemodialysis or hemoperfusion is available because it may be useful as an initial procedure.
• methanol, ethylene glycol, salicylate, and theophylline intoxication when other methods are not available.

Contraindications and Adverse Effects

• There is a risk of peritonitis, bowel injury, fluid and electrolyte disturbance, hypotension, and volume overload.
• Previous abdominal surgery or adhesions may make insertion of a peritoneal catheter difficult.
• Contraindicated in pregnancy.

Pitfalls

• It is important to anticipate the need and obtain consultation early because the initiation of peritoneal dialysis may require the involvement of other specialists.
• It is ineffective in severely hypotensive patients, and it should be initiated before intoxication becomes life threatening.

URINARY ALKALINIZATION

Mechanism of Action

Sodium bicarbonate is administered to raise the urine pH above 7.5. Drugs in which the parent compound is a weak acid with a pKa below 7.0 and which undergo significant urinary excretion become ionized in the kidney tubular fluid and are "trapped" because ionized forms do not readily cross cell membranes.

Drug Interactions

This procedure eliminates other therapeutic drugs with similar characteristics.

Indications

Urinary alkalinization is generally performed in cases of:

• mild to moderate salicylate intoxication.
• increasing elimination of phenobarbital, chlorpropamide, and 2,4-dichlorophenoxyacetic acid. However, it has not been shown to affect the outcome of any of these poisonings.
• preventing nephrotoxicity with a high dose of methotrexate.

Contraindications and Adverse Effects

• Urinary alkalinization is contraindicated in renal failure.
• Complications include volume overload, congestive heart failure, alkalosis, hypokalemia, and hypomagnesemia.

Pitfalls

Urinary alkalinization should be used for **mild to moderate intoxication** only. **Hemodialysis** is the preferred procedure in patients with serious intoxication.

URINARY ACIDIFICATION

Mechanism of Action

Urine pH is manipulated below the pKa of compounds that are weak bases. The ionized molecule is "trapped" in the kidney tubule because ionized forms do not readily cross cell membranes.

Indications

There are no indications to use this procedure. The risk of systemic acidemia, worsening acute tubular necrosis from precipitation of hemoglobin, or myoglobin in tubules far outweighs any benefits.

See also: Chapter for each poison (e.g., ethylene glycol, methanol, lithium, theophylline, salicylate) or poisoning presentation (e.g., anion gap metabolic acidosis). Also see SECTION III, Activated Charcoal chapter.

RECOMMENDED READING

Garrettson LK, Geller RJ. Acid and alkaline diuresis: when are they of value in the treatment of poisoning? Drug Saf 1990;5:220–232.

Pond SM. Techniques to enhance elimination of toxic compounds. In: Goldfrank's toxicologic emergencies. 6th Ed., Norwalk, CT: Appleton & Lange, 1998.

Authors: Steven A. Seifert and Katherine M. Hurlbut

Reviewer: Rivka H. Horowitz

Basics

DESCRIPTION

• A drug screen tests for a wide range of substances. It may be performed on urine or blood, depending on the specific drugs and techniques that are used. Unfortunately, the substances detected by a drug screen vary among hospitals.
• The drug screen is an adjunct to the history and physical examination in the evaluation of the poisoned patient. It rarely provides critical information but may be useful to evaluate patients in whom clinical information fails to provide a working diagnosis.

FORMS

Urine Drug Screening

• Urine is the sample of choice for drug screens because most drugs and their metabolites are excreted and concentrated in the urine.
• The two major methods used in drug screens are immunoassay and chromatography. Mass spectrometry can be used in conjunction with chromatography to verify drug identity more precisely.

Immunoassay

• A drug-specific antibody binds to the target drug. The antibody-drug complex formed is then detected by one of several techniques (enzymatic reaction, fluorescence, or radioisotope labeling).
• The advantages of using this method include rapid turnaround and the need for minimal specimen preparation and handling. This keeps time and costs relatively low.
• This is the method used in most laboratories. However, several bedside assays also use this method (e.g., Triage and Verdict).

Chromatography

• The differential solubility of drugs in polar and nonpolar solutions is used to separate the different compounds in a sample. The most common technique is thin-layer chromatography (Toxilab), but liquid or gas chromatography columns are used as well, depending on the drug to be identified.
• After separation, the compounds are then detected by color development.
• Chromatography can detect a wide array of substances but has several drawbacks. The process involves substantial specimen preparation, and interpretation requires well-trained and experienced technicians. In addition, cross-reactivity among compounds may occur, thus providing only probable identification of drugs in the urine.

Mass Spectrometry

• Mass spectrometry (MS) is usually combined with gas chromatography (GC/MS) and is used to confirm the drugs identified by other methods.
• The drug molecule is bombarded, breaking it into fragments. These fragments are then identified by comparison with a computer database of fragments of known compounds.
• The advantage of this system is high accuracy in identification. However, this process is relatively time consuming and expensive and requires experienced technicians.

Serum Drug Screening

For some substances (acetaminophen, anticonvulsants, ethyl alcohol, ethylene glycol, isopropyl alcohol, lithium, methanol, salicylate, theophylline), screening is best performed on a serum sample.

INDICATIONS

There are no absolute indications for toxicology screens. Routine urine toxicology screening in overdose patients is expensive and should be discouraged.

Recommended Uses of Drug Screening

• The patient has an altered mental status of undetermined etiology. Testing in this scenario may provide information and confirm the etiology of altered mental status.
• Reported ingestants do not correspond to clinical findings. For example, if a patient has reportedly ingested a benzodiazepine, but has a heart rate of 120 beats/min, further evaluation should include a drug screen to assess for the presence of stimulants, tricyclic antidepressants, or other drugs.

Other

• Athletics. Drug screening is used in athletics to detect illegal methods of enhancing performance.
• Brain Death. Declaration of brain death should not be made until the presence of CNS depressants has been excluded.
• Poisoning. Drug screens may be helpful if intentional poisoning is suspected.
• Pregnancy. If drug abuse is suspected, drug testing of pregnant women at the time of delivery may pave the way for a social service intervention.
• Psychiatric. Drug screening in patients with psychiatric symptoms may reveal a toxic cause.
• Treatment Programs. Drug screens may be helpful if noncompliance with drug treatment programs is suspected.
• Workplace. Drug screening in the workplace is used to detect high-risk potential employees and to reduce risk of occupational accidents.

METHOD OF USE

Preparation

- It should be determined how long it will take for test results to return. In order to have a meaningful impact on immediate patient care, results should be available within 1 hour.
- Drug screens should be ordered only after the treating physician has determined what actions will be taken when the results are obtained. For example, serum drug levels of unusual compounds are rarely of clinical use because the correlation of blood level to toxicity or prognosis is unknown. Furthermore, these test results may not be available for several days.
- Contacting a medical toxicologist for advice concerning the usefulness of drug screening should be considered.
- Prior to collecting the specimen, consider contacting the laboratory to assure that the specimen is correctly collected and handled.

Collection

Urine

- Specimen Collection. A urine sample of 20 to 100 cc should be obtained and sent to the laboratory. Be alert to techniques used to obscure the presence of drugs in urine. Ambulatory patients providing a sample for analysis should be observed to prevent tampering or substitution of another sample.
- Specimen Handling. The specific drug being sought or the clinical situation should be communicated to the laboratory. This will allow the technician to better interpret the results or to inform the clinician that the drug may not be detected by the assays that are available.

Blood

- Specimen Collection. Prior to collecting the specimen, consider contacting the laboratory to assure that the appropriate type of collection tube is used.
- Specimen Handling. The specific drug being sought or the clinical situation should be communicated to the laboratory. This will allow the technician to better interpret the results or to inform the clinician that the drug may not be detected by the assays that are available.

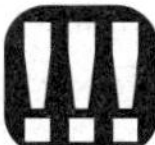

Pitfalls

DIAGNOSIS

- "Negative" drug screen. The inability to detect a drug does not mean that it is not present.

—The drug of interest may not be tested on the panel used.
—The urine may be too dilute for detection.
—The urine may have been collected before the drug was excreted.
—The sample may have been tampered with (rare in the acute illness setting but common in work-related drug screening).

- Detection of a drug in urine does not provide information about the clinical effects of the drug. Most drug assays will detect drugs days after the clinical effects are resolved.

IMMUNOASSAYS

- Immunoassays are limited to detection of the specific drugs covered in the panel. Other drugs with similar effects may not be detected (e.g., most opiate screens do not detect methadone or fentanyl).
- Immunoassay also may cross-react with drugs that are structurally similar but cause different clinical effects. If a drug test is reported as positive for an illegal drug, it is important that the test is confirmed by GC/MS for legal purposes.
- Thin-layer chromatography results are very operator dependent, and a high volume of tests are required to maintain proficiency.
- Bedside tests have been shown to be less accurate when used in nonlaboratory settings. A negative bedside test should be repeated by a laboratory if definitive results are required. Positive results are generally reliable but subject to the limitations for immunoassay listed above.
- Some drugs are **not** detected by most drug screens. These include iron, lithium, heavy metals, toxic alcohols, LSD, cyanide, hydrocarbons, and many less common substances.

ICD-9-CM 977

Poisoning by other and unspecified drugs and medicinal substances.

RECOMMENDED READING

Brett AS. Implications of discordance between clinical impression and toxicology analysis drug in drug overdose. Arch Intern Med 1988;148:437–441.

Pincus MR, Abraham NZ. Toxicology and therapeutic drug monitoring. In: Henry JB, ed. Clinical diagnosis and management by laboratory methods. Philadelphia: WB Saunders, 1991:349–356.

Author: Kennon Heard

Reviewer: Luke Yip

SECTION II

Patient Presentations with Toxicologic Causes

Acute Renal Failure

Basics

DESCRIPTION

- Acute renal failure (ARF) or insufficiency is an abrupt decline in renal function.
- Azotemia is an elevation of BUN and/or creatinine levels.
- Acute tubular necrosis (ATN) is renal tubule dysfunction and patchy tubular necrosis.
- Acute interstitial nephritis (AIN) is clinically similar to ATN.
- Nephrotic syndrome is proteinuria above 3.5 g/day associated with albumin less than 2.5 g/dl, hyperlipidemia, and edema

PATHOPHYSIOLOGY

Prerenal factors account for 40% to 80% of all cases of ARF.

EPIDEMIOLOGY

- Most common nephrotoxic lesions are intrinsic renal injuries (i.e., acute tubular necrosis and acute interstitial nephritis).
- Nephrotoxic effects are usually mild to moderate, but irreversible renal failure may occur.

RISK FACTORS

- Pre-existing renal disease
- Simultaneous exposure to multiple nephrotoxic agents

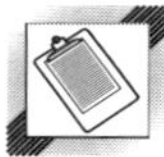

Diagnosis

DIFFERENTIAL DIAGNOSIS

Prerenal

- Volume depletion

—Dehydration is caused by many drugs.
—Caustic gastrointestinal injury.
—Hemorrhage.

- Cardiac dysfunction can be caused by doxorubicin, β-blockers, calcium channel blockers, and cardiac glycosides.
- Decreased renal artery perfusion can be caused by nonsteroidal antiinflammatory drugs (NSAIDs), cyclosporine, angiotensin-converting enzyme (ACE) inhibitors, ergot alkaloids, clonidine, β-blockers, and antihypertensive medications, as well as hepatorenal syndrome.
- Other drugs, such as amphotericin and methotrexate, can cause renal dysfunction.

Renal Parenchymal Disorders

- ATN can be caused by: acyclovir, allopurinol, aminoglycosides, amphotericin, amyl nitrite, aniline, arsenic, arsine, barium, bismuth, borates, bromides, captopril, carbamazepine, cephaloridine, cephalothin, chlorates, chromium, cisplatin, cortinarius mushrooms, cyclosporine, dapsone, diquat, elemental mercury, fluorinated anesthetics, glycols, halogenated hydrocarbons, insect venoms, methylbromide, methotrexate, mithramycin, naphthalene, neuroleptics, paraquat, phenazopyridine, radiocontrast media, snake venom, sulfonamides, rifampin, trichloroethylene, tetrachloroethylene, yellow phosphorus, and heme pigments.
- AIN has been associated with allopurinol, NSAIDs, cephalosporins, penicillins (especially methicillin, penicillin, and ampicillin), rifampin, sulfonamides, and vancomycin.
- Acute glomerular nephritis has been caused by captopril, heavy metals, heroin, amphetamines, hydralazine, NSAIDs, yellow phosphorous, penicillamine, rifampin, and sulfonamides.
- Nephrotic syndrome suggests use of an ACE inhibitor, dapsone, heroin, gold, mercury, NSAIDs, penicillamine, phenolphthalein, probenecid, trimethadione, or paramethadione.
- An unknown mechanism of a renal parenchymal disorder is associated with fluoride.

Acute Urinary Tract Obstruction

- Tubular. Obstruction can be caused by ethylene glycol, diethylene glycol, fluorinated anesthetics, myoglobin, and phenylbutazone.
- Ureteral. Obstruction can be caused by bromocriptine, methylsergide, LSD, milk alkali syndrome from milk or calcium-containing antacids, sulfonamides, vitamin C (chronic ingestion), vitamin D (chronic ingestion), and uric acid deposition.
- Bladder. Obstruction can be caused by anticholinergics and tricyclic antidepressants.

SIGNS AND SYMPTOMS

Vital Signs

Fever suggests a hypersensitivity reaction, metal fume fever, or cadmium fume pneumonitis.

Dermatologic

- Dermatitis, stomatitis, alopecia, and hypersensitivity pneumonitis suggest exposure to gold salts or gold-containing drugs.
- A "boiled lobster" appearance and desquamation associated with nausea and vomiting suggests exposure to borates.
- Burns suggest exposure to yellow phosphorus.
- Poor peripheral perfusion may indicate volume depletion or ingestion of clonidine, β-blockers, or antihypertensive medications or ergot alkaloids.

Cardiovascular

Cardiac dysfunction suggests ingestion of doxorubicin, a β-blocker, a calcium channel blocker, or a cardiac glycoside.

Pulmonary

- Pneumonitis associated with stomatitis and gingivitis suggests exposure to elemental mercury vapor.
- Pneumonitis involving a progressive fibronodular interstitial process suggests exposure to beryllium.
- Pulmonary fibrosis following episodes of bloody vomiting and diarrhea suggests paraquat.

Gastrointestinal

Nausea, mucosal burns, hematemesis, diarrhea, and abdominal pain suggest exposure to iron, arsenic, inorganic mercury, or other caustics.

Hepatic

Jaundice, hepatitis, and hepatic failure suggest exposure to acetaminophen, carbon tetrachloride, tetrachloroethylene, isoniazid, yellow phosphorus, or a cyclopeptide-containing mushroom.

Renal

- Diabetes insipidus suggests lithium, furosemide, ethacrynic acid, propoxyphene.
- Hemoglobinuria suggests a venom, phenol, aniline, arsine, or methylchloride exposure.

Hematologic

- Coagulopathy suggests exposure to anticoagulants or crotalid snake venom.
- Hypochromic, microcytic anemia and basophilic stippling suggests chronic lead toxicity.
- Hemolysis associated with generalized weakness, headache, "bronze" skin, and abdominal pain suggests exposure to arsine or stibine gas.
- Hemolysis suggests any cause of methemoglobinemia, as well as exposure to naphthalene, phenazopyridine, copper sulfate, or brown recluse spider bite in a child.

Fluids and Electrolytes

- Electrolyte abnormality suggest diuretic abuse; hyperkalemia suggests potassium-sparing diuretic.
- Anion gap metabolic acidosis with or without crystalluria suggests exposure to ethylene glycol or diethylene glycol.
- Severe hypokalemia suggests diuretics or barium.
- Hypercalcemia suggests vitamin D.
- Hypokalemia and hyperchloremia, with normal or increased anion gap metabolic acidosis, suggests toluene exposure.

Musculoskeletal

- Rhabdomyolysis suggests exposure to sympathomimetic agents, barbiturates, PCP, sedative-hypnotics (with coma), cyanide, carbon monoxide, zinc phosphate, copper sulfate, CNS stimulants, or snake and insect venoms.
- Teeth discoloration, painful microfractures due to osteomalacia, anemia, and generalized pain suggest cadmium exposure.
- Gout suggests chronic lead toxicity.

Neurologic

- Tremor, hyperreflexia, clonus, and altered mental status suggest lithium ingestion.
- CNS depression is associated with trichloroethylene.
- Altered mental status and ataxia suggest lead exposure.

Genitourinary

Retroperitoneal fibrosis suggests exposure to methysergide, LSD, or bromocriptine.

PROCEDURES AND LABORATORY TESTS

Renal dysfunction can be diagnosed by means of laboratory findings:

- ATN. Muddy-brown pigmented cellular casts or renal tubular cells are found on urine analysis.
- AIN. Eosinophiluria, hematuria, leukocyturia, a mononuclear cell infiltrate separating tubular structures on renal biopsy, and eosinophilia are diagnostic.
- Acute Glomerular Nephritis. Findings include hematuria, red blood cell casts, and proteinuria.

Microscopic Analysis of Urinary Sediment

Casts

- Hyaline casts suggest prerenal azotemia or obstructive nephropathy.
- Red blood cell casts suggest glomerulonephritis.
- Broad casts (diameter greater than 2 to 3 white cells) suggest chronic renal failure.
- Brown pigmented granular casts and positive dipstick for blood, but without red cells suggests hemoglobinuria or myoglobinuria.

Cells

- Red cells without casts suggest calculi
- Predominantly polymorphonuclear leukocytes suggest diffuse interstitial nephritis or papillary necrosis.

Crystals

- Urate crystals suggest uric acid nephropathy.
- Oxalate and hippurate crystals suggest ethylene glycol exposure.

Chemical Analysis of Urine (Prior to Intravenous Fluid or Diuretics)

Prerenal Azotemia

- Urine sodium is less than 20 mmol/L.
- Urine osmolality is greater than 500 mOsm/kg.
- Urine analysis is normal.
- Urine to plasma creatinine ratio is greater than 40.
- BUN is elevated out of proportion to the plasma creatinine concentration.
- The fractional excretion of sodium (FENa) is less than 1.

ATN or AIN

- Urine sodium is greater than 40 mmol/L.
- Urine osmolality is less than 400 mOsm/kg.
- The urine to plasma creatinine ratio is less than 20.
- FENa is greater than 1.
- Uric acid nephropathy. Urinary uric acid to urinary creatinine ratio is greater than 1, and serum uric acid is in excess of 20 mg/dl.

Serum Electrolytes, BUN, Creatinine, Calcium, Phosphate, and Magnesium

- Elevations in both the BUN and creatinine concentrations are common in all forms of renal failure. A disproportionately high creatinine may suggest rhabdomyolysis, due to the conversion of muscle creatine to creatinine.
- Hyperkalemia due to decreased elimination is common. A high potassium level suggests hemolysis or rhabdomyolysis.
- Serum uric acid level is usually higher than 20 mg/dl in acute uric acid nephropathy.
- Complete blood count. Anemia may indicate chronic renal failure. Leukocytosis is consistent with infection.
- Serum ethylene glycol level should be determined if metabolic acidosis is present.
- Quantitation of the appropriate toxin (aminoglycoside, heavy metal) should be determined as appropriate.
- Postvoid residual catheter volume greater than 100 cc suggests postrenal obstruction.

Imaging

- Intravenous pyelography (IVP) should be performed with caution in patients with evidence of renal insufficiency.
- CT scan should be considered in situations where IVP is contraindicated.

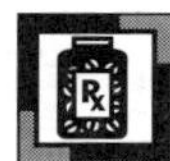

Treatment

DIRECTING PATIENT COURSE

Monitor fluid intake and output. Correct electrolyte abnormalities as needed.

DECONTAMINATION

If acute renal failure is present, decontamination would not be expected to be effective.

ANTIDOTES

There is no specific antidote for most causes.

ADJUNCTIVE TREATMENT

- Hypocalcemia and metabolic acidosis associated with ATN rarely require treatment.
- Allopurinol can be used to treat gouty nephropathy. Allopurinol prior to administration of cytotoxic drugs may prevent acute uric acid nephropathy.
- Aluminum hydroxide can be used to treat hyperphosphatemia.
- Calcium chloride, sodium bicarbonate, insulin and glucose, and sodium polystyrene sulfonate can be used to treat hyperkalemia.
- Life-threatening hyperkalemia and hyperphosphatemia should be corrected with dialysis.
- Urine alkalinization may limit methotrexate nephrotoxicity.

Oliguria

- In the oliguric patient in whom prerenal causes have been excluded, the administration of a loop diuretic or mannitol may be useful.
- Administration of renal doses of dopamine (1 to 3 μg/kg/min) may increase renal blood flow and allow a diuretic response.

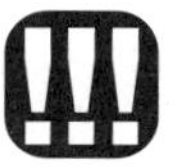

Pitfalls

- BUN or serum creatinine concentration at the upper end of the laboratory normal range may represent significant renal impairment.
- Trimethoprim and cimetidine block renal creatinine secretion, resulting in a reversible increase in serum creatinine.
- Elevated levels of serum acetone may artifactually increase the serum creatinine.
- Administration of diuretics or crystalloid fluid may interfere with urine analysis.

See also: SECTION IV, Hyperkalemia chapter, and chapters on specific poisons.

RECOMMENDED READING

Feinfeld DA. Principles of nephrotoxicity. In: Goldfrank LR, et al., eds. Goldfrank's toxicologic emergencies, 6th ed. Norwalk, CT: Appleton & Lange, 1998.

Author: Edwin K. Kuffner

Reviewer: Richard C. Dart

Anion Gap Metabolic Acidosis (Unexplained)

Basics

DESCRIPTION

• A metabolic acidosis (serum bicarbonate less than 24 mEq/L) may be associated with an increased anion gap.
• Anion gap is defined as the difference of measured cations and anions. Calculation: [serum sodium] − [serum chloride + serum bicarbonate] = anion gap.
• Normal anion gap is less than 16 mEq/L.

PATHOPHYSIOLOGY

• Blood is neutral in charge, with anions equaling cations. However, not all anions and cations are measured using standard laboratory tests. In a healthy, normal patient, the standard serum electrolyte panel appears to have an anion gap because there are more unmeasured anions than cations in the blood.
• In an increased anion gap metabolic acidosis, an anion (e.g., lactic acid), which is not measured in the electrolyte panel, accumulates in the blood. Serum bicarbonate decreases as it is consumed during neutralization of the acid thereby increasing the calculated anion gap above 16 mEq/L.

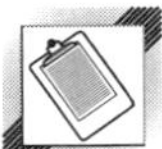

Diagnosis

DIFFERENTIAL DIAGNOSIS

Toxicologic Causes

• Further information on each poison is available in SECTION IV, CHEMICAL AND BIOLOGICAL AGENTS.
• MUDPILES is a mnemonic for common causes of increased anion gap metabolic acidosis:

M	Methanol
U	Uremia, hepatorenal syndrome
D	Diabetic ketoacidosis
P	Phenformin, Paraldehyde
I	Iron, isoniazid
L	Lactic acidosis: carbon monoxide, cyanide, hydrogen sulfide, seizure, hypotension caused by a toxicant
E	Ethylene glycol
S	Salicylates

Some authors include toluene and theophylline. Metabolic acidosis caused by toluene is often of nonanion gap type. Theophylline may produce mild anion gap without hypotension. Massive acetaminophen overdose may cause coma and metabolic acidosis.

Nontoxicologic Causes

Nontoxic causes of increased anion gap acidosis include any cause of acid accumulation. The most common cause is lactic acid arising from anaerobic glycolysis (ischemic tissue, hypoxia, severe agitation or seizure).

SIGNS AND SYMPTOMS

Associated physical signs may help reveal the poison involved when they occur in the setting of increased anion gap metabolic acidosis.

Vital Signs

Any cause of hypotension or hyperthermia may cause anion gap acidosis from lactic acid.

HEENT

• Blindness or blurred vision may indicate methanol poisoning.
• Unusual odors can identify cyanide (bitter almonds), hydrogen sulfide (rotten eggs), toluene (paint)

Dermatologic

• Diaphoresis is associated with β-receptor agonist, stimulants.
• Eyanosis is caused by hypoxia or methemoglobinemia.
• Paint may indicate toluene abuse.

Cardiovascular

See SECTION II, Bradycardia Toxidrome, Tachycardia, and Ventricular Dysrhythmia chapters.

Pulmonary

Acidosis will cause compensatory tachypnea unless coingestant causes respiratory depression.

Gastrointestinal

• Vomiting is associated with acetaminophen, iron, salicylate, or theophylline intoxication.
• Hematemesis may indicate iron ingestion.

Hepatic

Hepatic damage may be caused by acetaminophen or salicylates and most causes of hyperthermia.

Renal

Renal damage is most likely caused by ethylene glycol, occasionally by acetaminophen or rhabdomyolysis.

Musculoskeletal

Rhabdomyolysis may be secondary to direct muscle injury, muscle compression during coma, excercise, agitation, β-receptor agonists, seizures, or hyperthermic syndromes.

Neurologic

Toxicant-induced severe agitation or seizure may produce transient lactic acidosis.

PROCEDURES AND LABORATORY TESTS

See chapter on individual poisons for more detailed information.

Essential

Serum Electrolytes, Glucose, BUN, and Creatinine

- Hypokalemia may be caused by β-receptor agonist, caffeine, or theophylline.
- Anion gap of 16 to 19 mEq/L should raise concern. Repeat anion gap determination in 2 hours to determine if worsening.
- Anion gap is greater than 19 mEq/L.

—If possible cause is present (e.g., recent seizure), repeat anion gap determination in 1 to 2 hours and reevaluate.
—If source of gap unclear or osmolal gap is elevated, test for serum lactate, serum methanol, ethlyene glycol levels, serum iron. Cyanide level may be needed rarely.

- Anion gap of greater than 30 mEq/L usually indicates lactic acidosis or ketoacidosis.

Serum Acetaminophen and Salicylate Levels

- Salicylate causes an increased anion gap acidosis.
- Severe acetaminophen poisoning (serum level greater than 800 μg/ml) may cause anion gap acidosis.

Recommended

- ECG and continuous cardiac monitoring are used in overdose setting to detect occult poisoning with cardiotoxic medication.
- Arterial blood gas with cooximetry is used to detect poisoning by carbon monoxide.
- Serum osmolality.

—An elevated osmolal gap not accounted for by ethanol should initiate a workup for ethylene glycol or methanol.
—Acetone also produces increased osmolal gap, but not an increased anion gap.
—Due to variability in laboratories, a normal osmolal gap cannot be used to exclude the presence of methanol or ethylene glycol.

- Abdominal radiograph imaging may reveal radiopaque pills or material: bismuth subsalicylate, enteric coated tablets, iron sulfate, body packers.

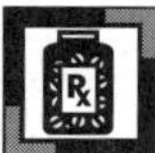

Treatment

- Focus management on decontamination and supportive care while determining cause of acidosis. If identity of poison is known, see chapter on specific agent. Correct hypoxia and electrolytes as clinically indicated.
- Determine dose and time for all substances involved.

DECONTAMINATION

- The presence of an anion gap metabolic acidosis indicates that absorption and toxic effects are already present.
- Induction of emesis is not recommended unless the specific agent is known (iron, sustained-release preparation, salicylate).
- Gastric lavage should be performed in pediatric (tube size 24–32 French) or adult (tube size 36–42 French) patients for large ingestion presenting within 1 hour of ingestion or if serious effects are present.
- One dose of activated charcoal (1–2 g/kg) should be administered without a cathartic if a substantial ingestion has occurred within the previous few hours.

ANTIDOTES

- Administer antidotes for altered mental status: oxygen, thiamine, glucose, and naloxone. See chapter on specific toxicant for other appropriate antidotes.
- Ethanol. Often the diagnosis of increased anion gap acidosis will be delayed while waiting for a methanol or ethylene glycol level. It is often prudent to begin treatment with fomepizole or ethanol until poisoning with either of these substances can be excluded.
- The use of sodium bicarbonate ($NaHCO_3$) for treatment of lactic acidosis is not recommended because it is not well supported by current medical evidence.

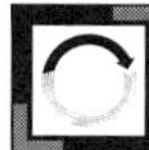

Follow-Up

PATIENT MONITORING

Serial evaluation of serum electrolytes and arterial blood gases is needed until diagnosis is established.

ADMISSION CRITERIA

All patients with persisent, unexplained, increased anion gap acidosis should be admitted.

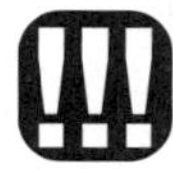

Pitfalls

- False depression of pCO_2 and calculated bicarbonate on the arterial blood gas from excess heparin (insufficient filling of tubes).
- Failure to decontaminate patients who have unknown or inapparent ingestion.
- Failure to perform endotracheal intubation before aspiration or respiratory arrest occurs.
- Failure to repeat electrolytes and recalculate anion gap in a patient with acidosis and slightly elevated anion gap.
- Failure to maintain compensatory hyperventilation in an intubated patient with metabolic acidosis and compensatory respiratory alkalosis who is placed on mechanical respiration.

ICD-9-CM

No code is available.

RECOMMENDED READING

Emmet M, Narins RG. Clinical use of the anion gap. Medicine 1977;56:38–54.

Author: Steven A. Seifert

Reviewer: Richard C. Dart

Anticholinergic Syndrome

Basics

DESCRIPTION

A syndrome of tachycardia, mydriasis, dry mucous membranes, decreased bowel sounds, urinary retention, hallucinations and warm, dry, and flushed skin caused by a blockade of the acetylcholine receptors.

PATHOPHYSIOLOGY

- Anticholinergic compounds competitively block acetylcholine at the postsynaptic muscarinic acetylcholine receptor. The result is decreased stimulation of the muscarinic acetylcholine receptor.
- Anticholinergic compounds do not have an effect on the postsynaptic nicotinic acetylcholine receptor.

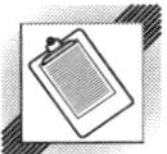

Diagnosis

- Numerous agents antagonize the effects of acetylcholine at the postsynaptic muscarinic receptor; therefore, medication and occupational histories are important in determining the cause of this syndrome.
- Most patients will not exhibit all the classic anticholinergic symptoms simultaneously. Some agents may produce more subtle clinical syndromes in which some signs or symptoms are more prominent than others.
- Antimuscarinic effects may be remembered as "mad as a hatter" (altered mental status, hallucinations), "hot as hell" (hyperthermia), "dry as a bone" (dry mucous membranes), "blind as a bat" (mydriasis, blurred vision), "red as a beet" (flushed skin), and "seizing like a squirrel" (seizures).

DIFFERENTIAL DIAGNOSIS

Further information on each poison is available in SECTION IV, CHEMICAL AND BIOLOGICAL AGENTS.

Toxicologic Causes

- Antihistamines (most commonly diphenhydramine)
- Phenothiazines
- Anticholinergic plants
- Cyclic antidepressants
- Antispasmodic agents (clidinium, dicyclomine, flavoxate, hyoscine, oxybutynin, propantheline, scopolamine)
- Mucous membrane drying agents (glycopyrrolate)
- Mydriatic agents (atropine, cyclopentolate, homatropine, tropicamide)
- Bronchodilator agents (ipratropium)
- Skeletal muscle relaxants (cyclobenzaprine, orphenadrine)
- Anti-parkinsonian medications (benztropine, biperiden)

Other Compounds that Produce Similar Clinical Effects

- Sympathomimetic amines may produce tachycardia, dry mucous membranes, mydriasis, hyperthermia, delirium, and seizures. They generally cause diaphoresis, and bowel sounds are usually present.
- Hallucinogenic drugs or mushrooms may cause delirium and mydriasis.

SIGNS AND SYMPTOMS

Vital Signs

- Tachycardia is common due to the antimuscarinic blockade of the vagus nerve. Its absence should question the diagnosis of anticholinergic toxicity.
- Hyperthermia is usually mild unless environmental factors exacerbate the effect.
- Hypertension and tachypnea may be caused by psychomotor agitation.

HEENT

- Mydriasis and dry mucous membranes are common. Blurred vision occurs as a result of mydriasis.
- Isolated mydriasis and anisocoria have occurred after instillation of an ophthalmic mydriatic or other anticholinergic agent into one eye.
- Ophthalmic instillation can produce systemic anticholinergic toxicity.

Dermatologic

- Warm, dry, and flushed skin is common.
- Dry axillae in an agitated patient with psychomotor agitation suggests anticholinergic effects or severe dehydration.

Cardiovascular

- Tachycardia is common due to antimuscarinic effects that block vagal stimulation of the sinoatrial node.
- Hypertension may be related to psychomotor agitation.
- Hypotension can occur following seizures and may be associated with hypovolemia. Life-threatening dysrhythmias are rare.

Pulmonary

Bronchodilation may occur as a result of therapeutic use of antimuscarinic agents but is not a reliable marker of toxicity.

Gastrointestinal

- Ileus and decreased bowel sounds are common.
- Constipation is a common side effect of medications with anticholinergic effects.

Musculoskeletal

Psychomotor agitation may produce rhabdomyolysis.

Neurologic

- Agitation with altered mental status is common. Toxic psychosis with anxiety, paranoia, and hallucinations is well documented.
- CNS depression with drowsiness and lethargy progressing to coma is less common.
- Seizures may occur.
- Dystonic reactions and movement disorders also have been reported.

Genitourinary

Urinary retention with bladder distension is common.

Psychiatric/Psychological

Toxic psychosis with hallucinations is well documented.

PROCEDURES AND LABORATORY TESTS

Essential Tests

Testing may not be needed in minimally symptomatic patients.

Recommended Tests

• Serum electrolytes, BUN, creatinine to assess dehydration and potential renal injury from myoglobin.
• Creatine kinase may be elevated if rhabdomyolysis occurs.
• Urinalysis to assess dehydration or myoglobin-induced renal injury.
• ECG, serum acetaminophen and aspirin levels, urine toxicology screen to detect occult overdose. Sinus tachycardia is common. Malignant dysrhythmia is rare.
• Lumbar puncture, bacterial cultures, head CT, and other tests as indicated to assess altered mental status of unknown etiology.

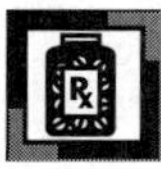

Treatment

• In the agitated patient, focus treatment on control of agitation and protection from self-harm. In the patient with CNS depression, focus treatment on airway management.
• Supportive care should be provided while evaluating source of poisoning.
• Dosage and time of exposure should be determined for all substances involved.

DIRECTING PATIENT COURSE

The health-care provider should call the poison control center when:

• the source of anticholinergic effects is unclear.
• coingestant, drug interaction, or underlying disease presents an unusual problem.

DECONTAMINATION

Out of Hospital

Ipecac should be administered to induce emesis within 1 hour of ingestion for an alert pediatric or adult patient if health-care evaluation will be delayed.

In Hospital

• Ipecac should be administered to induce emesis within 1 hour of ingestion for the alert patient who is too small to have effective gastric lavage.
• Gastric lavage should be performed in pediatric (tube size 24–32 French) or adult (tube size 36–42 French) patients for large ingestion presenting within 1 hour of ingestion or if serious effects are present. Lavage may be reasonable even 4 to 6 hours after ingestion due to the gastrointestinal slowing effects of anticholinergic agents.
• One dose of activated charcoal (1–2 g/kg) should be administered without a cathartic if a substantial ingestion has occurred within the previous few hours.
• Irrigate eyes, skin, and mucous membranes with copious amounts of water following exposure to those areas.

ANTIDOTES

Antidotes should be administered for altered mental status: oxygen, thiamine, glucose, and naloxone.

Physostigmine

Physostigmine may be administered as a diagnostic agent to distinguish altered mental status due to anticholinergic toxicity from other causes of agitation and hallucination. A positive response to this test may obviate the need for a head CT and lumbar puncture for evaluation of altered mental status.

Contraindications

• Known allergy to cholinergic agonist or sulfites
• Tricyclic antidepressant overdose, or ECG findings suggestive of tricyclic antidepressant overdose (QRS widening, R wave in ECG lead aVR)
• History of asthma, heart disease, diabetes, seizure disorder, inflammation of iris or ciliary body

Method of Administration

• Place the patient on a cardiac monitor and have atropine available at the bedside.
• Adult dose is 0.5 to 2.0 mg slow push intravenously over 5 minutes. Repeat dose intravenously once after 5 to 10 minutes if needed.
• Pediatric dose is 0.02 mg/kg up to 2.0 mg slow push intravenously over 5 minutes. Repeat dose intravenously once after 5 to 10 minutes if needed.

Potential Adverse Effects

• Adverse effects are more common with larger doses and faster rates of administration.
• Muscarinic effects are nausea, vomiting, diarrhea, sweating, bronchorrhea, bradycardia, hypotension. Cardiac dysrhythmia may occur.
• Nicotinic effects (weakness, fasciculation) also may occur.
• Seizures may occur.

ADJUNCTIVE TREATMENT

• Treat psychomotor agitation with benzodiazepines. Tachycardia and hyperthermia may improve with both benzodiazepines and intravenous hydration.
• Support blood pressure and perfusion as clinically indicated.
• Hypertension usually resolves with sedation and rarely requires specific treatment.

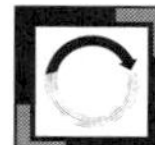

Follow-Up

EXPECTED COURSE AND PROGNOSIS

• The onset of anticholinergic syndrome is often gradual and may be delayed due to decreased gastrointestinal motility.
• The effects usually resolve over a period of 24 to 36 hours but may persist for days following large ingestions.

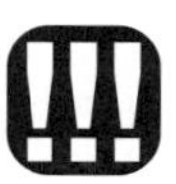

Pitfalls

• The administration of physostigmine to patients with known exposure to an anticholinergic agent and presentation consistent with anticholinergic toxicity is not useful because the diagnosis is already known.
• The administration of repeat doses of physostigmine to control psychomotor agitation increases the likelihood of an adverse effect. Benzodiazepines are the preferred agents.

ICD-9-CM 971.1

Poisoning by drugs primarily affecting the autonomic nervous system: parasympatholytics (anticholinergics and antimuscarinics) and spasmotics.

See also: SECTION II, Hypertension, Hypotension, and Tachycardia chapters; SECTION III, Physostigmine chapter; and SECTION IV, Anticholinergic Compounds and Plants—Anticholinergic chapters.

RECOMMENDED READING

Ellenhorn MJ. Antimuscarinic drugs. In: Medical toxicology: diagnosis and treatment of human poisoning. Baltimore: Williams & Wilkins, 1997:840–861.

Author: Edwin K. Kuffner

Reviewer: Richard C. Dart

Ascending Paralysis

Basics

DESCRIPTION

- Flaccid paralysis begins in the lower limbs and progresses upward to involve arms as well as respiratory and facial muscles.
- Peripheral neuropathy, tetrodotoxin, and tick paralysis are also addressed in separate chapters.

PATHOPHYSIOLOGY

- Guillain-Barré syndrome (GBS) is the demyelinating disease of peripheral and cranial nerves, which causes ascending paralysis.
- Tick-borne paralysis involves a neurotoxin that causes ascending paralysis by inhibiting acetylcholine and thereby motor neuron transmission.
- The fruit of Karwinskia humboldtiana (buckthorn, coyotillo, tullidora) causes ascending paralysis by demyelination of motor nerves.
- Tetrodotoxin is a neurotoxin that blocks sodium channels and neuromuscular transmission.
- Severe arsenic toxicity results in diffuse axon destruction, which, in severe cases, may result in ascending paralysis.
- Acute intermittent porphyria (AIP) is a multisystem disease that involves motor neuropathy, occasionally including ascending flaccid paralysis.

EPIDEMIOLOGY

- GBS is the most common type of acute ascending paralysis.

—Most cases are associated with antecedent infections (e.g., Campylobacter jejuni, HIV, cytomegalovirus, mycoplasma, and Epstein-Barr virus, among others).
—Other precipitants include neoplasms, surgical procedures, autoimmune disorders, and vaccinations.

- Tick-borne paralysis (see SECTION IV, Tick Paralysis chapter) in North America primarily occurs during the spring and summer in the Rocky Mountains and the Northwestern United States or Canada. Most cases occur in girls.
- Ingestion of the fruit of K. humboldtiana (buckthorn, coyotillo, tullidora) may cause ascending paralysis. Most cases are reported in the southwestern United States.
- AIP is a genetically transmitted disorder.

—Acute attacks usually require an additional trigger because over one third of patients with this enzyme deficiency never develop disease.
—Therapeutic doses of barbiturates, anticonvulsants, estrogens, contraceptives, and alcohol may trigger acute attacks. Fasting or infection also may trigger AIP.

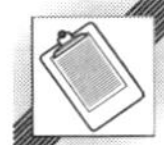

Diagnosis

DIFFERENTIAL DIAGNOSIS

See SECTION II, Peripheral Neuropathy chapter for related discussion.

Toxicologic Causes

- Further information on each poison is available in SECTION IV, CHEMICAL AND BIOLOGICAL AGENTS.
- Tick-borne paralysis. Symmetric, ascending flaccid paralysis progresses over hours to days. Decreased deep tendon reflexes (DTRs). Sensory symptoms and mental status changes are usually absent.
- Tetrodotoxin poisoning. Rapid-onset headache, cranial nerve palsies, paresthesia of face, hands, and feet, nausea, vomiting, dysphagia, weakness, fasciculation, and ascending paralysis may occur within an hour of ingesting puffer fish.
- Organophosphate toxicity. Acute or chronic exposure may result in lower extremity weakness, ataxia, and paresthesia, which may ascend to the upper extremities.
- Arsenic. Pain and paresthesia are prominent features of arsenic-associated peripheral neuropathy. Nausea, vomiting, diarrhea, and anorexia are common. Rash and alopecia also may occur. Sensory loss, decreased DTRs, weakness, and ascending paralysis are later findings of severe poisoning.
- Chronic solvent abuse results in ataxia, cranial nerve palsies, and cognitive impairment. Reflexes are usually preserved. Ascending flaccid paralysis occurs rarely in patients with massive exposure.
- Botulism. Botulism typically causes a descending paralysis, beginning with the cranial nerves.
- Severe lead poisoning

—Wrist or foot drop and encephalopathy may develop.
—Anemia and gastrointestinal symptoms usually develop before neurologic effects.
—Ascending paralysis does not occur.

Nontoxicologic Causes

- GBS

—Required diagnostic criteria include ascending paralysis and areflexia.
—Minor diagnostic criteria include symmetrical weakness, mild sensory symptoms, and facial weakness.
—Progression may be rapid or gradual.

- AIP is characterized by recurrent attacks of abdominal pain, nausea, vomiting, hypertension, tachycardia, psychiatric symptoms, and neuropathy, sometimes associated with ascending paralysis.
- Conversion reactions may result in weakness and sensory deficits inconsistent with neurologic anatomy.
- Spinal cord compression, trauma, or inflammation may present with symmetric lower-extremity weakness and decreased reflexes.

SIGNS AND SYMPTOMS

Flaccid paralysis begins in the lower limbs and progresses upward to the trunk, arms, and respiratory and facial muscles. Depending on the cause of paralysis, other systemic symptoms may develop.

Vital Signs

- Ascending paralysis from any cause may result in hypoventilation and respiratory arrest.
- GBS may cause hemodynamic instability, hyper- and hypotension, and brady- and tachydysrhythmias as a result of autonomic dysfunction.

HEENT

- Cranial nerve involvement with facial weakness is seen in 50% of patients with GBS. Papilledema, bilateral facial weakness, diplopia, ptosis, and oculomotor weakness may occur.
- Cranial nerve palsies may be found in tetrodotoxin poisoning or botulism.

Dermatologic

A tick may be found attached to the skin or scalp of patients with tick-borne paralysis. Arsenic poisoning may show rash, alopecia, and Mee's lines.

Pulmonary

Pulmonary manifestations from any cause include respiratory muscle weakness and paralysis.

Gastrointestinal

- Dysphagia may be seen in GBS and tetrodotoxin poisoning.
- Oral dysesthesia may precede ascending paralysis in tetrodotoxin poisoning.
- Nausea, vomiting, anorexia, abdominal pain, and diarrhea may be seen in AIP and arsenic or tetrodotoxin poisoning.

Renal

Urinary retention may develop in GBS.

Fluids and Electrolytes

Hyponatremia from inappropriate secretion of antidiuretic hormone may develop in AIP.

Musculoskeletal

Ascending muscle weakness begins in the lower extremities and progresses to the trunk and upper extremities.

Neurologic

- Ascending paralysis occurs, with areflexia and mild numbness or paresthesia of the feet and hands.

• Ataxia may occur with GBS, tick-borne paralysis, AIP, K. humboldtiana fruit ingestion, and tetrodotoxin poisoning.

PROCEDURES AND LABORATORY TESTS

Essential

• Serum electrolytes, blood urea nitrogen, creatinine, calcium, and magnesium determinations assess electrolyte-mediated causes.
• Arterial blood gases, pulse oximetry, and serial vital capacity measurements assess respiratory function and the need for intubation.
• Electrocardiography and monitoring assess rhythm and conduction defects.
• Lumbar puncture is performed to determine the absence or minimal number of lymphocytes in the presence of elevated levels of CSF protein, which suggests GBS.

Recommended

• Complete blood count is taken to determine anemia and basophilic stippling associated with lead poisoning. The whole blood lead level will confirm the diagnosis.
• A 24-hour urine collection for arsenic and other heavy metals supports the diagnosis of specific metal toxicity.
• Urinary concentrations of δ-aminolevulinic acid and porphobilinogen are elevated during acute attacks of AIP.
• Red cell and plasma cholinesterase levels are depressed in organophosphate poisoning.
• Nerve conduction studies help differentiate GBS, botulism, and other neuropathies.

Imaging

Radiographs of the spine and CT and MRI scans of the spinal column and brain can help detect underlying disease.

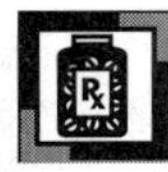

Treatment

• Treatment should be focused on assuring adequate ventilation and assessment of etiology (e.g., the tick should be sought and removed).
• Supportive care with appropriate airway management is vital. Specific treatment should be initiated while continuing supportive care.
• The dose and time of exposure must be determined for all substances involved.

DIRECTING PATIENT COURSE

The health care provider should call the poison control center when:

• The diagnosis of ascending paralysis is considered.
• A coingestant, drug interaction, or underlying disease presents unusual problems.

Admission Considerations

The health-care provider should consider referral to a health-care facility when:

• The patient has ascending paralysis, in which case, the patient should be admitted to an ICU.
• A coingestant, drug interaction, or underlying disease presents unusual problems.

DECONTAMINATION

Decontamination is necessary if acute ingestion is suspected.

Out of Hospital

Induction of emesis is not recommended; effects develop after the toxin has been absorbed.

In Hospital

• Gastric lavage should be performed in pediatric (tube size 24–32 French) or adult (tube size 36–42 French) patients for large ingestion presenting within 1 hour of ingestion or if serious effects are present.
• One dose of activated charcoal (1–2 g/kg) should be administered without a cathartic if a substantial ingestion has occurred within the previous few hours.

ANTIDOTES

• There is no specific antidote for the causes of ascending paralysis.
• In some cases, heavy metal chelation may be indicated.

ADJUNCTIVE TREATMENT

Patients with a declining vital capacity or a vital capacity of 10 to 12 ml/kg may require endotracheal intubation and mechanical ventilation.

GBS

• GBS is typically treated with immune globulin (0.4 g/kg/day intravenously for 5 days).
• Plasmapheresis may be beneficial for GBS if started within the first 2 weeks of the onset of symptoms.

AIP

• AIP is treated with glucose (a minimum of 300 g/day at rates of up to 20 g/hour).
• Intravenous heme (lyophilized hematin or hydroxyheme at 4 mg/kg every 12 hours for 3 to 6 days) inhibits porphyrin synthesis and ameliorates symptoms, if given early.

Hypotension

• Saline (0.9%) should be administered at 10 to 20 ml/kg, and the patient should be placed in the Trendelenburg position.
• Further fluid therapy should be guided by central pressure monitoring to avoid volume overload. A vasopressor should be added, if needed.

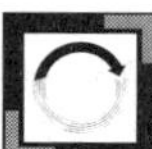

Follow-Up

PATIENT MONITORING

Ventilatory function must be assessed continuously. Patients should be monitored in an ICU setting until hemodynamically and neurologically stable and improving.

EXPECTED COURSE AND PROGNOSIS

• The mortality rate associated with GBS is 3% to 5%. Most patients recover in weeks to months but may have residual deficits. Relapse occurs in 5% to 9% of patients.
• Tick-borne paralysis reverses rapidly after tick removal.
• AIP attacks usually resolve within 2 to 3 days.
• Tetrodotoxin poisoning has a rapid onset. Recovery often requires prolonged mechanical ventilation.

DISCHARGE CRITERIA/INSTRUCTIONS

• From the emergency department. Patients with possible ascending paralysis should not be discharged.
• From the hospital. Patients whose vital signs are normal and neurologic status is improving can be discharged.

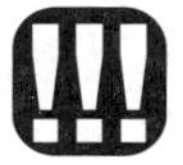

Pitfalls

• Early findings of ascending paralysis may be subtle, and the patient may be inappropriately discharged.
• Patients with AIP are often misdiagnosed with psychosis.

ICD-9-CM 989

Toxic effect of other substances, chiefly nonmedicinal as to source.

See also: SECTION II, Hypotension and Peripheral Neuropathy chapters, as well as SECTION IV, Arsenic, Tetrodotoxin, and Tick Paralysis chapters.

RECOMMENDED READING

Awong IE, Dandurand KR, Keeys CA, et al. Drug-associated Guillain-Barré syndrome: a literature review. Ann Pharmacother 1996;30:173–180.

Author: Robin Millin

Reviewer: Richard C. Dart

Asymptomatic Patient Presentation

Basics

DESCRIPTION

Despite consuming a life-threatening ingestion, a patient may be initially asymptomatic or have minimal symptoms that resolve and thereby mislead the health-care provider.

Diagnosis

DIFFERENTIAL DIAGNOSIS

Further information on each poison is available in SECTION IV, CHEMICAL AND BIOLOGICAL AGENTS.

TOXIC EXPOSURES THAT OFTEN SHOW NO INITIAL EFFECTS

Acetaminophen

- 12 to 48 hours: Hepatic failure associated with nausea, vomiting, right upper quadrant pain, and laboratory abnormalities consistent with hepatotoxicity may become apparent.
- Renal and pancreatic injury also may develop.

Anticoagulants

Anticoagulants (brodifacoum, chlorophacinone, diphacinone, pivalyn, pindone, valone, warfarin). 24 hours to several days: Clinical signs of bleeding (epistaxis, hematemesis, bleeding gums) associated with an elevated prothrombin time on laboratory studies may develop.

Arsenic or Thallium

- Days to months: Gastrointestinal effects usually occur within 1 to 2 hours in acute overdose.
- Repeated small doses will lead to delayed effects days or weeks later (water contamination, homicidal acts).

Body Packers

- Hours to days: The type of symptoms depends on the drug ingested; heroin and cocaine are the most common.
- Time of symptom onset varies with the packaging used; body packers wrap drugs carefully, but the packets contain large amounts of drug per package, resulting in rapid and severe development of symptoms once a package leaks or breaks.

Button (Disk) Battery

- Hours to days: Battery may split during transit through the gastrointestinal system.
- Symptoms may develop unpredictably at any time when the battery breaks and allows the caustic contents to leak.

Diphenoxalate

- Atropine (present in combination with diphenoxalate in most products) may delay absorption.
- 2 to 10 hours: CNS depression and coma may occur up to 10 hours after ingestion.

Ethylene Glycol

- 8 to 24 hours: Severe metabolic acidosis, tachycardia, tachypnea, and renal failure may develop after an initial asymptomatic period following ingestion.
- The acidosis takes several hours to develop.
- If the patient has ingested ethanol as well, symptoms may be delayed further still until the ethanol has been metabolized.

Hydrofluoric Acid

- Immediate to 12 hours: Low-concentration (6%–8%) dermal hydrofluoric acid injury may present hours after exposure to low-concentration compounds.
- Skin findings can appear minimal even when injury and pain are severe.

Lead

Hours to weeks: Acute ingestion of lead curtain weights, sinkers, etc. may produce delayed encephalopathy and death in a child.

Methanol

- 8 to 24 hours: Severe metabolic acidosis with a depressed mental status, tachycardia, tachypnea, and blindness may develop after an initial asymptomatic period following ingestion.
- The acidosis takes at least 9 to 12 hours to develop.
- If the patient has ingested ethanol as well, symptoms may be delayed further still until the ethanol has been metabolized.

Methylene Chloride

- Methylene chloride is metabolized to carbon monoxide, carbon dioxide, and formic acid.
- 8 to 12 hours: Although absorption of methylene chloride is rapid, toxicity from carbon monoxide may be delayed several hours following ingestion as the parent compound is metabolized.
- Carboxyhemoglobin levels peak several hours after exposure.

Mercury

Hours to months: A single exposure to mono- or dimethyl mercury (either dermal or through ingestion) has resulted in delayed neurologic and renal toxicity.

Monoamine Oxidase Inhibitors

- Immediately to 32 hours: Following acute overdose, the onset of tachycardia, hypertension, hypotension, hyperpyrexia, agitation, confusion, coma, and rigidity may be delayed.
- Patients should be observed for at least 24 hours following overdose.

Mushrooms

- 6 hours to days: Hepatotoxicity following mushroom ingestion from the cyclopeptide-producing group of mushrooms (Amanita, Gallerina, Lepiota, Conocybe species) produces severe hepatic injury with a high fatality rate.
- This group includes the "death cap" mushroom (Amanita phalloides).
- Hepatic injury typically manifests 1 to 6 days following ingestion, although vomiting and diarrhea typically occur within 24 hours, with a delay of at least 6 hours.
- Following ingestion of Coprinus mushrooms, the acute symptoms, characterized by tachycardia, flushing, and vomiting, usually occur within 0.5 to 2 hours of ingestion; however, an interaction with alcohol also typically occurs if alcohol is ingested within 72 hours of Coprinus ingestion.

Naphthalene

- 1 to 7 days: Hemolysis with fever, vomiting, abdominal pain, diarrhea, lethargy, jaundice, and dark urine are typically delayed after ingestion as naphthalene is metabolized to its hemolytic metabolite.

Oral Hypoglycemic

- Oral hypoglycemic agents (acetohexamide [Dymelor], chlorpropamide [Diabinase], glipizide [Micronase, DiaBeta], glyburide [Glucotrol], tolazamide [Tolinase], tolbutamide [Orinase, Orinade]).
- 2 to 12 hours: The onset of hypoglycemic symptoms may be delayed, particularly with long-acting agents such as chlorpropamide, which may have a delay in peak levels of up to 36 hours.
- It is recommended that the glucose level be monitored for 12 to 24 hours following ingestion of an unknown oral hypoglycemic.

Quinine

- Up to 12 hours: Delayed cardiotoxicity following ingestion developed 25 hours following overdose in a patient who did not develop nausea, vomiting, lethargy, and ataxia until 11.5 hours following ingestion.
- Delayed blindness also may occur.

Snakebite (Coral Snake, Rattlesnake)

- Immediate to 12 hours: Neurologic symptoms following coral snake envenomation may be delayed.
- Swelling, tenderness, ecchymosis, and coagulopathy of rattlesnake bite toxicity may be delayed 4 to 12 hours.
- Dependent positioning of an envenomated limb may delay toxin absorption and the onset of symptoms.

Sustained-Release Products

• Includes products such as (e.g., aspirin, lithium, propranolol, theophylline, and verapamil.)
• Up to 24 hours: Delayed absorption and toxicity may occur due to the formulation of these products.
• Symptoms vary with the specific toxin.

Sodium Monofluoroacetate (SMFA)

2 to 20 hours: Nausea, anxiety, cardiac dysrhythmias, seizures, and coma may be delayed following ingestion due to the conversion of nontoxic fluoroacetate to fluorocitric acid, which blocks function of the tricarboxylic acid cycle.

TOXIC EXPOSURES IN WHICH INITIAL SYMPTOMS MAY BE PRESENT

Acetonitrile

• Up to 14 hours: Gastrointestinal irritation may develop after ingestion, but toxicity may be delayed as the nitrile is metabolized and releases cyanide.
• Any patient with a history of ingestion should be hospitalized for observation.

Antineoplastic agents

Hours to days: Most agents will cause some gastrointestinal effects within several hours of exposure; however, bone marrow suppression, the major toxicity of most agents, may not develop for several days.

Cadmium

Up to 96 hours: After the resolution of initial symptoms, including cough, chest pain, dyspnea, malaise, and fever, a patient inhaling cadmium fumes during welding may develop delayed pulmonary edema.

Carbon Tetrachloride

• 1 to 3 days: Nausea and headache may occur initially.
• Hepatic necrosis develops 1 to 3 days after exposure.

Cement

• 12 to 24 hours: Dermal exposure to wet cement (calcium hydroxide) may result in skin injury and ulceration as cement leaks around boots or gloves.
• Symptoms do not develop for several hours.

Chlorine

• Up to 24 hours: After initial symptoms of airway irritation abate, pulmonary edema may develop following significant inhalation exposure.
• Some symptoms such as an intermittent cough are likely to persist in these cases.

Colchicine

• 2 to 12 hours: Gastroenteritis usually develops within hours.
• Bone marrow suppression develops 4 to 5 days following ingestion.

Hydrocarbons

• Up to 6 hours: Aspiration pneumonitis may occur following hydrocarbon ingestion.
• The results of an initial chest radiograph may be normal with the development of infiltrates several hours later accompanied by increasing respiratory distress.
• A persistent cough may be the only sign of aspiration during the otherwise asymptomatic period.

Iron

6 to 24 hours: Following a gastrointestinal phase involving vomiting, diarrhea, and abdominal pain, patients may appear to improve for several hours following ingestion before developing systemic symptoms, including shock, pallor, lethargy, metabolic acidosis, and coagulopathy.

Nitrogen Dioxide

• Immediately to 36 hours: Initial dyspnea and hypoxemia following nitrogen dioxide inhalation may progress to pulmonary edema despite improvement in symptoms and an initially normal chest radiograph.
• Bronchiolitis obliterans may occur 2 to 3 weeks later.

Paraquat

• Immediately to days: High-concentration ingestion causes initial caustic gastrointestinal symptoms.
• Lower concentration ingestion or dermal exposure may present with renal failure over 3 to 5 days and pulmonary fibrosis over 1 to 2 weeks.

Phosgene

• Up to 72 hours: Initial irritative symptoms of cough, dyspnea, and anxiety may be delayed following exposure to concentrations of less than 3 ppm.
• Pulmonary edema may be delayed for as long as 72 hours following inhalation.

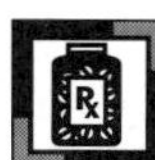

Treatment

• A common approach to poisoning involves patient observation and ancillary testing.
• Knowledge of the specific toxin helps determine an appropriate length of observation as well as indicating appropriate laboratory tests. See SECTION IV, CHEMICAL AND BIOLOGICAL AGENTS, for chapters on individual toxins.

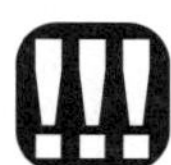

Pitfalls

TREATMENT

• Due to the low prevalence of late complications of toxic ingestion, some health-care providers develop a false sense of security.
• Asymptomatic patients may be discharged before more serious symptoms appear.
• Patients who have been exposed to an agent with the potential for delayed complications should undergo prolonged monitoring as indicated for that agent.

ICD-9-CM

No code is available.

See also: SECTION II, Body Packer/Body Stuffer chapter; and SECTION IV, Acetaminophen, Acetonitrile and Aliphatic Nitriles, Antineoplastic Agents, Arsenic, Brown Recluse Spider, Button Battery, Cadmium Fume Fever, Chlorine, Colchicine, Diphenoxylate, Ethylene Glycol, Hydrocarbons—General, Hydrofluoric Acid and Ammonium Bifluoride, Iron, Lead Poisoning, Lithium, MAO Inhibitors, Mercury—Organic, Methanol, Mothballs, Mushrooms, Nitrogen Oxides, Oral Hypoglycemic Agents, Paraquat/Diquat, Quinine, Snakebite—North American Coral Snakes, Snakebite—North American Crotalids, and Theophylline chapters.

Author: Lada Kokan

Reviewer: Katherine M. Hurlbut

Body Packer/Body Stuffer

Basics

DESCRIPTION

"Body packer" refers to the intentional transport of narcotics or contraband inside a body cavity, usually the gastrointestinal tract, specifically to elude detection by law enforcement authorities.

- Typically, the material is well-packaged for gastrointestinal transit in multiple layers of latex, condoms, or tape.
- If leaking occurs, toxic effects may be delayed from hours to days and are more likely to be life threatening than the effects experienced by a body stuffer.
- Package contents can include heroin, cocaine paste or powder, crack cocaine, hashish, marijuana, marijuana oil, 3,4-methylenedioxymethamphetamine (MDMA; "ecstacy"), or amphetamines.
- Body sites include the gastrointestinal tract, vagina, ears, and rectum (antegrade route).
- The number of packages varies, but can exceed 200; each package can contain 3 to 30 g of drug, and the total drug weight may exceed 1 kg.
- The individual may use anticholinergic agents to decrease gastrointestinal motility.

"Body stuffer" refers to impulsive drug ingestion to evade prosecution by "swallowing the evidence" or by concealing the drugs in the vagina or rectum.

- Due to time pressure, the drug(s) are usually unwrapped or wrapped poorly in plastic, cellophane, balloons, paper, or foil.
- Packages are likely to leak, and symptoms are generally milder and develop earlier than with body packers.
- Ingestion of large quantities of drug is unusual.

PATHOPHYSIOLOGY

- Direct toxic effects of the ingested drug or adulterant may develop if the package leaks.
- Mechanical bowel obstruction may occur, particularly in the body packer.
- Local trauma to the esophagus, gastrointestinal tract, vagina, or rectum may occur during insertion.

EPIDEMIOLOGY

- Body stuffing is common; its toxic effects are common, but severe effects are rare.
- Body packing is uncommon; its toxic effects are uncommon but severe when they develop.

RISK FACTORS

- Body packing should be suspected in cases of recent international travel or incarceration.
- Body stuffing should be suspected in cases of recent arrest or witnessed ingestion by law enforcement authorities.

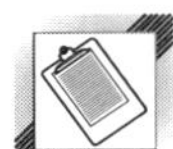

Diagnosis

DIFFERENTIAL DIAGNOSIS

Common Toxicologic Causes

- Body Packer. Heroin, cocaine paste or powder, or crack cocaine
- Body Stuffer. Any drug of abuse

Uncommon Toxicologic Causes

- Body Packer. Marijuana, hashish, marijuana oil, MDMA, or amphetamines
- Body Stuffer. Adulterants in drugs of abuse, including caffeine, lidocaine, procaine, ephedrine, strychnine, or quinine

Other Causes

- Bezoars, surgical abdomen, and constipation may mimic obstructive symptoms, and bowel ischemia may cause similar effects.
- Psychosis, infection, meningitis, hyperthyroidism, and pheochromocytoma may mimic sympathomimetic excess.

SIGNS AND SYMPTOMS

- Symptoms are determined by the ingested drug.
- Toxicity may develop rapidly if packets rupture.
- Rupture of packet should be suspected in a patient with abrupt deterioration.
- Abdominal pain or vomiting suggests obstruction or perforation.

Vital Signs

- Sympathomimetic drugs may cause tachycardia, hypertension, and hyperthermia, followed by cardiovascular collapse.
- Bradypnea and hypothermia may indicate opioid toxicity.

HEENT

- Dilated pupils indicate sympathomimetic ingestion or effects of anticholinergic drugs.
- Pinpoint pupils indicate opioid ingestion.
- Drooling or subcutaneous air suggests esophageal obstruction or perforation.

Cardiovascular

- Tachycardia and palpitations suggest cocaine or amphetamine effects.
- Bradycardia suggests opioid ingestion.
- Dysrhythmia or hypotension in body packer suggests that a life-threatening overdose is developing.
- Myocardial infarction, aortic dissection, bowel ischemia, and arterial spasm may occur.

Pulmonary

- Pulmonary edema may develop with heroin ingestion.
- Respiratory depression suggests opioid ingestion.

Gastrointestinal

- Abdominal tenderness or palpable mass may indicate obstruction, perforation, or abscess.
- Decreased bowel sounds indicate ileus due to anticholinergic drugs, opioids, or mechanical obstruction.

Hepatic

Severely hyperthermic patients may develop hepatic necrosis.

Renal

Acute renal failure may follow rhabdomyolysis, seizures, or hypotension.

Musculoskeletal

Rhabdomyolysis may develop in patients with seizures or hyperthermia.

Neurologic

- Seizures or stupor indicate significant toxicity in body stuffers and impending lethal deterioration in body packers.
- Agitation suggests sympathomimetic drug effects.
- Cerebrovascular accident may occur in severe overdose of sympathomimetics.

Psychiatric/Psychological

Hallucinations and paranoid behavior may indicate stimulants.

PROCEDURES AND LABORATORY TESTS

Testing is directed largely by the history and circumstances of presentation.

Essential Tests

- Body Stuffer. No tests may be needed in asymptomatic patients.
- Body Packer. Urine screen is used for drugs of abuse; a positive urine test result for drugs of abuse on presentation correlates well with the presence of drug packets in a body packer, regardless of findings on abdominal films. It is less useful to assess the course of evacuation of packets for body packers.

Recommended Tests

- ECG is used in symptomatic or tachycardic patients.

—Tachycardia is common in mild sympathomimetic intoxication.
—Other dysrhythmias suggest severe overdose.

- Arterial blood gases or pulse oximetry is used in cases involving bradypnea, hypoxia, or hypoventilation.
- Serum electrolytes, BUN, and creatinine should be measured in symptomatic patients; metabolic acidosis or renal injury suggests serious intoxication.

Imaging for Body Stuffer

- Abdominal radiograph is generally not indicated, unless mechanical obstruction is suspected.
- Transabdominal ultrasonography may be useful for noninvasive vaginal evaluation.
- Chest radiography is used in patients with pulmonary symptoms.

Imaging for Body Packers

- Abdominal radiography is diagnostic in 70% to 90% of cases.
- A falsely positive abdominal radiograph may occur due to constipation.
- Water-soluble contrast may increase sensitivity of abdominal films but requires a several hour delay. It is useful for evaluating complete passage of packets and mildly promotes gastrointestinal motility.
- CT scan may be indicated for a case with a negative abdominal series but a high suspicion of ingestion.
- Ultrasonography is useful for noninvasive vaginal evaluation, but does not improve detection of abdominal packages.

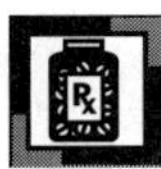

Treatment

- Supportive care with appropriate airway management is vital; specific treatment is initiated while supportive care continues.
- Dose and time of exposure should be determined for all substances involved.
- Emergent surgical consultation is indicated for symptomatic body packers or stuffers.

DIRECTING PATIENT COURSE

The health-care provider should call the poison control center when:

- hypoxia, seizures or other serious effects are present.
- coingestant, drug interaction, or underlying disease presents an unusual problem.

The patient should be referred to a health-care facility if a history of body packing or stuffing is obtained.

Admission Considerations

- Patients who are suspected body packers should be admitted to complete decontamination, which often requires several hours.
- Body stuffers should be admitted if persistent toxic effects develop.

DECONTAMINATION

- Do not induce emesis due to the risk of rupturing a drug packet and potential for aspiration or esophageal obstruction.
- Gastric lavage or manual removal of packets are not recommended due to the potential for rupture.
- One dose of activated charcoal (1–2 g/kg) should be administered if a substantial ingestion has occurred within the previous few hours.
- Whole bowel irrigation is recommended for body stuffers or packers.

—2 L/h of polyethylene glycol solution should be administered until passage of two packet-free stools.
—Water-soluble contrast abdominal series is useful for evaluating complete passage of packets in body packer.
—Gastrointestinal decontamination may require several days of close observation.

ANTIDOTES

Naloxone is used for opioid toxicity.

- Indication. Respiratory depression
- Contraindications. Documented naloxone allergy
- Method of administration

—Naloxone is administered as a 2.0-mg intravenous push, and the response should be observed.
—If no response, the dose is repeated in 2.0-mg increments to a total dose of 10 mg.
—Although less desirable, naloxone also may be administered by endotracheal, intramuscular, intralingual, intraosseous, or subcutaneous injection.

- Patients with persistent or recurrent effects may be treated with constant infusion of naloxone.

ADJUNCTIVE TREATMENT

- Respiratory depression. Endotracheal intubation is used for patients with respiratory depression who do not respond to naloxone.

—Body packers should be intubated early if toxic effects develop due to high risk of lethal overdose.
—Intravenous access, cardiac monitoring, and oxygen administration should be performed on all patients.

- Hyperthermia. Aggressive cooling measures are used for hyperthermic patients.
- The endoscopic removal of drug packages is contraindicated due to the risk of rupture.

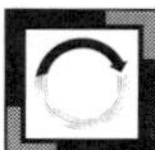

Follow-Up

EXPECTED COURSE AND PROGNOSIS

- Body stuffers usually manifest toxicity early and then recover rapidly with appropriate treatment.
- Body packers usually manifest toxicity days after ingestion and afterward have a stormy medical course with serious toxicity from whatever drug was used.

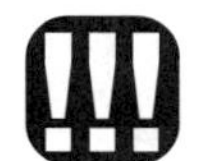

Pitfalls

DIAGNOSIS

The health-care professional should consider adulterants used to manufacture or dilute the drug.

TREATMENT

Early endotracheal intubation should be performed immediately in a deteriorating body packer.

ICD-9-CM 965.0

Poisoning by analgesics, antipyretics, and antirheumatics: opiates and related narcotics.

See also: SECTION III, Naloxone and Nalmephene and Whole Bowel Irrigation chapters; and SECTION IV, Cocaine chapter.

RECOMMENDED READING

McCarron M. The cocaine "body packer" syndrome. JAMA 1983;250:1417–1420.

Sporer KA. Clinical course of crack cocaine body stuffers. Ann Emerg Med 1997;29:596–601.

Utrecht MJ. Heroin body packers. J Emerg Med 1993;11:33–40.

Author: Michael Stackpool

Reviewer: Katherine M. Hurlbut

Bradycardia Toxidrome

Basics

DESCRIPTION

Bradycardia, or decreased heart rate at rest, is defined as follows:

- Adults and adolescents: fewer than 60 beats/min
- Children 5 to 10 years of age: fewer than 65 beats/min
- Children 1 to 5 years of age: fewer than 75 beats/min
- Newborns and infants less than 1 year of age: fewer than 110 beats/min

PATHOPHYSIOLOGY

- Common toxicologic mechanisms for persistent bradycardia include β-adrenergic receptor blockade, blockade of myocardial sodium or calcium channels, cholinergic effect, and increased vagal tone.
- Other mechanisms for bradycardia involve myocardial infarction; electrolyte abnormalities; cerebral edema; and physiologic response to hypoxia, hypothermia, and hypertension are other possible causes.
- Geriatric patients with underlying cardiovascular disease may be less tolerant of bradycardia than other populations.

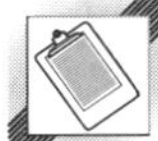

Diagnosis

DIFFERENTIAL DIAGNOSIS

Toxicologic Causes

Associated findings may help confirm the identity of the poison involved in the patient with bradycardia. Further information on each poison is available in SECTION IV, CHEMICAL AND BIOLOGICAL AGENTS.

- β-receptor blocking drugs also produce hypotension, hyperglycemia, atrioventricular (AV) block, ventricular dysrhythmia, CNS depression, and seizures.
- Calcium channel blocking drugs may produce hypotension, CNS depression, AV block, and ventricular dysrhythmia.
- Clonidine or imidazoline drugs (tetrahydrozoline) may produce small pupils, CNS depression, apnea, and hypotonia.
- Opioid drugs also may produce small pupils, CNS depression, and apnea perhaps with evidence of intravenous drug abuse.
- Digitalis glycosides frequently cause nausea and vomiting, visual complaints and halos, atrial and ventricular dysrhythmias, and AV block.
- Cholinergic agents (organophosphate or carbamate pesticides, bromocriptine, acetylcholine, physostigmine, pyridostigmine) cause vomiting, diarrhea, salivation, lacrimation, urination, bronchorrhea, small pupils, and sweating; nicotinic effects such as fasciculation and muscle weakness that are present in addition to the cholinergic effects suggest organophosphate or carbamate pesticide exposure.
- Ergot alkaloids, baclofen, skeletal muscle relaxants, lithium, lidocaine, flecainide, quinidine, amiodarone, bretylium, encainide, methyldopa, bufotoxin, mushrooms (inocybe, clitocybe), tetrodotoxin, and saxitoxin, all may be associated with bradycardia.

Nontoxicologic Causes

- All causes of hypotension or hypoxia may produce bradycardia.
- Hypothermia, electrolyte abnormalities (hyperkalemia, hypermagnesemia), hypoxia, increased intracranial pressure, myocardial infarction, congenital heart disease, and uncal herniation all can cause bradycardia.

SIGNS AND SYMPTOMS

If hypotension is not present, the heart rate may be appropriate for the patient even if it meets the definition for bradycardia.

Vital Signs

- Hypotension is common with severe bradycardia.
- Hypertension may be present if bradycardia is a reflex physiologic response.
- Hypothermia commonly produces bradycardia.

HEENT

- Dilated pupils suggest hypoxia.
- Pinpoint pupils suggest an opioid, clonidine, or imidazoline drug.
- Blurred or yellow vision or halos may indicate digitalis toxicity.
- Lacrimation suggests a cholinergic agent.

Dermatologic

Cyanosis suggests hypoxia or methemoglobinemia.

Pulmonary

- Bronchorrhea suggests a cholinergic agent (carbamate or organophosphate).
- Congestive heart failure may develop as a result of bradycardia from any cause.

Gastrointestinal

- Nausea and vomiting are common with digitalis and cholinergic agents.
- Decreased bowel sounds suggest opioids or β-receptor blockers.

Renal

- Hyperkalemia suggests digitalis poisoning.
- Hyperglycemia may be caused by β-receptor blockers
- Recurrent urination may be caused by cholinergic agents.

Neurologic

- Mental status depression or seizures may be caused by β-receptor blockers, cholinergic agents, and numerous other medications.

PROCEDURES AND LABORATORY TESTS

Essential Tests

- ECG and continuous cardiac monitoring should be obtained in all patients with bradycardia.

—Digitalis may cause any type of dysrhythmia.
—β-receptor blockers and calcium channel blocking drugs cause sinus bradycardia, AV block, and asystole.
—Myocardial ischemia may cause, or be produced by, bradycardia.

- Pulse oximetry or arterial blood gases should be performed to evaluate other possible causes of bradycardia.
- Serum electrolytes should be obtained to evaluate for hyperkalemia, hypermagnesemia, hypocalcemia, and hypoglycemia.

Recommended Tests

- Serum cholinesterase is used to assess organophosphate or carbamate poisonings.
- Serum acetaminophen and aspirin levels should be obtained in overdose settings to detect occult overdose with analgesic medications.
- Urine toxicology screen should be obtained in patients with persistent bradycardia of unknown cause.

• Arterial pressure monitoring (A line) may be helpful in management of bradycardia associated with hypotension.
• Swan-Ganz catheterization may be helpful to assess hemodynamic function.
• Chest radiograph may be obtained to evaluate hypoxia.
• Head CT may be ordered to evaluate for evidence of intracranial structural lesion or increased intracranial pressure.

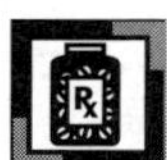

Treatment

• Intravenous access should be established.
• If hypotension unresponsive to initial intravenous isotonic fluid bolus is present, the patient should be intubated endotracheally until the cause can be determined and treated.
• The dose and time of exposure should be determined for all substances involved.
• Specific treatment (e.g., naloxone for mental status depression) should be initiated while continuing supportive care.

DIRECTING PATIENT COURSE

The health-care provider should call the poison control center when:

• cause of bradycardia is unclear.
• coingestant, drug interaction, or underlying disease presents unusual problems.

Admission Considerations

Patients with bradycardia should be admitted unless a reversible, physiologic cause is identified.

DECONTAMINATION

• Induction of emesis is not recommended for patients with bradycardia.
• Gastric lavage should be performed in pediatric (tube size 24–32 French) or adult patients (tube size 36–42 French) in most cases because bradycardia represents a serious toxic effect.
• One dose of activated charcoal (1 to 2 g/kg) should be administered without a cathartic if a substantial ingestion has occurred within the previous few hours.

ANTIDOTES

• Calcium chloride is used primarily for bradycardia or hypotension secondary to calcium channel blocker overdose; the optimal calcium chloride dose is unknown.
• Glucagon is used primarily for bradycardia and hypotension secondary to β-blocker overdose.

ADJUNCTIVE TREATMENT

• Hypoxia and electrolytes should be corrected as clinically indicated.
• If bradycardia is associated with hypotension, atropine should be administered.

—Adult dose is 0.5 to 1.0 mg intravenously, repeated in 5 minutes if necessary to a maximum of 2 mg.
—Pediatric dose is 0.02 mg/kg intravenously, repeated every 5 minutes as needed to a maximum dose of 1 mg in children, 2 mg in adolescents.

• If bradycardia and hypotension are unresponsive to atropine, isoproterenol should be considered.

—Adult dose is 5 μg/min infusion, titrated to effect.
—Pediatric dose is 0.1 μg/kg/min, titrated to effect.

• Intravenous fluid

—In patients with hypotension and no evidence of volume overload, 10 to 20 ml/kg 0.9% saline may be administered.
—If pressure is unresponsive to the initial bolus, further fluid therapy should be guided by central pressure measurement.
—Volume overload should be avoided because many agents that cause bradycardia are also myocardial depressants.

• Dopamine, 2 to 5 μg/kg/min, may be administered by intravenous infusion and titrated to desired effect; doses above 20 μg/kg/min are unlikely to have any further effect. If the patient is unresponsive to dopamine, 0.1 to 0.2 μg/kg/min of norepinephrine may be administered by continuous infusion and titrated to desired effect.
• Cardiac pacing may be considered if the patient is unresponsive to other attempts at treatment.

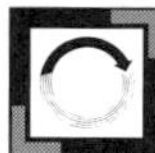

Follow-Up

EXPECTED COURSE AND PROGNOSIS

The duration of bradycardia is related to the underlying cause; drugs with prolonged absorption or half-life may produce prolonged bradycardia, whereas bradycardia secondary to increased vagal tone is generally short lived.

DISCHARGE CRITERIA/INSTRUCTIONS

Discharge only asymptomatic patients whose bradycardia was transient and not caused by a poisoning.

See also: SECTION III, Calcium Gluconate and Chloride, and Glucagon chapters; and SECTION IV, β-Receptor Blocking Drugs, Calcium Channel Blocking Drugs, Clonidine, Digoxin and Cardiac Glycosides, and Organophosphate Insecticides chapters.

ICD-9-CM 427.89

Other specified cardiac dysrhythmias.

RECOMMENDED READING

Goldfrank LR, Flomenbaum NE, Weisman RS, Lewin NA. Vital signs and toxic syndromes. In: Goldfrank LR, et al., eds. Goldfrank's toxicologic emergencies, 6th ed. Norwalk, CT: Appleton & Lange, 1998.

Author: Katherine M. Hurlbut

Reviewer: Richard C. Dart

Bradypnea

Basics

DESCRIPTION

Bradypnea, or decreased rate of respiration at rest, is defined as follows:

- Adults and adolescents: fewer than 12 respirations/min
- Children 6 to 12 years of age: fewer than 12 respirations/min
- Children 1 to 6 years of age: fewer than 20 respirations/min
- Infants 1 month to 1 year of age: fewer than 24 respirations/min

Hundreds of agents can cause depressed respiration; this discussion will focus on major agents that produce depressed respiration directly.

PATHOPHYSIOLOGY

- Bradypnea may be caused directly by depression of the medullary respiration center.
- Bradypnea may be caused indirectly by insensitivity of carotid body CO_2 detection.
- Muscular dysfunction may make an adequate respiratory rate unachievable.
- Neonatal patients or patients with underlying cardiovascular disease do not tolerate hypoxia well.

EPIDEMIOLOGY

Poisoning is common, usually as a therapeutic misadventure.

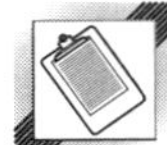

Diagnosis

The diagnosis of bradypnea is based on decreased respiratory rate.

DIFFERENTIAL DIAGNOSIS

Associated findings assist in determining the cause of bradypnea.

Common Toxicologic Causes

Further information on each poison is available in SECTION IV, CHEMICAL AND BIOLOGICAL AGENTS.

- Opioids often are associated with miosis, decreased bowel sounds, and depressed mental status.
- Cholinergic agonist drugs such as pilocarpine, bethanechol, and the organophosphate insecticides are associated with salivation, lacrimation, urination, defecation, and muscle weakness.
- Benzodiazepines, barbiturates, ethanol, or hypnotic agents (e.g., chloral hydrate, gamma hydroxybutyrate [GHB], or rohypnol ["roofies"]) are usually associated with midposition pupils and depressed mental status.
- Ethanol intoxication is associated with history and odor of intoxication.
- Nicotine poisoning may be associated with small pupils, nausea, vomiting, and tremors and fasciculations.
- α_2-receptor agonists (clonidine, tetrahydrozoline) produce depression of respiratory drive associated with small pupils and depressed mental status.
- Tricyclic antidepressant toxicity is usually associated with cardiac dysrhythmia in serious cases; anticholinergic effects are often absent.

Uncommon Toxicologic Causes

- Nearly any toxic agent may cause bradypnea as a preterminal event.
- Lomotil (diphenoxylate/atropine) may produce depressed respiration.
- Paralytic agents and diseases (succinylcholine, curare, strychnine, botulism, Guillain-Barré syndrome, polio, rabies, etc.) may produce depressed respiration.

Nontoxicologic Causes

- Altered mental status with localizing neurologic deficits indicates the probable presence of an intracranial lesion.
- Altered mental status without localizing findings may indicate the presence of hypoglycemia, or another metabolic abnormality.
- Any cause of hypotension or hypoxia may lead to bradypnea; for example, asthma, diabetic ketoacidosis, and pneumonia may all produce tachypnea that is followed by bradypnea as the patient tires.
- Many causes of muscle weakness also can cause bradypnea; however, these are generally also preceded by transient tachypnea with falling tidal volume (due to respiratory muscle weakness).
- Many nontoxicologic causes of mental status depression, such as severe electrolyte abnormalities or intracranial events, produce bradypnea when severe.

SIGNS AND SYMPTOMS

- Often the patient is unaware of bradypnea due to concurrent depression of mental status.
- Onset and duration of bradypnea may be extremely rapid or slow, depending on the toxic agent.

Vital Signs

Bradypnea often is associated with initial tachycardia that is followed by bradycardia as the patient's condition worsens.

HEENT

- Pinpoint pupils indicate an opioid as a probable cause; mid-position or dilated pupils may be present in an opioid overdose, however, if a concomitant substance that antagonizes the effect of the opioid has been ingested.
- Dilated pupils may indicate concurrent hypoxia, sympathomimetic effects, or anticholinergic effects.

Dermatologic

Peripheral and central cyanosis may be apparent if the patient is hypoxic.

Cardiovascular

- Tachycardia is a typical initial response to hypoxia; if hypoxia persists, tachycardia is followed by bradycardia.
- Hypotension, cyanosis, and cardiac ischemia or dysrhythmia may develop in severe cases.

Pulmonary

The chest is usually clear on examination unless aspiration has occurred.

Gastrointestinal

- Increased bowel sounds may be present with cholinergic stimulants.
- Decreased bowel sounds are consistent with opioids and sedative and hypnotic agents.

Fluids and Electrolytes

No abnormalities are expected, unless a coingestant complicates the course of bradypnea.

Musculoskeletal

Muscle weakness may contribute to bradypnea in conditions such as botulism and cholinergic poisoning.

Neurologic

Rapid onset of depressed mental status is common but reversible if detected and treated promptly.

PROCEDURES AND LABORATORY TESTS

Essential Tests

Oxygenation (pulse oximetry or arterial blood gas) should be assessed; hypoxia indicates clinically significant disease, and hypercarbia indicates hypoventilation.

Recommended Tests

- If bradypnea persists after initial measures, ventilation should be assessed with an arterial blood gas.

—Hypoxia indicates clinically significant disease.
—Elevated pCO_2 indicates hypoventilation.

- ECG should be obtained to detect the presence of tricyclic antidepressants or cardiac complications of hypoxia.
- Negative inspiratory force or other pulmonary function test findings assist in determining the need for endotracheal intubation and in establishing the source of hypoventilation.
- Serum levels of acetaminophen, salicylates, opioids, or other drugs should be obtained as needed to detect coingestions and help guide treatment if they are present.
- Blood, urine, and spinal fluid cultures, urine toxicology screen, and serum levels of specific drugs should be obtained as needed to determine other nontoxicologic causes of bradypnea.
- Chest radiograph should be obtained to assess potential intrathoracic causes of hypoxia and bradypnea.
- Head CT may be needed to evaluate the possibility of an intracranial event.

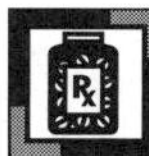

Treatment

- Supportive care with oxygen and appropriate airway management is vital, with specific treatment initiated as supportive care continues.
- The dose and time of exposure should be determined for all substances that could be involved.

DIRECTING PATIENT COURSE

The health-care provider should call the poison control center when:

- cause of bradypnea is unknown.
- coingestant, drug interaction, or underlying disease presents unusual problems.

DECONTAMINATION

- Emesis should not be induced because of the likelihood of depressed mentation.
- Gastric lavage is recommended for all critically ill patients with possible toxic ingestion who are unresponsive to naloxone.
- One dose of activated charcoal (1–2 g/kg) should be administered without a cathartic if a substantial ingestion has occurred within the previous few hours.

ANTIDOTES

Naloxone

- Indications. Any patient with depressed mental status.
- Contraindications. None.
- Method of administration. A 2.0-mg intravenous push, which may be repeated for refractory cases or recurrence of adverse effects.
- Potential adverse effects

—Naloxone may induce withdrawal syndrome.
—Reversal of opioid effects may unmask a coexistent toxicity, such as cocaine.

Dextrose

- Indications. Treatment of altered mental status.
- Contraindications. None.
- Method of administration

—Adult dose, D_{50}, 50 ml (25 g), in an intravenous push.
—Pediatric dose, D_{25}, 2 to 4 ml/kg (0.5–1.0 g/kg), in an intravenous push.

ADJUNCTIVE TREATMENT

- If serious respiratory depression or difficulty protecting the airway is present, the patient should be intubated endotracheally until the cause can be determined and treated.
- Intravenous access and cardiac monitor should be established, and naloxone should be administered.

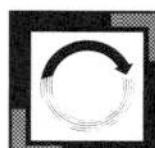

Follow-Up

EXPECTED COURSE AND PROGNOSIS

- The duration of the illness depends on the cause of bradypnea.
- Complications may develop rapidly; a few minutes of severe hypoxia may produce permanent cardiac or CNS injury or allow aspiration to occur.
- Most patients become bradypneic as the preterminal event.
- Death usually occurs only if the airway is not adequately managed.

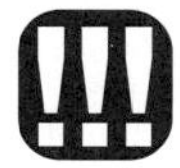

Pitfalls

- The airway should be managed aggressively; if clinically significant bradypnea develops, the patient should be intubated immediately.
- If vomiting is present, the health-care professional must ensure that aspiration has not occurred.

See also: SECTION II, Bradycardia and Coma chapters; and SECTION III, Naloxone chapter.

ICD-9-CM 786.09

Author: Richard C. Dart

Reviewer: Katherine M. Hurlbut

Cholinergic Syndrome (Unexplained)

Basics

DESCRIPTION

- A syndrome of salivation, lacrimation, urination, defecation, vomiting, diarrhea, and increased bronchial secretions caused by overstimulation of acetylcholine receptors.
- Altered mental status, fasciculation, weakness, and seizure occur in severe cases.

PATHOPHYSIOLOGY

- Cholinergic compounds inhibit the activity of the enzyme acetylcholinesterase, which results in the accumulation of acetylcholine and the overstimulation of the acetylcholine receptor.
There are two types of cholinergic effects, depending on the set of automatic nervous system receptors affected.

—Nicotinic effects are manifested by muscle weakness, fasciculation, hypertension, and tachycardia.
—Muscarinic effects involve pupillary constriction, bronchoconstriction, secretory functions, and bradycardia.

- Carbamate compounds (insecticides, physostigmine, neostigmine, pyridostigmine, edrophonium) are reversible inhibitors of acetylcholinesterase, and organophosphates are irreversible inhibitors of acetylcholinesterase.
- Organophosphate and carbamates bind to the acetylcholinesterase enzyme located in the synaptic junctions. The binding inactivates the acetylcholinesterase, preventing the breakdown of acetylcholine. Carbamates spontaneously disassociate from the acetylcholinesterase. The organophosphate-acetylcholinesterase bond eventually becomes permanent and inactivates the acetylcholinesterase. Natural recovery involves the synthesis of new acetylcholinesterase.

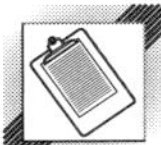

Diagnosis

- Numerous agents increase the concentration of acetylcholine in the synapse; therefore, medication and occupational histories are important in determining the cause of this syndrome.
- Organophosphates and carbamates often produce muscarinic symptoms that are clinically apparent. Other agents may produce more subtle clinical syndromes in which some symptoms or signs are more prominent than others.
- Muscarinic effects are manifested by the DUMBELS syndrome (Diaphoresis and diarrhea, Urination, Miosis, Bradycardia and bronchospasm, Emesis and excess of Lacrimation and salivation, and Seizures).
- Absence of symptoms or signs at presentation does not rule out potentially fatal ingestion.

DIFFERENTIAL DIAGNOSIS

Toxicologic Causes

- Further information on each poison is available in SECTION IV, CHEMICAL AND BIOLOGICAL AGENTS.
- Carbachol, methacholine, and arecholine are direct-acting parasympathomimetics, mimicking the action of acetylcholine.
- Arecoline produces both nicotinic and muscarinic effects associated with an elevation of acetylcholine in the CNS.
- Bethanechol produces primarily muscarinic effects.
- Pilocarpine used in the treatment of closed-angle glaucoma may produce systemic cholinergic effects.
- Numerous mushroom species produce cholinergic effects; both nicotinic and muscarinic effects occur, but muscarinic effects predominate.

Other Compounds that Produce Similar Clinical Effects

- Sympathomimetic amines may produce sweating, tachycardia, and hypertension.
- Nicotine overdose may be clinically indistinguishable from effects of agents that inhibit acetylcholinesterase.
- Beta-blockers, calcium channel blockers, and digoxin may produce bradycardia, atrioventricular (AV) block, and hypotension, mimicking some cholinergic effects.
- Muscle weakness and fasciculation of nicotinic agents may be mistaken for conditions that result in impaired neuromuscular transmission such as snake or scorpion envenomations, heavy metal poisoning, botulism, and Eaton-Lambert syndrome.
- Pulmonary irritants may produce nausea, vomiting, and bronchorrhea; these effects can usually be differentiated by the patient's medical history.
- Botulism is associated with descending muscle weakness or paralysis.

SIGNS AND SYMPTOMS

The examiner should check for unusual odors.

Vital Signs

- Bradycardia and hypotension are muscarinic effects.
- Ventricular dysrhythmias may result in hypotension.
- Tachycardia and hypertension are nicotinic effects.
- Tachypnea is common secondary to bronchorrea.

HEENT

- Miosis, excessive salivation, and lacrimation are common.
- Blurred vision, fasciculation of periorbital muscles, and eye pain may occur.

Dermatologic

Profuse diaphoresis is common.

Cardiovascular

- Cardiac depression or cardiovascular collapse may occur.
- Atrial fibrillation, atrioventricular blocks, and asystole may occur.

Pulmonary

Bronchospasm, bronchorrhea, and pulmonary edema are common.

Gastrointestinal

Nausea, vomiting, abdominal pain, diarrhea, and involuntary defecation occur.

Neurologic/Musculoskeletal

- Muscle fasciculation, weakness, and paralysis may occur.
- Seizures may occur.

Genitourinary

Urinary incontinence is common, especially in severe cases.

Other

Unusual odors may be perceived by the healthcare professional; some organophosphate insecticides have a garlic-like odor.

PROCEDURES AND LABORATORY TESTS

Essential Tests

• Red blood cell cholinesterase and plasma cholinesterase are both decreased when toxic effects of organophosphate or carbamate insecticide are present. Serum cholinesterase is often more readily available at most laboratories.
• Serum electrolytes, glucose, BUN, and creatinine are measured to detect other causes of dysrhythmia or decreased kidney function.
• ECG and continuous cardiac monitoring assess other potential causes of dysrhythmia and blood pressure abnormalities.

Recommended Tests

• Serum acetaminophen and aspirin levels in overdose setting are ordered to detect occult ingestion.
• Arterial blood gases are ordered to detect acidosis or hypoxia.
• Blood levels of specific agents are rarely useful during the acute episode. Blood levels may be useful during forensic investigations.
• Abused drugs, especially cocaine, may contain contaminants such as organophosphate insecticides.
• Head CT, lumbar puncture, bacterial cultures, and other tests are ordered as indicated in patients with altered mental status of unknown etiology.
• Chest radiography is used to assess pulmonary edema if clinically indicated.

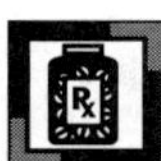

Treatment

• The health-care provider should provide supportive care while evaluating the source of poisoning and while treating with atropine and pralidoxime, if indicated.
• Dose and time of exposure should be determined for all substances involved.

DIRECTING PATIENT COURSE

The health-care provider should call the poison control center when:

• the source of cholinergic effects is unclear.
• coingestant, drug interaction, or underlying disease present unusual problems.

DECONTAMINATION

• Out of hospital. Emesis should not be induced.
• In hospital

—Gastric lavage in pediatric (tube size 24–32 French) or adult (tube size 36–42 French) patients is used for substantial ingestion presenting within 1 hour of ingestion or if serious effects are present.
—Endotracheal intubation before lavage should be considered if CNS depression, hydrocarbon carriers, or bethanechol is involved.
—One dose of activated charcoal (1–2 g/kg) is administered without a cathartic if a substantial ingestion has occurred within the previous few hours.

ANTIDOTES

Antidotes should be administered for altered mental status: oxygen, thiamine, glucose, and naloxone.

Atropine Sulfate

Treats the muscarinic effects by acting as a competitive inhibitor of acetylcholine at the acetylcholine receptor. Atropine is indicated for patients with severe bronchorrhea and/or bradycardia.

• Method of administration

—Adult dose is 1 to 4 mg intravenously initially, then every 1 to 10 minutes as needed to control bronchorrhea or to treat bradycardia.
—Pediatric dose is 0.01 to 0.04 mg/kg intravenously initially, then every 1 to 10 minutes to control bronchorrhea or to treat bradycardia.
—In severe cases (both adult and pediatric), the atropine requirement may exceed tens or hundreds of milligrams over the first 24 hours.

Pralidoxime (2-PAM)

Treats both nicotinic and muscarinic effects by removing organophosphate or carbamates from the cholinesterase binding site.

• Method of administration

—Adult dose is 1 to 2 g intravenously over 15 to 30 minutes. Repeat doses of 1 to 2 g intravenously every 2 to 4 hours or a continuous intravenous infusion at 500 mg/h is commonly required for organophosphates.
—Pediatric dose is 20 to 40 mg/kg intravenously over 15 to 30 minutes. Repeat doses of 20 to 40 mg/kg intravenously every 2 to 4 hours or an intravenous infusion of 10 mg/kg is commonly required for organophosphates.

ADJUNCTIVE TREATMENT

• Hypoxia and electrolytes should be corrected as clinically indicated.
• Tachycardia or bradycardia should be treated if clinically indicated.
• Hypertension should be treated if clinically indicated; short-acting and easily reversible agents should be used because most hypertensive effects of drugs are transient and may be followed by hypotension.

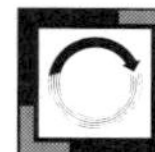

Follow-Up

EXPECTED COURSE AND PROGNOSIS

• Onset is often rapid, but may be delayed after dermal exposure.
• Effects peak in the first day, but may persist for days or weeks if not treated.

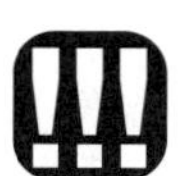

Pitfalls

The most common problem in treatment is the failure to administer adequate amounts of atropine, allowing respiratory effects to interfere with oxygenation.

ICD-9-CM 971

Poisoning by drugs primarily affecting the autonomic nervous system.

See also: SECTION II, Bradycardia Toxidrome, Hypotension, and Tachycardia chapters; SECTION III, Atropine and Pralidoxime chapters; and SECTION IV, Carbamate Insecticide, Nicotine, and Organophosphate Insecticide chapters.

RECOMMENDED READING

Aaron CK, Howland MA. Insecticides: organophosphates and carbamates. In: Goldfrank LR, et al., eds. Goldfrank's toxicologic emergencies, 6th ed. Norwalk, CT: Appleton & Lange, 1998.

Author: Steven A. Seifert

Reviewer: Richard C. Dart

Coma

Basics

DESCRIPTION

Coma is defined as markedly depressed mental status, generally without appropriate response to verbal stimuli.

PATHOPHYSIOLOGY

- Depressed mental status may be produced by hundreds of agents.
- General causes of coma include substrate insufficiency (hypoxia, ischemia, or hypoglycemia), effect of a chemical agent (e.g., gamma hydroxybutyrate acid [GHB] or opioid agonist), electrolyte abnormality (e.g., hyper- or hyponatremia), environmental disturbance (hyper- or hypothermia), or systemic infection.

EPIDEMIOLOGY

- Coma is common in poisonings and usually results from intentional ingestion or substance abuse.
- Elderly patients may develop CNS depression at therapeutic doses of some drugs, especially if more than one drug with a sedative effect is ingested.
- Death usually occurs only if adequate airway is not maintained.

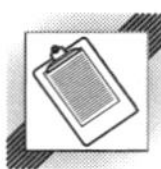

Diagnosis

DIFFERENTIAL DIAGNOSIS

Associated findings in the presence of coma assist in determining its cause.

Toxicologic Causes

Numerous commonly used toxicologic agents can cause coma. Further information on each poison is available in SECTION IV, CHEMICAL AND BIOLOGICAL AGENTS.

- Opioids also cause miosis, decreased bowel sounds, and respiratory depression.
- Cholinergic agonist drugs, such as pilocarpine, bethanechol, organophosphate, or carbamate insecticide, are associated with bradycardia, salivation, lacrimation, urination, defecation, and muscle weakness.
- Benzodiazepine drug overdose is usually associated with mid-position pupils and respiratory depression; coma is unusual in these cases unless the benzodiazepine is combined with other sedative agents or administered parenterally.
- Neuroleptic or other dopamine agonist or serotonin agonist ingestion, either chronic or recent, may suggest neuroleptic malignant syndrome (NMS) or serotonin syndrome, two similar entities that result in altered mental status, hyperthermia, muscle rigidity, and autonomic instability.
- Barbiturate overdose is usually associated with mid-position pupils and respiratory depression.
- Sedative-hypnotic agent overdose, such as with chloral hydrate, GHB, and rohypnol ("roofies"), is usually associated with mid-position pupils and respiratory depression.
- Clonidine and tetrahydrozoline produce respiratory depression with small pupils, bradycardia, and hypotension.
- Tricyclic antidepressant (TCA) overdose is usually associated with cardiac dysrhythmia, often with seizures; a QRS complex width of ≥ 0.10 seconds may be present, as may anticholinergic effects.
- Anticonvulsants commonly cause nystagmus, ataxia, and slurred speech prior to the onset of coma; carbamazepine may cause hallucinations, hyponatremia, and seizures.
- Carbon monoxide, cyanide, or hydrogen sulfide cause nausea, headache, and rapid onset of coma; metabolic acidosis is common. Multiple victims may be involved.
- Methanol is associated with nausea, ataxia, and slurred speech, followed by metabolic acidosis, visual complaints, or blindness.
- Ethylene glycol causes nausea, ataxia, and slurred speech, followed by metabolic acidosis, proteinuria, hematuria, calcium oxalate crystalluria, and renal failure.
- Isopropyl alcohol causes marked mental status depression and occasionally hemorrhagic gastritis without metabolic acidosis.
- Hydrocarbons such as toluene may cause metabolic acidosis and renal tubular acidosis.

A few less common agents also may cause coma:

- Nearly any toxic agent may cause CNS depression or coma as a preterminal event.
- Diphenoxylate/atropine (Lomotil) can cause anticholinergic effects initially, followed by narcotic effect.
- Ethchlorvynol (Placidyl) causes profound coma that may persist for days.

Nontoxicologic Causes

- Coma is nondiagnostic in itself; it is important to determine whether localizing neurologic signs are present. Localizing signs often indicate a focal intracranial infection, bleed, or other structural abnormality; lack of lateralization, however, does not exclude an intracranial process.
- All nontoxic causes of hypotension, hypoxia, or hypoglycemia may lead to coma.
- Specific nontoxic causes of mental status depression include severe electrolyte abnormalities, hypo- or hypernatremia, hypoglycemia, or intracranial events (infection, bleed, embolus).

SIGNS AND SYMPTOMS

Physical signs that occur in the patient with coma may help reveal the poison involved.

Vital Signs

- Tachycardia suggests poisoning by a TCA, phenothiazine, cyclobenzaprine, or sympathomimetic or anticholinergic drug.
- Bradycardia may indicate β-receptor or calcium channel blocker, baclofen, clonidine, imidazoline, cholinergic agent, or decongestant.
- Hypotension suggests TCA, phenothiazines, β-receptor or calcium channel blocker, clonidine, imidazolines, or late course of monoamine oxidase (MAO) inhibitor.
- Hypertension is typical early in the course of phenylpropanolamine, sympathomimetic, or anticholinergic poisoning.
- Hyperthermia is common in sympathomimetic or anticholinergic overdose, NMS, serotonin syndrome, overdose of salicylate or hallucinogen, and alcohol withdrawal.
- Environmental hypothermia may develop from any cause of prolonged coma.

HEENT

- Pinpoint pupils suggest opioid, clonidine, imidazoline, or cholinergic agent involvement.
- Mydriasis may indicate hypoxia or poisoning with sympathomimetic or anticholinergic agent, phenothiazine, TCA, or carbamazepine.
- Nystagmus suggests ethanol, carbamazepine, phenytoin, phencyclidine, phenobarbital, or sedative-hypnotic toxicity.

Dermatologic

- Dry, flushed skin suggests anticholinergic toxicity.
- Cyanosis suggests hypoxia or methemoglobinemia.
- "Track marks" may indicate heroin, cocaine, or amphetamine abuse.

Cardiovascular

- QRS widening or an R wave in the ECG lead aVR suggests TCA, phenothiazine, or severe carbamazepine overdose.
- β-receptor blockers also produce hypotension, hyperglycemia, bradycardia atrioventricular (AV) block, ventricular dysrhythmia, and seizures.
- Calcium channel blockers may produce hypotension, CNS depression, bradycardia, AV block, and ventricular dysrhythmia.

Pulmonary

- Respiratory depression may indicate opioid, sedative-hypnotic, TCA, phenothiazines, β-receptor or calcium channel blocker, clonidine, or imidazoline.
- Hyperpnea is typical with salicylates and agents that cause metabolic acidosis (e.g., isoniazid, ethylene glycol, or methanol), and with hypoxia or hyperthermia from any cause.

Gastrointestinal

- Increased bowel sounds and diarrhea may be present with cholinergic stimulant (organophosphate or carbamate insecticides) toxicity.
- Decreased bowel sounds are consistent with anticholinergic, opioid, or sedative-hypnotic agents.

Fluids and Electrolytes

- Increased anion gap metabolic acidosis suggests lactic acid, methanol, ethylene glycol, iron, isoniazid, salicylate, carbon monoxide, cyanide, metformin, paraldehyde, or toluene toxicity.
- Decreased anion gap suggest lithium or bromides.

• Hypoglycemia suggests hypoglycemic agents, ethanol (particularly in children), or severe hepatic injury from any cause.

Musculoskeletal

Rhabdomyolysis may develop from seizures or prolonged coma.

Neurologic

• Prolonged or recurrent seizures may develop with isoniazid, cocaine or other sympathomimetic agents, lithium, TCA, or carbamazepine toxicity among many others.
• Myoclonus and tremor may occur with lithium, methaqualone, carbamazepine, phenytoin, valproate, barbiturates, chloral hydrate, ethanol, glutethimide, ethanol, or phenothiazines.
• Myoclonus without tremor may occur with anticonvulsants, benzodiazepines, TCAs, ethanol, or sedative-hypnotics.
• Fasciculation may occur with lithium, amphetamines, cholinergic agents, cocaine, nicotine, and phencyclidine or hypoglycemia from any cause.

PROCEDURES AND LABORATORY TESTS

Essential Tests

• Oxygenation should be assessed (pulse oximetry or arterial blood gas); hypoxia and hypercarbia are treatable causes of CNS depression.
• Blood glucose should be measured.

—Hyperglycemia is a reversible cause of coma that may cause permanent neurologic injury if not promptly treated.
—Hypoglycemia should be treated presumptively with a bolus of D_{50} if bedside testing is not immediately available.

• ECG and continuous cardiac monitoring should be performed; these tests may reveal evidence of TCA intoxication (tachycardia, QRS widening, R wave in lead aVR), β-adrenergic antagonist (bradycardia, AV block), or calcium channel antagonist (bradycardia, AV block).
• Serum electrolytes, calcium, magnesium, BUN, and creatinine should be obtained to assess for anion gap metabolic acidosis and severe electrolyte abnormalities (hypo- or hypernatremia), and renal injury.

Recommended Tests

• Urine toxicology screen should be ordered to assess persistent coma of undetermined etiology; the presence of acetaminophen, salicylate, opioid, or other drugs will help guide treatment.
• Serum or breath ethanol level should be obtained to assess for this common cause of mental status depression.
• Serum acetaminophen and aspirin levels should be obtained in overdose settings to detect occult ingestion.
• Lumbar puncture; blood, urine, spinal fluid cultures; and specific drug levels (e.g., anticonvulsant) should be obtained as needed to evaluate for differential diagnoses.
• Head CT may be needed to investigate the possibility of intracranial disease.

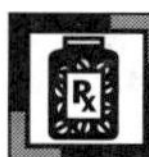

Treatment

• If serious respiratory depression or difficulty in protecting the airway is present, the patient should be intubated endotracheally until the cause can be determined and treated.
• Intravenous access should be established, cardiac monitor should be placed, and reversible causes of coma should be treated empirically with immediate administration of oxygen, 2 mg of naloxone, 50 ml of $D_{50}W$ (unless immediate glucose determination is available), and 100 mg of thiamine.
• Reversible causes of coma must be treated empirically.
• The dose and time of exposure should be determined for all substances involved.

DIRECTING PATIENT COURSE

The health-care provider should call poison control center when:

• the cause of the coma is unknown.
• coingestant, drug interaction, or underlying disease presents unusual problems.

Admission Considerations

Nearly all cases of coma require admission with exception of quickly reversible causes that have not caused permanent injury (e.g., transient hypoglycemia).

DECONTAMINATION

• Syrup of ipecac should never be administered to a patient with CNS depression.
• If toxic ingestion is possible, gastric lavage should be performed in pediatric (tube size 24–32 French) or adult (tube size 36–42 French) patients with altered mental status; in the comatose patient, lavage should be performed even if the ingestion occurred several hours previously.
• One dose of activated charcoal (1–2 g/kg) should be administered without a cathartic.

ANTIDOTES

Naloxone

• Indications. Altered mental status of undetermined etiology.
• Contraindications. None.
• Method of administration

—Adult or pediatric dose is 2 to 10 mg administered in 2-mg increments.
—A cumulative dose of 10 to 20 mg may be needed for propoxyphene, nalbuphine, or butorphanol poisonings.
—If more than 10 mg is needed or produces only partial response, suspect the influence of another toxicant.

• Potential adverse effects

—Naloxone may induce withdrawal syndrome.
—Reversal of opioid effects may unmask another coexistent toxicity, such as cocaine.

Dextrose

• Indications. Altered mental status.
• Contraindication. None.
• Method of administration

—Adult dose is 50 to 100 ml (25–50 g) of D_{50} administered by intravenous push.
—Pediatric dose is 2 to 4 ml/kg (0.5–1 g/kg) of D_{25} administered by intravenous push.

Flumazenil

• Indications. Depressed mental status requiring intubation and extensive diagnostic assessment.
• Contraindications. Patients with a history of seizures, history or ECG evidence of TCA overdose (QRS widening, R wave in ECG lead aVR), or known benzodiazepine dependence.
• Method of administration

—Adult dose is 0.2 mg administered intravenously and repeated every 1 to 2 minutes up to 2 mg; if effective, the dosage may be repeated every 30 minutes or more as needed.
—Pediatric dose is 10 μg/kg administered intravenously; if effective, the dose may be repeated every 30 minutes or more as needed.

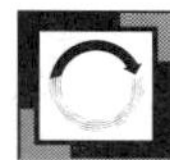

Follow-Up

PATIENT MONITORING

Cardiovascular and respiratory functions should be monitored continuously.

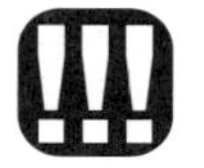

Pitfalls

DIAGNOSIS

Brain death cannot be diagnosed by EEG alone in comatose patients with drug intoxication (e.g., barbiturates).

TREATMENT

• Airway should be managed aggressively; many toxicologic deaths occur simply because endotracheal intubation was not performed early.
• If vomiting is present, it is important to ensure that aspiration has not occurred.

See also: SECTION II, Bradycardia Toxidrome chapter; and SECTION III, Dextrose, Flumazenil, and Naloxone and Nalmephene chapters.

ICD-9-CM 780.01

Alterations of consciousness: coma.

RECOMMENDED READING

Galliger EJ. Neurologic principles. In: Goldfrank LR, et al., eds. Goldfrank's toxicologic emergencies, 6th ed. Norwalk, CT: Appleton & Lange, 1998.

Author: Katherine M. Hurlbut

Reviewer: Luke Yip

Extravasation of Drugs

Basics

DESCRIPTION

Extravasation, or infiltration, is the leakage of intravenously infused fluids from the vein.

PATHOPHYSIOLOGY

- Hyperosmolar Agents. Hypertonic cation-containing solutions (e.g., potassium chloride or calcium chloride), high-concentration dextrose solutions (10% or greater), hyperalimentation, and radiographic contrast media are thought to cause damage due to hyperosmolality.
- Vasoconstriction. Vasopressors (e.g., dopamine or epinephrine) cause vasoconstriction-induced ischemic necrosis.
- Direct Cytotoxicity. Chemotherapeutic drugs and some antibiotics (e.g., nafcillin, tetracycline) are directly cytotoxic to subcutaneous tissue.
- Mechanical Compression. Large-volume extravasation of nontoxic solutions can cause mechanical compression.
- pH. Tissue injury can result from the high pH of an infiltrate (e.g., acyclovir pH 10.5–11.6, aminophylline pH 9, phenytoin pH 10–12.3).
- Infection. Tissue injury may predispose to infection and secondary tissue damage.

EPIDEMIOLOGY

- Extravasation is common; the incidence ranges from 0.1% to 6%.
- Extravasation incidence rates are higher for children and infants: 11% and 57% to 63%, respectively.
- About 2% of patients with extravasation develop serious injury.
- Extravasation occurs more often during surgery or cardiac resuscitation than in other settings.

CAUSES

- The primary cause of extravasation injury is phlebitis.
- Other causes of extravasation are mechanical: metal needles (e.g., butterfly needles), poor insertion technique, pressurized infusion pumps, or improper immobilization of the catheter or needle.

RISK FACTORS

- Noncommunicative (very young or old, unconscious) patients are at risk for extravasation.
- Severely debilitated or chronically ill patients (e.g., marked weight loss or extensive metastatic disease) are also at risk.
- Patients with abnormal limb circulation (e.g., vascular disease, connective tissue disease, venous thrombosis or insufficiency, tourniquets, prior radiation to the limb or regional lymph node dissection) are at increased risk.
- Multiple punctures of the same vein increase the risk for extravasation.
- Injections on the ankle or the dorsum of the foot or hand also increase the extravasation risk.
- Use of indwelling intravenous lines increases the risk for extravasation.
- Injections through needles, as opposed to plastic catheters, increase extravasation risk.
- Patients with underlying disease have greater risk of developing serious injury if extravasation occurs.

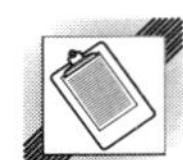

Diagnosis

DIFFERENTIAL DIAGNOSIS

Further information on each poison is available in SECTION IV, CHEMICAL AND BIOLOGICAL AGENTS.

- Antineoplastic agents that cause extravasation injury include aclacinomycin, amsacrine (M-AMSA), bisantrene, bleomycin, carmustine (BCNU), chlorzotocin, cyclophosphamide, cytarabine (Ara-C), dacarbazine (DTIC), dactinomycin (actinomycin D), daunorubicin (DNR), doxorubicin (ADR), etoposide (VP-16), fluorouracil (5-FU), mechlorethamine (nitrogen mustard), mitomycin (mitomycin-C), mitoxantrone, PALA, plicamycin (mithramycin), rubidazone, streptozocin, teniposide, vinblastine (VBL), vincristine (VCR), and vindesine (VDS).
- Other agents that cause extravasation injury include acyclovir, aminophylline, hyperosmolar agents (urea 30%, dextrose solutions greater than 10%, mannitol, parenteral nutrition solutions), calcium salts, methylene blue, nafcillin, phenytoin, potassium salts, radiography contrast media, radiopharmaceuticals, sodium bicarbonate, sympathomimetic vasopressors (dopamine, dobutamine, epinephrine, metaraminol, methoxamine, norepinephrine, phenylephrine), tetracycline, thiopental, thrombolytic agents (streptokinase, urokinase, alteplase), heparin, and vasopressin.
- Flares

—Local reactions called "flares" (pruritic, raised, red streaks 6–8 cm long along the course of the injected vein) should be differentiated from extravasation. Flares occur in the extremity through which an agent (doxorubicin, crotalid snake antivenom) is injected; these reactions develop within minutes and generally resolve in 30 to 90 minutes.
—Flares are distinguished from extravasation by lack of pain or swelling.
—If flares develop, the health-care provider should ensure that the catheter is functioning normally and extravasation has not occurred.

SIGNS AND SYMPTOMS

- The patient may be minimally symptomatic if the extravasated fluid is isotonic, or if the total extravasated volume is small.
- More severe symptoms include local irritation, erythema, edema, paresthesia, pain, altered tissue perfusion (e.g., change in skin color, decreased pulses, or capillary refill), change in sensation, skin ulceration, blistering, tissue necrosis, and damage to adjacent tendons, blood vessels, and nerves.
- Necrosis may be the first sign that extravasation has occurred.

PROCEDURES AND LABORATORY TESTS

Appropriate laboratory studies for the drug involved should be obtained.

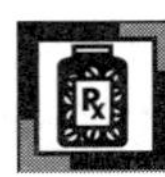

Treatment

- The severity of extravasation should be assessed.
- Nonpharmacologic treatment should be initiated while the need for pharmacologic therapy is determined.

ANTIDOTES

Phentolamine, an α-receptor antagonist, is the specific antidote for vasopressor extravasation.

- Therapeutic dose is 5 to 10 mg diluted in 10 ml of normal saline, infiltrated into the ischemic area within 12 hours of extravasation.
- In infants, no more than 5 mg should be used.

ADJUNCTIVE TREATMENT

Nonpharmacologic Treatment

- Needle aspiration of fluid from the site removes only minimal amounts; nonetheless, many clinicians recommend attempting fluid aspiration via the needle through which the extravasation occurred, before the needle is removed.
- The affected extremity should be elevated above the level of the heart.
- Heat or cold application. The use of either heat or cold packs remains debatable and some clinicians discourage their use. Heat is thought to enhance vasodilation and resorption; locally induced hyperthermia, however, could cause the chemical to spread and potentially increase tissue damage. Cold is thought to produce vasoconstriction, localizing the effect of extravasation.
- Cold packs

—An ice pack may be applied for 15 to 60 minutes three to four times a day for 1 to 3 days or until symptoms resolve.
—Cold packs should be avoided in vinca alkaloid extravasation.
—Moist towels or soaks should be avoided because moisture may cause maceration of the skin.

- Heat

—Specific protocols for heat application are not well described; application of dry, moderate heat has been used.
—Heat is recommended if extravasation involves vinca alkaloids, and it should be avoided with doxorubicin.

Pharmacologic Treatment

- When blistering occurs, silver sulfadiazine has been recommended to prevent local superinfection.

—Silver sulfadiazine should be applied twice daily beneath a gauze dressing.
—The wound should be cleansed with soap and water to remove old silver sulfadiazine before reapplication.

- Saline injection to dilute the extravasated fluid may decrease concentration and potentially reduce toxicity.

—A study involving saline injections of 20 to 90 ml between three and six times over several days into the sites of various chemotherapeutic drug extravasations found that the majority of patients healed without the need for surgery. (This study also used local cooling and systemic antiinflammatory drugs.)
—Local dilution is not uniformly recommended because of concern that administration of additional fluid could cause or worsen mechanical trauma.

- Hyaluronidase hydrolyzes hyaluronic acid (a component of connective tissue).

—Subcutaneous administration decreases local tissue damage by allowing the irritant material to disperse through a larger area, facilitating absorption into the vascular and lymphatic systems.
—Hyaluronidase is most effective if given within 1 hour of extravasation, and works within minutes of injection; connective tissue returns to normal after 24 to 48 hours.
—Doses of 150 to 300 U diluted in 1.5 to 6.0 ml of fluid have been used in most studies.
—Hyaluronidase is potentially effective in treating extravasation injuries caused by hypertonic saline, calcium salts, nafcillin, penicillin, aminophylline, potassium salts, mannitol, sodium bicarbonate, many chemotherapeutic agents (doxorubicin, vincristine, vinblastine), and radiographic contrast material.

- Dimethyl sulfoxide (DMSO) is a free oxygen radical scavenger and an excellent solvent (penetrates through tissue planes, conceivably carrying toxic agent with it); DMSO possibly produces antibacterial, vasodilatory, antiinflammatory, and analgesic effects.

—DMSO use is controversial, but the drug may have utility in the treatment of extravasation injury due to anthracycline chemotherapeutic agents (e.g., doxorubicin) because of its free radical scavenging activity.
—DMSO 15 ml (50% to 99% solution) has been used topically every 2 to 4 hours for about 3 days with or without concurrent use of α-tocopherol.

- Topical proteolytic enzymes

—Fibrinolysin/deoxyribonuclease (Elase) ointment may be an alternative to surgical debridement of partial- or full-thickness skin damage due to extravasation injury; after removal of loose tissue, Elase is applied every 8 hours for about 1 week.

—Travase ointment also may have a role in this capacity, although further study is needed.

- Vasodilators other than phentolamine. Nitroglycerin paste (2%) dilates vascular smooth muscle.

—Nitroglycerin paste has chiefly been studied in infants; good results were seen after application of nitroglycerin paste topically (4 mm/kg).
—Topical nitroglycerin exhibits effects for 3 to 6 hours after administration, which could be a theoretical advantage over the shorter acting phentolamine.

- Corticosteroids (e.g., hydrocortisone or dexamethasone) have been used to blunt the inflammatory response of extravasation; although results are conflicting, most studies have failed to show that steroid injections are of value in treating extravasation injury.
- Corticotropin releasing factor (CRF) has demonstrated effectiveness in decreasing the acute inflammatory reaction associated with experimental eyelid injection of doxorubicin.

—Doses of 75 to 150 μg reduced the acute influx of monocytes and macrophages and protected the skin overlying the injection site.

- Sodium thiosulfate is used for the treatment of injury produced by nitrogen mustard agents.

—The dose is 6.2 ml of a 1 g/10 ml solution, diluted with sterile water to a volume of 15 ml, injected into the infiltration site.
—Sodium thiosulfate is thought to prevent tissue necrosis by inactivation of free radicals.
—Infiltration with 8.4% sodium bicarbonate solution may decrease toxicity by increasing local pH and possibly preventing drug/DNA complexing; sodium bicarbonate, however, is itself toxic when extravasated and should not be used routinely.
—*N*-acetylcysteine and granulocyte/macrophage colony-stimulating factor (GM-CSF) have been beneficial in treating extravasation injury due to chemotherapeutic agents in some studies but not in others.
—Ineffective agents. Published studies have failed to demonstrate benefit from locally injected α-tocopherol, cimetidine, diphenhydramine, heparin, lidocaine, or procaine in alleviating the severity of chemotherapeutic agent extravasation.

Surgical Treatment

- Surgical treatment of an extravasation injury is generally effective.
- Surgical drainage has been recommended when radiographic contrast material is involved.
- Early excision may be of benefit for chemotherapeutic agents.
- Saline flushout and liposuction have been used successfully in recent studies.

Pitfalls

- The severity of extravasation injury is often underestimated initially.
- Scarring around nerves, tendons, or joints may occur despite intact skin.

ICD-9-CM

No code is available.

RECOMMENDED READING

Bertelli G, Gozza A, Forno GB, et al. Topical dimethylsulfoxide for the prevention of soft tissue injury after extravasation of vesicant cytotoxic drugs: a prospective clinical study. J Clin Oncol 1995;13:2851–2855.

Cohan RH, Ellis JH, Garner WL. Extravasation of radiographic contrast material: recognition, prevention, and treatment. Radiology 1996;200:593–604.

Levinson ML. Management of extravasation injuries due to non-cytotoxic drugs. Clin Trends Pharm Pract 1994;8:77–81.

Martin PH, Carver N, Petros J. Use of liposuction and saline washout for the treatment of extensive subcutaneous extravasation of corrosive drugs. Br J Anaesth 1994;72:702–704.

Author: Jana Vander Leest

Reviewer: Richard C. Dart

Gulf War Syndrome

Basics

DESCRIPTION

- Gulf War syndrome is an unexplained symptom complex among members of the military following deployment in the Persian Gulf War (August 1990 to June 1991).
- Gulf War syndrome is a previously unrecognized and unanticipated symptom complex that does not fit into a traditional diagnostic category.
- Synonyms for Gulf War syndrome include Gulf War illness, Desert Storm illness, and Persian Gulf War illness.

PATHOPHYSIOLOGY

A plausible biological mechanism for Gulf War syndrome has not yet been conclusively identified.

Toxicologic Causes

Some proponents maintain that the syndrome is caused by a combination of several toxicants. Possible exposures include hydrocarbons, depleted uranium, pyridostigmine, pesticides, chemical agent resistant coatings, chemical warfare agents, and vaccines.

Hydrocarbon Products

- During the Persian Gulf War, hundreds of oil well fires were set as the Iraqi military moved out of Kuwait; exposures could include the particulates, vapors, solvents, and combustion products of petroleum.
- The primary route of exposure was inhalation, with less likely dermal or ingestion exposure.
- Sulfur dioxide, nitrogen oxide, carbon monoxide, hydrogen sulfide, and reduced sulfur compounds may have been encountered. Although there were no reported measures of air-borne inorganic compounds during this time, prolonged exposure or acute high-dose exposure could result in pulmonary irritation, pneumonitis, asthma, and mucosal irritation.

Depleted Uranium

- Uranium was present in aerosolized forms from the impact of ammunition in certain areas; the radioactivity associated with these shells was considered to be within acceptable standards.
- Uranium metal may accumulate in the lungs and kidneys; the symptoms reported, however, do not seem to be related to this metal.

Pyridostigmine

- All U.S. personnel were provided with pyridostigmine bromide, 30 mg tablets in blister packs of 21 tablets each, to be ingested upon order of the commanding officer if an attack was considered imminent: one tablet was to be taken every 8 hours for up to 7 days or until discontinued by order of the commanding officer.
- Other troops in the coalition were also provided with pyridostigmine; it is likely that most ground forces received at least one dose of this agent, and some may have received multiple doses.
- Pyridostigmine inhibits acetylcholinesterase and causes cholinergic effects similar to an organophosphate insecticide; it should be noted that pyridostigmine (Mestinon) is widely used in the treatment of myasthenia gravis at dosages of up to 1,500 mg/day for years without long-term side effects reported.

Pesticides

- Many different pesticides, including insecticides and rodenticides, were used in the Persian Gulf War; all were approved by the Environmental Protection Agency.
- The use of pesticides was unrestricted, and no application records exist; relative quantities provided were large.
- Common pesticides included: d-phenothrin, chlorpyrifos, resmethrin, malathion, methomyl, lindane, pyrethroids, azamethiphos, and diethyltoluamide (DEET); acute symptoms consistent with organophosphate toxicity were not reported, and chronic effects from pesticides are not likely because of the absence of polyneuropathy among examined veterans.

Chemical Agent–Resistant Coatings

Much of the equipment in the Persian Gulf War was coated with chemical-resistant paints, either prior to shipment or upon arrival at the port of Dhahran, Saudi Arabia.

- The most significant toxicant used was toluene diisocyanate (TDI) which may lead to reactive airways disease if inhaled.
- Troop exposure to TDI was limited to a very small number of veterans and is not consistent with symptoms reported.

Chemical Warfare Agents

Chemical warfare agents remain one of the most controversial possibilities for etiology of Gulf War syndrome; both sarin and nitrogen mustard gas were apparently detected during the conflict, but the exposure was not confirmed by the U.S. Department of Defense.

- Sarin is a potent anticholinesterase agent that produces intense cholinergic stimulation.
- Nitrogen mustard causes severe skin and mucous membrane injury.

Although the possibility of exposure to chemical warfare agents remains unconfirmed, no evidence of mustard gas burns or acute or chronic organophosphate toxicity have been reported.

Vaccines

- Persian Gulf War participants were vaccinated against many infectious agents, including anthrax and botulinum toxins.
- The botulinum vaccines were manufactured by the Michigan State Health Department and have been widely available for many years; no long-term effects have been reported in people other than Persian Gulf War veterans receiving these vaccines.

Nontoxicologic Causes

Leishmaniasis

- Several cases of confirmed leishmaniasis by parasite identification have been reported among Persian Gulf War participants; many of the confirmed cases had nonspecific symptoms.
- Leishmaniasis may remain subclinical; typical symptoms include fever, weight loss, hepatosplenomegaly, pancytopenia, fatigue, and gastrointestinal symptoms.

Sand Dust

Troops were exposed at times to high concentrations of particulate matter, which at times measured a few milligrams per cubic meter; such exposures may result in bronchopulmonary irritation or exacerbation of asthma, but long-term effects are not likely.

Psychological Stressors

Stress following participation in military conflict is not unique to the Persian Gulf War but has been reported following many conflicts and wars and is known as posttraumatic stress disorder (PTSD); the Gulf War was somewhat different from previous conflicts because chemical and biological warfare tactics were predicated prior to deployment.

EPIDEMIOLOGY

- Approximately 697,000 troops were deployed in the Persian Gulf conflict.
- The exact prevalence of the Gulf War syndrome is unknown; the Veterans Administration Persian Gulf Health Registry, however, has evaluated 43,000 veterans for the syndrome.
- Of those 43,000, 3,000 veterans have an unexplained illness; several hundred additional veterans had unexplained symptoms and remained on active duty.
- There have been no reported cases of death related to this syndrome.
- Currently, several ongoing epidemiologic studies are being undertaken to address this syndrome.

PREGNANCY AND LACTATION

There are isolated reports of birth defects among children born to Persian Gulf War veterans; upon further evaluation, the total number was not greater than expected based on general population estimates.

RISK FACTORS

Participation in the Persian Gulf conflict in the only known risk factor.

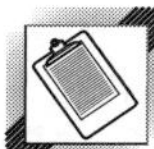

Diagnosis

The possible diagnosis of Gulf War syndrome is currently based on subjective complaints.

DIFFERENTIAL DIAGNOSIS

- Many toxic compounds can cause health effects similar to the myriad complaints reported by the veterans.
- Symptoms possibly caused by psychological stressors of the Persian Gulf War are not easily distinguished from other multisystem symptom complexes such as chronic fatigue, fibromyalgia, and somatoform disorders.
- Because the etiology of Gulf War syndrome is unknown, it is important to consider other common illnesses that have plagued veterans, such as shell shock, PTSD, and regional infectious illnesses.

SIGNS AND SYMPTOMS

- The most frequent complaints reported to the Persian Gulf Health Registry have been fatigue, rash, headache, muscle and/or joint pain, neuropsychological complaints, shortness of breath, sleep disturbances, diarrhea and other gastrointestinal complaints, cough, choking sensation, sneezing, and mouth breathing; these complaints typically tend to be chronic.
- No consistent abnormalities were identified among the patients upon standardized physical examination or by review of medical records and accompanying laboratory tests preformed by the U.S. Veterans Administration.

PROCEDURES AND LABORATORY TESTS

There are no consistent laboratory abnormalities in Gulf War syndrome.

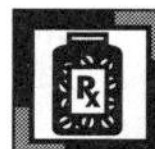

Treatment

No specific therapies for Gulf War syndrome have been tested; treatment is symptomatic and supportive.

DECONTAMINATION

Because the exposure is now remote in time, no decontamination should be performed.

ANTIDOTES

There is no specific antidote for Gulf War syndrome.

ADJUNCTIVE TREATMENT

Support groups for victims of Gulf War syndrome are available through veterans organizations and hospitals.

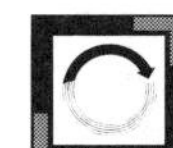

Follow-Up

EXPECTED COURSE AND PROGNOSIS

- Symptoms may be transient but are more likely reported to be persistent.
- An increase in mortality rate has not been found among Persian Gulf War veterans.
- There have been isolated reports of unexplained symptoms among spouses of Persian Gulf War veterans; person-to-person transmission, however, is unlikely from the information that is currently known.

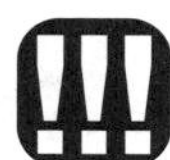

Pitfalls

Dismissing the patient without taking a thorough history and physical examination leads to a frustrated, angry patient and perhaps a missed diagnosis; it is important to be informative and to explore for other likely diagnoses.

ICD-9-CM

No code is available.

RECOMMENDED READING

Gray GC, Coate BD, Anderson CM, et al. The postwar hospitalization experience of U.S. veterans of the Persian Gulf War. N Engl J Med 1996;335:1505–1513.

Haley RW, Kurt TL, Hom J. Is there a Gulf War syndrome? Searching for syndromes by factor analysis of symptoms. JAMA 1997;277:215–222.

Hyams KC, Wignall FS, Roswell R. War syndromes and their evaluation: from the U.S. civil war to the Persian Gulf War. Ann Intern Med 1996;125:398–405.

Kang HK, Bullman TA. Mortality among U.S. veterans of the Persian Gulf War. N Engl J Med 1996;335:1498–1504.

Kizer K, Joseph S, Moll M, Rankin JT. Unexplained illness among Persian Gulf War veterans in an air national guard unit. MMWR 1995;44:443–447.

Persian Gulf Veterans Coordinating Board. Unexplained illness among desert storm veterans: a search for causes, treatment, and cooperation. Arch Intern Med 1995;155:262–268.

Presidential Advisory Committee on Gulf War Veterans Illness. www.gwvi.gov/toc-f.html

Author: Scott D. Phillips

Reviewer: Richard C. Dart

Hearing Abnormalities

Basics

DESCRIPTION

Poisons sometimes cause hearing abnormalities, such as tinnitus or decreased ability to hear.

PATHOPHYSIOLOGY

Physiology of Normal Hearing

- Sound waves stimulate the tympanic membrane, which activates the middle ear ossicles (malleus, incus, and stapes).
- Movement of the stapes causes a fluid wave to move through the cochlea and results in movement of hair cells in the organ of Corti.
- Movement of the hair cells creates an action potential that is transmitted to the cortex via the cochlear nerve and interpreted as sound.

Hearing Abnormalities

- Conduction abnormalities affect the external auditory canal or the middle ear and may be caused by inflammation, infections, otosclerosis or neoplasms.
- Sensorineural abnormalities affect the inner ear, including the cochlea (organ of Corti and stria vascularis) and the cochlear nerve (cranial nerve VIII).

—Abnormalities of sensorineural function affecting the inner ear may result from damage to hair cells of the organ of Corti caused by noise, infections, drugs, or chemicals; temporal bone fractures; meningitis; cochlear otosclerosis; Meniere's disease; aging; or vascular disease.

—Abnormalities of sensorineural function affecting cranial nerve VIII may result from cerebellar tumors (acoustic neuromas), demyelination, infections, or vascular insufficiency.

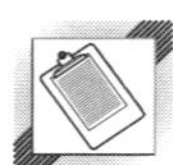

Diagnosis

DIFFERENTIAL DIAGNOSIS

Further information on each poison is available in SECTION IV, CHEMICAL AND BIOLOGICAL AGENTS.

Toxicologic Causes

- Tinnitus may be caused by aminoglycosides, amphotericin B, antihistamines, aspirin, benzene, bromates, bumetanide, caffeine, carbamazepine, chloroquine, cisplatin, clindamycin, dapsone, deferoxamine, dihydrostreptomycin, doxycycline, erythromycin, ethacrynic acid, furosemide, haloperidol, local anesthetics (lidocaine, bupivacaine, mepivacaine), metaproterenol, metoprolol, metronidazole, nonsteroidal antiinflammatory drugs (NSAIDs), naproxen, oral contraceptives, procaine penicillin, quinidine, quinine, salbutamol, streptomycin, tetracycline, theophylline, trialkyl tin, and tricyclic antidepressants.
- Hearing loss or abnormality may be caused by aminoglycoside antibiotics (neomycin, kanamycin, gentamicin, vancomycin, streptomycin, dihydrostreptomycin, tobramycin), azithromycin, bromates, bumetanide, carbon disulfide, carbon monoxide, carbon tetrachloride, chlorate, chlorhexidine, chloroquine, cisplatin, cobalt, cyanide, deferoxamine, erythromycin, ethacrynic acid, furosemide, lead, metronidazole, NSAIDs, organic mercury, quinine, quinidine, salicylate, toluene, trialkyl tin, trichloroethylene, vinblastine, and vincristine.

Nontoxicologic Causes

- Infections that cause hearing abnormalities include meningitis, otitis media, herpes simplex virus, herpes zoster, Lyme disease, syphilis, HIV, Rocky Mountain spotted fever, epidemic typhus, scrub typhus, mumps, mastoiditis, and botulism.
- Inflammation disorders that cause hearing loss include temporal arteritis, Kawasaki disease, and otosclerosis.
- Trauma, such as tympanic membrane perforation, head trauma, and hemotympanum, may cause hearing abnormalities.
- Idiopathic and other causes of hearing abnormalities include Meniere's disease, myxedema coma, Guillain-Barré syndrome, foreign bodies (e.g., cotton tips, pebbles, seeds, beads, buttons, food, and insects), cerumen, stenosis, and neoplasms.

SIGNS AND SYMPTOMS

Physical signs may help reveal the poison involved when they occur in a patient with a hearing abnormality.

HEENT

- Visual deficits, ECG conduction abnormality or dysrhythmia, and tinnitus suggests quinine or chloroquine.
- Visual abnormalities, headache, nausea, and paresthesia with tinnitus suggests trialkyl tin.
- Foreign bodies may be detected within the external auditory canal.
- Isolated hearing loss during intravenous diuretic treatment suggests furosemide, bumetanide, or ethacrynic acid; permanent hearing abnormalities have been reported with these agents.
- Hearing loss during intravenous antimicrobial therapy suggests aminoglycoside therapy.
- Bleeding and discharge from the ear canal may indicate trauma as a cause.
- Acute otitis externa or otitis media may impair hearing.
- Local instillation of chlorhexidine into the external auditory canal, especially in patients with tympanic membrane perforation, may cause sensorineural hearing abnormalities.
- Tinnitus or sensorineural hearing loss during the treatment of iron toxicity suggests an adverse reaction to deferoxamine.

Cardiovascular

- Chronic exposure to a substance with the odor of rotten eggs with ototoxicity and polyneuropathy suggests carbon disulfide toxicity.
- QRS prolongation, ventricular dysrhythmias, and tinnitus suggest quinidine.

Pulmonary

Conjunctivitis, rhinitis, interstitial fibrosis, or hypersensitivity pneumonitis with bilateral sensorineural hearing loss may indicate cobalt poisoning.

Gastrointestinal

- Vomiting, metabolic acidosis, tachypnea, and dehydration with tinnitus suggest salicylate intoxication.
- Vomiting, gastrointestinal bleeding, or interstitial nephritis and tinnitus suggest NSAID toxicity.
- Nausea, vomiting, and abdominal pain with tinnitus or decreased hearing during antimicrobial therapy suggests erythromycin, azithromycin, or metronidazole; hearing abnormalities are more common at higher doses and in patients with hepatic or renal insufficiency.

Renal

- Concurrent renal injury and tinnitus or hearing loss is associated with aminoglycoside therapy; neomycin and kanamycin are the most ototoxic.
- Renal injury with vomiting and diarrhea may implicate bromates; hearing loss from bromate toxicity may be irreversible.
- Renal injury and hearing loss in a chemotherapy patient suggest cisplatin; high-frequency hearing impairment is reported in approximately one third of patients receiving a single dose of cisplatin.
- Chronic analgesic abuse or aminoglycosides can cause renal insufficiency.

Fluids and Electrolytes

- An increased anion gap metabolic acidosis can be seen with salicylates, cyanide, and carbon monoxide.
- Hypokalemic metabolic acidosis (distal renal tubular acidosis) is associated with chronic toluene exposure.

Neurologic

- Either carbon monoxide or cyanide exposure may cause hearing loss, but the hearing loss is typically noted after initial recovery from the poisoning.
- Dysarthria, ataxia, tremor, or constricted visual fields with hearing loss suggests organic mercury toxicity.
- Initial CNS depression and cardiac dysrhythmias followed by pulmonary edema, hepatotoxicity, nephrotoxicity, and hearing loss suggests trichloroethylene.

Hematologic

Microcytic hypochromic anemia associated with anorexia, vomiting, weight loss, abdominal pain, and neurobehavioral abnormalities suggests lead toxicity.

PROCEDURES AND LABORATORY TESTS

Both the Weber and Rinne tests should be performed on all patients during the initial evaluation of a hearing abnormality because conductive and sensorineural hearing abnormalities may be differentiated by comparing the threshold of hearing from air conduction and from bone conduction.

Weber Tuning Fork Testing

In Weber tuning fork testing, the stem of a vibrating 256-Hz tuning fork is placed on the skull in the midline, and the patient is asked whether the sound is heard better in either ear or equally in both.

- Unilateral conductive hearing abnormality causes the sound to be heard better in the affected ear.
- Unilateral sensorineural hearing abnormality causes the sound to be heard better in the unaffected ear.

Rinne Tuning Fork Testing

In Rinne tuning fork testing, a vibrating 256-Hz tuning fork is first placed near the external auditory canal, and then the stem of the still-vibrating tuning fork is placed on the mastoid process; the patient is asked at which time the sound was louder.

- Normally, the sound is louder when the tuning fork is held next to the external auditory canal.
- Conductive hearing abnormality causes the sound to be louder when the tuning fork is placed on the mastoid process.
- Sensorineural hearing loss causes the sound to be heard best next to the external auditory canal.

By performing both tests, the hearing abnormality usually can be classified as conductive or sensorineural.

Other Procedures

- Serum electrolytes, BUN, and creatinine should be obtained to assess renal function and electrolyte status.
- Increased serum lactate can be seen with cyanide, carbon monoxide, and seizures associated with local anesthetic toxicity.
- Serum salicylate level is increased with aspirin or methyl salicylate toxicity.
- Blood levels of specific suspected toxicants and therapeutic medications should be obtained when available and appropriate.
- Arterial blood gas analysis may be helpful in evaluating acid base status and systemic oxygenation.
- Speech audiometry and tympanometry can provide additional information when evaluating hearing abnormalities.
- Sensorineural hearing abnormality is often an indication for electronystagmography and caloric testing.
- Unexplained conductive hearing abnormality usually warrants a head CT with focus on the temporal lobes and temporal bones.
- Unexplained unilateral sensorineural hearing abnormality often warrants MRI of the brain with gadolinium enhancement.

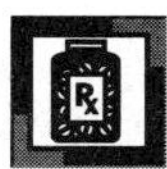

Treatment

- The dose and time of exposure should be determined for all substances involved.
- Initiate specific treatment while continuing supportive care.

DIRECTING PATIENT COURSE

The health-care provider should call the poison control center when:

- cause of hearing abnormality is unclear.
- coingestant, drug interaction, or underlying disease presents unusual problems.

DECONTAMINATION

- Inhalational Exposures. Patients should be removed from the source of the exposure, and appropriate measures should be taken to protect both rescue personnel and health-care workers.
- Ingestions. The decision to perform gastrointestinal decontamination with syrup of ipecac, gastric lavage, activated charcoal, or whole-bowel irritation should be based on the suspected toxicant and the clinical status of the patient.
- Dermal Exposures. The exposed areas should be irrigated with copious amounts of water, and appropriate measures should be taken to protect both rescue personnel and health-care workers.
- External Auditory Canal Foreign Bodies. The ear should be irrigated gently with warm tap water; irrigation should be avoided, however, if there is any suspicion of tympanic membrane perforation.

—Suction is particularly helpful for removing small spherical objects or when irrigation is contraindicated.
—Direct instrumentation is useful for removing larger objects close to the opening of the external auditory canal.

ANTIDOTES

Specific antidotes should be administered as indicated by patient presentation and suspected toxicant.

ADJUNCTIVE TREATMENT

The use of adjunctive treatment is based on the underlying toxic cause.

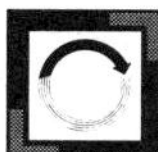

Follow-Up

The decision to admit or discharge the patient is based on the underlying toxic agent and the toxic effects.

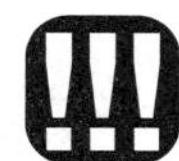

Pitfalls

In salicylate toxicity, the resolution of tinnitus does not necessarily correlate with a decreasing salicylate level and clinical improvement.

RECOMMENDED READING

Chiang W. Otolaryngolic principles. In: Goldfrank LR, et al., eds. Goldfrank's toxicologic emergencies, 6th ed. Norwalk, CT: Appleton & Lange, 1998.

Author: Edwin K. Kuffner

Reviewer: Richard C. Dart

Hyperkalemia

Basics

DESCRIPTION

- The normal extracellular fluid concentration of potassium is typically 3.5 to 4.8 mEq/L.
- Serum potassium concentration of greater than 5.5 mEq/L is hyperkalemia.

PATHOPHYSIOLOGY

- Hyperkalemia creates a steady subthreshold depolarization of the cell, which inactivates sodium channels essential to the production of action potentials and thereby prevents myocardial contraction.
- Even small increases in extracellular potassium cause excitable cells, especially in the heart, to partially depolarize.
- Hemolysis of drawn blood, tight tourniquet, leukocytosis, or thrombocytosis may cause elevated levels of K+ in a sample of blood that are **not** elevated in the patient.
- The pathophysiology is closely tied to causes of hyperkalemia, including:

—Pseudohyperkalemia
—Impaired excretion
—Effective circulating volume depletion
—Renal failure
—Pharmacologic intervention
 —Potassium-sparing diuretics
 —Prostaglandin synthesis inhibitors (ibuprofen and ketorolac)
 —angiotensin-converting enzyme (ACE) inhibitors
 —Trimethoprim-sulfamethozaxole
 —Pentamidine
 —Heparin
 —Digitalis
 —Aldosterone resistance/hypoaldosteronism
 —Addison's disease, sickle cell anemia, systemic lupus erythematosus, kidney transplant, amyloidosis, obstructive uropathy/tubulointerstitial disease, or type IV distal renal tubular acidosis

- Increased entry of K+ into the serum caused by hemolysis/rhabdomyolysis, potassium-rich foods or supplements, trauma, or tumor lysis syndrome
- Shifts of potassium from intracellular to extracellular fluid caused by digitalis intoxication, acidemia (especially nonanion gap metabolic acidosis), insulin deficiency, muscle overuse injury from agitation or straining, or hyperosmolality

EPIDEMIOLOGY

- True hyperkalemia is uncommon outside of the setting of renal failure, although it is associated with severe poisonings (e.g., digoxin).
- Hyperkalemia in the setting of decreased renal function is usually accompanied by an excess intake of potassium or by a pharmacologic intervention with potassium-sparing diuretics, β-receptor blockers, or ACE inhibitors.

RISK FACTORS

- Acute or chronic renal failure
- Diabetes mellitus
- Pharmacologic interventions
- Myopathy or trauma
- Malignant disease

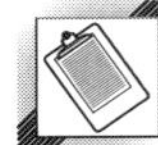

Diagnosis

DIFFERENTIAL DIAGNOSIS

- Common toxicologic causes of hyperkalemia include digoxin intoxication and acidemia or rhabdomyolysis from any source (e.g., sympathomimetic toxicity and seizures).
- Common nontoxicologic causes include pseudohyperkalemia or renal failure from any cause.

SIGNS AND SYMPTOMS

- Hyperkalemia primarily causes cardiac conduction abnormalities that may quickly deteriorate to ventricular fibrillation.
- ECG changes with hyperkalemia, especially with a widened QRS complex, constitute a medical emergency.
- Physical signs may help reveal the poison involved when they occur in a patient with hyperkalemia.

Vital Signs

Hypotension and bradycardia are common in severe cases.

HEENT

Blurred vision and colored halos may indicate digitalis toxicity.

Cardiovascular

- ECG effects range from a peaked T wave, decreased R wave, prolonged P-R interval, through a widened QRS complex, and degenerating into a sine wave in the most severe form.
- High-grade atrioventricular block may indicate digoxin or β-blocker toxicity.
- Sudden ventricular fibrillation or cardiac arrest is possible at any stage.

Gastrointestinal

Nausea and vomiting suggest digitalis toxicity.

Renal

Renal function tests often reveal transient or chronic renal insufficiency.

Fluids and Electrolytes

Hyperkalemia must be present for a diagnosis.

Musculoskeletal

Weakness progresses to paralysis in severe cases.

Neurologic

Paresthesia and decreased deep tendon reflexes may be present.

PROCEDURES AND LABORATORY TESTS

Essential Tests

- Serum electrolytes, BUN, and creatinine are needed to determine hyperkalemia and assess renal function.
- Pseudohyperkalemia must be excluded.

—A second sample may exclude hemolysis due to blood draw technique.
—True hyperkalemia is usually associated with other abnormal laboratory values.
—True hyperkalemia exists if serum and plasma values for potassium differ by less than 0.2 mEq/L.

- CBC is needed to determine whether hemolysis, leukocytosis, or thrombocytosis could be the cause of pseudohyperkalemia.
- ECG and continuous monitoring are needed; any changes in the ECG, especially QRS widening, constitute a medical emergency.
- A serum creatine kinase assay is needed to determine the contribution of muscle injury.

Recommended Tests

- A digoxin level may be needed to evaluate cardiac glycoside toxicity.
- Urine electrolytes, osmolality, and a 24-hour urine K+ excretion test are recommended to determine whether abnormal renal handling is responsible for the disorder. (Extrarenal hyperkalemia is associated with renal excretion of more than 200 mEq/day of potassium.)
- Determining morning serum cortisol levels is a useful first step to rule out Addison's disease in a case of mild elevation in potassium, hypotension, and hyponatremia.
- A cortrosyn stimulation test should be considered if cortisol levels are low.

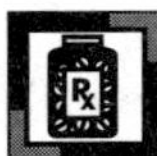

Treatment

- It is necessary to determine the urgency of the situation by evaluating the potassium level and performing an ECG; any ECG changes mandate immediate therapy, as does a true K+ level greater than 7.5 mEq/L.

—Immediate therapy usually consists of an intravenous calcium infusion, followed by glucose/insulin, sodium bicarbonate, or β-receptor agonist.

- If the total body load of potassium is increased (rather than shifted from an intracellular to extracellular location), sodium polysterene sulfonate (Kayexelate) is also administered to remove excess potassium from the body.
- Internal shifts in K+ are assessed by evaluating the patient for acidemia, digitalis, adrenergic agents, or hyperosmolar state.
- The state of renal potassium excretion should be assessed by presence of renal failure, hypoaldosteronism, K+-sparing diuretics or ACE inhibitors.
- The rate of potassium entry into serum should be assessed by the presence of muscle injury, overdose with potassium supplements, intravenous infusion rate supplemental potassium, dietary intake, or use of salt substitutes.

SEVERE HYPERKALEMIA (EMERGENCY TREATMENT)

Hyperkalemia in the setting of ECG changes, especially a widened QRS complex, or serum levels greater than 7.5 mEq/L, is considered a medical emergency. In severe cases, intervention should begin with immediate calcium administration, followed by administration of glucose and insulin or sodium bicarbonate, or both.

- Calcium chloride is administered first because it has the most rapid onset of action.

—Available as a 10% solution, the adult dose is 5 ml intravenously over 5 minutes during continuous ECG monitoring, repeated in 5 to 6 minutes as occasion requires; the pediatric dose is 0.2 to 0.3 ml (20–30 mg/kg/dose) up to 5 ml using the same infusion technique.
—Calcium should be avoided if digoxin toxicity is possible because calcium may increase the cardiac toxicity of cardiac glycosides.

- Glucose and insulin. This regimen redistributes potassium into the cell.

—Regular insulin 10 units, and 25 g of dextrose (1 ampule of D_{50}) should be administered immediately by intravenous push.
—Onset of action occurs in 15 to 30 minutes.

- β-receptor agonists. Like glucose/insulin, β-receptor agonists redistribute potassium into the cell.

—Onset of action occurs in 15 to 30 minutes.
—A large dose of an immediately available nebulized form (e.g., albuterol 10 mg nebulizer) should be used in addition to other measures.

- Sodium bicarbonate also redistributes potassium into cells. The adult dose is 2 ampules (88–100 mEq) by intravenous push every 1 to 2 hours as guided by potassium level; the pediatric dose is 1 to 2 mEq/kg.
- Following the above measures and if the total body stores of potassium are increased, sodium polystyrene sulfonate (Kayexelate) or hemodialysis should be used to increase potassium elimination.

—Sodium polystyrene sulfonate (Kayexelate) is an ion exchange resin used to enhance the gastrointestinal excretion of potassium. Its onset of action is 2 to 12 hours.
—Because it may cause anorexia, nausea, vomiting, and constipation, a suspension in 70% sorbitol (5 g resin/20 ml suspension) is used.
—The patient should be given 20 to 40 ml orally four times daily, or until the serum K+ is less than 5.5 mEq/L. A maintenance dose of 20 ml may be given orally two or three times daily if further treatment is needed.
—It also may be administered as a retention enema.

- Dialysis. Although dialysis effectively removes excess potassium from the body and is essential in patients with acute renal failure or end-stage renal failure, the process takes time to set up and should not be used alone under emergency situations.

DIGITALIS TOXICITY

- Digoxin immune Fab is indicated for ventricular dysrhythmia, hyperkalemia above 5.5 mEq/L, significant ingestion (more than 10 mg in adults, more than 4 mg in children), or when patient is unresponsive to conventional therapy.
- The use of calcium to treat hyperkalemia in the setting of digitalis intoxication may exacerbate the toxic effects of the cardiac glycosides.

MILD TO MODERATE HYPERKALEMIA (NONEMERGENCY)

- In hyperkalemia that does not constitute a medical emergency, management is focused on treating the cause of excess hyperkalemia.
- In a low-K+ diet, salt substitutes should be avoided.
- Drugs that may cause hyperkalemia should be discontinued.
- Sodium polystyrene sulfonate (Kayexelate) therapy may be used as described earlier.
- Other causes of hyperkalemia should be evaluated and treated, such as aldosterone resistance, hypoaldosteronism, or Addison's disease.

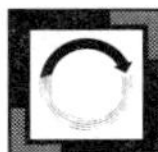

Follow-Up

PATIENT MONITORING

- Hyperkalemia should be monitored with serial electrolyte determinations, ECG, and cardiac monitoring.
- The patient should be evaluated to determine the cause of hyperkalemia; the evaluation should include drugs, diet, comorbidity, and endocrine causes.

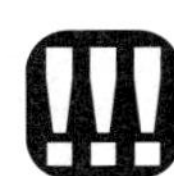

Pitfalls

DIAGNOSIS

- Pseudohyperkalemia must be differentiated from true hyperkalemia.
- True hyperkalemia is usually associated with more than one abnormal laboratory value.

ICD-9-CM 964

Poisoning by agents primarily affecting blood constituents.

See also: SECTION III, Digoxin Immune Fab chapter, and SECTION IV, β-Receptor Blockers, and Digoxin and Cardiac Glycosides chapters.

RECOMMENDED READING

Mandal AK. Hypokalemia and hyperkalemia. Med Clin North Am 1997;81:611–639.

Authors: Nirmal K. Veeramachaneni and Charles B. Cairns

Reviewer: Katherine M. Hurlbut

Hypertension

Basics

DESCRIPTION

Increased diastolic and/or systolic blood pressure at rest defines hypertension.

- Adults and adolescents: greater than 160 mm Hg systolic or 90 mm Hg diastolic
- Children 5 to 10 years of age: systolic blood pressure greater than 120 mm Hg
- Children 1 to 5 years of age: systolic blood pressure greater than 110 mm Hg
- Infants 6 months to 1 year of age: systolic blood pressure greater than 100 mm Hg

PATHOPHYSIOLOGY

- Common toxicologic mechanisms for persistent hypertension include excessive stimulation of α- and/or β-adrenergic receptors.
- The hypertensive response may result from direct receptor stimulation by a toxicant, stimulation of endogenous catecholamine release, or production of a generalized physiologic response (e.g., pain) that produces hypertension.

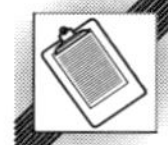

Diagnosis

DIFFERENTIAL DIAGNOSIS

Toxicologic Causes

Further information on each poison is available in SECTION IV, CHEMICAL AND BIOLOGICAL AGENTS.

- Cocaine. Additional findings may include tachycardia, hyperthermia, agitation, delirium, seizures, track marks, nasal septum erosion or perforation, and rhabdomyolysis.
- Amphetamines. Additional findings may include tachycardia, hyperthermia, agitation, psychosis, seizures, track marks, and rhabdomyolysis.
- Other sympathomimetic agents (ephedrine, phenylpropanolamine, β-agonist bronchodilator, theophylline). Additional findings may include headache, hypokalemia, tremor, tachycardia, and agitation.
- Anticholinergic agents (diphenhydramine, scopolamine, jimsonweed, hydroxyzine, phenothiazine, dramamine, etc.). Additional findings include tachycardia, dry flushed skin, dilated sluggish pupils, diminished bowel sounds, hyperthermia, hallucinations, agitation, and delirium.
- An α_2-adrenergic agonist (clonidine, imidazoline decongestants) may cause initial hypertension, bradycardia, and CNS depression, followed by apnea and hypotension.
- Monoamine oxidase (MAO) inhibitors may cause hyperthermia, hypertension, and altered mental status.
- LSD, phencyclidine, or hallucinogens of any type may cause rhabdomyolysis.
- Ergot alkaloids (ergotamine and dehydroergotamine) often cause signs of vasoconstriction such as pallor or cyanosis of lips and extremities.
- Nicotine causes initial hypertension, usually associated with vomiting, tachycardia, urinary incontinence, lethargy, seizures, and coma.
- Mushrooms may produce hallucinogenic or anticholinergic effects.
- Withdrawal from alcohol, opioids, or sedative-hypnotic agents is associated with a history of abstinence, tachycardia, and hypertension.

Nontoxicologic Causes

Nontoxicologic causes of hypertension include essential hypertension, secondary hypertension (e.g., renal artery stenosis and pheochromocytoma), anxiety (a diagnosis of exclusion), and severe pain.

SIGNS AND SYMPTOMS

Physical signs may help reveal the poison involved when they occur in the setting of hypertension.

Vital Signs

- Tachycardia may indicate sympathomimetic or anticholinergic toxicity, or withdrawal from alcohol or a sedative-hypnotic agent.
- Bradycardia may develop as a physiologic compensation.
- Hyperthermia may indicate intoxication with sympathomimetic, anticholinergic, or MAO inhibitor, drugs, or agents that cause prolonged seizures.

HEENT

- Dilated pupils suggest sympathomimetic, anticholinergic, or hallucinogen toxicity.
- Small pupils may indicate clonidine or nicotine effect.
- Nystagmus may indicate phencyclidine intoxication.
- A perforated nasal septum may indicate chronic drug abuse.

Dermatologic

- Flushed dry skin suggests an anticholinergic agent.
- Pale, sweaty skin may be associated with sympathomimetic drugs or cholinergic agents.
- Track marks suggest chronic parenteral drug abuse.
- Marked peripheral vasoconstriction may indicate ergot alkaloid toxicity.

Cardiovascular

- Tachydysrhythmia may be a sign of toxicity from sympathomimetic drugs, anticholinergic agents, or MAO inhibitors.
- Bradycardia and hypertension may occur early in the course of clonidine or imidazoline decongestant intoxication.
- Transient hypertension followed by hypotension may occur secondarily to severe intoxication with bretylium, cocaine, amphetamines, MAO inhibitors, tricyclic antidepressants, anticholinergic drugs, β-adrenergic agonists, and nicotine.

Pulmonary

Respiratory depression may indicate clonidine or imidazoline decongestant intoxication.

Gastrointestinal

Diminished bowel sounds suggest an anticholinergic agent.

Renal

Urinary retention suggests an anticholinergic agent.

Fluids and Electrolyte

Hypokalemia suggests a β-receptor agonist.

Musculoskeletal

Rhabdomyolysis often indicates stimulant or hallucinogen abuse.

Neurologic

- Hallucinations and delirium suggest an anticholinergic agent or abuse of a stimulant or hallucinogen.
- Anxiety, tremor, and seizures suggest theophylline or withdrawal from alcohol or sedative-hypnotic drugs.
- Coma and seizures suggest MAO inhibitors, nicotine, or possible intracranial bleeding due to hypertension.

PROCEDURES AND LABORATORY TESTS

Essential Tests

ECG and continuous cardiac monitoring should be done to detect:

- tachydysrhythmia, caused by sympathomimetic and anticholinergic drugs.
- bradycardia, which may occur as a reflex effect, or with clonidine or imidazoline decongestant poisoning.
- myocardial ischemia.

Recommended Tests

- Serum electrolytes, BUN, and creatinine assist in the assessment of metabolic acidosis and renal insufficiency; hypokalemia is associated with adrenergic agents such as β-agonist or theophylline.
- A urine toxicology screen should be obtained from patients with persistent hypertension of unknown cause.
- Serum acetaminophen and aspirin levels in an overdose setting should be measured to detect an occult overdose with analgesic medications.

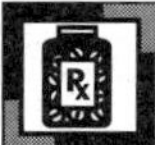

Treatment

- Intravenous access should be established.
- The dose and time of exposure should be determined for all substances involved.
- Specific treatment (e.g., sedation, nitroprusside) should be initiated while continuing supportive care.

DIRECTING PATIENT COURSE

Health-care provider should call the poison control center when:

- cause of hypertension is unknown.
- coingestant, drug interaction, or underlying disease presents unusual problem.

Admission Considerations

Nearly all patients with hypertension need hospitalization to assess effectiveness of treatment and underlying cause.

DECONTAMINATION

Out of Hospital

Induction of emesis is not recommended because altered mental status may develop.

In Hospital

- Gastric lavage should be performed in pediatric (tube size 24–32 French) or adult patients (36–42 French) for substantial ingestion presenting within 1 hour of ingestion or if serious effects are present.
- One dose of activated charcoal (1–2 g/kg) should be administered without a cathartic if a substantial ingestion has occurred within the previous few hours.

ADJUNCTIVE TREATMENT

Control of Blood Pressure

Often blood pressure will respond favorably to control of agitation. A benzodiazepine familiar to the clinician should be administered while monitoring the patient's airway closely.

- Diazepam. Adult dose is 5 to 10 mg intravenously, pediatric dose is 0.2 to 0.5 mg/kg intravenously, repeating doses at 5-minute intervals, titrating to effect.
- Lorazepam. Adult dose is 1 to 2 mg intravenously, pediatric dose is 0.05 mg/kg, with doses repeated at 5-minute intervals, titrating to effect.

In general, antihypertensive treatment should be avoided with the following poisons because hypertension is usually not life threatening and resolves with supportive care and hypotension may develop rapidly: clonidine, imidazoline decongestants, bretylium, cocaine, amphetamine, MAO inhibitors, tricyclic antidepressants, anticholinergics, β-adrenergic agonists, or nicotine.

To control hypertension that is severe and persistent (diastolic pressure more than 130 mm Hg not responsive to sedation) or complicated by end organ effects (CNS bleed, congestive heart failure, myocardial ischemia, or aortic dissection), a short-acting titratable agent such as nitroprusside is recommended.

- Adult and pediatric dose is 0.5 μg/kg/min by continuous infusion, which should be increased by 0.25 to 0.5 μg/kg/min every 5 minutes, titrating the dose until the desired effect is reached.
- An infusion rate over 10 μg/kg/min is rarely required and may produce cyanide toxicity.
- Nitroprusside should be tapered gradually in order to avoid rebound hypertension.
- Intraarterial pressure monitoring is recommended for persistent hypertension requiring nitroprusside treatment.

If hypertension is accompanied by marked tachycardia, refer to SECTION II, Tachycardia chapter.

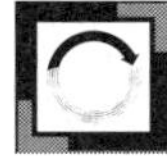

Follow-Up

PATIENT MONITORING

Cardiac and respiratory function should be monitored continuously.

EXPECTED COURSE AND PROGNOSIS

Toxic causes of hypertension usually respond to treatment without sequelae unless intracranial hemorrhage occurs before treatment.

DISCHARGE CRITERIA/INSTRUCTIONS

Asymptomatic patients with transient, mild hypertension may be discharged after decontamination and a 6-hour observation period and psychiatric evaluation, if needed.

ICD-9-CM 972

Poisoning by agents primarily affecting the cardiovascular system.

See also: SECTION II, Tachycardia chapter, and SECTION III, Nitroprusside chapter.

RECOMMENDED READING

Hessler R. Cardiovascular principles. In: Goldfrank LR, et al., eds. Goldfrank's toxicologic emergencies, 6th ed. Norwalk, CT: Appleton & Lange, 1998.

Author: Katherine M. Hurlbut

Reviewer: Richard C. Dart

Basics

DESCRIPTION

- The normal body temperature is 35.8° to 37.2°C (96.5°–99°F).
- Elevation of the temperature above 38°C (100.4°F) should be considered hyperthermia.

PATHOPHYSIOLOGY

Hyperthermia occurs when normal thermoregulation mechanisms are overwhelmed by increased motor activity, impairment of normal heat dissipation mechanisms, increased environmental heat, impairment of behavior to avoid increased environmental temperature, or impaired hypothalamic thermoregulation.

EPIDEMIOLOGY

- Hyperthermia related to drug use is common.
- Toxic effects following exposure are typically mild.
- Individuals with severe hyperthermia who do not receive timely supportive care may die.

PREGNANCY AND LACTATION

Hyperthermia in the pregnant patient is associated with an increased risk of congenital anomalies.

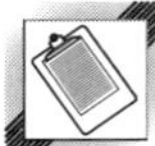

Diagnosis

The patient's temperature should be taken rectally to confirm hyperthermia.

DIFFERENTIAL DIAGNOSIS

Further information on each poison is available in SECTION IV, CHEMICAL AND BIOLOGICAL AGENTS.

Toxicologic Causes

- Neuroleptic malignant syndrome (NMS) consists of autonomic dysfunction (fever, tachycardia, hyper- or hypotension), movement disorder (rigidity, tremors, Parkinson-like symptoms, myoclonus), and an altered mental status following the use of neuroleptic drugs.
- Serotonin syndrome (SS) resembles NMS but occurs with use or overdose agents that increase serotonergic activity in the CNS.
- Monoamine oxidase (MAO) inhibitors. Agitation, tachycardia, hyper- and hypotension may accompany an MAO inhibitor overdose; phenelzine and tranylcypromine are included.
- Many drugs or foods interact with MAO inhibitors and produce a syndrome that involves autonomic dysfunction, an altered mental status, and rigidity.
- Malignant hyperthermia is a rare inherited disorder typified by fever, autonomic dysfunction, and severe muscular rigidity in patients undergoing general anesthesia.
- Anticholinergics and antihistamines cause fever in overdose and exacerbate hyperthermia by inhibiting the ability to cool evaporation; antihistamines and plant alkaloids found in jimsonweed and other plants, cyclic antidepressants, atropine, and phenothiazines are included.
- Aspirin and salicylates. Hyperthermia may accompany tachypnea, tinnitus, metabolic acidosis, and an altered mental status.
- Hallucinogens (LSD, PCP, peyote). Agitation associated with hallucinations may cause hyperthermia.
- Sympathomimetic drugs. Agitation, delirium, seizures, diaphoresis, tachycardia, hypertension, mydriasis, and seizure may occur with cocaine, caffeine, theophylline, methylphenidate (Ritalin), and amphetamines, including diet pills such as Fen-Phen (fenfluramine and phentermine), and methamphetamine intoxication.
- Withdrawal from ethanol, benzodiazepines, or barbiturates causes a sympathomimetic surge with delirium, diaphoresis, and agitation, such as that described for sympathomimetic overdose; seizures also may occur and contribute to hyperthermia.

Uncommon Toxicologic Causes

- Arsenic. Hyperthermia may occur with acute arsenic toxicity.
- Isoniazid may cause multiple seizures that contribute to hyperthermia.
- Thyroid hormones may cause agitation associated with hyperthermia as well as tachycardia, hypertension, tremors, goiter, and many other symptoms.

Other Causes

- Seizures, agitation, and inappropriate behavior in response to heat (overexertion, overswaddling of infants, or remaining in hot, unventilated rooms) due to any cause may bring on hyperthermia.
- Heat stroke and heat exhaustion also may present with dehydration, altered mental status, and organ failure, making them difficult to distinguish from drug-induced hyperthermia.
- Infection commonly causes hyperthermia but is usually identifiable.
- Thyroid storm may present with hyperthermia, tachycardia, hypertension, agitation, tremors, and other symptoms.
- Neoplasms, connective tissue disease, and granulomatous disease are associated with hyperthermia, but often have other diagnostic signs.

SIGNS AND SYMPTOMS

- Physical signs may help reveal the poison involved when they occur in the setting of hyperthermia.
- Delirium, agitation, coma, hypotension, seizures, and multiorgan failure may develop in severe cases.

Vital Signs

Extreme hypertension may occur with neuroleptic malignant syndrome, serotonin syndrome, or MAO inhibitor poisoning.

HEENT

- Tinnitus often accompanies salicylate toxicity.
- Dilated pupils are associated with anticholiergic or sympathomimetic toxicity, or hypoxia.

Dermatologic

- Flushed dry skin suggests an anticholinergic agent.
- Pale, sweaty skin may be associated with sympathomimetic drugs, cholinergic agents, or hypotension.

Cardiovascular

- QRS widening or presence of an R wave in the ECG lead aVR suggests tricyclic antidepressant poisoning.
- Severe tachydysrhythmia may indicate theophylline, sympathomimetic agent, NMS, SS, or MAO inhibitor toxicity.

Pulmonary

Tachypnea is produced by salicylates or any cause of metabolic acidosis.

Gastrointestinal

- Nausea and vomiting are common with aspirin and theophylline.
- Bowel sounds are commonly decreased with anticholinergic agents.

Fluids and Electrolytes

Dehydration is common due to increased insensible water losses.

Musculoskeletal

Rigidity, myoclonus, and tremors may indicate development of NMS, SS, or MAO inhibitor toxicity.

Neurologic

- Hallucinations may indicate anticholinergic poisoning or abuse of hallucinogens or stimulants.
- The triad of altered mental status, autonomic dysfunction, and movement disorder may indicate NMS, SS, or MAO inhibitor toxicity.

PROCEDURES AND LABORATORY TESTS

Essential Tests

No tests may be needed for mild hyperthermia (e.g., transient, mild, and environmental) that does not worsen.

Recommended Tests

- Serum electrolytes, glucose, BUN, and creatinine

—Dehydration with hypernatremia is common.
—Hyperkalemia may occur if renal failure or rhabdomyolysis is present. Hyperglycemia may occur. Metabolic acidosis is the rule in severe cases, sometimes preceded by respiratory alkalosis.
—Hypophosphatemia and hypocalcemia may also occur.

- Urinalysis. Blood and protein may be seen with the development of rhabdomyolysis.
- Serum aspartate aminotransferase, alanine aminotransferase, and lactic dehydrogenase in a hepatocellular pattern may occur.
- Creatine kinase may be elevated due to agitation or seizures causing muscle breakdown.
- Prothrombin time, partial thromboplastin time, fibrinogen, and fibrin split products may help to evaluate potential disseminated intravascular coagulation.
- An ECG may reveal various nonspecific findings.
- Arterial blood gases may show respiratory alkalosis followed by respiratory acidosis if the condition worsens.
- Serum acetaminophen and aspirin levels are advised in an overdose setting to detect an occult overdose with analgesic medications.
- A urine toxicology screen is recommended for patients with hyperthermia of unknown cause.

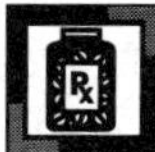

Treatment

- Intravenous access should be established, and cooling measures should begin immediately if temperature is above 40°C, particularly in the presence of altered mental status.
- The dose and time of exposure should be determined for all substances involved.
- Specific treatment (e.g., naloxone for mental status depression) should be initiated while continuing supportive care.

DIRECTING PATIENT COURSE

The health-care provider should call the poison control center when:

- cause of hyperthermia could be toxic.
- coingestant, drug interaction, or underlying disease presents unusual problems.

DECONTAMINATION

Out of Hospital

- Induction of emesis is not recommended.

In Hospital

- Gastric lavage should be performed in pediatric (tube size 24–32 French) or adult (36–42 French) patients for large ingestion presenting within 1 hour of ingestion or if serious effects are present.
- One dose of activated charcoal (1–2 g/kg) should be administered without a cathartic if substantial ingestion has occurred within the previous few hours.

ADJUNCTIVE TREATMENT

Aggressive supportive care is vital to avoid sequelae from severe hyperthermia.

- To control agitation, the provider should administer a benzodiazepine with which he has experience, while monitoring the patient's airway closely.

—Diazepam. The adult dose is 5 to 10 mg intravenously; the pediatric dose is 0.2 to 0.5 mg/kg intravenously, with doses repeated at 5-minute intervals, titrating to effect.
—Lorazepam. The adult dose is 1 to 2 mg intravenously; the pediatric dose is 0.05 mg/kg, with doses repeated at 5-minute intervals, titrating to effect.

- To reduce body temperature, all clothing should be removed, intravenous infusion of isotonic crystalloid should begin, and agitation should be controlled.

—Fluid losses may be severe and should be replenished until a urine output of 1 to 2 ml/kg/h is reached.
—Electrolyte abnormalities due to the initial insult or from iatrogenic changes should be corrected.
—Fluid administration should be carefully monitored to avoid fluid overload in predisposed patients, such as those with congestive heart failure, adult respiratory distress syndrome, or renal failure.
—Cooling fans and wet sheets are effective, especially in dry climates. Cooling blankets or application of ice may be needed in severe cases.
—Sedation and neuromuscular paralysis/mechanical ventilation may also assist decrease of temperature in agitated patients.
—Central temperature should be frequently monitored, and cooling should be discontinued when the body temperature decreases to 39°C.

- Tachycardia that persists after treatment of hyperthermia may be due to a toxic agent, hypovolemia, or a myocardial injury.

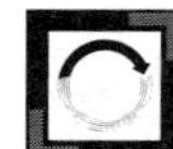

Follow-Up

PATIENT MONITORING

Temperature, respiratory, and cardiac function should be monitored continuously.

EXPECTED COURSE AND PROGNOSIS

Mild hyperthermia resolves without sequelae, but victims of severe hyperthermia may die immediately from multiorgan failure or survive the initial insult and die days later as a result of complications.

DISCHARGE CRITERIA/INSTRUCTIONS

Asymptomatic patients who experienced only mild hyperthermia may be discharged after monitoring for 6 hours and psychiatric evaluation, if needed.

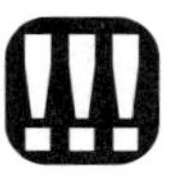

Pitfalls

TREATMENT

- Dehydration may be severe; adequate rehydration should be provided.
- Large amounts of benzodiazepines may be needed to treat agitation, particularly with ethanol, benzodiazepine, or barbiturate withdrawal.

ICD-9-CM 780.6

General symptoms: pyrexia of unknown origin. Certain adverse effects: hyperthermia following anesthesia.

See also: SECTION II, NMS and Serotonin Syndrome, and Tachycardia chapters; and SECTION IV for chapters on specific agents.

RECOMMENDED READING

Goldfrank LR, Flomenbaum NE, Weisman RS, Lewin NA. Vital signs and toxic syndromes. In: Goldfrank LR, et al., eds. Goldfrank's toxicologic emergencies, 6th ed. Norwalk, CT: Appleton & Lange, 1998.

Author: Lada Kokan

Reviewer: Richard C. Dart

Hypotension

Basics

DESCRIPTION

• Decreased systolic blood pressure defines hypotension.

—Adults and adolescents: less than 90 mm Hg systolic
—Children 5 to 10 years of age: less than 90 mm Hg systolic
—Children 1 to 5 years of age: less than 70 mm Hg systolic
—Infants up to 1 year of age: less than 60 mm Hg systolic

• Shock refers to hypotension combined with evidence of inadequate tissue perfusion (e.g., pale, cool extremities, altered mentation).

PATHOPHYSIOLOGY

• Common toxicologic mechanisms for persistent hypotension include α- or β-adrenergic receptor blockade, blockade of myocardial calcium channels, vasodilation, or increased fluid loss leading to hypovolemia (insensible, gastrointestinal, urinary, or redistribution).
• Myocardial infarction, dysrhythmia, electrolyte abnormality, physiologic response to hypoxia, and hypothermia are other possible causes.

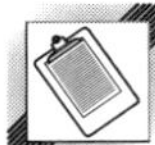

Diagnosis

DIFFERENTIAL DIAGNOSIS

Further information on each poison is available in SECTION IV, CHEMICAL AND BIOLOGICAL AGENTS.

Toxicologic Causes

• β-receptor blocker drugs may produce hypotension, hyperglycemia, atrioventricular (AV) block, ventricular dysrhythmia, CNS depression, and seizures.
• Calcium channel blockers may produce hypotension, CNS depression, sinus bradycardia, AV block, asystole, and ventricular dysrhythmia.
• Clonidine or imidazoline drugs (tetrahydrozoline) may produce miosis, CNS depression, apnea, hypotonia, and initial hypertension followed by hypotension.
• Digitalis glycosides frequently cause nausea and vomiting, visual distortion and halos, atrial and ventricular dysrhythmia, and AV block.
• Cholinergic agents (organophosphate and carbamate pesticides, bromocriptine, acetylcholine, physostigmine, pyridostigmine) cause vomiting, diarrhea, salivation, lacrimation, urination, bronchorrhea, small pupils, and sweating. Nicotinic effects such as fasciculation and muscle weakness suggest organophosphate or carbamate pesticide exposure.
• Opioids may cause miosis and respiratory depression and may be associated with track marks.
• Sympathomimetics (cocaine, amphetamines) may cause early hypertension, tachycardia, tachydysrhythmia, hyperthermia, agitation, seizures, and rhabdomyolysis.
• Iron often causes nausea, vomiting, diarrhea, gastrointestinal bleeding, CNS depression, anion gap metabolic acidosis, leukocytosis, hyperglycemia, and radiopacities on abdominal films.
• Tricyclic antidepressants often cause tachycardia, CNS depression, coma, seizures, QRS widening, and R wave in lead aVR.
• Theophylline may cause nausea, vomiting, tachydysrhythmia, hypokalemia, mild metabolic acidosis, and seizures.
• Sedative agents may cause CNS depression, coma, and hypothermia.
• Vasodilators usually cause tachycardia.

Nontoxicologic Causes

• All causes of dysrhythmia or hypoxia other than poisoning.
• Hypothermia, hypoxia, sepsis, spinal cord injury, myocardial infarction, blood loss, and severe fluid loss from any cause.

SIGNS AND SYMPTOMS

Physical signs may help reveal the poison involved when they occur in the setting of hypotension.

Vital Signs

• Severe bradycardia or atrioventricular block suggests β-adrenergic blocker, calcium channel blocker, cardiac glycoside, cholinergic agent, or α_1- or α_2-adrenergic agonists.
• Tachydysrhythmia suggests sympathomimetic or anticholinergic drugs, theophylline, tricyclic antidepressants, or phenothiazine.
• Hypothermia may produce bradycardia.
• Marked hyperthermia suggests severe sympathomimetic poisoning, neuroleptic malignant syndrome, monoamine oxidase (MAO) inhibitor overdose, or serotonin syndrome.

HEENT

• Dilated pupils suggest hypoxia.
• Pinpoint pupils suggest opioid, clonidine, or imidazoline drugs.
• Blurred or yellow vision or halos may indicate digitalis toxicity.
• Salivation, lacrimation, and small pupils suggest cholinergic agents or nicotine.

Dermatologic

• Cyanosis indicates hypoxia or methemoglobinemia.
• Diaphoresis may be caused by a cholinergic agent.
• Dry, flushed skin suggests an anticholinergic agent.

Cardiovascular

• QRS prolongation suggests tricyclic antidepressants, phenothiazine, antihistamine, procainamide, quinidine, or propoxyphene.
• Bradycardia or atrioventricular block suggests β-adrenergic blocker, calcium channel blocker, cardiac glycoside, α_1- or α_2-adrenergic agonists, or cholinergic agents.

Pulmonary

• Bronchorrhea may be caused by a cholinergic agent (carbamate or organophosphate insecticide).
• Respiratory depression can occur with opioids, sedatives, clonidine, or imidazoline drugs.

Gastrointestinal

• Vomiting is common with digitalis, iron, and cholinergic agents.
• Iron also may cause hematemesis or hematochezia.
• Decreased bowel sounds suggest anticholinergics, opioids, or β-receptor blockers.

Renal

• Recurrent urination may be caused by cholinergic agents.
• Urinary retention may develop with anticholinergic agents.

Fluids and Electrolytes

- Hyperkalemia suggests digitalis poisoning.
- Hyperglycemia may be caused by β-receptor blockers.
- Increased anion gap acidosis may be due to lactic acidemia induced by hypoperfusion or by iron toxicity.

Neurologic

- Mental status depression or seizures may be caused by β-receptor blocker, cholinergic agent, opioid, sedative-hypnotic, clonidine, and numerous other medications.
- Hypotonia may indicate clonidine or imidazoline drug.

PROCEDURES AND LABORATORY TESTS

Essential Tests

- ECG and continuous cardiac monitoring
- Pulse oximetry or arterial blood gas is used to evaluate other possible causes of hypotension.
- Serum electrolytes are measured to evaluate for metabolic acidosis, hypoglycemia, hypokalemia, and renal function.

Recommended Tests

- Serum cholinesterase assesses organophosphate or carbamate poisoning.
- Serum acetaminophen and aspirin levels in an overdose setting are measured to detect occult overdose with analgesic medications.
- Urine toxicology screen may be useful in patients with persistent hypotension of unknown cause.
- Creatine kinase is used to detect muscle injury when seizures, agitation, or prolonged hypotension may have occurred.
- Chest radiography is used if hypoxia is present.
- Abdominal radiography is used to evaluate for radiopaque pills, suggesting iron overdose.
- Swan-Ganz catheterization may be useful in assessing hemodynamic function and volume status.

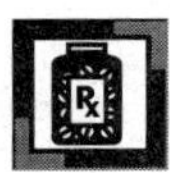

Treatment

- Intravenous access should be established; if hypotension is unresponsive to treatment or is worsening, the patient should be intubated endotracheally until the cause can be determined and treated.
- Dose and time of exposure should be determined for all substances involved.
- Specific treatment (e.g., naloxone for mental status depression) should be initiated while supportive care continues.

DECONTAMINATION

- Induction of emesis is not recommended.
- Gastric lavage should be performed in pediatric (tube size 24–32 French) or adult (36–42 French) patients for large ingestion presenting within 1 hour of ingestion or if serious effects are present.
- One dose of activated charcoal (1–2 g/kg) should be administered without a cathartic if a substantial ingestion has occurred within the previous few hours.

ANTIDOTES

- Calcium chloride has been used for bradycardia or hypotension secondary to calcium channel blocker overdose; optimal dose is unknown.
- Glucagon is used for bradycardia and hypotension secondary to β-blocker or calcium channel blocker overdose.
- Sodium bicarbonate has been used to treat QRS widening and ventricular dysrhythmia secondary to myocardial sodium channel blocking agents (tricyclic antidepressant, quinidine, propoxyphene): 1 to 2 mEq/kg intravenous bolus, repeated as needed without exceeding an arterial pH of 7.55.

ADJUNCTIVE TREATMENT

Hypoxia and electrolytes should be corrected as clinically indicated.

Hypotension

- Intravenous fluid

—Patients with no evidence of volume overload can receive 10 to 20 ml/kg 0.9% saline.
—If pressure is unresponsive to initial bolus, further fluid therapy should be guided with central pressure measurement.
—Volume overload should be avoided because many agents that cause hypotension are also myocardial depressants.

- Dopamine. The initial dosage is 2 to 5 μg/kg/min by intravenous infusion, titrated to effect; dosages above 20 μg/kg/min are unlikely to have further effect.
- Norepinephrine. If hypotension is unresponsive to dopamine, 0.1 to 0.2 μg/kg/min continuous infusion, titrated to effect, can be administered.
- Hypotension due to α blockade may, in theory, be more receptive to reversal by α agonists; phenylephrine (0.25 mg/ml in NaCl 0.9%) can be administered at 40 μg/min, titrated to effect.

Bradycardia

- Atropine. Adult dose is 0.5 to 1 mg intravenously, repeated in 5 minutes if necessary to a maximum of 2 mg; pediatric dose is 0.02 mg/kg intravenously, repeated every 5 minutes as needed to a maximum dose of 1 mg in children, 2 mg in adolescents.
- Isoproterenol. If bradycardia and hypotension are unresponsive to atropine, isoproterenol should be considered; adult dose, 5 μg/min infusion, titrated to effect; pediatric, 0.1 μg/kg/min, titrated to effect.
- Cardiac pacing may be needed in bradycardic patients unresponsive to the above measures.

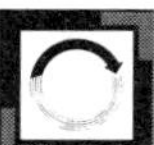

Follow-Up

PATIENT MONITORING

- Cardiac and respiratory function should be monitored continuously.
- Arterial pressure monitoring (A line) may be helpful in management of persistent hypotension.

EXPECTED COURSE AND PROGNOSIS

- Duration of hypotension is related to the underlying cause.
- Drugs with prolonged absorption or half-life may produce prolonged hypotension.
- Hypotension secondary to intravascular volume loss or dysrhythmias generally resolves when these are effectively treated.

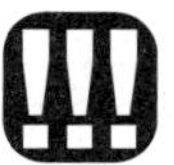

Pitfalls

If clinical evidence of hypoperfusion is not present, blood pressure may be appropriate for patient.

ICD-9-CM 972

Poisoning by agents primarily affecting the cardiovascular system.

See also: SECTION II, Bradycardia chapter; SECTION III, Calcium Gluconate, Chloride, and Sodium Bicarbonate chapters; and SECTION IV, Amphetamines, Antidepressants—Tricyclic, Calcium Channel Blocking Drugs, Clonidine, Cocaine, Digoxin, Glucagon, Iron, MAO Inhibitors, Organophosphate Insecticide, and Phenothiazine chapters.

RECOMMENDED READING

Hessler R. Cardiovascular principles. In: Goldfrank LR, et al., eds. Goldfrank's toxicologic emergencies, 6th ed. Norwalk, CT: Appleton & Lange, 1998.

Author: Katherine M. Hurlbut

Reviewer: Richard C. Dart

Hypothermia

Basics

DESCRIPTION

- Mild hypothermia is characterized by core temperature of 32° to 35°C (89.6°–95°F), tachypnea, tachycardia, ataxia, and dysarthria; shivering generates heat.
- Moderate hypothermia occurs when core temperatures range from 28° to 32°C (82.4°–89.6°F); the patient exhibits loss of shivering, dysrhythmias, Osborn J waves on ECG, and depressed mentation.
- Severe hypothermia occurs below 28°C (82.4°F), and is characterized by loss of reflexes, coma, hypotension, acidemia, ventricular fibrillation, and asystole.
- Profound hypothermia is reached at 14° to 20°C (57.2°–68°F); virtually all patients are asystolic.

PATHOPHYSIOLOGY

- Temperature regulation in humans occurs via the hypothalamic-pituitary system, regulating vasoconstriction, muscle tone, and metabolism.
- Below a core temperature of about 30°C, humans lose the ability to produce and conserve heat.

EPIDEMIOLOGY

When related to poisoning, hypothermia is usually the result of low ambient temperature combined with the victim's inability to leave the environment (e.g., depressed mental status and poorly heated apartment).

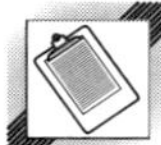

Diagnosis

DIFFERENTIAL DIAGNOSIS

Further information on each poison is available in SECTION IV, CHEMICAL AND BIOLOGICAL AGENTS.

- Toxicologic causes are numerous.

—Ethanol intoxication may be assessed using blood alcohol level.
—Carbon monoxide is associated with coma, acidosis, and increased carboxyhemoglobin level.
—Opioids cause small pupils and respiratory depression; evidence of chronic drug abuse may be apparent.
—Sedative-hypnotic agents can usually be detected on urine drug screen.
—Phenothiazines produce ECG abnormalities and perhaps anticholinergic effects.
—Hallucinogens or over-the-counter antihistamines are often abused by minors and may facilitate development of environmental hypothermia.
—Oral hypoglycemic agents impair response to hypothermia.

- Most cases of nontoxicologic hypothermia are environmental and have an apparent cause.
- Any condition that causes altered mental status may lead to hypothermia by preventing the patient from leaving the hypothermic environment.

SIGNS AND SYMPTOMS

Physical signs may help reveal the poison involved when they occur in the setting of hypothermia.

Vital Signs

Initial tachycardia is followed by bradycardia and hypotension.

HEENT

- Pinpoint pupils suggest an opioid, clonidine, or imidazoline drug.
- Dilated pupils indicate hypoxia, cold, or anticholinergic effect.

Dermatologic

Bullae may develop with coma associated with carbon monoxide or sedative-hypnotic agents.

Pulmonary

Loss of protective airway reflexes may allow aspiration.

Gastrointestinal

- Ileus usually develops.
- Opioids or anticholinergic drugs are other causes of decreased bowel sounds.

Hematologic

- Hemoconcentration is common.
- Disseminated intravascular coagulation may be present in severe cases.

Fluids and Electrolytes

- Acute hypothermia causes a "cold diuresis," resulting in volume depletion.
- Respiratory alkalosis may occur initially but will become respiratory acidosis if hypothermia is severe.
- Metabolic acidosis resulting from lactic acid accumulation is common.
- Hyper- or hypoglycemia may occur; hypoglycemia may indicate oral hypoglycemic ingestion.
- Hypokalemia occurs due to reversible redistribution of potassium into muscle; supplementation should be avoided.

Neurologic

- Mental status. Initial CNS stimulation is followed by depression, causing a progressive depressed mentation with ataxia and dysarthria; many patients are comatose below 30°C.
- Reflexes. Hyperreflexia is present at core temperatures from 32°C to 35°C, hyporeflexia from 26°C to 32°C; reflexes are absent below 26°C, the knee jerk being the last to go.

PROCEDURES AND LABORATORY TESTS

Essential Tests

- Rectal temperature should be taken to confirm hypothermia.
- Mild hypothermia requires no special laboratory testing in itself; appropriate laboratory tests are determined by the drugs involved.

Recommended Tests

- Serum electrolytes, glucose, BUN, creatinine. Hypokalemia and hypoglycemia are common. Hypoglycemia may indicate oral hypoglycemic ingestion.
- Complete blood count. Hemoconcentration is common.
- Arterial blood gases. Respiratory alkalosis followed by respiratory acidosis may occur.
- Amylase to check for hyperamylasemia in severe cases.
- ECG with continuous monitoring:

—ECG effects may obscure conduction abnormalities caused by toxicant.
—Severity of conduction abnormality is related to severity of hypothermia: bradycardia, QRS widening, prolonged QT, repolarization abnormalities with variable effects on the ST segment and T wave.
—The Osborn wave (J wave) is a hump at the J point immediately after the QRS complex, the size increasing with temperature depression.
—J waves are also associated with CNS lesions, focal cardiac ischemia, and sepsis; they may be present in young healthy persons.

- Serum acetaminophen and aspirin levels and urine drug screen in an overdose setting to detect occult overdose with analgesic medication and to screen for poisoning with sedative-hypnotic or drugs of abuse as cause.

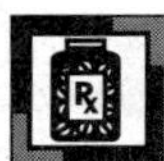

Treatment

- Treatment is directed toward preventing further heat loss, rewarming, and to preventing complications, especially cardiac dysrhythmias.
- Volume resuscitation should be performed with warmed dextrose 5% and normal saline, or with normal saline alone.
- Rewarming and specific treatments should be initiated while supportive care continues.
- Dose and time of exposure should be determined for all substances that could be involved.

DIRECTING PATIENT COURSE

Health-care provider should call poison control center when:

- cause of hypothermia is unclear.
- coingestant, drug interaction, or underlying disease presents unusual problems.

DECONTAMINATION

- Emesis should not be induced if patient is hypothermic.
- Gastric lavage can be performed in pediatric (tube size 24–32 French) or adult (tube size 36–42 French) patients for large ingestion presenting within 1 hour of ingestion or if serious effects are present.
- One dose of activated charcoal (1–2 g/kg) should be administered without a cathartic if a substantial ingestion has occurred within the previous few hours.

ADJUNCTIVE TREATMENT

Indications for Rewarming

- Mildly hypothermic patients (above 32°C) can be rewarmed with external noninvasive methods such as a blanket, heated humidified oxygen, and warm intravenous fluids.
- Moderate hypothermia (28°–32°C) should be treated with airway rewarming and warm intravenous fluids for all patients, possibly supplemented by gastric or peritoneal lavage if rewarming is proceeding at less than 1°C per hour.
- Severe hypothermia (below 28°C) mandates aggressive therapy and active core rewarming.
- If the core temperature is less than 25°C, femoral-femoral bypass should be considered if the facilities are available.
- For patients in cardiac arrest, femoral-femoral bypass is the rewarming method of choice.
- Open pleural lavage for direct cardiac rewarming should be considered if the core temperature remains below 28°C after 1 hour of bypass.

Methods for Rewarming

- Passive external rewarming consists of insulation of the patient.
- Active external rewarming uses convective blankets or other external heat sources for rewarming; radiant warmers work only if the patient is fully uncovered.
- Active core rewarming

—Airway warming: nebulizer or ventilator is modified to give 100% humidified air warmed to 40° to 45°C.
—Warm intravenous fluid (40°–42°C) is administered.
—Body cavity lavage should be considered; peritoneal lavage and pleural lavage with tube thoracostomy can be useful in patients with severe effects.
—Gastrointestinal or bladder irrigation also may rewarm central organs but are associated with risks of electrolyte imbalance.

Pharmacologic Treatment

- Target organs become progressively less responsive to medications as the core temperature decreases.
- Excessive pharmacologic manipulation of the vasoconstricted and depressed cardiovascular system should be avoided.
- Large doses of exogenous insulin or digoxin are ineffective at lower temperatures but can produce a toxic reaction as rewarming progresses.
- Infusion of low doses of catecholamine are indicated in patients who have lower blood pressure than would be expected for that degree of hypothermia and who are not responding to crystalloid infusion and rewarming.

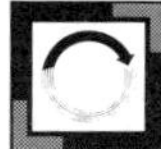

Follow-Up

PATIENT MONITORING

- Continuous cardiac and respiratory monitoring should be performed.
- Arterial pressure monitoring (A line) may be needed in severe cases.

EXPECTED COURSE AND PROGNOSIS

- Failure to restore a circulating cardiac rhythm within about 30 minutes after rewarming to 32° to 35°C makes further efforts unlikely to be successful.
- Disseminated intravascular coagulopathy, cardiac dysrhythmia, rhabdomyolysis, and other complications may become apparent during rewarming of patients with moderate to severe hypothermia.

DISCHARGE CRITERIA/INSTRUCTIONS

Asymptomatic patients who suffered mild hypothermia may be discharged following a 6-hour observation period, decontamination, and psychiatric evaluation, if needed.

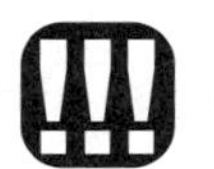

Pitfalls

TREATMENT

- Cardiovascular depression can persist on rewarming.
- Volume redistribution (to the core blood vessels) and cold diuresis can lead to decrease in blood pressure with rewarming and peripheral vasodilation.
- Jostling or vigorously moving the patient should be avoided as this may trigger ventricular fibrillation.

ICD-9-CM 780.9

General symptoms: hypothermia (not associated with environment).

See also: SECTION II, Bradycardia and Hypotension chapters, and SECTION IV, Chapters on individual agents.

RECOMMENDED READING

Danzl DF, Pozos RS. Accidental hypothermia. N Engl J Med 1994;331:1756–1760.

Danzl DF, Pozos RS, Hamlet MP. Accidental hypothermia. In: Auerbach PS, ed. Wilderness medicine, 3rd ed. St. Louis: Mosby, 1995:51–103.

Jolly BT, KT Ghezzi. Accidental hypothermia. Emerg Med Clin North Am 1992;10:311–319.

Author: Gayle E. Long

Reviewer: Richard C. Dart

Metal Fume Fever

Basics

DESCRIPTION

- Metal fume fever is an acute occupational self-limited illness that follows the inhalation of metal oxide fumes.
- The most common metals that cause metal fume fever are zinc, copper, brass (copper-zinc alloy), and magnesium.
- Less common are manganese, antimony, silver, tin, selenium, aluminum, nickel, chromium, vanadium, and stainless steel.
- Synonyms include brass chills, brazier's disease, galvanizer shakes, foundry ague or fever, metal malaria, Monday morning fever, solderer's fever, smelter shakes, welder's ague, welder's fever, zinc shakes, and "the smothers."
- Cadmium fume pneumonitis is discussed in SECTION IV, Cadmium Fume Fever.

PATHOPHYSIOLOGY

- When zinc or its alloys are heated above 930°F, particles of up to 1 micron in diameter are formed.
- Inhalation of particles less than 1 micron in diameter may result in metal fume fever, an acute febrile illness.

The exact etiology of metal fume fever is unknown; theories include:

- Modification of lung proteins because of absorption of metal oxide, reaction to foreign proteins, endotoxins, or a nonspecific response to interleukin-1
- Immune complex disease
- Interference of phagocytosis by metal particles accumulating in alveolar macrophages
- Hypersensitivity pneumonitis
- Delayed immunoglobulin E reaction

EPIDEMIOLOGY

- Toxic effects are common and underreported due to the benign nature.
- Death is not expected from this syndrome.

CAUSES

This is a disease of occupational exposure with high incidence in a select group of industries, most often the metal reclamation industry.

RISK FACTORS

- Employment as a welder is a risk factor.
- Metal fume fever also may occur among zinc smelters, brass solderers, brass foundry workers, chrome electroplaters, chrome welders, iron galvanizers, molten metal fabricators, metal grinders, manufacturers of steel alloys, workers near electric furnaces that are used to melt metals, and steel alloy manufacturers.
- Patients with previous pulmonary disease do not appear to be predisposed to metal fume fever and do not demonstrate unusual complications.

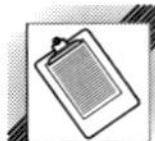

Diagnosis

DIFFERENTIAL DIAGNOSIS

- Further information on each poison is available in SECTION IV, CHEMICAL AND BIOLOGICAL AGENTS.
- Toxicologic causes of acute fever and respiratory complaints include salicylism, acute irritant gas inhalation (e.g., chlorine), chemical pneumonitis, polymer fume fever, occupational asthma due to metal oxides exposure, and nitrogen dioxide.
- Other causes include viral illness, malaria, pneumonia, sepsis, hypersensitivity pneumonitis, and pulmonary embolus.
- A careful occupational history is important to uncover exposure to metal oxide fumes. Chest discomfort and dyspnea with normal respiratory function and adequate oxygenation help to differentiate between infectious etiology and pulmonary embolism.

SIGNS AND SYMPTOMS

- Signs and symptoms develop rapidly and simultaneously within 4 to 12 hours of exposure to metal fumes. The symptoms disappear with only slight residual discomfort within 48 hours after removal from the source.
- Tachyphylaxis to the effect of metal fumes develops with repeated exposure; thus, symptoms improve during the work week. Symptoms resolve completely over the weekend, but recur with reexposure to the metal fumes (Monday morning fever).
- Generalized fatigue and chills are universal complaints.

Vital Signs

Fever and tachypnea are common.

HEENT

Sweet or metallic taste in the mouth, nasal irritation, sore throat, hoarseness, thirst, and headache may occur.

Dermatologic

Diaphoresis may occur, as may macular rash (rarely).

Pulmonary

- Chest tightness, wheezing, pleuritic chest pain, dyspnea, and nonproductive cough are common.
- Hemoptysis occurs rarely.

Gastrointestinal

Nausea, vomiting, and diffuse abdominal pain may occur.

Musculoskeletal

- Generalized arthralgia and myalgia occur.
- Fatigue and chills are common.

Neurologic

Weakness and lethargy may occur, as may paresthesia (rarely).

PROCEDURES AND LABORATORY TESTS

Essential Tests

There are no essential tests.

Recommended Tests

- Complete blood count may demonstrate leukocytosis.
- Arterial blood gases may show hypoxemia in severe cases.
- Spirometry may reveal lowered forced vital capacity (restrictive); it is rarely obstructive.
- Serum lactate dehydrogenase may be increased.
- Urinary or serum metals are often elevated but are of little help in the diagnosis.
- ECG, serum creatine kinase, and cardiac enzymes may be indicated based on signs and symptoms of chest pain and hypoxia.
- Chest radiograph is usually normal, but may show pneumonitis or pulmonary edema after severe exposure.

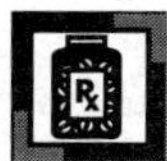

Treatment

- Exposure must be terminated and oxygen administered.
- Pulmonary supportive care is the basis of therapy.
- The exact composition of the metal and exposure time should be determined for all substances involved.

DIRECTING PATIENT COURSE

The health-care provider should call the poison control center when:

- cause of metal fume fever is unclear.
- drug interaction or underlying disease presents unusual problems.

DECONTAMINATION

The patient must be removed from exposure, undressed completely, and showered to remove any metal contaminants in the hair or on the skin.

ANTIDOTES

There is no specific antidote for metal fume fever.

ADJUNCTIVE TREATMENT

- Antipyretics are used to control fever; 1,000 mg of acetaminophen is administered every 4 to 6 hours, or 600 mg of ibuprofen is administered every 6 hours.
- The patient should be rehydrated either orally or intravenously.
- Analgesics are used to control pain.
- Bronchospasm

—Oxygen is administered, followed by albuterol 0.15 mg/kg (maximum 10 mg) in saline with humidified oxygen via nebulizer every 20 to 30 minutes. If the peak expiratory flow rate is greater than 90% after an initial dose, additional doses may not be needed. Response should be monitored.
—Methylprednisolone 60 to 125 mg (1.0–1.5 mg/kg) is administered intravenously every 6 to 8 hours. This may be decreased to a single daily dose and tapered rapidly.
—Initiation of prednisone should be considered, 2 mg/kg orally for several days.

- Not recommended therapies. Prophylactic antibiotics are not proven to be of value.

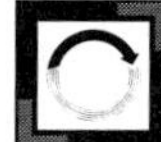

Follow-Up

EXPECTED COURSE AND PROGNOSIS

- Symptoms begin 4 to 12 hours after exposure; duration of illness is less than 48 hours; a temporary asymptomatic period may occur for 1 to 2 days afterward.
- Reexposure to metal oxide fumes will often cause recurrent metal fume fever, but is believed to be relatively benign, and long-term complications are not expected.

DISCHARGE CRITERIA/INSTRUCTIONS

The patient may be discharged when symptoms resolve and evaluation does not reveal a more serious process.

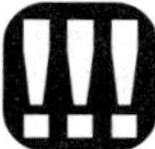

Pitfalls

DIAGNOSIS

- Because there are no specific physical or laboratory findings in metal fume fever, it is important to obtain a careful occupational history.
- Diagnosis may not be apparent on initial presentation because of the latent time from exposure to symptoms (symptoms usually occur after work) and delay in seeking medical evaluation.
- It is important to include cadmium fume pneumonitis, nickel carbonyl exposure, and nitrogen dioxide in the differential diagnosis of metal fume fever.
- It is important also to consider chemical pneumonitis, hypersensitivity pneumonitis, and occupational asthma due to metal oxides exposure.

ICD-9-CM 987

Toxic effect of other gases, fumes, or vapors.

RECOMMENDED READING

Behrman A. In: Greenberg M, Phillps S, et al., eds. Occupational, industrial and environmental toxicology. St. Louis: Mosby, 1997:303–309.

Farrell FJ. Metal oxides. In: Sullivan JB Jr, Krieger GR, eds. Hazardous materials toxicology. Baltimore: Williams & Wilkins, 1992:921–927.

Offerman PV, Finley CJ. Metal fume fever. Ann Emerg Med 1992;21:872.

Author: Gerald F. O'Malley

Reviewer: Luke Yip

Methemoglobinemia

Basics

DESCRIPTION

- Methemoglobin is hemoglobin in which the iron molecule has been oxidized from the normal ferrous state (Fe^{2+}) to the ferric state (Fe^{3+}).
- Methemoglobinemia is the clinical condition in which more than the normal amount of hemoglobin (2%) has been oxidized.

PATHOPHYSIOLOGY

- Under normal conditions, the methemoglobin level is less than 2%.
- A methemoglobin molecule cannot carry oxygen.
- Methemoglobin also increases the affinity of normal hemoglobin for oxygen, shifting the oxygen hemoglobin dissociation curve to the left, which results in reduced ability of normal hemoglobin to release oxygen; this reduces oxygen delivery to the tissues.
- Normally, the enzyme NADH methemoglobin reductase reduces methemoglobin back to hemoglobin; however, when large amounts of methemoglobin are produced, this pathway is overwhelmed.
- Another enzyme, NADPH methemoglobin reductase, also reduces a small amount of methemoglobin under normal conditions; unlike NADH methemoglobin reductase, this enzyme system can be accelerated when supplied with an exogenous electron carrier, such as methylene blue.
- Elevated methemoglobin levels can be produced by oxidizing agents, hemoglobin M (heterozygous), deficiency of NADH or NADPH methemoglobin reductase, and by oxidative stress in individuals with glucose-6-phosphate dehydrogenase (G6PD) deficiency.

EPIDEMIOLOGY

- Poisoning is uncommon.
- Toxic effects are typically mild to moderate.
- There is a higher incidence of comorbid diseases in the elderly population that may increase methemoglobin toxicity.
- Death is unusual, occurring in untreated cases with methemoglobin levels greater than 70%.

CAUSES

Most cases are secondary to adverse medication reaction, therapeutic misadventure, or recreational abuse of amyl nitrites ("poppers").

RISK FACTORS

- The heterozygous form of hemoglobin M, deficiencies in NADPH or NADH methemoglobin reductase, and G6PD deficiency may lead to methemoglobinemia.
- Fetal hemoglobin is oxidized to methemoglobin more easily than normal hemoglobin is; NADH methemoglobin reductase is not fully active until 4 months of age.
- Infants also have increased skin permeability to aniline compounds, which can cause methemoglobinemia.
- Patients with underlying heart disease, pulmonary disease, or anemia may develop symptoms at lower methemoglobin levels.

PREGNANCY AND LACTATION

- Because fetal hemoglobin is more susceptible to oxidation, the threshold for treatment of methemoglobinemia in pregnant patients should be lower.
- Anilines and some other drugs and chemicals can cross the placental barrier.

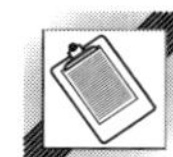

Diagnosis

DIFFERENTIAL DIAGNOSIS

Further information on each poison is available in SECTION IV, CHEMICAL AND BIOLOGICAL AGENTS.

Common Toxicologic Causes

Acetanilid, amyl nitrite, aniline dyes, antipyrine, benzocaine, chloroquine, dapsone, methylene blue, mothballs (more common with naphthalene), nitrates (including contaminated well water), nitrites (most commonly abused inhaled amyl nitrites), nitroglycerin, phenacetin, phenols, prilocaine, primaquine, pyridium, sulfonamides, toluidine, trinitrotoluene.

Uncommon Toxicologic Causes

Chlorates, dimethylamine, dimethyl aniline, dinitrobenzene, dinitrophenol, dinitrotoluene, hydroxylamine, marking inks, lidocaine, methanol, nitrobenzene, nitrofurans, nitrophenol, phenytoin, silver nitrite.

SIGNS AND SYMPTOMS

- Symptoms are related to decreased oxygen delivery to tissues and often correlate with methemoglobin concentration.
- Cyanosis of noncardiac and nonpulmonary etiologies that is unresponsive to oxygen therapy is suggestive of methemoglobinemia.
- Neonates are at risk for acute diarrheal syndrome caused by nitrite-producing bacteria; occult methemoglobinemia develops, causing acidemia, hyperchloremia, and low pO_2.

Vital Signs

- Tachycardia and tachypnea are common.
- Hypotension may develop in severe methemoglobinemia secondary to tissue hypoxia and acidosis.

Dermatologic

- Cyanosis occurs when methemoglobin concentrations exceed 1.5%.
- The cyanosis is typically more brown ("chocolate cyanosis") than blue in color, and is unresponsive to oxygen therapy.

Cardiovascular

- Dysrhythmias may occur in severe cases.
- Cardiac arrest and myocardial infarction have been reported.
- Hypotension may occur in severe cases from acidosis and hypoxia.
- Hypotension also may be due to nitrates and related compounds that are vasodilators, in addition to causes of methemoglobinemia.

Pulmonary

- Shortness of breath is common.
- Acute respiratory arrest has been reported.

Gastrointestinal

Nausea and vomiting may be present.

Hematologic

- Blood will have a chocolate brown color that does not change to red when oxygen is bubbled through it.
- Methemoglobin has been associated with hemolysis.

Neurologic

Lethargy, confusion, syncope, seizures, and coma may develop at high methemoglobin concentrations.

PROCEDURES AND LABORATORY TESTS

Essential Tests

- Methemoglobin level should be determined.

—Normal methemoglobin level is less than 2%.
—With 15% to 20% methemoglobin, cyanosis is present and the patient is generally asymptomatic.
—With 20% to 45% methemoglobin, anxiety, headache, dizziness, fatigue, syncope, and dyspnea occur.
—With 45% to 55% methemoglobin, CNS depression occurs.
—With 55% to 75% methemoglobin, coma, seizures, dysrhythmias, and shock occur.
—With more than 70% methemoglobin, death may occur if the condition is untreated.

- Blood color comparison. A drop of the patient's blood should be placed on a white sheet and compared with that from a normal control; blood with methemoglobinemia has a characteristic chocolate brown color.

Recommended Tests

- Arterial blood gases should be determined in symptomatic patients.

—This should be performed using a cooximeter to measure methemoglobin, carboxyhemoglobin, and pO_2 because calculated oxygen saturations may be inaccurate.
—Pulse oximetry readings may not be accurate.

- Serum G6PD determination is used to determine etiology (not helpful in acute management).

- Serum electrolytes, BUN, and creatinine assess for elevated anion gap acidosis.
- Complete blood count with smear and haptoglobin level are used to look for evidence of hemolysis.
- ECG, serum acetaminophen, and aspirin levels in an overdose setting can detect occult ingestion.

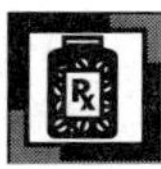

Treatment

- Supportive care with appropriate airway management is vital.
- Dose and time of exposure should be determined for all substances involved.
- Specific treatment should be initiated while supportive care continues.
- Methylene blue should be administered in severe cases.
- Many patients with mild methemoglobinemia require no specific therapy other than humidified oxygen and removal of the inciting drug or chemical.

DIRECTING PATIENT COURSE

The health-care provider should call the poison control center when:

- cause of cyanosis or methemoglobinemia is unclear.
- coingestant, drug interaction, or underlying disease presents unusual problems.

Admission Considerations

Patients with severe methemoglobinemia and those unresponsive to therapy should be admitted.

DECONTAMINATION

Out of Hospital

- Following acute ingestion, emesis should be induced with ipecac for alert pediatric or adult patient, if health-care evaluation will be delayed, especially if the patient is known to be G6PD deficient.
- Exposed skin areas should be washed to limit further toxin absorption.

In Hospital

- Ipecac-induced emesis is not recommended.
- Gastric lavage should be performed in pediatric (tube size 24–32 French) or adult (tube size 36–42 French) patients for large ingestion presenting within 1 hour of ingestion or if serious effects are present.
- One dose of activated charcoal (1–2 g/kg) should be administered if a substantial ingestion has occurred within the previous few hours.
- Exposed skin area should be washed to limit further toxin absorption.

ANTIDOTES

Methylene blue is a specific antidote for methemoglobinemia.

Methylene Blue

Indications

- Methemoglobin level above 20% to 25% and increasing in an asymptomatic patient
- Symptomatic patient with any elevation of methemoglobin level
- Symptomatic patient with cyanosis that does not correct with administration of 100% oxygen (before methemoglobin level is available)
- Any evidence of CNS or cardiac hypoxia (anxiety, confusion, hypotension, chest pain, etc.)

Contraindications

- Known allergy to methylene blue
- Known NADPH methemoglobin reductase deficiency or G6PD deficiency

Method of Administration

- Dose is 1 to 2 mg/kg of 1% solution intravenously over 5 minutes; clinical improvement should be apparent shortly after.
- Methemoglobin level is assessed 30 to 60 minutes later; if it is still elevated and patient is still symptomatic, dose is appropriate.

Potential Adverse Effects

- Hemolysis in patients with G6PD deficiency
- Paradoxical worsening of methemoglobinemia with extremely large doses of methylene blue (unlikely with cumulative dose less than 7 mg/kg)

Ascorbic Acid

Ascorbic acid works very slowly and is not recommended; it is used in cases of heterozygous hemoglobin M and NADH deficiency.

ADJUNCTIVE TREATMENT

Exchange transfusion and hyperbaric oxygen are used rarely for life-threatening methemoglobinemia refractory to methylene blue therapy or in patient with severe G6PD deficiency.

Hypotension

- Use atropine to correct hypotension related to bradycardia.
- Patient should receive 10 to 20 ml/kg 0.9% saline and be placed in Trendelenburg position.
- Further fluid therapy should be guided by central pressure monitoring to avoid volume overload.
- Vasopressor may be added if needed.

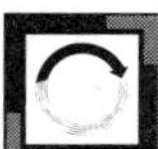

Follow-Up

PATIENT MONITORING

Monitor respiratory and cardiac function continuously.

EXPECTED COURSE AND PROGNOSIS

The reconversion rate of methemoglobin in normal patients is about 15% per hour, assuming no further methemoglobin production.

DISCHARGE CRITERIA/INSTRUCTIONS

Patients who have known cause and become asymptomatic following therapy may be discharged following a psychiatric evaluation, if needed.

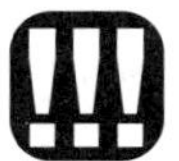

Pitfalls

DIAGNOSIS

- Other causes of cyanosis may be mistaken for methemoglobinemia.
- Some of the chemicals require transformation to toxic metabolites to produce methemoglobinemia; thus, signs and symptoms may be delayed for several hours or days.
- Sulfhemoglobinemia produces effects indistinguishable from methemoglobinemia and should be suspected when methemoglobinemia fails to respond to methylene blue treatment.

TREATMENT

Overdosing methylene blue, especially in patients with G6PD deficiency, can lead to worsening methemoglobinemia, cyanosis, and hemolysis.

ICD-9-CM 964

Poisoning by agents primarily affecting blood constituents.

See also: SECTION II, Hypotension chapter; SECTION III, Methylene Blue chapter; and SECTION IV, chapters on specific agents.

RECOMMENDED READING

Curry S. Methemoglobinemia. Ann Emerg Med 1982;11:214–221.

Price D. Methemoglobinemia. In: Goldfrank LR, Flomenbaum NE, Lewin NA, et al, eds. Goldfrank's toxicologic emergencies, 6th ed. Norwalk, CT: Appleton & Lange, 1998.

Authors: Christopher R. DeWitt and Kennon Heard

Reviewers: Luke Yip and G. O'Malley

Movement Disorders

Basics

DESCRIPTION

The presence of a movement disorder may help identify the cause of poisoning.

Akathisia

- Involuntary motor restlessness renders the patient unable to remain still and may resemble psychotic agitation.
- A history of increasing medication dose may help identify akathisia.
- Toxic causes include the use of neuroleptic, antiemetic, sympathomimetic, or antiparkinsonian medications.

Asterixis and Myoclonus

- Transient loss of postural tone in a muscle group results in jerking movements as tone is regained.
- It is difficult to distinguish these entities on examination: myoclonus results from contractions, and asterixis results from loss of tone in a muscle group.
- Medications causing asterixis and myoclonus include anticonvulsant, sedative-hypnotic, and cyclic antidepressant medications.
- Other toxic causes include lead or mercury exposures; a history of exposure and a urinary metal testing may reveal the cause.
- Nontoxic causes include metabolic encephalopathy, hepatic or renal failure, hyperosmolarity, or anoxia.

Ataxia

- This disorder involves loss of muscular coordination (e.g., an inability to maintain an upright posture while standing or attempting to walk in a straight line).
- Common toxic causes include ethanol, sedative-hypnotic agents, anticonvulsants, cyclic antidepressants, selective serotonin reuptake inhibitors (SSRIs), or antihistamine medications.
- Nontoxic causes include somnolence from various causes and sensory neuropathy.
- Alcoholic cerebellar degeneration may exacerbate ataxia resulting from other causes.

Chorea

- This involves a variety of sudden erratic random limb movements, often described as "waving" or, when movements are forceful, "ballismus."
- Medication causes include sedative-hypnotic, antihistamine, cyclic antidepressant, anticonvulsant, anti-parkinsonian, sympathomimetic, opioid, neuroleptic, and steroid medications.
- Other toxic causes include carbon monoxide, toluene, lithium, manganese, or thallium; the serum lithium level may be elevated, and the results of urine tests for manganese or thallium may show elevated levels.
- Metabolic causes include hyper- or hypoglycemia, hyper- or hyponatremia, hypocalcemia, hypomagnesemia, hyperthyroidism, and thiamine deficiency.
- Neurologic diseases include Huntington's chorea and Wilson's disease.

Dystonia

- This term covers a variety of movement disorders due to muscle spasm: blepharospasm, dysarthria, dysphagia, involuntary tongue movements, oculogyric crisis, opisthotonos, retrocollis, and torticollis.
- It usually involves the head and neck and only rarely involves the trunk or airway.
- Toxic causes include neuroleptic, antiemetic, or anti-parkinsonian drugs.
- Neuroleptics and antiemetics are the most common medications that cause dystonia.

Dysarthria

- This disorder, slurred speech, results from poor control of the speech muscles.
- Toxic causes include sedative-hypnotic agents, anticonvulsants, cyclic antidepressants, SSRIs, antihistamines, and many other medications.

Fasciculation

- Spasm of the fibers in a single motor unit of a muscle results in discrete twitching.
- Medication causes include sympathomimetic, cholinergic, and hypoglycemic drugs.
- Other toxic causes include a variety of animal venoms, strychnine, lithium, lead, mercury, or manganese.
- Nontoxic causes. Fatigue and cold may result in fasciculation.
- Pathologic fasciculation may result from a variety of neurologic disorders that affect the motor nerve.

Nystagmus

- Rapid eye movements appear to jerk the eyes in a given direction after a slow component in the opposite direction.
- Toxic causes include sedative-hypnotic agents, phencyclidine (PCP), lithium, anticonvulsants, and several other medications.
- A variety of neurologic causes such as intracranial lesions or labyrinthitis may cause nystagmus.

Parkinsonism

- This disorder is characterized by tremor, rigidity (classically cogwheel type), slow movements, and postural instability.
- Lack of facial expression, shuffling gait, drooling, and micrographia also may be seen both with Parkinson's disease and following toxic insults that may result in a parkinsonian syndrome.
- Toxic causes include MPTP (methyl-gamma-phenyl-1,2,3,6, tetrahydropyridine), which destroys the substantia nigra, resulting in parkinsonism.
- Medication causes. Parkinsonism also may result from the use of a number of drugs that antagonize dopamine: neuroleptic, alphamethyldopa, metoclopramide, prochlorperazine, reserpine, and tetrabenazine medications.
- Other toxic causes. Parkinsonism also may occur as sequelae of toxicity from carbon disulfide, carbon monoxide, cyanide, methanol, or manganese.

Rigidity

See also SECTION II, NMS and Serotonin Syndrome chapter.

- Malignant hyperthermia, neuroleptic malignant syndrome (NMS), and serotonin syndrome are characterized by muscle rigidity, fever, altered mental status, and autonomic dysfunction; tremor, dystonia, and chorea also may occur.
- Toxic causes include monoamine oxidase (MAO) inhibitor overdose or food or drug interaction with MAO inhibitors; these may be indistinguishable from NMS except by drug history.
- Similar syndromes include heat stroke, catatonia, and infection.

Tardive Dyskinesia

Tardive dyskinesia is not an uncommon complication of neuroleptic therapy. It is felt to be due to upregulation of dopamine receptors. Tardive dyskinesia commonly manifests as lip smacking, facial movements, or tongue protrusion. It can occur with changing doses or withdrawal of therapy. It is often not reversible. Anticholinergic agents may worsen symptoms. Toxic causes include phenothiazines and butyrophenones. Tardive dystonia is a delayed complication of the chronic use of neuroleptic, metoclopramide, or anti-parkinsonian drugs.

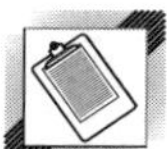

Diagnosis

Further information on each poison is available in SECTION IV. Types of compounds and their clinical manifestations are listed as follows:

- Alphamethyldopa. Parkinsonism
- Amantadine. Chorea, akathisia
- Amiodarone. Tremors (resting, postural, and kinetic), ataxia
- Amphetamine. Fasciculation, postural tremor, chorea, dystonia, akathisia
- Antiemetic. Dystonia, chorea, akathisia
- Antihistamine. Chorea
- Arsenic. Fasciculation, postural tremor
- Barbiturate. Tremor (postural, kinetic, and resting), myoclonus, asterixis, ataxia, nystagmus, chorea
- Barium. Fasciculation
- Benzodiazepine. Kinetic tremor, ataxia, myoclonus, asterixis, dysarthria, nystagmus
- Benztropine. Chorea
- Bismuth. Postural tremor, myoclonus, asterixis
- β-adrenergic agonist. Postural tremor
- Black widow spider venom. Fasciculation
- Bromocriptine. Chorea, dystonia
- Caffeine. Fasciculation, postural tremor, chorea
- Camphor. Fasciculation
- Carbamazepine. Kinetic tremor, myoclonus, asterixis, chorea, dystonia
- Carbon disulfide. Postural tremor, parkinsonism
- Carbon monoxide. Chorea, parkinsonism, postural tremor
- Chloral hydrate. Kinetic tremor, ataxia, asterixis, nystagmus, dysarthria
- Chloroquine. Dystonia
- Cholinergic agent. Fasciculation
- Cocaine. Chorea, dystonia, postural tremor, fasciculation, akathisia
- Colistin. Kinetic tremor
- Corticosteroid. Postural tremor, chorea
- Cyanide. Parkinsonism
- Cyclic antidepressant. Postural tremor, myoclonus, asterixis, chorea, dystonia
- DDT. Myoclonus, asterixis
- Ethanol. Ataxia, chorea, myoclonus, asterixis, kinetic tremor, dystonia, dysarthria, nystagmus
- Ethchlorovynol. Kinetic tremor, dysarthria, nystagmus, ataxia, asterixis
- Ergotamine. Fasciculation, postural tremor
- Fluoride. Fasciculation
- Glutethimide. Kinetic tremor, nystagmus, dysarthria, ataxia, asterixis
- Hypoglycemic agent. Fasciculation, tremor
- Insulin. Fasciculation, tremor
- Lead. Postural tremor, myoclonus, asterixis, fasciculation
- Levodopa. Myoclonus, asterixis, postural tremor, akathisia, chorea, dystonia
- Lithium. Fasciculation, tremors (postural, resting, and kinetic), chorea, dystonia, nystagmus
- MAO inhibitors. Postural tremor, rigidity
- Manganese. Parkinsonism, chorea, fasciculation
- Mercury. Myoclonus, fasciculation, postural and kinetic tremor, asterixis
- Metaldehyde. Dystonia
- Methanol. Parkinsonism
- Methaqualone. Ataxia, dysarthria, nystagmus, kinetic tremor, asterixis
- Methyl bromide. Postural tremor, myoclonus, asterixis
- Methyl mercury. Ataxia, kinetic tremor
- Methylphenidate. Chorea, akathisia, postural tremor
- Metoclopramide. Dystonia, chorea, akathisia, parkinsonism
- Monosodium glutamate. Postural tremor
- MPTP. Parkinsonism
- Neuroleptic drugs. Neuroleptic malignant syndrome, rigidity, tardive dyskinesia, dystonia, akathisia, chorea, parkinsonism
- Nicotine. Fasciculation
- Opioid drug. Chorea
- Oral contraceptive. Postural tremor, chorea
- Pergolide. Chorea, myoclonus, asterixis, akathisia, dystonia
- Phencyclidine (PCP). Fasciculation, dystonia, postural tremor, nystagmus
- Phenytoin. Dystonia, myoclonus, asterixis, chorea, postural and kinetic tremor, dysarthria, nystagmus, ataxia
- Piperazine. Kinetic tremor
- Prochlorperazine. Parkinsonism
- Rattlesnake venom. Fasciculation
- Reserpine. Parkinsonism
- Saxitoxin. Fasciculation
- Scorpion toxin. Fasciculation
- SSRI. Rigidity, myoclonus, chorea, tremor, dystonia, myoclonus
- Strychnine. Fasciculation, dystonia
- Tetrodotoxin. Fasciculation
- Thallium. Chorea
- Theophylline. Chorea, postural tremor, fasciculation
- Thyroid drug. Fasciculation, resting tremor, chorea
- Toluene. Chorea
- Valproate. Tremor (postural, resting, and kinetic), myoclonus, asterixis
- Water hemlock. Dystonia
- Withdrawal from ethanol, benzodiazepine, barbiturates. Postural tremor, ataxia

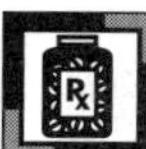

Treatment

Refer to specific toxicant chapters.

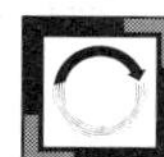

Follow-Up

Refer to specific toxicant chapters.

See also: SECTION II, NMS and Serotonin Syndrome chapter, and SECTION IV, chapters on individual poisons.

ICD-9-CM 975

Poisoning by agents primarily acting on the smooth and skeletal muscles and respiratory system.

Author: Lada Kokan

Reviewer: Kennon Heard

Multiple Chemical Sensitivity

Basics

DESCRIPTION

- Multiple chemical sensitivity (MCS) has been defined as an acquired disorder with several characteristics.
- Symptoms develop following a documentable environmental exposure, insult, or illness.
- Symptoms involve more than one organ system.
- Symptoms recur and abate in response to predictable stimuli.
- Symptoms are elicited by exposure to chemicals of diverse structural classes and toxicologic modes of action.
- Symptoms are elicited by exposures that are at a very low level (below levels known to cause direct toxic effects).

PATHOPHYSIOLOGY

No traditionally recognized pathophysiologic mechanism has been shown to cause MCS. Immunologic, neurotoxic, and psychiatric etiologies have been proposed; the exact cause remains controversial. There are four major theories of etiology:

- MCS is a physical or psychophysiologic response to multiple environmental chemicals.

—The most widely proposed mechanism is interaction of the environmental agent with the victim's immune system.
—However, no widely accepted study has yet demonstrated a definable, measurable, or reproducible biochemical or immunologic pattern.
—Other attempts to apply a psychophysiologic mechanism to MCS have relied on using conditions such as agoraphobia as a model.

- MCS symptoms may be precipitated by low-level environmental chemical exposures, but the underlying increased sensitivity is initiated primarily by psychologic stress.
- MCS is a misdiagnosis, and chemical exposure is not the cause of the symptoms; they may be due to misdiagnosis of other physical or psychologic illness.
- MCS is simply a belief system instilled by certain practitioners, the media, or others in society; MCS is therefore a culturally shaped illness behavior.

EPIDEMIOLOGY

- The frequency and prevalence is unknown.
- Most studies find that women comprise the majority of patients (70%–88%).
- Toxic effects are typically mild.
- Death has not been reported with this syndrome.

CAUSES

Usually an accidental environmental or occupational exposure triggers this illness. Subsequent exposure to different chemical classes then trigger recurrence of symptoms.

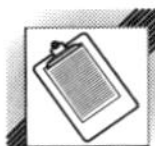

Diagnosis

DIFFERENTIAL DIAGNOSIS

- Further information on each poison is available in SECTION IV, CHEMICAL AND BIOLOGICAL AGENTS.
- Any infectious, allergic/immunologic, or rheumatologic process, or chemical or environmental pollutant, capable of causing a variety of nonspecific symptoms affecting multiple organ systems can cause symptoms similar to those of MCS.
- In some cases, an underlying disease is found: for example, multiple sclerosis, various types of malignancy, Alzheimer's or Parkinson's disease, thyroid disease, or systemic lupus erythematosus.
- A wide variety of potential toxicologic causes exist:

—The evaluation often involves heavy metals, formaldehyde, solvents, pesticides, insecticides, and irritant gases.
—In many cases, the suspected chemicals have either a distinct odor or are irritants.

SIGNS AND SYMPTOMS

Multiple nonspecific symptoms related to several organ systems are usually reported. Neurologic, immunologic, and respiratory symptoms predominate. Myriad physical findings have been reported, but no consistent abnormalities on examination have been identified; some of the more common ones follow.

- HEENT. Headache, visual disturbances, decreased visual acuity, decreased hearing, nasal congestion, noxious odors, aversion to perfume fragrances or auto or truck exhaust (particularly to odors present at the presumed initiating event), metallic taste, gum swelling, mouth ulcers, or difficulty in swallowing
- Dermatologic. Skin rashes, dermatitis, excessive dryness, or pruritus
- Cardiac. Palpitations or chest pain
- Pulmonary. Asthma, dyspnea, cough with or without sputum production, hemoptysis, or chest tightness
- Gastrointestinal. Weight loss, weight gain, increased or decreased appetite, bowel pattern changes, diarrhea with or without blood, colitis, gingivitis, stomatitis, dysphagia, hematemesis, nausea, vomiting, or abdominal pain
- Neurologic. Lack of concentration, poor attention span, fatigue, general malaise, irritability, memory loss (recent and past), confusion, depression, personality change, anxiety, emotional instability, insomnia, tremor, weakness, or paresthesia
- Genitourinary. Dysuria, menstrual irregularities, or changes in libido

PROCEDURES AND LABORATORY TESTS

Essential Tests

- A thorough physical examination is necessary to detect potential underlying diseases or effects of unrecognized toxic exposure.
- No specific laboratory tests may be needed for minimally symptomatic patients.

Recommended Tests

- Baseline complete blood count, serum electrolytes, BUN, glucose, creatinine, liver enzymes, urinalysis, thyroid profile, and rheumatologic screen are recommended.
- If a specific poison is in question (e.g., heavy metal or hydrocarbon solvent), laboratory studies are necessary to document exposure.
- Appropriate diagnostic tests should be performed to rule out medical problems such as collagen vascular disease or underlying inflammatory disease.
- Neuropsychiatric testing is often helpful, but is very operator dependent; if an experienced professional is available, the testing can isolate subtle neurologic deficits and assess the role of some other psychiatric conditions (e.g., depression).

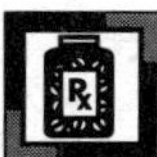

Treatment

- Focus therapy on symptomatic and supportive care.
- If an underlying medical illness is found, it should be treated.
- Dose and time of exposure should be determined for all substances that could be involved.
- Various treatment regimens have been proposed, including dietary changes, unorthodox desensitization techniques, strict avoidance of common low-level chemical exposures, psychological counseling, and biofeedback; there has been no objective evaluation of these interventions.

DIRECTING PATIENT COURSE

The health-care provider should call the poison control center when:

- assistance is desired in interpretation of patient's complaints.
- coingestant, drug interaction, or underlying disease presents unusual problems.

Admission Considerations

Unless a specific medical illness or psychiatric emergency is present, admission is usually not required.

DECONTAMINATION

Gastric decontamination is generally not necessary unless acute overdose could have occurred.

ANTIDOTES

There is no antidote for this illness.

ADJUNCTIVE TREATMENT

- No specific treatments have been consistently found to be useful for the treatment of this syndrome unless an underlying cause is found; specific treatment is then based on underlying cause (e.g., hyper- or hypothyroidism).
- Neuropsychiatric evaluation and therapy (e.g., desensitization to certain environmental stimuli) has been useful in selected cases.

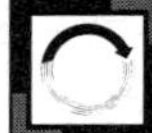

Follow-Up

EXPECTED COURSE AND PROGNOSIS

- Symptoms may be transient but are more likely to be relapsing or persistent.
- Commonly the patient notes worsening that is not reflected in the physical examination or laboratory testing.
- The overall system complaints, although nonspecific in nature, may become debilitating.

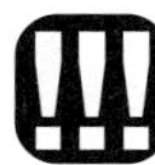

Pitfalls

DIAGNOSIS

Clinical symptoms should be correlated with history; it should not be assumed that the patient has been exposed to a chemical agent until history has been verified.

TREATMENT

- Patients typically visit multiple physicians; because of the physicians' inability to make a firm diagnosis, patients may be distrustful of their health-care providers.
- In many cases, because of lack of traditional or classical medical treatment modalities for this nonspecific symptom complex, patients become distrustful of the physician, thus decreasing the odds of successful therapeutic outcome; this scenario sometimes pushes the patient to alternative health-care providers.

ICD-9-CM 989

Toxic effect of other substances, chiefly nonmedicinal as to source.

See also: SECTION II, Gulf War Syndrome chapter.

RECOMMENDED READING

Bronstein AC. Multiple chemical sensitivities—new paradigm needed [Editorial]. Clin Toxicol 1995;33:92–93.

Cullen MR. The worker with multiple chemical sensitivities: an overview. In: Cullen MR, ed. Occupational medicine: state of the art reviews. Philadelphia: Hanley & Belfus, 1987:655–662.

Simon GE, Daniell W, Stockbridge H, et al. Immunologic, psychological, and neuropsychological factors in multiple chemical sensitivity. Ann Intern Med 1993;119:97–113.

Sparks J, Daniell W, Black DW, et al. Multiple chemical sensitivity syndrome: a clinical perspective. I. Case definition, theories of pathogenesis, and research needs. J Occup Med 1994;36:719–730.

Author: Alvin C. Bronstein

Reviewer: Katherine M. Hurlbut

Neuroleptic Malignant Syndrome and Serotonin Syndrome

Basics

DESCRIPTION

Neuroleptic malignant syndrome (NMS) and serotonin syndrome (SS) are similar syndromes that involve muscle rigidity, extrapyramidal signs, autonomic instability, and altered mental status. Several diagnostic strategies have been published. For NMS, four major criteria plus three minor criteria must be present for diagnosis.

Major Criteria for NMS

- Patient has recently used neuroleptic or other dopamine antagonist or discontinued use of a dopamine agonist (e.g., levodopa).
- Muscular rigidity.
- Hyperthermia above 38°C occurs without another cause.
- Altered mental status (e.g., confusion, delirium, mutism, stupor, coma).
- Creatine kinase is more than three times normal without other obvious causes.

Minor Criteria for NMS

- Other signs of extrapyramidal syndrome (tremor, cogwheeling, acute dystonic reaction, choreiform movement).
- Other signs of autonomic dysfunction exist (e.g., urinary incontinence, dysrhythmia, sweating, pulse above 100 beats/min, blood pressure higher than 150/100 mm Hg or lower than 90/60 mm Hg not counted above).
- Respiratory signs occur (e.g., tachypnea, severe dyspnea, hypoxemia, respiratory failure).
- Leukocytosis is greater than 12,000/mm^3.

SS Criteria

- SS has a presentation similar to that of NMS.
- Autonomic instability may include hyperthermia, hyper- or hypotension, salivation, or diarrhea.
- Muscular dysfunction includes shivering, myoclonus, tremor, or rigidity.
- Altered mental status may include confusion, agitation, seizures, or coma.
- SS has been reported after simultaneous use of monoamine oxidase (MAO) inhibitors and clomipramine, lithium, meperidine, tricyclic antidepressants, and selective serotonin reuptake inhibitors (SSRIs), as well as with the simultaneous use of SSRIs and tricyclic antidepressants, trazodone, or dextromethorphan.

PATHOPHYSIOLOGY

- NMS is believed to be related to CNS dopamine blockade.
- SS is believed to be caused by excessive stimulation of serotonin 1A and 2 receptors.

EPIDEMIOLOGY

- NMS and SS are uncommon.
- Toxic effects with SS are typically mild to moderate.
- Severity of NMS is variable, with death occurring in patients with delayed diagnosis or inadequate management of hyperthermia and rigidity.

Diagnosis

DIFFERENTIAL DIAGNOSIS

Further information on each poison is available in SECTION IV, CHEMICAL AND BIOLOGICAL AGENTS.
Initially, NMS and SS may be indistinguishable; diagnosis is based on the history and course of disease.

Toxicologic Causes of Symptoms Similar to NMS or SS

- Overdose with MAO inhibitors or drug and food interactions

—Agitation, tachycardia, and hyper- and hypotension may accompany MAO inhibitor overdose.
—Many drugs or foods interact with MAO inhibitors and produce a syndrome that involves autonomic dysfunction, altered mental status, and rigidity.

- Malignant hyperthermia is a rare inherited disorder typified by fever, autonomic dysfunction, and severe muscular rigidity that occurs in patients undergoing general anesthesia.
- Anticholinergics and antihistamines cause fever, agitated delirium, altered mental status, tachycardia, and hypertension.
- Sympathomimetics. Severe overdose may cause hyperthermia, tachycardia, and hypertension followed by hypotension, agitation, coma, seizures, and rhabdomyolysis.
- Hallucinogens (LSD, PCP, peyote) may cause agitation associated with hallucinations, hyperthermia, tachycardia, hypertension, and hypotension.
- Withdrawal from ethanol, benzodiazepines, or other sedative hypnotic drugs

—Withdrawal may cause delirium, diaphoresis, and agitation similar to sympathomimetic overdose.
—Seizures also may occur and contribute to hyperthermia.

Other Causes of NMS and SS Symptoms

- Heat stroke and heat exhaustion may present with dehydration, altered mental status, and organ failure.
- Meningitis or other infection causes fever, but is usually identifiable.
- Thyroid storm.
- Neoplasms, connective tissue disease, and granulomatous disease.

SIGNS AND SYMPTOMS

Delirium, agitation, coma, hypotension, multiorgan failure, and death may develop in severe cases.

Vital Signs

- Extreme hypertension, hypotension, and tachycardia may occur with NMS.
- Hypertension and tachycardia are common with SS.
- Hyperthermia may develop with either syndrome and become life threatening with NMS.

HEENT

Dysarthria and salivation may occur.

Dermatologic

Diaphoresis may occur.

Cardiovascular

- Tachycardia is common with NMS or SS.
- Hypertension or hypotension may occur with NMS or SS.

Pulmonary

Tachypnea and respiratory failure may develop with NMS.

Gastrointestinal

Diarrhea is common with SS.

Fluids and Electrolytes

Dehydration is common.

Musculoskeletal

- Rigidity ("lead pipe"), myoclonus, and tremors may occur with NMS or SS.
- Rigidity may affect lower extremities primarily in SS.
- Rhabdomyolysis may develop.

Neurologic

- Seizures may occur.
- Altered mental status occurs in nearly all cases.
- Muscle rigidity, tremor, and myoclonus may occur with either NMS or SS.
- Cogwheeling, dystonic reactions, and choreiform movements may occur with NMS.

PROCEDURES AND LABORATORY TESTS

Essential Tests

- Rectal temperature should be taken to confirm hyperthermia.
- Serum electrolytes, BUN, creatinine, and creatine kinase should be assayed to assess metabolic acidosis and rhabdomyolysis.
- Complete blood count often reveals increased white blood cell count.
- Arterial blood gases may show respiratory alkalosis, respiratory acidosis, or metabolic acidosis.
- Urinalysis may reveal blood and protein if rhabdomyolysis develops.
- Liver and pancreatic tests often reveal elevation of aspartate aminotransferase, alanine aminotransferase, and lactic dehydrogenase in a hepatocellular pattern.
- ECG may reveal various nonspecific findings.

Recommended Tests

- Serum lithium level should be checked to rule out lithium toxicity.
- Serum acetaminophen and aspirin levels should be checked in an overdose setting to detect occult overdose.
- Urine toxicology screen should be performed in patients with hyperthermia, altered mental status, or autonomic dysfunction of unknown cause.

• Other tests (blood cultures, lumbar puncture, head CT, thyroid functions) should be ordered as needed to evaluate other causes of fever and altered mental status.

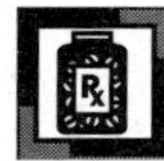

Treatment

• Focus therapy on airway management, aggressive cooling measures if temperature exceeds 40°C, and general supportive care.
• Dose and time of exposure should be determined for all substances involved.
• Specific treatment should be initiated while supportive care continues.

DIRECTING PATIENT COURSE

The health-care provider should call the poison control center when:

• the cause of hyperthermia syndrome is unclear.
• coingestant, drug interaction, or underlying disease presents unusual problems.

Admission Considerations

All patients with NMS or SS require admission to an intensive care setting.

DECONTAMINATION

• Gastric decontamination may not be necessary unless acute overdose could have occurred.
• Induction of emesis is not recommended.
• Gastric lavage should be performed in pediatric (tube size 24–32 French) or adult (tube size 36–42 French) patients for substantial ingestion presenting within 1 hour of ingestion or if serious effects are present.
• One dose of activated charcoal (1–2 g/kg) may be administered without a cathartic if a substantial ingestion has occurred within the previous few hours.

ANTIDOTES

There is no specific antidote for NMS or SS.

ADJUNCTIVE TREATMENT

• Initial therapy is expectant and supportive.
• Complications are common and repeated physical and laboratory examination of the patient are crucial.
• Early endotracheal intubation of the patient is strongly advised.

Control of Agitation

A benzodiazepine with which the provider has experience should be administered; the airway must be monitored closely.

• Diazepam. Adult, 5 to 10 mg intravenously; pediatric, 0.2 to 0.5 mg/kg intravenously; doses repeated at 5-minute intervals, titrated to effect
• Lorazepam. Adult, 1 to 2 mg intravenously; pediatric, 0.05 mg/kg intravenously; doses repeated at 5-minute intervals, titrated to effect

Muscle Rigidity and Body Temperature

• Patient's clothing should be removed and intravenous infusion of isotonic crystalloid begun.
• Fluid losses should be replenished, while fluid administration is monitored carefully to avoid fluid overload.
• Cooling fans and wet sheets are effective, especially in a dry climate.
• Cooling blankets or application of ice may be needed in severe cases.
• Sedation and neuromuscular paralysis/mechanical ventilation are important in severe cases and will also help control temperature; in cases of NMS, a nondepolarizing neuromuscular blocking agent should be used and succinylcholine avoided.
• Core temperature should be monitored frequently and cooling discontinued when body temperature decreases to 39°C.
• Agents used to antagonize CNS and musculoskeletal effects of NMS or SS

—Dantrolene
 —Dantrolene is used for NMS, but supporting evidence is anecdotal; aggressive supportive care may be equally effective.
 —Initial dose is 2 mg/kg intravenously, repeated as needed up to total dose of 10 mg/kg.
 —Maintenance dose is 2.5 mg/kg intravenously every 6 hours or 1 mg/kg orally every 12 hours, up to 50 mg/dose.
—Bromocriptine
 —Bromocriptine is used in NMS, but supporting evidence is anecdotal.
 —Initially the dose is 5 mg orally three times a day; if response is inadequate, the dose may be increased rapidly to a maximum of 20 mg orally four times a day.
 —If NMS remits, the medication should be continued for 10 days.
—Cyproheptadine
 —This medication has been used for treatment of SS.
 —The dose is 4 mg to 8 mg orally and is repeated up to a total dose of 32 mg if signs persist.
 —Pediatric dose is 0.25 mg/kg/day in four divided doses; maximum dosage is 12 mg/day.

Tachycardia

• Specific therapy is rarely required.
• Symptoms may improve with control of hyperthermia, agitation, and muscle rigidity.

Hypotension

• Patient should receive 10 to 20 ml/kg 0.9% NaCl and be placed in Trendelenburg position.
• If hypotension is unresponsive, a vasopressor such as dopamine can be administered at an initial rate of 2 to 5 μg/kg per minute, titrated to effect; rates above 20 μg/kg/min are unlikely to provide further benefit.
• High rate of infusion may cause tissue ischemia.

Hypertension

• This often improves with control of agitation.
• If persistent hypertension (higher than 130 mm Hg diastolic, not responsive to sedation) or end-organ injury develops (worsening altered mental status, congestive heart failure, myocardial ischemia, or aortic dissection), a short-acting titratable agent such as nitroprusside can be administered.

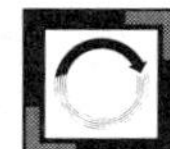

Follow-Up

PATIENT MONITORING

Respiratory, cardiac, temperature, and severity of muscle injury should be monitored continuously.

EXPECTED COURSE AND PROGNOSIS

• NMS typically begins gradually with rapid progression over the day or two before presentation.
• SS usually begins more abruptly but is less severe and resolves without sequelae with supportive care.
• Severe NMS may be fatal if not promptly diagnosed and treated; some patients sustain permanent neurologic injury.

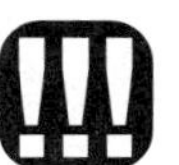

Pitfalls

TREATMENT

• Both NMS and SS are dynamic processes that will remit and worsen while gradually improving over several days.
• Dehydration may be severe; adequate rehydration is important.
• Large amounts of benzodiazepines may be needed.

ICD-9-CM

No code is available.

See also: SECTION II, Hypertension, Hyperthermia, Hypotension, and Tachydysrhythmia (Unexplained) chapters; SECTION III, Dantrolene and Nitroprusside chapters; and SECTION IV, chapters on specific agents.

RECOMMENDED READING

Martin T. Serotonin syndrome. Ann Emerg Med 1996;28:520–526.

Mills KC. Serotonin syndrome. Med Toxicol 1997;13:763–783.

Author: Katherine M. Hurlbut

Reviewer: Luke Yip

Odors

Basics

DESCRIPTION

The odor of certain compounds may be used to identify the poison.

PATHOPHYSIOLOGY

- Olfactory receptors are located in the superior nasal turbinates near the nasal septum; axons from these receptors cross the cribriform plate and join the olfactory bulb.
- The olfactory bulb is connected to the olfactory cortex and other sites within the CNS.
- Primary olfaction for most substances is via the olfactory nerve (cranial nerve I).
- Olfaction for ammonia and acetone is via the trigeminal nerve (cranial nerve V).
- Human olfaction usually cannot distinguish more than four substances simultaneously.
- Olfactory fatigue is a process by which an individual rapidly develops tolerance to an odor (e.g., hydrogen sulfide); within a few minutes, the person can no longer smell the compound, even though it is still present.

RISK FACTORS

Individuals who have impaired olfaction may not be able to identify odors associated with a particular poison; for example, only 55% to 60% of the population can smell cyanide.

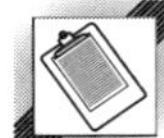

Diagnosis

DIFFERENTIAL DIAGNOSIS

Further information on each poison is available in SECTION IV. Characteristic odors and the toxicants associated with them are listed as follows:

- Ammonia. Ammonia or uremia
- Bananas. Amyl acetate
- Bitter almond. Cyanide
- Burning rope. Marijuana
- Cereal. Nystatin
- Charcoal/smoke. Cyanide or carbon monoxide (through smoke inhalation)
- Chlorine. Chlorine or other halogen such as bromine
- Decaying fish. Phosphine
- Fruity. Isopropyl alcohol, acetone, amyl nitrite, butyl nitrite, isobutyl nitrite, diabetic ketoacidosis, alcoholic ketoacidosis, or chloroform
- Garlic. Organophosphates, selenium, arsenic, thallium, tellurium, phosphorus, or phosphine
- Hay. Phosgene
- Mothballs. Naphthalene, paradichlorobenzene, or camphor
- Paint. Toluene
- Peanuts. Vacor
- Pear-like/acrid. Paraldehyde or chloral hydrate
- Peppermint. Methylsalicylate (oil of wintergreen)
- Raw fish/must. Zinc phosphide, aluminum phosphide, or calcium phosphide
- Rotten eggs. Hydrogen sulfide, disulfiram, succimer, carbon disulfide, dimethyl sulfoxide (DMSO), mercaptan or sulfur. Mercaptans are nontoxic agents with an easily detectable odor and are often added to toxic substances as a warning odor; the odor of natural gas is produced by mercaptans.
- Shoe polish. Nitrobenzene or aniline
- Tobacco. Nicotine
- Vinegar. Acetic acid
- Vinyl/"new car." Ethchlorvynol (Placidyl)
- Violets. Urine following turpentine ingestion

SIGNS AND SYMPTOMS

Physical signs may help reveal the poison involved when they occur in conjunction with an odor.

HEENT

- Miosis and garlic odor suggest organophosphate.
- Mucous membrane irritation and mothball odor suggest paradichlorobenzene.
- Mucous membrane irritation and coughing with vinegar odor suggests acetic acid; with acrid smell suggests ammonia; with bleach smell suggests chlorine or other halogen.
- Dermal and mucous membrane irritation, headache, CNS depression, and a banana odor suggest amyl acetate.

Dermatologic

- Skin flushing, headache, tachycardia, abdominal pain, vomiting, and anxiety following ethanol ingestion accompanied by a rotten egg odor suggest disulfiram.
- Rash, nausea, headache and a garlic-onion-oyster smell suggest DMSO.

Pulmonary

- Bronchorrhea, wheezing, progressive respiratory failure, and an odor of garlic or petroleum may indicate organophosphate.
- Dyspnea, cough, mucous membrane irritation, pleuritic chest pain, frothy sputum, pulmonary edema, and cyanosis with the odor of hay suggest phosgene.
- Cough, mucous membrane irritation, altered mental status, and delayed pulmonary edema with the musty odor of fish or raw liver suggest zinc, aluminum, or calcium phosphide (all liberate phosphine gas when exposed to water).

Gastrointestinal

- Hematemesis, abdominal pain, CNS depression, and a fruity acetone-like odor suggest isopropyl alcohol ingestion.
- Nausea, abdominal pain, gastrointestinal bleeding, and a garlic odor may indicate arsenic, thallium, or selenium.
- Luminescent or fluorescent smoking stools combined with hepatic and renal injury after ingestion of a substance with a garlic odor suggest phosphorus.

Hematologic

- Methemoglobinemia or hemolysis and the odor of mothballs suggest exposure to naphthalene.
- Hemolysis and the odor of garlic suggest arsine poisoning.

Fluids and Electrolytes

- An anion gap metabolic acidosis and a peppermint odor on the breath or of the gastric contents suggest oil of wintergreen (methyl salicylate).
- Proteinuria, hematuria, distal renal tubular acidosis, and odor of paint suggest toluene.

Neurologic

Altered mental status may involve the following relationships:

- Bitter almond odor and increased anion gap lactic acidosis suggest pure cyanide toxicity.
- The odor of smoke or burned flesh suggests cyanide or carbon monoxide toxicity.
- The odor of rotten eggs suggests hydrogen sulfide toxicity.
- Odor of paint with hypokalemia, abnormal urinalysis, and perhaps paint on face or hands indicates toluene abuse.
- The odor of burned leaves or rope with bloodshot eyes, somnolence, and mild euphoria suggests marijuana.
- A shoe polish odor associated with hypoventi-

lation, nausea, headache, and occasionally methemoglobinemia suggests nitrobenzene.
• A "new car" vinyl odor on the breath associated with hypoventilation, nystagmus, slurred speech, ataxia, and occasionally coma suggests ethchlorvynol (Placidyl).
• A pear-like odor on the breath associated with CNS depression, hypoventilation, and ventricular dysrhythmias suggests chloral hydrate.

Seizures

• The odor of moth balls associated with nausea, vomiting, and abdominal pain suggests camphor.
• A tobacco odor, salivation, nausea, vomiting, and abdominal pain suggest nicotine.

Peripheral Neuropathy

A chronic exposure to a substance with the odor of rotten eggs suggests carbon disulfide.

Other Neurologic Effects

Inhalation of a substance with a fruity odor associated with tachycardia, hypotension, mucous membrane irritation, nausea, lightheadedness, headache, and occasionally methemoglobinemia suggests amyl, butyl, or isobutyl nitrite.

Endocrine

Ingestion of a rodenticide with a peanut odor associated with new onset diabetes mellitus suggests vacor.

Procedures and Laboratory Tests

• Serum electrolytes, BUN, and creatinine
—An increased anion gap metabolic acidosis can be seen with exposure to methyl salicylate, paraldehyde, cyanide, carbon monoxide, or hydrogen sulfide; uremia; diabetic ketoacidosis; and seizures produced by water hemlock or other agents.
—Normal anion gap metabolic acidosis with hypokalemia and low serum bicarbonate may indicate toluene exposure.
—Hyperglycemia may be produced by PNU (Vacor) or diabetic ketoacidosis.
• Serum lactate. Increased serum lactate can develop with poisoning from cyanide, carbon monoxide, hydrogen sulfide, or seizures, hypotension, or hypoxia from any cause.
• Serum ketones are seen with acetone or isopropyl alcohol poisoning or diabetic ketoacidosis.
• Serum osmolality is increased with ethanol, acetone, isopropyl alcohol, and diabetic ketoacidosis until metabolism has occurred.
• Salicylate level is increased with methyl salicylate poisoning.
• Arterial blood gas analysis may be helpful in evaluating acid-base status and systemic oxygenation.
• Chest radiograph may demonstrate infiltrates and noncardiogenic pulmonary edema that may be delayed following severe exposures to ammonia, chlorine, phosphine, organophosphate, or phosgene.
• Abdominal radiograph. Paradichlorobenzene-containing mothballs are more densely radiopaque when compared with naphthalene-containing mothballs; chloral hydrate is radiopaque.

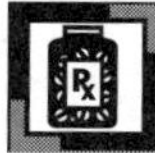

Treatment

• Management should be focused on removal of the patient from the source of the exposure, decontamination, and supportive care.
• Appropriate airway management is vital.
• Dose and time of exposure should be determined for all substances involved.

DIRECTING PATIENT COURSE

The health-care provider should call the poison control center when:

• assistance with odor identification is needed.
• coingestant, drug interaction, or underlying disease presents unusual problems.

DECONTAMINATION

• Inhalational Exposure. Patient should be removed from the source of the exposure; appropriate measures must be taken to protect both rescue personnel and health-care workers.
• Ingestion. The decision to perform gastrointestinal decontamination is based on the suspected toxicant, the time of ingestion, and the clinical status of the patient.
• Dermal Exposure. Exposed areas should be washed by copious irrigation with water; appropriate measures must be taken to protect both rescue personnel and health-care workers.

ANTIDOTES

Specific antidotes are not available for most poisons; thus, the decision to administer an antidote should be based on the suspected toxicant and the clinical status of the patient.

ADJUNCTIVE TREATMENT

• Specific treatment is based on the suspected toxicant.
• Dysrhythmias, blood pressure abnormalities, and electrolyte abnormalities should be corrected as clinically indicated.

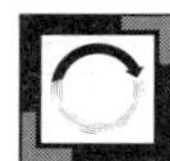

Follow-Up

PATIENT MONITORING

• Vital signs and cardiac rhythm should be monitored continuously.
• Appropriate airway management is vital; 100% oxygen should be administered.

EXPECTED COURSE AND PROGNOSIS

Complications should be anticipated based on the suspected toxicant and the clinical status of the patient.

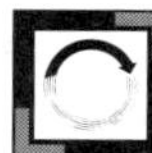

Follow-Up

EXPECTED COURSE AND PROGNOSIS

Delayed pulmonary edema is a complication of poorly water-soluble inhalants, such as phosgene and phosphine.

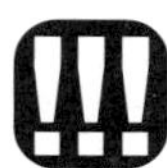

Pitfalls

DIAGNOSIS

• Lack of an odor does not rule out the presence of toxic substances; many toxic substances are odorless, and some individuals have anosmia for specific toxic substances.
• Odors of extremely toxic substances may be masked by odors of less toxic substances; human olfaction usually cannot detect more than four substances at any given time.
• The disappearance of an odor does not mean that the concentration is decreasing; olfactory fatigue may produce a false sense of security and leads to poisoning.
• Other life-threatening causes of an altered mental status should always be ruled out before attributing the effects to ethanol.

ICD-9-CM 987

Toxic effect of other gases, fumes, or vapors.

See also: SECTION II, Bradycardia, Hypertension, Hypotension, Tachycardia, and Ventricular Dysrhythmia chapters; and SECTION IV, chapters on individual agents.

RECOMMENDED READING

Chiang W. Otolaryngolic principles. In: Goldfrank LR, Flomenbaum NE, Lewin NA, et al., eds. Goldfrank's toxicologic emergencies, 6th ed. Norwalk, CT: Appleton & Lange, 1998.

Goldfrank LR, Weisman R, Flomenbaum N. Teaching the recognition of odors. Ann Emerg Med 1982;11:684–686.

Author: Edwin K. Kuffner

Reviewer: Katherine M. Hurlbut

One Pill Can Kill

Basics

DESCRIPTION

Certain chemicals and drugs can produce life-threatening toxicity in a 10-kg toddler following a small ingestion (one or a few pills or one to two gulps).

PATHOPHYSIOLOGY

Because so many compounds are labeled as toxic, it is difficult for parents or other caregivers to differentiate between compounds with minimal toxicity and those likely to cause major toxicity or death.

EPIDEMIOLOGY

- Ingestion of pills and foreign objects by toddlers is very common.
- Nearly all events produce minimal or no toxicity; however, at least 25 to 50 infant or toddler deaths occur each year in the United States.

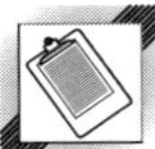

Diagnosis

DIFFERENTIAL DIAGNOSIS

- Further information on each poison is available in SECTION IV, CHEMICAL AND BIOLOGICAL AGENTS.
- For the purposes of this review, it is assumed that the victim has not yet experienced clinical effects; clinical effects should be treated as noted in the appropriate chapter for that manifestation (e.g., seizure).
- Based on ingestion by a 10-kg child, the following compounds may result in death of a toddler after ingestion of a few pills or one to two gulps.

Common Toxicologic Causes

- Antimalarial agents

—Chloroquine. One 500-mg tablet may cause death.
—Hydroxychloroquine. One 200-mg tablet is potentially lethal.
—Quinine. One or two 650-mg tablets are potentially lethal.

- Tricyclic antidepressants

—Imipramine. One tablet of 150 mg is potentially lethal.
—Desipramine. Two 75-mg tablets are potentially lethal.
—It is likely that other tricyclic antidepressants possess similar toxicity.

- Theophylline. One 500-mg tablet can be lethal.
- Phenothiazines

—Thioridazine. One 200-mg tablet is potentially lethal.
—Chlorpromazine. One 200-mg tablet is potentially lethal.
—It is likely that other phenothiazines possess similar toxicity.

- Sulfonylurea oral hypoglycemic agents. One tablet of a sulfonylurea oral hypoglycemic agent (acetohexamide, carbutamide, chlorpropamide, glibenclamide, glibornuride, gliclazide, glimepiride, glipizide, glyburide, glymidine, metahexamide, tolazamide, or tolbutamide) can cause severe hypoglycemia in a nondiabetic child.
- Toxic alcohols. A gulp or two of either ethylene glycol or methanol may produce severe manifestations.
- Narcotic medications

—Codeine. One 30-mg tablet can produce opioid toxicity.
—Methadone. One 10-mg tablet has been associated with death in a toddler.
—Hydrocodone. Less than 5 ml of elixir has been associated with death in an infant.

- Calcium channel blockers

—Verapamil. Four 240-mg sustained-release tablets may produce severe toxicity.
—Nifedipine. A single tablet has been reported to be fatal in a 14-month-old child.

- Cocaine and amphetamines. Depending on purity, one handful, "a rock," or a few pills can cause seizures and other severe effects.

Uncommon Toxicologic Causes

- Camphor. Potentially lethal amount is 5 ml (1 teaspoon).
- Methyl salicylate. Less than 5 ml (1 teaspoon) can be fatal.
- Clonidine. One 0.1-mg tablet can produce respiratory depression in a toddler.
- Lomotil (diphenoxylate). A few tablets may cause respiratory depression in a toddler.
- Organophosphate insecticides. A single sip of a commercial agricultural product can produce severe effects; household products are less toxic, but may still produce toxicity with a few swallows.
- Hydrogen peroxide 30% ("food grade"). Death has resulted from an ingestion of 4 to 6 oz through widespread oxygen embolization.
- Coral snake, rattlesnake bite, or bite from one of numerous venomous snakes available around the world can cause death.
- Lindane, 1% solution or pellets. Ingestion of more than 5 ml may produce toxicity.
- Corrosives. A single sip of an acid or alkaline corrosive can produce serious esophageal injury; poison center consultation to identify product components is recommended.
- Hydrofluoric acid or ammonium bifluoride. A single sip of commercial product may produce life-threatening hypocalcemia.
- Lead foreign bodies (e.g., one curtain weight, fishing weight) may cause lethal lead poisoning.
- Paraquat. Death can result from ingestion of 5 to 10 ml.
- Amanita phalloides mushroom. A single mushroom can cause death.
- Eucalyptus oil. Severe effects may result from 10 to 15 ml.
- Encainide. Ventricular dysrhythmias occurred in a 6-month-old after ingesting one 25-mg pill.
- Quinidine. Five grams caused death in a toddler.
- Copper sulfate. One swallow produces severe gastrointestinal effects and potentially death.

PROCEDURES AND LABORATORY TESTS

These should be ordered as clinically indicated by the product ingested.

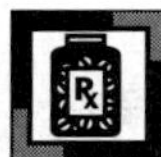

Treatment

- Supportive care with oxygen administration and appropriate airway management is vital.
- Dose and time of exposure should be determined for all substances involved.
- Many of these compounds lead to abrupt clinical deterioration.

DIRECTING PATIENT COURSE

The health-care provider should call the poison control center when:

- there has been ingestion of any of these compounds.
- coingestant, drug interaction, or underlying disease present unusual problems.

Admission Considerations

Prolonged observation or admission will usually be needed for all of these agents.

DECONTAMINATION

- Ipecac-induced emesis is generally not recommended in the management of ingestion of these medications as abrupt clinical deterioration may develop rapidly.
- Gastric lavage should be performed in pediatric (tube size 24–32 French) or adult (tube size 36–42 French) patients for substantial ingestion if repeated vomiting has not already developed.
- One dose of activated charcoal (1–2 g/kg) should be administered without a cathartic if a substantial ingestion has occurred within the previous few hours.

ANTIDOTES

Naloxone

- Indications. Altered mental status of undetermined etiology.
- Contraindications. None.
- Method of administration

—Adult or pediatric dose is 2 to 10 mg administered in 2-mg increments.
—Cumulative dose of 10 to 20 mg may be needed for treatment of poisoning from propoxyphene, nalbuphine, and butorphanol.
—If more than 2 mg is needed or produces only partial response, the influence of another toxicant is possible.

- Potential adverse effects

—Naloxone may induce withdrawal syndrome.
—Reversal of opioid effects may unmask another coexistent toxicity such as cocaine.

Dextrose

- Indications. Treatment of altered mental status.
- Contraindications. None.
- Method of administration

—Adult. D_{50}, 50 to 100 ml (25–50 g) intravenous push
—Pediatric. D_{25} 2 to 4 ml/kg (0.5–1.0 g/kg) intravenous push

ADJUNCTIVE TREATMENT

In many cases it is prudent to insert an intravenous line and prepare for endotracheal intubation if mental status alteration, respiratory depression, or difficulty in protecting airway develops.

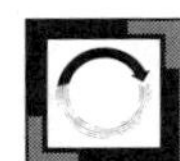

Follow-Up

PATIENT MONITORING

Respiratory and cardiovascular function should be monitored continuously.

DISCHARGE CRITERIA/INSTRUCTIONS

Discharge asymptomatic patients after 6-hour observation period and following decontamination.

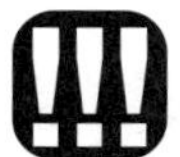

Pitfalls

DIAGNOSIS

- A careful history of ingestion is critical; often it is discovered that more than one pill or type of medication was available.
- It is often useful to insist on the caregiver returning to the home to retrieve a pill bottle to determine other agents that could be involved.

TREATMENT

Airway should be managed aggressively; many toxicologic deaths occur simply because endotracheal intubation was not performed early.

ICD-9-CM 989

Toxic effect of other substances, chiefly nonmedicinal as to source. See also codes in SECTION IV, chapters on individual agents.

See also: SECTION III, Dextrose and Naloxone chapters; and SECTION IV chapters on individual agents.

RECOMMENDED READING

Koren G. Medications which can kill a toddler with one tablet or teaspoonful. J Toxicol Clin Toxicol 1993;31:407–413.

Author: Richard C. Dart

Reviewer: Katherine M. Hurlbut

Osmolar Gap

Basics

DESCRIPTION

• The osmolar gap is the difference in the measured and calculated serum osmolarity (measured osmolarity minus calculated osmolarity).

—The measured osmolarity is measured by the clinical laboratory.
—The calculated osmolarity is determined as follows: 2 × [Na (mEq/L)] + [BUN (mg/dl)/2.8] + [glucose (mg/dl)/18].
—The normal osmolar gap is less than 10 mEq/L.

• An elevated osmolar gap suggests the presence of an unmeasured solute; the primary toxic compounds of medical interest are ethylene glycol, methanol, and isopropyl alcohol (isopropanol).
• For clinical purposes, the terms osmolal gap, osmolar gap, and osmol gap are equivalent.

PATHOPHYSIOLOGY

• The main osmotically active compounds normally found in the body are sodium, glucose, bicarbonate, urea, chloride, and potassium; these are measurable and are accounted for in the calculation of serum osmolarity.
• The cause of the normal gap is serum proteins and lipids that contribute slightly to serum osmolarity, but they are typically not measured by clinical laboratories.
• Other compounds that are not usually measured include mannitol, ethanol, isopropyl alcohol, methanol, ethylene glycol, propylene glycol, and acetone.
• The osmolarity of serum should be measured by freezing point depression (vapor pressure methods [i.e., boiling point evaluation] do not accurately detect volatile compounds such as the alcohols and thus should not be used).

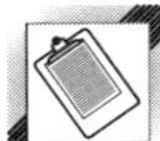

Diagnosis

DIFFERENTIAL DIAGNOSIS

Further information on each poison is available in SECTION IV, CHEMICAL AND BIOLOGICAL AGENTS.

• Common toxicologic causes of an elevated osmolar gap include ethanol, methanol, isopropyl alcohol, and ethylene glycol.
• Uncommon toxicologic causes include acetone and propylene glycol (usually detected after administration of a medication that uses this agent as a diluent).
• Nontoxicologic causes of increased osmolar gap include renal failure, hyperlipidemia, hyperparaproteinemia, and the therapeutic administration of mannitol or glycerol.

SIGNS AND SYMPTOMS

Associated physical signs may help reveal the poison involved when they occur in the setting of increased osmolar gap. The presence of an osmolar gap produces no symptoms itself, but specific agents that cause an osmolar gap may result in symptoms.

Vital Signs

• Tachypnea suggests a metabolic acidosis as seen with ethylene glycol or methanol.
• Hypotension may occur with very large methanol, ethanol, ethylene glycol, or isopropyl alcohol toxicity.

HEENT

• Blurred vision, perception of peering through a "snowstorm," and other visual complaints, including blindness and optic disk pallor, can occur with methanol ingestion.
• Sweet odor of the patient's breath suggests acetone, ethanol, or isopropyl alcohol ingestion.

Cardiovascular

Hypotension may occur with very large methanol, ethanol, ethylene glycol, or isopropyl alcohol ingestion.

Pulmonary

Tachypnea suggests a metabolic acidosis as seen with ethylene glycol or methanol.

Gastrointestinal

• Abdominal pain, nausea, and vomiting may occur with methanol, ethanol, ethylene glycol, or isopropyl alcohol ingestion.
• Hemorrhagic gastritis is common with isopropyl alcohol ingestion.

Hepatic

Chronic ethanol ingestion can cause hepatitis and cirrhosis.

Renal

Hematuria, proteinuria, and renal insufficiency are associated with ethylene glycol.

Fluids and Electrolytes

Profound increased anion gap metabolic acidosis can result from methanol or ethylene glycol poisoning.

Musculoskeletal

Rhabdomyolysis can occur with ethylene glycol ingestion or prolonged coma.

Neurologic

Initial intoxication followed by CNS depression and coma is associated with ethanol, methanol, isopropyl alcohol, or ethylene glycol intoxication.

PROCEDURES AND LABORATORY TESTS

• The presence of an osmolar gap produces no symptoms; precise identification of the cause requires specific laboratory testing.
• Serum osmolarity should be measured using the freezing point depression method.
• Serum electrolytes, BUN, and glucose should be measured to allow determination of the calculated serum osmolarity.
• If osmolar gap is elevated, serum ethanol, methanol, ethylene glycol, and isopropyl alcohol should be determined on the same blood sample; it is possible to estimate the contribution of each compound to the osmolar gap.

—Ethanol contribution = serum ethanol concentration (mg/dl) ÷ 4.6.
—Methanol contribution = serum methanol concentration (mg/dl) ÷ 3.2.
—Ethylene glycol contribution = serum ethylene glycol (mg/dl) ÷ 6.2.
—Acetone contribution = serum acetone concentration (mg/dl) ÷ 5.8.
—Isopropyl alcohol contribution = isopropyl alcohol concentration ÷ 6.

• Anion gap calculation should also be performed

—[Serum sodium] − [serum chloride + serum bicarbonate]. Normal is less than 16 mEq/L.
—If elevated, it is likely that significant metabolism of ethylene glycol or methanol has occurred.
—If not elevated, these toxic alcohols cannot be excluded because they may not yet have been metabolized.

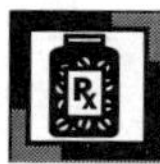

Treatment

- Supportive care with appropriate airway management is vital.
- Dose and time of exposure should be determined for all substances involved.
- Treatment with fomepizole should be considered while supportive care continues.

DECONTAMINATION

- Causes of an increased osmol gap involve liquids composed of small-molecular-weight molecules; thus, decontamination is rarely an option.
- Nasogastric aspiration using a nasogastric tube within the first 30 to 60 minutes following a large ingestion may be beneficial.
- If there is concern for a coingestant, gastric lavage with a large-bore orogastric tube may be indicated.
- If there is concern for a coingestant, one dose of activated charcoal (1–2 g/kg) can be administered.

ANTIDOTES

- 4-methylpyrazole (fomepizole) is the preferred antidote for methanol and ethylene glycol poisoning, the most dangerous causes of an increased osmolar gap.
- Ethanol is much more difficult and dangerous to use and should only be used if fomepizole is unavailable.

Fomepizole

- Indications: Ethylene glycol or methanol level greater than 20 mg/dl, reliable history of significant ingestion, unexplained anion gap metabolic acidosis, or unexplained osmol gap.
- Dose: 15 mg/kg loading dose followed by 10 mg/kg every 12 hours as a maintenance dose until ethylene glycol or methanol level is less than 20 mg/dl.

Ethanol 10%

- Indications: Ethylene glycol or methanol level above 20 mg/dl (if levels are not immediately available, therapy should be instituted for a reliable history of significant ingestion, unexplained anion gap acidosis, or unexplained osmolar gap).
- Contraindications: Preexisting ethanol level greater than 100 mg/dl obviates need for the ethanol loading dose.
- Administration: loading dose

—10 ml/kg of a 10% ethanol solution infused intravenously over 1 hour; if intravenous route is not possible, four 1-oz "shots" of a 40% (80 proof) ethanol beverage should be administered. This dose is based on a 70-kg adult. Dosing should be adjusted for patient's weight.
—Determine ethanol level upon completion of loading dose; target serum ethanol level is 100 to 150 mg/dl.

- Maintenance dose

—1 to 2 ml/kg/h of a 10% ethanol solution should be administered intravenously; use 2.0 ml/kg/h for alcoholic patients.
—Rate should be adjusted to maintain an ethanol level above 100 mg/dl; if an intravenous route is not possible, one 1-oz "shot" of a 40% (80 proof) ethanol should be given orally every hour. This dose is based on a 70-kg patient and should be adjusted accordingly.
—Ethanol level should be checked each hour initially, decreasing the frequency as the ethanol level stabilizes between 100 and 150 mg/dl.
—During hemodialysis, the maintenance 10% ethanol infusion should be increased to 3.0 ml/kg/h.

- Potential adverse effects. Hypotension or hypoglycemia may develop, especially in children.

ADJUNCTIVE TREATMENT

Hemodialysis is used to treat methanol poisoning, ethylene glycol poisoning, or very severe isopropyl alcohol poisoning.

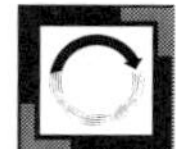

Follow-Up

EXPECTED COURSE AND PROGNOSIS

- Intoxication develops soon after ingestion; however, toxic effects are delayed until metabolism of the toxic alcohol occurs, which usually requires several hours.
- Patients with ethanol, isopropyl alcohol, and acetone ingestion do well with supportive care. Patients with isopropyl ingestion may develop hemorrhagic gastritis.
- Patients with methanol or ethylene glycol poisoning may have significant effects if untreated, but do well if the ingestion is detected early and proper treatment is instituted.

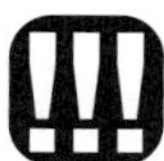

Pitfalls

DIAGNOSIS

- Due to inherent inaccuracies in its measurement, the absence of an osmolar gap does not exclude a significant ethylene glycol or methanol ingestion.
- Osmometers that measure vapor pressure (i.e., boiling point elevation) commonly underestimate the osmotic contribution of methanol and sometimes ethylene glycol.

TREATMENT

The osmolar gap will decrease as the ingested product is metabolized; however, toxic metabolites may still be present even though the osmolar gap has resolved.

ICD-9-CM 980

Toxic effect of alcohol.

See also: SECTION III, Ethanol and Fomepizole chapters, and SECTION IV, Ethylene Glycol, Isopropyl Alcohol, and Methanol chapters.

RECOMMENDED READING

Hoffman RS, Smilkstein MJ, Howland MA, et al. Osmol gaps revisited: normal values and limitations. J Toxicol Clin Toxicol 1993;31:81–93.

Glaser DS. Utility of the serum osmol gap in the diagnosis of methanol or ethylene glycol ingestion. Ann Emerg Med 1996;27:343–346.

Author: Kennon Heard

Reviewer: Katherine M. Hurlbut

Peripheral Neuropathy

Basics

DESCRIPTION

Peripheral neuropathy is a disorder of a peripheral nerve that causes abnormal sensory, motor, or autonomic function.

Sensory Complaints

- Paresthesia (tingling, prickling, burning, or stinging) often starts in the fingers and toes and progresses proximally in a symmetrical fashion.
- Symptoms may start unilaterally but eventually become symmetrical in a "stocking-glove" distribution.
- Lower extremity involvement usually precedes involvement of the upper extremities.

Motor Complaints

- Weakness often progresses from distal to proximal in a symmetrical fashion.
- Lower extremities are often affected more than the upper extremities.
- Decreased deep tendon reflexes occasionally progress to diffuse areflexia.

PATHOPHYSIOLOGY

- Peripheral neuropathy can be divided into three general categories based on the part of the nerve affected:

—Neuronopathy occurs when the cell body of the anterior horn (motor), dorsal root ganglion (sensory), or autonomic nervous system is affected.
—Axonopathy, the most common form of drug-induced peripheral neuropathy, occurs when the axon is affected.
—Myelinopathy is demyelination that involves large-diameter axons more than small axons; proprioception, vibration, and light touch are involved to a greater extent than smaller fibers that mediate pain and temperature.

- Mononeuropathy occurs when there is involvement of just one isolated peripheral nerve.
- Polyneuropathy

—Polyneuropathy is the involvement of multiple areas of the peripheral nervous system.
—Most toxic peripheral neuropathies are diffuse, symmetric, and involve many different nerves and nerve roots.

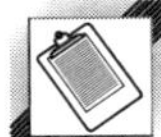

Diagnosis

DIFFERENTIAL DIAGNOSIS

Further information on each poison is available in SECTION IV, CHEMICAL AND BIOLOGICAL AGENTS.

Toxicologic Causes of Predominantly Sensory Neuropathy

- Axonopathy. Colchicine, ethambutol, ethionamide, glutethimide, nitrous oxide, nucleosides (dideoxyinosine), cisplatin, and taxol
- Neuronopathy. Pyridoxine
- Unknown Lesion Location. Dimethylamino propionitrile, thalidomide, nalidixic acid, colistin, thiamphenicol, chloramphenicol, sulthiame, phenelzine, ergotamine, and methysergide

Toxicologic Causes of Combined Sensory and Motor Neuropathy

- Axonopathy. Acrylamide, ethanol, allyl chloride, arsenic, disulfiram, carbon disulfide, gold, ethylene oxide, hydralazine, isoniazid, methylbromide, metronidazole, misonidazole, nitrofurantoin, organophosphates, polychlorinated biphenyls, phenytoin, podophyllin, thallium, vincristine, hexacarbons (n-hexane and methyl n-butyl ketone are both metabolized to 2,5-hexanedione), and triorthocresyl phosphate
- Myelinopathy. Ethanol, amiodarone, diphtheria, gold, lead, trichloroethylene, and arsenic
- Unknown Lesion Location. Aurothioglucose, perhexilene, allopurinol, streptomycin, amitriptyline, penicillamine, indomethacin, phenylbutazone, clofibrate, disopyramide, chlorambucil, chlorpropamide, and tolbutamide

Toxicologic Causes of Predominantly Motor Neuropathy

- Axonopathy. Dapsone, mercury, and vacor
- Neuronopathy. Doxorubicin
- Myelinopathy. Buckthorn and lead
- Unknown Lesion Location. Benzene, bismuth, chloramphenicol, chlorphenoxy herbicides, chloroquine, organochlorines, dinitrophenols, emetine, paralytic shellfish poisoning, styrene, amphotericin B, sulfonamide, and cimetidine

Nontoxicologic Causes of Peripheral Neuropathy

- Common Causes. Diabetes mellitus, direct nerve trauma, compression or entrapment, Guillain-Barré syndrome, uremia, vitamin B_{12} deficiency, thiamine deficiency, carcinoma, carpal tunnel syndrome, mononeuropathy multiplex, small vessel disease vasculitis, rheumatoid arthritis, systemic lupus erythematosus, sarcoidosis, multiple sclerosis, frostbite, herpes zoster neuritis, leprous neuritis, and Bell's palsy
- Uncommon Causes. Porphyria, primary biliary cirrhosis, amyloidosis, hypothyroidism, acromegaly, polycythemia vera, lymphoma, multiple myeloma, celiac disease, mononucleosis, macroglobulinemia, diphtheria, Friedreich's ataxia, neurofibroma, leprosy, immune-mediated acquired demyelinating neuropathy (acute hemorrhagic leukoencephalitis and smallpox or measles infection), genetically determined demyelinating neuropathy, progressive multifocal leukoencephalopathy, peripheral nerve tumors (usually either schwannoma or neurofibroma), collagen vascular disease, hysteria, malingering, and psychogenic numbness

Neuromuscular Problems Misdiagnosed as Peripheral Neuropathy

Botulism, myasthenia gravis, drug-induced muscular weakness (polymyxin, propranolol, procainamide, phenytoin, chlorpromazine, aminoglycosides, d-penicillamine), Eaton-Lambert syndrome, tick paralysis, Lyme disease, hypokalemia, strychnine, tetanus, and coral snake envenomation

SIGNS AND SYMPTOMS

Associated physical signs may help reveal the poison involved when they occur in a patient with peripheral neuropathy.

Vital Signs

Orthostatic hypotension is common in autonomic neuropathy.

HEENT

- Cranial nerve palsies following a sore throat suggest diphtheria, but this is unlikely if immunization status is up to date.
- Optic neuropathy during tuberculosis (TB) treatment suggests ethambutol poisoning.
- Stomatitis and gingivitis suggest elemental mercury vapor poisoning.

Dermatologic

- Alopecia suggests arsenic or thallium poisoning.
- Hyperhidrosis and cool cyanotic limbs suggest acrylamide toxicity.
- Allergic dermatitis, stomatitis, alopecia, and hypersensitivity pneumonitis suggest exposure to gold salts or gold drugs.

Pulmonary

Pulmonary fibrosis suggests amiodarone poisoning.

Hepatic

- Elevated hepatic transaminase during TB treatment suggests isoniazid poisoning.
- Increased liver function tests and glomerulonephritis suggest exposure to allyl chloride.

Renal

Renal insufficiency with predominant loss of vibration and proprioception suggests cisplatin toxicity.

Hematologic

• Hypochromic microcytic anemia suggests chronic lead toxicity.
• Aplastic anemia developing during chelation therapy suggests penicillamine or arsenic poisoning.

Musculoskeletal

• Bilateral foot and wrist drop suggests exposure to lead.
• Muscle weakness during treatment of gout suggests colchicine poisoning.
• Muscle atrophy suggests that neuropathy is chronic.

Neurologic

• Recurrent exacerbations of focal or multifocal neurologic dysfunction suggest multiple sclerosis.
• Onset of neuropathy one to several days following exposure suggests acrylamide poisoning.
• Paresthesia in hands preceding that in feet suggests vincristine poisoning.
• Predominantly vision and hearing deficits suggest trichlorethylene exposure.

PROCEDURES AND LABORATORY TESTS

Essential Tests

Complete neurologic examination includes mental status; cranial nerves; sensory including pain, temperature, light touch, vibration, and position sense; muscle strength; cerebellar function; and deep tendon reflexes.

Recommended Tests

• Complete blood count is used to check for hypochromic microcytic anemia and basophilic stippling (lead), or pancytopenia (arsenic, thallium, or colchicine).
• Serum electrolytes, BUN, and creatinine are measured to check for hypokalemia, a common cause of muscle weakness.
• Urinalysis is used to detect concurrent renal injury.
• Lumbar puncture

—Elevated protein without an increased number of cells suggests Guillain-Barré syndrome.
—Increased immunoglobin gamma G with relatively normal protein and oligoclonal bands on protein electrophoresis suggest multiple sclerosis.

• Blood lead level is usually elevated in lead neuropathy.
• 24-hour urine collection for mercury, arsenic, or thallium should be ordered as indicated by history of exposure.
• Electrodiagnostic studies are used to differentiate demyelinating disorders from axonal disorders.
• Spirometry, which checks for decreases in negative inspiratory flow, may be the earliest finding of respiratory muscle weakness and should be used on patients with muscle weakness.
• Chest radiograph detects amiodarone-induced pulmonary fibrosis.
• Magnetic resonance imaging is used for screening the brain and spinal cord for metastatic disease and detecting multiple sclerosis.

Not Recommended Tests

Nerve biopsy is usually of limited value in confirming a toxic neuropathy.

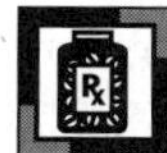

Treatment

• Dose and time of exposure should be determined for all substances involved.

DIRECTING PATIENT COURSE

The health-care provider should call the poison control center when:

• peripheral neuropathy may have potential toxic cause.
• coingestant, drug interaction, or underlying disease present unusual problems.

DECONTAMINATION

Owing to the time required for a neuropathy to develop, decontamination is not usually helpful.

ANTIDOTES

There are no specific antidotes for peripheral neuropathy.

ADJUNCTIVE TREATMENT

Symptomatic therapy should be provided to treat pain.

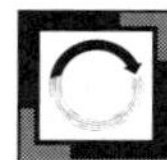

Follow-Up

EXPECTED COURSE AND PROGNOSIS

• Neurologic deficits may continue to worsen for days to weeks after therapy is initiated before either stabilizing or improving.
• Although motor or sensory function may not return to baseline, the peripheral neuropathy will usually improve.
• It is difficult to predict which patients will have full recovery.

DISCHARGE CRITERIA/INSTRUCTIONS

Most patients can be discharged following evaluation and if concurrent toxic effects of poison are not present.

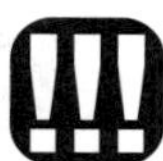

Pitfalls

• Failure to remove a patient from potential sources of exposure may lead to irreversible neurologic dysfunction.
• Following removal from a source of exposure, the neurologic deficits may continue to worsen for days to a few weeks before either stabilizing or improving.

ICD-9-CM 971

Poisoning by drugs primarily affecting the autonomic nervous system.

RECOMMENDED READING

POISINDEX Editorial Staff. Peripheral neuropathy. In: Rumack BH, Sayre NK, Gelman CR, eds. POISINDEX System. Englewood, CO: MICROMEDEX, Inc.

Author: Edwin K. Kuffner

Reviewer: Richard C. Dart

Pulmonary Edema

Basics

DESCRIPTION

Pulmonary edema is the accumulation of fluid within the interstitial spaces and alveoli of the lung.

PATHOPHYSIOLOGY

- As fluid for pulmonary edema accumulates in the lung, the exchange of gas within the lung is impaired, resulting in hypoxia.
- The accumulation of fluid within the lung tissue also decreases lung elasticity and further impairs ventilatory function and gas exchange.

Pulmonary edema is classified as cardiogenic and noncardiogenic:

- Cardiogenic pulmonary edema results from left ventricular failure.

—The fluid "backs up" into the pulmonary vasculature, resulting in increased pulmonary capillary pressure and transudation of fluid into the alveoli.
—The increase in left atrial pressure is most commonly caused by poor systolic function of the left ventricle but also may result from valvular dysfunction, impaired relaxation of the left ventricle, or increased systemic resistance.

- Noncardiogenic pulmonary edema (adult respiratory distress syndrome) results from increased permeability of the capillaries within the pulmonary vasculature and can result from a direct toxic insult to the lungs (e.g., phosgene inhalation), from systemic drug toxicity (e.g., heroin), or from a systemic inflammatory response (e.g., sepsis).

EPIDEMIOLOGY

Elderly patients are more likely to have cardiac disease, which may increase their susceptibility to cardiogenic edema.

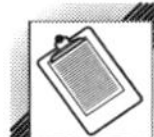

Diagnosis

Diagnosis is based on symptoms of shortness of breath and clinical findings of rales, or wheezing, and tachypnea.

- Major symptoms include shortness of breath, chest pain, cough, dyspnea on exertion, production of frothy pink sputum, and air hunger.
- Other symptoms may be related to underlying causes (e.g., lethargy from narcotic overdose), and associated physical signs may help identify the poison involved.

DIFFERENTIAL DIAGNOSIS

Nearly all toxicologic etiologies produce noncardiogenic pulmonary edema. Further information on each poison is available in SECTION IV, CHEMICAL AND BIOLOGICAL AGENTS.

Common Toxicologic Causes

- Opioids are associated with pinpoint pupils and CNS and respiratory depression. Opioid-induced pulmonary edema responds to naloxone, although pulmonary edema also has occurred after naloxone treatment.
- Salicylate is associated with tachypnea, tinnitus, increased anion gap metabolic acidosis, and altered mental status.
- Cocaine or amphetamine use (both intravenous and inhalational) is associated commonly with tachycardia, agitation, and the possible development of hyperthermia, seizures, and dysrhythmia.
- Hydrocarbon aspiration is more common with low-viscosity agents. It is associated with initial persistent cough followed by fever and worsening pulmonary function over several hours.
- Inhalation injury from smoke, acrolein, ammonia, chlorine, chloramine, hydrochloric acid, isocyanates, nitrogen dioxide, ozone, or phosgene usually presents with symptoms of upper airway irritation; symptoms may be delayed with agents that have low water solubility.
- Metal fume or polymer fume fever is associated with fever, myalgia, malaise, and headache following inhalation exposure.
- Tricyclic antidepressants. Pulmonary edema may occur in up to 15% of admitted cases; tricyclic antidepressant toxicity is associated with altered mental status, seizures, widening of the QRS complex, dysrhythmia, and hypotension.
- Organophosphate or carbamate insecticides are associated with lacrimation, bradycardia, vomiting, and diarrhea.

Uncommon Toxicologic Causes

- Hydrochlorothiazide diuretic. Idiosyncratic cases of noncardiogenic pulmonary edema may occur after suicidal ingestion.
- β-blockers or calcium channel blockers. Cardiac depression can result in cardiogenic pulmonary edema; bradycardia and widened QRS should be evident.
- Colchicine poisoning can result in myocardial depression, which can cause cardiogenic pulmonary edema, and is associated with nausea, vomiting, abdominal pain, and diarrhea.
- Nickel carbonyl, ethchlorvynol, or nitrogen dioxide and cadmium fume poisoning also can result in pulmonary edema.

Other Causes

- Cardiac disease. Myocardial depression from ischemic heart disease, cardiomyopathy, or myocarditis, among other diseases, may result in pulmonary edema.
- Systemic inflammatory syndromes are associated with sepsis, burns, or multisystem trauma, among other conditions.
- Aspiration of gastric contents may result in pulmonary edema.

SIGNS AND SYMPTOMS

- Pulmonary edema results in hypoxia, which is the main cause of signs and symptoms.
- Patients with cardiogenic edema may have findings of congestive heart failure such as a third heart sound, peripheral edema, jugular venous distention, or pulsus alternans.
- Patients with noncardiogenic pulmonary edema should have no evidence of cardiac dysfunction but may have signs caused by the precipitating poison.

Vital Signs

Tachycardia, tachypnea, and hypertension develop initially, followed by bradycardia and hypotension as hypoxia progresses.

HEENT

- Nasal flaring may occur.
- Jugular venous distention may develop in cardiogenic heart failure.

Dermatologic

- Diaphoresis is common.
- Cyanosis may occur as hypoxia worsens.
- Peripheral edema may develop with cardiogenic failure.

Cardiovascular

- Cardiogenic pulmonary edema

—Patient may have signs of underlying heart disease: S3 and S4 signs of ventricular hypertrophy, pulsus alternans, ventricular lifts, or heart murmurs.
—Pulmonary artery pressure will be elevated.

- Noncardiogenic pulmonary edema

—Cardiac function and pulmonary artery pressure are generally normal.

Pulmonary

• Isolated tachypnea may be the first sign of pulmonary edema.

—As fluid accumulates, rales and wheezing may develop.
—Further accumulation may produce signs of consolidation such as bronchial breath sounds and egophony.

• Pleural effusions may develop, causing decreased breath sounds and dullness to percussion.
• Hypoxia and hypercarbia may develop as respiratory failure worsens.

Neurologic

Patients will initially be restless and agitated, with progression to CNS depression as hypoxia progresses.

PROCEDURES AND LABORATORY TESTS

Essential Tests

• Arterial blood gases or pulse oximetry are used to assess oxygenation.
• Cardiac enzyme levels are used to assess contribution of myocardial ischemia, as is ECG, which may show evidence of acute or old myocardial infarction, nonspecific changes of myocarditis, or changes consistent with ventricular hypertrophy.
• Serum electrolytes, BUN, creatinine, and glucose detect presence of acidosis and other toxic effects.
• Chest radiographs

—Cardiogenic edema. Radiographs classically show a butterfly distribution around the hilum, which is associated with Kerley B lines, increased heart size, and cephalization of pulmonary vessels.
—Noncardiogenic edema. Radiograph may be normal initially, but as the toxicity progresses, septal lines develop, consolidation may occur, and pleural effusions may occur in the presence of normal heart silhouette.

Recommended Tests

• Serum levels of acetaminophen, aspirin, and ethanol are measured, and urine toxicology screen in overdose setting is used to detect occult ingestion.
• Urinalysis and serum creatine kinase are performed on comatose patients to evaluate for rhabdomyolysis.
• Head CT, lumbar puncture, cultures, and other tests are used as needed to assess CNS depression.
• Pulmonary artery catheterization is indicated if the etiology is uncertain and if the procedure may assist in patient management. Increased pulmonary wedge pressures typically indicate a cardiac etiology while normal wedge and pulmonary artery pressures indicate noncardiogenic causes.

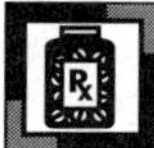

Treatment

• Therapy should be focused on the rapid treatment of hypoxia and the underlying cause of pulmonary edema.
• Supportive care with appropriate airway management is vital, with specific treatment initiated while supportive care continues.
• Dose and time of exposure should be determined for all substances involved.

DIRECTING PATIENT COURSE

The health-care provider should call the poison control center when:

• cause of pulmonary edema is unclear.
• coingestant, drug interaction, or underlying disease presents unusual problems.

Admission Considerations

All patients with pulmonary edema warrant inpatient treatment.

DECONTAMINATION

• Induced emesis is not recommended.
• Gastric lavage should be performed in pediatric (tube size 24–32 French) or adult (tube size 36–42 French) patients for large ingestion presenting within 1 hour of ingestion or if serious effects are present.
• One dose of activated charcoal (1–2 g/kg) should be administered without cathartic if a substantial ingestion has occurred within the previous few hours.

ADJUNCTIVE TREATMENT

• If serious respiratory depression, difficulty in protecting the airway, or inadequate oxygenation on 100% oxygen develops, the patient should be intubated endotracheally.
• Intravenous access should be established and the patient should be placed on a cardiac monitor.
• Hypotension should be treated with a small isotonic fluid bolus.

—Overly aggressive fluid administration should be avoided.
—If the patient does not respond to fluid, vasopressors should be initiated early.
—Early pulmonary artery catheterization should be considered to optimize therapy.

• Treatment of cardiogenic pulmonary edema includes morphine, furosemide, and nitrates.

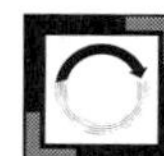

Follow-Up

PATIENT MONITORING

The patient's pulmonary and cardiovascular function should be monitored continuously.

EXPECTED COURSE AND PROGNOSIS

Most toxic causes of pulmonary edema respond well to therapy. Sequelae are determined by underlying cause, however, and permanent pulmonary dysfunction may occur.

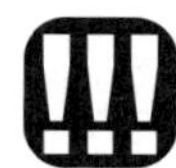

Pitfalls

DIAGNOSIS

Chest radiographs may be normal initially.

TREATMENT

Overadministration of fluid may worsen pulmonary edema.

See also: SECTION IV, chapters on individual poisons.

ICD-9-CM 975

Poisoning by agents primarily acting on the smooth and skeletal muscles and respiratory system.

RECOMMENDED READING

Albertson TE, Walby WF, Derlet RW. Stimulant induced pulmonary toxicity. Chest 1995;108:1140–1149.

Reed CR, Glauser FL. Drug induced noncardiogenic pulmonary edema. Chest 1991;100:1120–1124.

Author: Kennon Heard

Reviewer: Luke Yip

Seizures

Basics

DESCRIPTION

- Seizure is an abrupt onset of involuntary muscle activity associated with loss of consciousness, possibly associated with a toxic exposure.
- See also the chapter on movement disorders.

PATHOPHYSIOLOGY

- Most seizures associated with toxic causes are generalized, tonic-clonic seizures.
- Typically, a seizure of toxic origin is caused by metabolic changes or alteration in the neurotransmitter levels within the brain (e.g., inhibition of gamma aminobutyric acid activity).

EPIDEMIOLOGY

- Seizures are a common toxic effect of drugs.
- Permanent sequelae or death may occur if prolonged, repeated seizures occur.

RISK FACTORS

Patients with an underlying seizure disorder are more likely to develop seizures as a toxic effect.

PREGNANCY AND LACTATION

Seizure in a pregnant patient should always suggest eclampsia.

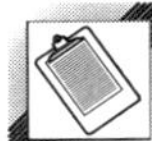

Diagnosis

DIFFERENTIAL DIAGNOSIS

Common Toxicologic Causes

- Antihistamines/anticholinergic agents. Associated with dry mouth, tachycardia, decreased bowel activity, and delirium
- Buproprion. Self-limited seizures and, often, tachycardia
- Camphor. Usually occurring in children and associated with a "mothball" odor
- Carbon monoxide. Headache and nausea; often, simultaneous multiple victims
- Cocaine/amphetamines. Agitation, tachycardia, hypertension, and hyperthermia
- Ergotamine. Peripheral vasospasm, cyanosis, and vomiting
- Hydrocarbons. Strong "solvent" odor; pulmonary edema if toxin is aspirated
- Isoniazid. Seizures refractory to standard therapy; often involving patient under treatment for tuberculosis
- Lithium. Vomiting, altered mental status, fasciculations, hyperactive reflexes, and clonus
- Meperidine or propoxyphene. CNS depression, miosis, and respiratory depression
- Oral hypoglycemic agents or insulin. Hypoglycemia, delirium, and diaphoresis
- Organophosphate or carbamate insecticide. Salivation, vomiting, diarrhea, diaphoresis, and pulmonary edema
- Phencyclidine. Nystagmus, marked agitation, and delirium
- Phenothiazines. Dry mouth, tachycardia, decreased bowel activity, and history of psychiatric illness
- Salicylate. Tachypnea and, prior to seizure, anion gap acidosis
- Theophylline. Tachycardia (often marked), vomiting, hypokalemia, and tremors
- Tricyclic antidepressants (TCAs). Tachycardia, QRS widening, coma, and hypotension

Uncommon Toxicologic Causes

- Butyrophenones. Somnolence and history of psychiatric illness
- DEET. Usually a small child treated with mosquito repellent
- Chloroquine. Cardiovascular collapse and wide complex tachycardia
- Lindane. History of recent treatment for scabies
- Lead. Anemia, encephalopathy, or abdominal pain
- Local anesthetics. Seizures often preceded by tingling and flushing
- Monoamine oxidase (MAO) inhibitors. Hyperthermia, autonomic instability, coma, and muscular rigidity
- Strychnine. Intermittent severe muscular spasms with normal mental status (not true seizures)
- Water hemlock. History of ingestion of a plant root found near water

Nontoxicologic Causes

- CNS infections, including meningitis, encephalitis, and abscess
- Structural abnormalities, including subdural hematoma, epidural hematoma, intracerebral bleed, cerebral contusion, CNS tumors, stroke, subarachnoid hemorrhage, and cerebral edema
- Metabolic, including hypoxia, hypoglycemia, and electrolyte abnormalities
- Idiopathic, including epilepsy
- Withdrawal from ethanol or sedative-hypnotic agents, which may also present with tremor, hypertension, tachycardia, low-grade fever, and hallucinosis
- Pseudoseizures should be suspected in patients with a psychiatric history, atypical seizures, asynchronous extremity movement, eyes rolled back into the head or a lack of postictal period; however, this diagnosis can rarely be made in the emergency department.

SYMPTOMS AND SIGNS

Associated physical signs may help reveal the poison involved when they are associated with a seizure.

Vital Signs

- Tachycardia, hypertension, and hyperthermia suggest cocaine, amphetamines, other stimulants, MAO inhibitor, neuroleptic malignant syndrome, serotonin syndrome, or withdrawal from benzodiazepines, ethanol, or barbiturates.
- Tachycardia and hypotension suggest TCAs, theophylline, quinidine, or chloroquine.
- Bradycardia and hypotension suggest propranolol, organophosphate, or carbamate insecticides.

HEENT

- Dry mucous membranes and large pupils suggest anticholinergic drugs, antihistamines, or TCAs.
- Small pupils suggests meperidine, propoxyphene, organophosphate, or carbamate insecticide.
- Nystagmus suggests PCP, carbamazepine, or other anticonvulsants.

Dermatologic

- Diaphoresis suggests cocaine, amphetamines, organophosphate, or carbamate insecticide, or withdrawal from agents such as benzodiazepines, ethanol, or barbiturates.
- Dermatitis and excoriations may suggest that the patient received lindane therapy for scabies.

Cardiovascular

- Tachycardia, QRS greater than 100 msec (0.1 sec), and hypotension suggest TCAs, type 1 antidysrhythmic agents, quinine, or chloroquine.
- Peripheral vasospasm and cyanosis suggest ergot toxicity.

Pulmonary

- Increased pulmonary secretions and pulmonary edema suggest exposure to organophosphate or carbamate insecticide or nicotine, or mushroom ingestion.
- Noncardiogenic pulmonary edema suggests hydrocarbon aspiration, salicylate, or camphor.

Gastrointestinal

Recurrent vomiting or diarrhea suggests organophosphates, carbamates, lithium, or mushrooms.

Hepatic

Hepatic injury suggests chlorinated hydrocarbons.

Renal

Diabetes insipidus suggests lithium.

Fluids and Electrolytes

Hypokalemia suggests theophylline.

Musculoskeletal

- Rhabdomyolysis may occur with any cause of seizures.
- Fasciculation and tremor suggests theophylline, lithium, organophosphates, or carbamates.
- Muscular rigidity suggests MAO inhibitors, neuroleptic malignant syndrome, or serotonin syndrome.
- Opisthotonos suggests strychnine.

Neurologic

- Agitation and psychosis are seen with cocaine, amphetamines, hypoxia from any cause, PCP or other hallucinogens, or withdrawal from agents such as benzodiazepines, ethanol, or barbiturates.
- Seizures refractory to standard therapy suggest isoniazid exposure.
- Ataxia, coma, and somnolence suggest propoxyphene, meperidine, carbamazepine, chlorinated hydrocarbons, carbon monoxide, butyrophenones, or phenothiazines.

Endocrine

Hypoglycemia suggests insulin, oral hypoglycemics, or propranolol.

PROCEDURES AND LABORATORY TESTS

Essential Tests

- Serum electrolytes, BUN, creatinine, and rapid glucose test should be obtained in all patients. An increased anion gap acidosis that clears promptly over 2 to 3 hours may follow seizures.
- ECG is used to evaluate QRS duration for possible ingestion of TCA, phenothiazine, or antidysrhythmic agent.
- Arterial blood gases and pulse oximetry assess oxygenation and effects on respiration.

Recommended Tests

- Serum acetaminophen and aspirin levels and urine toxicology screen are used to detect occult ingestion.
- Serum levels of anticonvulsants are measured to assess potential noncompliance or seizure induced by anticonvulsant toxicity.
- Carboxyhemoglobin level is measured if inhalation exposure to carbon monoxide was possible.
- Serum drug levels are measured as indicated: salicylate, theophylline, red blood cell or plasma cholinesterase.
- Head CT, lumbar puncture, bacterial cultures, and other tests are used as needed to assess altered mental status.

Treatment

- Focus therapy on appropriate airway management and immediate treatment of seizures.
- Dose and time of exposure should be determined for all substances involved.

DECONTAMINATION

Out of Hospital

- Emesis should be avoided.

In Hospital

- Gastric lavage should be performed in pediatric (tube size 24–32 French) or adult (tube size 36–42 French) patients for large ingestion presenting within 1 hour of ingestion or if serious effects are present.
- One dose of activated charcoal (1–2 g/kg) should be administered without a cathartic if a substantial ingestion has occurred within the previous few hours.

ADJUNCTIVE TREATMENT

- Endotracheal intubation may prevent pulmonary aspiration.
- It is vital to determine glucose and oxygen concentrations rapidly.
- Supplemental oxygen should be administered.
- Benzodiazepine is administered for initial control, while monitoring the airway closely.

—Diazepam. Adult, 5 to 10 mg intravenous push over 2 to 5 minutes, repeated every 10 minutes as needed; pediatric, 0.2 to 0.5 mg/kg every 10 minutes as needed.
—Lorazepam. Adult, 2 to 4 mg intravenous push over 2 to 5 minutes, repeated every 10 minutes as needed; pediatric, 0.1 mg/kg intravenous push over 2 to 5 minutes (not to exceed 4 mg/dose), repeated every 10 minutes as needed.

- Seizure unresponsive to benzodiazepine

—Phenobarbital should be given (after intubation due to respiratory depression).
—Pediatric and adult dose is 18 mg/kg intravenously.
—Rate of infusion should not exceed 60 to 100 mg/min.
—Rapid infusion may cause hypotension.

- Seizure unresponsive to phenobarbital

—Patient must be intubated.
—Neuromuscular blockade is performed with a nondepolarizing agent to prevent ongoing acidosis and muscle injury.
—Paralyzed patients should have continual EEG monitoring as nonconvulsive status epilepticus can result in ongoing brain injury.
—Patients with ongoing EEG evidence of seizures should receive intravenous bolus of pentobarbital, 5 to 6 mg/kg at 25 mg/min, followed by 1.0 to 3.0 mg/kg/hr infusion, titrated to EEG effect.

- Phenytoin is considered less effective for seizure of toxic origin but is not contraindicated.

ANTIDOTES

Pyridoxine

- Indications. Seizures of unknown etiology that are refractory to standard measures
- Dosage and method of use. Pyridoxine should be administered empirically. The dose is 5 g administered intravenously. If needed, the dose is repeated once in 30 minutes. Unless the patient received a known isoniazid overdose (in which case a gram-for-gram treatment is used) the treatment should not exceed 10 g.

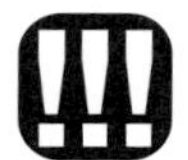

Pitfalls

DIAGNOSIS

It is vital to consider nontoxic causes of seizures.

TREATMENT

Aggressive airway management is critical to successful outcome.

FOLLOW-UP

Additional complications should be anticipated (e.g., dysrhythmias).

See also: SECTION II, Movement Disorders and Pulmonary Edema chapters; SECTION III, Pyridoxine chapter; and Section IV, Isoniazid chapter.

RECOMMENDED READING

Pollack CV, Pollack ES. Seizures. In: Rosen P, ed. Emergency medicine. St. Louis: Mosby, 1998:2150–2165.

Author: Kennon Heard

Reviewer: Katherine M. Hurlbut

Tachycardia

Basics

DESCRIPTION

Tachycardia, or increased heart rate at rest, is defined as follows:

- Adults and adolescents: more than 100 beats/min
- Children 5 to 10 years of age: more than 120 beats/min
- Children 1 to 5 years of age: more than 130 beats/min
- Newborns and infants less than 1 year of age: more than 150 beats/min

PATHOPHYSIOLOGY

- Common toxicologic mechanisms for persistent tachycardia include excessive β-adrenergic receptor stimulation and anticholinergic effects.
- Physiologic responses to hypotension, hyperthermia, hypoxia, and volume depletion are other possible causes of tachycardia.

Diagnosis

DIFFERENTIAL DIAGNOSIS

Toxicologic Causes

- Further information on each poison is available in SECTION IV, CHEMICAL AND BIOLOGICAL AGENTS.
- Cocaine, amphetamines, and other sympathomimetic agents (ephedrine, phenylpropanolamine, β_2-agonist bronchodilators, and many others). Additional clinical and laboratory findings may include hypertension, hyperthermia, agitation, delirium, seizures, track marks, nasal septum erosion or perforation, and rhabdomyolysis.
- Tricyclic antidepressants (TCAs). Additional clinical and laboratory findings might include seizure, hypotension, dysrhythmias, QRS widening, presence of an R wave in ECG lead aVR, and coma.
- Type Ia antiarrhythmic agents (quinidine, procainamide, disopyramide) all cause prolongation of ECG intervals (PR, QRS, QT) and may be associated with ventricular dysrhythmias and torsade de pointes.
- Anticholinergic agents (diphenhydramine, scopolamine, jimsonweed, hydroxyzine, phenothiazines, Dramamine, etc.). Additional clinical and laboratory findings include flushing, dilated and sluggish pupils, diminished bowel sounds, hyperthermia, hallucinations, agitation, delirium, and dry skin.
- Theophylline. Additional clinical and laboratory findings may include tremor, vomiting, seizures, dysrhythmias, hypokalemia, mild metabolic acidosis, or preexisting diagnosis of chronic obstructive pulmonary disease.
- Selective serotonin reuptake inhibitors (SSRI) cause depressed mental status and seizure without dysrhythmia (other than tachycardia) or hypotension.
- Digitalis may produce tachycardia with heart block, vomiting, hyperkalemia (acute), or hypokalemia (chronic intoxication).
- Monoamine oxidase (MAO) inhibitors may cause hyperthermia, hypertension, and altered mental status.
- Carbamazepine is associated with coma, hyponatremia, and nystagmus.
- Marijuana causes dilated pupils and conjunctival injection.
- Cholinergic agents (organophosphate or carbamate pesticides) may cause vomiting, diarrhea, salivation, lacrimation, urination, bronchorrhea, small pupils, and sweating.
- Hallucinogens of any type (LSD, phencyclidine) may cause rhabdomyolysis.
- Mushrooms may produce hallucinogenic or anticholinergic effects.
- Substances that produce methemoglobinemia (e.g., dapsone, nitrates). Methemoglobinemia often causes cyanosis.
- Thyroid hormones may be associated with history of thyroid disease, tremor, and fever.
- Vasodilators (nifedipine, hydralazine, etc.) primarily cause hypotension.
- Withdrawal (from alcohol, opiates, or sedative-hypnotics) is associated with a history of abuse and abstinence, and hypertension.

Nontoxicologic Causes

- All causes of hypotension or hypoxia produce tachycardia, which may be followed by bradycardia as disease worsens.
- Common nontoxic causes of tachycardia include anxiety (a diagnosis of exclusion), anemia, fever, hypoxia, hypotension, pulmonary embolus, renal failure, vasodilation (sepsis, neurogenic shock), volume depletion, and metabolic acidosis.

SIGNS AND SYMPTOMS

Associated physical signs may help to reveal the poison involved when they are associated with tachycardia.

Vital Signs

Hypertension may indicate sympathomimetic toxicity or withdrawal from alcohol, sedative-hypnotics, or MAO inhibitors.

HEENT

- Dilated pupils suggest anticholinergic or sympathomimetic toxicity.
- Conjunctival injection and dilated pupils suggest marijuana.
- Perforated nasal septum may indicate chronic drug abuse.

Dermatologic

- Flushed, dry skin suggests an anticholinergic agent.
- Pale, sweaty skin may be associated with sympathomimetic drugs, cholinergic agents, or hypotension.
- Cyanosis suggests hypoxia or methemoglobinemia.

Cardiovascular

- Tachycardia with no other cardiovascular findings may indicate theophylline toxicity.
- See also SECTION II, Ventricular Dysrhythmias chapter.

Pulmonary

- Mucous membrane irritation and wheezing may result from smoke inhalation or hydrocarbon aspiration.
- Cholinergic agonists may produce bronchorrhea and wheezing.

Gastrointestinal

- Vomiting is commonly associated with iron, salicylate, or theophylline intoxication.
- Diminished bowel sounds suggest an anticholinergic agent.

Renal

Urinary retention suggests an anticholinergic agent.

Fluids and Electrolytes

Hypokalemia suggests a β-receptor agonist or theophylline.

Musculoskeletal

Rhabdomyolysis often indicates stimulant or hallucinogen abuse.

Neurologic

- Hallucinations and delirium suggest an anticholinergic agent or abuse of stimulants or hallucinogens.
- Anxiety, tremor, and seizures suggest theophylline or withdrawal from alcohol or sedative-hypnotic drugs.
- Coma and seizures suggest tricyclic antidepressant toxicity.
- CNS depression or coma, nystagmus, ataxia, diminished bowel sounds, and hyponatremia suggest carbamazepine.

PROCEDURES AND LABORATORY TESTS

Essential Tests

- ECG should be obtained and continuous cardiac monitoring established.

—QRS widening, an R wave in ECG lead aVR, and hypotension suggest tricyclic antidepressant poisoning or other type Ia antidysrhythmic agents.
—Digitalis produces a wide variety of tachydysrhythmias and heart blocks.

- A complete blood count should be obtained to rule out anemia.

Recommended Tests

- Serum electrolytes, BUN, and creatinine should be obtained to assist in assessment of metabolic acidosis and renal insufficiency; acute digitalis toxicity often causes hyperkalemia, and theophylline or β-agonists produce hypokalemia.
- Arterial blood gases should be performed to assess the contribution of hypoxia to tachycardia.
- Urine toxicology screen should be obtained in patients with persistent tachycardia of unknown cause.
- Metabolic acidosis of unknown etiology with tachycardia should prompt testing of salicylate level, methanol level, ethylene glycol level, serum iron level, lactate level, and carboxyhemoglobin.
- Serum acetaminophen and aspirin levels should be obtained in overdose settings to detect occult overdose.
- CT and LP cultures may be needed to evaluate other causes.
- Orthostatic vital signs should be assessed and central venous pressure monitoring established to evaluate for other possible causes of tachycardia.

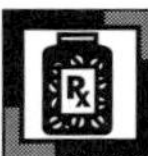

Treatment

- An intravenous line should be established.
- Treatment of specific effects (e.g., sodium bicarbonate for QRS widening) should be initiated while continuing supportive care.
- The dose and time of exposure should be determined for all substances involved.

DIRECTING PATIENT COURSE

- The need for consultation with a poison center or other specialists should be evaluated.
- A poison center or toxicology consultant should be consulted for patients with metabolic acidosis of unknown etiology with tachycardia, unless the etiology can be determined quickly.

The health-care provider should call the poison control center when:

- cause of persistent tachycardia is unclear.
- coingestant, drug interaction, or underlying disease presents unusual problems.

Admission Considerations

The decision to admit a patient is based on the underlying cause of tachycardia.

DECONTAMINATION

- Induction of emesis is not recommended.
- Gastric lavage should be performed in pediatric (tube size 24–32 French) or adult (36–42 French) patients for large ingestion presenting within 1 hour of ingestion, or if serious effects are present.
- One dose of activated charcoal (1–2 g/kg) should be administered without a cathartic if a substantial ingestion has occurred within the previous few hours.

ADJUNCTIVE TREATMENT

Control of Heart Rate

- The general approach of Advanced Cardiac Life Support guidelines should be followed.
- Often, agitation is an important contributor to tachycardia; in such cases, a benzodiazepine (diazepam or lorazepam) should be administered in small doses and titrated to effect, and the airway should be monitored closely.
- Tachycardia due to hypoxia, anemia, or electrolyte disorder is corrected by treating the underlying cause.
- β-receptor blockade may be indicated if other measures are unsuccessful.

—Esmolol may be administered in an intravenous bolus of 500 μg/kg infused over 1 minute, followed by an infusion of 50 μg/kg/min for 4 minutes.
—If response to initial esmolol therapy is inadequate, the loading dose should be repeated and 100 μg/kg/min infused for 4 minutes; this titration may be repeated as needed until heart rate is controlled or toxicity (hypotension) develops.
—Unopposed α-receptor stimulation is a theoretical concern during β blockade; if heart rate or blood pressure increase dangerously during esmolol infusion, α-receptor stimulation may be the cause.

Hypotension

- The health-care provider should administer 10 to 20 ml/kg of 0.9% saline and place the patient in the Trendelenburg position.

—Further fluid therapy should be guided by central monitoring or right heart catheter to avoid volume overload.
—If hypotension is unresponsive to saline, a vasopressor should be administered.

Hypertension

If hypertension is not responsive to benzodiazepines, or if end organ damage (aortic dissection, CNS bleed, myocardial infarction) develops, a short-acting, titratable agent may be administered (see SECTION II, Nitroprusside chapter).

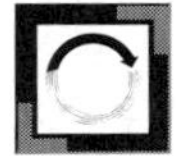

Follow-Up

PATIENT MONITORING

Respiratory and cardiac function should be monitored continuously.

DISCHARGE CRITERIA/INSTRUCTIONS

The asymptomatic patient may be discharged after the tachycardia resolves, the underlying cause is corrected, decontamination is complete, and a psychiatric evaluation, if needed, has been performed.

ICD-9-CM 785.0

Symptoms involving the cardiovascular system: tachycardia, unspecified.

See also: SECTION II, Hypotension, Pulmonary Edema, Ventricular Dysrhythmias, Cholinergic Syndrome, Withdrawal, Methemoglobinemia, and Anion Gap Metabolic Acidosis chapters; SECTION III, Nitroprusside chapter; and SECTION IV, Anticholinergic Compounds chapter.

RECOMMENDED READING

Goldfrank LR, Flomenbaum NE, Weisman RS, et al. Vital signs and toxic syndromes. In: Goldfrank LR, et al., eds. Goldfrank's toxicologic emergencies, 6th ed. Norwalk, CT: Appleton & Lange, 1998.

Author: Katherine M. Hurlbut

Reviewer: Richard C. Dart

Tachypnea

Basics

DESCRIPTION

Tachypnea, or increased rate of respiration at rest, is defined as follows:

- Adults and adolescents: more than 20 respirations/min
- Children 5 to 10 years of age: more than 25 respirations/min
- Children 1 to 5 years of age: more than 30 respirations/min
- Newborns and children less than 1 year of age: more than 40 respirations/min

Hyperpnea is defined as breathing that is deeper and more rapid than usual. Hyperventilation refers to increased alveolar ventilation which lowers the alveolar CO_2.

PATHOPHYSIOLOGY

- Tachypnea may be caused directly by stimulation of the medullary respiration center or airway receptors.
- Indirect causes of tachypnea include metabolic acidosis, hypoxia, hypotension, or uncoupling of oxidative phosphorylation; each of these conditions produces tachypnea as a compensatory physiologic response.

EPIDEMIOLOGY

Neonatal patients or patients with underlying cardiovascular disease will not tolerate many of the conditions associated with tachypnea, especially hypoxia.

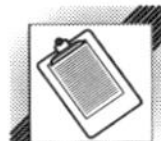

Diagnosis

DIFFERENTIAL DIAGNOSIS

Further information on each poison is available in SECTION IV, CHEMICAL AND BIOLOGICAL AGENTS.

Toxicologic Causes

- Salicylates are also associated with tinnitus, metabolic acidosis, and altered mental status.
- Stimulants such as amphetamines or cocaine often cause tachycardia, hypertension, restlessness, agitation, and hyperthermia.
- Cholinergic agents such as organophosphate or carbamate insecticides may be associated with nausea, vomiting, salivation, lacrimation, and urination.
- Anticholinergic agents often cause tachycardia, mydriasis, and decreased bowel sounds.
- Substances and conditions that produce metabolic acidoses (methanol, ethylene glycol, toluene, renal failure, metformin, ketoacidosis, isoniazid, iron, and others) are usually associated with acidosis, tachycardia, and depressed serum bicarbonate level.
- Irritant gases (chloramine, chlorine, hydrochloric acid [HCl], isocyanates, nitrogen dioxide [NO_2], ozone, phosgene, and others) also are associated with cough, mucous membrane irritation, and bronchorrhea.
- Theophylline or caffeine also may cause nausea, vomiting, tachycardia, tremors, or seizure.
- Pentachlorophenol and dinitrophenols are associated with fever and depressed mentation.
- Nicotine also causes small pupils, nausea, and vomiting.
- Substances and conditions that produce hypoxia (cyanide, carbon monoxide, methemoglobinemia, and others) are associated with tachycardia metabolic acidosis, cyanosis, tachycardia, and depressed mentation.
- Substances that produce noncardiogenic pulmonary edema (salicylates, inhaled smoke, irritant gases, cocaine, ethchlorvynol, opioids) often are associated with cough, dyspnea, diffuse lung infiltrates, and tachycardia.
- Metal fume fever is associated with chills, cough, and lung infiltrates in serious cases.
- Substances that produce hyperthermic syndromes (neuroleptic malignant syndrome [NMS], serotonin syndrome) often are associated with confusion, tachycardia, and muscle rigidity.
- Substances that produce acute hemolysis may produce relative hypoxia and tachypnea.
- Withdrawal (from alcohol, opiates, sedative-hypnotics) is associated with history of abuse and abstinence, tachycardia, and hypertension and hallucination in serious cases.

Nontoxicologic Causes

- All causes of hypotension or hypoxia produce tachypnea, which may be followed by bradypnea as disease progresses.
- There are many nontoxicologic causes of tachypnea, which generally are related to anxiety (a diagnosis of exclusion), fever, hypoxia, hypotension, pulmonary embolus, renal failure, increased intracranial pressure, or compensation for metabolic acidosis.

SIGNS AND SYMPTOMS

Physical signs may help reveal the poison involved when they occur in the setting of tachypnea.

Vital Signs

Hypertension may indicate sympathomimetic toxicity, monoamine oxidase (MAO) inhibitor, or alcohol withdrawal.

HEENT

- Tinnitus suggests salicylate intoxication.
- Dilated pupils suggest an anticholinergic or sympathomimetic agent.

Dermatologic

- Cyanosis may be associated with methemoglobinemia or with hypoxia of any cause.
- Pale, sweaty skin may be associated with sympathomimetic drugs, cholinergic agents, or hypotension.
- Flushed, dry skin suggests an anticholinergic agent.

Cardiovascular

- Profound cardiogenic shock is most commonly caused by digoxin, β-blocking drugs, or calcium channel blocking drugs; all serious poisonings, however, may produce shock as a terminal effect.
- See also SECTION II, Bradycardia, Tachydysrhythmia, and Ventricular Dysrhythmias chapters.

Pulmonary

- Pulmonary infiltrates suggest chemical pneumonitis (e.g., smoke inhalation, hydrocarbon aspirator) or noncardiogenic pulmonary edema (e.g., salicylates, opioids).
- Fever, chills, headache, myalgia, fatigue, and cough that occurs after inhalation of metal oxides indicates metal fume fever.

Gastrointestinal

Vomiting is commonly associated with iron, salicylate, nicotine, or theophylline intoxication.

Renal

- Prolonged hyperventilation may produce a compensatory increase in serum bicarbonate.
- Hyperventilation may cause carpopedal spasm from an acute decrease in ionized calcium concentration.

Fluids and Electrolytes

- Volume depletion often occurs because of increased insensible loss of respiration; these losses are often underestimated.

- Volume depletion is also possible from hemorrhage in iron, anticoagulant, or snake venom poisonings.
- Metabolic acidosis suggests salicylate, toxic alcohol (methanol, ethylene glycol), theophylline, iron, or toluene exposure.
- Hypokalemia suggests theophylline intoxication.

Musculoskeletal

Tachypnea and decreased tidal volume may result from conditions that reduce respiratory muscle function, such as botulism, organophosphate intoxication, and others. Tachypnea may be followed by bradypnea as respiratory muscle function fails.

Neurologic

- Appearance of intoxication suggests toxic alcohol poisoning.
- Hallucinations and delirium suggest an anticholinergic agent, abuse of stimulants or hallucinogens, or withdrawal from alcohol or sedative-hypnotics.
- Anxiety, tremor, and seizures suggest theophylline toxicity.
- Coma and seizures suggest tricyclic antidepressant poisoning.

PROCEDURES AND LABORATORY TESTS

Essential Tests

- Arterial blood gases should be obtained to determine the presence of hypoxia or acidosis.
- Pulse oximetry should be performed for continuous respiratory status monitoring.

Recommended Tests

- Serum electrolytes, BUN, and creatinine should be obtained to assist in assessment of metabolic acidosis or renal insufficiency.
- Salicylate level, methanol level, ethylene glycol level, serum iron level, lactate level, and carbon monoxide are used to determine the cause of metabolic acidosis.
- Serial peak flow determination should be determined to evaluate bronchoconstriction.
- Serum cholinesterase should be obtained to assess organophosphate or carbamate poisoning.
- Urine toxicology screen should be considered in patients with persistent tachypnea of unknown cause.
- Serum acetaminophen and aspirin levels should be obtained in overdose settings to detect occult overdose of analgesic medications.
- Chest radiograph should be obtained to assess potential intrathoracic causes of tachypnea.

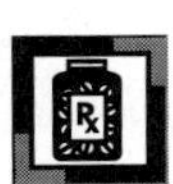

Treatment

- If serious respiratory depression is present, or if protecting the airway is difficult, the patient should be intubated endotracheally until the cause can be determined and treated.
- It is important to maintain the intubated patient's respiratory rate to prevent worsening of acidosis.
- Intravenous access should be considered for all patients with tachypnea.
- The dose and time of exposure should be determined for all substances involved.
- Treatment for specific effects (e.g., naloxone for mental status depression) should be initiated while continuing supportive care.

DIRECTING PATIENT COURSE

The health-care provider should call the poison control center when:

- The cause of tachypnea is unclear.
- Coingestant, drug interaction, or underlying disease presents unusual problems.
- A patient presents with metabolic acidosis of unknown etiology with tachypnea, unless the etiology can be determined quickly.

Admission Considerations

The decision to admit depends on the underlying cause of tachypnea.

DECONTAMINATION

- Induction of emesis in not recommended.
- Gastric lavage should be performed in pediatric (tube size 24–32 French) or adult (36–42 French) patients for large ingestion presenting within 1 hour of ingestion, or if serious effects are present.
- One dose of activated charcoal (1–2 g/kg) should be administered without a cathartic if a substantial ingestion has occurred within the previous few hours.

ADJUNCTIVE TREATMENT

Bronchospasm

- Oxygen should be administered, followed by albuterol 0.15 mg/kg (maximum of 10 mg) in saline with humidified oxygen via nebulizer every 20 to 30 minutes. If the peak expiratory flow rate is greater than 90% after the initial dose, additional doses may not be needed.
- Methylprednisolone 60 to 125 mg (1–1.5 mg/kg in adults, 1–2 mg/kg in children) may be given intravenously every 6 to 8 hours; the dosage may be decreased to a single daily dose and tapered.
- Initiation of prednisone, 1.0 mg/kg orally for several days, should be considered.

Hypotension

- The health-care provider should administer 10 to 20 ml/kg 0.9% saline and place the patient in the Trendelenburg position.
- Further fluid therapy should be guided by central monitoring or right heart catheter to avoid volume overload.
- If hypotension is unresponsive to saline, a vasopressor should be administered.

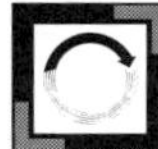

Follow-Up

PATIENT MONITORING

Respiratory and cardiovascular function should be monitored continuously.

DISCHARGE CRITERIA/INSTRUCTIONS

The asymptomatic patient may be discharged after tachypnea resolves, the underlying cause has been established and treated, decontamination is complete, and psychiatric evaluation, if needed, has been performed.

Pitfalls

DIAGNOSIS

Tachypnea and hyperpnea may be clinically subtle, especially in young adults who may increase minute ventilation without tachypnea or other obvious clinical effects.

TREATMENT

- Airway should be managed aggressively; if hypoxia develops or pCO_2 begins to increase, indicating progressive respiratory failure, the patient should be promptly intubated endotracheally.
- Often, hyperventilation is a necessary compensation for metabolic acidosis.

—If the ability to hyperventilate is eliminated by mechanical ventilation, acidemia may develop rapidly.
—In such cases, the patient's increased ventilation rate or minute ventilation volume should be maintained during mechanical ventilation.

FOLLOW-UP

Patients exposed to some poisons (nitrogen dioxide, metal fumes, cadmium) may worsen after an initial period of minimal effects.

ICD-9-CM 786.09

Symptoms involving respiratory system and other chest symptoms: dyspnea and respiratory abnormality.

See also: SECTION II, Anion Gap Metabolic Acidosis, Bradycardia, Hyperthermia, Hypotension, Metal Fume Fever, Methemoglobinemia, NMS and Serotonin Syndrome, Pulmonary Edema, Tachydysrhythmia, Ventricular Dysrhythmias, and Withdrawal chapters; and SECTION IV, Anticholinergic Compounds chapter.

Author: Richard C. Dart

Reviewer: Katherine M. Hurlbut

Unknown Ingestion

Basics

DESCRIPTION

- This discussion covers patient presentations in which it is known that a suicidal or other potentially toxic ingestion has occurred, but the substances involved are uncertain or unknown.
- If the ingestion is presumed to be nontoxic, see SECTION I, Nontoxic Ingestion chapter.

PATHOPHYSIOLOGY

An unknown ingestion may involve agents that are:

- Nontoxic
- Toxic, but not ingested in sufficient dose to cause toxicity
- Toxic and ingested in sufficient dose to produce toxicity

Causes

- Child neglect should be considered if the patient is less than 1 year of age.
- Attempted suicide should be considered if the patient is over 6 years of age.

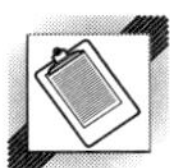

Diagnosis

- Careful and persistent attention to history taking is essential to reaching an accurate diagnosis.
- If the patient is unwilling or unable to provide information, other sources of information should be pursued aggressively; family members and the pharmacy the patient typically has used should be contacted to obtain medical and medication history.
- The health-care provider should request that emergency medical personnel search the scene and bring all potential poisons to the emergency department because evidence is often found in rooms other than the one in which the patient was found.

DIFFERENTIAL DIAGNOSIS

Many patients with toxic ingestions have no symptoms upon presentation, or have effects that initially appear to be manifestations of infectious, inflammatory, neoplastic, or even traumatic origin.

- A toxidrome is a collection of physical signs that identifies a type of poison. The presence of a toxidrome can help narrow the diagnosis and identify the poison involved; unfortunately, toxidromes are usually not present, even in poisoned patients.

—Opioid toxidrome consists of small (often pinpoint) pupils with CNS and respiratory depression.
—Cholinergic toxidrome consists of small pupils, salivation, lacrimation, diaphoresis, vomiting, diarrhea, and muscle fasciculation or weakness.
—Sympathomimetic toxidrome consists of dilated pupils, tachycardia, hypertension, diaphoresis, and possibly seizure or dysrhythmia.
—Sedative-hypnotic toxidrome consists of nystagmus, depressed mentation and respirations; hypothermia may complicate the course.
—Anticholinergic toxidrome consists of dilated pupils, tachycardia, flushed skin, dry mucous membranes, agitation, and hallucinosis.
—Withdrawal syndromes. See SECTION II, Withdrawal—Depressants and Stimulants chapter.

- Common toxic substances involved in unknown overdose

—Over-the-counter drugs include acetaminophen, salicylate, diphenhydramine, phenylpropanolamine, and ibuprofen.
—Substances found in the home include cleaning agents (especially bleach), caustics, ethanol, ethylene glycol, methanol, isopropanol, insecticides, and weed killers.
—Prescribed drugs include tricyclic antidepressants (TCAs), benzodiazepines, noncyclic antidepressants, phenothiazine and other antipsychotics, anticonvulsants, antihypertensives, and hypoglycemic agents.
—Street drugs include heroin and other opiates, cocaine, amphetamines, phencyclidine, barbiturates, and jimsonweed; gamma hydroxybutyrate (GHB) is rapidly gaining popularity.

SIGNS AND SYMPTOMS

The absence of symptoms or signs at presentation does not rule out potentially serious or fatal ingestion.

Vital Signs

- Bradypnea/apnea is most commonly caused by opioid and sedative-hypnotic medications.
- Hyperpnea is associated with any substance that causes stimulation, hypoxia, or metabolic acidosis; most common among these substances are carbon monoxide, ethylene glycol, methanol, salicylates, sympathomimetic drugs, and theophylline.
- Hypertension, hypotension, hypothermia, hyperthermia, tachycardia or bradycardia may be present. See individual chapters for more information.

HEENT

- Decreased or blurred vision may indicate methanol, botulism, carbon monoxide, digitalis, or quinine.
- Miosis may be caused by opioids, organophosphate or carbamate insecticides, chloral hydrate, or topical miotic agents.
- Mydriasis is associated with any substance that produces hypoxia or anticholinergic effects, and may also be caused by LSD, marijuana, or a topical mydriatic.
- Nystagmus is most commonly caused by sedative-hypnotic toxicity and occasionally by phencyclidine (PCP).
- Papilledema suggests vitamin A or severe lead poisoning.
- Ptosis or ocular motor palsy may be caused by botulism, diphtheria, lead, phenytoin, thallium, neurotoxic snake venom poisoning, or Wernicke-Korsakoff syndrome.

Dermatologic

- Bullae may be associated with prolonged coma resulting from barbiturates, carbon monoxide, ethchlorvynol, or baclofen.
- Burns may be caused by alkalis or acids.
- Cyanosis is most commonly caused by hypoxia or methemoglobinemia.
- Desquamation may be caused by arsenic or boric acid.
- Diaphoresis may be caused by organophosphates, carbamates, cocaine, amphetamines, sympathomimetics, or muscarinic mushrooms.
- Petechiae or purpura may be caused by anticoagulants, rodent poison bait, salicylates, or crotalid snakebite.
- Red skin may be caused by anticholinergics, boric acid, niacin, or carbon monoxide (postmortem).

Cardiovascular

- Prolonged QRS duration may result from severe anticholinergic overdose, type 1 antidysrhythmic agents, β-receptor blockers, TCAs, digitalis, phenothiazine, or hypokalemia.
- Prolonged QTc interval may result from amiodarone, type 1 antidysrhythmic agents, arsenic, TCAs, fluoride, organophosphates, quinidine, procainamide, propoxyphene, thioridazine, or hypocalcemia.
- Atrioventricular block may be caused by digitalis glycoside, β-receptor blockade, and calcium channel blocker.

Pulmonary

- Pulmonary edema is a separate chapter.
- Bronchospasm may be caused by known medication allergens, β-blockers taken by patients with underlying reactive airway disease, carbamate or organophosphate insecticides, caustics, or irritant gases.
- Bronchorrhea may be caused by carbamate or organophosphate insecticides or nicotine.

Gastrointestinal

- Abdominal pain may be caused by isopropyl alcohol, black widow spider (rigidity), cathartics, caustics, cholinergics, drug withdrawal, erythromycin, food poisoning, iron, or mushrooms.
- Decreased bowel sounds suggest anticholinergic or opioid effects.
- Hypermotility or diarrhea may indicate carbamate or organophosphate insecticides or nicotine.
- Repetitive nausea and vomiting may be caused by cholinergic agents, iron, theophylline, caustics, heavy metals, or ipecac.

Hepatic

Striking liver enzyme elevation is usually caused by acetaminophen toxicity but also may be caused by chlorinated hydrocarbons such as carbon tetrachloride, or may occur as an idiosyncratic reaction to many drugs.

Renal

- Renal failure is most commonly caused by hypotension associated with poisoning.
- Urinary retention suggests atropine and other anticholinergic agents, isoniazid, neuroleptics, or TCAs.
- Myoglobinuria may indicate cocaine, PCP, or any toxic agent that produces coma or repeated seizures.

Fluids and Electrolytes

- Hypernatremia may be caused by lactulose, lithium, mannitol, severe gastroenteritis, or sodium chloride; hypernatremia is also associated with volume contraction caused by repeated administration of sorbitol.
- Hyponatremia suggests polydipsia or syndrome of inappropriate secretion of antidiuretic hormone, which may be caused by lithium, amitriptyline, clofibrate, or phenothiazine toxicity.
- Hyperkalemia may indicate alpha adrenergic agonists, angiotensin-converting enzyme (ACE) inhibitors, potassium-sparing diuretics, β-receptor blockers, digitalis, fluoride, lithium, or potassium tablets; hyperkalemia also may be caused by severe acidosis from any cause.
- Hypokalemia may be caused by barium, β-receptor agonists, caffeine, digitalis (chronic use), potassium-wasting diuretics, or theophylline.
- Increased anion gap acidosis indicates certain poisons.

Musculoskeletal

Rhabdomyolysis may be caused by amphetamines, barbiturates, multiple bee stings, β-receptor stimulation, cocaine, cyanide, ethanol, fenfluramine, glutethimide, hydrogen sulfide, lithium, monoamine oxidase inhibitors, mercuric chloride, NMS or serotonin syndrome, paraquat, PCP, phenobarbital, snake bite, strychnine, or toluene.

Neurologic

- Ataxia. Ethanol, phenytoin, or other anticonvulsants are the most common causes; other causes include arsenic, barbiturates, lithium, benzodiazepines, nicotine, and sedative hypnotics.
- Delirium suggests amphetamines, anticholinergics, antidepressants, antihistamines, cocaine, ethanol, hallucinogens, opiates, salicylate, or alcohol or benzodiazepine withdrawal.
- Dystonia or dyskinesia may occur.
- Mental status depression or coma may occur.
- Psychosis may indicate amphetamines, cocaine, PCP, anticholinergics, antihistamines, LSD, methamphetamines, or TCAs.
- Seizures may occur.

Endocrine

- Hyperglycemia may be caused by caffeine, dextrose, glucagon, steroids, thiazides, or iron.
- Hypoglycemia suggests any alcohol (especially in children), insulin, oral hypoglycemics, or salicylate toxicity.

PROCEDURES AND LABORATORY TESTS

Essential Tests

- Serum electrolytes, BUN, creatinine, and glucose should be obtained to evaluate renal, fluid and electrolyte status.
- ECG, cardiac monitoring, and serum acetaminophen and salicylate levels should be ordered to detect occult ingestion.

Recommended Tests

- Blood levels of specific suspected toxic agents and therapeutic medications should be obtained when immediately available and appropriate.
- Urine toxicology screen as described in SECTION I, Urine Drug Screening chapter.
- Serum calcium and magnesium and liver function tests should be performed.
- Head CT, lumbar puncture, bacterial cultures, and other tests may be needed to evaluate altered mental status.
- Abdominal radiographs may reveal radiopaque pills or material such as bismuth subsalicylate, calcium carbonate, chloral hydrate, enteric coated tablets, iron, lead, lithium, metallic foreign bodies, potassium tablets, phenothiazine, phosphorus, or zinc sulfate; the absence of radiopacities, however, does not rule out toxic ingestion.
- Chest radiograph should be obtained to assess pulmonary complaints.

Treatment

- Supportive care should be provided while performing diagnostic evaluation and continued while initiating treatment for specific toxic ingestions.
- The dose and time of exposure should be determined for all substances involved.

DIRECTING PATIENT COURSE

The health-care provider should call the poison control center when:

- any toxic effects are present.
- coingestant, drug interaction, or underlying disease presents unusual problems.

Admission Considerations

The decision to admit depends on the specific toxic agent (if discovered) and any manifestations that develop.

DECONTAMINATION

- Out of Hospital

—Induced emesis is not recommended when the toxic agent is unknown.

- In hospital

—Gastric lavage should be performed in pediatric (tube size 24–32 French) or adult (tube size 36–42 French) patients for large ingestion presenting within 1 hour of ingestion or if serious effects are present.
—One dose of activated charcoal (1–2 g/kg) should be administered without a cathartic if a substantial ingestion has occurred within the previous few hours.

ANTIDOTES

Antidotes to specific toxins should be used as indicated by evaluation (see SECTIONS III and IV).

ADJUNCTIVE TREATMENT

- Hypoxia and electrolytes should be corrected as clinically indicated.
- Tachy- or bradycardia should be treated if clinically indicated.
- Blood pressure and perfusion should be supported as clinically indicated.
- Hypertension should be treated if clinically indicated; short-acting and easily reversible agents should be chosen because most hypertensive effects of drugs are transient and may be followed by hypotension.

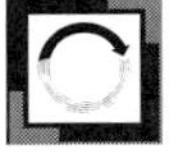

Follow-Up

DISCHARGE CRITERIA/INSTRUCTIONS

Asymptomatic patients may be discharged following decontamination, a 6-hour observation period, and psychiatric evaluation if needed.

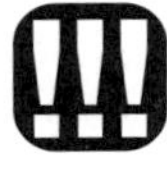

Pitfalls

Toxic ingestion should always be considered as a cause of altered mental status or vital signs.

See also: SECTION I, Urine Drug Screen chapter; SECTION II, Acute Renal Failure, Anion Gap Metabolic Acidosis, Bradycardia, Coma, Hyperthermia, Hypotension, Hypothermia, Movement Disorders, Nontoxic Ingestion, Odors, Pulmonary Edema, Tachysdysrhythmia, and Withdrawal—Depressants and Stimulants chapters.

Author: Steven A. Seifert

Reviewer: Katherine M. Hurlbut

Urinary Color Change

Basics

DESCRIPTION

A variety of urinary color changes may occur due to excretion of parent chemical or its metabolites in the urine.

PATHOPHYSIOLOGY

- The yellow color of urine is due to a number of pigments, predominantly urochrome.
- Urine concentration affects its color; more concentrated urine usually is deeper in color than less concentrated urine.

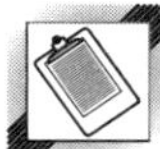

Diagnosis

DIFFERENTIAL DIAGNOSIS

Further information on each poison is available in SECTION IV, CHEMICAL AND BIOLOGICAL AGENTS.

- Bright yellow urine may be caused by:

—Bilirubin (unconjugated bilirubin can be differentiated from urobilin by shaking; bilirubin produces yellow foam when shaken)
—Fluorescein dye
—Phenacetin, an analgesic
—Riboflavin (vitamin B_2)

- Orange urine may be caused by:

—Bilirubin (unconjugated bilirubin can be differentiated from urobilin by shaking; bilirubin produces yellow foam when shaken)
—Carrots
—Dehydration
—Phenazopyridine (Pyridium), which produces orange foam, the color of which is heightened by hydrochloride
—Rifampin, which may discolor all body fluids
—Sulfasalazine, in alkaline urine
—Vitamin A
—Warfarin, an anticoagulant, in alkaline urine

- Red urine may be caused by:

—Heme pigments, specifically erythrocytes, hemoglobin, or myoglobin
—Aminosalicyclic acid, an antituberculous agent, which causes red urine when hypochlorite bleach (found in toilet cleaners) is added
—Aniline dyes
—Bile
—Carbon tetrachloride, a solvent
—Chloroquine, an antimalarial agent
—Chlorzoxazone, a muscle relaxant
—Doxorubicin, a chemotherapeutic agent
—Heparin, an anticoagulant that may cause hemoglobinuria
—Ibuprofen, an analgesic and antipyretic
—Phenacetin, an analgesic
—Phenothiazine, a class of antipsychotics that includes chlorpromazine, thioridazine, fluphenazine, and trifluoperazine
—Phensuximide, an anticonvulsant
—Phenytoin, an anticonvulsant
—Porphyrins, which darken urine upon standing
—"Red diaper syndrome," which may occur from a nonpathogenic chromobacterium, Serratia marcescens
—Rhodamine B, a nontoxic, vegetable-based food dye
—Rifampin, which may discolor all body fluids
—Trinitrophenol, a pesticide and insecticide
—Warfarin, an anticoagulant that may cause hemoglobinuria
—Acidic red urine, due to beets (which contain anthocyanin pigments), blackberries, methemoglobin, or metronidazole (an antibiotic)
—Alkaline red urine due to aloe laxatives, anthraquinone laxatives (cascara, rhubarb), eosin (a laboratory stain pigment), levodopa (an anti-parkinsonian agent), methyldopa (Aldomet, an anti-parkinsonian agent), phenazopyridine (Pyridium, which turns orange when hydrochloride is added), phenolphthalein (the chemical used in acid-base test strips and as a laxative, which is red-purple in alkali and clear in acid), and senna laxatives

- Purple urine may be caused by:

—Chlorzoxazone, a muscle relaxant
—Porphyrins, which darken urine upon standing
—Phenolphthalein, the chemical used in acid-base test strips (turning red-purple in alkali and clear in acid) and used as a laxative
—Senna laxatives, in alkaline urine

- Blue-green urine may be caused by:

—Amitriptyline (Elavil), an antidepressant
—Bile
—Biliverdin, which causes a positive dipstick for bile, produces green foam when shaken, and may accumulate with chronic obstructive jaundice
—Boric acid, an insecticide
—"Blue diaper syndrome," which occurs in infants with a metabolic defect of tryptophan absorption and, possibly, hypercalcemia and nephrocalcinosis
—Carbolic acid, an antiseptic
—Evans blue dye
—Guaiacol, which is found in some cough remedies
—Indigo-carmine dye
—Indomethacin, an analgesic
—Magnesium salicylate (Doan's pills), an analgesic
—Methocarbamol (Robaxin), which darkens urine upon standing.
—Methylene blue, a diagnostic medicinal dye and antidote for methemoglobinemia
—Propofol (Diprivan), a sedative, when used as infusion
—Pseudomonas bacteriuria
—Thymol, which is found in Listerine
—Triamterene, a potassium-sparing diuretic, which fluoresces blue in acidic urine

- Yellow-green urine may be caused by:

—Biliverdin, which causes a positive dipstick for bile, produces green foam when shaken, and may accumulate with chronic obstructive jaundice
—Cresol (Chloraseptic), which darkens urine upon standing
—Methocarbamol (Robaxin), which darkens urine upon standing
—Phenol, which darkens upon standing and is found in cleaners such as Chloraseptic

• Brown urine may be caused by:

—Heme pigments, specifically erythrocytes, hemoglobin, or myoglobin
—Aloe laxatives
—Anthraquinone laxatives (cascara, rhubarb)
—Aniline dyes
—Bile
—Carbon tetrachloride, a solvent
—Chloroquine, an antimalarial agent
—Cresol (Chloraseptic), which darkens urine upon standing.
—Doxorubicin, a chemotherapeutic agent
—Eosin, a laboratory pigment that appears green under fluorescent light
—Homogentisic acid, which becomes blue-green when ferric chloride is added and accumulates in patients with alkaptonuria
—Ibuprofen, an analgesic
—Levodopa, an anti-parkinsonian agent
—Melanin, which blackens urine upon standing and with the ferric chloride test, and becomes red with the sodium nitroprusside test
—Melanogen, which blackens urine upon standing and with the ferric chloride and sodium nitroprusside tests, and which may be found in patients with melanoma
—Methemoglobin
—Methocarbamol (Robaxin), which darkens urine upon standing
—Methyldopa (Aldomet), an anti-parkinsonian agent
—Metronidazole, an antibiotic
—Naphthol, which is used in the manufacture of dyes and perfumes
—Naphthalene, a type of mothball
—Nitrofurantoin, an antibiotic often used for urinary tract infection (UTI)
—Phenacetin, an analgesic
—Phenazopyridine (Pyridium), which produces orange foam, and the color of which is heightened by hydrochloride
—Phenol, which may be found in dyes and cleaners such as Chloraseptic
—Phenothiazine, a class of antipsychotics that includes chlorpromazine, mesoridazine, thioridazine, fluphenazine, and trifluoperazine
—Phensuximide, an anticonvulsant
—Phenytoin, an anticonvulsant
—Porphyrins, which darken urine upon standing and fluoresce with ultraviolet light
—Povidone-iodine, an antiseptic
—Quinine
—Senna laxatives, in acidic urine
—Sulfamethoxazole, an antibiotic often used for UTI
—Thymol, which is found in Listerine
—Triamterene, a diuretic that fluoresces blue in acidic urine.

• White urine may be caused by:

—Chyle, which may be found with defects of lymphatic circulation
—Lipids, which may be associated with hyperlipidemia, nephrotic syndrome, or trauma of large, marrow-containing bones
—Neutrophils, which may cause a cloudy urinary appearance with UTI
—Oxalic acid
—Phosphates
—Radiographic dyes, which may cause a cloudy urinary appearance

SIGNS AND SYMPTOMS

• Dermatologic

—Hepatic failure that turns urine yellow may be associated with jaundice.
—Ecchymoses and petechiae with red or brown urine may occur with overcoagulation.
—Cyanosis with blue or brown urine may occur with methemoglobinemia.
—Porphyria (red or purple urine) causes dermatologic lesions.

• Pulmonary. Dyspnea and blue or brown urine may accompany methemoglobinemia.
• Gastrointestinal. Episodic abdominal pain with red or purple urine may accompany porphyria.
• Hepatic

—Hepatic failure may cause urine to appear bright yellow from increased bilirubin.
—Bilirubin also may be present in the urine with biliary obstruction or obstructive hepatic disease.
—Early hepatitis, cirrhosis, or hemolytic jaundice may produce urobilin (bright yellow urine).

• Renal. Renal failure may be associated with hemoglobinuria, proteinuria, and pyuria.
• Neurologic

—Ataxia and sedation may accompany the use of phenytoin (red or brown urine).
—Delirium and other neuropsychiatric symptoms may occur from porphyria (red or purple urine).

PROCEDURES AND LABORATORY TESTS

• O-tolidine urine dipstick test. A few drops of urine placed on this commonly available dipstick test helps differentiate hemoglobinuria from myoglobinuria or other causes of urinary color change.

—Hemoglobinuria causes a positive dipstick (O-tolidine) test result for blood.
—Myoglobinuria causes a negative dipstick (O-tolidine) test result for blood.
—Bilirubin causes a positive dipstick (O-tolidine) test result for bile; bilirubin produces yellow foam when shaken, which differentiates it from urobilin.
—Biliverdin causes a positive dipstick (O-tolidine) test result for bile; biliverdin is a green bile pigment formed from cholesterol breakdown that produces green foam when shaken.

• Light microscopy

—Red blood cells may be seen with hemoglobinuria.
—A positive urine dipstick test result for blood, but no red cells on microscopy, is typically seen with myoglobinuria or hemoglobinemia.
—White blood cells may be seen following urinary tract infection.

ICD-9-CM

No specific code available.

RECOMMENDED READING

Cone TE Jr. Diagnosis and treatment: some syndromes, diseases and conditions associated with abnormal coloration of the urine or diaper. Pediatrics 1968;41:654–658.

Raymond JR, Yarger WE. Abnormal urine color: differential diagnosis. South Med J 1988;81:837–841.

Authors: Lada Kokan and Kennon Heard

Reviewer: Richard C. Dart

Ventricular Dysrhythmias

Basics

DESCRIPTION

This discussion covers abnormal ventricular rhythms or conductions arising from toxic causes.

PATHOPHYSIOLOGY

Ventricular dysrhythmias caused by toxic agents may involve several mechanisms.

- Myocardial ischemia may be due to vessel spasm, hypotension or hypoxia; hypoxia can be caused by direct lung injury, alteration of hemoglobin, or hypoventilation.
- Electrolyte abnormalities, especially hyperkalemia, hypocalcemia, or hypomagnesemia, can cause ventricular dysrhythmias.
- Blockade of ion channels in the myocardium, particularly sodium or calcium channels, may result in ventricular dysrhythmias.

RISK FACTORS

Underlying cardiovascular disease may predispose to development of dysrhythmias.

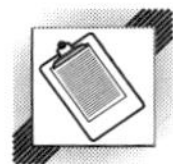

Diagnosis

DIFFERENTIAL DIAGNOSIS

Further information on each poison is available in SECTION IV, Chemical and Biological Agents.

Toxicologic Causes

Associated findings with ventricular dysrhythmias may help confirm the identity of the poison involved.

- Tricyclic antidepressants (TCAs)

—Dysrhythmia is usually heralded by a QRS complex of 100 msec or more and altered mental status.
—Additional findings may include seizure, hypotension, and presence of an R wave in ECG lead aVR.
—Phenothiazines produce similar effects.

- Cocaine, amphetamines, and other sympathomimetic agents (ephedrine, phenylpropanolamine, β_2 receptor agonists) present with sinus tachycardia or ventricular tachydysrhythmias and are often associated with hypertension, hyperthermia, agitation, delirium, seizures, and rhabdomyolysis.
- Antihistamine and anticholinergic agents (diphenhydramine, scopolamine, jimsonweed weed, hydroxyzine, phenothiazine, dramamine, etc.) present with sinus tachycardia or ventricular dysrhythmias and may be indicated by flushing, dilated pupils, diminished bowel sounds, hyperthermia, hallucination, agitation, and delirium. Widening of the QRS complex and prolongation of the QT interval occur in a severe overdose.
- Theophylline is associated with tremor, vomiting, seizures, dysrhythmias, hypokalemia, mild metabolic acidosis, and preexisting diagnosis of chronic obstructive pulmonary disease. Sinus tachycardia and atrial and ventricular ectopy are most common. Ventricular tachycardia is rare, although ventricular fibrillation may occur following a single massive overdose.
- Type Ia antiarrhythmic agents (quinidine, procainamide, disopyramide) all cause QT interval prolongation.
- Digitalis may produce visual complaints, heart block, vomiting, hyperkalemia (acute), or hypokalemia (chronic intoxication). Premature ventricular contractions are the most common digitalis-induced dysrhythmias, although any dysrhythmia, even tachydysrhythmias, may result from digitalis toxicity.
- Monoamine oxidase (MAO) inhibitors may cause hyperthermia, hypertension, muscle rigidity and altered mental status. Ventricular tachydysrhythmias are often the presenting cardiovascular effect of MAO inhibitor ingestion.
- Carbamazepine is associated with coma, hyponatremia, and nystagmus. In a large overdose, carbamazepine may produce cardiac effects similar to TCAs.
- Organophosphate or carbamate pesticides also may cause vomiting, diarrhea, salivation, lacrimation, urination, bronchorrhea, small pupils, and sweating. Classically, organophosphates has been reported to cause bradydysrhythmias, but in reality, sinus tachycardia is often the presenting dysrhythmia.
- Substances that produce methemoglobinemia often cause cyanosis.
- Thyroid hormones generally cause supraventricular tachycardia; ventricular dysrhythmia may complicate severe cases. They are associated with history of thyroid disease, tremor, and fever.

NONTOXICOLOGIC CAUSES

Nontoxicologic causes include primarily coronary artery disease, congenital cardiac abnormalities, intracranial bleed, hypoglycemia, electrolyte abnormalities, or hypoxia.

SIGNS AND SYMPTOMS

- Patients may develop weakness, dizziness, chest pain, palpitations, or any symptom of hypoxia.
- Syncope, seizure, or cardiac arrest may occur precipitously in severe cases; syncope should be considered a sign of ventricular dysrhythmia until proven otherwise.

Vital Signs

Hypertension may indicate sympathomimetic toxicity or withdrawal from alcohol, sedative-hypnotic agents, or MAO inhibitors.

HEENT

Dilated pupils suggest anticholinergic or sympathomimetic toxicity.

Dermatologic

- Flushed, dry skin suggests an anticholinergic agent.
- Pale, sweaty skin may be associated with sympathomimetic drugs, cholinergic agents, or hypotension.
- Cyanosis suggests hypoxia or methemoglobinemia.

Cardiovascular

- QRS widening prior to ventricular tachycardia suggests poisoning by type 1 antiarrhythmics, TCAs, phenothiazine, antihistamine, chloroquine, quinine, sotalol and several others.
- "Slow VT" suggests digitalis or calcium channel blocker toxicity.

Pulmonary

Cholinergic agonists may produce bronchorrhea and wheezing.

Gastrointestinal

- Vomiting is commonly associated with digitalis, iron, salicylate, or theophylline intoxication.
- Diminished bowel sounds suggest an anticholinergic agent.

Renal

Urinary retention suggests an anticholinergic agent.

Fluids and Electrolytes

- Hypokalemia suggests a β-receptor agonist or theophylline.
- Hyperkalemia may indicate acute digitalis intoxication.

Neurologic

- Hallucinations and delirium suggest an anticholinergic agent or abuse of stimulants or hallucinogens.
- Anxiety, tremor, and seizures suggest theophylline or withdrawal from alcohol or sedative-hypnotic drugs.
- Coma and seizure suggest TCAs or type 1 antidysrhythmic drugs.
- CNS depression or coma, nystagmus, ataxia, diminished bowel sounds, or hyponatremia suggest carbamazepine.

PROCEDURES AND LABORATORY TESTS

Essential Tests

- ECG and continuous cardiac monitoring should be performed to assess conduction abnormalities and evaluate underlying cardiac disease or ischemia.
- Arterial blood gases should be obtained in patients with clinical effects or who are receiving bicarbonate therapy.
- Serum electrolytes, glucose, BUN, creatinine, calcium, magnesium, and phosphorus levels should be obtained to evaluate for other causes of dysrhythmia.

Recommended Tests

• Serum salicylate, methanol, ethylene glycol, iron, lactate, and carboxyhemoglobin levels should be obtained in cases of metabolic acidosis of unknown etiology with tachycardia.
• Serum acetaminophen and aspirin levels should be obtained in overdose settings to detect an occult overdose.
• Urine toxicology screen should be performed in patients with dysrhythmia of unknown cause.

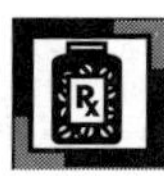

Treatment

• Supportive care with appropriate airway management is vital; many patients require endotracheal intubation. Specific treatment should be initiated while supportive care continues.
• The dose and time of exposure should be determined for all substances involved.

DIRECTING PATIENT COURSE

The health-care provider should call the poison control center when:

• The cause of dysrhythmia is unclear.
• Coingestant, drug interaction, or underlying disease presents unusual problems.

Admission Considerations

All patients with new ventricular dysrhythmia should be admitted to an intensive care unit.

DECONTAMINATION

• Emesis should not be induced because coma or seizures may develop abruptly.
• Gastric lavage should be performed in pediatric (tube size 16–28 French) and adult (tube size 36–42 French) patients for large ingestion presenting within 1 hour of ingestion or if serious effects are present.
• One dose of activated charcoal (1–2 g/kg) should be administered without a cathartic if a substantial ingestion has occurred within the previous few hours.

ANTIDOTES

• There is no antidote specific to ventricular dysrhythmias.
• Antidotes to specific toxins should be used as indicated by evaluation (see SECTIONS III and IV).

ADJUNCTIVE TREATMENT

Hypoxia and Electrolyte Abnormalities

Hypoxia and electrolyte abnormalities should be corrected as clinically indicated.

Bradydysrhythmia

Standard agents, including atropine and isoproterenol, are usually ineffective; early use of specific antidotes followed by a pacemaker is recommended.

Ventricular Dysrhythmias

For stable patients, drug therapy may be begun without delay; for unstable patients, the Advanced Cardiac Life Support algorithm should be used.

Sodium Bicarbonate

• Indication: Widening of the QRS complex to more than 0.16 seconds. Some authorities recommend treatment at the QRS complex to more than 0.12 seconds.
• Dosage: A dose of 1 to 2 mEq/kg should be administered in an intravenous bolus and repeated as needed but should not raise the arterial pH above 7.55.
• Simultaneous hyperventilation and bicarbonate therapy must be undertaken cautiously because they may cause severe alkalemia.

Lidocaine

• Indication: Frequent premature ventricular contractions or ventricular tachycardia.
• Adult dose is 1.0 to 1.5 mg/kg in an intravenous push, and infusion should be titrated from 1 to 4 mg/min to maintain suppression; doses of 0.50 to 0.75 mg/kg boluses may be repeated and maintenance infusions increased every 5 to 10 minutes until ventricular tachycardia resolves or a total of 3 mg/kg has been given.
• Pediatric dose is 1 mg/kg intravenously, intraosseously, or endotracheally, and the same dose may be repeated in 10 to 15 minutes; if a second dose is required, infusion should be started at 20 to 50 μg/kg/min.
• Lidocaine dosage should be reduced in patients with hepatic insufficiency, congestive heart failure, or cardiogenic shock and in patients over 70 years of age.

Phenytoin or Fosphenytoin

• Indication: Ventricular dysrhythmia unresponsive to other agents.
• Dosage: Phenytoin loading dose for adults and children is 15 to 20 mg/kg intravenously, and the rate of infusion should not exceed 50 mg/min (adults) or 1.5 mg/kg/min (children); maintenance dose for adults is 100 mg every 6 to 8 hours, and ECG and blood pressure should be monitored during infusion, which should be stopped if dysrhythmia or hypotension occurs.
• Fosphenytoin loading dose is 15 to 20 mg of phenytoin equivalents/kg, given at a rate of 100 to 150 mg phenytoin equivalents/min.
• Bretylium should be avoided, because alpha-blocking effects may worsen hypotension; other class IA antiarrhythmic agents should also be avoided because they may worsen dysrhythmias.

Torsade de pointes

• Electrolyte abnormalities, if present, should be corrected first.
• Quinidine, disopyramide, procainamide, amiodarone, and bretylium should be avoided because they prolong the QT interval.
• In adults, 1 to 2 g of magnesium sulfate should be administered in an intravenous push, and the dose may be repeated in 10 to 15 minutes; intravenous infusion should begin at 2 to 10 mg/min and titrated to antidysrhythmic effect.
• In children, 25 to 50 mg/kg of magnesium sulfate should be administered intravenously over 5 minutes.
• Isoproterenol should be administered 2 to 4 μg/ml, initially 0.5 to 1.0 μg/min, and titrated to effect; in children, 0.1 μg/kg/min may be administered and titrated to effect.
• Overdrive pacing may be used for unresponsive patients.

Hypotension

The primary treatment of hypotension is correction of the dysrhythmia; in addition, 10 to 20 ml/kg of 0.9% saline should be administered, the patient placed in the Trendelenburg position, and a vasopressor administered if needed.

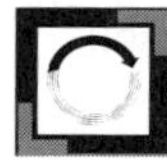

Follow-Up

PATIENT MONITORING

Respiratory and cardiac monitoring should be performed continuously in an intensive care setting.

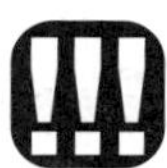

Pitfalls

The airway must be managed aggressively; many toxic deaths are due to hypoxic injury or aspiration.

ICD-9-CM 427.89

Other specified cardiac dysrhythmias: other.

See also: SECTION II, Hypertension and Seizures chapters; and SECTION IV, specific toxic agents.

RECOMMENDED READING

Hessler R. Cardiovascular principles. In: Goldfrank LR, et al., eds. Goldfrank's toxicologic emergencies, 6th ed. Norwalk, CT: Appleton & Lange, 1998.

Author: Richard C. Dart

Reviewer: Katherine M. Hurlbut

Visual Loss Complaints

Basics

DESCRIPTION

This discussion covers acute changes in vision clarity or acuity that may be associated with a toxic exposure.

PATHOPHYSIOLOGY

- Visual loss may result from damage to the ocular structures (cornea, lens, and aqueous and vitreous humors) or to nerves radiating from the retina or the ocular cortex.
- Distorted or blurred vision may arise from an ocular injury or a drug effect on extraocular muscles.

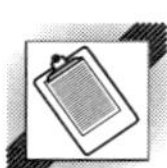

Diagnosis

DIFFERENTIAL DIAGNOSIS

Further information on each poison is available in SECTION IV, Chemical and Biological Agents.

Common Toxicologic Causes

- Methanol poisoning may cause complaints of "snowstorm" or blurred vision, abdominal pain, altered mental status, vomiting, increased anion gap metabolic acidosis, and pale optic disk.
- Quinine, chloroquine, and quinidine are also associated with mydriasis, tachycardia, tinnitus, dizziness, vomiting, and dysrhythmias.
- Acidic or basic caustic substances splashed in an eye (acids, alkali, phenol) may produce severe corneal pain, ulceration, edema, and opacification, unless highly dilute in form.
- Excessive lacrimation and irritation are associated with ocular irritants (e.g., mace, pepper spray, tear gas).
- Anticholinergic agents (topical ophthalmologic ingestion) may cause blurred vision due to extreme pupil dilation.
- Digitalis and cardiac glycosides may cause photophobia, yellow-green visual distortion (xanthopsia), halos, and cardiac dysrhythmia.

Uncommon Toxicologic Causes

- Botulism may produce blurred vision or difficulty focusing, as well as dysphagia, weakness, and bulbar palsies.
- Cisplatin may rarely cause reversible visual loss with alteration of color vision, papilledema, and retrobulbar neuritis.
- Corneal damage, or "crack eye," has been described following exposure during inhalation crack cocaine use. These symptoms may be delayed due to the local anesthetic effects of cocaine.
- Cataracts and glaucoma have been reported with chronic use of systemic corticosteroids.
- Decreased vision, visual fields, and color vision have been associated with chronic deferoxamine therapy; in most cases, visual symptoms are reversible.
- Visual symptoms of ergot toxicity may occur because of vasospasm or clot formation.
- Visual changes, including tunnel vision, may result from significant exposures to elemental or organic mercury.
- Pitch fumes may cause photosensitization keratitis.
- Talc retinopathy has been associated with chronic intravenous drug abuse.
- Chronic toluene abuse may cause optic nerve atrophy.
- Hydroxychloroquine may produce neurotoxicity with subacute myelo-optic neuropathy, potentially leading to loss of vision.
- Ethambutol may cause optic neuropathy (with chronic use), color vision disturbance, or blindness.
- Ciguatera toxins may rarely cause extraocular paresis, blurred vision, dilated pupils, and transient blindness.
- Vitamin A may produce diplopia, headache, desquamation, papilledema, and increased liver enzymes.
- Thallium may rarely cause optic neuritis, decreased visual acuity, and impaired color vision.

Nontoxicologic Causes

- Binocular visual loss may result from acute angle closure glaucoma, blunt head trauma, electrical injury, high altitude illness, papilledema from any cause, or porphyria.
- Monocular visual loss may result from central retinal artery occlusion, migraine headache, orbital cellulitis, retinal detachment or hemorrhage, subarachnoid hemorrhage, temporal arteritis, thromboembolic stroke, or transient ischemic attack.

SIGNS AND SYMPTOMS

Associated physical signs may help identify the poison involved when they occur in a patient with decreased visual clarity or acuity.

History

- Patients may note diminished visual fields (tunnel vision), complete absence of light and shadow, or blurred or otherwise distorted vision.
- Methanol toxicity is typically described as looking through a snowstorm.

Vital Signs

Tachycardia, and in severe cases hypotension, may occur with severe methanol, quinine, or chloroquine poisoning.

HEENT

- During direct examination of the eye, careful attention should be directed to the pupil size, shape, and reactivity; any conjunctival hemorrhage or hyperemia; foreign objects; ptosis; clouding of the lens or vitreous; or retinal hyperemia or changes in the optic disk.
- Acute corneal and conjunctival irritation or caustic injury may be caused by direct injury from acid or alkaline corrosives, irritant gases (chlorine, nitrogen dioxide, or many others), or lacrimators (tear gas or pepper spray).
- Blurred or snowstorm visual complaints with optic disc hyperemia and retinal edema progressing to dilated, unreactive pupils indicate methanol poisoning.
- Blurred vision, scotomata, and decreased vision with retinal edema and dilated, unreactive pupils may indicate quinine toxicity.
- Markedly dilated pupils may indicate an anticholinergic agent.

Dermatologic

Evidence of marked vasoconstriction (peripheral pallor or cyanosis) may indicate ergotamine toxicity.

Cardiovascular

Cardiac dysrhythmias may indicate digitalis, quinine, chloroquine, or quinidine poisoning.

Pulmonary

Cough, shortness of breath, or other symptoms of mucous membrane irritation may indicate irritant gas or mist.

Gastrointestinal

- Nausea and vomiting are features of cinchonism from quinine, chloroquine, or quinidine toxicity.
- Abdominal pain and vomiting are common with methanol poisoning.

Fluids and Electrolytes

- Increased anion gap metabolic acidosis with loss of vision may indicate methanol poisoning.
- Hypocalcemia may be associated with hydrogen fluoride (direct eye contact injury).

Neurologic

CNS depression and coma may result from ingestion of methanol, quinine, chloroquine, or quinidine toxicity.

PROCEDURES AND LABORATORY TESTS

- Visual acuity should be measured using the Snellen eye chart.
- Ocular pH testing should be performed after topical exposure; the pH should return to the normal range of 6.5 to 7.5 after decontamination.
- Elevated serum methanol levels confirm exposure; peak levels higher than 20 mg/dl may cause serious retinal toxicity if not treated appropriately.
- Serum electrolytes should be obtained to detect increased anion gap metabolic acidosis.
- Serum quinine levels higher than 15 μg/ml in the first 10 hours following exposure are associated with a risk of permanent blindness.
- Serum digoxin levels confirm exposure.
- Slit-lamp examination with fluorescein is essential to document corneal damage following topical ocular exposure.
- Determination of intraocular pressure should be performed to rule out glaucoma.

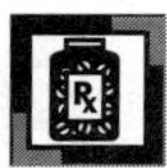

Treatment

- Supportive care with immediate irrigation for ocular and dermal exposures is vital.
- The dose and time of exposure should be determined for all substances involved.

DIRECTING PATIENT COURSE

The health-care provider should call the poison control center when:

- Cause of visual complaints is unclear.
- Coingestant, drug interaction, or underlying disease presents unusual problems.

Admission Considerations

The need for admission is based on identity of the toxicant and clinical effects.

DECONTAMINATION

Out of Hospital

Copious irrigation with tap water or isotonic saline for 15 to 30 minutes is recommended for nearly all topical ocular exposures.

In Hospital

Copious irrigation with isotonic saline or Ringer's lactate is recommended following ocular and dermal exposure.

- At least 2 liters per affected eye is recommended.
- Continuous irrigation may be needed for an hour or more following severe alkali burns involving concentrated or large amounts of alkali or agents that are strong bases (e.g., sodium hydroxide) or that penetrate tissue readily (e.g., ammonium hydroxide).
- If a caustic agent is involved, the ocular pH should be tested after 2 liters of irrigation and every 15 minutes thereafter to ensure that a normal ocular pH (6.5–7.5) is achieved.
- The eyelids should be retracted for thorough irrigation, and a topical anesthetic may be needed if severe pain limits access to the cornea.
- A scleral irrigator (Morgan lens) may be used to aid irrigation.

ANTIDOTES

- Fomepizole

—Indication. Methanol poisoning.
—Contraindications. None.
—Method of administration. Loading dose of 15 mg/kg followed by maintenance dose of 10 mg/kg every 12 hours until methanol level is less than 20 mg/dl.
—Alternative antidote is ethanol. See fomepizole and ethanol chapters for further information.

ADJUNCTIVE TREATMENT

- Topical antibiotics effective against Staphylococcus and Pseudomonas organisms may be used prophylactically for corneal and mucosal injuries.
- Cycloplegics may reduce pain and decrease the likelihood of formation of synechiae following corneal injury.
- Systemic analgesics and an eye patch also may reduce pain; topical anesthetics can be used initially in the emergency department to aid irrigation if intense pain and blepharospasm make irrigation difficult, but topical anesthetics should never be dispensed to a patient, nor should they ever be used repeatedly.
- Polyethylene glycol (PEG-400, Golytely) may be effective after phenol exposure; water or saline, however, are more readily available, and irrigation with either should not be delayed while the PEG solution is sought.

—Contraindications. None.
—Method of administration. Copious irrigation with at least 2 to 4 liters of polyethylene glycol per affected eye is the goal.
—Potential adverse effects. None.

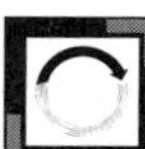

Follow-Up

EXPECTED COURSE AND PROGNOSIS

- Recovery from visual disturbances from methanol or quinine toxicity varies from full recovery to loss of visual fields or complete blindness.
- The prognosis following alkali injury may become evident 48 to 72 hours after exposure, but severe scarring and blindness is much more common than with other caustic agents.
- Recovery from other direct corneal poisons is typically rapid and complete once corneal epithelialization occurs.

DISCHARGE CRITERIA/INSTRUCTIONS

- Patients with corneal injury caused by topical exposure can usually be discharged with ophthamologic follow-up.
- Patients with visual effects from systemic poison often require admission.

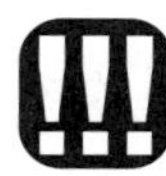

Pitfalls

- Failure to recognize that methanol or quinine poisoning is involved in a visual complaint may lead to inadequate treatment, resulting in blindness.
- Lack of pain should not be mistaken for a sign of minimal damage; ocular exposures that cause serious injury in which nerve endings are severely damaged may be painless.

ICD-9-CM 976

Poisoning by agents primarily affecting skin and mucous membrane, ophthalmologic, otorhinolaryngologic, and dental drugs.

See also: SECTION III, Ethanol chapter; and SECTION IV, Anticholinergic Compounds, Caustics—Acidic, Caustics—Basic, Methanol, Quinine, and Fomepizole chapters.

RECOMMENDED READING

Grant WM. Toxicology of the eye. Springfield, IL: Charles C. Thomas, 1986.

Smilkstein MJ. Ophthalmologic Principles. In: Goldfrank LR et al., eds. Goldfrank's toxicologic emergencies, 6th ed. Norwalk, CT: Appleton & Lange, 1998.

Smilkstein MJ, Kulig KW, Rumack BH. Acute toxic blindness: unrecognized quinine poisoning. Ann Emerg Med 1987;16:98–101.

Authors: Lada Kokan and Gerald F. O'Malley

Reviewers: Katherine M. Hurlbut and Kennon Heard

Withdrawal—Depressants and Stimulants

Basics

DESCRIPTION

- Withdrawal is characterized by physical or psychological signs and symptoms that occur following discontinuation of a drug.
- This discussion covers withdrawal from alcohol, benzodiazepine, opioid, stimulant, and sedative-hypnotic classes of drugs.

PATHOPHYSIOLOGY

Alcohol and Sedative-Hypnotic Withdrawal

Chronic ethanol or sedative-hypnotic use produces downward regulation of inhibitory CNS receptors and a suppression of gamma-aminobutyric acid (GABA) production; withdrawal states are characterized by a relative GABA deficiency. Sedative-hypnotic withdrawal is caused by cessation of any of numerous compounds, including benzodiazepines (diazepam, chlordiazepoxide, clonazepam, lorazepam, and many others), intermediate-acting barbiturates (phenobarbital, pentobarbital, and many others), chloral hydrate, ethchlorvynol, glutethimide, meprobamate, and methaqualone and gammahydroxybutyric acid (GHB).

Opioid Withdrawal

Chronic opioid use produces downward regulation of CNS opioid receptors. Substances capable of producing opioid withdrawal upon cessation include codeine, alphaprodine, buprenorphine, butorphanol, diamorphine, diphenoxylate, fentanyl, sufentanil, remifentanil, dihydrocodeine, hydrocodone, hydromorphone, levorphanol, meperidine, methadone, morphine, nalbuphine, opium, oxycodone, oxymorphone, pentazocine, and propoxyphene.

Stimulant Withdrawal

Chronic stimulant use produces CNS dopaminergic excess; withdrawal states are characterized by a relative dopamine deficiency. Substances capable of producing stimulant withdrawal upon cessation include caffeine, nicotine, cocaine, amphetamines, methamphetamine, and phenylpropanolamine.

PREGNANCY AND LACTATION

- Neonatal withdrawal syndromes have been reported in infants born to mothers addicted to opioids, stimulants, ethanol, or sedative hypnotic agents.

CAUSES

- Withdrawal syndrome may result from abrupt cessation or from decreasing the dosage of a drug.
- Administration of an antagonist or partial antagonist may precipitate withdrawal symptoms in addicted patients.

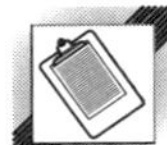

Diagnosis

DIFFERENTIAL DIAGNOSIS

Further information on each poison is available in SECTION IV, Chemical and Biological Agents.

Alcohol or Sedative-Hypnotic Withdrawal

- Toxicologic causes of symptoms that resemble alcohol or sedative-hypnotic withdrawal include neuroleptic malignant syndrome, malignant hyperthermia, serotonin syndrome, monoamine oxidase inhibitor toxicity, sympathomimetic toxicity, anticholinergic toxicity, clonidine withdrawal, theophylline toxicity, thyroid hormone toxicity, and nicotine toxicity.
- Nontoxicologic causes of symptoms that resemble alcohol or sedative-hypnotic withdrawal include hyperthyroidism, pheochromocytoma, heat stroke, intracranial hemorrhage, cerebral vascular accident, intracranial infection, seizures, and acute or chronic psychosis.
- Withdrawal from sedative-hypnotic agents may be life threatening in elderly patients.

Stimulant Withdrawal

- Toxicologic causes of symptoms that resemble stimulant withdrawal include opioid toxicity, sedative-hypnotic toxicity, and toxicity caused by agents capable of producing CNS depression.
- Nontoxicologic causes of symptoms that resemble stimulant withdrawal include intracranial infection, cerebral vascular accident, intracranial hemorrhage, acute depression, and seizure with postictal period.

SIGNS AND SYMPTOMS

Withdrawal syndromes generally result in findings that are the opposite of the usual drug effects.

Vital Signs

Alcohol or sedative-hypnotic withdrawal produces low-grade fever, tachycardia, and hypertension.

HEENT

- Sneezing, yawning, rhinorrhea, and lacrimation are common in cases of opioid withdrawal.
- Dilated pupils are common in cases of alcohol or sedative-hypnotic, opioid, or stimulant withdrawal.

Dermatologic

- Diaphoresis is common in cases of alcohol or sedative-hypnotic withdrawal.
- Piloerection is common in cases of opioid withdrawal.

Cardiovascular

- Tachycardia and hypertension are the hallmarks of both alcohol and sedative-hypnotic withdrawal.
- Tachycardia related to agitation and dehydration may accompany opioid withdrawal.
- Cocaine withdrawal may produce ST segment elevation.

Gastrointestinal

- Nausea, vomiting, abdominal cramping, increased bowel sounds, and diarrhea are common in cases of opioid withdrawal
- Nausea and vomiting also may accompany ethanol and sedative-hypnotic withdrawal.

Fluids and Electrolytes

- Dehydration with hypokalemic metabolic alkalosis may accompany severe opioid withdrawal.
- In cases of alcohol or sedative-hypnotic withdrawal, seizures may cause lactic acidosis.

Musculoskeletal

- In cases of alcohol or sedative-hypnotic withdrawal, seizures can cause rhabdomyolysis.
- Opioid withdrawal commonly produces myalgias.

Neurologic

- Seizures are common in cases of alcohol or sedative-hypnotic withdrawal.
- Seizures may be associated with opioid withdrawal in neonates born to mothers addicted to opioids, but such seizures are not associated with isolated opioid withdrawal in adults.
- Delirium tremens is the most severe form of alcohol withdrawal and is characterized by hyperthermia, tachycardia, hypertension, altered mental status, persistent hallucinations, and seizures.
- Stimulant withdrawal may produce generalized fatigue, dysphoria, irritability, and depression.
- Although stimulant withdrawal can cause extreme sleepiness that responds to verbal and tactile stimulation, it does not produce true alteration of mental status.

PROCEDURES AND LABORATORY TESTS

- No test may be needed in asymptomatic patients.
- Serum electrolytes, BUN, creatinine, and glucose levels should be obtained to evaluate other causes of seizures and altered mental status.
- Serum liver enzymes, coagulation studies, and creatine kinase may be elevated in patients with hyperthermia or agitation, or in patients with liver injury from previous ethanol abuse.
- Head CT, lumbar puncture, and toxicology studies should be performed as needed to evaluate other causes of seizure or altered mental status.

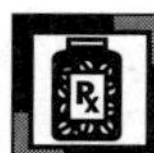

Treatment

Supportive care with appropriate airway management is vital, with specific treatment initiated while supportive care continues.

DIRECTING PATIENT COURSE

The health-care provider should call the poison control center when:

- Cause or management of withdrawal is unclear.
- Drug interaction or underlying disease presents unusual problems.

Admission Considerations

Patients in withdrawal from ethanol or sedative-hypnotics should be admitted.

DECONTAMINATION

Decontamination is usually unnecessary for a patient experiencing withdrawal, unless the patient has self-medicated in an attempt to prevent or treat withdrawal.

ADJUNCTIVE TREATMENT

- Because patients experiencing any type of withdrawal are at risk for dehydration, intravenous fluids should be administered to maintain a urine output of 1 to 2 ml/kg/h.
- Patients experiencing withdrawal may be a danger to themselves or others and should be placed in a protected, monitored setting.

Alcohol or Sedative-Hypnotic Withdrawal

- A long-acting sedative that will be eliminated slowly should be provided in the treatment of tachycardia, hypertension, hyperthermia, agitation, tremor, altered mental status, or seizure.
- A long-acting benzodiazepine is the drug of choice; although any benzodiazepine will be effective in large doses, short-acting agents should be avoided.

—Diazepam. Adult dosage is 5 to 10 mg by intravenous push, repeated every 5 to 10 minutes as needed; pediatric dosage is 0.2 to 0.5 mg/kg, up to 5 to 10 mg by intravenous push, repeated every 5 to 10 minutes as needed.
—Lorazepam. Adult dosage is 1 to 2 mg by intravenous push, repeated every 5 to 10 minutes as needed; pediatric dose is 0.05 mg/kg by intravenous push, repeated every 5 to 10 minutes as needed.

- Phenobarbital is also effective in cases of alcohol or sedative-hypnotic withdrawal.

Opioid Withdrawal

- Clonidine has been used to ameliorate the symptoms of narcotic withdrawal; the adult dose of 0.1 to 0.2 mg orally every 4 to 6 hours until withdrawal symptoms resolve, usually in 7 to 10 days.
- Paregoric is the drug of choice for symptoms of neonatal opioid withdrawal, which can be life threatening

—Dosage is 0.2 ml orally every 3 to 4 hours, increased by 0.05 ml every dose until symptoms are controlled and tapered over 7 to 10 days.
—Side effects include sedation and respiratory depression.

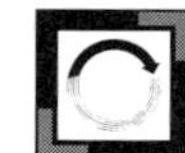

Follow-Up

EXPECTED COURSE AND PROGNOSIS

- Ethanol withdrawal begins 8 to 36 hours following discontinuation or decrease of ethanol intake, peaks within 36 to 72 hours, and subsides over 1 week. Death occurs occasionally and is usually associated with significant comorbid states.
- The course of sedative-hypnotic withdrawal varies substantially with the specific agent, but usually begins within 1 to 2 days following cessation of drug or decrease in dosage, peaks within 36 to 72 hours, and subsides over 1 week; withdrawal may, however, occur up to 1 to 2 weeks following discontinuation or decreasing drug administration. Death occurs occasionally and is usually associated with significant comorbid states.
- The course of opioid withdrawal varies substantially with the specific agent, but usually begins within 8 to 48 hours following discontinuation or decrease of drug administration, peaks within 36 to 72 hours, and subsides over 1 week. Opiate withdrawal is not considered life threatening in adults. Neonatal withdrawal seizures have resulted in fatalities.
- Stimulant withdrawal usually begins within 1 to 5 days following discontinuation or decrease of drug administration, peaks within the first 1 to 3 days, and subsides gradually over 1 to 3 weeks. Stimulant withdrawal is not life threatening.

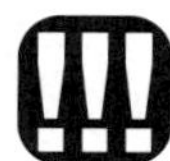

Pitfalls

- It is important to determine whether drug toxicity rather than withdrawal may be the cause of symptoms. For example, the toxic effects of a stimulant may be similar to ethanol withdrawal.
- In chronic alcoholic patients, alcohol withdrawal symptoms may occur at declining blood ethanol levels that are still in the referenced range for intoxication.
- Withdrawal does not require abstinence but may occur after decreasing the dose.
- Discontinuation of long-acting sedative hypnotic agents may produce signs and symptoms of withdrawal as late as 1 to 2 weeks following the last use.
- Neuroleptic agents, clonidine, and β-blockers may be used as adjunctive therapy, but they are not useful for primary treatment of ethanol or sedative-hypnotic withdrawal.
- Phenytoin is not useful in treating withdrawal seizures.
- Patients may claim to be in withdrawal in an effort to gain access to drugs for abuse; this claim is especially common for opioid abusers.

ICD-9-CM 965.0

Poisoning by analgesics, antipyretics, and antirheumatics: opiates and related narcotics.

See also: SECTION IV, Cocaine Coma chapter.

RECOMMENDED READING

Mayo-Smith MF, et al. The pharmacologic management of alcohol withdrawal. JAMA 1997;278:144–151.

Author: Edwin K. Kuffner

Reviewers: Kennon Heard and Richard C. Dart

SECTION III

Antidotes

Activated Charcoal

Basics

DESCRIPTION

Activated charcoal binds a wide array of compounds and thereby prevents their absorption.

FORMS AND USES

- Substances included are activated charcoal (Actidose, Actidose-Aqua, Insta-Char, Liqui-Char), activated carbon, and adsorbent charcoal. Some products are premixed with a cathartic.
- Activated charcoal is used in gastrointestinal decontamination to bind adsorb poison.
- It is also used to enhance elimination of some drugs (e.g., phenobarbital).

MECHANISM OF ACTION

- Activated charcoal is created by steam or chemical activation of wood pulp (heating in the presence of an oxidizing gas or dehydrating agent). The result is a highly porous material with a very large surface area. Surface area varies in commercial products from 950 to 1,500 m^2/g.
- Most drugs and other chemicals bind to the walls of the pores in activated charcoal, thereby reducing the material available for adsorption into the bloodstream. Adsorption is reversible, but desorption occurs slowly.
- Nondissociated salts and low-water soluble compounds are best adsorbed. Small, ionized compounds and highly water-soluble compounds are the most poorly adsorbed.
- Substances that undergo enterohepatic circulation or are secreted into the gastrointestinal tract may undergo enhanced elimination by repeated-dose activated charcoal.

DRUG AND DISEASE INTERACTIONS

- Charcoal will adsorb some orally administered antidotes.
- Repeat-dose activated charcoal may remove significant quantities of therapeutic medications from the body (e.g., anticonvulsants).

PREGNANCY AND LACTATION

Activated charcoal is not absorbed into the body and should not have any effect on pregnancy.

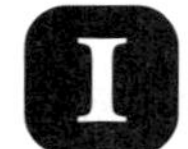

Indications

SINGLE-DOSE THERAPY

- Agents bound by charcoal

—Nearly all chemicals and drugs are bound by activated charcoal. Thus, activated charcoal should be administered unless it is known that the drug ingested is not bound by charcoal.
—Patients often ingest multiple agents. Activated charcoal is usually indicated if any of the drugs are adsorbed by charcoal (e.g., a lithium and phenytoin ingestion).

- Substances for which activated charcoal administration has not been shown to be clinically effective include mineral acids, mineral bases, ethanol, arsenic, boric acid, bromide, fluoride, iron, iodide, ipecac, lithium, and potassium.
- The appropriate time to administer activated charcoal is controversial. In general, a single dose is recommended if a substantial ingestion has occurred within the previous few hours. It is also recommended even later, if the patient has clinical manifestations. This suggests that adsorption is ongoing and activated charcoal may limit further absorption.

MULTIPLE-DOSE THERAPY

- Although the elimination of several substances is increased by activated charcoal, there is no drug for which clinical efficacy has been proven.
- In general, multiple-dose therapy is recommended in cases of phenobarbital and theophylline intoxication.
- Other commonly proposed indications for multiple-dose therapy include ingestion of sustained-release formulations and when bezoar formation is suspected (e.g., rising salicylate levels despite appropriate decontamination and urinary alkalinization).
- Enhanced elimination, but not clinical efficacy, has been demonstrated for carbamazepine, chlordecone, cyclosporine, dapsone, digitoxin, meprobamate, nadolol, phenylbutazone, phenytoin, quinine, salicylate, and valproic acid.
- Owing to the increased frequency of complications and lack of proven clinical efficacy, multiple-dose therapy is discouraged.

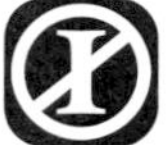

Contraindications and Adverse Effects

CONTRAINDICATIONS

- Repeat-dose activated charcoal is contraindicated in patients with known bowel obstruction or ileus.
- It should be used with caution in patients with diminished bowel sounds or following ingestion of agents known to produce ileus.

ADVERSE EFFECTS

- Emesis occurs in about 15% of cases but is not usually recurrent; however, it may lead to further complications:

—Pulmonary injury may result if hydrocarbons have been ingested and aspiration occurs.
—Esophageal injury may be increased when corrosives have been ingested.
—Aspiration pneumonitis may occur.

- Aspiration of charcoal may cause airway obstruction and bronchiolitis obliterans.
- Activated charcoal may obscure the endoscopic visualization of gastroesophageal injury.
- Constipation, bowel obstruction, and charcoal bezoars have been reported in patients who have ingested agents that decrease gastrointestinal motility. However, this appears to occur more commonly during multiple-dose administration.
- Bowel perforation has occurred.
- Corneal abrasions may occur following eye contamination with activated charcoal.

Dosage and Method of Administration

SINGLE-DOSE USE

- A dose of 1 to 2 g/kg administered orally is recommended. If patient is unable to drink, activated charcoal may be administered via nasogastric tube. Patients who are obtunded or have a depressed gag reflex should be intubated prior to administration.
- A second dose of activated charcoal administered 2 to 3 hours after the initial dose may be advisable in some circumstances in order to assure binding as much of the ingested toxicant as possible. This may include:

—Drugs with prolonged absorption phase or slow dissolution (sustained-release or enteric-coated medications)
—Agents with anticholinergic effects (tricyclic antidepressants, phenothiazine, and some plants)
—Drugs that form concretions or bezoars (salicylate and carbamazepine).

- Activated charcoal is administered as a slurry of 30 g of activated charcoal in 240 cc of liquid.
- A saline cathartic or sorbitol may be used with the first dose, although there is no reported evidence that this increases effectiveness. Cathartics that have been used with activated charcoal include:

—Magnesium or sodium sulfate: Adult 20 to 30 g/dose; child 250 mg/kg/dose
—Magnesium citrate: adult or child 4 cc/kg/dose, up to 300 cc/dose
—Sorbitol: adult 1 to 2 g/kg/dose, up to 150 g/dose; child: 1 to 1.5 g/kg/dose, up to 50 g/dose

- If the patient vomits charcoal within 1 hour, half of the original dose should be administered. Aggressive antiemetic therapy may be required for repetitive vomiting:

—Adult: metoclopramide 1.0 to 2.0 mg/kg intravenously plus prochlorperazine 10 mg intravenously or droperidol 1.25 to 2.5 mg intravenously.
—Diphenhydramine 25 to 50 mg intravenously may be added to this regimen.

MULTIPLE-DOSE USE

- When the decision has been made to use multiple-dose activated charcoal, a repeat dose may be administered every 2 to 6 hours. A uniform dose has not been established. Suggested regimens include:

—0.5 g/kg every 2 to 4 hours
—20 g every 2 hours, 40 g every 4 hours, or 60 g every 6 hours.

- The duration of therapy has not been established. A typical approach is to continue it for 24 to 48 hours.
- Continuous nasogastric instillation of activated charcoal, 0.25 to 0.5 g/kg/h, has been advocated to reduce the incidence of emesis.
- When the first dose of activated charcoal is combined with a cathartic, subsequent doses should not be given with a cathartic because of the risk of fluid and electrolyte disorders. Note that some charcoal products already contain a cathartic.

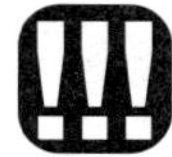

Pitfalls

PEDIATRIC

- Children are more susceptible to the fluid and electrolyte disorders that can result from cathartic use.
- Small airway size increases the risk of airway compromise following aspiration.

GERIATRIC

- Older patients are more likely to have gastrointestinal motility disorders.
- They are also more likely to be on therapeutic medications that may be removed from the body by repeat-dose activated charcoal.

ICD-9-CM 973

Poisoning by agents primarily affecting the gastrointestinal system.

RECOMMENDED READING

Al-Shareef AH, Buss DC, Allen EM, et al. The effects of charcoal and sorbitol (alone and in combination) on plasma theophylline concentrations after sustained-release formulation. Hum Exp Toxicol 1990;9:179–182.

Chin L, Picchioni AL, Duplisse BR. Action of activated charcoal on poisons in the digestive tract. Toxicol Appl Pharmacol 1970;16:786.

Neuvonen PJ, Olkolla KT. Oral activated charcoal in the treatment of acute toxic ingestions. Ann Emerg Med 1989;18:101–104.

Author: Steven A. Seifert

Reviewer: Katherine M. Hurlbut

Adenosine

Basics

DESCRIPTION

Adenosine is an ultra short-acting antidysrhythmic agent.

FORMS AND USES

- Adenosine is used to interrupt tachydysrhythmics such as supraventricular tachycardias that are associated with conditions such as:

—Thyrotoxicosis
—Theophylline intoxication
—Wolff-Parkinson-White syndrome
—Lown-Ganong-Levine syndrome

- Adenosine for intravenous injection: 6 mg/2 ml and 12 mg/4 ml vials.
- Adenoscan for intravenous injection: 90 mg/30 ml vials.

MECHANISM OF ACTION

- Adenosine binds to adenosine-specific receptors that activate acetylcholine-sensitive potassium channels in the sinoatrial and atrioventricular (AV) nodes, as well as atrial myocardial tissue.
- Interference with the potassium current results in transient slowing of the sinus rate with slowing of the AV nodal conduction velocity and increasing AV nodal refractoriness.
- Adenosine has no direct effects on ventricular myocardium.
- The major advantage of adenosine is its ultra-short half-life (seconds). Thus, adverse events should resolve quickly.

DRUG AND DISEASE INTERACTIONS

- Dipyridamole and carbamazepine potentiate adenosine effects.
- Methylxanthines, such as theophylline and caffeine, are adenosine antagonists.

PREGNANCY AND LACTATION

US FDA Pregnancy Category C. Studies have shown that the drug exerts animal teratogenic or embryocidal effects, but there are no controlled studies in women, or no studies are available in either animals or women.

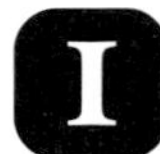

Indications

- Paroxysmal supraventricular tachycardia that is refractory to nonpharmacologic therapy.
- Toxic causes of supraventricular tachycardia may be refractory to adenosine therapy because the initiating stimulus usually persists beyond the half-life of adenosine.

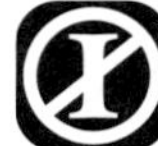

Contraindications and Adverse Effects

CONTRAINDICATIONS

- Adenosine is contraindicated for second- or third-degree AV block unless an artificial pacemaker is present.
- It also should not be used for sick sinus syndrome due to the potential for prolonged asystole with loss of consciousness.

ADVERSE EFFECTS

- Adenosine may induce bronchospasm and therefore should be used with caution in patients with reactive airway disease.
- Hypotension may occur occasionally.
- Patients have reported:

—chest tightness (1%)
—lightheadedness (2%)
—nausea (3%)
—dyspnea (12%)
—facial flushing (18%)

Dosage and Method of Administration

• Adult: Initial dose should be 6 mg as a rapid intravenous bolus.
• Child: The initial dose in infants and children is 50 μg/kg.
• The patient must be closely monitored, and resuscitation equipment should be available during adenosine therapy.
• Due to its half-life of only 10 seconds, adenosine will be inactivated before reaching the heart if infused slowly via a peripheral intravenous route. Therefore, it should be pushed via rapid bolus through a central intravenous line.
• If the dysrhythmia does not respond within 1 to 2 minutes, a dose of 12 mg should be pushed via rapid intravenous bolus.
• The 12-mg dose may be repeated in 1 to 2 minutes. If the third dose of adenosine does not eliminate the dysrhythmia, then alternative therapies should be pursued and the diagnosis reconsidered.
• The second and third doses in infants and children should be 100 and 150 μg/kg, respectively.

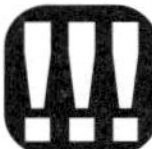

Pitfalls

• The clinician must push adenosine rapidly, thereby avoiding inactivation of the drug before it reaches the heart.
• It is important to identify paroxysmal supraventricular tachycardia correctly. Adenosine will be ineffective in converting other tachydysrhythmias, such as atrial fibrillation, atrial flutter, or ventricular tachycardia, into a sinus rhythm.
• No controlled studies exist regarding the safety and efficacy in pediatric patients.

ICD-9-CM 972

Poisoning by agents primarily affecting the cardiovascular system.

RECOMMENDED READING

Faulds D, Chrisp P, Buckley MM-T. Adenosine: an evaluation of its use in cardiac diagnostic procedures and in the treatment of paroxysmal supraventricular tachycardia. Drugs 1991;41:596–624.

Till J, Shinebourne EA, Rigby ML, Clarke B, Ward DE, Rowland E. Efficacy and safety of adenosine in the treatment of supraventricular tachycardia in infants and children. Br Heart J 1989;62:204–211.

Author: Gerald F. O'Malley

Reviewer: Richard C. Dart

Atropine

Basics

DESCRIPTION

- Atropine is an anticholinergic agent used as an antidote for various toxic and anticholinesterase agents.
- It is also an antisecretory, mydriatic, and cycloplegic drug.

FORMS AND USES

Atropine sulfate injection is available in:

- 400 μg/ml vials and ampules
- 1 mg/ml dosette vials
- 0.5 mg/5 ml and 1 mg/10 ml prefilled syringes

MECHANISM OF ACTION

- Atropine is an antimuscarinic agent because it is a competitive antagonist of acetylcholine at the muscarinic receptors on autonomic synapses.
- The decreased activity of acetylcholine at the muscarinic receptor site explains characteristic symptoms of atropism, which are anticholinergic by definition: mental status changes, hyperthermia, visual disturbances, mydriasis, urinary retention, flushing, constipation, and absence of sweat or secretions.
- Atropine has little effect on nicotinic receptor sites.

DRUG AND DISEASE INTERACTIONS

- The anticholinergic properties of atropine are potentiated by the sympathomimetic drugs:

—Catecholamines: epinephrine, norepinephrine, isoproterenol, dopamine, and dobutamine
—Noncatecholamines: amphetamine, methamphetamine, ephedrine, and phenylephrine
—Selective β-adrenergic agonists: metaproterenol, terbutaline, albuterol, and ritodrine

- The anticholinergic effects of atropine can be reversed by the cholinergic effects of bethanechol, methacholine, and, more commonly, physostigmine.

PREGNANCY AND LACTATION

US FDA Pregnancy Category C: The drug exerts animal teratogenic or embryocidal effects, but there are no controlled studies in women, or no studies are available in either animals or women.

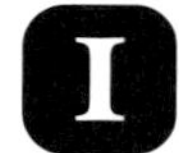

Indications

- Conditions involving symptomatic bradycardia, such as hypotension, lightheadedness, nausea, and vomiting
- Cholinergic poisoning that produces bronchospasm or bronchorrhea, such as organophosphate, carbamate, and edrophonium intoxication
- As a preinduction agent in pediatric sedation to prevent vagally mediated bradycardia
- Production of mydriasis and cycloplegia for examination of the retina and in the management of inflammatory conditions of the iris and uveal tract

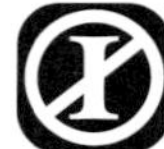

Contraindications and Adverse Effects

CONTRAINDICATIONS

Ophthalmic preparations are contraindicated in known or suspected acute angle closure glaucoma because of the likelihood of increasing intraocular pressure. This is especially true for the elderly.

ADVERSE EFFECTS

- Anticholinergic effects (tachycardia, pupillary dilation, fever, etc.) may develop.
- Irritation, hyperemia, and edema of the eye may occur after prolonged use.
- Ophthalmic application has been associated with systemic absorption and generation of cardiac dysrhythmias.
- High environmental temperatures may precipitate heat-related illness in patients treated with anticholinergic medications such as atropine.
- Atropine should be used with extreme caution in patients who are already tachycardic or hypertensive because these conditions may be exacerbated.

Dosage and Method of Administration

- Symptomatic bradycardia

—The initial adult dose is 0.5 to 1.0 mg intravenously. The initial dose for a child is 0.01 mg/kg.
—The dose may be repeated every few minutes until the heart rate increases.
—Administer in the emergency department or intensive care unit with continuous cardiac monitoring.

- Bronchospasm or bronchorrhea from organophosphate, carbamate, or other cholinesterase inhibitor intoxication (e.g., nerve agents)

—Administration should begin with a full vagolytic dose of a 2-mg intravenous push.
—The dose should be repeated at 5-minute intervals until the bronchial secretions are attenuated.
—Doses in excess of a gram have been required over 24 hours for severe poisoning.
—When treating severe bronchorrhea secondary to cholinergic toxicity or organophosphate poisoning, the clinical endpoint is resolution of bronchial hypersecretion.

- Cycloplegia

—A 0.6-mg (approximately one drop of a 1% solution) dose will act as an effective cycloplegic and mydriatic for as long as 1 to 2 weeks.

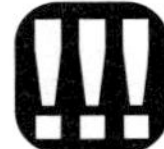

Pitfalls

The health-care provider should:

- Provide atropine in vagolytic doses during bradycardia.
- Provide enough atropine to reverse muscarinic effects of cholinergic poisoning (e.g., by an organophosphate or carbamate). Significant poisoning by these agents may require the entire atropine stores of a hospital for one patient.

Discontinuation of atropine based on development of tachycardia may not provide control of bronchial secretions.

ICD-9-CM 971.1

Poisoning by drugs primarily affecting the autonomic nervous system: parasympatholytics (anticholinergics and antimuscarinics) and spasmolytics.

RECOMMENDED READING

Brown JH, Taylor P. Muscarinic receptor agonists and antagonists. In: Gilman A, Goodman LS, Rall TW, et al., eds. Goodman and Gilman's the pharmacologic basis of therapeutics, 9th ed. New York: McGraw-Hill, 1996:149.

Kaiser SC, McClain PL. Atropine metabolism in man. Clin Pharmacol Ther 1970;11:214–227.

Lahdes K, Kaila T, Hunponen R, et al. Systemic absorption of topically applied ocular atropine. Clin Pharmacol Ther 1988;44:310–314.

Author: Gerald F. O'Malley

Reviewer: Katherine M. Hurlbut

Black Widow Spider Antivenom

Basics

DESCRIPTION

Black widow spider antivenom is an antidote to black widow spider venom.

FORMS AND USES

The formulation is ANTIVENIN (Latrodectus mactans), USP (Merck).

- Each package contains 6,000 units of powdered antivenom.
- The powder is reconstituted with a 2.5-ml vial of water for injection (included in package).
- Also included is a 1-ml vial of normal horse serum (1:10 dilution) for sensitivity testing.
- The inactive ingredient is thimerosal 1:10,000.

MECHANISM OF ACTION

- This antivenom contains immunoglobulin G from the serum of horses hyperimmunized to the venom of Latrodectus mactans (black widow spider); it confers passive immunity by binding constituents of black widow spider venom.
- Due to cross-reactivity with the venom of other subspecies, the antivenom is considered effective treatment for all Latrodectus subspecies.

PREGNANCY AND LACTATION

- US FDA Pregnancy Category C. The drug exerts animal teratogenic or embryocidal effects, but there are no controlled studies in women, or no studies are available in either animals or women.
- Black widow antivenom should be used in pregnant women as it is in other patients.

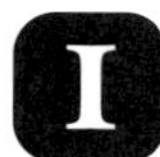

Indications

Owing to adverse effects to this product, black widow antivenom is recommended only in cases of severe bites when any of the following occur:

- Severe hypertension
- Persistent pain not controlled by opioids and muscle relaxants
- Respiratory failure
- Suspected myocardial ischemia
- Premature labor

Contraindications and Adverse Effects

CONTRAINDICATIONS

Known hypersensitivity to horse serum or black widow spider antivenom precludes its use.

ADVERSE EFFECTS

Acute Allergic Reactions (Rash, Bronchospasm)

- Frequency of acute reactions is unknown, but occurs in 20% to 25% of patients receiving other equine antivenoms.
- Antivenom infusion should be discontinued.
- Patient should receive antihistamine such as diphenhydramine; adult, 25 to 50 mg intravenously or orally every 6 to 8 hours; pediatric, 1 mg/kg intravenously or orally up to 50 mg every 6 to 8 hours.
- Bronchospasm should be treated with a bronchodilator, such as albuterol 0.15 mg/kg (maximum of 10 mg), in saline with humidified oxygen via nebulizer every 20 to 30 minutes.

Anaphylaxis

- Frequency is unknown; one death has been reported from anaphylaxis induced by the horse serum skin test.
- Patient should receive 100% oxygen, and a secure airway and intravenous access should be maintained.
- H_1 and H_2 antihistamines should be administered.

—Diphenhydramine. Adult, 25 to 50 mg intravenously every 6 to 8 hours; pediatric, 1 mg/kg intravenously up to 50 mg every 6 to 8 hours.
—Cimetidine. Adult, 300 mg intravenously every 6 hours; pediatric, 40 mg/kg per day intravenously divided every 6 hours up to 300 mg/dose.

Bronchospasm

Bronchospasm is treated with a bronchodilator, such as albuterol 0.15 mg/kg up to 10 mg, in saline with humidified oxygen via nebulizer every 20 to 30 minutes; use of epinephrine 1:1,000 should be considered in refractory cases: adult, 0.3 to 0.5 ml subcutaneously; pediatric, 0.01 ml/kg subcutaneously up 0.5 ml.

Hypotension

If hypotension develops, crystalloid should be administered in an initial bolus of 0.9% NaCl, 10 to 20 ml/kg; epinephrine can be added if needed.

- Initial bolus of epinephrine 1:10,000 diluted 10:1 is administered.

—Adult. Intravenous push 3 to 5 ml over 5 to 10 minutes.
—Pediatric. Intravenous push 0.1 ml/kg up to 5 ml over 5 to 10 minutes.

- Bolus should be followed with infusion if necessary: 1 mg of 1:1,000 epinephrine in 250 ml D5W; 1 μg/min initially should be titrated to desired blood pressure.

Methylprednisolone

Methylprednisolone 60 to 125 mg (1–1.5 mg/kg) should be given intravenously (pediatric, 1–2 mg/kg) every 6 to 8 hours.

Type IV Hypersensitivity (Serum Sickness)

- Frequency after use of black widow antivenom is unknown.
- Serum sickness typically begins 3 to 14 days after antivenom infusion as malaise and diffuse arthralgia and progresses to diffuse rash, pruritus, and (rarely) pericarditis and glomerulonephritis.
- Antihistamine such as diphenhydramine should be administered.

—Adult, 25 to 50 mg orally every 6 to 8 hours
—Pediatric, 1 mg/kg orally up to 50 mg every 6 to 8 hours

- Prednisone should be administered to most symptomatic patients.

—Adult, 40 to 60 mg/day orally for 7 to 10 days
—Pediatric, 1 mg/kg per day orally for 7 to 10 days
—Tapering regimen acceptable, but not needed, in patients not treated chronically with steroids

- Antipyretics and pain control

—Acetaminophen. Adult, 1 g orally every 4 to 6 hours, up to 4 g/day; pediatric, 10 mg/kg every 4 to 6 hours up to 4 g/day.
—Ibuprofen. Adult, 600 to 800 mg orally every 8 hours; pediatric, 5 to 10 mg/kg every 6 to 8 hours.

Dosage and Method of Administration

- Skin test should be performed with 0.02 ml of the horse serum provided.

—Serum should be injected intradermally.
—Patient should be observed for 10 to 20 minutes for wheal and flare reaction; the test should be read using the same parameters as for the tuberculin skin test (wheal and erythema larger than 10 mm in diameter).

- If the skin test is negative, one vial of antivenom should be reconstituted with 2.5 ml sterile water for injection (included), and then diluted in 50 to 100 ml intravenous fluid (D5W or 0.9% NaCl).
- The infusion should begin slowly (10–25 ml/h) using an infusion controller; in the absence of reaction, the rate can slowly be increased every few minutes while observation for evidence of acute allergic reaction continues.

—Infusion should be completed over 20 to 30 minutes as tolerated.
—Patient should be monitored continuously during administration; airway management and anaphylaxis treatment may be required.
—If reaction occurs, infusion should be terminated immediately.

- Clinical improvement is usually evident within 30 to 60 minutes.
- If patient shows no response or partial response, one additional vial can be administered.
- If there is no clinical response after the administration of two vials of antivenom, the diagnosis should be reconsidered.

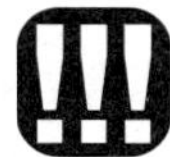

Pitfalls

- Rapid intravenous bolus administration may produce an anaphylactoid reaction.
- Antivenom use is generally not indicated in minor envenomation syndromes because the risk of anaphylaxis outweighs the potential benefits.
- Inadequate monitoring may allow anaphylaxis to develop without treatment.

ICD-9-CM 989.5

Toxic effect of venom.

See also: SECTION IV, Black Widow Spider chapter.

RECOMMENDED READING

Clark RF, Wethern-Kestner S, Vance MV, et al. Clinical presentation and treatment of black widow spider envenomation: a review of 163 cases. Ann Emerg Med 1992;21:782–787.

Moss HS, Binder LS. A retrospective review of black widow spider envenomation. Ann Emerg Med 1987;16:188–191.

Author: Katherine M. Hurlbut

Reviewer: Richard C. Dart

Botulinum Antitoxin

Basics

DESCRIPTION

Botulinum antitoxin is used to counter the effects of a toxin produced by Clostridium botulinum, an anaerobic bacterium that can cause botulism.

FORMS AND USES

- Botulinum antitoxin is used in the treatment of food-borne or wound types of botulism; it is usually not recommended for infant-type botulism.
- Botulinum antitoxin is available in monovalent (against A, B, or E toxins), bivalent (A and B), trivalent (A, B, and E), and septavalent (A, B, C, D, E, F, and G) forms.
- Trivalent botulinum antitoxin contains 7,500 IU against type A, 5,500 IU against type B, and 8,500 IU against type E toxin.
- U.S. Food and Drug Administration (FDA)-approved antitoxin is available only from the Centers for Disease Control and Prevention (CDC).

—Each state health department has a designated contact person for the CDC; the appropriate state health department should be contacted first and will then facilitate procurement of antitoxin.
—If the state contact person cannot be reached in a timely manner, the CDC can be contacted directly at (404) 639-3311 days, and at (404) 639-2888 nights, weekends, and holidays.

- An experimental septavalent (A, B, C, D, E, F, and G) antitoxin is in clinical trials and available through the U.S. military.

MECHANISM OF ACTION

- FDA-approved botulinum antitoxin is an equine whole immunoglobulin G (IgG) preparation derived from the serum of immunized horses.
- Botulinum antitoxin acts by binding to botulinum toxin that has not yet bound to tissue; it slows or stops progression of the disease, but does not reverse symptoms because binding of toxin to nerve endings is irreversible.
- Patients treated within the first 24 hours have shortened clinical courses; mortality, however, is comparable with that of patients receiving delayed antitoxin.
- Antitoxin specific to one serotype will not be effective against other serotypes.
- Peak serum levels of antitoxin following the administration of two to four vials (10 ml/vial) were 10 to 1,000 times higher than the amount needed to neutralize toxin measured in the serum of botulism patients.
- Antitoxin levels do not appear to be affected by route of administration; both intravenous and intramuscular routes produce similar levels.

PREGNANCY AND LACTATION

The pregnancy category is undetermined; however, its use is recommended to shorten the course of illness in the mother.

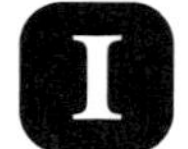

Indications

EXPOSURE TO BOTULISM

- Adult and pediatric patients with suspected botulism
- Adult and pediatric patients who have ingested food strongly suspected of containing botulinum toxin

ESTABLISHED DISEASE

Adult and pediatric patients with confirmed food-borne botulism, regardless of time since onset of symptoms.

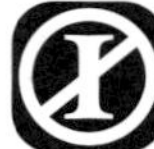

Contraindications and Adverse Effects

CONTRAINDICATIONS

- Botulinum antitoxin has not been shown to be effective in infant botulism.
- Known hypersensitivity to horse serum or to previous administration of antitoxin is a relative contraindication.

ADVERSE EFFECTS

Mild Allergic Reactions (Rash, Bronchospasm)

- The frequency is unknown, but is possible with infusion of any protein-containing product.
- Antihistamine (diphenhydramine) should be administered; adult dose is 25 to 50 mg intravenously or orally every 6 to 8 hours; pediatric dose is 1 mg/kg intravenously or orally every 6 to 8 hours.
- For bronchospasm, albuterol 0.15 mg/kg (maximum of 10 mg) should be administered in saline with humidified oxygen via nebulizer every 20 to 30 minutes.
- H_1 and H_2 receptor blocking drugs are used by some clinicians.

Anaphylaxis or Shock

- These occur rarely, but the true frequency is unknown.

—Anaphylaxis (IgE-mediated reaction) occurs in approximately 2% of patients treated.
—Anaphylactoid (non-IgE mediated) reaction is partially rate dependent, and its incidence may be reduced by further dilution and slowing of the infusion rate.

- Initial treatment involves administration of 100% oxygen and securing of the airway.
- The patient also should receive epinephrine 1:1,000 (adult 0.3–0.5 ml subcutaneously; child 0.01 ml/kg subcutaneously).
- Antihistamine should be administered to block both H_1 and H_2 receptors.

—Diphenhydramine should be administered; adult dose is 25 to 50 mg intravenously every 6 to 8 hours; pediatric dose is 1 mg/kg intravenously every 6 to 8 hours.
—Cimetidine should be given as well; adult dose is 300 mg intravenously every 6 hours; pediatric dose is 10 mg/kg intravenously every 6 hours.
—Bronchospasm should be treated with albuterol 0.15 mg/kg (maximum of 10 mg) in saline with humidified oxygen via nebulizer every 20 to 30 minutes.

- Hypotension is treated with crystalloid and epinephrine.

—Crystalloid should be administered in an initial bolus of 0.9% NaCl 10 to 20 ml/kg.
—Epinephrine should also be administered.
  —The subcutaneous dose as described above may be used. If life-threatening hypotension is present, the initial dose is 3 to 5 ml of

epinephrine 1:10,000 diluted 10:1 and administered by slow intravenous push over 5 to 10 minutes.
—Children should receive 0.1 ml/kg diluted 10:1 by slow intravenous push over 5 to 10 minutes.
—The initial dose should be followed with infusion if necessary; 1 mg of epinephrine 1:1,000 should be diluted in 250 ml D5W in water and infused at 1 μg/minute, titrated to desired blood pressure.
—Methylprednisolone 60 to 125 mg (1–1.5 mg/kg) should be given to adults intravenously (pediatric dose is 1–2 mg/kg) every 6 to 8 hours.

Type IV Hypersensitivity

- Serum sickness begins 3 to 14 days after antitoxin infusion as malaise and diffuse arthralgia, and progresses to diffuse rash, pruritus, and (rarely) pericarditis and glomerulonephritis.
- Serum sickness may occur more frequently in persons who receive more than 40 ml of antitoxin; the frequency of serum sickness is reported to be 5% to 10%.

Treatment

- Antihistamine (diphenhydramine). Adult, 25 to 50 mg orally every 6 to 8 hours; pediatric, 1 mg/kg orally every 6 to 8 hours.
- Prednisone. Adult 40 to 60 mg/day orally for 7 to 10 days; child 1 mg/kg per day orally for 7 to 10 days.
- Antipyretics and pain control

—Acetaminophen is recommended; adult 1 g every 4 to 6 hours, not to exceed 4 g/day; pediatric, 10 mg/kg every 4 to 6 hours not to exceed 90 mg/kg/day
—Ibuprofen is an alternative; adult, 600 mg every 8 hours; pediatric, 5 to 10 mg/kg every 6 to 8 hours

Dosage and Method of Administration

- Patients who have ingested food suspected of containing botulinum toxin or patient with suspected disease

—If the serotype is unknown, trivalent antitoxin (A, B, E) should be used.
—If the serotype is known, serotype-specific antitoxin should be used.
—The initial dose is two vials intravenously; alternatively, one vial may be administered intravenously and one intramuscularly.
—In cases of pediatric botulism (not infant botulism), the initial dose of antitoxin is the same as for adults because it is based on estimated toxin load, not body weight.
—Subsequent doses may be given every 2 to 4 hours if clinical effects develop or progress.
—When giving antitoxin for prevention of botulism only, some clinicians suggest giving the antitoxin intramuscularly to decrease allergic potential.
—If the intravenous route is chosen, the technique is the same as described below.

- Adult and pediatric patients with confirmed food-borne botulism, regardless of delay from onset of symptoms

—If the serotype is unknown, trivalent antitoxin (A, B, E) should be used.
—If the serotype is known, the serotype-specific antitoxin should be used.
—Patients should be skin-tested, using 0.1 ml intradermal injection of a 1:10 dilution of the treatment medication, and observed for reaction for 15 minutes; patients with a known history of horse-serum sensitivity should not be skin-tested and should be pre-treated with H_1 and H_2 receptor blockers, if the decision to use the antitoxin is made.
—The initial dose is two vials intravenously; alternatively, one vial may be administered intravenously and one intramuscularly.
—In cases of pediatric botulism (not infant botulism), the initial dose of antitoxin is the same as for adults because it is based on estimated toxin load, not body weight.
—Antitoxin should be administered intravenously over at least 30 minutes as a 1:10 vol/vol dilution in normal saline.
—Subsequent doses may be given every 2 to 4 hours if clinical effects continue to worsen.
—Clinician must be prepared for possible allergic reaction to antitoxin; if allergic reaction is anticipated (e.g., patient history of horse serum allergy), patient should be pretreated with H_1 and H_2 blockers and possibly steroids.
—Epinephrine should be at the bedside and clinician prepared to treat anaphylaxis.
—Instructions that accompany the product regarding skin testing and administration of antitoxin should be used.

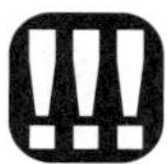

Pitfalls

Antitoxin should not be withheld for fear of a hypersensitivity reaction. Rather, pretreatment, cautious antitoxin administration, and appropriate measures to treat hypersensitivity should be available.

ICD-9-CM 005.1

Other food poisoning (bacterial): botulism.

See also: SECTION IV, Botulism chapter.

RECOMMENDED READING

Goldfrank LR. Botulinum antitoxin. In: Goldfrank LR, Flomenbaum NE, Lewin NS, et al., eds. Goldfrank's toxicologic emergencies, 6th ed. East Norwalk, CT: Appleton & Lange, 1998.

Author: Steven A. Seifert

Reviewer: Katherine M. Hurlbut

British Anti-Lewisite

Basics

DESCRIPTION

British anti-Lewisite (dimercaprol, BAL) is a heavy metal chelating agent used in the treatment of arsenic, mercury, lead, or gold toxicity.

FORMS AND USES

- Each milliliter of BAL in oil contains 100 mg dimercaprol, 200 mg benzyl benzoate, and 700 mg peanut oil.
- The chemical structure of dimercaprol, the active ingredient in BAL, is $CH_2(SH)CH(SH)CH_2OH$ (dithiol).
- BAL is highly lipid soluble but has limited water solubility.
- It is a colorless liquid with a sulfur odor, similar to rotten eggs.

MECHANISM OF ACTION

Sulfhydryl groups bind heavy metals, thereby preventing or possibly removing metal from binding sites on enzymes or other physiologic proteins.

DRUG AND DISEASE INTERACTIONS

- Iron supplementation should not be given to patients receiving BAL due to the potential for increased toxicity of the BAL-iron complex.
- BAL administration to patients on gold therapy for rheumatoid arthritis may lead to an exacerbation of the arthritis.

PREGNANCY AND LACTATION

- The safety of BAL in human pregnancy has not been established.
- BAL is teratogenic in animal models; therefore, it should be used during pregnancy only to treat life-threatening toxicity.

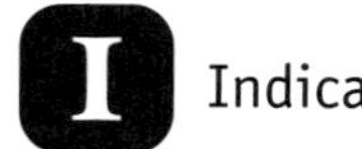

Indications

ACUTE INORGANIC ARSENIC TOXICITY

- BAL use is indicated if oral agents, such as succimer, cannot be used.
- BAL therapy has not been proven effective for chronic arsenic or arsine toxicity.

MERCURY TOXICITY (ACUTE INORGANIC, ELEMENTAL, OR NON–SHORT-CHAIN ORGANIC MERCURY)

- BAL should be used if oral agents, such as succimer, cannot be used.
- BAL therapy has not been proven effective for chronic organic mercury toxicity or short-chain organic mercury (methylmercury) toxicity.
- BAL is not routinely recommended for chelation of short-chain organic mercury compounds such as methylmercury due to a theoretical concern that chelation may facilitate the redistribution of mercury into the CNS.

LEAD TOXICITY

- BAL is recommended for acute poisoning associated with encephalopathy. It is commonly used in combination with calcium disodium EDTA ($CaNa_2EDTA$).
- BAL therapy is not recommended for symptomatic lead toxicity without encephalopathy or in asymptomatic children or adults with elevated blood lead levels.
- Potential benefits of BAL chelation prior to chelation with $CaNa_2EDTA$ include limiting the redistribution of lead into the CNS, mobilizing lead from the CNS, and making it more accessible to the water-soluble $CaNa_2EDTA$.

GOLD TOXICITY

- BAL has been used for hematologic effects resulting from gold toxicity.

OTHER PROPOSED USES

- Toxicity resulting from antimony, bismuth, chromium, copper, nickel, tungsten, or zinc.

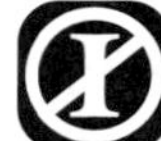

Contraindications and Adverse Effects

CONTRAINDICATIONS

- Patients with peanut allergy should not receive BAL because of its peanut oil base.
- Patients with glucose-6-phosphate deficiency should not receive BAL due to its potential for hemolysis.
- In the case of iron toxicity, the BAL-metal complex may be more toxic than the iron itself.
- BAL should not be given to patients with hepatic insufficiency unless the insufficiency is related to postarsenical jaundice.

ADVERSE EFFECTS

- Allergic reactions may occur in patients with peanut or other nut allergies.
- Pain at the injection site is common; it may be reduced by using a local anesthetic prior to or with the injection.
- Abscess formation at the injection site is possible.
- Other adverse reactions are dose related; administration of more than 5 mg/kg frequently produces serious adverse events.

—Viral syndrome–like symptoms are common: fever, headache, chest pain, nausea, vomiting, diaphoresis, rhinorrhea, lacrimation, salivation, sore throat, myalgia, abdominal pain, dental pain, and urticaria; the effect peaks soon after administration and resolves in an hour.
—Paresthesia, anxiety, and apprehension are common; the effect peaks soon after administration and resolves in an hour.
—Tachycardia and hypertension occur, more commonly in patients with underlying hypertension.
—Increased excretion of essential metals such as copper and zinc may occur.
—Nephrotoxicity related to the metal chelate may occur.

Dosage and Method of Administration

ACUTE ARSENIC POISONING

- BAL should be administered if vomiting or other conditions preclude the administration of an oral antidote.
- In potentially serious poisoning, BAL should be administered as soon as poisoning is suspected.
- The adult and pediatric dose is 2.5 to 5.0 mg/kg intramuscularly every 4 hours for 24 hours, tapering over 1 to 2 days at intervals of every 6 to 12 hours until an oral antidote can be tolerated. An alternative pediatric dose is 300 to 450 mg/m^2/day divided four times per day.
- BAL dosing may be discontinued when signs and symptoms of arsenic toxicity resolve, when the 24-hour urinary arsenic concentration is less than 50 to 100 μg/ml, or when chelation with an oral agent such as succimer or 2,3-dimercapto-1-propanesulfonate (DMPS) is instituted.

MERCURY TOXICITY

Acute Inorganic Mercury

- BAL should be administered if vomiting or other conditions preclude the administration of an oral chelating agent.
- The dose for adult or pediatric patients is 2.5 to 5.0 mg/kg intramuscularly every 4 hours, tapering over 1 to 2 days at intervals of every 6 to 12 hours until an oral antidote can be tolerated. An alternative pediatric dose is 300 to 450 mg/m^2/day in four divided doses.
- BAL dosing may be discontinued when signs and symptoms of mercury toxicity resolve or chelation with an oral agent such as D-penicillamine, succimer, or DMPS is instituted.

Elemental Mercury

- This exposure rarely requires chelation unless mercury vapor is inhaled.
- A parenteral agent is rarely required, because oral administration is feasible.
- The same dosing regimen should be followed as for acute inorganic mercury poisoning.

Acute Organic Mercury (Excluding Methylmercury)

- A parenteral agent is rarely required, because oral administration is feasible.
- The same dosing regimen should be followed as for acute inorganic mercury poisoning.

LEAD TOXICITY

- The dose for adult or pediatric patients is 2.5 to 5.0 mg/kg intramuscularly every 4 hours prior to the first dose of $CaNa_2EDTA$; BAL should be administered at least 4 hours prior to the administration of $CaNa_2EDTA$. An alternative pediatric dose is 300 to 450 mg/m^2/day in four divided doses.
- Administration of BAL should rarely be continued for more than 24 hours.
- BAL dosing may be discontinued when signs and symptoms of lead encephalopathy resolve or chelation with another chelating agent such as succimer is instituted.

GOLD TOXICITY

- The dose for pediatric or adult patients is 2.5 to 5.0 mg/kg intramuscularly every 4 hours, tapering over 1 to 2 days at intervals of every 6 to 12 hours until an oral antidote can be tolerated. An alternative pediatric dose is 300 to 450 mg/m^2/day in four divided doses.
- BAL dosing may be discontinued when signs and symptoms of gold toxicity resolve.

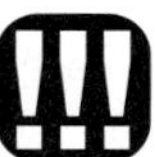

Pitfalls

- BAL is often continued unnecessarily after the patient has regained the ability to tolerate an oral agent.
- Dosage of BAL should be reduced or treatment discontinued if renal insufficiency develops during therapy.
- Hemodialysis may be indicated in order to remove the metal-BAL complex in patients with renal insufficiency or oliguric renal failure.

ICD-9-CM 963.8

Poisoning by other specified systemic agents.

See also: SECTION IV, Arsenic, Gold, Lead, and Mercury chapters.

RECOMMENDED READING

Howland MA. Dimercaprol (BAL). In: Goldfrank LR, Flomenbaum NE, Lewin NS, et al., eds. Goldfrank's toxicologic emergencies, 6th ed. East Norwalk, CT: Appleton & Lange, 1998.

Woody NC, Kometani JT. BAL in the treatment of arsenic ingestion of children. Pediatrics 1948;1:372–378.

Author: Edwin K. Kuffner

Reviewer: Richard C. Dart

Basics

DESCRIPTION

Calcium is used to treat calcium channel blocker poisoning, local or systemic hydrogen fluoride poisoning, black widow spider envenomation, and potassium or magnesium toxicity, as well as other toxic causes of hypocalcemia (sodium fluoride, ammonium bifluoride, ethylene glycol, sodium or potassium phosphate).

FORMS AND USES

- Calcium chloride 10% (100 mg/ml). One ampule contains 10 ml (1 g calcium chloride; 13.6 mEq calcium ion).
- Calcium gluconate 10% (100 mg/ml). One ampule contains 10 ml (1 g calcium gluconate; 4.5 mEq calcium ion).

MECHANISM OF ACTION

- Hyperkalemia. Calcium directly antagonizes the membrane effects of excess potassium.
- Hydrogen fluoride poisoning

—Fluoride ions bind calcium and magnesium, thereby inducing cellular and plasma electrolyte abnormalities that lead to cell death.
—Administration of exogenous calcium binds the fluoride before this damage can occur and replenishes calcium that has already been bound by fluoride.

- Hypermagnesium. Calcium directly antagonizes the effect of magnesium on the level of the skeletal membrane.
- Calcium channel blocker toxicity. Calcium administration is used to simply overwhelm the blockade induced by the calcium channel blocker.
- Latrodectus mactans (black widow) spider bites. Increasing extracellular calcium levels may transiently counteract the calcium permeability derangements caused by black widow venom.

DRUG AND DISEASE INTERACTIONS

- Calcium use in the presence of digitalis has been reported to cause cardiac tetany.
- Calcium binds to some drugs (e.g., fluoroquinolones), but this effect is not considered clinically important during acute therapy.

PREGNANCY AND LACTATION

Calcium is generally accepted as safe in pregnancy.

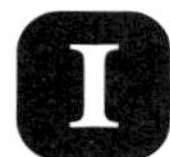

Indications

- Calcium channel blocker overdose. Calcium administration is recommended at the first sign of bradycardia, hypotension, heart block, or any other serious signs of toxicity.
- Hydrogen fluoride poisoning

—Local injury. Topical calcium administration is recommended for any symptomatic skin exposure to hydrogen fluoride. Dermal burns caused by hydrogen fluoride at a concentration of less than 20% can often be treated simply with calcium gluconate gel. Burns caused by higher concentrations of hydrogen fluoride may require tissue infiltration or other measures.
—Systemic effects. Intravenous calcium administration is recommended at the first sign of hypocalcemia, usually evidenced by prolongation of the QTc interval.

- Calcium is used to treat hypocalcemia caused by other poisonings, for example, sodium fluoride or ammonium bifluoride, ethylene glycol, or phosphates such as sodium or potassium phosphate. The presence of hypocalcemia alone indicates the need for calcium treatment. Muscular twitching, QTc interval prolongation on the ECG, dysrhythmia, or seizure indicates the need for urgent infusion.
- Hyperkalemia. Intravenous calcium administration is recommended if ECG changes such as wide QRS or peaked T waves occur.
- Magnesium poisoning. Intravenous calcium administration is recommended if bradycardia, QTc interval prolongation, or muscular weakness develops (unless these effects need to be tolerated in order to administer high-dose magnesium antidotal therapy).
- Black widow envenomation. Calcium may be indicated as first-line therapy along with musculoskeletal agents and opioids.

Contraindications and Adverse Effects

CONTRAINDICATIONS

Digitalis toxicity is a contraindication.

ADVERSE REACTIONS

- Transient hypercalcemia may cause cardiac dysrhythmia, hypertension, muscle weakness, and lethargy.
- Calcium chloride can cause venous thrombosis after intravenous infusion.
- Skin necrosis can result if calcium chloride is used intradermally, subcutaneously, or topically.

Dosage and Method of Administration

Intravenous or intraarterial calcium should always be administered to a patient on a cardiac monitor in an intensive care setting.

CALCIUM CHANNEL BLOCKER OVERDOSE

- Calcium chloride 10% is preferred over calcium gluconate.
- Calcium should be administered intravenously over 5 minutes to avoid cardiac effects of transient hypercalcemia.

—Initial dose for adults is one ampule (10 ml of 10% solution) infused over 5 minutes.
—The pediatric dose is 10 to 25 mg/kg up to one ampule per dose.
—The dose may be repeated every 10 minutes as needed; however, if more than two additional treatments are needed, consultation with a poison center or medical toxicologist is strongly recommended.

- Calcium gluconate 10% may alternatively be used.

—The adult dose is 10 to 30 ml (i.e., 1–3 g) intravenously over 5 minutes.
—The pediatric dose is 30 to 75 mg/kg over 5 minutes, with a maximum of 1 g/dose.
—The dose may be repeated every 10 minutes as needed; however, if more than two additional treatments are needed, consultation with a poison center or medical toxicologist is strongly recommended.

- ECG should be monitored continuously during therapy.
- Serum calcium, preferably ionized calcium, should be monitored frequently during therapy.
- In severe calcium channel blocker overdose, large doses of calcium (producing significant hypercalcemia) may be required.

HYDROGEN FLUORIDE POISONING: LOCAL EFFECTS

- Poisoning from hydrogen fluoride at a concentration of less than 20% can often be treated with topical application of 2.5% calcium gluconate gel.

—The gel can be extemporaneously prepared in the pharmacy using 3.5 g calcium gluconate powder in 150 ml of water-soluble lubricant such as K-Y Jelly.
—The gel may be kept in contact with the burned area using a latex glove or other occlusive dressing.

- Poisoning from hydrogen fluoride at a concentration of more than 20% or any burn unresponsive to topical gel application is often treated with calcium gluconate infiltration.

—The use of calcium chloride must be avoided intradermally.

—The initial therapy is intradermal injection of 10% calcium gluconate solution.

—Standard calcium gluconate 10% solution is injected intradermally in the affected area with a 30-gauge needle to administer 0.5 ml/cm^2.

—This use of this method is limited because most dermal exposures involve areas such as the fingers where significant volume cannot be injected.

- Persistent pain in fingers or toes despite calcium gluconate gel or infiltration may be treated with regional perfusion or intraarterial calcium gluconate. These methods should be chosen in consultation with a medical toxicologist.

Regional perfusion method

—Using a technique similar to Bier block, an intravenous line is placed in the dorsum of the affected hand. The veins are emptied by elevating the arm.

—A double-cuffed pneumatic tourniquet is applied above the elbow, inflated to 100 mm Hg above the systolic blood pressure, and 10 cc of 10% calcium gluconate infused. The cuff is maintained for 25 minutes and then deflated over 5 minutes.

—Intraarterial method

—This method should be chosen in consultation with a medical toxicologist.

—A proximal artery (e.g., brachial or radial) is cannulated with a 20-gauge needle, and 20 ml of 10% calcium gluconate (2 g) in 40 ml of normal saline is infused intraarterially over 4 hours with an infusion pump.

—If pain persists, the dose may be repeated.

HYDROGEN FLUORIDE POISONING: SYSTEMIC EFFECTS

- Calcium chloride 10% is preferred over calcium gluconate.
- Calcium should be administered intravenously over 5 minutes to avoid cardiac effects of transient hypercalcemia.

—Initial dose for adults is one ampule (10 ml of 10% solution) infused over 5 minutes.
—For children the infused dose is 10 to 25 mg/kg up to one ampule per dose
—The dose may be repeated every 10 minutes as needed; however, if more than two additional treatments are needed, consultation with a poison center or medical toxicologist is strongly recommended.

- Calcium gluconate 10% may be used.

—Adult dose is 10 to 30 ml (i.e., 1–3 g), administered intravenously over 5 minutes; the pediatric dose is 30 to 75 mg/kg, administered intravenously over 5 minutes, with a maximum pediatric amount of 1 g/dose.
—The dose may be repeated every 10 minutes as needed.

- ECG should be monitored continuously during therapy.
- Serum calcium, preferably ionized calcium, should be monitored frequently during therapy.

HYPOCALCEMIA CAUSED BY OTHER POISONINGS (SODIUM FLUORIDE, AMMONIUM BIFLUORIDE, ETHYLENE GLYCOL, PHOSPHATES)

- Calcium chloride 10% is preferred over calcium gluconate.
- Calcium should be administered intravenously over 5 minutes to avoid the cardiac depressant effects of transient hypercalcemia.

—The initial adult dose is one ampule of calcium chloride (10 ml of 10% solution) infused over at least 5 minutes.
—The initial pediatric dose is 10 to 25 mg/kg of calcium chloride (10 ml of 10% solution) up to one ampule per dose.
—The dose may be repeated every 10 minutes as needed; however, if more than two additional treatments are needed, consultation with a poison center or medical toxicologist is strongly recommended.

- Calcium gluconate 10% also may be used; adult, 10 to 30 ml (i.e., 1–3 g) intravenously over 5 minutes; pediatric, 30 to 75 mg/kg intravenously over 5 minutes; the maximum pediatric amount is 1 g/dose. The dose may be repeated every 10 minutes as needed.
- ECG should be monitored continuously during therapy.
- Serum calcium, preferably ionized calcium, should be monitored frequently during therapy.

HYPERKALEMIA

- The adult dose is 10 ml (i.e., 1 g) of calcium chloride administered intravenously over 5 minutes.
- The pediatric dose is 0.5 to 1 mg/kg of calcium chloride administered intravenously over 5 minutes, with a maximum pediatric amount of 1 g/dose.
- The dose may be repeated in 5 minutes or as needed, guided by the ECG.

MAGNESIUM TOXICITY

- The adult dose is 10 ml (i.e., 1 g) of calcium gluconate 10%, administered intravenously over 5 minutes.
- The pediatric dose is 20 mg/kg of calcium gluconate 10%, administered intravenously over 5 minutes, with a maximum pediatric amount of 1 g/dose.
- The dose may be repeated in 5 minutes.

BLACK WIDOW ENVENOMATION

- Initial dose in adults is 10 ml (1 g) of 10% calcium chloride intravenously over 5 minutes.
- Initial dose in children is 10 mg/kg of 10% calcium chloride intravenously over 5 minutes.
- The dose may be repeated in 15 minutes if no effects are seen. If no improvement is seen with calcium chloride, muscle relaxants, and narcotics, then consideration should be given to the use of Latrodectus antivenom.

Pitfalls

- The onset of life-threatening toxicity from hypocalcemia may be abrupt; for example, cardiac arrest due to dysrhythmia may occur precipitously following hydrofluoric acid ingestion or severe hyperkalemia.
- Patients with a significant overdose of calcium channel blocker overdose should be monitored at least 24 hours because signs and symptoms may be delayed following poisoning with sustained-release preparations.
- Large amounts of calcium may be needed to treat hypocalcemia from severe fluoride or calcium channel blocker poisoning.
- Myocardial depression from transient hypercalcemia may occur if intravenous calcium is administered too rapidly.
- In patients with renal failure, systemic calcium administration must be individually tailored.

ICD-9-CM

None.

See also: SECTION IV, Calcium Channel Blocking Drugs, Hydrofluoric Acid and Ammonium Bifluoride, Black Widow Spider chapters.

RECOMMENDED READING

Graudins A, Burns MJ, Aaron CK. Regional intravenous infusion of calcium gluconate for hydrofluoric acid burns of the upper extremity. Ann Emerg Med 1997;30:604–607.

Vance MV, Curry SC. Digital hydrofluoric acid burns: treatment with intra-arterial calcium infusion. Ann Emerg Med 1986;15:890–896.

Author: Lada Kokan

Reviewer: Katherine M. Hurlbut

Cholestyramine

Basics

DESCRIPTION

Cholestyramine is a medication used to reduce cholesterol levels by binding bile acids. It also binds other chemicals.

FORMS AND USES

- Cholestyramine (Questran, Questran Light) is provided as a 4-g packet of powder for dissolution in liquid.
- It is also available as bars (cholybar) containing 4 g of cholestyramine and in cans (Questran)

MECHANISM OF ACTION

- Cholestyramine adsorbs bile acids in the intestine to form an insoluble complex that is excreted in the feces.
- Increased fecal loss of bile acids leads to an increased oxidation of cholesterol to bile acids, a decrease in beta-lipoprotein or low-density lipoprotein plasma levels, and a decrease in serum cholesterol levels.
- Cholestyramine is used occasionally in toxicology to interfere with the absorption of ingested drugs.

DRUG AND DISEASE INTERACTIONS

Cholestyramine interferes with the absorption of many drugs, including acetaminophen, amiodarone, bezafibrate, cephalexin, chloroquine, chlorothiazide, cholecalciferol, dicumarol, digitoxin, digoxin, doxepin, fluvastatin, folic acid, furosemide, glipizide, hydrochlorothiazide, hydrocortisone, iron, levothyroxin, liothyronine, methotrexate, metronidazole, mofentil, mycophenolate, penicillin G, phenobarbital, phenprocoumon, phenylbutazone, piroxicam, povastatin, sulindac, temoxicam, tetracycline, trimethoprim, ursodiol, vitamin A, vitamin E, vitamin K, and warfarin.

PREGNANCY AND LACTATION

- US FDA Pregnancy Category C. The drug exerts animal or embryocidal effects, but there are no controlled studies in women, or no studies are available in either animals or women.
- Cholestyramine is not excreted in breast milk, but it does bind fat soluble vitamins; therefore, its use is not recommended in nursing mothers.

Indications

There are no widely accepted indications for the use of cholestyramine in the treatment of poisoning. The following proposed uses are considered investigational.

ORGANOCHLORINE PESTICIDE POISONING

- Cholestyramine enhances fecal elimination but has not been shown to affect outcome.
- Routine use is not recommended.

CARDIAC GLYCOSIDE TOXICITY

- Cholestyramine enhances elimination of digoxin and digitoxin but has not been shown to affect outcome.
- Routine use is not recommended.

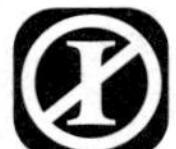

Contraindications and Adverse Effects

CONTRAINDICATIONS

- Known hypersensitivity to bile acid sequestering resins is a contraindication.
- Complete biliary obstruction.

ADVERSE EFFECTS

- Gastrointestinal. Most common adverse effects include constipation, abdominal pain, bloating, flatulence, anorexia, nausea, vomiting, diarrhea, indigestion, steatorrhea, and, rarely, gastrointestinal obstruction.
- Hematologic. Hypoprothrombinemia may occur secondary to decreased vitamin K absorption with chronic use.

Dosage and Method of Administration

The adult dose for hypercholesterolemia is 4 to 16 g/day orally in two to four divided doses. However, the dose for potential use in poisoning is unknown.

PEDIATRIC

- Experience is limited.
- In children 6 to 12 years of age, a dose of 80 mg/kg three times a day has been used.
- A dose of 2 g twice daily for 3 days, has been used for outpatient treatment of acute diarrhea in infants 4 to 36 months of age.

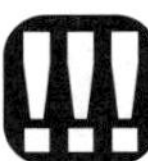

Pitfalls

Although cholestryamine may increase excretion of some compounds, the time course is not likely to be clinically meaningful.

Author: Katherine M. Hurlbut

Reviewer: Richard C. Dart

Cyanide Antidote Package

Basics

DESCRIPTION

The cyanide antidote package contains antidotes for cyanide and hydrogen sulfide toxicity.

FORMS AND USES

The cyanide antidote package (also known as cyanide kit) contains:

- 12 pearls of amyl nitrite for inhalation
- two ampules of sodium nitrite 300 mg in 10 cc of sterile water for injection
- two vials of sodium thiosulfate 12.5 g in 50 cc of sterile water for injection

MECHANISM OF ACTION

- Cyanide binds ferric iron (Fe^{3+}) contained in cytochrome oxidase, thereby impairing adenosine triphosphate (ATP) production and resulting in anoxic tissue injury.
- Cyanide does not significantly bind to hemoglobin (ferrous iron, Fe^{2+}).
- The cyanide antidote package works by producing methemoglobinemia.

—Amyl nitrite is used as a temporizing measure until sodium nitrite can be infused.
—Sodium nitrite oxidizes the ferrous iron in hemoglobin to ferric iron, producing methemoglobin.
—Methemoglobin binds cyanide avidly and is thought to reverse cyanide toxicity by removing cyanide from cytochrome oxidase; the resulting complex of cyanide and methemoglobin is termed cyanmethemoglobin.
—Cyanmethemoglobin may subsequently dissociate slowly to cyanide and methemoglobin, allowing cyanide toxicity to continue or recur.
—Sodium thiosulfate is used to complete the elimination of cyanide; the enzyme rhodanese catalyzes the reaction of thiosulfate and cyanmethemoglobin to produce thiocyanate, a water-soluble product that is excreted in urine.

- Toxicity often develops more slowly with cyanide ingestion than with inhalation because absorption takes longer.

DRUG AND DISEASE INTERACTIONS

Use of the cyanide kit in a patient with preexisting methemoglobinemia may produce overwhelming methemoglobinemia.

PREGNANCY AND LACTATION

The effect in pregnancy is unknown, but the benefits are thought to outweigh the risks.

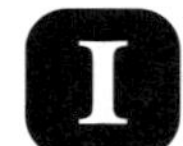

Indications

CYANIDE POISONING

- Patients with known cyanide poisoning and with serious clinical effects (hypotension, hyperkalemia, metabolic acidosis, altered mental status) should receive the antidote.
- In the case of a patient with known cyanide exposure, but in whom clinical effects have not developed, treatment with the sodium thiosulfate component of the kit alone is recommended. This scenario would be most common after ingestion of a cyanide-containing product.
- In cases of suspected cyanide poisoning (e.g., altered mental status and metabolic acidosis in a smoke inhalation victim), treatment with the sodium thiosulfate component of the kit alone is recommended. In these cases, addition of methemoglobin (which would result from sodium nitrite injection) to carboxyhemoglobin may further decrease the oxygen-carrying capacity of hemoglobin.
- Cyanide toxicity associated with nitroprusside infusion.

HYDROGEN SULFIDE POISONING

Administration of the sodium nitrite component of the kit alone in conjunction with supportive therapy within 15 to 20 minutes of exposure is supported by anecdotal reports.

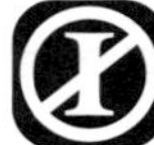

Contraindications and Adverse Effects

CONTRAINDICATIONS

- Sodium nitrite should not be used in clinical situations where the methemoglobin level is already 20% to 30%, in order to avoid compromise of oxygen delivery to tissues.
- If time allows, smoke inhalation victims should have their carboxyhemoglobin level measured when use of the sodium nitrite component is anticipated; the use of sodium thiosulfate alone should be considered because it will increase cyanide excretion without inducing methemoglobinemia.
- There are no known contraindications for the sodium thiosulfate component alone.

ADVERSE EFFECTS

- Hypotension induced by rapid infusion of sodium nitrite may be treated by reducing the infusion rate and administering crystalloid intravenous fluid and pressors.
- Cyanosis or hypoxia may occur if methemoglobinemia exceeds 30%.

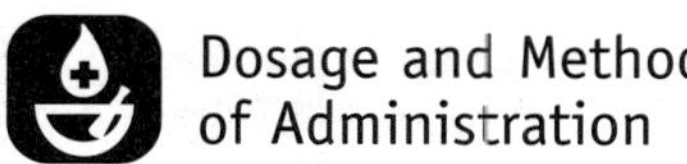

Dosage and Method of Administration

KNOWN CYANIDE POISONING WITH SERIOUS CLINICAL EFFECTS

Amyl Nitrite Ampules

Until vascular access is obtained, a crushed ampule is held to the nose or mouth, or in front of ventilation bag intake valve for 30 seconds of each minute.

Sodium Nitrite Injection

- This should be administered as soon as intravenous access has been established.
- Adult dose is 10 ml (300 mg of 3% solution) diluted to 100 ml with 0.9% sodium chloride and infused intravenously over 20 minutes; the infusion should be slow to prevent hypotension.
- Pediatric dose is 0.15 to 0.30 ml/kg of a 3% solution diluted to 100 ml with 0.9% sodium chloride and infused intravenously over 20 minutes; infusion should be slow to prevent hypotension.
- Methemoglobin level should be obtained 30 minutes after administration.
- If anemia complicates interpretation of the methemoglobin level, the hemoglobin concentration can be used to guide therapy.

—If the hemoglobin level is 8 g, the initial dose of sodium nitrite should be 0.22 ml/kg (6.6 mg/kg), and the initial dose of sodium thiosulfate should be 1.1 ml/kg.
—If the hemoglobin level is 10 g, the initial dose of sodium nitrite should be 0.27 ml/kg (8.3 mg/kg), and the initial dose of sodium thiosulfate should be 1.35 ml/kg
—If the hemoglobin level is 12 g, the initial dose of sodium nitrite should be 0.33 ml/kg (10 mg/kg), and the initial dose of sodium thiosulfate should be 1.65 ml/kg
—If the hemoglobin level is 14 g, the initial dose of sodium nitrite should be 0.39 ml/kg (11.6 mg/kg), and the initial dose of sodium thiosulfate should be 1.95 ml/kg

Sodium Thiosulfate

- Adult dose is sodium thiosulfate 50 ml (12.5 g of 25% solution) over several minutes.
- Pediatric dose is sodium thiosulfate 1.65 ml/kg up to 50 ml (25% solution) over several minutes.

If clinical evidence of cyanide poisoning persists for 30 minutes or recurs after an initial response to treatment, sodium nitrite and sodium thiosulfate doses may be repeated; some authorities suggest that half of the initial dose be used.

KNOWN CYANIDE EXPOSURE, BUT CLINICAL EFFECTS HAVE NOT DEVELOPED

Use of sodium thiosulfate alone should be considered in patients with cyanide ingestion.

SUSPECTED CYANIDE POISONING

Many practitioners use sodium thiosulfate injection alone in cases in which the oxygen-carrying capacity of blood is impaired, for example, in a victim of smoke inhalation (carbon monoxide poisoning).

CYANIDE TOXICITY ASSOCIATED WITH NITROPRUSSIDE INFUSION

- Prevention of cyanide toxicity.
- Concomitant infusion of both nitroprusside and sodium thiosulfate has been used.
- Administer infusion containing 10 mg of thiosulfate for every 1 mg of nitroprusside (10 ml of 0.1% solution of nitroprusside and 50 ml of 1% sodium thiosulfate); the admixture is stable up to 8 days.
- If cyanide toxicity has already occurred, use the full cyanide package as directed for symptomatic cyanide poisoning.

HYDROGEN SULFIDE POISONING

- Sodium nitrite should be administered within 15 to 20 minutes of exposure.

—Adult dose is 10 ml (300 mg of 3% solution) diluted to 100 ml with 0.9% NaCl intravenously over 20 minutes, infused slowly to prevent hypotension.
—Pediatric dose is 0.15 to 0.30 ml/kg of a 3% solution diluted to 100 ml with 0.9% NaCl intravenously over 20 minutes, infused slowly to prevent hypotension.

- Methemoglobin level should be checked 30 minutes after administration.

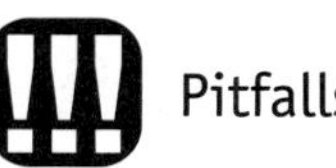

Pitfalls

- The most common error is the failure to consider a diagnosis of cyanide poisoning.
- Amyl nitrite pearls are inefficient producers of methemoglobin; it is more important to adequately ventilate and oxygenate the patient than to administer amyl nitrite by inhalation.
- The administration of an entire ampule (10 cc) of 3% sodium nitrite to a small child may produce lethal methemoglobinemia; total hemoglobin and methemoglobin concentrations should be measured before repeating sodium nitrite to ensure that dangerous methemoglobinemia will not occur, especially in children.
- The opportunity to administer sodium thiosulfate to unconscious fire victims is commonly overlooked.
- In the presence of renal failure, thiocyanate will accumulate instead of being excreted, resulting in nausea, vomiting, and muscle aches and cramps. Hypotension and altered mental status may also develop.
- Hospitals usually stock insufficient amounts to treat more than one victim for cyanide poisoning.

ICD-9-CM 989.0

Toxic effect of other substances, chiefly nonmedicinal as to source: hydrocyanic acid and cyanides.

See also: SECTION II, Methemoglobinemia chapter; and SECTION IV, Cyanide and Hydrogen Sulfide chapters.

RECOMMENDED READING

Curry SC: Hydrogen cyanide and inorganic cyanide salts. In: Sullivan JB, Krieger GR, eds. Hazardous materials toxicology, ed 1. Baltimore, Maryland: Williams & Wilkins, 1994.

Hall AH, Rumack BH. Clinical toxicology of cyanide. Ann Emerg Med 1986;15:1067–1074.

POISINDEX Editorial Staff. Cyanide (Management/Treatment Protocol). In: Rumack BH, Hess AJ, Gelman CR, eds. POISINDEX System. Englewood, CO: MICROMEDEX, Inc. (Edition expires May 31, 1998).

Author: Luke Yip

Reviewer: Richard C. Dart

Dantrolene

Basics

DESCRIPTION

Dantrolene is a medication used in the treatment of malignant hyperthermia and proposed for some poisonings complicated by hyperthermia and muscle rigidity.

FORMS AND USES

Dantrolene (Dantrium, Dantamacrin) is available as:

- A suspension of 5 mg/ml
- Capsules containing 25, 50, or 100 mg of dantrolene
- A 70-ml vial of lyophilized powder for reconstitution and intravenous injection (lyophilized dantrolene 20 mg, mannitol 3000 mg, reconstituted with water for injection 60 ml)

MECHANISM OF ACTION

- Dantrolene acts directly on skeletal muscle; it does not affect central or peripheral nerves.
- It decreases calcium release from the sarcoplasmic reticulum, thereby decreasing the strength of skeletal muscle contraction.
- Dantrolene may inhibit the cellular inward calcium activator current, thereby decreasing the amount of calcium available to trigger intracellular calcium release.
- It does not produce complete muscle paralysis therapeutically or in overdose.
- Dantrolene is highly protein bound; elimination occurs via both liver and kidney clearance.

DRUG AND DISEASE INTERACTIONS

Dantrolene may potentiate the effects of CNS depressants and may further impair respiratory or cardiovascular function in patients with respiratory or cardiac muscle weakness.

PREGNANCY AND LACTATION

- US FDA Pregnancy Category C. The drug exhibits animal teratogenic or embryocidal effects, but there are no controlled studies in women, or no studies are available in either animals or women.
- Dantrolene appears safe when administered in the third trimester to women at risk for developing malignant hyperthermia related to anesthetics administered at the time of delivery.

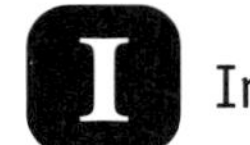

Indications

TOXIC CONDITIONS

Dantrolene may be useful in the treatment of muscle rigidity syndromes associated with the following conditions.

- Malignant hyperthermia
- Prophylaxis for malignant hyperthermia
- Neuroleptic malignant syndrome (NMS)
- Serotonin syndrome
- Amphetamine or cocaine toxicity
- Carbon monoxide poisoning
- Monoamine oxidase (MAO) inhibitor poisoning
- Dantrolene also has been used in the treatment of lethal catatonia or tremors induced by amphotericin refractory to other therapy.

NONTOXIC CONDITIONS

- Multiple sclerosis
- Spasticity
- Muscle cramping and spasm

Contraindications and Adverse Effects

CONTRAINDICATIONS

- Chronic use in patients with hepatic insufficiency, especially active hepatitis or cirrhosis
- When spasticity or muscle tone is required for function

ADVERSE EFFECTS

- Most adverse effects occur during chronic therapy.
- Adverse reactions are very uncommon during short-term therapy of a few days for malignant hyperthermia, NMS, or serotonin syndrome.

Pulmonary

Pulmonary edema, possibly related to large crystalloid volume required to administer dantrolene

Cardiovascular

Tachycardia, hypertension, hypotension, and pericarditis

Gastrointestinal

Nausea, vomiting, diarrhea, abdominal pain, gastrointestinal hemorrhage, constipation, and ileus with functional bowel obstruction

Hepatic

- Increased transaminase (aspartate aminotransferase and alanine aminotransferase), bilirubin, and alkaline phosphatase have been reported.
- Incidence of hepatotoxicity is increased with high dose (more than 300 mg), longer duration of therapy (more than 2 months), older age (more than 30 years old), and female gender.

Neurologic

CNS depression, muscle weakness, ataxia, hallucinations, and fatigue

Genitourinary

Increased urinary frequency, crystalluria, hematuria, incontinence, and impotence

Dermatologic

Rash, acne, and photosensitivity

Musculoskeletal

Myalgia and subjective muscle weakness

Dosage and Method of Administration

• Malignant hyperthermia, NMS, serotonin syndrome, prophylaxis for malignant hyperthermia, amphetamine toxicity, carbon monoxide poisoning, and MAO inhibitor poisoning

—The first action should be to discontinue all agents that may cause the syndrome.
—The preparation should be reconstituted with sterile water because dantrolene may be incompatible with dextrose 5% in water, normal saline, or any acidic solution.
—The dose for either adult or pediatric patients is a minimum of 1 mg/kg, administered by rapid intravenous injection.
—After the first dose, the patient should receive repeated 1 mg/kg dosing until symptoms resolve or a cumulative dosage of 10 mg/kg has been administered.
—Most patients respond to 2 to 5 mg/kg; however, the use of 40 mg/kg has been reported in the control of malignant hyperthermia.
—Following intravenous treatment, patients should receive 4 to 8 mg/kg per day orally divided four times a day for 1 to 3 days following the acute event to reduce the probability of recurrence.
—In the treatment of NMS or serotonin syndrome, it is often necessary to administer 5 to 10 mg/kg because the response is often not dramatic.

• Prophylaxis of malignant hyperthermia

—Adult or pediatric patient should receive dantrolene 4 to 8 mg/kg per day orally, divided four times a day, for 1 to 2 days prior to surgery.
—The last dose should be administered 3 to 4 hours prior to surgery.

• Syndromes with muscle spasticity

—Adult patients should receive 25 to 100 mg orally two to four times a day; doses above 400 mg/day are rarely required.
—Pediatric patients should receive 0.5 mg/kg, up to 3 mg/kg, orally two to four times a day.
—Treatment may be required for 1 to 2 weeks to produce clinical improvement.

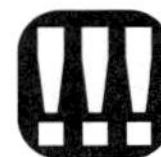

Pitfalls

• Dantrolene administration is not a substitute for aggressive supportive care and cooling measures when treating malignant hyperthermia, NMS, or serotonin syndrome.
• Dantrolene is not likely to be effective for treating hyperthermia caused by disorders of impaired heat dissipation (e.g., anticholinergic syndromes), increased metabolic rate (e.g., salicylate toxicity), or environment stress (e.g., heat stroke).
• Liver function tests should be monitored, especially in patients with advanced age, history of hepatic disease, large daily doses, or prolonged therapy.
• Older patients are more prone to develop hepatotoxicity.

ICD-9-CM 975

Poisoning by agents primarily acting on the smooth and skeletal muscles and respiratory system.

See also: SECTION II, Hyperthermia and Neuroleptic Malignant Syndrome and Serotonin Syndrome chapters.

RECOMMENDED READING

Granato JE, Stern BJ, Ringel A, et al. Neuroleptic malignant syndrome: successful treatment with dantrolene and bromocriptine. Ann Neurol 1983;14:89–90.

May DC, Morris SW, Stewart RW, et al. Neuroleptic malignant syndrome: response to dantrolene sodium. Ann Intern Med 1983;98:183–184.

Rosebush PI, Stewart T, Mazurek MF. The treatment of neuroleptic malignant syndrome: Are dantrolene and bromocriptine useful adjuncts to supportive care? Br J Psych 1991;159:709–712.

Author: Edwin K. Kuffner

Reviewer: Katherine M. Hurlbut

Deferoxamine

Basics

DESCRIPTION

Deferoxamine mesylate (Desferal) is an antidote for iron poisoning.

FORMS AND USES

- Each vial contains 500 mg of lyophilized powder.
- Deferoxamine is used therapeutically for:

—Acute iron poisoning.
—Chronic iron overload from multiple transfusions.
—Chronic aluminum overload from treatment with dialysis or total parenteral nutrition.

MECHANISM OF ACTION

- Free iron in the ferric (Fe^{+3}) form causes iron toxicity by directly injuring the intestinal mucosa and creating oxygen free radicals.
- Deferoxamine chelates ferric iron, to form ferrioxamine, a less toxic compound than ferric iron.
- Deferoxamine does not remove iron from transferrin, ferritin, hemoglobin, hemosiderin, or cytochrome enzymes.
- Ferrioxamine is not metabolized and is excreted unchanged in the urine.
- One mole of deferoxamine binds 1 mole of iron; therefore, 100 mg of deferoxamine binds 9.35 mg of iron.

DRUG AND DISEASE INTERACTIONS

Concurrent administration of deferoxamine with ascorbic acid is not recommended for treating either acute or chronic iron overload because it may mobilize iron, which both enhances excretion and allows further tissue deposition.

PREGNANCY AND LACTATION

- US FDA Pregnancy Category C. Studies have shown that the drug exerts animal teratogenic or embryocidal effects, but there are no controlled studies in women, or no studies are available in either animals or women.
- Deferoxamine crosses the placenta poorly; however, its use is recommended in acute maternal iron poisoning to optimize the mother's condition.

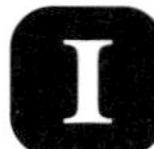

Indications

- Treatment of acute iron toxicity

—Signs of iron toxicity, including protracted vomiting or diarrhea, persistent tachycardia, hypotension, altered mental status, increased anion gap metabolic acidosis, acidemia, or hematochezia
—Serum iron greater than 500 μg/dl on blood drawn 4 to 6 hours after ingestion

- Chronic iron overload from multiple transfusions
- Chronic aluminum overload states in patients on chronic dialysis

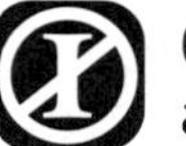

Contraindications and Adverse Effects

CONTRAINDICATIONS

- Renal insufficiency or oliguric renal failure are relative contraindications
- Ferrioxamine complex is renally eliminated; therefore, combined deferoxamine and hemodialysis treatment may be useful in the treatment of iron poisoning.

ADVERSE EFFECTS

Hypotension

- Dose-related hypotension occurs commonly with rapid intravenous infusion or following the intramuscular administration of a large dose.
- Hypotension is avoided by using continuous intravenous infusion instead of bolus intramuscular administration.
- If hypotension due to deferoxamine occurs, the rate of infusion should be decreased.

Anaphylactoid Reactions

- The risk of reaction is increased with large dose or rapid infusion rate.
- Anaphylactoid reactions increase the risk of hypotension in patients who are already volume depleted.

Infections

- Yersinia enterocolitica infection. Yersinia enterocolitica is a siderophore and thrives in a high iron environment as provided by the iron-deferoxamine complex.
- Fungal infection (mucormycosis, Rhizopus, phycomycosis) is associated rarely with treatment of iron or aluminum toxicity.

Ocular Toxicity

- Decreased visual acuity, decreased visual fields, impairment of night vision, altered color vision, retrobulbar optic neuropathy, and cataracts have been reported.
- The risk increases with larger doses and long-term therapy for chronic iron overload.

Auditory Toxicity

- Tinnitus and sensorineural hearing loss have been reported.
- There is an increased risk with larger doses and chronic therapy for states of chronic iron overload.

Adult Respiratory Distress Syndrome

- Pulmonary edema has been reported after prolonged use (more than 24 hours) of deferoxamine treatment of acute iron overdose.
- Deferoxamine can usually be tapered or discontinued within 24 hours.

Renal Insufficiency

Renal insufficiency may be related to hypotension produced by severe iron toxicity.

Dosage and Method of Administration

ACUTE IRON TOXICITY

Intravenous Dose

- The initial adult or pediatric dose is 15 mg/kg/hour by continuous infusion. This dose is adequate for most patients.
- The dose should be titrated to signs of iron toxicity, the serum iron concentration, and severity of acidosis. Rates of 20 to 25 mg/kg/h are usually adequate to treat severe poisoning, although rates as high as 40 mg/kg/h have been used when treating life-threatening iron toxicity.
- As the patient improves, the hourly dose of deferoxamine can be tapered.
- Although the package labeling indicates that 6 g is the recommended maximum 24-hour dose, this limit is based on intramuscular administration. Much larger doses are often needed. Intravenous doses of more than 25 g/day are commonly administered without adverse effect.
- Only severe cases of iron toxicity require more than 24 hours of continuous infusion.

Intramuscular Dose

Intramuscular treatment is not usually recommended for the treatment of acute iron toxicity due to erratic absorption and the increased incidence of adverse events. Pain and induration at the injection site may occur if an intramuscular route of administration is used. It has been used to begin therapy in some cases where intravenous access is difficult. However, intravenous administration is needed for crystalloid resuscitation, and this approach is discouraged.

- The initial adult dose is 1 g followed by 500 mg every 4 to 12 hours.
- The initial pediatric dose is 50 mg/kg followed by 50 mg/kg every 4 to 6 hours.

CHRONIC IRON OVERLOAD

Intravenous Dose

- Concurrent with blood transfusions or dialysis. Doses of 15 mg/kg/h to a dose of 2 g have been administered with each unit of blood or during each dialysis session.
- Deferoxamine should not be administered in the same intravenous line as blood.
- Intramuscular dose. The adult or pediatric dose is 500 mg to 1 g per day.
- Subcutaneous infusion has been reported useful.
- Rectal administration is not recommended due to decreased excretion of iron compared with intravenous administration.

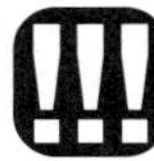

Pitfalls

- Following deferoxamine administration, the serum iron level becomes uninterpretable.
- A deferoxamine challenge test is not recommended.
- Absence of a vin rosé discoloration of the urine following the administration of deferoxamine does not exclude iron toxicity.
- In the treatment of acute iron toxicity deferoxamine should be administered by the intravenous route, not intramuscularly.
- The health-care provider should not delay deferoxamine while awaiting iron levels in severely symptomatic patients.
- Hemodialysis may be useful in patients with renal insufficiency or renal failure and iron toxicity to remove the ferrioxamine complex, which is normally renally excreted.
- Oral administration is contraindicated because it may increase the absorption of iron.
- The total iron-binding capacity (TIBC) measured at a time of concurrent deferoxamine administration may be falsely elevated (the TIBC is not clinically useful when managing acute iron toxicity).

ICD-9-CM 985.8

Toxic effect of other metals: other specified metals.

See also: SECTION IV, Aluminum and Iron chapters.

RECOMMENDED READING

Goldfrank LR. Iron. In: Goldfrank LR, et al., eds. Goldfrank's toxicologic emergencies, 6th ed. Norwalk, CT: Appleton & Lange, 1998.

Author: Edwin K. Kuffner

Reviewer: Katherine M. Hurlbut

Dextrose

Basics

DESCRIPTION

Dextrose is D-glucose, a six-carbon sugar used to supplement or restore blood glucose levels.

FORMS AND USES

- Dextrose is available as 5%, 10%, 20%, 25%, or 50% (D5, D10, D20, D25, D50).
- It is used to treat hypoglycemia or presumed hypoglycemia, or hyperkalemia resulting in ECG abnormalities.

MECHANISM OF ACTION

- Glucose provides a substrate for oxidative metabolism and adenosine triphosphate production.
- Metabolism of glucose causes potassium to enter cells and thereby decreases serum potassium concentration.
- Thiamine is a required cofactor in glucose utilization.

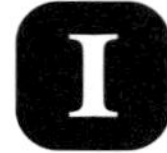

Indications

- Symptoms of hypoglycemia or glucose level less than 60 mg/dl

—The most commonly encountered cause of hypoglycemia is insulin reaction from exogenous insulin.
—Other toxic causes of hypoglycemia include ingestion of sulfonylurea oral hypoglycemic agents, salicylate, alcohol, or agents that cause fulminant hepatic failure.
—Diabetic patients who are chronically hyperglycemic may develop hypoglycemic symptoms at "normal" glucose levels.

- Altered mental status of unknown cause
- Hyperkalemia with ECG abnormality (in conjunction with insulin)

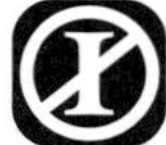

Contraindications and Adverse Effects

CONTRAINDICATIONS

- Some data indicate that hyperglycemia worsens the outcome in stroke patients.
- It is reasonable to withhold dextrose in patients with a history and examination consistent with stroke if a glucose level can be btained within 5 minutes.
- Known preexisting hyperglycemia.

ADVERSE EFFECTS

- Dextrose 10%, 20%, or 50% may cause burning and thrombophlebitis at the infusion site.
- Hypokalemia may develop after dextrose administration in patients with preexisting low or low-normal serum potassium levels.
- Prolonged infusion without close monitoring may result in hyperglycemia.
- Dextrose solutions may cause volume overload in patients with congestive heart failure.
- Poorly monitored infusion can cause hyperosmolar coma in diabetic patients.

Dosage and Method of Administration

- Symptoms of hypoglycemia or glucose level less than 60 mg/dl

—Dose for adults and adolescents
—Bolus. Initial treatment is 50 cc of 50% dextrose solution (25 g) as an intravenous bolus. Profoundly hypoglycemic patients may require multiple doses. Patients with mild hypoglycemia may be treated with oral administration.
—Continuous infusion. Patients with recurrent hypoglycemia should be treated with a 10% dextrose infusion. Adult dose is 250 cc/h and titrated to maintain blood glucose above 100 mg/dl. Occasionally patients may require continuous infusion of 20% dextrose. This requires central venous access and should be started at 100 cc/h and titrated to maintain blood glucose above 100 mg/dl.
—The dose for neonates is 2 to 4 cc/kg of 10% dextrose by intravenous bolus).
—The initial pediatric dose is 2 to 4 cc/kg of 25% dextrose by intravenous bolus.
—The infusion should not be discontinued abruptly; hypoglycemia may result. The infusion should be tapered over several hours with hourly glucose determinations.
—The glucose level should initially be monitored hourly in all patients.

- Altered mental status of unknown cause

—The adult and adolescent dose is 50 cc of 50% dextrose solution (25 g), administered as an intravenous bolus for symptomatic hypoglycemia.
—The dose for neonates is 2 to 4 cc/kg of 10% dextrose.
—The pediatric dose is 2 to 4 cc/kg of 25% dextrose.
—If repeated doses are needed, it is preferable to administer them using a large-bore intravenous line or central line.
—Glucose levels should be checked hourly.
—If no response is achieved, the diagnosis should be reconsidered; for example, evaluation of altered mental status or coma.

- Hyperkalemia with ECG changes

—The adult and adolescent dose is 50 cc of 50% dextrose (25 g) and 10 units of regular insulin administered intravenously as adjunct therapy for hyperkalemia.
—Concurrent therapy with bicarbonate and calcium also should be given.
—The pediatric dose is 0.5 to 1.0 g/kg (5–10 cc/kg) intravenously followed by 1 unit of insulin intravenously.

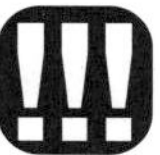

Pitfalls

- Supplemental glucose should not be administered prophylactically to patients with oral hypoglycemic overdose before hypoglycemia develops.

—This practice may delay the onset of hypoglycemia and obscure the diagnosis.
—Instead, the glucose level should be monitored hourly and dextrose administered if the glucose level drops below 60 mg/dl or the patient develops symptoms of hypoglycemia.

- Severe hypoglycemia (less than 20 mg/dl) may require more than one dose for initial response.
- Hypoglycemia may recur after bolus administration.
- Continuous dextrose infusion can rapidly cause hyperglycemia if not closely monitored.
- Neonates and infants have very limited glycogen stores, and hypoglycemia recurs readily.
- Geriatric patients have limited glycogen stores and exaggerated responses to medications, resulting in hypoglycemia.

ICD-9-CM 962.3

Poisoning by hormones and synthetic steroids: insulins and antidiabetic agents.

See also: SECTION IV, Insulin, Metformin and Biguanide Hypoglycemic Agents, and Oral Hypoglycemic Agents chapters.

RECOMMENDED READING

POISINDEX Editorial Staff. Sulfonylurea and related drugs. In: Rumack BH, Sayre NK, Gelman CR, eds. POISINDEX System. Englewood, CO: MICROMEDEX, Inc. (Edition expires November 30, 1997).

Author: Kennon Heard

Reviewer: Katherine M. Hurlbut

Digoxin Immune Fab (Digibind)

Basics

DESCRIPTION

- Digoxin immune Fab is an antidote used for toxicity from cardiac glycosides.
- Digoxin Fab is a purified Fab antibody that specifically binds the cardiac glycosides, digoxin, and digitoxin, forming a Fab-digoxin complex that terminates the activity of digoxin. It also binds cardiac glycosides from some plants and animals.

FORMS AND USES

Digoxin immune Fab (Digibind) is provided lyophilized in vials containing 40 mg of Fab/vial.

MECHANISM OF ACTION

- The concentration of free digoxin in the intravascular compartment becomes virtually zero since any free digoxin becomes bound to digoxin Fab.
- Toad toxins contain compounds similar to digitalis glycosides and have been successfully treated in some cases by digoxin Fab.

DRUG AND DISEASE INTERACTIONS

Depending on the dose, digoxin immune Fab also terminates the desired therapeutic effects of digoxin or digitoxin and may allow recurrence of underlying rapid ventricular response or congestive heart failure.

PREGNANCY AND LACTATION

- US FDA Pregnancy Category C. The drug exerts animal teratogenic or embryocidal effects, but there are no controlled studies in women, or no studies are available in either animals or women.
- Digoxin Fab should be used in pregnant women as it is used in other adult patients.

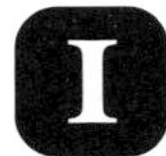

Indications

DIGOXIN OR DIGITOXIN TOXICITY

- Signs of cardiovascular instability, including hypotension, symptomatic bradycardia, and other potentially unstable dysrhythmias.
- Rapid progression of toxicity, including gastrointestinal or cardiovascular symptoms.
- Hyperkalemia greater than 5.5 mEq/L without other major effects (associated with a poor prognosis).

OTHER CARDIAC GLYCOSIDES (PLANT, APHRODISIAC, OR TOAD SECRETIONS)

- Digoxin immune Fab has been useful for cardiac toxicity induced by plant cardiac glycosides (e.g., oleander and lanatoside C), certain aphrodisiacs (e.g., Rock Hard and Love Stone), and some abused animal products (Bufo toad species).
- A therapeutic trial in patients with cardiac effects following ingestion of these products is warranted (see SECTION IV, Plants—Cardiac Glycosides chapter).

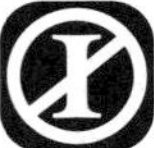

Contraindications and Adverse Effects

CONTRAINDICATIONS

Allergy to sheep products contraindicates use (a history of skin irritation to wool products does not constitute an allergy).

ADVERSE EFFECTS

- Allergic reactions to digoxin Fab may occur; however, they have been rare and mild.
- Hypokalemia may develop rapidly; patients with a low or borderline potassium level should receive supplemental potassium during treatment with digoxin immune Fab.
- Loss of digoxin effect may occur; for example, loss of rate control in atrial fibrillation could occur.

Dosage and Method of Administration

Dosage of digoxin immune Fab can be calculated in three ways.

• If both the amount ingested and the serum digoxin levels are unknown, digoxin immune Fab can be administered empirically.

—Acute single ingestion. The manufacturer recommends that 20 vials be administered for acute adult or pediatric overdoses. However, most authorities recommend 10 vials as the initial dose with subsequent therapy as needed.
—Chronic digitalis intoxication. The recommended empiric dose is two to three vials for adults and 1/4 to 1/2 vial for a small child.

• If only the amount of digoxin ingested is known.

—The following calculation is used:
  —Amount ingested (mg) × [bioavailability/0.6 mg] = dose of Fab in vials
  —The bioavailability of digoxin tablets is 0.8, but is 1.0 for the capsule (Lanoxicaps) and varies for other preparations. If the bioavailability is unknown, the value of 0.8 should be used. Each vial of digoxin immune Fab neutralizes 0.6 mg of digoxin.
  —For example, the dose for ingestion of ten 0.25 mg tablets is: 2.5 mg × (0.8/0.6) = 3.3 vials.

• If a 6-hour or greater postingestion serum concentration is available.

—The following calculation is used:
  —[serum concentration of digoxin (μg/ml) × 6 L/kg × patient weight (kg)]/[1,000 × 0.6 mg] = number of vials
  —The volume of distribution of digitalis is 6 L/kg.
  —The serum level should be drawn at least 6 hours postingestion.
  —If the patient is dependent on digitalis for cardiac stability, this calculation can be modified to maintain the serum level of unbound digitalis at 1.0. In this modified calculation, the "serum concentration of digoxin" is then reduced to 1.0 μg/ml.

• If other cardiac glycoside, plant, aphrodisiac, or food secretion has been ingested, the dose is unknown.

—In case reports treatment has typically started with 5 to 10 vials.
—Additional doses may be necessary. However, it is unlikely that all cardiac glycosides in these products are neutralized by digoxin immune Fab; therefore, if no apparent response is obtained, there should be no delay in using alternative treatments.

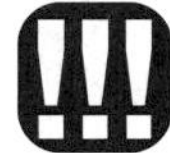

Pitfalls

• When calculating the required dose of digoxin immune Fab from the serum digoxin concentration, a serum digoxin level drawn earlier than 6 hours after the last digoxin dose is difficult to interpret. Distribution of digoxin requires at least 6 hours, and levels drawn earlier than this will be higher than the actual blood concentration and should not be used in calculating digoxin immune Fab doses.
• Patients who rely on digoxin for medical reasons, such as rate control of atrial fibrillation, should probably not have their entire serum digoxin load reversed with digoxin immune Fab.

—Doing so could make the patient medically unstable.
—Thus, partial neutralization may be a safer method to reverse a specific amount of digoxin.

• Digoxin toxicity has recurred in patients with renal failure who received digoxin immune Fab.

—The Fab-digoxin complex begins to dissociate about 3 days after administration of digoxin immune Fab.
—If a significant portion of the complex remains unexcreted a week after administration due to renal insufficiency, toxicity may recur.

• If the initial dose of digoxin immune Fab is inadequate, digoxin toxicity may recur within a few hours of the administration of digoxin immune Fab. This is not dangerous if it is anticipated and monitored. Additional digoxin immune Fab should be administered if clinical effects recur.
• Digoxin-like immunoreactive substances are endogenous substances that may be detected by digoxin assays.

—They have been reported in neonates, and rarely in pregnant women or patients with renal or hepatic failure.
—Although it produces a high apparent digoxin level, clinically apparent toxic effects should not be present.

• The elderly with cardiac problems may be more likely to succumb to digoxin toxicity and should therefore be more readily treated.

See also: SECTION IV, Digoxin and Plants—Cardiac Glycosides chapters.

ICD-9-CM 972.1

Poisoning by agents primarily affecting the cardiovascular system: cardiotonic glycosides and drugs of similar action.

RECOMMENDED READING

Taboulet P, Baud FJ, Bismuth C. Clinical features and management of digitalis poisoning: rationale for immunotherapy. Clin Tox 1993;31:247–260.

Woolf AD, Wenger T, Smith TW, et al. The use of digoxin-specific Fab fragments for severe digitalis intoxication in children. N Engl J Med 1992;326:1739–1744.

Authors: Lada Kokan and Kennon Heard

Reviewer: Richard C. Dart

Edrophonium

Basics

DESCRIPTION

Edrophonium is a medication used in the diagnosis of myasthenia gravis and occasionally in the treatment of snakebite.

FORMS AND USES

Edrophonium chloride (Tensilon, Enlon, Reversol)

MECHANISM OF ACTION

- Edrophonium is a reversible inhibitor of the enzyme acetylcholinesterase in the synaptic junction.
- Inhibition of acetylcholinesterase in the synaptic junction increases the concentration of acetylcholine, thereby overcoming the effect of blockade of the acetylcholine receptor.
- The onset of action is 30 to 60 seconds, and its duration is 10 to 30 minutes.

DRUG AND DISEASE INTERACTIONS

- Synergistic cholinergic effects can occur in patients with pre-existing cholinergic inhibition (neostigmine, pyridostigmine, physostigmine, organophosphate, or carbamate insecticides).
- Increased dysrhythmias may occur with digoxin, calcium channel blockers, or β-blockers.
- Quinidine may antagonize the effects of edrophonium and may mask diagnostic response in patients with myasthenia gravis.
- Procainamide may antagonize the effects on skeletal muscle.

PREGNANCY AND LACTATION

US FDA Pregnancy Category C. Studies have shown that the drug exerts teratogenic or embryocidal effects, but there are no controlled studies in women, or no studies are available in either animals or women.

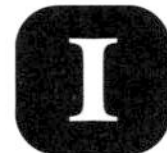

Indications

- Edrophonium acts as an antagonist to nondepolarizing, neuromuscular blockers:

—It is used for postoperative, postprocedure reversal of paralysis.
—It is used for bites of the Philippine cobra (Naja naja phillippinesis), as well as some other snakebites with neurotoxicity, especially if antivenom is unavailable.

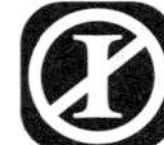

Contraindications and Adverse Effects

CONTRAINDICATIONS

- Known hypersensitivity to cholinergic agonists
- Known adequate anticholinesterase therapy
- Organophosphate or carbamate poisoning

ADVERSE EFFECTS

- Acute overdose or oversensitivity reactions are usually manifested by symptoms of muscarinic cholinergic receptor stimulation: nausea, vomiting, diarrhea, sweating, increased bronchial and salivary secretions, bradycardia, and hypotension.
- Bradycardia and cardiac standstill may occur.
- Respiratory weakness may occur.
- Airway obstruction by secretions may occur.

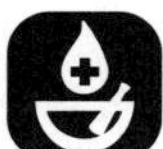

Dosage and Method of Administration

- As an antagonist to nondepolarizing, neuromuscular blockers. The dose for adults is 10 mg given intravenously over 30 to 45 seconds, repeated as necessary to a maximum of 40 mg. The pediatric dose is 233 μg/kg.
- Bite by Philippine cobra, or some other snakebites with neurotoxicity if antivenom is unavailable

—Atropine is administered intravenously (0.6 mg for adults, 50 μg/kg for children).
—Then edrophonium is administered.
 —The adult test dose is 2 mg given intravenously over 15 to 30 seconds. If there is no reaction in 45 seconds, another 8 mg (total 10 mg) is injected.
 —For children over 75 pounds, the test dose is 1 mg given intravenously over 15 to 30 seconds. If there is no reaction in 45 seconds, the remainder of up to 5 mg is injected.
 —For children under 75 pounds, the dose is 2 mg given intramuscularly.
 —The effect of each dose should be carefully assessed before giving additional edrophonium.

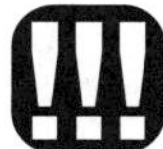

Pitfalls

- Cholinergic symptoms of excessive respiratory secretions and bradycardia from edrophonium are common.
- Symptoms of cholinergic excess in patients already on anticholinesterases may complicate therapy.
- Hypoxia may result if inadequate airway management is provided when cholinergic effects occur.
- Neurotoxicity from snakebite may produce respiratory paralysis indistinguishable from that seen as an adverse reaction to edrophonium.
- Hypotension may occur and should be managed with isotonic fluid infusion, Trendelenburg position, and, if needed, dopamine.
- Seizures may occur and should be controlled with benzodiazepine administration; phenytoin and phenobarbital are second-line treatments.
- Cardiac rhythm should be monitored continuously until the dysrhythmia resolves, the airway is controlled, and the patient is stable.
- Geriatric patients have an increased susceptibility to dysrhythmia and greater likelihood of underlying renal failure and drug-drug interactions.

ICD-9-CM 971.0

Poisoning by drugs primarily affecting the autonomic nervous system: parasympathetics (cholinergics).

See also: SECTION II, Hypotension, Seizure, and Bradycardia chapters; SECTION III, Atropine chapter; and SECTION IV, Edrophonium chapter.

RECOMMENDED READING

Gilman AG, Rall TW, Nies AS, et al., eds. Goodman and Gilman's the pharmacological basis of therapeutics, 8th ed. New York: Pergamon, 1990.

Osserman KE, Kaplan LI. Rapid diagnostic test for myasthenia gravis: increased muscle strength, without fasciculations, after intravenous administration of edrophonium (TensilonR chloride). JAMA 1952;150:265–268.

Youngberg JA. Cardiac arrest following treatment of paroxysmal atrial tachycardia with edrophonium. Anesthesiology 1979;50:234–235.

Author: Steven A. Seifert

Reviewer: Luke Yip

Ethanol

Basics

DESCRIPTION

Ethanol is a short-chain alcohol used for the treatment of ethylene glycol or methanol poisoning.

FORMS AND USES

Ethanol (ethyl alcohol USP) is available in a 95% concentration in vials or in dilute forms (5% or 10%) ready for administration. The preferred agent for ethylene glycol or methanol poisoning is fomepizole, owing to ease of administration and reduced costs for ancillary and ICU care.

MECHANISM OF ACTION

- Ethanol, methanol, and ethylene glycol are all metabolized by the enzyme alcohol dehydrogenase.
- The products of metabolism from methanol and ethylene glycol are responsible for their toxicity.
- The affinity of alcohol dehydrogenase for ethanol is much higher than for methanol or ethylene glycol; by providing ethanol in sufficient quantity to saturate alcohol dehydrogenase, the metabolism and therefore the toxicity of methanol or ethylene glycol can be blocked.

DRUG AND DISEASE INTERACTIONS

- The effects of CNS depressant drugs is increased by ethanol.
- Ethanol may produce acute flushing, vomiting, and hypotension when the patient has taken disulfiram, metronidazole, or numerous other antimicrobials; oral sulfonylurea agents (chlorpropamide, glipizide, others); several industrial agents (carbon disulfide, trichloroethylene, ethylene dibromide, thiuram, etc.); chloral hydrate, monamine oxidase inhibitors (tranylcypramine, procarbazine); or Coprinus mushrooms ("inky caps"). See also SECTION IV, Disulfiram chapter.

PREGNANCY AND LACTATION

- US FDA Pregnancy Category X. Studies have demonstrated fetal abnormalities or there is evidence of fetal risk based human risk and the risk clearly outweighs any possible benefit.
- However, ethanol therapy should not be withheld in pregnant patients because the risk of methanol and ethylene glycol toxicity outweigh the risk of ethanol therapy.

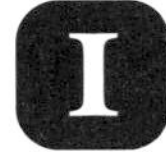

Indications

- Ethylene glycol ingestion

—Ethanol therapy should be instituted for an ethylene glycol level over 20 mg/dl or for any degree of metabolic acidosis or other toxic effect (coma, renal injury) in the setting of possible ethylene glycol ingestion.
—If levels are not immediately available, therapy should be instituted for a reliable history of ingestion while further evaluation is performed.

- Methanol ingestion

—Ethanol therapy should be instituted for a methanol level over 20 mg/dl or for any degree of metabolic acidosis or other toxic effect (coma, visual complaints) in the setting of possible methanol ingestion.
—If levels are not immediately available, therapy should be instituted for a reliable history of ingestion while further evaluation is performed.

- Unexplained increased anion gap acidosis not improving with hydration while further evaluation is performed
- Unexplained osmolar gap while further evaluation is performed

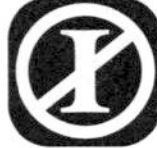

Contraindications and Adverse Effects

CONTRAINDICATIONS

Preexisting ethanol intoxication. Patients with a measurable blood ethanol level should have ethanol dosing adjusted as directed in the section on "Dosage and Method of Administration."

ADVERSE EFFECTS

- Patients may have significant CNS depression and require airway management.
- Ethanol is very irritating to vessels and may cause phlebitis.
- Hypoglycemia may occur, especially in children or diabetic patients; glucose should always be added to intravenous fluid and serum glucose levels followed closely.
- Because large volumes of water are infused with ethanol, fluid overload and hyponatremia may occur.
- Ethanol infusion may exacerbate gout.
- Ethanol impairs cardiovascular function and may compromise hemodynamic status in seriously ill patients.

Dosage and Method of Administration

The goal of therapy for methanol or ethylene glycol ingestion is to maintain a blood ethanol level of 100 to 150 mg/dl.

Loading Dose

- The patient should be treated with 10 cc/kg of 10% ethanol infused intravenously over 30 minutes.
- A loading dose is not needed if the preexisting serum ethanol level is greater than 100 mg/dl.

Maintenance Dose

The maintenance dose is 1 cc/kg/h infusion of 10% ethanol; the chronic alcoholic should be treated with 2 cc/kg/h infusion of 10% ethanol.

Oral Dosages

- If an intravenous formulation is not available, oral loading using the same amount is acceptable.
- To load, the patient should ingest four 1-ounce "shots" of a 40% (80 proof) ethanol.
- For maintenance, the patient should ingest one 1-ounce shot orally every hour.
- Ethanol level should be monitored hourly.

Ethanol Levels and Repeat Boluses

- Ethanol levels should be obtained immediately after the loading dose infusion and followed hourly until stable for 4 hours, and then obtained every 4 hours until the ethylene glycol or methanol level is below 20 mg/dl.
- If low ethanol levels are detected, the patient should receive a repeat bolus of ethanol in addition to increasing the rate.

—Patients with a blood ethanol level of 0 to 50 mg/dl should receive a bolus of 10 cc/kg of 10% ethanol and have the infusion rate doubled.
—Patients with levels of 50 to 80 mg/dl should receive a bolus of 5 cc/kg of 10% ethanol and have the rate increased by 50%.
—Patients with ethanol levels of 80 to 100 mg/dl should receive a bolus of 2.5 cc/kg of 10% ethanol and the rate increased by 25%.

Dialysis Patients

- The infusion rate should be doubled or tripled during the dialysis session.
- Ethanol levels should be followed hourly.

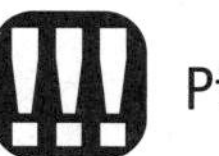

Pitfalls

- If clinical suspicion is high, ethanol therapy should not be withheld while awaiting ethylene glycol or methanol levels.
- Ethanol levels should be followed closely to assure therapeutic levels.
- Children may be more prone to hypoglycemia.
- Elderly patients may be more prone to CNS depression from ethanol.

ICD-9-CM 980.1

Toxic effect of alcohol: ethylene glycol or methanol.

See also: SECTION IV, Disulfiram chapter.

RECOMMENDED READING

Bryson PD. Ethylene glycol/methanol. In: Comprehensive review in toxicology. Washington, DC: Taylor & Francis, 1996:394–408.

Author: Kennon Heard

Reviewer: Katherine M. Hurlbut

Ethylenediaminetetraacetic acid (EDTA)

Basics

DESCRIPTION

EDTA (ethylenediaminetetraacetic acid) is a medication used to chelate several different metals.

FORMS AND USES

Calcium disodium edetate (calcium disodium versenate) contains calcium disodium EDTA. It is provided as a solution (200 mg/ml) for intravenous administration.

MECHANISM OF ACTION

- The calcium component of EDTA is displaced by lead to form a stable lead-containing chelate.
- The chelate is then excreted in the urine, thereby preventing injury. EDTA may remove lead from binding sites on enzymes and other physiologic proteins.

DRUG AND DISEASE INTERACTIONS

- EDTA also increases the excretion of zinc and iron.
- Only calcium disodium EDTA should be used. Forms without calcium may cause hypocalcemia when administered.

PREGNANCY AND LACTATION

- The safety of EDTA in human pregnancy has not been established.
- EDTA is teratogenic in animal models; therefore, it should be used during pregnancy only to treat serious toxicity.

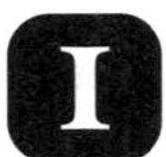

Indications

The use of EDTA in lead poisoning is evolving rapidly due to the introduction of newer and better agents. Consultation with a physician experienced in the treatment of lead poisoning is recommended. EDTA is indicated for treatment of:

- Lead toxicity without CNS toxicity

—EDTA is used as a single-drug regimen in pediatric or adult patients who typically have blood lead levels of less than 100 μg/dl and who cannot tolerate oral medication (e.g., succimer)

- Severe lead toxicity or lead encephalopathy

—EDTA should be used in conjunction with British anti-Lewisite (BAL).
—Severe lead poisoning is defined as:
  —Lead level of greater than 100 μg/dl in a child.
  —Evidence of CNS toxicity (seizure, altered mental status, or encephalopathy).
  —Severe gastrointestinal effects precluding oral administration (severe abdominal pain episodes and dehydration from recurrent vomiting) in an adult or child.

EDTA is also used as an "alternative" health technique for the treatment of atherosclerotic heart disease and other unproven indications. Acceptable evidence of efficacy is lacking and its use is discouraged.

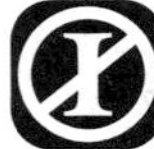

Contraindications and Adverse Effects

CONTRAINDICATIONS

- Renal failure

—The EDTA dose should be reduced in renal insufficiency.
—EDTA should not be used in anuric patients unless hemodialysis will be performed.

- Known hypersensitivity to calcium disodium edetate

ADVERSE EFFECTS

- Injury to proximal and distal renal tubules occurs rarely.

—It is more common in dehydrated patients.
—It is managed by supportive care and is usually reversible unless doses larger than recommended have been used.

- Because redistribution of lead from blood to brain has been reported in animal models, use of EDTA for lead encephalopathy should be avoided or delayed 4 hours or more after BAL has been administered.
- Other adverse effects include rashes, malaise, fatigue, chills, fever, myalgia, headache, anorexia, urinary frequency and urgency, nasal congestion and sneezing, lacrimation, glycosuria, anemia, hypotension, prolonged prothrombin time, and inverted T waves. These effects resolve after infusion is discontinued.
- Extravasation may cause painful local calcinosis.

Dosage and Method of Administration

LEAD TOXICITY WITHOUT CNS EFFECTS IF ORAL AGENTS CANNOT BE USED

- EDTA may be used if vomiting or other conditions preclude the administration of an oral antidote for an asymptomatic patient or a symptomatic patient without encephalopathy and a blood lead level less than 100 μg/dl.

—The dose for adults or children is a continuous intravenous infusion of 50 mg/kg/day or 1,000 mg/m^2/day over 24 hours or as a divided dose every 8 to 12 hours; a dosage of 50 mg/kg/day should not be exceeded. The therapy continues for 5 days and is then interrupted for 2 days, and the need for further chelation is reassessed.
—The blood lead level should be reassessed several days after completion of each course of chelation and every 2 to 4 weeks thereafter until the level stabilizes. If the blood lead level increases substantially, the possibility that a repeat exposure could have occurred in the interim should be investigated. If a repeat exposure has not occurred, the course of chelation should be repeated. If repeat exposure has occurred, the patient should be moved to lead-free environment before chelation therapy is repeated.

- The treatment should change to an oral chelator as early as possible. Succimer is the preferred oral agent.
- If renal insufficiency is present, the dose should be reduced to 500 mg every 12 hours in adults and 10 to 15 mg/kg/day in pediatrics.
- Continuous infusion is preferred. If intermittent infusion is used, each dose should be administered over 2 hours or more.
- The manufacturer recommends diluting one 5-ml ampule (1 g) with 250 to 500 ml of isotonic sodium chloride or sterile 5% dextrose solution in water.
- Adequate urine output (1–2 cc/kg/h) should be maintained throughout the therapy.
- Although intramuscular administration has been used, it is not recommended due to local pain and complications.

SEVERE LEAD TOXICITY OR LEAD ENCEPHALOPATHY

- First, BAL therapy must be initiated.
- The EDTA dose is 1,500 mg/m^2/day, administered as a continuous infusion over 24 hours. A total dose of 75 mg/kg/day should not be exceeded. Therapy continues for 5 days; then it is interrupted for 2 days, and the need for further chelation is reassessed.
- Testing of the blood lead level should be repeated several days after completion of therapy and every 2 to 4 weeks thereafter until the level stabilizes. If the blood lead level increases substantially, the possibility that a repeat exposure could have occurred in the interim should be investigated. If a repeat exposure has not occurred, the course of chelation should be repeated. If a repeat exposure has occurred, the patient should be moved to lead-free environment before chelation is repeated.
- Continuous infusion of EDTA is preferred. If intermittent infusion is used, each dose should be administered over 2 hours or more.
- Adequate urine output (1–2 ml/kg/h) should be maintained throughout the therapy.

EDTA PROVOCATION TEST

A single dose of EDTA may be administered to determine the need for chelation in patients with blood levels between 25 and 45 μg/dl. The EDTA provocation test is no longer used in most centers.

Procedure

Intravenous EDTA, 1 g, is administered intravenously to adult patients (50 mg/kg intravenously up to 1 g in pediatric patients). All urine is collected for the following 24 hours after EDTA infusion. If the ratio of lead in the urine to EDTA administered [(total lead excreted in μg)/(EDTA dose in mg)] is greater than 0.7, the test result is positive and a course of chelation is indicated. A ratio between 0.6 and 0.69 is indeterminate, and a ratio below 0.6 is considered negative.

Single Daily Dose Technique

EDTA has also been used as an outpatient treatment in asymptomatic lead-poisoned children. A single daily dose of 1,000 mg/m^2/day is administered intravenously over 15 to 20 minutes for 5 days.

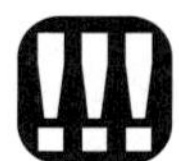

Pitfalls

- Unnecessary patient discomfort should be avoided; use of EDTA should be discontinued after patient has regained the ability to tolerate an oral agent.
- Dose of EDTA should be reduced or treatment discontinued if renal insufficiency develops during therapy.
- Prior to the initiation of EDTA, the patient should be hydrated; during therapy, good urine output should be maintained to lessen the chance of nephrotoxicity.
- Use of EDTA alone in lead encephalopathy is not recommended.

ICD-9-CM 984

Toxic effect of lead and its compounds.

See also: SECTION III, British Anti-Lewisite and Succimer chapters.

RECOMMENDED READING

Centers for Disease Control. Preventing lead poisoning in young children. A statement by the Centers for Disease Control, Atlanta, GA, October 1991.

Howland MA. Calcium disodium edetate. In: Goldfrank LR, et al., eds. Goldfrank's toxicologic emergencies, 6th ed. East Norwalk, CT: Appleton & Lange, 1998.

Author: Katherine M. Hurlbut

Reviewer: Luke Yip

Flumazenil

Basics

DESCRIPTION

Flumazenil is a medication that blocks benzodiazepine receptors.

FORMS AND USES

Flumazenil is used to diagnose benzodiazepine overdose or to reverse benzodiazepine-induced conscious sedation. Flumazenil (Romazicon, Anexate) is available in 5- and 10-ml vials with concentration solution of 0.1 mg/ml.

MECHANISM OF ACTION

- Flumazenil is a specific benzodiazepine receptor antagonist that inhibits the CNS effects of benzodiazepine drugs by competing for the benzodiazepine receptor.
- It is structurally related to the short-acting benzodiazepine midazolam (Versed).
- The elimination half-life is short (approximately 1 hour), and the duration of action varies from 15 to 140 minutes.
- The pharmacokinetics of flumazenil do not change with age, gender, or renal insufficiency.
- Clearance of flumazenil is greatly reduced in patients with mild to moderate liver disease, prolonging its effect.

DRUG AND DISEASE INTERACTIONS

Reversal of benzodiazepine effect should be undertaken cautiously in patients who have also ingested drugs that lower the seizure threshold (tricyclic antidepressants, cocaine, haloperidol). Abrupt termination of benzodiazepine effect may precipitate seizures.

PREGNANCY AND LACTATION

- US FDA Pregnancy Category C. The drug exerts animal teratogenic or embryocidal effects, but there are no controlled studies in women, or no studies are available in either animals or women.
- Flumazenil should be used in pregnancy as it is in other adult patients.

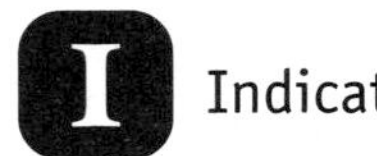

Indications

DIAGNOSIS OF BENZODIAZEPINE OVERDOSE

If a marked improvement of CNS depression follows administration of flumazenil to a patient with depressed mentation, the diagnosis of benzodiazepine intoxication is likely. This may allow some tests or procedures to be avoided (endotracheal intubation, head CT, lumbar puncture).

REVERSAL OF CONSCIOUS SEDATION

Flumazenil is used to treat patients who develop undesired respiratory or CNS depression during benzodiazepine administration for therapeutic procedures such as fracture reduction.

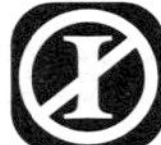

Contraindications and Adverse Effects

CONTRAINDICATIONS

- Tricyclic antidepressant overdose (especially if QRS duration is greater than 100 msec), due to the possibility of ventricular dysrhythmia
- Chronic benzodiazepine treatment for seizure control, due to the likelihood of inducing withdrawal
- Known hypersensitivity reaction to benzodiazepines
- Patients who are potentially dependent upon benzodiazepines due to chronic use or high-dose administration in the intensive care unit (this may develop after only 2–3 days of treatment)
- Mixed overdose with agents known to cause seizures

—Substances may include cocaine, lithium, methylxanthines, isoniazid, propoxyphene, monoamine oxidase inhibitors, bupropion, and cyclosporine.
—Flumazenil treatment may eliminate benzodiazepine suppression of seizures and thus "unmask" seizures induced by the coingestant.

- Known seizure disorder
- Head injury patients receiving benzodiazepines (because antidote may alter blood flow and induce seizures)

ADVERSE EFFECTS

- Anxiety, vertigo, nausea, vomiting (which may lead to aspiration in obtunded patients), tremor, discomfort, dyspnea, and headache may occur.
- Hypotension and ventricular dysrhythmia have occurred in seriously ill patients, usually with preexisting severe acidosis or tricyclic antidepressant overdose.
- Seizures and the precipitation of an acute withdrawal reaction may occur in chronic benzodiazepine users. Because of the potential for complications of withdrawal (including seizures), it is suggested that small doses be used initially, with additional incremental doses given as needed.

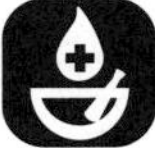

Dosage and Method of Administration

DIAGNOSIS OF BENZODIAZEPINE OVERDOSE

- Flumazenil should be administered as a series of small injections, not as a bolus.
- Adult. Initial dose of 0.2 mg (2.0 ml) is administered intravenously over 30 seconds. If there is no response, an additional 0.3 mg is administered. Repeated dosing with 0.5 mg can be used, administered every 1 to 2 minutes, up to a total of 3 mg (10 mg has been used in exceptional cases).
- The pediatric dose of 0.01 mg/kg (0.1 ml/kg) is administered intravenously, titrated to effect with a maximum dose of 1 mg.
- If there is no effect within 5 minutes, the cause of altered mental status is unlikely to be benzodiazepine and another cause should be sought.
- Patients should be monitored for recurrent sedation, respiratory depression, and signs of withdrawal. Recurrent sedation may occur within 30 minutes, but does not occur in all patients.
- Flumazenil should be administered in a setting, such as an emergency department or intensive care unit, where seizures can be promptly and effectively managed.
- Patients who have ingested longer acting benzodiazepines may require multiple doses or continuous infusion (0.1–0.2 mg/h). This should be attempted only if it offers a substantial benefit (e.g., if it avoids endotracheal intubation).

REVERSAL OF CONSCIOUS SEDATION

- Adult dose is 0.2 mg (2.0 ml), administered intravenously over 15 seconds. If there is no response, the dose should be repeated every 1 minute, up to a total dose of 1 mg.
- Pediatric dose is 0.01 mg/kg, administered intravenously with a maximum dose of 1 mg.
- The patient should be monitored for recurrent sedation or respiratory depression.

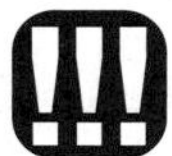

Pitfalls

- Flumazenil is not recommended for patients with agitation, tachycardia, tachypnea, or other signs of adrenergic stimulation because they are unlikely to have benzodiazepine toxicity as a major component of their condition. Thus, reversal may place the patient at risk of adverse effects without likely benefit.
- Patients should not be discharged soon after reversal because recurrent sedation has occasionally occurred 2 to 3 hours after flumazenil administration.

ICD-9-CM 969.4

Poisoning by psychotropic agents: benzodiazepine-based tranquilizers.

RECOMMENDED READING

Geller E, Crome P, Schaller MD, et al. Risks and benefits of therapy with flumazenil (Anexate) in mixed drug intoxications. Eur Neurol 1991;31:241.

Hojer J, Baehrendtz S, Matell G, Gustafsson LL. Diagnostic utility of flumazenil in coma with suspected poisoning: a double blind, randomised controlled study, BMJ 1990;301:1308.

Spivey WH, Roberts JR, Derlet RW. A clinical trial of escalating doses of flumazenil for reversal of suspected benzodiazepine overdose in the emergency department. Ann Emerg Med 1993;22:1813.

Authors: Jeffrey S. Peterson and Charles B. Cairns

Reviewer: Katherine M. Hurlbut

Basics

DESCRIPTION

Folic acid is a water-soluble, essential vitamin used in the treatment of methanol or methotrexate poisoning and proposed for the treatment of ethylene glycol poisoning.

FORMS AND USES

Folic Acid

- Oral. It is available alone or in combination with other vitamins. It is also available in foods such as leafy vegetables, yeast, and liver in the form of reduced polyglutamates.
- Parenteral. Folic acid (sodium folate, Folvite) is available in 5 and 10 mg/ml in 10-ml vials.

Folinic Acid (Leucovorin, Citrovorum Factor, Wellcovorin)

- Oral. The 5-mg tablet contains 5 mg of leucovorin and inactive ingredients (cornstarch, dibasic calcium phosphate, magnesium stearate, and pregelatinized starch). The 15-mg tablet contains 15 mg of leucovorin and inactive ingredients (lactose, magnesium stearate, microcrystalline cellulose, pregelatinized starch, and sodium starch glycolate).
- Parenteral. Solution contains leucovorin (as the calcium salt) 10 mg/ml. Inactive ingredients include 80 mg of sodium chloride per vial and sodium hydroxide or hydrochloric acid to adjust the pH to 8.1. The dry product has no preservatives. It should be diluted with bacteriostatic water for injection (USP), which contains benzyl alcohol, or with sterile water for injection (USP).

MECHANISM OF ACTION

- Folic acid is actively transported into cells and converted to its biologically active form, tetrahydrofolate, by a two-step enzymatic reduction involving dihydrofolate reductase.
- Tetrahydrofolate has several biologically active forms that are cofactors in biochemical reactions and synthesis of DNA and RNA precursors and several amino acids.
- In methanol poisoning, the administration of folic acid or leucovorin enhances the metabolism and elimination of formic acid, the toxic end-product of methanol metabolism to carbon dioxide and water.
- In ethylene glycol poisoning, a minor metabolic pathway may produce formic acid.

—Theoretically, administration of folic acid or leucovorin will enhance the elimination of formic acid.
—The clinical usefulness of folate in this scenario has not been tested.

- Methotrexate is a folate analog and a potent inhibitor of dihydrofolate reductase.

—Administration of leucovorin bypasses the inhibited dihydrofolate reductase system, displaces methotrexate from dihydrofolate reductase, competes with methotrexate for intercellular transport, and increases efflux of methotrexate from the cell.

DRUG AND DISEASE INTERACTIONS

- Death from severe enterocolitis, diarrhea, and dehydration have been reported in elderly patients receiving leucovorin and fluorouracil.
- Folic acid in large amounts may counteract the antiepileptic effect of phenobarbital, phenytoin, and primidone.

PREGNANCY AND LACTATION

- US FDA Pregnancy Category C. Studies have shown that the drug exerts animal teratogenic or embryocidal effects, but there are no controlled studies in women, or no studies are available in either animals or women.
- It is unknown whether leucovorin is excreted in human milk.

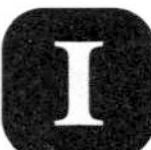

Indications

- Methanol poisoning. Folic acid or leucovorin may be used. Patients treated with fomepizole or ethanol should also receive folic acid or leucovorin.
- Ethylene glycol poisoning. Although the use of leucovorin has theoretical application, it is not routinely recommended.
- Methotrexate overdose. Typically, this involves patients in whom an inadvertent, iatrogenic overdose is discovered after methotrexate administration. Leucovorin (not folic acid) is the only effective treatment.

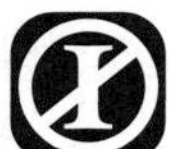

Contraindications and Adverse Effects

CONTRAINDICATIONS

There are no known contraindications.

ADVERSE EFFECTS

- Rare allergic reactions to folic acid preparations include erythema, rash, itching, malaise, and wheezing.
- Gastrointestinal effects, anorexia, nausea, and abdominal distention, may occur.
- CNS effects, including altered sleep patterns, difficulty in concentrating, irritability, depression, and confusion, have been reported rarely in patients receiving 15 mg of folic acid daily for 1 month. Minimal daily intake is estimated to be 0.1 to 0.2 mg, and usual dietary intake is 0.5 to 1.0 mg/day.
- Decreased serum vitamin B_{12} concentrations may occur in patients receiving prolonged folic acid therapy.
- Because of the benzyl alcohol contained in certain diluents, when doses greater than 10 mg/m^2 are administered, leucovorin calcium should be reconstituted with sterile water instead and used immediately.
- Because of the calcium content of the leucovorin solution, no more than 160 mg per minute (16 ml/min) of leucovorin should be injected intravenously.

Dosage and Method of Administration

Leucovorin is preferred to folic acid for all indications.

METHANOL POISONING

- Leucovorin. A dose of 1 to 2 mg/kg is administered intravenously every 4 to 6 hours until methanol is eliminated and acidosis resolves. If hemodialysis is indicated, a dose of leucovorin should be administered at the completion of dialysis.
- Folic acid. A dose of 50 to 75 mg is administered intravenously every 4 to 6 hours until methanol is eliminated and acidosis resolves.

METHOTREXATE TOXICITY

- Folic acid is not an effective antidote.
- Intravenous leucovorin is administered immediately in a dose equal to or greater than the ingested dose of methotrexate.

—The dose is repeated every 6 hours until methotrexate level is less than 10^{-8} molar.
—If the methotrexate dose is unknown, 10 mg/m^2 of leucovorin is administered every 6 hours until the methotrexate level is less than 10^{-8} molar.
—The duration of leucovorin therapy typically ranges from 12 to 72 hours.
—The pediatric dose for an unknown methotrexate dose is 10 mg/m^2.

- Serum creatinine and methotrexate levels should be determined at 24-hour intervals.

—If serum creatinine has increased 50% over baseline, if the 24-hour methotrexate level is greater than 5×10^{-6} molar, or if the 48-hour level is greater than 9×10^{-7} molar, intravenous leucovorin dosage should be increased to 100 mg/m^2 every 6 hours until the methotrexate level is less than 10^{-7} molar at 24 hours or 10^{-8} molar at any time.
—If the 24-hour methotrexate level is greater than 5×10^{-5} molar or if the 48-hour level is greater than 9×10^{-6} molar, the intravenous leucovorin dose should be increased to 1,000 mg/m^2 every 6 hours until the methotrexate level is less than 10^{-7} molar at 24 hours or 10^{-8} molar at any time.

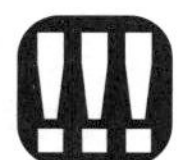

Pitfalls

- Intravenous administration is preferred, especially if gastrointestinal symptoms are present or if more than 50 mg is to be given, because intestinal cellular transport mechanisms for leucovorin become saturated at this amount.
- Because both folic acid and leucovorin are highly water soluble and will be removed during hemodialysis, an additional dose of folic acid or leucovorin should be administered following dialysis.
- Folic acid should not be substituted for leucovorin in methotrexate overdose.

ICD-9-CM 964.1

Poisoning by liver preparations and other antianemic agents.

See also: SECTION IV, Antineoplastic Medications, Ethylene Glycol, and Methanol chapters.

RECOMMENDED READING

Howland MA. Folic acid and leucovorin (folinic acid). In: Goldfrank LR, Flomenbaum NE, Lewin NA, et al., eds. Goldfrank's toxicologic emergencies, 6th ed. Norwalk, CT: Appleton & Lange, 1998.

Jacobsen D, McMartin K. Methanol and ethylene glycol poisonings—mechanism of toxicity, clinical course, diagnosis and treatment. Med Toxicol 1986;1:309–334.

Osterloh JD, Pond SM, Grady S, et al. Serum formate concentrations in methanol intoxication as a criterion for hemodialysis. Ann Intern Med 1986;104:200–203.

Author: Luke Yip

Reviewer: Rivka S. Horowitz

Fomepizole (Antizol)

Basics

DESCRIPTION

Fomepizole (Antizol) is an antidote for ethylene glycol and methanol poisoning.

FORMS AND USES

Fomepizole is provided in vials containing 1.5 ml of 1,000 mg/ml (total 1.5 g/vial)

MECHANISM OF ACTION

- Both ethylene glycol and methanol are metabolized by alcohol dehydrogenase to toxic metabolites.
- Before the development of fomepizole, the standard treatment of ethylene glycol or methanol poisonings involved the infusion of ethyl alcohol (ethanol), which blocks the formation of toxic metabolites by competing with ethylene glycol and methanol for metabolism by alcohol dehydrogenase.
- Fomepizole uses the same mechanism as ethanol and is a potent inhibitor of alcohol dehydrogenase; however, it produces more constant inhibition than ethanol and is simpler and safer to use.
- Because metabolism has been blocked, elimination occurs via urine (ethylene glycol) or breath (methanol).
- Patients with large body burdens of either ethylene glycol or methanol may require hemodialysis because the half-life is prolonged.

DRUG AND DISEASE INTERACTIONS

- Fomepizole will block metabolism of ethanol.
- Other drugs metabolized by the cytochrome P450 system may be similarly affected, although they have not been studied (phenytoin, carbamazepine, ketoconozole).

PREGNANCY AND LACTATION

- US FDA Pregnancy Category C. The drug exhibits animal teratogenic or embryocidal effects, but there are no controlled studies in women, or no studies are available in either women or men.
- It is not known if fomepizole is excreted in breast milk.

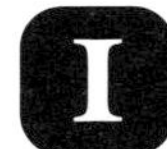

Indications

ETHYLENE GLYCOL POISONING

- History of possible ethylene glycol ingestion and evidence of toxicity (increased anion gap metabolic acidosis, hematuria, proteinuria)
- Serum ethylene glycol level above 20 mg/dl
- Preparation for dialysis of ethylene glycol poisoning

METHANOL POISONING

- History of possible methanol ingestion and evidence of intoxication or another effect of methanol (visual complaints, increased anion gap metabolic acidosis)
- Serum methanol level above 20 mg/dl
- Preparation for hemodialysis of methanol poisoning

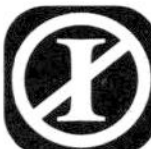

Contraindications and Adverse Effects

CONTRAINDICATIONS

- History of allergic response to fomepizole or other agents with pyrazole structure
- Concurrent infusion with ethanol because of accumulation and potential toxicity of ethanol

ADVERSE EFFECTS

- Administration of this compound has been generally free of any serious side effects.
- High doses (50 to 100 mg/kg) are associated with nausea, dizziness, diarrhea, headache, and vertigo; the dose should be decreased or the infusion slowed.
- Low doses (3 mg/kg) for 4 days may cause a slight increase in blood pressure and liver enzymes.

Dosage and Method of Administration

ETHYLENE GLYCOL OR METHANOL POISONING

- Loading dose. Adult or pediatric dose is 15 mg/kg.
- Maintenance dose. Adult and pediatric dose is 10 mg/kg every 12 hours for four doses, then 15 mg/kg every 12 hours thereafter until ethylene glycol or methanol level is less than 20 mg/dl (increase in rate is due to self-induction of cytochrome P450 system).
- Method of administration. Each dose should be diluted in 100 cc of normal saline or D5W and infused slowly over 30 minutes. After dilution, fomepizole should be used within 24 hours.

USE OF FOMEPIZOLE IN PATIENTS UNDERGOING HEMODIALYSIS

- Dose at beginning of hemodialysis:

—If less than 6 hours since last fomepizole dose, do not administer another dose.
—If more than 6 hours since last dose, administer 10 mg/kg at beginning of dialysis.

- Dosing during hemodialysis:

—Increase frequency of maintenance dose infusion to every 4 hours instead of 12 hours.

- Dosing at the end of hemodialysis session:

—If less than 1 hour since last fomepizole dose, do not administer dose at end of hemodialysis session.
—If 1 to 3 hours since last dose, administer half of next dose.
—If more than 3 hours since last dose, administer next scheduled dose.

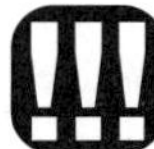

Pitfalls

- If clinical suspicion is high, fomepizole therapy should not be witheld while awaiting ethylene glycol or methanol levels.
- Overly rapid administration should be avoided; the rate of dose delivery does not affect outcome.

ICD-9-CM 980.1

Toxic effect of alcohol: ethylene glycol, methyl alcohol.

See also: SECTION II, Increased Anion Gap Metabolic Acidosis; SECTION IV, Ethylene Glycol and Methanol chapters.

RECOMMENDED READING

Baud FJ, Galliot M, Astier A, et al. Treatment of ethylene glycol poisoning with intravenous 4-methylpyrazole. N Engl J Med 1988;319:97–100.

Brent J, McMartin K, Phillips S, et al. Fomepizole for the treatment of ethylene glycol poisoning. N Eng J Med 1999;340:832–838.

McMartin KE, Heath A. Treatment of ethylene glycol poisoning with intravenous 4-methylpyrazole. N Engl J Med 1989;320:125.

Author: Scott D. Phillips

Reviewer: Richard C. Dart

Glucagon

Basics

DESCRIPTION

Glucagon is a naturally occurring hormone that is secreted in response to hypoglycemia.

FORMS AND USES

- Lyophilized powder is available in 1- or 10-mg vials, but it is most commonly supplied in 1-mg vials. The diluent may contain phenol 2 mg/ml as a preservative.
- A glucagon emergency kit contains 1 mg in an autoinjector syringe.

MECHANISM OF ACTION

- Glucagon increases blood sugar by stimulating hepatic gluconeogenesis and glycogenolysis. It also stimulates cyclic adenosine monophosphate (cAMP) production, which increases intracellular calcium and leads to increased heart rate and contractility.
- Because a β-receptor agonist also increases cAMP concentration, it is thought that glucagon may bypass the receptor blockade caused by β-receptor blocking drugs.

DRUG AND DISEASE INTERACTIONS

- Glucagon may increase anticoagulation of patients treated with warfarin.
- The hypoglycemic effects of both insulin and oral hypoglycemic agents are antagonized.

PREGNANCY AND LACTATION

US FDA Pregnancy Category B. Animal studies indicate no fetal risk and there are no controlled human studies, or animal studies show an adverse fetal effect but well-controlled studies in pregnant women do not.

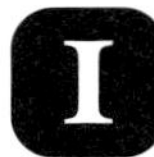

Indications

- Treatment is indicated for cardiac toxicity from β-blockers or calcium channel blockers.
- Specific indications:

—Bradycardia, which is refractory to standard interventions including administration of atropine (see SECTION IV, β-Receptor Blocking Drugs and Calcium Channel Blocking Drugs chapters for standard interventions).
—Hypotension, which is refractory to standard interventions including administration of isotonic saline, atropine, calcium (in the case of calcium channel blockers), and vasopressor (dopamine, norepinephrine or epinephrine).
—Glucagon is typically used after atropine has been administered and an infusion of vasopressor (e.g., dopamine, norepinephrine) has been initiated.

- Nontoxicologic indications include hypoglycemia, esoophageal food impaction, premedication for gastrointestinal endoscopy or radiographic procedures, asthma, acute biliary colic, colonic spasm secondary to acute diverticulitis, refractory congestive heart failure, and refractory anaphylaxis.

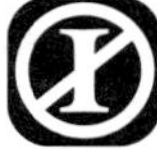

Contraindications and Adverse Effects

CONTRAINDICATIONS

- Hypersensitivity to glucagon.
- Hypoglycemia caused by severe insulin or oral hypoglycemic should be treated with infusion of dextrose instead of glucagon.

ADVERSE EFFECTS

- Nausea and vomiting are common
- Anaphylactoid or anaphylactic reactions
- Hyperglycemia
- Hypoglycemia, produced by paradoxical insulin release in a patient with an insulinoma
- Catecholamine release and hypertension may occur in a patient with pheochromocytoma
- Hypokalemia, due to hyperglycemia and intracellular shift of both glucose and potassium
- Toxicity from phenol diluent (contains 2 mg/ml)

—Thrombophlebitis and metabolic acidosis occur, due to effects of the phenol diluent.
—If the dose of glucagon to be administered is greater than 2 mg, it should be reconstituted with normal saline or D5W to avoid phenol toxicity.

Dosage and Method of Administration

BOLUS DOSE

- The adult dose is an initial bolus of 5 to 10 mg intravenously over 1 minute; if there is no effect within 5 minutes, a repeat dose, up to 10 to 20 mg, can be administered.
- The pediatric dose is 50 μg/kg bolus over 1 minute; if there is no effect within 5 minutes, a repeat dose, up to 10 mg, can be administered.

MAINTENANCE INFUSION

- The phenol diluent should not be used when reconstituting glucagon for continuous infusions; instead, it should be reconstituted with normal saline or D5W.
- The adult dose is 2 to 10 mg/h, titrated to the desired effect on heart rate and blood pressure.
- The pediatric dose is 0.07 mg/kg/h, titrated to the desired effect on heart rate and blood pressure.

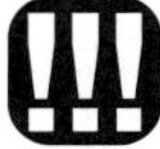

Pitfalls

- When toxicity to a β-receptor or calcium channel blocker develops, the pharmacy should be immediately alerted.

—Many pharmacies do not stock enough glucagon to manage even one severely poisoned patient, and it is not uncommon that an initial bolus infusion of glucagon would consume the glucagon supply for an entire health-care facility.
—More glucagon can often be found in the radiology and gastrointestinal departments or can be obtained from another institution.

- If metabolic acidosis develops, the phenol-containing diluent should not be used to reconstitute glucagon.
- Vomiting is very common with use of high-dose glucagon.

ICD-9-CM 962.3

Poisoning by hormones and synthetic substitutes: insulins and antidiabetic agents.

RECOMMENDED READING

Howland MA. Glucagon. In: Goldfrank LR, Flomenbaum NE, Lewin NS, et al. eds. Goldfrank's toxicologic emergencies, 6th ed. Norwalk, CT: Appleton & Lange, 1998.

Author: Edwin K. Kuffner

Reviewer: Richard C. Dart

Hyperbaric Oxygen

Basics

DESCRIPTION

Hyperbaric oxygen (HBO) is 100% oxygen delivered as pressure greater than 1 atmosphere.

FORMS AND USES

- HBO is used to deliver high concentrations of oxygen to tissues when hemoglobin cannot; this generally applies to carbon monoxide poisoning, but HBO also may be useful in other poisonings (e.g., cyanide, hydrogen sulfide, or severe methemoglobinemia).
- 100% oxygen is delivered by two basic types of hyperbaric chambers, mono-place and multi-place.
- Both types are capable of accommodating critical care devices, such as mechanical ventilators, arterial lines, central lines, Swan-Ganz catheters, and continuous ECG monitoring; however, only multi-place chambers allow direct patient access by the provider.

Mono-place Chambers

- These are 8 by 3 foot tubular chambers which accommodate one patient. Two patients may be treated in special circumstances (e.g., mother and small child).
- The entire chamber is pressurized with 100% oxygen, and no mask is worn by the patient.

Multi-place Chambers

- These are larger structures with benches or gurneys contained within the chamber, and can accommodate several patients at one time.
- A nurse or physician can accompany the patients.
- The chamber interior is pressurized with air (21% oxygen) and each patient wears a face mask or hood that delivers 100% oxygen.
- Multi-place chambers are expecially useful when an entire family needs HBO as in the case of household carbon monoxide exposure.

MECHANISM OF ACTION

- The primary action is to provide adequate oxygen delivery despite loss or dysfunction of hemoglobin.
- HBO increases the amount of oxygen physically dissolved in plasma; at 3 atmospheres absolute pressure, the amount of oxygen dissolved in the plasma (not carried by red cells) is sufficient to allow tissue respiration in the absence of hemoglobin.
- HBO also increases the rate of carbon monoxide elimination, thereby decreasing exposure.
- HBO also may have effects that decrease the inflammatory response to hypoxia produced by carbon monoxide; it decreases white blood cell activity and also inhibits lipid peroxidation.

DRUG AND DISEASE INTERACTIONS

- HBO may cause pain or barotrauma in patients with middle ear infection or from other causes.
- HBO also may exacerbate seizure disorder.

PREGNANCY AND LACTATION

Although concern about the potential teratogenic effect of HBO has been expressed, there is no clinical evidence to support this concern.

Indications

Widely accepted guidelines for determining which patients should receive HBO have not emerged; the following indications reflect a "middle-ground" approach to recommending HBO therapy, with the final decision based on availability of HBO and the exact clinical scenario.

- Carbon monoxide poisoning

—Definite indication for HBO
—Any patient with serious end-organ damage, including myocardial ischemia or infarction or serious neurologic effects (coma, loss of consciousness, focal deficits)
—Pregnant patient with carboxyhemoglobin level above 15%
—Conscious patient with neurologic effects, such as abnormal neuropsychiatric testing, but without other apparent end organ damage
—Carboxyhemoglobin above 25%, but without serious symptoms and signs

- Cyanide poisoning. Adjunctive therapy for metabolic acidosis caused by cyanide poisoning that does not respond adequately to administration of the cyanide antidote package.
- Hydrogen sulfide poisoning. Adjunctive therapy of critically ill patients.
- Carbon tetrachloride or chloroform poisoning. Adjunctive therapy to limit hepatic injury.
- Methemoglobinemia. HBO provides oxygen delivery in serious cases that do not respond to methylene blue.
- Osteoradionecrosis (radiation tissue damage)
- Other reported uses

—Air embolism, decompression sickness
—Wounds. Gas gangrene and other necrotizing soft tissue infections, diabetic foot ulcers, soft-tissue radiation injury, crush injury, osteomyelitis, skin grafts and flaps (compromised), thermal burns.
—Intracranial abscess. Adjunctive therapy.
—Severe blood loss anemia where other therapy is unavailable or ineffective

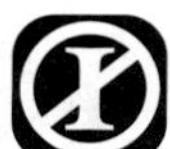

Contraindications and Adverse Effects

CONTRAINDICATIONS

- Recent chest surgery precludes use.
- Untreated pneumothorax precludes use.
- Hereditary spherocytosis is a relative contraindication.
- Patients unable to equalize ear/sinus pressures is a relative contraindication.
- HBO should be used cautiously in several patient groups:

—Comatose patients because barotrauma may not be apparent
—Patients at the extremes of age because of increased incidence of adverse effects
—Patients with head injury, history of seizure disorder, ethanol withdrawal due to possibility of seizure while in chamber
—Extreme claustrophobia

ADVERSE EFFECTS

- Acute oxygen toxicity (seizure) has been reported, but only at pressure higher than 2.8 atmospheric absolute (ATA).
- Rupture of tympanic membrane can occur.
- Some patients experience panic reaction due to confinement anxiety or claustrophobia.

Dosage and Method of Administration

- Consultation with a certified and experienced HBO provider is required.
- Chambers are widely distributed throughout the United States; to locate the nearest chamber, call the Divers Alert Network (DAN) at Duke University, 1-919-684-8111.
- Carbon monoxide poisoning

—The number of treatments, duration of treatment, and profile of pressure treatment vary substantially by institution.
—The initial treatment consists of 30 minutes of 100% oxygen at 3 ATA, then 60 minutes at 2 ATA or until a carboxyhemoglobin level less than 10% is achieved; another common regimen is 2.7 ATA for 30 minutes, then 2.2 ATA for 90 minutes.
—Recovery of consciousness often occurs during the treatment.
—Subsequent treatments depend on local practice and degree of recovery following first treatment.

- Cyanide, hydrogen sulfide, carbon tetrachloride, chloroform poisoning, or methemoglobinemia. There are no widely recognized regimens available. HBO is typically used in a manner similar to that used for carbon monoxide poisoning in patients refractory to other therapy.

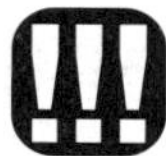

Pitfalls

Complications may be due to associated procedures or underlying disease rather than HBO itself (e.g., seizure can arise from carbon monoxide poisoning or oxygen toxicity).

ICD-9-CM 986

Toxic effect of carbon monoxide.

See also: SECTION IV, Carbon Monoxide, Cyanide, Hydrogen Sulfide, and Hydrocarbons—Chlorinated chapters; and SECTION II, Methemoglobinemia chapter.

RECOMMENDED READING

Ducasse JL, Celsis P, Marc-Vergnes JP, et al. Non-comatose patients with acute carbon monoxide poisoning: hyperbaric or normobaric oxygenation? Undersea Hyperbaric Med 1995;22:9–15.

Raphael JC, Elkharrat D, Jars-Guincestre MC, et al. Trial of normobaric and hyperbaric oxygen for acute carbon monoxide intoxication. Lancet 1989;2:414–419.

Thom SR, Taber RL, Mendiguren II, et al. Delayed neuropsychologic sequelae after carbon monoxide poisoning: prevention by treatment with hyperbaric oxygen. Ann Emerg Med 1995;25:474–480.

Author: Scott D. Phillips

Reviewer: Richard C. Dart

Ipecac Syrup

Basics

DESCRIPTION

Ipecac is an oral emetic agent.

FORMS AND USES

- Syrup of ipecac is composed of cephaeline and emetine in a 2.5:1 to 1.0:1 ratio.
- Typical doses are 10 cc for an infant 6 to 12 months of age, 15 cc for a child 1 to 5 years of age, and 30 cc for anyone over 5 years of age.
- It is available in 15- and 30-cc containers.

MECHANISM OF ACTION

- Cephaeline stimulates the central vomiting center, and emetine activates sensory receptors in the proximal small intestine.
- Time to vomiting: 88% of patients vomit in less than 30 minutes.
- Mean episodes of vomiting are three; the range is one to eight episodes.
- Duration of vomiting is 23 to 60 minutes.

DRUG AND DISEASE INTERACTIONS

Syrup of ipecac may be absorbed by charcoal, but no effect on time to initiation of vomiting has been demonstrated.

PREGNANCY AND LACTATION

- US FDA Pregnancy Category C. The drug exerts animal teratogenic or embryocidal effects, but there are no controlled studies in women, or no studies are available in either animals or women.
- Ipecac is relatively contraindicated during pregnancy due to potential mechanical effects on the uterus.

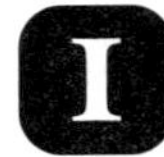

Indications

ADULT PATIENTS

- Prehospital care. Alert patients in whom health-care evaluation will not occur for an hour or more should be administered ipecac.
- Health-care facility. Gastric lavage should be used instead of ipecac, except for unusual conditions such as the ingestion of toxic plant material or tablets of a size that will not pass through the orogastric lavage tube.

PEDIATRIC PATIENTS

- Prehospital care. Alert patients in whom health-care evaluation will not occur for an hour or more should be administered ipecac.
- Health-care facility. Although gastric lavage is preferred, ipecac should be used within 1 hour of ingestion for patients who are too small to have effective gastric lavage due to orogastric tube size constraints.

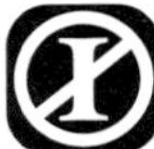

Contraindications and Adverse Effects

CONTRAINDICATIONS

- Ingestion of a substance that could cause further injury during emesis, for example, caustic substances or hydrocarbons
- Ingestion of a substance for which the antidote is administered orally (e.g., *N*-acetylcysteine or activated charcoal), because ipecac may delay administration greatly.
- Children under 6 months of age
- Ingestion of sharp object
- Patients whose ability to protect airway within subsequent 1 hour may deteriorate (e.g., anticipated seizure or coma)
- Ingestion of liquid with rapid absorption (aspiration with nasogastric tube is more rapid)

ADVERSE EFFECTS

- Persistent vomiting is the most common adverse reaction
- Aspiration of vomited substance (e.g., hydrocarbon)
- Vagal-induced bradycardia during emesis
- Esophageal injury, especially Mallory-Weiss tears
- Stomach herniation into chest
- Intracranial hemorrhage
- Pneumomediastinum

Dosage and Method of Administration

- Adult dose is 30 ml, administered orally; the dose may be repeated once if vomiting does not occur within 30 minutes.
- Dose for a child 1 to 5 years of age is 15 ml administered orally; the dose may be repeated once if vomiting does not occur within 30 minutes.
- Dose for a child 6 months to 1 year of age is 10 ml, administered orally; the dose may be repeated once if vomiting does not occur within 30 minutes.
- The use of a fluid, like water, to enhance vomiting has not been shown to alter the time to emesis but may increase patient or parent comfort with the procedure because "dry heaves" is considered more uncomfortable than vomiting water.
- Increasing the activity of the patient (e.g., walking) has been recommended to enhance the activity of ipecac; however, the data do not support this belief.
- Giving ipecac with milk products or activated charcoal may delay the onset of vomiting.

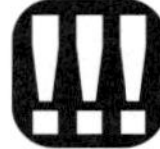

Pitfalls

Although it has been widely believed that ipecac is never useful in medical practice, this is incorrect: ipecac is of benefit to a patient who is more than an hour distant from a medical facility, when the patient is of small size, or when ingestion of plant material or large pills renders gastric lavage ineffective.

ICD-9-CM 973.6

Poisoning by agents primarily affecting the gastrointestinal system: emetics.

RECOMMENDED READING

Bond GR, Requa RK, Normann SA, et al. Influence of time until emesis on the efficacy of decontamination using acetaminophen as a marker in a pediatric population. *Ann Emerg Med* 1993;22:1403–1407.

Howland MA. Syrup of ipecac. In: Goldfrank LR, Flomenbaum NE, Lewin NA, et al., eds. *Goldfrank's toxicologic emergencies,* 6th ed. Norwalk, CT: Appleton & Lange, 1998.

Author: Richard C. Dart

Reviewer: Katherine M. Hurlbut

Magnesium Sulfate

Basics

DESCRIPTION

Magnesium sulfate is used to treat torsades de pointes and hydrofluoric acid toxicity.

FORMS AND USES

Each 20 ml solution of magnesium sulfate for intravenous infusion contains 2 g of magnesium sulfate (16.2 mEq magnesium), with sodium hydroxide or sulfuric acid added to adjust pH.

MECHANISM OF ACTION

- In treating polymorphic ventricular tachycardia (torsade de pointes), magnesium prolongs the PR interval, the atrioventricular nodal effective refractory period, and the sinoatrial conduction time, thereby preventing the early depolarization of the ventricle, which would otherwise cause ventricular tachycardia.
- In treating hydrofluoric acid burns to the skin, each magnesium ion binds two ions of fluoride, forming a salt (MgF_2); this action may prevent complexation of fluoride and calcium, which can cause burns and cell death.
- In the blood, fluoride ions induce life-threatening hypocalcemia by binding calcium ions (CaF_2); magnesium complexes these fluoride ions and thereby may prevent systemic hypocalcemia and the resultant ventricular dysrhythmias.

DRUG AND DISEASE INTERACTIONS

- The concomitant use of magnesium and aminoglycoside can produce weakness and paralysis.
- Magnesium sulfate potentiates the effects of neuromuscular blocking agents.

PREGNANCY AND LACTATION

- US FDA Pregnancy Category B. Animal studies indicate no fetal risk, and there are no controlled human studies, or animal studies show an adverse fetal effect but well-controlled studies in pregnant women do not.
- High-dose magnesium therapy has been used for many years in obstetrics with an excellent safety record.

Indications

- Polymorphic ventricular tachycardia (torsade de pointes) and hemodynamically stable dysrhythmias are indications for the use of magnesium sulfate; unstable ventricular dysrhythmias should be treated according to Advanced Cardiac Life Support guidelines.
- Hydrofluoric acid exposure to the skin is treated symptomatically by topical application or local infiltration of magnesium sulfate, which is the second-line agent after calcium gluconate gel.
- In the setting of hydrogen fluoride ingestion, laboratory-determined hypocalcemia or any degree of its clinical symptoms should be immediately treated with calcium chloride or magnesium sulfate to prevent ventricular dysrhythmia.
- A history of a large ingestion may indicate use of magnesium infusion to prevent hypocalcemia. (Immediate consultation with a poison control center or medical toxicologist is recommended.)

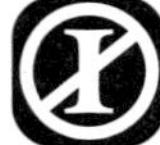

Contraindications and Adverse Effects

CONTRAINDICATIONS

- The dose should be reduced in renal insufficiency; magnesium should not be used in an anuric or dialysis-dependent patient unless dialysis is available.
- History of anaphylaxis to magnesium sulfate contraindicates use.

ADVERSE EFFECTS

- Weakness in or loss of deep tendon reflexes may progress to respiratory insufficiency if large doses are needed.
- Vasodilation and hypotension may develop.
- Other overdose effects include nausea, vomiting, flushing, CNS depression, bradycardia, QRS interval widening, and QT interval prolongation.

Dosage and Method of Administration

POLYMORPHIC VENTRICULAR TACHYCARDIA (TORSADE DE POINTES)

- An initial bolus of 2 to 4 g in adults, or 25 to 50 mg/kg in children, may be administered by intravenous push.
- The dose may be repeated in 10 to 15 minutes.
- A continuous infusion of 1 to 2 g/h should be started, titrated to antidysrhythmic effect.
- The patient should be monitored frequently for hyporeflexia and respiratory insufficiency.
- In reports of severe cases of refractory torsade de pointes, such large doses of magnesium were required to control the dysrhythmia that endotracheal intubation and mechanical ventilation were needed.

HYDROFLUORIC ACID EXPOSURE TO THE SKIN

- Magnesium salts have been used to treat dermal exposure to hydrofluoric acid, but there is less human experience than with calcium gluconate.
- Magnesium gluconate or acetate (10%) injected subcutaneously or intradermally has been effective in animal models
- Extemporaneous preparations of magnesium gluconate gel were less effective than calcium gluconate gels in animal studies.

HYDROFLUORIC ACID EXPOSURE VIA INGESTION

- Due to the potentially catastrophic deterioration of patients who have ingested hydrogen fluoride, pretreatment with magnesium is a reasonable therapeutic option.
- After suicidal ingestion by an adult, an initial intravenous bolus of 2 to 4 g may be administered.
- Maintenance infusion is 1 to 2 g/h, although higher rates may be needed if ECG evidence of hypocalcemia develops or persists.
- The infusion should be continued for 1 to 2 hours and then should be tapered slowly while monitoring ECG for evidence of QT interval prolongation.
- Serum calcium levels (levels of ionized calcium, if available) should be followed as well.

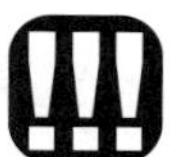

Pitfalls

- Renal function and urine output must be monitored in patients receiving high-dose magnesium.
- Frequent clinical monitoring of magnesium toxicity (decreased reflexes) should be used instead of serum magnesium levels.
- In severe cases, magnesium toxicity must be tolerated to reach the dose that suppresses ventricular dysrhythmia.

ICD-9-CM 985

Toxic effect of other metals.

See also: SECTION II, Ventricular Dysrhythmia chapter; and SECTION IV, Hydrofluoric Acid chapter.

RECOMMENDED READING

Vukmir RB. Torsade de pointes: a review. *Am J Emerg Med* 1991;9:250–255.

Author: Katherine M. Hurlbut

Reviewer: Luke Yip

Methylene Blue

Basics

DESCRIPTION

Methylene blue is a thiazine dye used to reverse drug-induced methemoglobinemia.

FORMS AND USES

- Methylene blue is produced as a dark green crystalline powder that stains blue.
- It is typically provided in an ampule of 1% (1 mg/ml) solution or as tablets containing up to 65 mg.
- It is used in the treatment of methemoglobinemia.
- It is also used to inject into joints, ducts, or tubes in the body to assess integrity.
- Methylene blue is occasionally used as a weak urinary antibiotic.

MECHANISM OF ACTION

- Normally, the methemoglobin level is less than 1%; a small amount of methemoglobin is produced by the body each day and converted to normal hemoglobin by the enzymes NADH and NADPH methemoglobin reductase.
- The NADH methemoglobin reductase cannot accommodate large increases in methemoglobin; if large increases occur, methemoglobin accumulates, producing cyanosis and hypoxia.
- The NADH methemoglobin reductase cannot be rapidly induced; however, action of NADPH methemoglobin reductase can be accelerated when an exogenous electron carrier such as methylene blue is provided.
- Following injection, methylene blue is rapidly reduced to leukomethylene blue by NADPH methemoglobin reductase; leukomethylene blue then reduces methemoglobin (Fe^{3+}) to hemoglobin (Fe^{2+}).

DRUG AND DISEASE INTERACTIONS

There is no known drug interaction with methylene blue.

PREGNANCY AND LACTATION

- US FDA Pregnancy Category C. The drug exerts animal teratogenic or embryocidal effects, but there are no controlled studies in women, or no studies are available in either animals or women.
- Mild methemoglobinemia does not appear to adversely affect pregnancy. In more severe cases, the physiologic (tissue hypoxia) condition of the mother should guide its use.

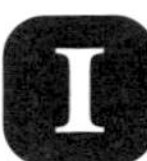

Indications

- Asymptomatic patient with methemoglobin level greater than 30% and rising
- Symptomatic patient with elevated methemoglobin level (some patients will develop symptoms at lower methemoglobin levels due to underlying disease or other factors)
- Symptomatic patient with cyanosis that does not correct with administration of 100% oxygen (administration of a single empiric dose is warranted before methemoglobin level is known, if the methemoglobin level is not immediately available)

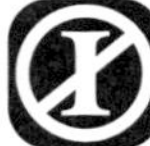

Contraindications and Adverse Effects

CONTRAINDICATIONS

A previous anaphylactic reaction to methylene blue is an absolute contraindication. Relative contraindications include:

- Glucose-6-phosphate dehydrogenase (G-6-PD) deficiency. Although methylene blue may paradoxically increase methemoglobinemia in G-6-PD–deficient patients, most patients will have some activity of the enzyme, and methylene blue may be used cautiously in symptomatic patients.
- Known NADPH methemoglobin reductase deficiency.

ADVERSE EFFECTS

- A cumulative dose of more than 7 mg/kg can result in a paradoxical increase in methemoglobin.
- Rapid infusion can cause flushing, shortness of breath, apprehension, and vomiting.
- Tissue necrosis can occur with extravasation.
- Large doses may cause nausea and vomiting, headaches, dizziness, confusion, sweating, chest pain, hyper- or hypotension, and dysrhythmias.
- Blue-green discoloration of urine and stools may occur.
- Delayed hemolysis may be noted in patients with G-6-PD deficiency.

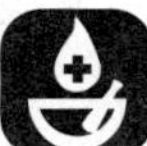

Dosage and Method of Administration

ASYMPTOMATIC PATIENT WITH METHEMOGLOBIN LEVEL GREATER THAN 30% AND RISING

- The initial dose is 1 to 2 mg/kg of a 1% solution (1 to 2 ml/kg) administered via intravenous push over 5 minutes for both adult and pediatric patients.
- The bolus infusion should be followed by administration of 15 to 30 ml of crystalloidal fluid flush.
- A second dose of 1 to 2 mg/kg can be given intravenously 30 to 60 minutes later if no clinical effect is noted.
- The maximum effect is expected within 30 minutes, after which the methemoglobin level should be checked again.
- If symptoms persist or methemoglobinemia recurs, repeated doses of methylene blue can be administered (the effectiveness of decontamination should also be reexamined).
- The cumulative dose of methylene blue should not exceed 7 mg/kg.

SYMPTOMATIC PATIENT WITH ELEVATION OF METHEMOGLOBIN LEVEL

- The dose and administration of methylene blue are the same as for a methemoglobin level greater than 30%.
- The reason that the patient has symptoms at a low level of methemoglobin should be carefully examined.

—If the patient is anemic or another underlying disease makes the patient susceptible, other therapy may be needed to achieve full response.
—These patients are also at increased risk of adverse effects (i.e., the paradoxical methemoglobin induced by large doses of methylene blue will compromise a larger portion of hemoglobin in an anemic patient).
—Repeat doses should be carefully considered. Consultation with a poison control center or medical toxicologist is recommended.

SYMPTOMATIC PATIENT WITH CYANOSIS THAT DOES NOT CORRECT WITH ADMINISTRATION OF 100% OXYGEN

- Dose and administration of methylene blue are the same as for a methemoglobin level greater than 30%.
- However, an accurate methemoglobin level should be determined as quickly as possible by cooximeter to guide further therapy.
- Failure to achieve response indicates possibility of enzyme deficiency or underlying disease causing cyanosis (G-6-PD deficiency, NADPH methemoglobin deficiency, cardiac shunting, other causes of hypoxia).

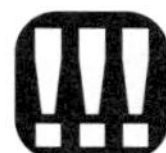

Pitfalls

DIAGNOSIS

- Patients with anemia or other underlying disease may have symptoms at methemoglobin levels much lower than 30%.
- Serial methemoglobin levels should be performed to assess response to therapy and possible recurrence of methemoglobin.

TREATMENT

- Patients with G-6-PD deficiency may have partial or no response due to lack of NADPH.
- Patients with hereditary G-6-PD deficiency are at an increased risk of developing methemoglobinemia and of having methemoglobinemia complicate methylene blue therapy.
- Patients with NADPH methemoglobin reductase deficiency may have no response to therapy.
- Doses over 7 mg/kg can result in paradoxical increase in methemoglobin.
- Inadvertent administration of adult doses of methylene blue to children may result in serious methemoglobinemia.
- Patients with no symptoms and methemoglobin levels lower than 30% do not require treatment unless they become symptomatic.
- Some hospital pharmacies fail to stock antidotes adequately, and it may be necessary to obtain methylene blue from another hospital.
- Sulfhemoglobinemia appears as methemoglobinemia, but does not respond to methylene blue therapy.

ICD-9-CM 964

Poisoning by agents primarily affecting blood constituents.

See also: SECTION II, Methemoglobinemia chapter.

RECOMMENDED READING

Avner JR, Henretig FM, McAneney CM. Acquired methemoglobinemia: the relationship of cause to course of illness. *Am J Dis Child* 1990;144:1229–1230.

Curry S. Methemoglobinemia. *Ann Emerg Med* 1982;11:214–221.

Author: Richard Chen

Reviewer: Luke Yip

N-Acetylcysteine

Basics

DESCRIPTION

N-acetylcysteine (NAC), an antidote for acetaminophen poisoning, was originally used as an inhalation mucolytic agent.

FORMS AND USES

- Pharmaceutical preparations include Mucomyst and Acetylcysteine Solution USP.
- NAC is available as a 10% or 20% solution for inhalation or oral administration.

MECHANISM OF ACTION

Several mechanisms of action have been proposed:

- NAC acts as a precursor of glutathione, which detoxifies the toxic metabolite of acetaminophen, *N*-acetyl-p-benzoquinoneimine (NAPQI).
- Providing NAC as a substrate for glutathione synthesis may prevent depletion of glutathione stores associated with acetaminophen toxicity and thereby prevent liver injury.
- The sulfhydryl group of NAC may bind and detoxify NAPQI directly.
- Donation of a sulfur group by NAC may drive the metabolism of acetaminophen toward the nontoxic sulfation pathway and away from its toxic pathway.
- NAC may improve hepatic microcirculation and reduce acetaminophen toxicity.
- NAC may be a hepatic antioxidant, attenuating oxidant-induced acetaminophen liver injury.

PREGNANCY AND LACTATION

- US FDA Pregnancy Category B. Animal studies indicate no fetal risk, and there are no controlled human studies, or animal studies show an adverse fetal effect but well-controlled studies in pregnant women do not.
- Pregnant women with toxic serum acetaminophen levels as determined by the Rumack-Matthew nomogram should receive a full course of NAC.
- An infant delivered to a woman receiving NAC for acetaminophen toxicity should receive a full course of NAC, typically by the intravenous route.

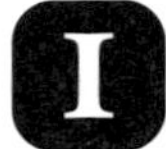

Indications

ACUTE SINGLE INGESTION

- The decision to treat with NAC is determined by plotting the patient's serum or plasma acetaminophen level on the Rumack-Matthew acetaminophen nomogram (see figure below).
- The acetaminophen level must be drawn between 4 and 24 hours after ingestion. If the level plots above the "possible toxicity" line, the patient should be treated with NAC.

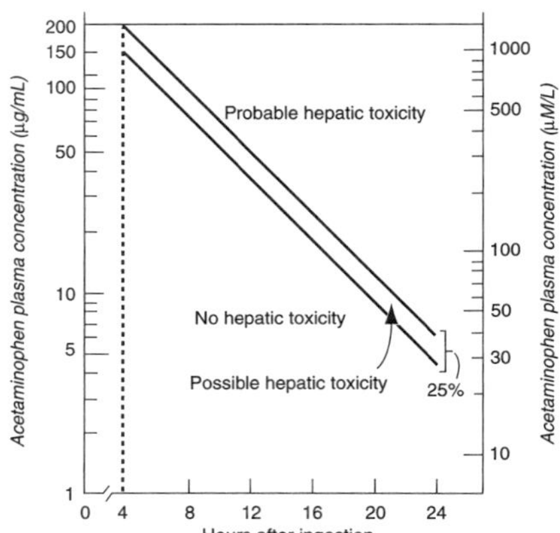

Semilogarithmic plot of plasma acetaminophen levels versus time. (Modified and reproduced, with permission, from Rumack BH, Matthew H. Acetaminophen poisoning and toxicity. *Pediatrics* 1975;55:871.)

ACETAMINOPHEN, ATYPICAL OVERDOSE CONDITIONS

- Known acute overdose, but the time of ingestion is uncertain or unknown.
- Possible acute overdose where elevated results on liver function tests are present; increase in levels of alanine aminotransferase (ALT) or aspartate aminotransferase (AST) indicate acetaminophen injury until proven otherwise.
- Known acute overdose patient that presents more than 48 hours after ingestion. NAC is not needed if liver enzymes are normal, but patient should receive NAC if liver enzymes are abnormal.
- Patients with a history of a single acute overdose between 24 and 36 hours prior to presentation should receive NAC therapy regardless of whether measurable acetaminophen is present or whether liver function tests are normal, because liver toxicity may not become apparent until 24 to 48 hours postingestion.
- Repeated ingestion of acetaminophen rather than single ingestion. If ALT or AST are abnormal, the patient should be treated with NAC. If ALT and AST are normal and acetaminophen level is undetectable, the patient does not need NAC therapy.

OTHER POISONINGS TREATED WITH NAC

- Chlorinated hydrocarbon poisoning (carbon tetrachloride, chloroform). NAC is the proposed therapy, but efficacy has not been studied.
- Amanita phalloides mushroom poisoning. NAC is the proposed therapy, but efficacy is unproven.
- Monochloroacetic acid. NAC is the proposed therapy, but efficacy is unproven.
- Cyclophosphamide. Severity of cyclophosphamide-induced hemorrhagic cystitis is reduced by NAC.
- Doxorubicin. Possible prevention by NAC of doxorubicin-induced cardiomyopathy.

Contraindications and Adverse Effects

CONTRAINDICATIONS

A history of allergy to NAC is a relative contraindication.

ADVERSE EFFECTS

- Oral administration. Nausea and vomiting are common; diarrhea and rash occur rarely.
- Intravenous administration. Allergic reactions ranging from rash to anaphylaxis occur rarely.

Dosage and Method of Administration

ORAL DOSAGE

- The loading dose for adult and pediatric patients is 140 mg/kg orally.
- The maintenance dose for adult and pediatric patients is 70 mg/kg orally every 4 hours for 17 additional doses (72 hour protocol).
- Health-care provider should be aware that some poison centers recommend a truncated treatment course under special conditions.
- To administer NAC, 10% or 20% NAC solution is diluted in water, juice, or soda to a 5% solution.

—Use of ice and a straw may diminish the unpleasant taste and odor, making NAC more palatable to drink.
—If the patient is unable to drink, NAC may be administered via small-bore nasogastric tube.
—If the patient vomits within 1 hour of any dose, the full dose should be readministered.

- Aggressive anti-emetic therapy may be required for repetitive vomiting.

—Adult regimen is metoclopramide 1.0 to 2.0 mg/kg intravenously, plus prochlorperazine 10 mg or droperidol 2.5 to 5.0 mg, administered intravenously.
—Diphenhydramine 25 to 50 mg intravenously may be added to this regimen.
—Ondansetron 8 mg intravenously may be used if the above medications fail.

- If liver or renal injury is not improving, NAC should be continued beyond the standard 72 hours (oral) or 48 hours (intravenous) protocol, until improvement of liver and renal function occurs.

ADMINISTRATION OF ORAL FORMULATION BY THE INTRAVENOUS ROUTE

- Occasionally, oral administration cannot be used because of intractable vomiting despite antiemetic therapy or medical conditions that contraindicate oral intake (gastrointestinal hemorrhage, acute abdomen, intestinal obstruction, or severe oral or esophagogastric burns).
- An intravenous NAC preparation is not available in the United States.

—Because the commercially available NAC solution is sterile (intended for nebulized or oral treatment), however, patients may be safely treated with the oral NAC formulation administered via the intravenous route.
—The Rocky Mountain Poison and Drug Center can provide medical consultation to health-care providers on the method of administration (800-525-6115).

- The United States intravenous protocol is as follows.

—If possible, informed consent should be obtained.
—Intravenous NAC should be administered in a monitored setting such as an emergency department or ICU.
—The loading dose is 140 mg/kg, followed by maintenance doses of 70 mg/kg intravenously every 4 hours for 12 additional doses (48-hour protocol).
—Some poison centers recommend truncated treatment course under special conditions.
—The 10% or 20% NAC solution should be diluted to 5% concentration with D5W.
—Each dose is infused over 30 to 60 minutes through a 0.2-μm in-line filter. Faster rates of infusion are associated with more frequent adverse effects.

- A 20-hour intravenous NAC protocol is approved for use in the United Kingdom, but it is not commonly used in the United States. The NAC dosage for the 20-hour protocol is 150 mg/kg in 200 ml D5W infused over 15 minutes, followed by 50 mg/kg in 500 ml D5W infused over 4 hours, followed by 100 mg/kg in 1 L D5W over 16 hours.

TREATMENT OF REACTIONS DURING NAC INFUSION

Dermatologic Reactions

- The infusion should be temporarily discontinued.
- Development of rash does not contraindicate further use of NAC.
- Diphenhydramine should be administered intravenously: adult, 25 to 50 mg; pediatric, 1 to 2 mg/kg up to adult dose.
- The rash typically resolves within 1 hour.
- The intravenous NAC may be restarted.
- Subsequent doses may require pretreatment with diphenhydramine.

Anaphylactoid Reaction (Hypotension, Angioedema, Bronchospasm)

- NAC should be discontinued and the anaphylactoid reaction treated in the standard manner.
- Further use of NAC intravenously is relatively contraindicated. Consultation with a poison center is recommended.

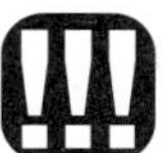

Pitfalls

- Although rare, serious adverse reactions are associated with intravenous NAC; therefore, one should maximize antiemetic therapy before abandoning NAC via the oral route.
- Rapid administration of intravenous NAC should be avoided because the rate of dose delivery does not affect outcome.
- No increase in oral NAC dose is required when it is coadministered with activated charcoal.
- Treatment of alcoholic patients with acetaminophen poisoning is the same as for nonalcoholic patients, and the standard Rumack-Matthew nomogram may be used in alcoholic patients to determine the need for NAC treatment.

ICD-9-CM 965

Poisoning by analgesics, antipyretics, and antirheumatics.

See also: SECTION IV, Acetaminophen—Acute Single Ingestion and Acetaminophen—Repeated Ingestion chapters.

RECOMMENDED READING

Dawson AH, Henry DA, Macewen J. Adverse reactions to *N*-acetylcysteine during treatment for paracetamol poisoning. *Med J Aust* 1989;150:329–331.

Flanagan RJ, Meredith TJ. Use of *N*-acetylcysteine in clinical toxicity. *Am J Med* 1991;91:131S–139S.

Smilkstein MJ, Bronstein AC, Linden C, et al. Acetaminophen overdose: a 48 hour intravenous *N*-acetylcysteine protocol. *Ann Emerg Med* 1991;20:1058–1063.

Smilkstein MJ, Knapp GL, Kulig KW, Rumack BH. Efficacy of oral *N*-acetylcysteine in the treatment of acetaminophen overdose: analysis of the national multicenter study (1976 to 1985). *N Engl J Med* 1988;319:1557–1562.

Yip L, Dart RC, Hurlbut KM. Intravenous administration of oral *N*-acetylcysteine. *Crit Care Med* 1998;26:40–43.

Author: Rivka S. Horowitz

Reviewer: Richard C. Dart

Naloxone and Nalmefene

Basics

DESCRIPTION

Naloxone and nalmefene are narcotic antagonists.

FORMS AND USES

- Substances include naloxone (Narcan) and nalmefene (Revex).
- These drugs are used for the reversal of narcotic toxicity.

—Naloxone hydrochloride is available in 0.02, 0.4, and 1.0 mg/ml injectable form.
—Nalmefene is available in 0.1- or 1.0-mg concentrations.

MECHANISM OF ACTION

- These drugs compete and displace opioid drugs from μ, κ, and σ opioid receptors, thereby reversing the effect of narcotic administration.
- Neither drug has agonist activity.
- At lower doses, naloxone and nalmefene have clinically indistinguishable durations of action.
- At higher doses, nalmefene has a longer duration; activity may extend up to 8 hours after a 2-mg dose.

DRUG AND DISEASE INTERACTIONS

- Naloxone and nalmefene prevent action of all opioid drugs.
- Patients may develop agitation, hypertension, or ventricular irritability when sympathomimetic drugs are also present.

PREGNANCY AND LACTATION

- US FDA Pregnancy Category B. Animal studies indicate no fetal risk, and there are no controlled human studies, or animal studies show an adverse fetal effect but well-controlled studies in pregnant women do not.
- Withdrawal may be precipitated in unborn children when the mother receives naloxone during labor.
- Narcotic antagonists should be used during pregnancy only when the mother's life is endangered by opioid toxicity.

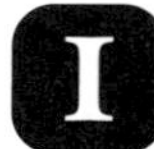

Indications

- Altered mental status of undetermined etiology
- Respiratory depression from known opioid overdose
- CNS depression from known opioid overdose without respiratory depression

—When treating known heroin overdose, it may be prudent to observe those patients who can maintain their airway and oxygenation rather than to treat them with naloxone.
—This may allow discharge of the patient without the concern of recurrent opioid toxicity or withdrawal.

- Reversal of opioid anesthesia
- Clonidine intoxication. Conflicting evidence exists concerning use of naloxone for clonidine intoxication, and it is not routinely recommended.

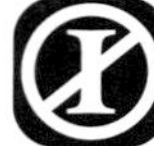

Contraindications and Adverse Effects

CONTRAINDICATIONS

Known hypersensitivity to naloxone or nalmefene contraindicates their use.

ADVERSE EFFECTS

- Withdrawal can occur in opioid-dependent patients.
- Withdrawal seizures in neonates of opioid-dependent mothers may be life threatening.
- Noncardiogenic pulmonary edema occurs rarely.

—High-dose opioid administration may reverse the pulmonary edema
—Generally, supportive care is sufficient.

Dosage and Method of Administration

ALTERED MENTAL STATUS OF UNDETERMINED ETIOLOGY

Naloxone

- Dose in adult or pediatric patients is 2.0 to 10.0 mg administered intravenously in 2.0-mg increments.
- If no response is observed after each 2.0-mg bolus, another 2.0 mg may be administered.
- A cumulative dose of 10 to 20 mg may be needed for intoxication with propoxyphene, nalbuphine, or butorphanol.
- Although these routes are less desirable, naloxone also may be administered by endotracheal, intramuscular, intralingual, intraosseous, or subcutaneous injection as circumstances demand.
- If reversal response occurs, patients should be observed for 4 hours after final dose; repeat bolus doses may be needed.
- A patient with persistent or recurrent effects may be treated with constant infusion of naloxone; naloxone should be mixed in D5W and administered at a rate that delivers two thirds of the initially effective bolus dose per hour, titrated to effect.

Nalmefene

- Patient can receive a cumulative dose of 0.5 to 1.5 mg.
- The recommended starting dose of 0.5 mg should be administered as an intravenous push; if the patient exhibits no response, an additional 1 mg should be given. However, some practitioners start with a dose of 1.0 mg followed by another dose of 1.0 mg, if needed.
- Higher doses of nalmefene appear to give prolonged activity; 1.5 mg of nalmefene was effective in blocking opioid activity up to 8 hours.
- If repeat dosing is required, the patient should be admitted.
- Nalmefene may be administered by intravenous, intramuscular, or subcutaneous administration. The dose is the same, but onset of effect may be delayed 10 to 15 minutes.

RESPIRATORY DEPRESSION FROM KNOWN OPIOID OVERDOSE

- Naloxone is the first choice; 2.0 to 10.0 mg is administered in 2.0-mg increments.
- A cumulative dose of 10 to 20 mg may be needed for propoxyphene, nalbuphine, or butorphanol, administered as described for altered mental status above.
- Nalmefene is effective but difficult to use appropriately unless the patient's likelihood of dependency is known; it should be administered as described above for altered mental status.

CNS DEPRESSION FROM KNOWN OPIOID OVERDOSE WITHOUT RESPIRATORY DEPRESSION

- Because time is less urgent, smaller doses (with lower risk of producing florid withdrawal) may be used.
- Treatment should begin with a bolus dose of naloxone of 0.1 to 0.4 mg, escalating to typical 2.0-mg dose as described for altered mental status above, if needed.

REVERSAL OF OPIOID ANESTHESIA

If anesthesia has resulted in depression of respiratory or CNS function, 0.4 to 2.0 mg naloxone can be administered in an intravenous push as dictated by the urgency of the situation. If serious respiratory depression has developed, the initial dose should be 2.0 mg.

CLONIDINE INTOXICATION

Conflicting evidence exists concerning use of naloxone for clonidine intoxication, and it is not routinely recommended.

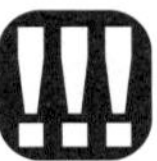

Pitfalls

- Because of the short duration of action for naloxone, opioid toxicity may recur after discharge of the patient.
- Precipitation of withdrawal in opioid-dependent patients may be severe, although not considered life-threatening; however, an agitated patient may disrupt or injure health-care personnel.
- Infants of dependent mothers may develop status epilepticus after naloxone administration.
- Withdrawal seizures in infants may be life-threatening.
- Withdrawal also may be life-threatening in geriatric patients with underlying cardiac diseases.
- Geriatric patients with chronic pain may be opioid dependent.

ICD-9-CM 970.1

Poisoning by central nervous system stimulants: opiate antagonists.

See also: SECTION IV, Clonidine and Narcotics chapters.

RECOMMENDED READING

Gal TJ, Difazio CA. Prolonged antagonism of opioid action with intravenous nalmefene in man. *Anesthesiology* 1986;64:175–180.

Weisman RS. Naloxone. In: Goldfrank L, Flomenbaum N, Lewin N, et al., eds. *Goldfrank's toxicologic emergencies,* 6th ed. East Norwalk, CT: Appleton & Lange, 1998.

Author: Kennon Heard

Reviewer: Katherine M. Hurlbut

Nitroprusside

Basics

DESCRIPTION

Nitroprusside is a short-acting parenteral antihypertensive agent.

FORMS AND USES

Most commonly used to treat hypertension. Sodium nitroprusside is available in 50-mg vials.

MECHANISM OF ACTION

- Nitroprusside is a direct-acting vasodilator.
- The onset of hypotensive effect occurs within 1 minute of intravenous administration.
- Hypotensive effects may persist from 3 to 5 minutes following discontinuation of the infusion.
- Oral administration does not produce hypotension.
- Nitroprusside contains five cyanide groups.

—Metabolism releases these groups slowly.
—Under normal conditions, the enzyme rhodanese can easily detoxify cyanide. However, cyanide and thiocyanate may accumulate and produce toxicity if the rate of cyanide production overwhelms the activity of rhodanese or if thiocyanate elimination is impaired.

DRUG AND DISEASE INTERACTIONS

- Nitroprusside can potentiate hypotension caused by other drugs.
- Geriatric patients need close monitoring for the development of cyanide toxicity due to age-related renal and hepatic insufficiency.
- Older patients may be more sensitive to hypotensive effects.

PREGNANCY AND LACTATION

- US FDA Pregnancy Category C. The drug exerts animal teratogenic or embryocidal effects, but there are no controlled studies in women, or no studies are available in either animals or women.
- Due to risk of cyanide toxicity, nitroglycerin is preferred in the treatment of life-threatening hypertension in pregnancy.

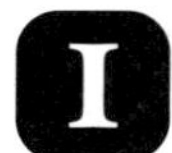

Indications

- Persistent severe hypertension (diastolic pressure greater than 130 mm Hg and not responsive to sedation) or hypertension complicated by end-organ effects (CNS bleed, chronic heart failure, myocardial ischemia, congestive heart failure, aortic dissection).
- Induction of controlled hypotension in surgery.
- Treatment of peripheral ischemia secondary to ergot alkaloids and sympathomimetic agents.
- Treatment of myocardial ischemia (may cause coronary steal syndrome), aortic stenosis, or pulmonary hypertension.

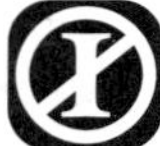

Contraindications and Adverse Effects

CONTRAINDICATIONS

Treatment of hypertension that is compensatory (ventricular septal defect, arteriovenous shunting, coarctation of the aorta) precludes use of nitroprusside.

ADVERSE EFFECTS

- Hypotension is common and usually responds promptly to discontinuation of infusion.
- Nausea, vomiting, muscle twitching, headache, and lightheadedness may occur.
- Cyanide toxicity may result.

—High-dose nitroprusside therapy (less than 2 μg/kg/min is not usually associated with toxicity) is a risk factor for cyanide toxicity, especially when treatment involves more than 3 to 4 μg/kg/min for 12 to 24 hours, more than 5 μg/kg/min for several hours, or more than 50 mg infused over 6 hours.
—Prolonged infusion over days is a risk factor for cyanide toxicity.
—Malnutrition may reduce endogenous levels of thiosulfate and thereby allow accumulation of cyanide.
—Whole-blood cyanide levels correlate poorly with toxicity because they may not accurately reflect tissue cyanide concentrations.
—Some clinicians recommend following cyanide levels as a general guide for toxicity:
 —Less than 0.2 μg/ml is unlikely to cause toxicity.
 —0.5 to 1.0 μg/ml may cause mild symptoms.
 —1.0 to 2.5 μg/ml is associated with change in mental status.
 —More than 2.5 μg/ml may produce life-threatening toxicity.
—Thiocyanate levels should be monitored during high-dose nitroprusside therapy.
 —More than 5 to 10 μg/ml is considered an elevated level.
 —More than 60 μg/ml is associated with an increased incidence of thiocyanate toxicity.

- Methemoglobinemia has been reported, with increased incidence in patients with hemoglobin M, hereditary methemoglobinemia (NADH-methemoglobin reductase deficiency), or concomitant exposure to other agents capable of causing methemoglobinemia.
- Hypothyroidism. Thiocyanate inhibits iodide production by thyroid and may produce hypothyroidism if used for prolonged periods.

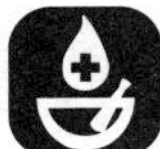

Dosage and Method of Administration

PREPARATION

- Nitroprusside solution needs protection from photodegradation with an opaque covering such as aluminum foil.

—Photodegradation will produce marked dark discoloration.
—Intravenous tubing does not need to be protected from light.

- Nitroprusside powder is initially reconstituted using 2 to 3 ml of D5W or sterile water (without bacteriostatic agents) and then diluted to 250 ml or greater volume with D5W.
- Blood pressure must be continuously monitored; intraarterial blood pressure monitoring is recommended.
- Baseline renal and hepatic function should be checked.

ADMINISTRATION

- Nitroprusside is administered by continuous intravenous infusion with an infusion pump to regulate the infusion rate.

—Direct intravenous push or gravity-driven infusion should not be used.
—The initial dose for adults and children is 0.5 μg/kg/min by continuous intravenous infusion.
—Infusion is increased by 0.25 to 0.50 μg/kg/min every 5 minutes, titrating dose to the desired effect.

- Cessation of nitroprusside therapy should be gradual in order to avoid rebound hypertension.
- Administration of large doses over prolonged periods carries the risk of cyanide toxicity.

—The risk of cyanide toxicity is dose-related, especially in patients with either renal or hepatic insufficiency.
—Concurrent administration of sodium thiosulfate may prevent cyanide toxicity.
 —For concurrent sodium thiosulfate therapy (see SECTION III, Cyanide Antidote Package chapter), each 100 mg of sodium nitroprusside should be mixed with 1 g of sodium thiosulfate (10 ml of 10% sodium thiosulfate).
 —Very high rates of nitroprusside infusion are possible by using this admixture.
 —The mixture is stable for 7 days if protected from light.

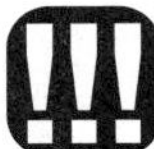

Pitfalls

- Ambient light will degrade nitroprusside solution if not protected from light.
- It is difficult to recognize the development of cyanide toxicity, especially in patients with renal insufficiency and in patients treated for a prolonged period.
- Because sodium thiosulfate has a very low rate of adverse effects, the clinician should not wait for laboratory confirmation of cyanide toxicity before administering sodium thiosulfate to the patient when cyanide toxicity is suspected.
- Failure to infuse sodium thiosulfate concurrently and prophylactically when patients are receiving high doses for prolonged durations increases the risk of cyanide toxicity.
- Tachyphylaxis to nitroprusside hypotensive effect is rare, but has been reported.

—If the hypotensive effect of nitroprusside diminishes, the clinician should ensure that the drug is actually infusing.
—If tachyphylaxis is suspected, treatment with another antihypertensive agent should be considered.

- If the patient has renal insufficiency, the nitroprusside infusion is administered in the standard manner; however, the patient is at increased risk of developing toxicity.

—The clinician must monitor closely for the development of cyanide toxicity because thiocyanate renal clearance is impaired.
—Thiocyanate can be removed by either hemodialysis or peritoneal dialysis.

- If the patient has hepatic insufficiency, nitroprusside is administered in the standard manner; however, the clinician must monitor closely for the development of cyanide toxicity because cyanide conversion to thiocyanate by hepatic rhodanese may be impaired.

ICD-9-CM 975

Poisoning by agents primarily acting in the smooth and skeletal muscles and respiratory system.

See also: SECTION III, Cyanide Antidote Package chapter; and SECTION IV, Cyanide chapter.

RECOMMENDED READING

Curry SC, Arnold-Capell P. Nitroprusside, nitroglycerin, and angiotensin converting enzyme inhibitors. *Crit Care Clin* 1991;7:555–581.

Rindone JP, Sloane EP. Cyanide toxicity from sodium nitroprusside: risks and management. *Ann Pharmacother* 1992;26:515–519.

Author: Edwin K. Kuffner

Reviewer: Katherine M. Hurlbut

Penicillamine

Basics

DESCRIPTION

Pencillamine is a medication that increases urinary excretion of some metals (copper, lead, mercury, and arsenic).

FORMS AND USES

- Pencillamine is primarily used in the treatment of chronic copper toxicity (Wilson's disease).
- It is a second-line therapy for lead, mercury, copper, or arsenic toxicity.
- It is also used in treating rheumatoid arthritis, Wilson's disease, and cystinuria.
- It is available as Cuprimine (125 mg, 250 mg capsules) or Depen (250 mg tablets).

MECHANISM OF ACTION

- Penicillamine is a chelating agent that directly binds several heavy metals.
- The drug-penicillamine complex is excreted in the urine, thereby decreasing the body burden of the metal.

DRUG AND DISEASE INTERACTIONS

Penicillamine may potentiate the effects of immunosuppressive therapy.

PREGNANCY AND LACTATION

- US FDA Pregnancy Category D. Evidence of human fetal risk exists, but benefits in certain situations (e.g., life-threatening situations or serious diseases) may make use of the drug acceptable despite its risks.
- Penicillamine is appropriate therapy during pregnancy for treatment of Wilson's disease.

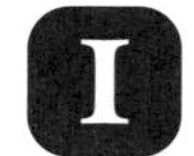

Indications

LEAD POISONING WITHOUT ENCEPHALOPATHY

Adults

- It is a second-line agent behind succimer for the treatment of lead poisoning without encephalopathy.
- In some cases it may be used with a parenteral chelator for treatment of lead poisoning with encephalopathy.

Pediatric

- Penicillamine has been used for treating asymptomatic or minimally symptomatic children.
- Succimer is the preferred agent.

MERCURY TOXICITY

- Penicillamine has been used for treatment of symptomatic acute or chronic elemental mercury poisoning or elevated urinary excretion of mercury.
- Penicillamine has been used for neuropathy induced by inorganic mercury.

COPPER TOXICITY

- Penicillamine is the mainstay of therapy for chronic copper toxicity in Wilson's disease but has not been well studied in acute copper poisoning.
- Penicillamine can be used in symptomatic chronic copper intoxication when levels remain elevated despite the discontinuation of exposure.

ARSENIC TOXICITY

Penicillamine has been used for symptomatic arsenic toxicity if BAL and succimer are not available.

Contraindications and Adverse Effects

CONTRAINDICATIONS

- Penicillin allergy precludes use.
- Renal insufficiency is a relative contraindicator because the metal-penicillamine complex is renally excreted.
- Penicillamine should not be used in conjunction with other drugs that cause bone marrow depression or in patients with abnormal bone marrow function.

ADVERSE EFFECTS

- Allergic reactions occur in 5% of patients.
- Penicillamine increases the need for pyridoxine. Pyridoxine therapy should be considered in long-term pencillamine therapy (e.g., Wilson's disease), but should not be needed for intermittent treatment of heavy metal poisoning.
- Chronic therapy has been associated with optic neuritis, myasthenia gravis, retinopathy, pulmonary alveolitis and hemorrhage, seizures, neuropathy, gastroenteritis, cholestasis, hepatitis, pancreatitis, polyarteritis nodosa, bone marrow suppression, thrombocytopenia, aplastic anemia, proteinuria, and nephrotic syndrome.
- There is no specific therapy for these adverse effects; symptomatic and supportive care should be provided.

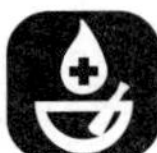

Dosage and Method of Administration

LEAD POISONING WITHOUT ENCEPHALOPATHY

- The clinician must first ensure that lead exposure has stopped.
- Adult dose is 15 to 40 mg/kg/day orally in four divided doses, up to a maximum of 250 to 500 mg, four times per day for 5 days, administered before meals.
- Pediatric dose is 20 to 30 mg/kg/day, given orally once or twice daily before meals.
- Blood lead levels should be measured.

—Levels should be repeated once several days after completion of each course of therapy and every 2 to 4 weeks thereafter until the level stabilizes.
—If the blood lead level rebounds to 45 μg/dl, the clinician should investigate whether repeat exposure could have occurred in the interim; if it has not, the course of chelation should be repeated.
—If repeat exposure has occurred, the patient should be moved to lead-free housing and the course of chelation repeated.
—If the level rebounds to 20 to 45 μg/dl, treatment recommendations are uncertain. Many centers would perform at least one more course of chelation. Serial blood lead levels should be followed to assess efficacy.

- If repeated courses of treatment are used, the white blood cell count should be monitored biweekly.

MERCURY TOXICITY

- Adult dose is 15 to 40 mg/kg/day orally, up to a maximum of 250 to 500 mg, given four times a day, before meals.
- Pediatric dose is 20 to 30 mg/kg/day, given orally once or twice daily before meals.
- The treatment should be administered for 5 to 10 days.
- Urinary excretion of mercury should be monitored.

—If urine mercury decreases rapidly, the body burden of mercury is probably small; after 10 days, the urine mercury level should be repeated.
—If urine mercury is elevated, another course of chelation may be needed.

COPPER TOXICITY

- For treatment of Wilson's disease, the adult dose is 15 to 40 mg/kg/day orally, up to a maximum of 250 to 500 mg, given four times a day, before meals.
- Pediatric dose is 20 to 30 mg/kg/day, given orally once or twice daily before meals.
- The dose for treatment of copper poisoning following acute ingestion is uncertain. Empiric use of the same dose as for lead or mercury poisoning may be used initially.

ARSENIC TOXICITY

- Adult dose is 15 to 40 mg/kg/day orally, up to a maximum of 250 to 500 mg, given four times a day for 5 days, before meals.
- Pediatric dose is 20 to 30 mg/kg/day, given orally once or twice daily before meals.
- The clinician should observe 24-hour urinary arsenic levels and stop therapy when levels are less than 50 μg/24-hour specimen.

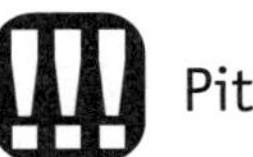

Pitfalls

- Prevention of ongoing exposure is critical for all types of heavy metal poisoning.
- Side effects are generally related to rapid increase in dose.

ICD-9-CM 963.8

Poisoning by primarily systemic agents: other specified systemic agents (heavy metal antagonists).

See also: SECTION IV, Arsenic, Copper, Lead, Mercury, and Succimer chapters.

RECOMMENDED READING

Shannon M, Graef J, Lovejoy FH. Efficacy and toxicity of D-penicillamine in low-level lead poisoning. *J Pediatr* 1988;112:799–804.

Author: Kennon Heard

Reviewer: Katherine M. Hurlbut

Physostigmine

Basics

DESCRIPTION

Physostigmine is used to reverse anticholinergic toxicity.

FORMS AND USES

- Used primarily to diagnose anticholinergic toxicity.
- Physostigmine salicylate (Antilirium) is provided in 2-ml ampules containing 1 mg/ml physostigmine salicylate; the vehicle contains sodium bisulfite 0.1% and benzyl alcohol 2.0%.

MECHANISM OF ACTION

- Physostigmine is a cholinergic agonist that reversibly binds to acetylcholinesterase, increasing the concentration and duration of action of acetylcholine at the nerve receptor.
- Tertiary amine structure permits penetration into the CNS, thereby allowing reversal of central anticholinergic effects (hallucinosis).
- Because of actions on the reticular activating system, it produces analeptic effects and may result in partial, nonspecific arousal of obtunded patients.
- The onset of action after intravenous administration is 3 to 8 minutes; the duration of action is 15 to 40 minutes.

DRUG AND DISEASE INTERACTIONS

- Synergistic cholinergic effects may develop in patients already taking carbamate or anticholinesterase agents (edrophonium, neostigmine, and pyridostigmine).
- Synergistic effect with other cholinergic agents such as organophosphate or carbamate insecticides.
- Use in tricyclic antidepressant overdose has been reported to result in seizures and asystole even when physostigmine is given properly in moderate doses.
- Geriatric patients have increased susceptibility to arrhythmias and greater likelihood of underlying renal failure and drug interactions.

PREGNANCY AND LACTATION

- US FDA Pregnancy Category C. Studies have shown that the drug exerts animal teratogenic or embryocidal effects, but there are no controlled studies in women, or no studies are available in either animals or women.
- The appropriate use of physostigmine in pregnant women has not been defined; in general, its use is discouraged due to low mortality of anticholinergic toxicity.

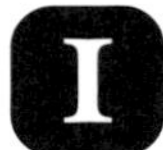

Indications

- To differentiate between anticholinergic and other organic causes of altered mental status with hallucinations and psychosis, through use of the "physostigmine challenge test."

—If dramatic reversal of anticholinergic effects is produced, it may be possible to avoid CT and lumbar puncture for evaluation of altered mental status.

- To reverse neuromuscular blockade after general anesthesia.
- To treat paraplegic anejaculation.
- To produce miosis through an ophthalmic preparation.

Contraindications and Adverse Effects

CONTRAINDICATIONS

- Known hypersensitivity to cholinergic agonists or sulfites precludes use of physostigmine.
- Ventricular dysrhythmia may occur with use of physostigmine in a known or suspected tricyclic antidepressant overdose.
- Underlying health problems such as asthma, heart disease, diabetes, inflammation of iris or ciliary body contraindicate use of physostigmine.
- Physostigmine is generally contraindicated in patients with significant cardiac conduction disturbances of anticholinergic overdoses.
- Physostigmine should not be used to reverse depolarizing blockers (e.g., succinylcholine, decamethonium) because blockade may be potentiated.

ADVERSE EFFECTS

- Acute overdose or oversensitivity reactions to physostigmine

—Muscarine-like sympathetic (cholinergic) effects, including nausea, vomiting, diarrhea, sweating, increased bronchial and salivary secretions, bradycardia, and hypotension
—Airway obstruction by secretions

Vital Signs

Bradycardia and increased respiratory rate secondary to pulmonary secretions

HEENT

Increased salivation and lacrimation; diplopia and pupillary constriction

Dermatologic

Diaphoresis

Cardiovascular

Tachydysrhythmia such as atrial fibrillation, ventricular tachycardia, and (rarely) asystole; cardiac standstill possible

Pulmonary

Increased pulmonary secretions, laryngospasm, bronchoconstriction, and central or peripheral paralysis of respiration

Gastrointestinal

Nausea, vomiting, diarrhea, abdominal cramps, and increased salivation and intestinal secretion

Musculoskeletal

Weakness or fasciculation

Neurologic

Seizures, dysarthria, dysphonia, and dysphagia

Dosage and Method of Administration

- Patient preparation

—Patient should have intravenous access and continuous cardiac monitoring prior to and during physostigmine administration.
—Atropine should be immediately available should excessive muscarinic side effects develop.
—Physostigmine challenge test is used to diagnose the presence of anticholinergic syndrome. Baseline assessment of hallucinosis and presence of anticholinergic signs should be recorded.

- Dose

—Adult dose is 1.0 to 2.0 mg; 2.0 mg is the most commonly used initial dose.
—Pediatric dose is 0.02 mg/kg up to 2.0 mg; physostigmine should be administered by slow intravenous push over 5 minutes.
—May be repeated once after 5- to 10-minute interval if needed.

- If symptoms and signs are truly the result of anticholinergic toxicity, reversal or attenuation of anticholinergic effects should be noted about 5 minutes after administration of physostigmine.
- If reversal of anticholinergic effects occurs, these effects may relapse approximately 30 minutes later.
- To reverse neuromuscular blockade, the patient should receive 0.5 to 1 mg, slow intravenous push, repeated as needed at intervals of 10 to 30 minutes.

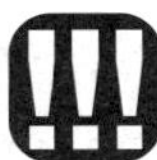

Pitfalls

- The use of physostigmine when there is no true need is common.
- Physostigmine is primarily a diagnostic tool; because of its short half-life, anticholinergic effects often recur. Fortunately most anticholinergic syndromes can be managed with supportive care.
- Mistaking nonspecific arousal for reversal of anticholinergic effects can lead to giving more physostigmine to a patient without true anticholinergic activity; this increases the risk of cholinergic crisis.
- Reversal of the central anticholinergic syndrome usually results in return to completely normal mentation for the duration of action. Partial response indicates the presence of another toxin or etiology that is not anticholinergic.
- Overly rapid administration is more likely to result in seizure or cardiac dysrhythmia, including asystole.
- Some patients exhibit an increased sensitivity to cholinergic agents and develop cholinergic crisis from very small doses.
- Sodium bisulfite, used as a preservative, may cause allergic reactions.
- Inadequate or excessive atropinization should be avoided in treating cholinergic crisis.

ICD-9-CM 971.1

Poisoning by drugs affecting the autonomic nervous system: parasympatholytics (anticholinergics and antimuscarinics) and spasmolytics.

See also: SECTION II, Anticholinergic Syndrome, Bradycardia Toxidrome, Hypotension, and Seizures (Unexplained) chapters; and SECTION III, Atropine chapter.

RECOMMENDED READING

Gilman AG, Fall TW, Nies AS, et al., eds. *Goodman and Gilman's the pharmacological basis of therapeutics,* 8th ed. New York: Pergamon, 1990.

Pentel P, Peterson CD. Asystole complicating physostigmine treatment of tricyclic antidepressant overdose. *Ann Emerg Med* 1980;9:588–590.

Author: Steven A. Seifert

Reviewer: Katherine M. Hurlbut

Pralidoxime

Basics

DESCRIPTION

Pralidoxime chloride (Protopam chloride, 2-PAM chloride) is an antidote for organophosphate or carbamate insecticide poisoning.

FORMS AND USES

- Each 20-cc vial contains 1 g of powder.
- The powder can be reconstituted with 0.9% sodium chloride solution.

MECHANISM OF ACTION

- Chemicals with organophosphate or carbamate activity inhibit plasma and erythrocyte cholinesterase and neurotoxic esterase by phosphorylating the serine esteratic site of the enzyme. Phosphorylation causes cholinergic toxicity by inhibiting the action of the cholinesterase.
- Pralidoxime can remove the phosphate group, thereby reactivating the enzyme and terminating cholinergic toxicity.
- Reactivation of erythrocyte cholinesterase occurs rapidly when pralidoxime is administered soon after exposure; delay in administration may allow the organophosphate-cholinesterase complex to bind covalently and thereby become irreversible.
- Reactivation of plasma cholinesterase is minimal.
- The most striking clinical effect is at nicotinic receptor sites as compared with muscarinic receptor sites.

DRUG AND DISEASE INTERACTIONS

Atropine and pralidoxime given together may act synergistically and may decrease atropine requirements.

PREGNANCY AND LACTATION

- US FDA Pregnancy Category C. Studies have shown that the drug exerts animal teratogenic or embryocidal effects, but there are no controlled studies in women, or no studies are available in either animals or women.
- In the presence of cholinergic symptoms, treatment is recommended for pregnant or lactating women.

Indications

- Clinically significant organophosphate insecticide poisoning

—Nicotinic effects (muscle and diaphragmatic weakness, fasciculation, muscle cramps, etc.) should be treated with pralidoxime.
—CNS effects (confusion, coma, and seizures) should be treated with pralidoxime in addition to atropine.

- Carbamate poisoning. Use of pralidoxime in the treatment of carbamate poisoning is controversial but recommended, particularly for severe cases. In an animal model, the use of pralidoxime with the carbamate carbaryl was associated with worsening. However, it has been used in humans with poisoning by other carbamates without ill effect.
- Toxicity of drugs used to treat myasthenia gravis. Neostigmine and pyridostigmine inhibit cholinesterase and may produce cholinergic effects.

Contraindications and Adverse Effects

CONTRAINDICATIONS

- A known previous anaphylactic reaction to pralidoxime contraindicates its use.
- Pralidoxime is not generally recommended in cases of known exposure to carbaryl (Sevin) due to exacerbation of toxicity in animal models, although its use/nonuse in such situations is still a matter of controversy.

ADVERSE EFFECTS

- Mild serum creatinine kinase enzyme elevation
- Neuromuscular blockade may develop with serum pralidoxime concentration above 400 μg/cc. Therapeutic use does not approach this level.

Cardiovascular

Tachycardia, hypertension, and, rarely, cardiopulmonary arrest have been associated with rapid infusion.

Neurologic

Dizziness, headache, drowsiness, and apprehension associated with rapid infusion.

Dermatologic

Rash.

Gastrointestinal

Nausea and hepatic enzyme elevation.

Visual

Blurred vision, diplopia, and mydriasis.

Pulmonary

Apnea, hyperventilation, and laryngospasm associated with rapid infusion.

Dosage and Method of Administration

- Adult

—Loading dose. 1 to 2 g in 0.9% sodium chloride solution should be infused intravenously over 30 minutes. Higher dose used for severe poisoning.
—Maintenance dose. Continuous intravenous infusion at 500 mg/h should be continued for 24 to 48 hours. Intermittent infusion of 1 g in 250 cc normal saline, administered every 6 to 12 hours has also been recommended.

- Pediatric

—Loading dose. 25 mg/kg (up to 1 g) in 0.9% sodium chloride solution should be infused intravenously over 30 minutes.
—Maintenance dose. Intravenous infusion at 10 to 20 mg/kg (up to 500 mg) per hour should be continued for 24 to 48 hours. Intermittent infusion also has been used.

- Because excretion is renal, the dose of pralidoxime should be reduced in patients with renal insufficiency.
- Oral dosing of pralidoxime has been described but is not typically used.
- See SECTION IV, Organophosphate Insecticides chapter, for monitoring procedures.

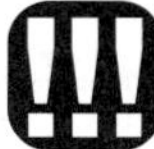

Pitfalls

- Rapid large intravenous bolus administration has produced sudden cardiac and respiratory arrest.
- Failure of treatment is usually a function of inadequate loading or maintenance dose.
- Treatment should be initiated as early as possible; administration more than 24 hours after exposure is thought to allow "aging" of the organophosphate-cholinesterase complex, rendering inactivation irreversible. However, treatment should be attempted in symptomatic patients even after 24 hours because reports of clinical response have been published.
- Treatment may require many days while residual organophosphate is metabolized or slowly cleared from body stores.
- Premature termination of treatment may result in recurrent signs and symptoms of organophosphate poisoning.
- Pralidoxime is not equally effective with all anticholinesterase agents.

ICD-9-CM 989.3

Toxic effect of other substances, chiefly nonmedicinal as to source: organophosphate and carbamate.

See also: SECTION III, Atropine chapter; and SECTION IV, Carbamate Insecticides, Organochlorine Pesticides, and Organophosphate Insecticides chapters.

RECOMMENDED READING

Farrar HC, Wells TG, Kearns GL. Use of continuous infusion of pralidoxime for treatment of organophosphate poisoning in children. *J Pediatr* 1990;116:658–661.

Howland MA, Aaron CK. Pralidoxime. In: Goldfrank LR, Flomenbaum NE, Lewin NA, et al., eds. *Goldfrank's toxicologic emergencies,* 6th ed. Norwalk, CT: Appleton & Lange, 1998.

Namba T, Hiraki K. PAM (Pyridine-2-aldoxime methiodide) therapy for alkylphosphate poisoning. *JAMA* 1958;166:1834–1839.

Thompson DF, Thompson GD, Greenwood RB, et al. Therapeutic dosing of pralidoxime chloride. *Drug Intell Clin Pharm* 1987;21:590–593.

Willems JL, De Bisschop HC, Verstraete AG, et al. Cholinesterase reactivation in organophosphorus poisoned patients depends on the plasma concentrations of the oxime pralidoxime methylsulphate and of the organophosphate. *Arch Toxicol* 1993;67:79–84.

Author: Luke Yip

Reviewer: Rivka S. Horowitz

Protamine Sulfate

Basics

DESCRIPTION

Protamine is used to reverse coagulopathy caused by heparin.

FORMS AND USES

• Protamine sulfate (10 mg/ml, 250 mg/25 ml) is derived from the sperm or testes of fish from the family Salmonidae.
• It is a low molecular weight protein that reverses the anticoagulant activity of heparin; 1 mg of protamine sulfate will neutralize approximately 100 U of heparin.
• Hexadimethrine (Polybrene) is a synthetic quaternary ammonium salt that can also neutralize the anticoagulant effects of heparin; hexadimethrine is not currently marketed in the United States but has been used successfully to treat heparin-induced anticoagulation in patients who had previously developed severe adverse reactions to protamine sulfate.

MECHANISM OF ACTION

• Protamine is a strongly basic protein and binds to the strongly acidic heparin molecule to form a stable, inactive heparin salt.
• It also may cause dissociation of the heparin-antithrombin III complex.
• Protamine is also a weak anticoagulant and may cause coagulopathy if administered in excess.

DRUG AND DISEASE INTERACTIONS

• Protamine sulfate may be incompatible with some penicillins and cephalosporins when administered concomitantly by the intravenous route.

PREGNANCY AND LACTATION

US FDA Pregnancy Category C. The drug exerts animal teratogenic or embryocidal effects, but there are no controlled studies in women, or no studies are available in either animals or women.

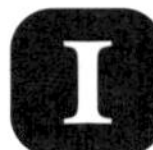

Indications

• Usage is indicated when the patient exhibits serious hemorrhage and markedly elevated activated partial thromboplastin time (APTT) or partial thromboplastin time (PTT) caused by heparin.
• Minor hemorrhage following heparin over-anticoagulation should not be treated with protamine sulfate; most cases of heparin-related over-anticoagulation with only minor bleeding can be managed conservatively.
• Oral, rectal, or sublingual exposure to heparin does not require protamine treatment; heparin is not absorbed by the gastrointestinal tract.

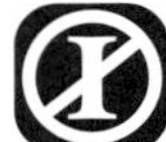

Contraindications and Adverse Effects

CONTRAINDICATIONS

• History of life-threatening protamine reaction precludes its use.

ADVERSE EFFECTS

• Anaphylactoid and anaphylactic reactions. These reactions are treated with crystalloidal isotonic fluid infusion, antihistamines, and, if needed, epinephrine.
• Allergic reactions are more common in the following patients:

—Those with prior exposure to protamine
—Diabetics exposed to insulin (neutral protamine Hagedorn insulin; NPH), which contains protamine.
—Patients who have a history of cardiac surgery, cardiac catheterization, or hemodialysis, and who may have had previous heparin neutralization with protamine
—Men with vasectomy or infertility who may have developed antiprotamine antibodies
—Patients with fish allergy, because protamine is derived from the sperm and testes of salmon

• Hypotension is commonly related to the rate of protamine sulfate infusion.

—Hypotension may resolve when the rate is decreased; if the patient does not immediately respond to slowing of infusion, the diagnosis of an allergic reaction should be considered.
—Hypotension also may occur as an idiosyncratic reaction.

- Flushing is reversible.
- Thrombocytopenia is reversible.
- Leukopenia is reversible.
- Paradoxical anticoagulation is a rare occurrence of unknown etiology that occurs under the following conditions:

—Protamine is administered in the absence of heparin.
—The protamine dose greatly exceeds the empiric dose, as calculated by the amount of heparin requiring neutralization.
—The protamine dose exceeds 3 mg/kg.
—The effects are rarely severe and resolve with discontinuation of therapy.

- Heparin rebound is the recurrence of anticoagulation following the administration of protamine sulfate after initial control of anticoagulation has been achieved.

—Its incidence can be decreased when a moderate excess of protamine is administered (1.5–2.0 mg per 100 U of heparin).
—Rebound most often occurs when heparin has been administered during extracorporeal bypass procedures, even when adequate initial neutralizing doses of protamine sulfate have been administered; it occurs within 30 minutes to 18 hours following initial neutralization.
—Its etiology is unclear, but it may be related to redistribution of heparin from extravascular spaces, liberation of heparin from intravascular surfaces, or a dissociation of the heparin-protamine complex.

- Acute overdose of protamine is generally well tolerated.

—The primary effect is mild anticoagulation.
—Doses up to 800 mg in adults have been tolerated without severe effects.

Dosage and Method of Administration

LIFE-THREATENING HEMORRHAGE AND MARKEDLY ELEVATED APTT OR AN ELEVATED PTT

Initial Dose

- One milligram of protamine sulfate neutralizes approximately 100 U of heparin.
- Empiric calculation of the initial dose of protamine sulfate required for complete neutralization should be made as follows:

—If the heparin injection was given within the preceding 15 minutes, 1 mg of protamine sulfate should be administered for each 100 U of heparin that the patient received.
—If the heparin injection was given 15 to 30 minutes earlier, 0.5 mg of protamine sulfate should be administered for each 100 U of heparin that the patient received.
—If the heparin injection was given 30 minutes to 2 hours earlier, 0.25 mg of protamine sulfate should be administered for each 100 U of heparin that the patient received.

Subsequent Doses

Subsequent doses of protamine sulfate should be guided by the following:

- Plasma heparin levels may be useful in guiding subsequent protamine dosing but are not widely available.
- If the APTT or PTT remains dangerously elevated following the initial dose of protamine sulfate, additional administration of protamine sulfate may be indicated.
- Dosing of additional protamine sulfate is empiric; a reasonable approach would be to administer half the initial dose, not to exceed 3 mg/kg.

Method of Administration

- Protamine sulfate should be administered by the intravenous route only.
- Protamine sulfate is compatible with either dextrose 5% in water or 0.9% normal saline.
- Intravenous infusion rate should not exceed 0.5 mg/min.
- An APTT or a PTT should be drawn every 15 minutes to guide subsequent protamine therapy.

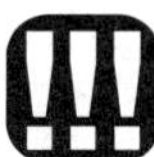

Pitfalls

- Because serum concentrations of heparin decrease rapidly (the half-life of heparin is 60–90 minutes) the amount of protamine sulfate needed to neutralize a given overdose of heparin will decrease as the interval from the time of administration of heparin increases.
- Although reactions to protamine are rare (fewer than 0.5% of cases), potentially lethal anaphylaxis may occur.
- Due to the short half-life of heparin, most cases of heparin-related over-anticoagulation can be managed conservatively and do not require the administration of protamine sulfate.

ICD-9-CM 964.5

Poisoning by agents primarily affecting blood constituents: anticoagulant antagonists and other coagulants.

See also: SECTION IV, Heparins, Standard and Fractionated chapter.

RECOMMENDED READING

Howland MA. Protamine. In: Goldfrank LR, Flomenbaum NE, Lewin NA, et al., eds. *Goldfrank's toxicologic emergencies,* 6th ed. Norwalk, CT: Appleton & Lange, 1998.

Author: Edwin K. Kuffner

Reviewer: Richard C. Dart

Pyridoxine

Basics

DESCRIPTION

Pyridoxine is a water-soluble B-complex vitamin that is an essential cofactor in many enzymatic reactions.

FORMS AND USES

- Pyridoxine is available in tablets (Beelith, Lurline PMS, Marlyn Formula, Mega-B, Aminoxin, Apatate) or in injection form at a concentration of 100 mg/ml.
- Pyridoxine is used for treatment of seizure associated with isoniazid (INH), Gyromitra mushroom [monomethylhydrazine (MMH)], or penicillamine poisoning.
- Pyridoxine is also used prophylactically to prevent development of peripheral neuropathy in patients taking INH.
- In ethylene glycol intoxication, pyridoxine therapy has been proposed to reduce levels of toxic metabolites.

MECHANISM OF ACTION

- Pyridoxine (after conversion to pyridoxal phosphate) is required for the synthesis of gamma-aminobutyric acid (GABA), the main inhibitory neurotransmitter of the CNS. A decreased level of GABA is believed to cause seizures due to loss of neural inhibition.
- INH and MMH interfere with the synthesis of pyridoxal phosphate, leading to a functional pyridoxine deficiency.
- As pyridoxine levels decrease, GABA production declines and seizure activity or coma may ensue.

DRUG AND DISEASE INTERACTIONS

- Pyridoxine levels can be depleted by penicillamine, cycloserine, and hydralazine.
- Pyridoxine enhances peripheral decarboxylation of levodopa, reducing its effectiveness against Parkinson's disease.

PREGNANCY AND LACTATION

- Pregnant women receiving INH should be given 25 mg/day of pyridoxine as prophylaxis against peripheral neuritis.
- Used as a vitamin within recommended daily allowance. US FDA Pregnancy Category A. Controlled studies in women fail to demonstrate a risk to the fetus in the first trimester, and the possibility of fetal harm appears remote.
- High-dose use. US FDA Pregnancy Category C. The drug exerts animal teratogenic or embryocidal effects, but there are no controlled studies in women, or no studies are available in either animals or women.

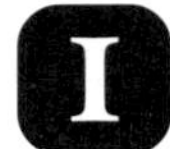

Indications

SEIZURES OF UNKNOWN CAUSE

INH or Gyromitra mushroom ingestion may be unrecognized; if patient does not respond to initial anticonvulsant therapy, pyridoxine should be administered.

KNOWN INGESTION OF INH

- In cases of suicidal ingestion of INH, prophylactic treatment before onset of seizure is recommended.
- Any INH ingestion associated with seizures should be treated with pyridoxine.

ETHYLENE GLYCOL TOXICITY

- Pyridoxine should be considered in the treatment of patients who have ingested ethylene glycol.
- Pyridoxine (and thiamine) are adjuncts to ethanol therapy and may reduce production of oxalic acid, a toxic metabolite of ethylene glycol.

MMH TOXICITY

- Ingestion of Gyromitra species of mushroom can produce seizures and should be treated with pyridoxine.

PENICILLAMINE-INDUCED SEIZURES

- Pencillamine-induced seizures have been reported to respond to pyridoxine 100 mg intravenously.

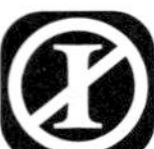

Contraindications and Adverse Effects

CONTRAINDICATIONS

Patients with known hypersensitivity reaction to pyridoxine.

ADVERSE EFFECTS

- Acute and or repeated supratherapeutic doses of pyridoxine have been associated with peripheral sensory neuropathy.

—Although the maximum nontoxic pyridoxine dose is unknown, acute single doses up to 10 to 15 g are well tolerated.
—In general, unless massive INH ingestion has occurred, the maximum pyridoxine dose is 10 to 15 g.

- Large, acute overdose of pyridoxine (5 g/kg) may cause tachypnea, postural hypotension, paralysis, or seizures.

Dosage and Method of Administration

SEIZURES OF UNKNOWN CAUSE

- Benzodiazepines should be administered initially.
- If seizures continue, 5 g of pyridoxine can be given intravenously over 10 minutes.
- Dose should be repeated in 30 minutes if needed for control of seizures.

KNOWN INGESTION OF INH

- In cases of suicidal ingestion of INH (unknown dose), 5 g of pyridoxine should be administered intravenously over 30 minutes.
- The pediatric dose is 70 mg/kg up to 5 g.
- When the amount of INH ingested is known and seizures or coma have occurred:

—The maximum total amount of INH that could have been ingested should be calculated.
—An equal amount of pyridoxine should be administered (e.g., if 10 tablets of 300 mg INH were ingested, patient should receive 3 g of pyridoxine) intravenously over 10 minutes.
—Pediatric dosage. The pyridoxine administered should be based on the amount of INH ingested, not the weight of the patient.
—Dose should be repeated in 15 to 30 minutes if seizures persist or recur.

- When the amount of INH ingested is unknown and seizures or coma have occurred:

—The patient should receive 5 g of pyridoxine intravenously over 10 minutes.
—Dose should be repeated in 15 to 30 minutes if seizures persist or recur.

ETHYLENE GLYCOL TOXICITY

- The adult dose is 50 to 100 mg pyridoxine intravenously every 6 hours until the ethylene glycol level is undetectable.
- The pediatric dose is 1 to 2 mg/kg every 6 hours until their ethylene glycol level is undetectable.
- The dose should be repeated after dialysis unless the ethylene glycol level is less than 20 mg/dl.

MMH TOXICITY

- Patients with coma or seizures from MMH should have 25 mg/kg pyridoxine administered intravenously over 10 minutes to a maximum dose of 10 g.

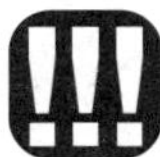

Pitfalls

- If no parenteral form of pyridoxine is available, pyridoxine tablets may be crushed and mixed with water to form a slurry, which should be administered orally or via an endogastric tube in a gram-for-gram dose for each gram of INH ingested, or according to above doses for MMH and ethylene glycol toxicities.
- Pyridoxine should be used in conjunction with a benzodiazepine for the synergistic effect exerted to control seizures induced by INH.
- If seizures are refractory to repeated dosing with pyridoxine and benzodiazepine, a loading dose of phenobarbital should be considered, possibly followed by neuromuscular blockade and general anesthesia (including endotracheal intubation).
- Seizures that remain unresponsive to high doses of pyridoxine may not be due to INH or MMH toxicity.
- Careful attention must be directed to the consideration of other potential causes of seizure in refractory patients (hypoxia, hypoglycemia, or other poisons).

ICD-9-CM 966

Poisoning by anticonvulsants and antiparkinsonism drugs.

See also: SECTION IV, Ethylene Glycol, Isoniazid, and Mushrooms chapters.

RECOMMENDED READING

Wason S, Lacouture PG, Lovejoy FH. Single high dose pyridoxine treatment for isoniazid overdose. *JAMA* 1981;246:1102–1104.

Author: Mark C. Goodman

Reviewer: Luke Yip

Snake Antivenom—Crotalid and Elapid Snakes

Basics

DESCRIPTION

The antivenoms described here are for use against bites by crotalid (pit viper) snakes (rattlesnakes, cottonmouths, and copperheads) and elapid snakes (coral snakes).

FORMS AND USES

Pit Viper (Crotalid Snakes) Antivenoms

- Antivenin (Crotalidae) Polyvalent, commonly referred to as Wyeth antivenom. Each antidote package contains one vial of lyophilized antivenom, one vial of horse serum for skin testing, and one vial of bacteriostatic water for injection.
- Affinity-purified, mixed monospecific crotalid antivenom ovine Fab is an investigational drug. It is currently under consideration by the U.S. Food and Drug Administration and should be approved by December 1999.
- Antivenin (Crotalidae) Polyvalent (Wyeth) and affinity-purified, and mixed monospecific crotalid antivenom ovine Fab are used for envenomation by North or South American rattlesnakes, cottonmouth, or copperhead snakes.

Coral Snake Antivenom (Micrurus fulvius) Merck

- Each antidote package contains one vial of lyophilized antivenom and one vial of bacteriostatic water for injection.
- It is used in the treatment of envenomation by the eastern or Texas coral snakes.

MECHANISM OF ACTION

- Wyeth antivenom and coral snake antivenom contain immunoglobulin G (IgG) isolated from horses immunized to snake venom; they act by conferring passive immunity to the components of snake venom.
- The Wyeth antivenom is produced by immunization with venom of eastern and western diamondback rattlesnakes, the tropical rattlesnake, and the fer-de-lance.
- Coral snake antivenom is produced by immunization with eastern coral snake venom.
- Affinity-purified, mixed monospecific crotalid antivenom ovine Fab is sheep derived and is composed of IgG fragments termed Fab. It is expected to produce fewer adverse reactions.

PREGNANCY AND LACTATION

Use of antivenom in pregnancy for crotalid snakebite is recommended and appears to decrease the likelihood of spontaneous abortion and bleeding complications.

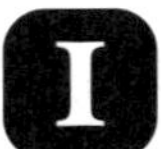

Indications

- Antivenin (Crotalidae) Polyvalent (Wyeth) or affinity-purified, mixed monospecific crotalid antivenom ovine Fab (investigational drug)

—Treatment is indicated when there is a progression of venom effects
  - —Local injury (pain or swelling)
  - —Coagulopathy [prolongation of prothrombin time (PT) or international normalized ratio (INR) or hypofibrinogenemia] or thrombocytopenia
  - —Systemic effects, including compartment syndrome, hypotension, altered mental status, or other evidence of progression.

—Bites without evidence of progression do not require antivenom treatment.

- Micrurus fulvius antivenin, Merck

—Physical evidence that coral snake bite has occurred: fang puncture marks, history of snake holding on and chewing
—Presence of clinical effects of envenomation: weakness, ptosis, respiratory deterioration

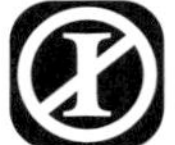

Contraindications and Adverse Effects

CONTRAINDICATIONS

Known hypersensitivity to horse serum or to antivenom are relative contraindications. If history of true acute allergic reaction is obtained, consultation with a medical toxicologist, poison control center, or other physician experienced in the use of antivenom is recommended.

ADVERSE EFFECTS

Mild Acute Allergic Reactions (Rash, Bronchospasm)

- These occur in 20% to 25% of patients treated with Wyeth antivenom; incidence for other products is unknown.
- Administration of H_1 and H_2 antihistamine is recommended. Diphenhydramine: adult dose is 25 to 50 mg (child, 1 mg/kg up to 50 mg) intravenously. Cimetidine: adult dose is 300 mg intravenously. Pediatric dose is 10 mg/kg up to 300 mg.
- Bronchospasm is treated with albuterol 0.15 mg/kg (maximum of 10 mg) in saline with humidified oxygen via nebulizer every 20 to 30 minutes.

Anaphylaxis or Shock

- This occurs rarely, but its true frequency is unknown; overwhelming anaphylaxis and death are possible within minutes of administration of Wyeth antivenom.
- First, the patient is administered 100% oxygen and the airway is secured.
- Epinephrine should be administered immediately. In severe cases an intravenous bolus of epinephrine 3 to 5 ml of 1:10,000 diluted 10:1 should be administered by slow intravenous push over several minutes. A continuous infusion may be started for persistent effects as described below.

Antihistamine

Both diphenhydramine and cimetidine (or other H_2 blocker) should be administered. The adult dose of diphenhydramine is 25 to 50 mg (child 1 mg/kg up to 50 mg) administered intravenously every 6 to 8 hours. The adult dose of cimetidine is 300 mg intravenously every 6 hours; pediatric dose is 10 mg/kg up to 300 mg every 6 hours.

Bronchospasm

- Albuterol 0.15 mg/kg (maximum of 10 mg) is administered in saline with humidified oxygen via nebulizer every 20 to 30 minutes.
- Epinephrine 1:1,000 is administered subcutaneously; adult dose is 0.3 to 0.5 ml (pediatric, 0.01 ml/kg up to 0.5 ml) subcutaneously.

Hypotension (Type I Hypersensitivity)

Crystalloid and epinephrine are administered.

- An initial bolus of 0.9% sodium chloride 10 to 20 ml/kg should be infused rapidly.
- If necessary, the initial epinephrine bolus is followed with an infusion; 1 mg of 1:1,000 epinephrine is diluted in 250 ml D5W; infusion starts at 1 μg/min and is titrated to desired blood pressure.
- Methylprednisolone is administered intravenously; adult dose is 60 to 125 mg (1.0–1.5 mg/kg); pediatric dose is 1 to 2 mg/kg up to 125 mg every 6 to 8 hours

Type IV Hypersensitivity (Serum Sickness)

- Serum sickness typically begins 3 to 14 days after the antivenom infusion as malaise and fever, and progresses to diffuse rash, arthralgia, pruritus, and (rarely) pericarditis and glomerulonephritis.
- It occurs in 70% to 75% of patients treated with Wyeth antivenom and 5% to 10% for Fab antivenom; the incidence is unknown for coral snake antivenom.
- Treatment consists primarily of antihistamines and steroids. Both should be administered except in the mildest of cases. The adult dose of diphenhydramine is 25 to 50 mg (child 1 mg/kg up to 50 mg) orally every 6 to 8 hours.
- The adult dose of prednisone is 40 to 60 mg/day (child 1 mg/kg per day up to 60 mg) orally for 7 to 10 days.
- Antipyretics and analgesics are used as guided by the patient's symptoms

—Acetaminophen. Adult, 1 g every 4 to 6 hours, not to exceed 4 g/day; pediatric, 10 mg/kg every 4 to 6 hours
—Ibuprofen. Adult, 200 to 600 mg every 8 hours; pediatric, 5 to 10 mg/kg every 6 to 8 hours

Dosage and Method of Administration

- Antivenom should be administered in an emergency department or intensive care unit.
- Clinician should be prepared to treat abrupt onset of airway obstruction and hypotension due to anaphylaxis; epinephrine and equipment for endotracheal intubation should be immediately available.

ANTIVENIN (CROTALIDAE) POLYVALENT, WYETH

- No antivenom is needed for patients without clinical effects.
- Initial dose of 20 vials should be administered to adult or pediatric patients with rapidly progressive swelling, severe coagulation abnormalities, presence of frank bleeding, or severe hypotension.
- All other patients should receive 10 vials initially.
- Additional rounds of antivenom (10 vials) are administered if venom effects persist or worsen after initial dose; common examples are continued swelling, any persistent coagulation abnormality despite antivenom, or recurrence of any toxic venom effect after antivenom therapy.
- For copperhead bite with progressive swelling, some physicians recommend an initial dose of five vials.
- Bite site should not be infiltrated locally with antivenom.
- Method of administration is as follows:

—Intravenous access should be established.
—Skin test should be performed with 0.02 ml of horse serum intradermally, and patient observed 20 to 30 minutes for wheal and flare reaction; the test should be read using same parameters as tuberculosis skin test (wheal and erythema larger than 10 mm).
—Ten vials of lyophilized antivenom powder should be prepared [each vial is reconstituted with 10 ml of sterile water (included) for injection]; dissolution may take 15 to 60 minutes (rolling vials between hands speeds dissolution; vials should not be shaken).
—Ten vials (100 ml) should be injected into 250- or 500-ml bag of D5W or 0.9% sodium chloride (an equivalent amount of fluid should be removed from the bag first).
—The infusion should begin slowly (10 to 25 ml/h) using infusion controller; rate can be increased slowly, while patient is observed for evidence of acute allergic reaction, until rate is reached that will infuse initial dose over a 1-hour period.

- Allergic reaction during infusion occurs in 25% of patients.

—The infusion should be halted, and the severity of reaction assessed; the reaction should be treated as described above under "Adverse Effects."
—The decision of whether to restart antivenom infusion requires a difficult risk-benefit analysis; severe or rapidly progressive effects generally warrant an attempt to restart the infusion.
—If the infusion is restarted, antivenom should be mixed in a more dilute solution (e.g., five vials in 1,000 cc diluent) and the patient should be pretreated with diphenhydramine and cimetidine (some clinicians would also administer an epinephrine or steroid dose).
—The infusion should be started very slowly and the rate titrated upward very slowly.
—Concurrent infusion of epinephrine has been used in difficult cases.

- The patient should be monitored continuously during antivenom infusion.

AFFINITY-PURIFIED, MIXED MONOSPECIFIC CROTALID ANTIVENOM OVINE FAB (INVESTIGATIONAL DRUG)

- Until greater experience is available, this antivenom should also be administered in an emergency department or ICU. However, no skin test is needed.
- The patient should be infused with four vials initially and assessed to determine whether initial control of venom effects has been achieved (four-vial dose may be repeated up to two times to achieve initial control).
- Thereafter, two vials should be administered every 6 hours for three additional doses; subsequent doses are administered at the physician's discretion.
- Each dose should be diluted in 250 cc of crystalloid and infused intravenously over 1 hour.
- Acute adverse effects occur during infusion in 15% to 20% of patients.

MICRURUS FULVIUS ANTIVENIN, MERCK

- An initial dose of three to five vials should be administered to adult or pediatric patient with evidence of coral snake bite.
- Coral snake venom binds irreversibly to presynaptic nerve terminals; therefore, antivenom should be administered before clinical effects develop.
- A skin test should be performed with 0.02 ml of horse serum intradermally, and the patient should be observed for 20 to 30 minutes for wheal and flare reaction; the test should be read with the same parameters as the tuberculosis skin test (wheal and erythema larger than 10 mm).
- If the skin test result is negative, three to five vials of lyophilized powder should be prepared [each vial is reconstituted with 10 ml of sterile water (included) for injection] and injected into 100- or 250-ml bag of dextrose 5% in water or 0.9% sodium chloride (an equivalent amount of fluid should be removed from the bag first).
- The infusion should begin slowly (10–25 ml/h) with an infusion controller; the rate should be increased slowly while the patient is observed for evidence of an acute allergic reaction.
- The initial dose (three to five vials) should be infused over a 1-hour period.
- The patient should be monitored continuously during administration; the clinician should be prepared to manage airway and treat anaphylaxis.

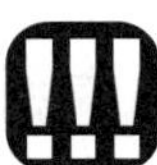

Pitfalls

- Adult and pediatric dosages of snake antivenoms are the same.
- Rapid intravenous bolus administration may produce severe anaphylactoid reactions, including death.
- Inadequate monitoring during antivenom infusion may allow anaphylaxis to develop without appropriate treatment.
- Allergic reaction to antivenom may be rate dependent; often antivenom can be infused successfully at a lower rate.

ICD-9-CM 989.5

Toxic effect of other substances, chiefly nonmedicinal as to source: venom.

See also: SECTION IV, Snakebite—North American Crotalids and Snakebite—North American Coral Snakes chapters.

RECOMMENDED READING

Horowitz R, Dart RC. Antivenins and immunobiologicals: immunotherapeutics of envenomation. In: Auerbach P, ed. *Management of wilderness emergencies.* Chicago: Mosby Year Book, 1995:731–741.

Kitchens CS, Van Mierop LHS. Envenomation by the eastern coral snake (*Micrurus fulvius fulvius*): a study of 39 victims. *JAMA* 1987;258:1615–1618.

Russell FE. *Snake venom poisoning.* New York: Scholium, 1983.

Author: Katherine M. Hurlbut

Reviewer: Luke Yip

Sodium Bicarbonate

Basics

DESCRIPTION

Sodium bicarbonate is a medication used to alkalinize the blood or urine.

FORMS AND USES

Sodium bicarbonate injection USP ($NaHCO_3$) is available at concentrations of 2.5%, 5%, 7.5% (44 mEq/50 ml ampule) or 8.4% (50 mEq/50 ml ampule).

MECHANISM OF ACTION

- Serum alkalinization

—$NaHCO_3$ bolus transiently increases serum sodium concentration and increases serum pH.
—Increased plasma sodium concentration antagonizes sodium channel blockade induced by agents with type 1 antidysrhythmic activity.

- Urinary alkalinization

—$NaHCO_3$ infusion is used to increase urinary pH above 7.5.
—For weak acids (salicylate; phenobarbital; chlorpropamide; 2,4-dichlorophenoxy acetic acid), increased pH produces charged species in the urine; charged species are reabsorbed poorly and urinary excretion is increased.

- Inhalation of $NaHCO_3$ may neutralize acid.

—This has been reported in uncontrolled studies to decrease pain and respiratory symptoms following chlorine inhalation.
—The proposed mechanism of action is unclear.

DRUG AND DISEASE INTERACTIONS

- Sodium load may exacerbate conditions with fluid overload (e.g., congestive heart failure).
- Hypernatremia may result from repeated administration.

PREGNANCY AND LACTATION

US FDA Pregnancy Category C. Studies have shown animal teratogenic or embryocidal effects, but there are no controlled studies in women, or no studies are available in either animals or women.

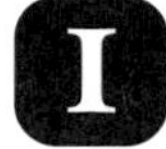

Indications

- Tricyclic antidepressant drug toxicity

—The purpose of $NaHCO_3$ administration is to narrow the QRS complex.
—The use of $NaHCO_3$ is based on the ECG, and is recommended for patients with a QRS interval at or above 120 msec (0.12 seconds).
—$NaHCO_3$ is not recommended for treatment of coma or hypotension alone because its efficacy is not well supported by current evidence.

- Type 1 antidysrhythmic drug toxicity

—The purpose of $NaHCO_3$ administration is to narrow the QRS complex.
—Case reports suggest that quinine, quinidine, encainide, and flecainide, as well as other drugs that block the sodium channel (e.g., propoxyphene, cocaine, diphenhydramine), respond to $NaHCO_3$.
—Use is recommended for patients with a QRS interval at or above 120 msec (0.12 seconds).

- Salicylate poisoning

—The purpose of administering $NaHCO_3$ is to produce urinary alkalinization.
—Use is recommended for the patient with clinically significant salicylate poisoning (systemic symptoms or signs).
—$NaHCO_3$ should be used with caution in cases of adult respiratory distress syndrome, renal failure, congestive heart failure, and states of volume overload.

- Phenobarbital poisoning

—The purpose of administering $NaHCO_3$ is to produce urinary alkalinization.
—Case reports and case series suggest that $NaHCO_3$ is helpful in increasing elimination, but they have not shown it to affect the course of illness; therefore, its use is not routinely recommended.

- Chlorpropamide toxicity

—The purpose of administering $NaHCO_3$ is to produce urinary alkalinization.
—Experimental evidence in normal volunteers suggests that $NaHCO_3$ increases excretion, but it has not been shown to affect the course of illness and is not routinely recommended.

- Chlorphenoxy herbicides (e.g., 2,4-dichlorophenoxyacetic acid) poisoning

—The purpose of administering $NaHCO_3$ is to produce urinary alkalinization.
—It has been recommended in symptomatic patients; however, adequate data are lacking and its use is not routinely recommended.

- Chlorine gas poisoning

—The purpose of having a patient inhale $NaHCO_3$ is to neutralize acid.
—Case reports and case series suggest that $NaHCO_3$ is helpful, but contradictory evidence exists and indications have not been established.
—The use of inhaled $NaHCO_3$ in the case of chlorine gas poisoning is questionable, but it has not been harmful.

- Lactic acidosis induced by a poison

—$NaHCO_3$ has been used for the patient with metabolic acidosis that cannot be promptly treated by another means.
—The use of $NaHCO_3$ for treatment of lactic acidosis is not recommended because it is not well supported by current experimental evidence.

- Rhabdomyolysis induced by a poison

—$NaHCO_3$ for treatment of rhabdomyolysis is recommended by some clinicians, but it is not well supported by experimental evidence and therefore is not recommended.
—Appropriate rehydration to maintain urine output at 1 to 2 ml/kg per hour by use of isotonic saline infusion should be the goal of therapy.

Contraindications and Adverse Effects

CONTRAINDICATIONS

- Relative contraindications. Preexisting volume overload syndrome (congestive heart failure, renal failure, etc.)
- Absolute contraindications. Serum pH above 7.55 (for serum alkalinization)

ADVERSE EFFECTS

- Paradoxical intracellular acidosis may develop in patients with lactic acidosis or diabetic ketoacidosis.
- Electrolyte abnormalities: Hypernatremia, hypokalemia, hypochloremia, hypocalcemia, or alkalosis may occur.
- Fluid overload may worsen congestive heart failure or other volume overload states.

Dosage and Method of Administration

TRICYCLIC ANTIDEPRESSANT DRUG TOXICITY

- Adult. Initial administration of $NaHCO_3$ should be one to two ampules (either 44 or 50 mEq) intravenous push; if the QRS duration does not narrow to less than 100 msec, dose should be repeated until arterial blood pH reaches 7.45 to 7.55.
- Pediatric. A dose of 1 to 2 mEq/kg intravenous push should be administered; if the QRS duration does not narrow to less than 100 msec, dose should be repeated until arterial blood pH reaches 7.45 to 7.55.
- Continuous intravenous infusion should not be initiated.

TYPE 1 ANTIDYSRHYTHMIC DRUG TOXICITY

- $NaHCO_3$ may be useful against quinine, quinidine, encainide, flecainide, propoxyphene, and diphenhydramine.
- The dose is unknown, but generally considered to be the same as for tricyclic antidepressant drugs.

SALICYLATE POISONING

- Adult

—$NaHCO_3$ should be administered as one to two ampules (either 44 or 50 mEq) intravenous push.
—In addition, three ampules of $NaHCO_3$ (either 44 or 50 mEq) should be mixed in 1 L D5W and infused at 200 ml/h.
—Urinary pH should be checked frequently; the rate of infusion can be increased within clinically reasonable boundaries (consider underlying medical conditions) to produce a urinary pH of 7.5 or greater.

- Pediatric

—One to two mEq/kg should be administered via intravenous push.
—In addition, one or two ampules (either 44 or 50 mEq) of $NaHCO_3$ should be mixed in 1 L D5W and infused at a rate within clinically reasonable boundaries (consider underlying medical conditions) to produce a urinary pH of 7.5 or above.
—Supplemental potassium administration should be considered.

PHENOBARBITAL, CHLORPROPAMIDE, OR CHLORPHENOXY HERBICIDE POISONING

- The use of $NaHCO_3$ is not routinely recommended.
- Adult

—$NaHCO_3$ should be administered as one to two ampules (either 44 or 50 mEq) intravenous push.
—Three ampules of $NaHCO_3$ should be mixed in 1 L D5W and infused at 200 ml/h.
—Urinary pH should be monitored frequently; the rate should be increased within clinically reasonable boundaries (considering underlying medical conditions) to produce a urinary pH of 7.5 or above.

- Pediatric

—One to two mEq/kg should be administered via intravenous push.
—One or two ampules (either 44 or 50 mEq) of $NaHCO_3$ should be mixed in 1 L D5W and infused at a rate within clinically reasonable boundaries (considering underlying medical conditions) to produce a urinary pH of 7.5 or above.

- Supplemental potassium administration should be considered.

CHLORINE GAS POISONING

- Adult or pediatric patients: Two cc $NaHCO_3$ (7.5% or 8.4%) should be mixed with 2 cc 0.9% normal saline USP.
- This $NaHCO_3$ inhalant should be administered to the patient by hand-held nebulizer.

METABOLIC ACIDOSIS INDUCED BY A POISON

- The use of $NaHCO_3$ is not routinely recommended.
- The most important treatment is to reverse the underlying cause of acidosis.

RHABDOMYOLYSIS INDUCED BY A POISON

The use of $NaHCO_3$ is not routinely recommended.

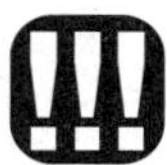

Pitfalls

- Poorly monitored infusion of maintenance $NaHCO_3$ may become excessive, producing a systemic pH above 7.6, which impairs cardiac contractility.
- Hypernatremia and fluid overload may occur.
- Pediatric patients

—Rapid administration of large amounts of $NaHCO_3$ to children under the age of 2 years has been associated with hypernatremia, decreased cerebrospinal fluid pressure, and intracranial hemorrhage.
—Use of the 4.2% solution (1:1 dilution of 8.4% solution) may be preferable.

- Geriatric patients may be susceptible to sodium and fluid overload.

See also: SECTION IV, Antidysrhythmic Agents, Barbiturates, Chlorine, Organochlorine Pesticides, Salicylates, Antidepressants—Tricyclic, and Oral Hypoglycemic Agents chapters.

RECOMMENDED READING

Stackpoole P. Lactic acidosis: the case against bicarbonate therapy. *Ann Intern Med* 1986;105:276–279.

Wax PM, Hoffman RS. Sodium bicarbonate. In: Hoffman RS, Goldfrank LR, eds. *Critical care toxicology.* New York: Churchill Livingstone, 1991:81–108.

Author: Richard C. Dart

Reviewer: Katherine M. Hurlbut

Sodium Polystyrene Sulfonate

Basics

DESCRIPTION

Sodium polystyrene sulfonate (Kayexalate) is a cation exchange resin used to increase excretion of potassium.

FORMS AND USES

- Sodium polystyrene sulfonate (SPS) is available as a suspension of 15 g of SPS, 14.1 g of sorbitol, and 0.1% ethanol per 60 ml for administration orally or as an enema.
- It is also supplied as a powder for reconstitution in water.

MECHANISM OF ACTION

In the intestines, sodium ions are released from the resin and replaced by other cations (potassium or lithium), which are subsequently eliminated in the stool.

DRUG AND DISEASE INTERACTIONS

- Simultaneous administration with nonabsorbable cation-donating antacids and laxatives may reduce the effectiveness of cation exchange or cause systemic alkalosis.
- Administration of SPS may cause hypokalemia.

PREGNANCY AND LACTATION

- US FDA Pregnancy Category C. The drug exerts animal teratogenic or embryocidal effects, but there are no controlled studies in women, or no studies are available in either animals or women.
- It is unknown whether SPS is excreted in breast milk.

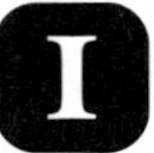

Indications

- Hyperkalemia

—SPS enhances fecal elimination of potassium over hours to days.
—It is used as an adjunct to other measures (insulin and dextrose, calcium, and sodium bicarbonate) in patients with life-threatening hyperkalemia.

- Lithium toxicity

—SPS has been shown to enhance elimination of lithium in human volunteer studies, but has not been shown to affect outcome in patients with lithium toxicity.
—Routine use is not recommended.

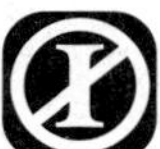

Contraindications and Adverse Effects

CONTRAINDICATIONS

- Known hypersensitivity to SPS
- Preexisting hypokalemia

ADVERSE EFFECTS

- Gastrointestinal

—The most common adverse effects include anorexia, nausea, vomiting, constipation, diarrhea, and fecal impaction.
—Colonic necrosis has occurred rarely.

- Fluids and electrolytes

—Hypokalemia
—Hypocalcemia
—Sodium retention

Dosage and Method of Administration

- Adult

—The dosage for hyperkalemia is 15 g orally one to four times daily.
—Alternatively, SPS may be given as a retention enema, 30 to 50 g every 6 hours.
—Serum electrolytes need to be monitored during therapy.

- Pediatric

—Experience is limited.
—The usual dose is 1 g/kg/dose up to 15 g every 6 hours orally or every 2 to 6 hours as a retention enema.
—The dose should be adjusted with 1 mEq potassium per gram of sodium polystyrene sulfonate resin as a guide.
—Multiple doses of sorbitol-containing suspension should not be given to children.
—Serum electrolytes need to be monitored frequently.

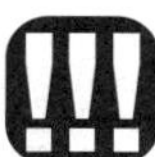

Pitfalls

Multiple doses may lead to sodium overload in susceptible patients (e.g., congestive heart failure).

ICD-9-CM 964

Poisoning by agents primarily affecting blood constituents.

See also: SECTION II, Hyperkalemia chapter.

RECOMMENDED READING

Belanger DR, Tierney MG, Dickinson G. Effect of sodium polystyrene sulfonate on lithium bioavailability. *Ann Emerg Med* 1992;21:1312–1315.

Tomaszewski C, Musso C, Pearson JR, et al. Lithium absorption prevented by sodium polystyrene sulfonate in volunteers. *Ann Emerg Med* 1992;21:1308–1311.

Author: Katherine M. Hurlbut

Reviewer: Richard C. Dart

Succimer

Basics

DESCRIPTION

Succimer (dimercaptosuccinic acid, DMSA, Chemet) is a metal-chelating agent with a strong sulfur odor similar to rotten eggs.

FORMS AND USES

- Succimer is primarily used for lead poisoning, occasionally for mercury or arsenic poisoning.
- Succimer is formulated in 100-mg capsules for oral use; capsules contain microspheres that may be mixed into food or drink for children.
- The sodium salt of succimer has been used parenterally but is not available in the United States.

MECHANISM OF ACTION

- Succimer binds lead, mercury, or arsenic, probably via sulfhydryl groups, thereby preventing toxic metal effect or possibly removing the metal from binding sites on enzymes or other physiologic proteins.
- The succimer–heavy metal complex is then excreted renally; succimer increases urinary excretion of lead, mercury, and arsenic and lowers blood lead levels in humans.
- Succimer use does not result in the elimination of clinically significant amounts of trace essential minerals such as zinc, copper, iron, magnesium, and calcium; it differs from other chelators such as British anti-Lewisite and ethylenediaminetetraacetic acid (EDTA) in this respect.
- In animal models, succimer does not appear to redistribute lead from the blood to the brain.

DRUG AND DISEASE INTERACTIONS

Unlike British anti-Lewisite, succimer can be administered concurrently with iron without detrimental effect.

PREGNANCY AND LACTATION

US FDA Pregnancy Category C. The drug exerts animal teratogenic or embryocidal effects, but there are no controlled studies in women, or no studies are available in either animals or women.

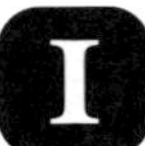

Indications

Succimer is a relatively new drug and its use is in transition; consultation with a practitioner experienced in its use is highly recommended.

- Oral treatment of lead poisoning

—FDA-approved use is for children with blood lead levels at or above 45 μg/dl.
—Succimer is also often used to treat children with blood lead level between 20 and 45 μg/dl when removing the child from the lead-contaminated environment does not decrease the blood lead level.
—Succimer is also used for adults with symptoms of lead poisoning or elevated blood lead level, but the exact level at which to chelate is controversial.

- Chelation of other heavy metals such as mercury and arsenic. Succimer is used for confirmed symptomatic mercury or arsenic poisoning or to prevent severe anticipated poisoning (e.g., ingestion of large amount and presentation to health care before toxic effects develop). However, precise criteria for treatment have not been established.

Contraindications and Adverse Effects

CONTRAINDICATIONS

History of allergy to succimer precludes its use.

ADVERSE EFFECTS

- Elevations of alanine aminotransferase and aspartate aminotransferase have occurred during succimer use but have resolved despite continued therapy.
- The drug imparts a sulfur-like odor to the patient's body fluids, which may decrease compliance, especially in adolescents.
- Other side effects of oral administration of succimer are rare and mild; they include gastrointestinal discomfort and mild pain, rashes, and eosinophilia, which have not required treatment.
- One case of hemolysis in a glucose-6-phosphate dehydrogenase–deficient patient has been reported.

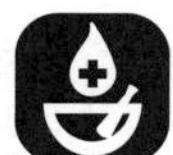

Dosage and Method of Administration

LEAD POISONING (ADULTS AND CHILDREN)

- Patient should be removed from lead exposure.
- Patient should receive 10 mg/kg (or 350 mg/m^2) orally three times a day for 5 days followed by 10 mg/kg twice a day for 14 days (capsules contain microspheres that may be poured into food or drink for consumption by small children).
- The blood lead level should be checked several days after completion of therapy and every 2 to 4 weeks thereafter until the level stabilizes.

—If the blood lead level rebounds to 45 μg/dl or above, interim repeat exposure to lead should be investigated; if repeat exposure has not occurred, the course of chelation should be repeated. If repeat exposure has occurred, the patient should be moved to lead-free housing and the course of chelation repeated.
—If the blood level rebounds to 20 to 45 μg/dl, treatment recommendations are uncertain; many treatment centers would perform at least one more course of chelation.

ARSENIC OR MERCURY POISONING (ADULTS AND CHILDREN)

- A baseline 24-hour urine collection should be performed for the metal of interest.
- Succimer should be administered; because the proper dose is unknown, most practitioners use the same dose as recommended for lead poisoning.
- It may be necessary to begin therapy with a parenteral chelator such as British anti-Lewisite or EDTA due to vomiting; the patient can often be switched to succimer after a day of parenteral therapy.
- Because arsenic and mercury are renally excreted, 24-hour urine collection should be repeated during the first day of therapy.

—If this collection does not demonstrate marked increase in metal excretion, succimer will probably not be clinically helpful.

- Repeated courses of chelation have been used in patients with persistent symptoms of arsenic or mercury toxicity and persistent elevation of urine metal excretion; however, the exact indications for repeat courses of therapy have not been established.

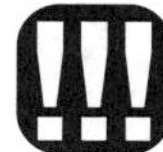

Pitfalls

- Succimer primarily chelates lead in blood and soft tissues; following discontinuation of therapy, blood lead levels often rebound to approximately two thirds of the original value.

—This phenomenon is affected by the duration of lead poisoning and repeated courses of chelation.
—Blood lead levels should be repeated every 2 to 4 weeks until stable; repeat chelation may be needed.

- Some patients find the sulfur odor objectionable and are noncompliant with therapy; the patient should be informed that a sulfur-like odor of the body and urine may occur (presence of this odor can be used to confirm compliance with therapy).

ICD-9-CM 984

Toxic effect of lead and its compounds.

See also: SECTION IV, Arsenic, Lead, and Mercury chapters.

RECOMMENDED READING

Fournier L, Thomas G, Garnier R, et al. 2,3-Dimercaptosuccinic acid treatment of heavy metal poisoning in humans. *Med Toxicol* 1988;3:499–504.

Graziano JH, Lolacono NJ, Moulton T, et al. Controlled study of meso-2,3-dimercaptosuccinic acid for the management of childhood lead intoxication. *J Pediatr* 1992;120:133–139.

Liebelt EL, Shannon M, Graef JW. Efficacy of oral meso-2,3-dimercaptosuccinic acid therapy for low-level childhood plumbism. *J Pediatr* 1994;124:313–317.

Author: Lada Kokan

Reviewer: Katherine M. Hurlbut

Thiamine

Basics

DESCRIPTION

Thiamine is a water-soluble vitamin (B1).

FORMS AND USES

- Thiamine is formulated as thiamine hydrochloride (Aneurine hydrochloride, vitamin B1, Betalin S, Biamine).
- It is used therapeutically as an adjunctive treatment of ethylene glycol toxicity.
- Other uses of thiamine are in the treatment of thiamine deficiency, beri-beri, and Wernicke's encephalopathy, and as a dietary supplement.

MECHANISM OF ACTION

- Thiamine is converted by thiamine pyrophosphokinase to the active cofactor thiamine pyrophosphate, which is a cofactor for carbohydrate metabolism.
- Thiamine pyrophosphate is a cofactor for:

—Pyruvate dehydrogenase, which links glycolysis to the Krebs cycle
—Alpha-ketoglutarate dehydrogenase in the Krebs cycle
—Transketolase in the pentose phosphate shunt, which allows the formation of NADPH

- Oxalic acid is a toxic metabolite produced by ethylene glycol metabolism. Thiamine is thought to partially divert metabolism of ethylene glycol to production of α-hydroxy-β-ketoadipic acid instead, which should reduce the production of oxalic acid (toxic to the kidney).

PREGNANCY AND LACTATION

- US FDA Pregnancy Category A. Controlled studies in women fail to demonstrate a risk to the fetus in the first trimester, and the possibility of fetal harm appears remote.
- Thiamine is excreted in breast milk.

Indications

- Adjunctive treatment of ethylene glycol toxicity
- Altered mental status, particularly in the setting of poor nutrition (e.g., history of alcoholism)
- Treatment of Wernicke's encephalopathy or beri-beri
- Other conditions that may exhibit thiamine deficiency: alcoholism, hyperemesis gravidarum, malabsorption syndromes, hyperalimentation without thiamine supplementation, anorexia nervosa, regional enteritis, and dialysis

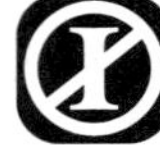

Contraindications and Adverse Effects

CONTRAINDICATIONS

Known hypersensitivity to thiamine contraindicates its use; patients with hypersensitivity should undergo intradermal sensitivity testing before thiamine is administered.

ADVERSE EFFECTS

Anaphylactoid reactions can occur following repeated thiamine administration over several days.

- The frequency of occurrence is the same by intravenous or intramuscular route.
- Treatment is the same as for any anaphylactoid reaction.

—Patient should receive 100% oxygen, a secure airway should be maintained, and intravenous access should be assured.
—Antihistamine should be administered to block both H_1 and H_2 receptors.
  —Diphenhydramine. Adult, 25 to 50 mg intravenously every 6 to 8 hours; pediatric, 1 mg/kg intravenously, up to 50 mg, every 6 to 8 hours
  —Cimetidine. Adult, 300 mg intravenously every 6 hours; pediatric, 40 mg/kg per day intravenously up to 300 mg/dose divided every 6 hours
—Bronchospasm can be treated with a bronchodilator, such as albuterol 0.15 mg/kg, up to 10 mg, in saline with humidified oxygen via nebulizer every 20 to 30 minutes.
—If hypotension develops, crystalloid should be administered in an initial bolus of 0.9% NaCl (10 to 20 ml/kg); epinephrine can be added if needed.

- Burning may occur during rapid intravenous infusion; the rate of infusion should be decreased.
- Local erythema, edema, and tenderness have been reported following subcutaneous and intramuscular administration.
- Contact dermatitis has been reported following occupational exposures.

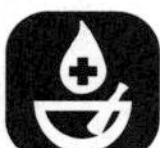

Dosage and Method of Administration

• Adjunctive treatment of ethylene glycol toxicity

—Adult dose is 100 mg intravenously or intramuscularly every 6 hours until ethylene glycol level is undetectable.
—Pediatric dose is 25 to 50 mg intravenously or intramuscularly every 6 hours until ethylene glycol level is undetectable.

• Altered mental status

—Adult. A dose of 100 mg thiamine should be administered upon establishment of intravenous line.
—Pediatric. A dose of 50 to 100 mg should be administered intravenously upon establishment of intravenous line.
—Thiamine should be administered before or simultaneously with the administration of glucose.

• Wernicke's encephalopathy

—Adult. A dose of 100 mg should be given intravenously or intramuscularly every hour until clinical response is seen or dosage of 1 g is reached.
—The patient may require 500 to 1,000 mg over the first 12 to 24 hours.

• Beri-beri

—Patient should receive 50 mg/day intravenously or intramuscularly for several days.
—Oral thiamine (5 mg/day) can be administered thereafter.

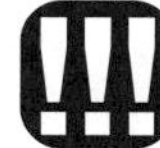

Pitfalls

• Rapid intravenous bolus administration may produce severe anaphylactoid reactions, including death.
• Patients with Wernicke's encephalopathy may require large amounts of thiamine in the first several hours of treatment.
• Decreased gastrointestinal absorption of oral thiamine may occur in patients with chronic liver disease, concurrent ethanol ingestion, steatorrhea, and folate deficiency.

ICD-9-CM 980

Toxic effect of alcohol.

See also: SECTION IV, Ethylene Glycol chapter.

RECOMMENDED READING

Goldfrank LR, Flomenbaum NE, Howland MA. Methanol, ethylene glycol, and isopropanol. In: Goldfrank LR, et al., eds. *Goldfrank's toxicologic emergencies,* 6th ed. Norwalk, CT: Appleton & Lange, 1998.

Hoffman RS. Thiamine. In: Goldfrank LR, et al., eds. *Goldfrank's toxicologic emergencies,* 6th ed. Norwalk, CT: Appleton & Lange, 1998.

Author: Edwin K. Kuffner

Reviewer: Richard C. Dart

Vitamin K

Basics

DESCRIPTION

Vitamin K is an antidote for anticoagulants that deplete vitamin K_1.

FORMS AND USES

- Phytonadione is a synthetic derivative identical to naturally occurring vitamin K_1.
- Phytonadione is used in the treatment of vitamin K deficiency.
- It is also used for coagulopathy induced by anticoagulants that deplete vitamin K–dependent clotting factors.
- Pharmaceutical formulations include:

—Oral preparation (Mephyton) 5 mg tablets
—Intramuscular preparation (Konakion) 1 mg or 10 mg/ampule, not to be administered intravenously
—Intravenous preparation (AquaMephyton) 2 mg/ml in 0.5-ml vial; 10 mg/ml in 1-ml, 2.5-ml, or 5-ml vials

MECHANISM OF ACTION

- Vitamin K_1 is an essential cofactor for the production of coagulation factors II (prothrombin), VII, IX, and X.
- During normal coagulation factor synthesis, vitamin K_1 is converted into an inactive metabolite, vitamin K1 2,3-epoxide; the epoxide can be converted back into the active form by a microsomal epoxide reductase.
- The warfarin types of oral anticoagulants interfere with the epoxide reductase and inhibit the reactivation of biologically inactive vitamin K_1 2,3-epoxide to biologically active vitamin K_1, thereby creating a coagulopathy.
- Following treatment with vitamin K_1, the time to reversal of anticoagulant effects depends on several factors:

—Individual variability in hepatic synthesis of factors II, VII, IX, and X.
—Potency of the anticoagulant agent
—Severity of anticoagulation
—Route of administration
  —Oral treatment may take 24 to 48 hours to increase levels of coagulation factors.
  —Intravenous treatment may take 2 to 8 hours to increase levels of coagulation factors.

DRUG AND DISEASE INTERACTIONS

Some compounds inhibit the reactivation of vitamin K_1 2,3-epoxide.

- Warfarin and super-warfarins (brodifacoum, difenacoum, bromadiolone, chlorophacinone, diphacinone, flocoumafen, pindone, valone, coumateralyl)
- Moxalactam
- Cefamandole
- Salicylate

PREGNANCY AND LACTATION

- US FDA Pregnancy Category C. The drug exerts animal teratogenic or embryocidal effects, but there are no controlled studies in women, or no studies are available in either animals or women.
- Newborns are at risk for vitamin K deficiency and hemorrhage because vitamin K crosses the placenta poorly and breast milk contains little vitamin K.
- It has been suggested that hyperbilirubinemia with the potential for kernicterus may occur with near-term maternal administration.
- In the treatment of poison-induced coagulopathy, vitamin K_1 should be used in pregnant women as it is in other adults.

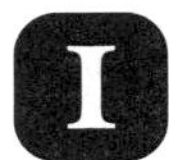

Indications

- Coagulopathy induced by long-acting products such as rodent poisons (brodifacoum and others)

—Marked prolongation of prothrombin time (PT) or international normalized ratio (INR) without bleeding: patients with an INR over 2 should receive therapy; oral route may be used.
—Severe prolongation of PT or INR and frank bleeding: vitamin K may be administered intravenously; fresh frozen plasma (FFP) should also be administered to reverse coagulopathy until response to vitamin K_1 develops.

- Coagulopathy produced by pharmaceutical product [warfarin (Coumadin)]

—Due to relatively short duration of action (days), vitamin K_1 therapy is often not used. Instead, patients with a prolonged PT or INR, but without frank bleeding, should have warfarin doses withheld until PT or INR improves.
—Patients with life-threatening bleeding should be completely reversed by treatment with FFP and vitamin K_1.

- Vitamin K deficiency

—Vitamin K_1 is prophylactically administered to all newborns
—Patients receiving total parenteral nutrition should receive supplementation.

Contraindications and Adverse Effects

CONTRAINDICATIONS

- Known hypersensitivity to vitamin K precludes its use.
- Patients with a known ingestion of an anticoagulant and a normal INR should not receive therapy before INR becomes elevated.
- Many patients will not develop coagulopathy; administration of vitamin K_1 prior to development of coagulopathy will make interpretation of PT/INR difficult.

ADVERSE EFFECTS

- Administration of large doses orally may cause mild gastrointestinal distress.
- Anaphylactoid and anaphylactic reactions may occur and are most common following a rapid intravenous administration of undiluted solution.
- Dermatologic lesions overlying the intramuscular injection site are rare but have been reported; lesions may develop 1 to 2 weeks following the injection and commonly consist of erythematous plaques.
- Patients with severe hepatic insufficiency may have a paradoxical decrease in prothrombin concentration following large doses of phytonadione.
- Patients who require anticoagulation may be refractory to oral anticoagulation following large doses of phytonadione.
- Hemolytic anemia and thrombocytopenia have been reported but are rare.
- Intramuscular administration in excessively anticoagulated patients may result in hematomas; oral or subcutaneous administration is preferred.

Dosage and Method of Administration

COAGULOPATHY INDUCED BY LONG-ACTING PRODUCT

Marked Prolongation of PT or INR without Bleeding

- Initial adult dose is 25 to 100 mg/day orally as a single or divided dose, depending on severity of PT/INR prolongation. Pediatric dose is 0.6 mg/kg or more, as a single or divided dose depending on severity of coagulopathy.
- INR and PT should be repeated daily and dose increased as needed to normalize INR or PT; dosage may reach more than 200 mg/day.
- Vitamin K_1 therapy may be needed for weeks or months; once the appropriate dose to normalize INR has been achieved, PT/INR should be monitored weekly.
- After 1 month of therapy the dose can be halved and the INR repeated in 3 to 5 days. If PT or INR increases, return to previous dose for 2 to 4 weeks. This process should be repeated until the patient no longer requires therapy.

Severe Prolongation of PT or INR and Bleeding

- Vitamin K_1 should be administered intravenously in a critical care setting.

—Phytonadione 25 to 50 mg should be diluted with dextrose 5% in water or 0.9% sodium chloride and infused slowly at a rate not to exceed 1 mg/minute.
—The dose should be repeated two to four times daily, depending on response of PT/INR to therapy.
—Parenteral vitamin K_1 in doses as high as 400 mg has been used.
—The clinician should be prepared to treat anaphylactoid reactions.

- After the coagulation abnormality is controlled, the patient should be switched to oral preparation.
- The dose should be titrated and gradually reduced as described above for PT prolongation without bleeding.
- Deaths from anaphylactoid reactions have occurred following intravenous administration; therefore patients without bleeding should be treated with oral or subcutaneous administration.
- Intravenous administration of vitamin K_1 should be performed in a critical care setting.

COAGULOPATHY PRODUCED BY PHARMACEUTICAL PRODUCT [WARFARIN (COUMADIN)]

- Patients with life-threatening bleeding should be completely reversed with FFP.
- Patients who require anticoagulation and are reversed to a normal PT or INR may require heparin therapy to prevent thrombosis.
- Adult. Small doses (1 to 5 mg/dose) of vitamin K1 should be administered intravenously to titrate patient to a normal PT or INR.
- Intravenous administration of vitamin K_1 should be performed in a critical care setting.
- Patients with a prolonged PT or INR, but without frank bleeding, should have warfarin doses withheld but usually do not require vitamin K_1 or blood component treatment.

VITAMIN K DEFICIENCY

- Newborns should receive 0.5 to 1.0 mg intramuscularly.
- Patients on total parenteral nutrition typically receive 2.5 mg/day intravenously.

Pitfalls

- FFP should be used in addition to vitamin K_1 for immediate reversal of life-threatening hemorrhage.
- Rapid intravenous infusion can result in an anaphylactoid reaction and has caused death.
- The health-care provider should avoid pretreatment of long-acting anticoagulants (before PT/INR becomes prolonged) with empiric vitamin K, because it obscures the meaning of the INR to assess toxicity and may result in unneeded therapy.
- Vitamin K_1 will not reverse the anticoagulant effects of heparin.
- Vitamin K_1 does not correct hypoprothrombinemia resulting from hepatic insufficiency.
- Other forms of vitamin K (vitamin K_2, K_3, K_4) should not be used as therapy.

ICD-9-CM 964.2

Poisoning by agents primarily affecting blood constituents: anticoagulants.

See also: SECTION IV, Brodifacoum, Coumadin, and Warfarin chapters.

RECOMMENDED READING

Hirsch J, Dalen JE, Deykin D, et al. Oral anticoagulants: Mechanism of action, clinical effectiveness and optimum therapeutic range. *Chest* 1992;102[suppl]:312–326.

Author: Edwin K. Kuffner

Reviewer: Katherine M. Hurlbut

Whole-Bowel Irrigation

Basics

DESCRIPTION

Whole-bowel irrigation (WBI) is a method to clear the gut by mechanical displacement of foreign substances.

FORMS AND USES

- WBI is used in gastrointestinal decontamination when the agent involved is not absorbed by activated charcoal or is in a form that may persist in the gastrointestinal tract (e.g., extended-release formulations).
- WBI is also used routinely for bowel evacuation in preparation for surgical and endoscopic procedures and in the treatment of constipation.
- WBI is performed by orally administering polyethylene-glycol–based bowel evacuation solutions, including Golytely and Colyte.

—These products are mixtures of polyethylene glycols with molecular weights of 3,000 to 3,700 daltons and electrolytes (sodium sulfate, sodium bicarbonate, sodium chloride, or potassium chloride).
—They are supplied as powders, to be mixed with water so that the final solution is 280 mOsm/kg, the same osmolarity as human plasma.

MECHANISM OF ACTION

- WBI involves the administration of a polyethylene-glycol–based solution to push intestinal contents through the gastrointestinal tract before they can be absorbed.
- WBI acts by mechanically displacing the bowel contents, which is thought to make it particularly appropriate for the treatment of drug bezoars or concretions.
- Because the solutions are isoosmolar, they do not induce the fluid and electrolyte shifts seen in patients treated with multiple doses of cathartics.

DRUG AND DISEASE INTERACTIONS

The absorption of therapeutic drugs probably is decreased during the course of WBI treatment.

PREGNANCY AND LACTATION

- Polyethylene glycol solutions are not absorbed from the gastrointestinal tract and are considered safe in pregnancy.
- US FDA Pregnancy Category C. The drug exerts animal teratogenic or embryocidal effects, but there are no controlled studies in women, or no studies are available in either animals or women.

Indications

- Precise recommendations for WBI have not yet emerged.
- Typical uses of WBI in gastrointestinal decontamination include:

—Substances that are not well adsorbed to activated charcoal (e.g., iron, lithium, and lead)
—Drugs that are designed for sustained or delayed release (many antidysrhythmic drugs, lithium, and theophylline); for example, in the case of an increasing theophylline level despite appropriate gastrointestinal decontamination
—Substances that form bezoars or concretions (salicylate, carbamazepine, or enteric-coated medications, etc.); for example, in the case of an increasing salicylate level despite appropriate gastrointestinal decontamination
—A history of ingestion of drug packets (body stuffers or body packers)
—Heavy metals (lead, arsenic, or mercury); for example, presence of radioopaque objects on abdominal radiographs
—Cases of ingestion of foreign bodies with potential toxic effects (batteries or lead objects); for example, presence of radioopacities on abdominal radiographs

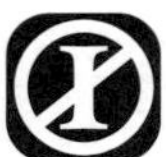

Contraindications and Adverse Effects

CONTRAINDICATIONS

- Ileus or mechanical bowel obstruction will lead to recurrent vomiting.
- WBI may increase intraabdominal contamination if perforation exists.
- Unprotected airway may allow pulmonary aspiration.

ADVERSE EFFECTS

- Diarrhea, bloating, nausea, vomiting, and anal discomfort secondary to diarrhea are all common; the rate of fluid ingestion can be decreased.
- Persistent emesis may make administration of polyethylene glycol solution difficult, especially in patients who have received ipecac or ingested drugs that cause emesis.

—Aggressive use of antiemetic agents may be necessary.
—Suggested combination regimens in adults include metoclopramide 0.5 to 1.0 mg/kg, diphenhydramine 25 to 50 mg, and prochlorperazine 10 mg or droperidol 2.5 mg intravenously; ondansetron 8 mg intravenously infused over 15 minutes is an alternative. Suggested regimens in children include diphenhydramine 1 mg/kg, maximum of 5 mg/kg/day; metoclopromide (dose is the same as adults); prochlorperazine should not be used in children; droperidol should not be used in children; ondansetron 0.15 mg/kg for three doses is an alternative (should not be used in children under 4 years of age).

- Pulmonary aspiration of pure polyethylene glycol solution is relatively nontoxic; however, if the aspirate is contaminated with stomach contents, infection and diffuse pulmonary injury may occur.

Dosage and Method of Administration

ADULTS AND ADOLESCENTS

- The initial dose is 2 L/h for 1 hour followed by 1 to 2 L/h; typical adult dose is 4 to 5 L ingested over 2 to 4 hours.
- Solution may be administered orally or by continuous infusion through a nasogastric tube.
- Administration should continue until rectal effluent becomes clear.
- For radioopaque substances or foreign bodies, abdominal radiographs may be useful in demonstrating disappearance of toxicant.

CHILDREN

- The initial dose is 20 ml/kg/h followed by 10 to 20 ml/kg/h, up to 1 L/h.
- Solution should be administered orally or by continuous infusion through nasogastric tube.
- Administration should continue until rectal effluent becomes clear.
- For radioopaque substances or foreign bodies, abdominal radiographs may be useful in demonstrating disappearance of toxicant.

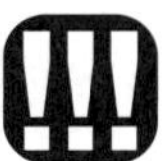

Pitfalls

- Patients with CNS depression, seizures, or other compromise in protecting airway require endotracheal intubation prior to WBI.
- Patients with partial ileus secondary to drug effects (anticholinergic, opioid, etc.) may not tolerate the large volume of fluid.
- Children may be less tolerant of the large volumes of fluid required.
- WBI may be difficult to administer in an uncooperative patient.
- WBI does not enhance elimination of toxicants that have already been absorbed; it should be administered early to maximize efficacy.
- Polyethylene glycol solutions decrease the adsorptive capacity of activated charcoal for some substances; administering a second dose of activated charcoal to patients receiving WBI should be considered.

RECOMMENDED READING

Howland MA. Whole-bowel irrigation. In: Goldfrank LR, Flomenbaum NE, Lewin NS, et al., eds. *Goldfrank's toxicologic emergencies.* 6th ed. Norwalk, CT: Appleton & Lange, 1998.

Author: Katherine M. Hurlbut

Reviewer: Richard C. Dart

SECTION IV

Chemical and Biological Agents

Acetaminophen—Acute Single Ingestion

Basics

DESCRIPTION

Acetaminophen is an oral analgesic available in many over-the-counter and prescription medications. It is also known as paracetamol in many countries.

FORMS AND USES

- Numerous brands contain acetaminophen alone, whereas others are combination products.
- Acetaminophen in all formulations is used for temporary relief of mild to moderate pain and for temperature reduction in febrile patients.
- Regular formulation acetaminophen. Dosage for adults and children 12 years and older is as follows:

—Oral: 325 to 650 mg every 4 to 6 hours, not to exceed 4 g in 24 hours; single doses of 1 g may be used in adults.
—Rectal: 325 to 650 mg every 4 to 6 hours as needed, not to exceed 4 g in 24 hours.

- Tylenol Arthritis Extended Relief Caplet is a bilayer of 325 mg immediate-release acetaminophen and 325 mg slow-release acetaminophen.

—Adults and children 12 years and older: 1.3 g every 8 hours as needed, not to exceed 3.9 g in 24 hours.

- Pediatric suspension, elixir, or drops (oral or rectal): 10 to 15 mg/kg every 4 to 6 hours, not to exceed 90 mg/kg in 24 hours.
- If the product packaging is available, the health-care professional should check the product label to determine whether the main ingredient is acetaminophen or acetylsalicylic acid (aspirin) and to identify other active constituents such as decongestants, stimulants, or opioids.

TOXIC DOSE

An acute ingestion of greater than 15 g in an adult often produces liver injury. The pediatric toxic dose of a single ingestion is unknown.

PATHOPHYSIOLOGY

- Acetaminophen is primarily metabolized to nontoxic products in the liver.
- An additional metabolic pathway, involving cytochrome P450, produces a toxic metabolite, *N*-acetyl-p-benzoquinoneimine (NAPQI), which causes liver injury if not detoxified.
- With therapeutic dosing, NAPQI is detoxified by liver glutathione and no liver injury occurs.
- However, high blood levels of acetaminophen deplete glutathione stores and allow NAPQI to bind to liver cells, producing cell injury and death.
- Acetaminophen toxicity also stimulates the release of inflammatory mediators such as cytokines, which further contribute to liver injury.

EPIDEMIOLOGY

- Intentional overdose is common.
- Toxicity is typically mild if the patient is treated early.
- Death is unusual, developing in patients who present after 24 hours or in whom treatment is mistakenly withheld.
- "Chronic" acetaminophen toxicity may result from repetitive, supratherapeutic dosing; such poisonings are usually unintentional and occur in adults with acute, persistent pain syndromes or in persistently febrile infants. Adults who ingest greater than 4 g/day for more than 1 day, and infants less than 2 years of age who are given more than 150 mg/kg/day for more than 1 day, may be at increased risk.

CAUSES

- Ingestion is usually with suicidal intent.
- Child neglect or abuse should be considered if the patient is less than 1 year of age, suicide attempt if the patient is older than 6 years of age.

DRUG AND DISEASE INTERACTIONS

- Adults with malnutrition or underlying liver disease (e.g., alcoholics) who ingest an overdose amount may be more susceptible to liver toxicity.
- Chronic ingestion of medications which induce cytochrome P450 enzymes, such as isoniazid and carbamazepine, may potentiate acetaminophen toxicity.

PREGNANCY AND LACTATION

- US FDA Pregnancy Category B. Animal studies indicate no fetal risk and there are no controlled human studies, or animal studies show an adverse fetal effect but well-controlled studies in women do not.
- Acetaminophen crosses the placenta, but documented fetal death or hepatotoxicity from maternal overdose is rare.
- In the absence of fetal distress, induction of labor or termination of pregnancy based on maternal acetaminophen toxicity is not indicated.
- Preliminary evidence indicates that the antidote, *N*-acetylcysteine (NAC), crosses the placenta and should be administered to a pregnant woman with the same indications as patients who are not pregnant.
- An infant born to a mother with acetaminophen toxicity should receive a 48-hour course of intravenous NAC.

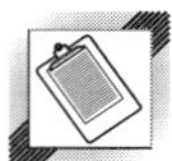

Diagnosis

DIFFERENTIAL DIAGNOSIS

- Toxicologic agents that cause nausea and vomiting for several hours followed by right upper quadrant pain and elevated liver function tests include amanita mushroom, carbamazepine, valproic acid, phenytoin, methyldopa, isoniazid, carbon tetrachloride, halothane, disulfiram, pennyroyal, procainamide, pyrrolizidine alkaloids, and methotrexate, among others.
- Nontoxicologic causes include biliary tract disease and viral or alcoholic hepatitis.

SIGNS AND SYMPTOMS

- Acute overdose is usually characterized by nausea, vomiting, and diffuse abdominal pain, beginning within hours after overdose and resolving within 24 hours.
- Right upper quadrant pain and laboratory evidence of liver injury usually develops between 24 to 48 hours.
- Severe toxicity may produce fulminant hepatic failure 3 to 5 days postingestion.
- Patients with "chronic" overdose resulting from repetitive, supratherapeutic dosing usually present with liver injury already established [elevated aspartate aminotransferase (AST), alanine aminotransferase (ALT), prothrombin time, and bilirubin levels].

Vital Signs

Vital signs are usually normal, although patients with dehydration from vomiting or anorexia may have tachycardia.

Dermatologic

Jaundice may occur if hepatic injury develops.

Gastrointestinal

- Nausea and vomiting are common over the first 24 hours after ingestion.
- Pancreatitis occurs rarely, 3 to 5 days after ingestion.

Hepatic

- Liver injury ranges from mild, asymptomatic disease to fulminant hepatic failure.
- Right upper quadrant pain and abnormal liver function tests typically develop between 24 and 48 hours postingestion, although liver injury may occasionally develop earlier.

Renal

Acute renal failure may develop 3 to 5 days postingestion and may occur independent of hepatic injury.

Hematologic

Thrombocytopenia has been reported.

Fluids and Electrolytes

Dehydration may occur from intractable vomiting and anorexia.

Neurologic

Hepatic encephalopathy and coma may complicate hepatic failure.

Acid-Base

Increased anion gap metabolic acidosis may occur after massive acute overdose, but more common causes of metabolic acidosis must be sought.

PROCEDURES AND LABORATORY TESTS

Essential Tests

Serum acetaminophen level drawn between 4 and 24 hours after ingestion of acute overdose. The optimal level is drawn at 4 hours after ingestion or as soon after 4 hours as possible.

- The serum level should be plotted on the Rumack-Matthew nomogram (see figure).

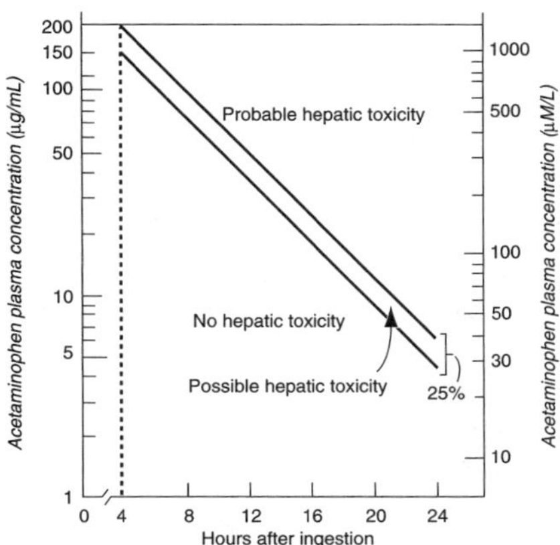

Semilogarithmic plot of plasma acetaminophen levels versus time. (Modified and reproduced, with permission, from Rumack BH, Matthew H. Acetaminophen poisoning and toxicity. *Pediatrics* 1975;55:871.)

—If the level is above the "possible toxicity" level (the lower of the two lines), NAC is administered.
—The Rumack-Matthew nomogram cannot be used when the time of ingestion is uncertain, if the ingestion occurred more than 24 hours before presentation, or if repeated ingestion has occurred.

—Tylenol Arthritis Extended Relief does not fulfill the assumptions of the Rumack-Matthew nomogram.
—The nomogram assumes that acetaminophen is completely absorbed within 4 hours of ingestion, but Tylenol Arthritis Extended Relief may be absorbed beyond this time.
—Thus, if the initial serum acetaminophen level falls into the nontoxic range, a second level should be obtained 4 to 6 hours later.
—If either level is on or above the nomogram's possible toxicity line, a full course of NAC should be administered.

- NAC therapy should be initiated empirically if the serum acetaminophen level is delayed or the patient presents more than 8 hours after ingestion. In these situations, the delayed administration of NAC may allow liver injury to occur, and NAC should be administered until it is found that the serum acetaminophen level is nontoxic.

—NAC can be discontinued if the acetaminophen level is later found to be nontoxic on the Rumack-Matthew nomogram.

- Serum electrolytes, BUN, creatinine, glucose

—Massive acetaminophen ingestion may produce metabolic acidosis 8 to 12 hours after ingestion.
—Hepatic failure may produce acidosis, electrolyte abnormalities, and hypoglycemia.

- Prothrombin time or international normalized ratio (PT/INR), AST, ALT, and bilirubin

—Elevated PT is the earliest sign of acetaminophen toxicity.
—Liver enzymes begin to increase at about 24 hours and peak at 72 hours.

Acetaminophen—Acute Single Ingestion

Recommended Tests

- Serum ammonia is elevated in hepatic encephalopathy.
- Arterial blood gases are used to assess the severity of acidemia.
- ECG and aspirin level in overdose setting are used to detect occult overdose.

Not Recommended Tests

- Once NAC therapy has been initiated, repeated serum acetaminophen levels are not useful.
- The only exception is for Tylenol Arthritis Extended Relief, as described above.

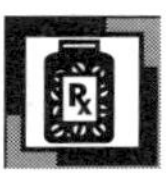

Treatment

- Treatment focuses on prevention of absorption, control of emesis, and administration of NAC within 8 hours of ingestion (as indicated by the Rumack-Matthew nomogram) if potentially toxic ingestion has occurred.
- Aggressive antiemetic therapy is important for patients with vomiting who require NAC therapy.
- The dose and time of exposure should be determined for all substances involved.

DIRECTING PATIENT COURSE

The health-care professional should call the poison control center when:

- Metabolic acidosis, renal insufficiency, encephalopathy, or hepatic failure develop.
- Ingestion involves Tylenol Arthritis Extended Relief Caplets, or patients presenting more than 24 hours postingestion.
- Oral NAC therapy cannot be successfully administered.
- Repeated (chronic) acetaminophen ingestion is suspected.
- Toxic effects are not consistent with acetaminophen poisoning.
- Coingestant, drug interaction, or underlying disease presents an unusual problem.

Patients should be referred to a health-care facility when:

- Attempted suicide or homicide is possible.
- Patient or caregiver seems unreliable.
- Toxic effects are apparent.
- Children with estimated ingestion greater than 150 mg/kg should be referred to an emergency department for charcoal and a 4-hour serum acetaminophen level.
- Coingestant, drug interaction, or underlying disease presents an unusual problem.

Admission Considerations

Inpatient management is warranted for:

- Patients who require treatment with NAC, present 24 to 36 hours after ingestion, or have an uncertain time of ingestion but have a measurable acetaminophen level or a history of acetaminophen overdose given by others.
- Patients with chronic toxicity.

Consultation with a liver transplant center is recommended when the following signs of poor prognosis are present:

- Arterial pH is less than 7.3.
- Encephalopathy is rated at grade III or IV.
- Creatinine level is greater than 3.4 mg/dl.
- PT is greater than 35 to 40 seconds, or PT is increasing rapidly.

DECONTAMINATION

Out of Hospital

Ipecac should be administered to induce emesis within 1 hour of ingestion for alert pediatric or adult patient, if health-care evaluation will be delayed.

In Hospital

- Ipecac should be administered to induce emesis within 1 hour of ingestion for the alert patient who is too small to have effective gastric lavage.
- Gastric lavage should be performed in pediatric (tube size 24–32 French) or adult (tube size 36–42 French) patients for large ingestion presenting within 1 hour of ingestion or if serious effects are present.
- One dose of activated charcoal (1–2 g/kg) should be administered without a cathartic if a substantial ingestion has occurred within the previous few hours.
- Simultaneous administration of activated charcoal and NAC will not affect outcome.

ANTIDOTES

NAC is a very effective antidote for acute acetaminophen ingestion.

Indications

- An acute overdose has occurred, and the serum acetaminophen level, drawn between 4 and 24 hours after ingestion, is plotted on or above the possible toxicity line (lower of the two lines) on the Rumack-Matthew nomogram.
- An acute ingestion has occurred, but the time of ingestion is uncertain or unknown.
- An acute overdose is possible and elevated liver function tests are already present. An increase in AST or ALT is considered to be due to an acetaminophen injury until proven otherwise.
- A patient presents with an acute overdose more than 48 hours after ingestion; the patient should receive NAC if liver enzymes are abnormal, but NAC is not needed if liver enzymes are normal.
- Because liver toxicity may not become apparent until 24 to 48 hours postingestion, patients with a history of a single acute ingestion 24 to 36 hours prior to presentation should receive NAC therapy regardless of whether measurable acetaminophen is present or whether liver function tests are normal.
- Chronic toxicity also indicates use (see SECTION IV, Acetaminophen—Repeated Ingestion chapter).

Contraindications

History of anaphylactic reaction to NAC precludes use.

Method of Administration

- Water, juice, or soda is used to dilute a 10% or 20% NAC solution to a 5% solution.
- A loading dose of 140 mg/kg is administered orally, followed by 17 maintenance doses of 70 mg/kg every 4 hours.
- If the patient vomits NAC within 1 hour of any dose, the dose is repeated.
- Administering NAC oral formulation via an intravenous route. On rare occasions, patients with acetaminophen toxicity cannot tolerate oral NAC; such patients may be treated with the oral formulation administered via the intravenous route.
- NAC is continued beyond 72 hours (oral) or 48 hours (intravenous protocol) if the liver or renal injury is not improving.
- Treatment of alcoholic patients is the same as for nonalcoholic patients.

Adverse Effects

- NAC has an unpleasant smell and taste.
- Urticaria and papular rashes occur rarely.
- Rarely, intravenous administration of NAC overdose has caused life-threatening allergic reactions.

ADJUNCTIVE TREATMENT

- Antiemetic therapy. Patients may require aggressive antiemetic therapy to ensure that NAC is retained.

—Metoclopramide, 1.0 to 2.0 mg/kg, intravenously plus prochlorperazine, 10 mg intravenously, or droperidol, 2.5 to 5.0 mg intravenously.
—Diphenhydramine, 25 to 50 mg intravenously, may be added to this regimen.
—Ondansetron, 8 mg intravenously, may be used if above regimen fails.

- Therapies not recommended

—Because PT is an important prognostic indicator, vitamin K1 or fresh frozen plasma administration is not recommended to correct PT of less than 40 seconds unless frank bleeding develops.
—Cimetidine is an unproven therapy and is not recommended.

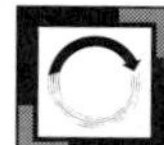

Follow-Up

PATIENT MONITORING

If the patient requires NAC treatment, PT or INR, AST, ALT, bilirubin, electrolytes, BUN, creatinine, and glucose should be repeated daily.

EXPECTED COURSE AND PROGNOSIS

Most patients who are treated with NAC recover without sequelae even if liver injury complicates the course. Prognosis is related to the time to treatment with NAC. Mild hepatotoxicity, or none, is expected if treated within 8 hours of ingestion, but the likelihood of liver injury increases if NAC is administered more than 8 hours after overdose. Fulminant hepatic failure may develop if NAC is started more than 24 hours after ingestion.

POSSIBLE COMPLICATIONS

- Fulminant hepatic failure is the main cause of death from acetaminophen toxicity; a liver transplant may be life saving.
- Renal injury occurs rarely, developing 3 to 5 days postingestion and after the onset of hepatotoxicity.
- Renal failure is usually reversible but may last for several weeks and require hemodialysis.

DISCHARGE CRITERIA/INSTRUCTIONS

- From the emergency department. Patients may be discharged if the time of ingestion is certain, the serum acetaminophen level is below the possible toxicity level, and a psychiatric evaluation has been performed.
- From the hospital. Patients may be discharged after a full course of NAC, if liver and renal function tests are normal or improving, and after a psychiatric evaluation, if needed.

PATIENT EDUCATION

- The health-care professional should educate patients on the potential dangers of over-the-counter medications.
- Patients should be cautioned that simultaneous use of more than one acetaminophen product may lead to inadvertent overdose.
- Substitution of inappropriate formulation (e.g., use of an adult acetaminophen suppository in a child instead of a pediatric one) may result in toxicity.

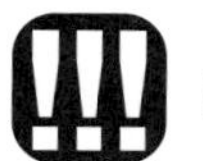

Pitfalls

DIAGNOSIS

Signs of poisoning may be minimal and overlooked during the first 24 hours.

TREATMENT

Failure to treat vomiting aggressively may result in substantial delays in NAC treatment and less favorable patient outcome.

ICD-9-CM 965.4

Poisoning by aromatic analgesics (acetaminophen).

See also: SECTION III, *N*-acetylcysteine chapter; and SECTION IV, Acetaminophen—Repeated (Chronic) Ingestion chapter.

RECOMMENDED READING

Keays R, Harrison P, Wendon, J, et al. Intravenous acetylcysteine in paracetamol induced fulminant hepatic failure: a prospective controlled trial. *Br Med J* 1991;303:1026–1029.

O'Grady JG, Alexander G, Hayllar KM, et al. Early indicators of prognosis in fulminant hepatic failure. *Gastroenterology* 1989;97:439–445.

Rumack BH, Matthew H. Acetaminophen poisoning and toxicity. *Pediatrics* 1975;55:871–876.

Smilkstein MJ, Knapp GL, Kulig KW, et al. Efficacy of oral *N*-acetylcysteine in the treatment of APAP overdose: analysis of the national multicenter study (1976 to 1985). *N Engl J Med* 1988;319:1557–1562.

Yip L, Dart RC, Hurlbut KM. Intravenous administration of oral *N*-acetylcysteine. *Crit Care Med* 1998;26:40–43.

Author: Rivka S. Horowitz

Reviewer: Richard C. Dart

Acetaminophen—Repeated (Chronic) Ingestion

Basics

DESCRIPTION

• Acetaminophen is a common over-the-counter pain reliever.
• "Chronic" or "repeated supratherapeutic" acetaminophen ingestion is defined as repetitive ingestion of more than the recommended maximum daily dose.

—Adult dose: Greater than 4 g over a 24-hour period
—Pediatric dose: Greater than 90/mg/kg over a 24-hour period

FORMS AND USES

• Numerous brands contain acetaminophen alone, whereas others are combination products.
• The product label should be checked carefully to determine whether the main ingredient is acetaminophen or acetylsalicylic acid (aspirin) and for other constituents such as decongestants, stimulants, or opioids.

TOXIC DOSE

• For repeated ingestions, the precise dose of acetaminophen and the time course of ingestion required to produce hepatotoxicity are unknown.
• In children, repeated ingestion of more than 150 mg/kg/day may lead to liver injury.

PATHOPHYSIOLOGY

• Acetaminophen is primarily metabolized to nontoxic products in the liver.
• An additional pathway, involving cytochrome P450, produces a toxic metabolite, *N*-acetyl-p-benzoquinoneimine (NAPQI), which causes liver injury if not detoxified.

—With therapeutic dosing, NAPQI is detoxified by liver.
—However, depletion of glutathione stores allows NAPQI to injure liver cells.

EPIDEMIOLOGY

Chronic acetaminophen poisonings are usually unintentional and occur in adults with acute, prolonged pain syndromes or in young children with persistent fever.

CAUSES

• Chronic supratherapeutic ingestion is common; patients may repeatedly ingest supratherapeutic doses of acetaminophen in the belief that no harm will result.
• Child abuse has been suspected in several cases of "chronic" acetaminophen toxicity in infants.

RISK FACTORS

In an overdose, adults with malnutrition and underlying liver disease (e.g., alcoholics) may be more susceptible to "chronic" acetaminophen toxicity.

DRUG AND DISEASE INTERACTIONS

Chronic ingestion of cytochrome P450 enzyme inducers, such as alcohol, isoniazid, and carbamazepine, may potentiate chronic supratherapeutic acetaminophen toxicity.

PREGNANCY AND LACTATION

• US FDA Pregnancy Category B. Animal studies indicate no fetal risk, and there are no controlled human studies, or animal studies show an adverse fetal effect, but well-controlled studies in women do not exist.
• Acetaminophen crosses the placenta, but documented fetal death or hepatotoxicity from maternal overdose is rare.
• In the absence of fetal distress, induction of labor or termination of pregnancy based on maternal acetaminophen toxicity is not indicated.
• Preliminary evidence indicates that *N*-acetylcysteine (NAC) crosses the placenta and should be administered to the mother according to the same indications as for patients who are not pregnant.
• An infant delivered to a woman with acetaminophen toxicity should receive a 48-hour course of intravenous NAC.

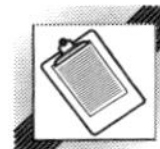

Diagnosis

DIFFERENTIAL DIAGNOSIS

• Toxicologic agents that cause right upper quadrant pain and elevated liver function tests include salicylate, carbamezapine, valproic acid, phenytoin, isoniazid, halothane, disulfuram, procainamide, and methotrexate, among many others.
• Nontoxicologic causes include biliary tract disease or viral or alcoholic hepatitis.

SIGNS AND SYMPTOMS

• Patients with chronic acetaminophen overdose often present with liver injury: elevated levels of alanine aminotransferase (ALT), aspartate aminotransferase (AST), and bilirubin, and prolonged prothrombin time (PT) or international normalized ratio (INR).
• Infants typically have a febrile illness and may present with lethargy and dehydration.

Vital signs

Patients with dehydration may have tachycardia.

HEENT

Scleral icterus occurs if hepatic injury develops.

Dermatologic

Jaundice occurs if hepatic injury develops.

Gastrointestinal

Nausea and vomiting may occur.

Hepatic

• Liver injury ranges from mild, asymptomatic liver injury to fulminant hepatic failure.
• Right upper quadrant pain and abnormal liver function test results may be observed days to weeks after initiation of repetitive, supratherapeutic ingestion.
• PT and INR elevation are sensitive indicators of liver injury and may precede the increase in AST and ALT.

Renal

Acute renal insufficiency and failure may occur in severe cases and may be independent of liver injury.

Hematologic

Thrombocytopenia may occur.

Fluids and Electrolytes

Dehydration is common.

Neurologic

Hepatic encephalopathy may be associated with liver failure.

PROCEDURES AND LABORATORY TESTS

Essential Tests

If a history of repetitive, supratherapeutic ingestion is elicited, the clinician should obtain:

• Serum acetaminophen level.
• Serum electrolytes, BUN, and creatinine are ordered to assess changes in electrolytes and kidney injury.
• AST, ALT, and PT or INR are used to determine whether liver injury has occurred.

Recommended Tests

• Glucose, amylase are assayed if evidence of liver injury exists.

—Fulminant hepatic failure may result in acidosis, electrolyte abnormalities, and hypoglycemia.
—Renal injury or pancreatitis also may develop.

• Serum ammonia may be elevated if hepatic encephalopathy develops.
• Arterial blood gases, if acidosis is suspected from low serum bicarbonate.

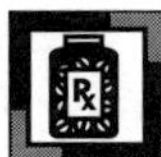

Treatment

- Treatment should focus on prevention of absorption, control of emesis, and administration of NAC if indicated.
- The dose and time of exposure must be determined for all substances involved.
- Aggressive anti-emetic therapy is important for patients with vomiting who require NAC.

DIRECTING PATIENT COURSE

The health-care professional should call the poison control center when:

- Metabolic acidosis, renal insufficiency, encephalopathy, or fulminant hepatic failure develops.
- Ingestion involves Tylenol Arthritis Extended Relief Caplets (a prolonged release formulation).
- Toxic effects are not consistent with acetaminophen poisoning.
- Coingestant, drug interaction, or underlying disease presents an unusual problem.

Patients should be referred to a health-care facility when:

- History of repetitive, supratherapeutic acetaminophen ingestion is obtained.
- Patient or caregiver seems unreliable.
- Any toxic effects are present.
- Coingestant, drug interaction, or underlying disease presents an unusual problem.

Admission Considerations

- Inpatient treatment is warranted for patients who are treated with NAC.
- Consultation with a liver transplantation center is recommended if the following signs develop:

—Acidosis. pH less than 7.3
—Encephalopathy. Grade III or IV
—Renal insufficiency. Creatinine higher than 3.4 mg/dl
—Coagulopathy. PT greater than 35 to 40 seconds (without treatment with coagulation factors), or rapidly rising

DECONTAMINATION

One dose of activated charcoal (1–2 g/kg) should be administered without a cathartic if a substantial ingestion has occurred within the previous few hours.

ANTIDOTES

NAC (N-Acetylcysteine) is the antidote for acetaminophen poisoning.

- Indications. Patients with a history of repetitive, supratherapeutic ingestion who have evidence of liver injury (elevated PT/INR, AST, or ALT, or right upper quadrant pain), or measurable acetaminophen level should be treated.
- Contraindications. History of anaphylactic reaction to NAC precludes use.
- Method of administration

—Patients who meet criteria for NAC treatment should be treated for a minimum of 36 hours after the last ingested dose.
—NAC should be discontinued if liver function test levels do not increase during this time, or if previously elevated liver function test results are near normal or at patient's baseline.
—Further details on administration of NAC are found in SECTION III, *N*-acetylcysteine chapter).

ADJUNCTIVE TREATMENT

- Antiemetic therapy. Patients may require aggressive antiemetic therapy to ensure that NAC is retained.

—Adult. Metoclopramide, 1.0 to 2.0 mg/kg is given intravenously, plus prochlorperazine 10 mg intravenously or droperidol 2.5 mg intravenously.
—Diphenhydramine, 25 to 50 mg given intravenously may be added to this regimen.
—Ondansetron, 2 to 8 mg given intravenously may be tried if the above regimen fails.

- Not recommended therapies

—Fresh frozen plasma administration is not recommended to correct PT of less than 40 seconds unless frank bleeding develops, because PT is an important prognostic indicator.
—Cimetidine is an unproven therapy and is not recommended.

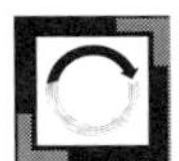

Follow-Up

PATIENT MONITORING

- PT/INR, AST, ALT, bilirubin, hematocrit, electrolytes, creatinine, and glucose tests should be repeated daily during NAC therapy.
- Ammonia and platelet count should be followed as clinically indicated.

EXPECTED COURSE AND PROGNOSIS

- Most patients who are treated with NAC recover without sequelae, even if liver injury complicates course.
- Renal failure is usually reversible but may last for several weeks and require hemodialysis.
- Fulminant hepatic failure is the main cause of death.
- Renal insufficiency or pancreatitis occur in a small number of patients.

DISCHARGE CRITERIA/INSTRUCTIONS

- From the emergency department

—Patients may be discharged if liver tests are normal or baseline, there is no right upper quadrant abdominal tenderness, and no acetaminophen is detectable in blood samples.
—A psychiatric evaluation should be obtained, if indicated.

- From the hospital

—Patients may be discharged when liver function test results, including PT, are normal or progressively decreasing and the course of NAC has been completed.
—A psychiatric evaluation should be obtained, if indicated.

PATIENT EDUCATION

- Patients should be cautioned that simultaneous use of more than one acetaminophen product may lead to inadvertent overdose.
- Repeated substitution of inappropriate formulation (e.g., use of an adult acetaminophen suppository in a child instead of a pediatric one) may result in toxicity.

Pitfalls

DIAGNOSIS

Chronic acetaminophen poisoning may be subtle; history of marked subacute pain syndrome such as tooth pain should elicit an evaluation.

TREATMENT

Failure to treat vomiting aggressively may result in delayed NAC treatment and less favorable outcome.

ICD-9-CM 965.4

Poisoning by analgesics, antipyretics, and antirheumatics: aromatic analgesics, not elsewhere classified.

See also: SECTION III, *N*-acetylcysteine chapter; and SECTION IV, Acetaminophen—Acute Single Ingestion chapter.

RECOMMENDED READING

Henretig FM, Selbst SM, Forrest C, et al. Repeated acetaminophen overdosing causing hepatotoxicity in children. *Clin Pediatr* 1989;28:525–528.

Author: Rivka S. Horowitz
Reviewer: Richard C. Dart

Acetonitrile and Aliphatic Nitriles

Basics

DESCRIPTION

Aliphatic nitriles are organic chemicals with the general formula R-CN.

FORMS AND USES

- Among the aliphatic nitriles are acetonitrile (synonyms are methyl cyanide, ethanenitrile, cyanomethane, ethyl nitrile, methane carbonitrile), acrylonitrile (synonyms are vinyl cyanide, cyanoethylene, propenenitrile), malonitrile, *n*-butyronitrile, succinonitrile, propionitrile, acetone cyanohydrin, and methylacrylonitrile.
- Common industrial uses of these chemicals are in the production of synthetic fibers, resins, plastics, and dyes; pharmaceuticals and vitamins; plasticizers, solvents, extractants, and elastomers; agricultural insecticide (acrylonitrile); and high-pressure lubricants.
- High-concentration acetonitrile has been available over the counter as a remover of the cyanoacrylate-based glues used for sculptured nails; ingestion of this product has resulted in pediatric deaths.

TOXIC DOSE

One swallow of acetonitrile-containing artificial nail glue remover can cause death in a toddler.

PATHOPHYSIOLOGY

- The aliphatic nitriles are readily absorbed by ingestion, inhalation, and dermal routes.
- Dermal absorption can continue even after appropriate dermal decontamination measures have been instituted.
- The cause of toxicity is cyanide poisoning.

—The mechanism and extent of cyanide liberation differ for the various aliphatic nitriles.
—Some parent compounds are metabolized by the hepatic P450 microsomal enzyme system to a cyanohydrin intermediate that is unstable and degrades spontaneously, liberating free hydrogen cyanide.
—Acetone cyanohydrin does not require metabolism, it slowly decomposes at room temperature to acetone and hydrogen cyanide; decomposition is increased by temperature, an increased pH, or by the addition of water.

EPIDEMIOLOGY

- Poisoning is rare, but toxic effects are often severe.
- Carcinogenesis. Acrylonitrile is a possible human carcinogen.

CAUSES

The cause of aliphatic nitrile poisoning is usually an accidental workplace exposure.

DRUG AND DISEASE INTERACTIONS

There are no drug and disease interactions of note.

PREGNANCY AND LACTATION

Acetonitrile is a probable teratogen and should be avoided by pregnant women.

WORKPLACE STANDARDS

Acetonitrile

- OSHA. PEL TWA is 40 ppm, 70 mg/m^3.
- NIOSH

—REL TWA is 20 ppm, 34 mg/m^3.
—IDLH is 500 ppm.

Acrylonitrile

- OSHA. PEL TWA is 2 ppm, 15-minute ceiling limit 10 ppm.

NIOSH.

—REL TWA is 1 ppm, 15-minute ceiling limit 10 ppm.
—IDLH is 85 ppm.

Acetone Cyanohydrin

- OSHA. None
- NIOSH. REL TWA ceiling limit is 1 ppm.

Malonitrile

- OSHA. None
- NIOSH. REL TWA is 3 ppm, 8 mg/m^3.

Methylacrylonitrile

- OSHA. None.
- NIOSH. REL TWA is 1 ppm, 3 mg/m^3.

Propionitrile

- OSHA. None.
- NIOSH. REL TWA is 6 ppm, 14 mg/m^3.

Succinonitrile

- OSHA. None
- NIOSH. REL TWA is 6 ppm, 20 mg/m^3.

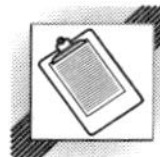

Diagnosis

DIFFERENTIAL DIAGNOSIS

- Other toxicologic chemicals that can produce severe metabolic acidosis include aspirin, ethylene glycol, methanol, iron, metformin, carbon monoxide, toluene, and isoniazid.
- Nontoxicologic causes include sepsis and other causes of seizures and altered mental status (CNS bleed or mass, meningitis, or electrolyte abnormalities).

SIGNS AND SYMPTOMS

- Signs and symptoms of aliphatic nitrile poisoning may develop within a few hours but may be delayed for 12 to 24 hours.
- Initial effects include nausea, vomiting, and mucous membrane irritation.
- If cyanide toxicity develops, tachycardia, hypotension, lactic acidosis, altered mental status, and seizures may occur.

Vital Signs

- Tachycardia, hypotension, tachypnea, and hyperpnea are common and suggest cyanide toxicity.
- Oxygen saturation is usually normal.

HEENT

- Mucous membrane irritation is common following inhalation.
- Splash exposure may cause corneal burns.

Dermatologic

- Cherry-red skin may develop as a terminal event.
- Cyanosis may develop secondary to hypoventilation or hypoperfusion.
- Dermatitis and burns may develop following dermal contact.

Pulmonary

- Tachypnea and hyperpnea, chest pain, and dyspnea are common.
- Both cardiogenic and noncardiogenic pulmonary edema have been reported in severe cases.

Gastrointestinal

- Nausea and vomiting are common following ingestion or inhalation.
- Abdominal pain and diarrhea are reported.

Fluids and Electrolytes

Increased anion gap metabolic (lactic) acidosis suggests cyanide toxicity.

Neurologic

- Headache and lightheadedness are common following inhalation.
- Agitation, anxiety, confusion, lethargy, altered mental status, tremor, ataxia, and seizures occur in severe cases.

PROCEDURES AND LABORATORY TESTS

Essential Tests

Serum electrolytes, BUN, and creatinine should be checked.

- An increased anion gap metabolic acidosis suggests cyanide toxicity.
- Renal insufficiency decreases renal clearance of thiocyanate and increases likelihood of cyanide toxicity.

Recommended Tests

- Arterial and venous blood gas analysis should be performed; metabolic acidosis and a decreased arteriovenous oxygen saturation gradient suggest cyanide toxicity.
- An increased serum lactate suggests cyanide toxicity.
- Blood or urine cyanide and thiocyanate determination should be made.

—Cyanide levels are difficult to assay and may be unreliable; thus, treatment should be determined by signs and symptoms.
—Levels may be useful to confirm the diagnosis but are rarely useful during acute management.
—Following exposure to aliphatic nitriles, blood cyanide levels in the range of 0 to 1 μg/ml have been associated with mild effects.
—Blood cyanide levels in the 3 to 10 μg/ml range have been reported in seriously ill patients and in patients who eventually died.
—Serum thiocyanate concentrations above 12 mg/dl have been associated with severe cyanide toxicity.

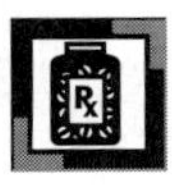

Treatment

- Treatment should focus on decontamination, airway management, 100% oxygen administration, and monitoring for the onset of cyanide poisoning, which may be delayed for 12 to 24 hours.
- Dose and time of exposure should be determined for all substances involved.

DIRECTING PATIENT COURSE

The health-care professional should call the poison control center when:

- Any known nitrile exposure has occurred.
- Patient exhibits unexplained increased anion gap metabolic acidosis.
- Toxic effects are not consistent with nitrile poisoning.
- Coingestant, drug interaction, or underlying disease presents an unusual problem.

The patient should be referred to a health-care facility when:

- Attempted suicide or homicide is possible.
- Patient or caregiver seems unreliable.
- Symptoms develop.
- Coingestant, drug interaction, or underlying disease presents an unusual problem.

Admission Considerations

Inpatient management is warranted for most patients with probable exposure to aliphatic nitriles; extended emergency department observation at least is required.

DECONTAMINATION

Out of Hospital

Ipecac should be administered to induce emesis within 1 hour of ingestion for alert pediatric or adult patient, if health-care evaluation will be delayed.

In Hospital

- Ipecac should be administered to induce emesis within 1 hour of ingestion for the alert patient who is too small to have effective gastric lavage.
- Gastric lavage should be performed in pediatric (tube size 24–32 French) or adult (tube size 36–42 French) patients for large ingestion presenting within 1 hour of ingestion or if serious effects are present.
- One dose of activated charcoal (1–2 g/kg) should be administered without a cathartic if a substantial ingestion has occurred within the previous few hours.
- Dermal decontamination should be performed by washing skin with soap and water.
- If ocular exposure has occurred, face and eyes should be irrigated with copious amounts of water.

ANTIDOTES

Cyanide Antidote Kit

- Its use is indicated in patients with known cyanide poisoning and clinical effects.
- In patients with mild effects, administration of sodium thiosulfate alone may be a reasonable first treatment; the full package should be administered if thiosulfate alone does not produce improvement.

—Adult treatment is sodium nitrite 300 mg (10 ml of 3% solution) intravenously over 5 minutes or more; intravenous administration of sodium thiosulfate 12.5 g (50 ml of 25% solution) should follow.
—Pediatric patients should receive an initial intravenous dose of sodium nitrite ($NaNO_2$) in ml/kg based on hemoglobin measurement (grams), followed by sodium thiosulfate 1.65 ml/kg up to 50 ml (25% solution) over several minutes.
—See SECTION III, Cyanide Antidote Package chapter for details.

ADJUNCTIVE TREATMENT

- If hypotension occurs, 10 to 20 ml/kg 0.9% saline should be administered and the patient placed in the Trendelenburg position; further fluid therapy should be guided by central venous pressure monitoring to avoid volume overload.
- If hypotension is unresponsive, a vasopressor may be administered.

—The dose of dopamine is 2 to 5 μg/kg/min, titrated to effect; rates above 20 μg/kg/min are unlikely to provide further benefit.
—If dopamine is ineffective, norepinephrine may be added at 0.1 to 0.2 μg/kg/min, titrated to effect.
—Tissue ischemia is possible with a high rate of infusion.

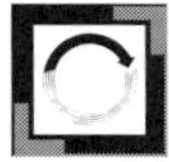

Follow-Up

PATIENT MONITORING

Respiratory and cardiac function should be monitored continuously.

EXPECTED COURSE AND PROGNOSIS

Toxic effects may be delayed for hours until compound is metabolized.

DISCHARGE CRITERIA/INSTRUCTIONS

- From the emergency department

—An asymptomatic patient with confirmed nonexposure or a low-concentration, short-duration exposure may be discharged after decontamination and 6 hours of observation.

- From the hospital

—An exposed patient who remains asymptomatic may be discharged after 24 hours of observation.
—Symptomatic patients may be discharged after metabolic acidosis, hemodynamic instability, and mental status changes have resolved.

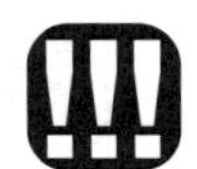

Pitfalls

DIAGNOSIS

- Failing to admit an asymptomatic patient with a known ingestion, inhalation, or dermal exposure for a 24-hour observation period can lead to serious complications.
- The presence of the classically described cherry-red skin color is an unreliable indicator of cyanide poisoning, and its absence should never be used to rule out cyanide toxicity.

ICD-9-CM 987

Toxic effect of other gases, fumes or vapors.

See also: SECTION II, Hypotension chapter; and SECTION III, Cyanide Antidote Package chapter.

RECOMMENDED READING

Ducatman AM, Liberman DF. Worker hazards in the biotechnology industry. In: Sullivan JB Jr, Krieger GR, eds. *Hazardous materials toxicology.* Baltimore: Williams & Wilkins, 1992:556–562.

Author: Edwin K. Kuffner

Reviewer: Katherine M. Hurlbut

Acrolein

Basics

DESCRIPTION

Acrolein (CH_2CHCHO) is a strong, volatile irritant liquid used as an herbicide and in industrial processes.

FORMS AND USES

Acrolein (acrylaldehyde, ethylene aldehyde) is a highly reactive chemical used to control weeds, algae, and plant growth and in the manufacture of numerous consumer products such as glycerin and other chemicals.

TOXIC DOSE

- A concentration of 2 ppm in air is considered immediately dangerous to life or health.
- Marked irritation of the eye, respiratory system, and mucous membranes may occur quickly, even at low air concentrations (less than 1 ppm).

PATHOPHYSIOLOGY

- Acrolein is a caustic agent that rapidly produces direct cellular injury on contact.
- Acrolein has no proven carcinogenic or teratogenic potential in humans.

EPIDEMIOLOGY

Poisoning is uncommon. Most exposures occur as a splash to skin or eyes during occupational use.

RISK FACTORS

The use of acrolein in an occupational setting.

PREGNANCY AND LACTATION

Embryotoxic and teratogenic effects occur in animals.

WORKPLACE STANDARDS

- ACGIH

—TLV TWA is 0.1 ppm (0.25 mg/m^3)
—STEL is 0.3 ppm.

- OSHA. PEL TWA is 0.1 ppm (0.25 mg/m^3).
- NIOSH

—PEL TWA is 0.1 ppm (0.25 mg/m^3).
—STEL is 0.3 ppm (0.8 mg/m^3).

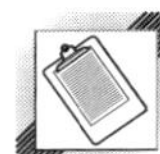

Diagnosis

DIFFERENTIAL DIAGNOSIS

Other causes of acute mucosal or pulmonary irritation include chlorine or other halogens, chloramine, hydrogen sulfide, ammonia, smoke inhalation, phosgene, and many others.

SIGNS AND SYMPTOMS

The primary effect is caustic injury; either locally to skin, eye, or to lungs from inhalation.

Vital Signs

Acute exposure causes tachycardia, tachypnea, and hypertension.

HEENT

- Mucous membrane irritation and erythema are the most common effects.
- Splash exposure may cause corneal burns.

Dermatologic

Prolonged contact or a high concentration may cause burns.

Pulmonary

- Injury may range from irritation (rhinorrhea, cough, or tachypnea) to frank bronchospasm and pulmonary edema (which may be delayed up to 24–72 hours).
- Pulmonary injury may lead to permanent dysfunction.

Gastrointestinal

Nausea, vomiting, and diarrhea are common following either inhalation or ingestion.

PROCEDURES AND LABORATORY TESTS

Essential Tests

No tests may be needed for asymptomatic patients.

Recommended Tests

- Arterial blood gases and pulmonary function tests may help evaluate injury.
- Chest x-rays may help evaluate injury, although they cannot rule out delayed pulmonary injury.
- A slit-lamp examination should be performed following ocular exposure. Patients with an ocular injury should be referred to an ophthalmologist immediately.

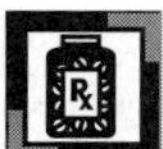

Treatment

DIRECTING PATIENT COURSE

Patients with a history of significant exposure or respiratory or systemic effects should be treated as inpatients.

The health-care professional should call the poison control center when:

- Severe or persistent effects develop.
- Coingestant, drug interaction, or underlying disease presents an unusual problem.

The patient should be referred to a health-care facility when:

- Toxic effects develop.
- Coingestant, drug interaction, or underlying disease presents an unusual problem.

DECONTAMINATION

- Exposure via inhalation. The patient should be removed from the source of exposure and 100% oxygen administered.
- Exposure to eyes. The eyes should be irrigated copiously with water.
- Exposure to skin. The skin should be irrigated copiously with water.

ANTIDOTES

There is no specific antidote for acrolein poisoning.

ADJUNCTIVE TREATMENT

- Exposure via inhalation. Supportive respiratory and cardiovascular care should be provided. For bronchospasm, oxygen should be administered followed by albuterol 0.15 mg/kg (maximum of 10 mg) in saline with humidified oxygen via nebulizer every 20 to 30 minutes.
- Exposure to the eyes

—The eyes should be irrigated with copious amounts of water.
—The pH of the cul-de-sac should be tested after irrigation to ensure neutral pH.

- Exposure to the skin

—The skin should be irrigated with copious amounts of water, washed with soap and water, and debrided as needed.
—A sterile dressing should be applied.

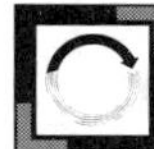

Follow-Up

PATIENT MONITORING

Respiratory and cardiac function should be monitored continuously in symptomatic patients.

EXPECTED COURSE AND PROGNOSIS

- Skin burns and ocular injury develop soon after exposure and resolve over several days unless high concentration or prolonged exposure produces a third-degree injury.
- Noncardiogenic pulmonary edema may be delayed up to 24 to 72 hours following extensive exposures.

DISCHARGE CRITERIA/INSTRUCTIONS

Patients may be discharged from the emergency department or hospital when:

- Patient with minimal inhalation exposure is asymptomatic following a 4- to 6-hour observation period. The patient should be cautioned to return if any difficulty in breathing develops.
- Patients with splash or ocular exposures may be discharged following decontamination and arrangement of follow-up wound care.

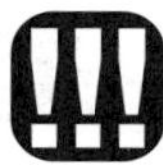

Pitfalls

In diagnosing the patient, the cause of the initial effect may be confused with other, more common industrial chemicals.

ICD-9-CM 987

Toxic effect of other gases, fumes, or vapors.

See also: SECTION II, Tachycardia, Tachypnea, and Hypertension chapters.

RECOMMENDED READING

POISINDEX editorial staff, Rumack BH, Hess AJ, Gelman CR, eds. POISINDEX System. Englewood, CO: Micromedex, Inc. (edition expires May 31, 1998).

Author: Edwin K. Kuffner

Reviewer: Richard C. Dart

Acrylamide

Basics

DESCRIPTION

Acrylamide (C_3H_5NO, vinyl amide) is a water soluble vinyl monomer that is used to make polyacrylamide.

FORMS AND USES

- Acrylamide is used mainly in the production of polyacrylamide, in the synthesis of dyes, and in construction of dam foundations, tunnels, and sewers.
- The polymerized form of the acrylamide monomer is relatively nontoxic and is used in the treatment of sewage and industrial waste, weather control (to dissipate fog), mining and timber operations, preparation of gels for chromatography, and grouting agents.

TOXIC DOSE

- Acute ingestion of 50 to 100 mg/kg can cause neurologic effects.
- Chronic ingestion of contaminated water (400 ppm) for 1 month can cause severe neurologic effects.

PATHOPHYSIOLOGY

- Exposure occurs via inhalation, dermal absorption, or ingestion.
- Acrylamide monomer is neurotoxic, producing progressive degeneration of axons in the peripheral, autonomic, and central nervous systems (e.g., dying-back polyneuropathy).
- Toxicity associated with the polymer form of acrylamide is thought to be related to the contamination of the product with acrylamide monomer.
- Acrylamide is a probable human carcinogen.

EPIDEMIOLOGY

- Poisoning is uncommon.
- The toxic effects following exposure range from mild to severe; incomplete recovery has been documented in a few cases.
- Death may occur after massive acute exposure.

CAUSES

Poisoning is usually associated with chronic occupational skin exposure. However, acute poisoning following the ingestion of contaminated underground water supply has been reported.

PREGNANCY AND LACTATION

Human data have not been compiled. Animal data suggest sperm changes and decrease in fertility, as well as DNA inhibition and mutagenicity.

WORKPLACE STANDARDS

Work place standards for acrylamide monomer:

- ACGIH. TLV is 0.03 mg/m^3.
- OSHA. PEL TWA is 0.3 mg/m^3.
- NIOSH. PEL TWA is 0.03 mg/m^3. IDLH is 60 mg/m^3.

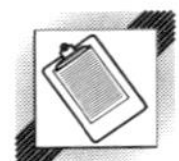

Diagnosis

DIFFERENTIAL DIAGNOSIS

- Toxicologic causes of peripheral neuropathy include alcoholism, carbon disulfide, heavy metals, hexane, *n*-butyl ketone, and organophosphates, among others.
- Nontoxicologic causes include diabetes, nutritional deficiency states, hand-arm vibration injury, as well as multiple sclerosis or other disease states causing combined central and peripheral neuropathy.

SIGNS AND SYMPTOMS

- Acute high-dose exposure may produce confusion, disorientation, ataxia, tremors, and seizures, with cardiovascular collapse after a delay of several hours. Peripheral neuropathy may begin 1 to 2 days later.
- First signs of chronic exposure are numbness and weakness of hands and feet and occur after weeks to months of exposure.
- Most toxic effects follow chronic exposure.

HEENT

Inhalation may produce irritation in the eyes and throat.

Dermatologic

- Abnormal sweating of the limbs may occur.
- Handling of acrylamide monomer causes erythema and peeling of the skin as well as red or blue discoloration where skin contact occurred.

Pulmonary

Persistent cough without parenchymal disease has been described.

Gastrointestinal

- Anorexia, constipation, and weight loss have been observed following chronic exposure.
- Liver injury has also occurred.
- Pancreatitis has been reported in one case.

Renal

Urinary retention and overflow urinary incontinence may develop if neuropathy develops.

Musculoskeletal

Weakness of the wrist and ankle extensor muscles, as well as loss of deep tendon and plantar reflexes, may occur as part of neuropathy.

Hematologic

Decreased platelet count may develop after large acute exposure.

Neurologic

- Acute CNS effects range from nervousness, sleeplessness, and difficulty in concentration to disorientation, confusion, hallucination, slurred speech, lethargy, and seizure.
- Peripheral signs include numbness, paresthesia, and weakness of the hands and feet (first signs of chronic exposure).
- Cerebellar effects may occur in severe cases.

Reproductive

Acrylamide is teratogenic in animal models.

PROCEDURES AND LABORATORY TESTS

Essential Tests

No tests may be needed for brief acute exposure or asymptomatic patients.

Recommended Tests

- Complete blood count, serum electrolytes, glucose, lipase BUN, creatinine and liver function tests are used to assess renal, hepatic, bone marrow, and pancreatic function in symptomatic patients.
- Lumbar puncture in the symptomatic patient may show increased protein levels.
- Heavy metal screens for arsenic, mercury, and thallium may be useful in the differential diagnosis.
- Serial nerve conduction studies may be used to document the extent and progression of peripheral neuropathy.
- The EEG may be abnormal in severe poisoning.

Not Recommended Tests

Acrylamide levels are not clinically useful.

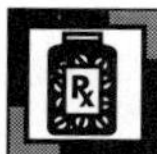

Treatment

- Treatment should focus on terminating exposure, performing decontamination (following acute exposure), and providing general supportive care.
- The dose and time of exposure should be determined for all substances involved.

DIRECTING PATIENT COURSE

The health-care professional should call the poison control center when:

- CNS toxicity or other severe effects are present.
- Toxic effects are not consistent with acrylamide toxicity.
- Coingestant, drug interaction, or underlying disease presents unusual problems.

The patient should be referred to a health-care facility when:

- The patient or caregiver seems unreliable.
- Any toxic effects are present.
- A coingestant, drug interaction, or underlying disease presents unusual problems.

Admission Considerations

Inpatient management is warranted for patients with CNS effects.

DECONTAMINATION

Out of Hospital

- Induction of emesis is not recommended.
- For inhalation exposure, move the patient to fresh air.
- For skin exposure, wash the skin with soap and water.
- For eye exposure, irrigate the eyes with room-temperature water for 15 to 20 minutes. Seek health-care evaluation if irritation or visual defect persists.

In Hospital

- Gastric lavage should be performed in pediatric (tube size 24–32 French) or adult (tube size 36–42 French) patients for large ingestion presenting within 1 hour of ingestion or if serious effects are present.
- One dose of activated charcoal (1–2 g/kg) should be administered without a cathartic if a large ingestion has occurred within the previous few hours.

ANTIDOTES

- A specific antidote is not available for acrylamide poisoning.

ADJUNCTIVE TREATMENT

- Seizures should be treated as explained in SECTION II, Seizures chapter.
- The patient should be ensured of an adequate airway and oxygenation.
- A benzodiazepine provides initial control.

—Cardiac and respiratory monitoring should be performed continuously.
—Diazepam
  —Adult dose is 5 to 10 mg intravenously initially, repeated every 10 minutes, as needed.
  —Pediatric dose is 0.2 to 0.5 mg/kg every 10 minutes, as needed.
—Lorazepam
  —Adult dose is 2 to 4 mg intravenous push over 2 to 5 minutes; this should be repeated every 10 minutes as needed.
  —Pediatric dose is 0.1 mg/kg intravenous push over 2 to 5 minutes, not to exceed 4 mg/dose. This dose should be repeated every 10 minutes as needed.

- If seizures persist or recur, the patient should be treated with an additional anticonvulsant, such as phenobarbital or phenytoin and neuromuscular blockade should be considered.

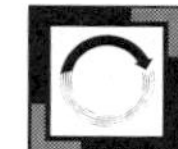

Follow-Up

PATIENT MONITORING

- Renal and hepatic function, complete blood count, amylase and serum glucose levels should be monitored in patients subjected to an extensive, acute exposure.
- Duration of monitoring in asymptomatic patients has not been investigated.
- Outpatient followup with occupational physician or clinical toxicologist is recommended.

EXPECTED COURSE AND PROGNOSIS

- Most patients develop mild effects and recover over several months. Patients with severe exposure often develop permanent sequelae and may die.
- Peripheral neuropathy often improves but may leave residual sensory and motor defects.

DISCHARGE CRITERIA/INSTRUCTIONS

- From the emergency department

—Asymptomatic patients can be discharged after gastrointestinal decontamination, if needed.
—Patients with transient respiratory symptoms may be monitored as outpatients.
—Patients with extensive, acute exposures should be observed for at least 6 to 12 hours.

- From the hospital. Patients may be discharged when toxic effects are improving, and they can care for themselves.

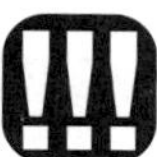

Pitfalls

- Detailed occupational history or examination of the workplace may be needed to detect acrylamide exposure.
- If a patient working with acrylamide develops a rash or becomes accident prone (for example, frequently dropping items or stumbling), he or she should be evaluated for peripheral neuropathy.
- Patients recovering from acrylamide intoxication may be more susceptible to repeat exposure.

ICD-9-CM 968

Poisoning by other central nervous system depressants and anesthetics.

RECOMMENDED READING

Donovan JW, Pearson R. Ingestion of acrylamide with severe encephalopathy, neurotoxicity and hepatotoxicity. *Vet Hum Toxicol* 1987;29:462.

Mulloy KB. Two case reports of neurological disease in coal mine preparation plant workers. *Am J Ind Med* 1996;30:56–61.

Tilson HA. The neurotoxicity of acrylamide: an overview. *Neurol Behav Toxicol Teratol* 1981;3:445–461.

Author: Martha M. Foley

Reviewer: Luke Yip

Akee Fruit

Basics

DESCRIPTION

Akee is the fruit of the tree *Blighia sapida* (soapberry).

TOXIC DOSE

The toxic dose is unknown because the concentration of the toxic component varies depending on the ripening of the fruit.

PATHOPHYSIOLOGY

- Akee fruit is edible when fully mature but is poisonous at all other times.
- The fruit contains hypoglycin A, a toxic amino acid. The immature fruit contains more than 12 times the hypoglycin A of mature fruit.
- Hypoglycin A causes hypoglycemia by inhibiting hepatic gluconeogenesis. A metabolite inhibits the oxidation of fatty acids.

EPIDEMIOLOGY

- *B. sapida* grows in western Africa, Jamaica, and southern Florida; however, the fruit is not commonly eaten outside Jamaica. Poisoning ("vomiting sickness") occurs with greater frequency in Jamaica, where the akee is a food staple, and generally among poor children.
- Toxic effects are typically severe, with death occurring in 40% to 80% of diagnosed cases.

CAUSES

Child neglect or abuse should be considered if the patient is less than 1 year of age, suicide attempt if the patient is older than 6 years of age.

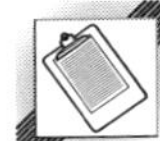

Diagnosis

DIFFERENTIAL DIAGNOSIS

Conditions that cause nausea, vomiting, liver injury, and seizures, such as Reye's syndrome or salicylate intoxication.

SIGNS AND SYMPTOMS

Initial nausea, vomiting, and central nervous system depression are followed by lethargy, seizures, coma, and death in severe cases. The typical disease course lasts less than 12 hours.

Gastrointestinal

Recurrent nausea and vomiting are usually present.

Hepatic

Acute hepatitis may develop.

Renal

Volume depletion due to vomiting often occurs.

Fluids and Electrolyte

Hypoglycemia is often present.

Neurologic

Initial lethargy is often followed by seizures and coma.

PROCEDURES AND LABORATORY TESTS

Essential Tests

Serum electrolytes, BUN, glucose, and creatinine should be measured in symptomatic patients. Hypoglycemia, electrolyte abnormalities, and volume depletion are common.

Recommended Tests

- Liver function tests should be performed to assess liver damage.
- Serum salicylate level may be useful for differential diagnosis.

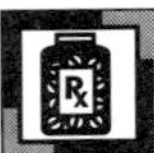

Treatment

Treatment should focus on supporting hemodynamic function and managing electrolyte, glucose, and pH balance.

DIRECTING PATIENT COURSE

The health-care professional should call the poison control center when:

- Severe or persistent effects develop.
- Coingestant, drug interaction, or underlying disease presents an unusual problem.

The patient should be referred to a health-care facility when:

- Toxic effects develop.
- Coingestant, drug interaction, or underlying disease presents an unusual problem.

Admission Considerations

Patients with hypoglycemia, seizures, or obtundation should be admitted.

DECONTAMINATION

Out of Hospital

Ipecac should be considered to induce emesis within 1 hour of ingestion for alert pediatric or adult patients if health-care evaluation will be delayed and vomiting has not already occurred.

In Hospital

- Gastric lavage should be performed in pediatric (tube size 24–32 French) or adult (tube size 36–42 French) patients for large ingestion presenting within 1 hour of ingestion or if serious effects are present.
- One dose of activated charcoal (1–2 g/kg) should be administered without a cathartic if a substantial ingestion has occurred within the previous few hours.

ANTIDOTES

There is no specific antidote for akee fruit poisoning.

ADJUNCTIVE TREATMENT

- Intravenous glucose should be administered immediately to hypoglycemic or obtundated patients.
- Adult dose is 50 mg/kg of D50W by intravenous push; pediatric dose is D25W 1 to 2 mg/kg.
- A continuous intravenous infusion of D10W or D20W should be initiated and the rate titrated to maintain serum glucose level of 100 to 150 mg/dl. It may then be gradually decreased over 12 to 24 hours depending on serum glucose level.

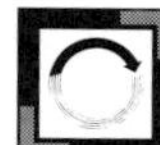

Follow-Up

PATIENT MONITORING

Respiratory and cardiac monitoring should be performed continuously in symptomatic patients.

EXPECTED COURSE AND PROGNOSIS

Toxicity peaks within hours. Outcome is good unless sequelae of prolonged hypoglycemia or seizures intercede.

DISCHARGE CRITERIA/INSTRUCTIONS

Asymptomatic patients may be discharged following decontamination and a 6-hour observation period.

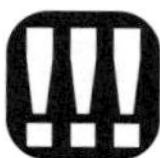

Pitfalls

Hypoglycemia may be severe and requires continuous glucose infusion.

ICD-9-CM 988.2

Toxic effects of noxious substances eaten as food: berries and other plants.

See also: SECTION III, Dextrose chapter.

RECOMMENDED READING

Centers for Disease Control and Prevention. Toxic hypoglycemia syndrome—Jamaica. *MMWR* 1992;41:53–55.

Author: Netti Riggs

Reviewer: Richard C. Dart

α_1-Adrenergic Antagonists

Basics

DESCRIPTION

α_1-Adrenergic antagonists are oral antihypertensive prescription medications.

FORMS AND USES

Pharmaceutical preparations include prazosin (Minipress), doxazosin (Cardura), and terazosin (Hytrin). These drugs are used in the treatment of hypertension and benign prostatic hypertrophy.

Hypertension

- Prazosin. Adult initial dose should not exceed 1 mg, given at bedtime; maintenance doses range from 3 to 20 mg/day in divided doses every 6 to 12 hours; pediatric dose is 5 μg/kg to a maximum of 25 μg/kg every 6 hours.
- Doxazosin. Adult initial dose is 1 mg/day (once daily) at bedtime; maintenance doses should be attained by increasing the daily dose by 2 to 4 mg every 2 weeks, titrated to antihypertensive effect.
- Terazosin. Adult initial dose is 1 mg/day (once daily) at bedtime; maintenance dose should be reached by increasing daily dose every 2 weeks, titrated to antihypertensive effect, up to 20 mg/day.

Benign Prostatic Hypertrophy

- Prazosin. Initial dose is 0.5 to 1.0 mg twice a day, titrated up to 2 mg twice a day.
- Doxazosin. Dose is 2 to 10 mg/day.
- Terazosin. Initial dose is 1 mg/day, titrated to 4 to 12 mg/day.

Other uses of these drugs include the treatment of Raynaud's syndrome, cirrhosis, congestive heart failure, pheochromocytoma, and autonomic dysreflexia.

TOXIC DOSE

Dangerous doses are poorly characterized, but death occurs rarely even in large overdose.

PATHOPHYSIOLOGY

- Blockade of peripheral α_1-receptors on arterioles results in vasodilatation and lowered blood pressure.
- Blockade of peripheral α_1-receptors on the prostatic urethra results in relaxation and increased urine flow.
- In overdose, profound vasodilatation may markedly decrease vascular resistance and cause hypotension.

EPIDEMIOLOGY

- Poisoning is uncommon.
- Toxic effects are typically mild to moderate.
- Death occurs most commonly following suicidal ingestion.
- None of the selective α_1-antagonists have been shown to be carcinogenic to humans.

CAUSES

- Toxic ingestion is usually intentional.
- Child abuse or neglect must be considered if the patient is less than 1 year of age, suicide attempt if the patient is over 6 years of age.

RISK FACTORS

Geriatric patients have an increased risk of orthostatic hypotension; thus, lower initial doses and slower increases in daily dosing are recommended.

DRUG AND DISEASE INTERACTIONS

- α_1-Adrenergic antagonists may potentiate the hypotensive effects of other antihypertensive agents, and dose reduction may be necessary.
- β-receptor or calcium channel blockers may exacerbate hypotension by blocking compensatory tachycardia.

PREGNANCY AND LACTATION

US FDA Pregnancy Category C. The drug exerts animal teratogenic or embryocidal effects, but there are no controlled studies in women, or no studies are available in either animals or women.

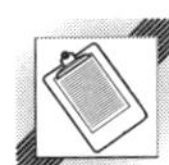

Diagnosis

DIFFERENTIAL DIAGNOSIS

- Toxicologic causes of hypotension include β-receptor blockers, calcium channel blockers, antidysrhythmics, tricyclic antidepressants, monoamine oxidase inhibitors, guanethidine, reserpine, clonidine, imidazolines, α-methyldopa, guanabenz, nitrates, minoxidil, and many others.
- Nontoxicologic causes include sepsis, adrenal insufficiency, thyrotoxicosis, autonomic dysfunction, alcohol, volume depletion, or other causes.

SIGNS AND SYMPTOMS

The predominant feature of overdose is hypotension.

Vital Signs

- Hypotension and reflex tachycardia are common.
- Orthostatic hypotension may develop during therapy or following overdose.

HEENT

Blurred vision is common during therapy.

Dermatologic

Rash develops infrequently.

Cardiovascular

- Postural hypotension is common within the first 30 to 90 minutes following the initial dose (first dose phenomenon).
- Chest pain, bradycardia, palpitations, and edema have been reported with therapeutic dosing but are rare.

Gastrointestinal

- Nausea is most common.
- Vomiting, diarrhea, and constipation have been reported.
- Abdominal pain and pancreatitis occur rarely.

Hepatic

Hepatotoxicity occurs rarely during chronic therapy.

Hematologic

- Inhibition of platelet aggregation occurs rarely.
- Doxazosin may rarely cause leukopenia and neutropenia.

Neurologic

Lightheadedness, dizziness, weakness, and syncope are commonly associated with therapeutic dosing and secondary to orthostatic hypotension.

Genitourinary

- Polyuria has been reported.
- Sexual dysfunction is a known side effect of chronic therapy.
- Priapism has occurred after prazosin overdose.

Endocrine

All of the selective α_1-antagonists lower serum low-density lipoprotein cholesterol and triglyceride levels and increase serum high-density lipoprotein cholesterol levels.

PROCEDURES AND LABORATORY TESTS

Essential Tests

No tests may be needed in minimally symptomatic patient.

Recommended Tests

- Serum electrolytes, BUN, creatinine, and glucose should be assayed to evaluate other causes of hypotension.
- ECG, serum acetaminophen, and aspirin levels should be performed in an overdose setting to detect occult ingestion.
- Dexamethasone suppression test should be performed in patients with suspected adrenal insufficiency.

Not Recommended Tests

Serum levels of the selective α_1-adrenergic antagonists are not clinically useful.

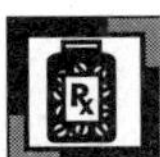

Treatment

- Treatment should focus on monitoring and maintaining blood pressure.
- Dose and time of exposure should be determined for all substances involved.

DIRECTING PATIENT COURSE

The health-care professional should call the poison control center when:

- Hypotension or other serious effects are present.
- Toxic effects are not consistent with selective α_1-antagonist toxicity.
- Coingestant, drug interaction or underlying disease presents an unusual problem.

The patient should be referred to a health-care facility when:

- Attempted suicide or homicide is possible.
- Patient or caregiver seems unreliable.
- Lightheadedness, dizziness, syncope, chest pain, altered mental status, or other severe effects are present.
- Toxic effects are not consistent with selective α_1-antagonist toxicity.
- Coingestant, drug interaction, or underlying disease presents an unusual problem.

Admission Considerations

Inpatient management is warranted if:

- Patient develops hypotension or persistent symptomatic orthostatic hypotension.
- Following a large ingestion, admitting an asymptomatic patient for 12 to 24 hours of observation should be considered, because hypotensive effects can be delayed.

DECONTAMINATION

Out of Hospital

Ipecac should be administered to induce emesis within 1 hour of ingestion for alert pediatric or adult patients if health-care evaluation will be delayed.

In Hospital

- Ipecac should be administered to induce emesis within 1 hour of ingestion for the alert patient who is too small to have effective gastric lavage.
- Gastric lavage should be performed in pediatric (tube size 24–32 French) or adult (tube size 36–42 French) patients for large ingestion presenting within 1 hour of ingestion or if serious effects are present.
- One dose of activated charcoal (1–2 g/kg) should be administered without a cathartic if a substantial ingestion has occurred within the previous few hours.

ANTIDOTES

There is no specific antidote for selective α_1-antagonist poisoning.

ADJUNCTIVE TREATMENT

- Hypotension is the primary effect of overdose.
- The patient should be treated with isotonic fluid infusion (0.9% saline 10 to 20 cc/kg), placed in the Trendelenburg position, and, if needed, given vasopressors.
- Dopamine may be started at 2 to 5 μg/kg/min, titrated upward to desired effect; rates above 20 μg/kg/min are unlikely to provide further benefit.
- Norepinephrine should be added for refractory hypotension.

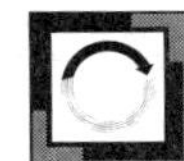

Follow-Up

PATIENT MONITORING

- Respiratory and hemodynamic parameters should be monitored continuously.
- Complications related to hypotension are rare when patients receive early and aggressive hemodynamic support; ischemic damage most commonly involves the CNS, myocardium, and kidneys.

EXPECTED COURSE AND PROGNOSIS

- Hypotension typically resolves over 12 to 24 hours; however, following large overdose, hypotension may persist for days.
- Doxazosin and terazosin have a longer duration of effect than prazosin.

DISCHARGE CRITERIA/INSTRUCTIONS

- From the emergency department. An asymptomatic patient with documented normal blood pressure during 6 to 10 hours of observation may be discharged, following psychiatric evaluation, if needed.
- From the hospital. Patients may be discharged after toxic effects resolve or stabilize and after psychiatric evaluation, if needed.

PATIENT EDUCATION

Patients should be warned about orthostatic hypotension, especially those beginning therapy.

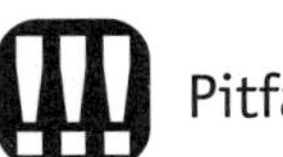

Pitfalls

DIAGNOSIS

Failure to check for orthostatic hypotension is a common cause of missed diagnosis.

TREATMENT

- Overdose patients with documented hypotension should be admitted for at least 24 hours of observation.
- Patients should not be treated with vasopressors before adequate fluid resuscitation has taken place.

FOLLOW-UP

Patients may develop delayed hypotension.

ICD-9-CM 971.3

Poisoning by drugs primarily affecting the autonomic nervous system: sympatholytics (antiadrenergics).

See also: SECTION II, Hypotension chapter.

RECOMMENDED READING

POISINDEX Editorial Staff. Vasodilators. In: Rumack BH, Sayre NK, Gelman CR, eds. *POISINDEX System*. Englewood, CO: MICROMEDEX, Inc. (edition expires May 31, 1997).

Author: Edwin K. Kuffner

Reviewer: Katherine M. Hurlbut

Amiodarone and the Class III Antidysrhythmics

Basics

DESCRIPTION

Amiodarone (Cordarone) and bretylium (Bretylol) are Vaughan-Williams class III antidysrhythmic agents.

FORMS AND USES

• Amiodarone is used in the treatment of recurrent or refractory supraventricular and ventricular dysrhythmias resistant to standard therapy.

—Adult dose is 400 to 2,000 mg/day taken orally.
—Pediatric dose is 5 to 10 mg/kg/day.

• Bretylium is used to treat ventricular dysrhythmias. Adult and pediatric dose is 5 mg/kg by intravenous push.
• Sotalol is covered in another chapter.

TOXIC DOSE

• Acute amiodarone ingestion of several grams produces little effect in adults.
• Chronic amiodarone ingestion producing levels greater than 2 to 3 μg/ml may produce toxicity.

PATHOPHYSIOLOGY

• Amiodarone and bretylium prolong the myocardial cell action potential by decreasing the slow outward potassium current without affecting phase 4 spontaneous depolarization.
• Amiodarone also causes inhibition of the atrioventricular node, delayed atrioventricular conduction, QT interval prolongation, and decreased atrial and ventricular automaticity.
• Amiodarone blocks both α- and β-adrenergic receptors, causing systemic and coronary vasodilatation.

EPIDEMIOLOGY

Poisoning is uncommon with either agent. Death has occurred only rarely, primarily in patients with chronic accumulation of amiodarone.

CAUSES

• Toxic amiodarone effects usually arise from chronic ingestion.
• Child neglect or abuse should be considered if the patient is less than 1 year of age, suicide attempt if the patient is over 6 years of age.

DRUG AND DISEASE INTERACTIONS

• β-receptor blocking drugs accentuate the effects of amiodarone.
• Cimetidine increases amiodarone blood levels.
• Drug levels of digoxin, quinidine, procainamide, warfarin, phenytoin, and diltiazem may be increased with the use of amiodarone.

PREGNANCY AND LACTATION

• Amiodarone. US FDA Pregnancy Category C. Studies have shown that the drug exerts animal teratogenic or embryocidal effects, but there are no controlled studies in women, or no studies are available in either animals or women.
• Bretylium has not been assigned a category.
• Amiodarone is excreted in breast milk in appreciable quantities.

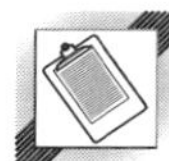

Diagnosis

DIFFERENTIAL DIAGNOSIS

Toxicologic causes of hypotension and cardiac dysrhythmia include tricyclic antidepressants, numerous other antidysrhythmic agents, calcium channel blocker, or β-receptor blocker, among others.

SIGNS AND SYMPTOMS

Amiodarone and bretylium may cause similar effects due to their mechanism of action; however, bretylium is not used chronically and therefore rarely causes toxicity.

Vital Signs

• Bradycardia and hypotension occur in overdose.
• Bretylium may rarely cause initial hypotension followed by cardiovascular collapse.

HEENT

Amiodarone may cause photosensitivity or corneal microdeposits.

Dermatologic

• Blue-gray skin pigmentation may occur with long-term amiodarone use.
• Photosensitivity reactions may occur during amiodarone use.

Cardiovascular

• Amiodarone induced hypotension unrelated to dysrhythmia is associated with intravenous use only and is believed to be related to the benzyl alcohol and polysorbate diluent.
• During chronic amiodarone therapy, there have been reports of QT interval prolongation and torsade de pointes. It is often associated with hypokalemia, hypomagnesemia, or concomitant use of a class I antidysrhythmic agent.
• Bretylium can cause marked QT interval prolongation.

Pulmonary

Chronic therapy with amiodarone may rarely be complicated by rapidly progressive acute respiratory distress syndrome and pulmonary fibrosis.

Gastrointestinal

Following acute amiodarone overdose, the patient may present with nausea and vomiting.

Hepatic

Transient increase in liver enzymes may occur during amiodarone therapy.

Endocrine

• Gynecomastia, hypothyroidism, or hyperthyroidism may develop during chronic amiodarone therapy.
• Thyrotoxicosis has been reported during chronic amiodarone therapy.

PROCEDURES AND LABORATORY TESTS

Essential Tests

No tests may be needed in asymptomatic patients.

Recommended Tests

• Serum electrolytes, BUN, and creatinine are tested to evaluate other causes of dysrhythmia.
• Liver function tests are used to determine if hepatic injury has developed.
• The ECG in acute overdose may indicate sinus bradycardia, first-degree atrioventricular block, QT interval prolongation, and a transient T-wave inversion that simulates a non–Q-wave myocardial infarction.
• ECG, serum acetaminophen, and aspirin levels are used in an overdose setting to detect occult ingestion.

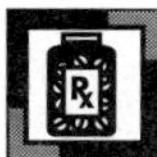

Treatment

- Therapy should focus on hypertension and bradydysrhythmias.
- Toxicity associated with long-term therapeutic use is much more common than that associated with acute overdose.

DIRECTING PATIENT COURSE

The health-care professional should call the poison control center when:

- Respiratory or cardiac effects are noted.
- Toxic effects are not consistent with amiodarone or bretylium toxicity.
- The coingestant, drug interaction, or underlying disease presents an unusual problem.

The patient should be referred to a health-care facility when:

- Attempted suicide or homicide is possible.
- Patient or caregiver seem unreliable.
- Any toxic effects develop.
- The coingestant, drug interaction, or underlying disease presents an unusual problem.

Admission Considerations

Inpatient management in an intensive care setting is warranted for patients with respiratory or cardiac effects.

DECONTAMINATION

Out of Hospital

Ipecac should be administered to induce emesis within 1 hour of ingestion for alert pediatric or adult patients if health-care evaluation will be delayed.

In Hospital

- Ipecac should be administered to induce emesis within 1 hour of ingestion for the alert patient who is too small to have effective gastric lavage.
- Gastric lavage should be performed in pediatric (tube size 24–32 French) or adult (tube size 36–42 French) patients for large ingestion presenting within 1 hour of ingestion or if serious effects are present.
- One dose of activated charcoal (1–2 g/kg) should be administered without a cathartic if a substantial ingestion has occurred within the previous few hours.

ADJUNCTIVE TREATMENTS

Bradycardia

- Standard agents including atropine and isoproterenol are usually ineffective.
- Early use of pacemaker is recommended.

Torsade de Pointes

- If electrolyte abnormalities are present, they should be corrected.
- Quinidine, disopyramide, procainamide, amiodarone, or bretylium should be avoided because they also prolong the QT interval.

—Adult initial dose is 1 to 2 g of magnesium sulfate intravenous push, repeated after 10 to 15 minutes, if needed. An intravenous infusion should be started at 2 to 10 mg/min, titrated to antidysrhythmic effect.
—Pediatric loading dose is 25 to 50 mg/kg intravenously over 5 minutes.

- Isoproterenol may be used to increase heart rate and thereby shorten the QTc interval.

—Adult dose is 2 to 4 μg/ml at an initial rate of 0.5 to 1.0 μg/min, titrated to effect.
—Pediatric dose is 0.1 μg/kg/min, titrated to effect.

- If condition is unresponsive, overdrive pacing may be necessary.

Hypotension

- The primary treatment is correction of the dysrhythmia.

Other

- Cardiac pacing may be useful in patients with bradycardia or an atrioventricular block not responsive to other measures.
- Bretylium is dialyzable, but there is no evidence to suggest that dialysis is effective in the treatment of any of the class III agents.

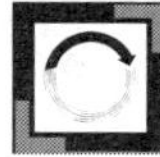

Follow-Up

PATIENT MONITORING

Respiratory and cardiac function should be monitored continuously throughout hospitalization.

EXPECTED COURSE AND TREATMENT

- Recovery is expected unless hypoxic injury intercedes.
- Sequelae of hypoxia may occur.

DISCHARGE CRITERIA/INSTRUCTIONS

- From the emergency department. Asymptomatic patients may be discharged after gastrointestinal decontamination, observation for 6 to 8 hours, and psychiatric evaluation, if needed.
- From the hospital. Asymptomatic patients may be discharged after toxic effects have resolved and psychiatric evaluation, if needed.

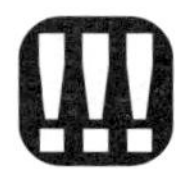

Pitfalls

DIAGNOSIS

- Failure to monitor the patient for 6 to 8 hours may allow toxicity to develop outside the health-care facility.
- Failure to realize that amiodarone causes thyrotoxicosis may lead to misdiagnosis.

ICD-9-CM 972.4

Poisoning by agents primarily affecting the cardiovascular system.

See also: SECTION II, Bradycardia, Hypotension, and Ventricular Dysrhythmia chapters; and SECTION IV, Sotalol chapter.

RECOMMENDED READING

Bigger JT, Hoffman BF. Antiarrhythmic drugs. In: *Gilman and Goodman's pharmacological basis of therapeutics.* New York: MacMillan, 1985:864–871.

Hruby K, Missliwetz J. Poisoning with oral antiarrhythmic drugs. *Int J Clin Pharmacol Ther Toxicol* 1985;23:253–257.

Authors: Gerald F. O'Malley and Edwin K. Kuffner

Reviewer: Richard C. Dart

Ammonia

Basics

DESCRIPTION

Anhydrous ammonia is a colorless alkaline gas, lighter than air, with a pungent choking odor.

FORMS AND USES

- Anhydrous ammonia (NH_3) is used in the production of fertilizers, dyes, plastics, synthetic fibers, and other chemicals and pharmaceuticals; commercial refrigerant gas; nitrogen fertilizer; and explosives.
- Aqueous ammonia is an ingredient in many household (usually at a concentration of 5% to 10%) and commercial (usually at concentrations above 25%) cleaning agents.

TOXIC DOSE

- Just a few drops of liquified anhydrous ammonia can cause severe airway burns and swelling.
- Large amounts of household ammonia (5% to 10%) must be ingested to produce injury.

PATHOPHYSIOLOGY

- Anhydrous ammonia is highly water soluble, forming highly caustic ammonium hydroxide when combined with water.
- Commercial aqueous solutions may cause severe alkali burns and liquefaction necrosis.
- Household products cause few effects unless very large amounts are involved.
- The combination of aqueous ammonia with hypochlorite bleaches may release chloramine and chlorine gases, which can cause irritant airway injury.

EPIDEMIOLOGY

- Ingestion of household products is common and typically accidental.
- Exposure to anhydrous or commercial strength aqueous ammonia is usually occupational.

CAUSES

Child neglect or abuse should be considered if the patient is less than 1 year of age, suicide attempt if the patient is over 6 years of age.

DRUG AND DISEASE INTERACTIONS

Ammonia may exacerbate reactive airway disease.

WORKPLACE STANDARDS

- ACGIH

—TLV TWA is 25 ppm.
—STEL is 35 ppm.

- OSHA

—PEL TWA is 50 ppm, 35 mg/m^3.

- NIOSH

—PEL TWA is 25 ppm, 18 mg/m^3.
—IDLH is 300 ppm.

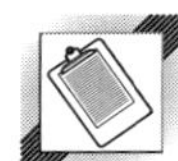

Diagnosis

SIGNS AND SYMPTOMS

- The severity of injury varies with the route, concentration, and duration of exposure.
- Inhalation of the anhydrous form causes rapid onset of respiratory symptoms, whereas inhalation of the household concentration typically produces no effect.

Vital Signs

- Tachycardia, tachypnea, and decreased pulse oximetry are common following inhalation.
- Hypertension has been reported.

HEENT

- Mucous membrane irritation is common (lacrimation, rhinorrhea, conjunctivitis, blepharospasm, drooling) from splash or inhalation exposure.
- Corneal burns, laryngeal edema, and laryngospasm may follow severe exposures.
- Oropharyngeal burns with epithelial desquamation may produce airway obstruction.

Dermatologic

- Erythema and dermatitis are common from contact exposure.
- Second- and third-degree burns are usually caused by contact with higher concentration commercial products.

Pulmonary

- Cough, chest pain, stridor, wheezing, bronchospasm, rhonchi and rales, chemical pneumonitis, and noncardiogenic pulmonary edema may occur following inhalation or aspiration.
- Pulmonary edema may be delayed following severe exposures.
- Upper airway edema may develop.

Gastrointestinal

- Nausea and vomiting are common following either inhalation or ingestion.
- Burns to the esophagus and stomach may follow ingestion of higher concentration commercial products or intentional large ingestion of lower concentration household products.

PROCEDURES AND LABORATORY TESTS

Essential Tests

No tests may be needed in asymptomatic patients following exposure to low-concentration products.

Recommended Tests

- Chest radiographs, arterial blood gases, and pulmonary function tests may help to evaluate injury.
- A chest radiograph is usually normal following mild to moderate exposures; infiltrates and pulmonary edema may not be evident for several hours.
- Bronchoscopy should be considered after a severe exposure because of the possibility of upper airway edema.
- Endoscopy should be performed to evaluate for burns within 24 hours following ingestion of high-concentration products or large amounts of lower concentration household products and in patients with oral burns, drooling, dysphagia, or abdominal pain.

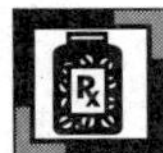

Treatment

• After exposure to high-concentration products, the focus should be placed on aggressive airway management and early endotracheal intubation of patients with airway injuries.
• Dose and time of exposure should be determined for all substances involved.

DIRECTING PATIENT COURSE

The health-care professional should call the poison control center when:

• Respiratory or gastrointestinal symptoms are present.
• Signs and symptoms are not consistent with ammonia exposure.
• Coingestant, drug interaction, or underlying disease presents an unusual problem.

The patient should be referred to a health-care facility when:

• Attempted suicide or homicide is possible.
• Patient or caregiver seem unreliable.
• Symptoms are present.
• Coingestant, drug interaction, or underlying disease presents an unusual problem.

Admission Considerations

Inpatient management is warranted if:

• Patient is symptomatic.
• Patient was exposed to anhydrous ammonia or other high-concentration commercial product.

DECONTAMINATION

• Inhalation. Remove from exposure and provide 100% oxygen.
• Ingestion

—Emesis should not be induced.
—Dilution with oral administration of 4 to 6 ounces of milk or water may be useful.

• Dermal exposure

—Skin should be irrigated with copious amounts of water, followed by thorough washing with soap and water.
—Burned area should be covered with a sterile dressing after irrigation.

• Eye exposure

—Exposed eyes should be irrigated with copious amounts of water; pH of cul-de-sac should be tested after irrigation to ensure neutral pH.
—Slit-lamp examination should be performed, and patients with an ocular burn should be referred to an ophthalmologist immediately.

ANTIDOTES

There is no antidote for ammonia poisoning.

ADJUNCTIVE TREATMENT

• Bronchospasm should be treated with nebulized β_2-receptor agonist (albuterol).
• Ingestion of high concentration products (anhydrous or industrial products) is managed as an alkaline corrosive.
• Corticosteroids may reduce the degree of pulmonary injury, but their efficacy has not been proven in clinical trials.
• Skin burns are treated in the same manner as thermal burns.

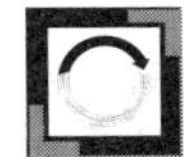

Follow-Up

PATIENT MONITORING

Respiratory and cardiac function should be monitored continuously in symptomatic patients.

EXPECTED COURSE AND PROGNOSIS

• Toxicity usually develops within minutes (inhalation or aspiration) to hours (ingestion or skin exposures).
• Course depends on concentration of product and duration of exposure.
• Inhalation of high-concentration products may result in permanent pulmonary dysfunction.
• Ingestion of high-concentration products may cause esophageal strictures.

DISCHARGE CRITERIA/INSTRUCTIONS

• From the emergency department. Patients who are asymptomatic after toxic ingestion and patients with documented absence of gastrointestinal burns or first-degree burns and tolerating oral intake may be discharged after 6 hours observation and psychiatric evaluation, if needed.
• From the hospital. Patients with second- or third-degree burns may be discharged when they are tolerating oral feeding, with follow-up evaluation scheduled to detect stricture formation.

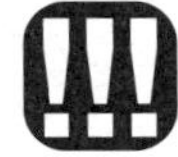

Pitfalls

DIAGNOSIS

Chest radiograph abnormalities may take hours to develop.

ICD-9-CM 983

Toxic effect of corrosive aromatics, acids, and caustic alkalis.

See also: SECTION IV, Caustics—Basic chapter.

RECOMMENDED READING

Close LG, Catlin FI, Cohn AM. Acute and chronic effects of ammonia burns of the respiratory tract. *Arch Otolaryngol* 1980;106:151–158.

Author: Edwin K. Kuffner

Reviewer: Richard C. Dart

Amoxapine and Loxapine

Basics

DESCRIPTION

Amoxapine is an oral antidepressant medication similar to the tricyclic antidepressant agents.

FORMS AND USES

- Pharmaceutical preparations include amoxapine (Asendin, Demolox, Moxadil) and loxapine (Loxapac, Loxitane).
- Amoxapine is used in the treatment of depression; adolescent dose is 25 to 100 mg/day; adult dose is 75 to 600 mg/day.
- Loxapine is used in the treatment of psychotic disorders; the adult dose is 60 to 100 mg/day in two to four divided doses.

TOXIC DOSE

Death has occurred after ingestion of 250 mg by a small child and 2 to 5 g in an adult.

PATHOPHYSIOLOGY

- Amoxapine and loxapine block the neuronal reuptake of norepinephrine, serotonin, and dopamine.
- Toxic effects may be caused by blockade of the myocardial sodium channel.
- Anticholinergic, adrenergic, and β-blocking effects also occur.

EPIDEMIOLOGY

- Poisoning is uncommon.
- Toxic effects following exposure are typically moderate.
- Death can occur in a severe overdose with uncontrolled seizures.
- Elderly patients and those with underlying cardiovascular and pulmonary disease may not tolerate prolonged seizures.

CAUSES

- Poisoning in adults is usually suicidal.
- Poisoning in children is usually accidental.
- Child neglect or abuse should be considered if the patient is less than 1 year of age, suicide attempt if the patient is over 6 years of age.

DRUG AND DISEASE INTERACTIONS

- Use with drugs that increase serotoninergic neurotransmission (e.g., MAO inhibitors, SSRIs) may produce serotonin syndrome.
- Amoxapine may potentiate the effects of sedative, hypnotic, or sympathomimetic drugs.

PREGNANCY AND LACTATION

- US FDA Pregnancy Category C. The drug exerts animal teratogenic or embryocidal effects, but there are no controlled studies in women, or no studies are available in either animals or women.
- Prolonged seizures compromise the fetus.

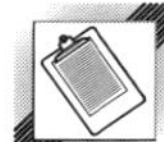

Diagnosis

DIFFERENTIAL DIAGNOSIS

- Other toxicologic causes of seizures include type 1A antidysrhythmics, sympathomimetic agents, theophylline, isoniazid, lindane, and mefenamic acid.
- Other causes of seizures include CNS tumor or bleed, meningitis, encephalitis, and withdrawal from ethanol or sedative-hypnotic agents, among others.

SIGNS AND SYMPTOMS

- Repeated seizures and CNS depression are common, and may be complicated by hyperthermia, tachycardia, metabolic acidosis, hypotension, rhabdomyolysis, and acute renal failure.
- Serious dysrhythmia is not common, but may develop after neurologic toxicity.

Vital Signs

- Tachycardia, respiratory failure, and hyperthermia may develop secondary to prolonged seizures.
- Hypotension may occur in severe overdose.

Cardiovascular

- Sinus tachycardia is common.
- Atrial and ventricular dysrhythmias (supraventricular tachycardia, atrial flutter, premature ventricular contractions, bradycardia, or electromechanical dissociation), prolonged QRS and QTc intervals, and hypotension have been reported.

Pulmonary

- Respiratory depression or aspiration pneumonitis may develop.
- Adult respiratory distress syndrome has developed after severe overdose.

Renal

Acute renal failure may develop due to rhabdomyolysis.

Fluids and Electrolytes

Metabolic acidosis may develop due to seizures.

Musculoskeletal

Rhabdomyolysis may develop due to seizures.

Neurologic

Altered mental status ranging from drowsiness, lethargy, and confusion to seizures and coma is common and may develop abruptly.

PROCEDURES AND LABORATORY TESTS

Essential Tests

ECG should be obtained and continuous cardiac monitoring instituted.

- Sinus tachycardia is common.
- Dysrhythmias are generally associated with severe neurologic toxicity.

Recommended Tests

- Serum electrolytes, BUN, and creatinine are measured to assess electrolytes, acid-base status, and renal function in patients with altered mental status, seizures, or cardiac effects.
- Serum creatine kinase is measured to assess muscle injury if seizures occur.
- A urinalysis is used to detect renal injury.
- Arterial blood gases detect metabolic acidosis, from prolonged seizures.
- Serum acetaminophen and aspirin levels in overdose setting are used to detect occult overdose.
- Head CT, lumbar puncture, and cultures are used as needed to evaluate other causes of coma or seizures.

Not Recommended Tests

Serum levels of amoxapine or loxapine are not clinically useful.

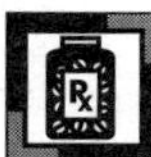

Treatment

- Treatment should focus on managing the airway, supporting blood pressure, and controlling seizures.
- The dose and time of exposure must be determined for all substances involved.

DIRECTING PATIENT COURSE

The health-care professional should call the poison control center when:

- Seizures, coma, dysrhythmia, hypotension, acidemia, or other severe effects are present.
- Signs and symptoms are not consistent with amoxapine or loxapine poisoning.
- Coingestant, drug interaction, or underlying disease presents an unusual problem.

The patient should be referred to a health-care facility when:

- Attempted suicide or homicide is possible.
- Patient or caregiver seems unreliable.
- Toxic effects are present.
- Signs and symptoms are not consistent with amoxapine or loxapine poisoning.
- Coingestant, drug interaction, or underlying disease presents an unusual problem.

Admission Considerations

Inpatient management in an intensive care setting is warranted for patients with altered mental status, seizure, hypotension, or dysrhythmia.

DECONTAMINATION

Out of Hospital

Emesis should not be induced because coma or seizures may develop abruptly.

In Hospital

- Emesis should not be induced because coma or seizures may develop abruptly.
- Gastric lavage should be performed in pediatric (tube size 24–32 French) or adult (tube size 36–42 French) patients for large ingestion presenting within 1 hour of ingestion or if serious effects are present.
- One dose of activated charcoal (1–2 g/kg) should be administered without a cathartic if a substantial ingestion has occurred within the previous few hours.
- A second dose of charcoal (0.5–1.0 g/kg) may be worthwhile 2 to 4 hours after the first dose.
- Evidence does not support the use of multiple-dose activated charcoal for amoxapine or loxapine poisoning.

ANTIDOTES

There is no specific antidote for amoxapine or loxapine poisoning.

ADJUNCTIVE TREATMENT

Seizure

- A benzodiazepine is administered for initial control.
- The airway must be monitored closely.
- Diazepam. Adult dose is 5 to 10 mg intravenously initially, repeated every 10 minutes if needed; pediatric dose is 0.2 to 0.5 mg/kg intravenously, repeated every 10 minutes if needed.
- Lorazepam. Adult dose is 2 to 4 mg intravenous push over 2 to 5 minutes, repeated every 10 minutes if needed; pediatric dose is 0.1 mg/kg intravenous push over 2 to 5 minutes, not to exceed 4 mg/dose, and repeated every 10 minutes if needed.
- If seizures persist or recur, another anticonvulsant, such as phenobarbital or phenytoin, should be added.

Hypotension

- A bolus infusion of 10 to 20 ml/kg 0.9% saline solution should be administered and the patient placed in the Trendelenburg position.
- Further fluid therapy should be guided by central pressure monitoring to avoid volume overload.
- If hypotension is unresponsive, a vasopressor should be administered.

—Dopamine is infused at 2 to 5 μg/kg/min, titrated upward to desired effect; rates above 20 μg/kg/min are unlikely to provide further benefit.
—If hypotension is unresponsive, norepinephrine may be added at an infusion rate of 0.1 to 0.2 μg/kg/min; titrated to desired effect.
—A high rate of infusion may cause tissue ischemia.

Ventricular Dysrhythmia or Conduction Abnormality

- Seizures must be controlled and acidemia corrected; if QRS interval widening or dysrhythmias persist, sodium bicarbonate is administered at 1 to 2 mEq/kg intravenous bolus, repeated as needed to narrow the QRS complex. Arterial pH should not exceed 7.55.
- Lidocaine is used for ventricular tachycardia or multifocal premature ventricular contractions.

—The adult dose is 50 to 100 mg by intravenous bolus, followed by an infusion of 2 to 4 mg/min, titrated to desired effect.
—The pediatric dose is 1 mg/kg bolus followed by infusion of 20 to 50 μg/kg/min, titrated to effect.
—The bolus dose may be repeated once in 10 to 15 minutes (dose should be ½ initial bolus).

Not Recommended Therapies

- Physostigmine is not recommended.
- Hemodialysis and hemoperfusion are not effective.

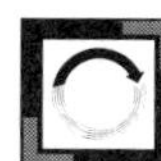

Follow-Up

PATIENT MONITORING

Cardiac and pulmonary function should be monitored continuously.

EXPECTED COURSE AND PROGNOSIS

- Toxicity usually develops within hours and peaks within 12 hours.
- Patients who do not develop repeated seizures do well.
- Repeated seizures are more likely result in permanent neurologic injury or death.

DISCHARGE CRITERIA/INSTRUCTIONS

- From the emergency department. Asymptomatic patients may be discharged after gastrointestinal decontamination is completed, when the ECG is normal at 6 hours after overdose, and after psychiatric evaluation, if needed.
- From the hospital. Patients may be discharged after mental status, ECG, and vital signs have returned to normal, and complications are stable.

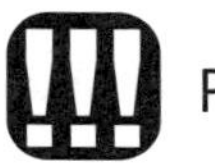

Pitfalls

DIAGNOSIS

Amoxapine and loxapine may produce the cardiac manifestations typical of tricyclic antidepressant overdose.

TREATMENT

Prompt seizure control is mandatory; general anesthesia or neuromuscular paralysis and EEG monitoring may be required.

ICD-9-CM 969.0

Poisonings by antidepressants.

See also: SECTION II, Hypotension, Seizure, and Ventricular Dysrhythmia chapters.

RECOMMENDED READING

Kulig K, Rumack BH, Sullivan JB, et al. Amoxapine overdose: coma and seizures without cardiotoxic effects. *JAMA* 1982;248:1092–1094.

Litovitz TL, Troutman WG. Amoxapine overdose: seizures and fatalities. *JAMA* 1983;250:1069–1071.

Author: Katherine M. Hurlbut

Reviewer: Richard C. Dart

Amphetamines

Basics

DESCRIPTION

- Amphetamines are commonly abused drugs.
- Slang terms include crank, crystal, ice, jeff, and speed.

FORMS AND USES

- Numerous illicit preparations are available.
- Amphetamine substances available by prescription include Adderall, benzphetamine (Didex), biphetamine, chlorphentermine, dextroamphetamine (Bontril, Dexedrine, Dextrostat), diethylpropion, ephedrone, mazindol, mephentermine, pemoline, phendimetrazine tartrate (Prelu-2 Timed Release), phenmetrazine, phentermine (Fastin, Ionanimin, Obenix, Oby-Cap, Zantryl), Oby-Trim, and Xtrozine.
- Methamphetamine and methylphenidate are covered in other chapters.
- Therapeutic uses include treatment of attention deficit disorder, narcolepsy, and obesity.
- Typical doses are:

—Adderall 50 to 60 mg/day
—Benzphetamine 25 to 50 mg one to three times daily
—Dextroamphetamine 5 to 60 mg/day in divided doses
—Phendimetrazine 105 mg/day
—Phenterimine 15 to 37.5 mg/day

TOXIC DOSE

- The toxic dose is variable; therefore, serial observation of the patient is used to assess severity.
- Repeated users develop tolerance; therefore, higher doses are needed to produce toxicity.

PATHOPHYSIOLOGY

Amphetamines are indirectly acting sympathomimetic drugs that stimulate norepinephrine release and have direct agonist effects on α- and β-adrenergic receptors.

EPIDEMIOLOGY

- Poisoning is common, with large regional variations in the incidence of abuse.
- Toxic effects following exposure are typically mild to moderate.
- Death occurs in patients abusing amphetamines at escalating doses.

CAUSES

- Poisoning usually results from recreational abuse.
- Child neglect or abuse should be considered if the patient is less than 1 year of age, suicide attempt if the patient is over 6 years of age.

DRUG AND DISEASE INTERACTIONS

- There is a synergistic effect with other sympathomimetic agents and tricyclic antidepressants.
- Use with monoamine oxidase inhibitors may produce severe toxicity.

PREGNANCY AND LACTATION

- Most amphetamine drugs. US FDA Pregnancy Category C. The drug exerts animal teratogenic or embryocidal effects, but there are no controlled studies in women, or no studies are available in either animals or women.
- Diethylpropion. US FDA Pregnancy Category B. Animal studies indicate no fetal risk, and there are no controlled human studies, or animal studies show an adverse fetal effect but well-controlled studies in women do not.
- Abruptio placentae may occur.
- Withdrawal syndrome has been reported in neonates.
- The fetus is at risk for premature delivery and low birth weight.

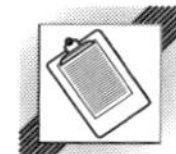

Diagnosis

DIFFERENTIAL DIAGNOSIS

- Toxicologic causes of agitation, seizures and hyperthermia include ingestion or abuse of other sympathomimetic agents (cocaine, ephedrine, and many others).
- Nontoxicologic causes include diseases with adrenergic excess: hyperthyroidism, manic behavior, alcohol withdrawal, and many others.

SIGNS AND SYMPTOMS

- Tachycardia, hypertension, diaphoresis, agitation, and seizures are common.
- Hyperthermia, dysrhythmia, shock, rhabdomyolysis, hepatic necrosis, and acute renal failure may develop in severe overdose.

Vital Signs

- Hypertension, tachycardia, and mild hyperthermia are common.
- Severe hyperthermia and hypotension may develop with life-threatening overdose.

HEENT

Mydriasis may develop.

Cardiovascular

- Dysrhythmia, hypotension, aortic dissection, myocardial infarction, or cardiomyopathy may occur.
- Arterial spasm and localized tissue ischemia may develop after arterial injection.

Pulmonary

Pulmonary edema and adult respiratory distress syndrome may develop with severe overdose.

Hepatic

Hepatic necrosis may develop in patients with severe hyperthermia.

Renal

Acute renal failure may complicate hypotension, seizures, and rhabdomyolysis.

Hematologic

Coagulopathy may develop in severe cases.

Fluids and Electrolytes

- Dehydration and hypokalemia are common.
- Lactic acidosis is common and may become severe if hypotension or hyperthermia develops.

Musculoskeletal

Rhabdomyolysis may develop due to hyperthermia or seizures.

Neurologic

- Headache, agitation, and seizures are common.
- Intracranial hemorrhage, ischemic infarcts, and cerebral vasculitis may occur.

Psychiatric

Paranoid delusions and psychosis may persist beyond the acute phase.

PROCEDURES AND LABORATORY TESTS

Essential Tests

- Laboratory testing may not be needed in asymptomatic patients.
- Serum electrolytes, BUN, and creatinine should be determined; metabolic acidosis and renal injury suggest severe intoxication.
- ECG and cardiac monitoring should be performed.

—Sinus tachycardia is common; other dysrhythmia suggests severe intoxication.
—Ischemia may occur.

Recommended Tests

- Liver function, coagulation studies, and serum creatine kinase may be abnormal in patients with hyperthermia or agitation.
- Serum acetaminophen and aspirin levels should be performed in overdose setting to detect occult ingestion.
- Head CT, lumbar puncture, and cultures should be performed in patients with altered mental status, headache, seizures, or fever.
- Chest radiograph should be taken in patients with hypoxia or pulmonary symptoms.
- Abdominal radiographs should be taken in patients suspected of ingesting packets.

Not Recommended Test

Serum levels of amphetamine are not available nor useful.

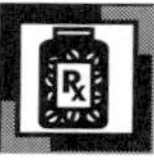

Treatment

- Treatment should be focused on controlling agitation, reversing hyperthermia, and supporting hemodynamic function.
- The dose and time of exposure should be determined for all substances involved.

DIRECTING PATIENT COURSE

The health-care professional should call the poison control center when:

- Severe effects such as shock, hyperthermia,

renal or hepatic injury, or coagulopathy are present.
• Toxic effects are not consistent with amphetamine.
• Coingestant, drug interaction, or underlying disease presents an unusual problem.

Patients should be referred to a health-care facility when:

• There has been inadvertent ingestion of more than a daily dose.
• Attempted suicide or homicide is possible.
• Patient or caregiver seems unreliable.
• Toxic effects are present.
• Coingestant, drug interaction, or underlying disease presents unusual problem.

Admission Considerations

Inpatient treatment is warranted for patients with refractory agitation, recurrent seizures, hyperthermia, persistent tachycardia, or other end-organ injury.

DECONTAMINATION

Out of Hospital

Induction of emesis is not recommended.

In Hospital

• Gastric lavage should be performed in pediatric (tube size 24–32 French) or adult (tube size 36–42 French) patients presenting within 1 hour of a large ingestion or if serious effects are present.
• One dose of activated charcoal (1 to 2 g/kg) should be administered without a cathartic if a substantial ingestion has occurred within the previous few hours.
• Whole-bowel irrigation should be considered in patients ingesting packets, 1 to 2 L/h until rectal effluent is clear.

ANTIDOTES

There is no specific antidote for amphetamine poisoning.

ADJUNCTIVE TREATMENT

Control of Agitation

A benzodiazepine with which the provider has experience should be administered.

• Diazepam

—Adult dose is 5 to 10 mg intravenously.
—Pediatric dose is 0.2 to 0.5 mg/kg intravenously.
—Doses are repeated at 10-minute intervals, titrating to effect.

• Lorazepam

—Adult dose is 2 to 4 mg intravenously.
—Pediatric dose is 0.1 mg/kg intravenously.
—Doses are repeated at 10-minute intervals, titrating to effect.

• The airway should be monitored closely.

Seizure

• An adequate airway and oxygenation should be ensured.
• A benzodiazepine should be administered for initial control.

—Diazepam
  —Adult dose is 5 to 10 mg by intravenous push, repeated every 10 minutes as needed.
  —Pediatric dose is 0.2 to 0.5 mg/kg, repeated every 10 minutes as needed.
—Lorazepam
  —Adult dose is 2 to 4 mg by intravenous push over 2 to 5 minutes, repeated every 10 minutes as needed.
  —Pediatric dose is 0.1 mg/kg by intravenous push over 2 to 5 minutes, not to exceed 2 mg/dose.
  —Doses are repeated at 10-minute intervals as needed.

• The airway should be monitored closely.
• If seizures persist or recur, another anticonvulsant such as phenobarbital or phenytoin should be added.
• The use of neuromuscular blockade and artificial ventilation should be considered in refractory patients, especially if hyperthermia is present.

Hypertension

If hypertension is not responsive to benzodiazepines or end-organ damage develops (aortic dissection, CNS bleed, myocardial infarction), a short-acting titratable agent (such as nitroprusside) should be administered.

Hypotension

• The patient should be given 10 to 20 ml/kg 0.9% saline and placed in the Trendelenburg position.
• Further fluid therapy should be guided by central pressure monitoring to avoid volume overload.
• If hypotension does not respond to treatment, a vasopressor is administered.

—Dopamine
  —Initial dosage for both children and adults is 2 to 5 μg/kg/min intravenously, titrated upward to effect.
  —Rates greater than 20 μg/kg/min are unlikely to provide further benefit.
—Norepinephrine
  —Initial dosage for both children and adults is 0.1 to 0.2 μg/kg/min, titrated upward to effect.
  —High rates of infusion may cause tissue ischemia.

Ventricular dysrhythmia

Treatment methods are discussed in SECTION II, Ventricular Dysthythmias chapter.

Rhabdomyolysis

• Adequate hydration and urine output (1 to 2 ml/kg/h) should be ensured.
• Urinary alkalinization has not been shown to be beneficial.

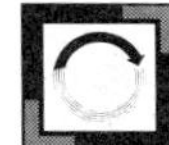

Follow-Up

PATIENT MONITORING

Symptomatic patients require continuous monitoring of respiratory and hemodynamic function and core temperature.

EXPECTED COURSE AND PROGNOSIS

• Patients generally recover quickly after oral amphetamine overdose.
• Complications are more common in patients with massive or chronic intravenous abuse.
• Possible complications include:

—End-organ injury from hypertension or seizures.
—Hepatic necrosis from severe hyperthermia.
—Acute renal failure from severe rhabdomyolysis or hypotension.
—Vasculitis and other sequelae of chronic intravenous abuse (endocarditis, abscess, HIV, sepsis, hepatitis, and tetanus).

DISCHARGE CRITERIA/INSTRUCTIONS

• From the emergency department

—Asymptomatic patients may be discharged after decontamination, observation for 4 to 6 hours, and psychiatric evaluation, if needed.
—Patients should be referred for substance abuse treatment.

• From the hospital

—Patients may be discharged after effects have resolved, mental status has returned to baseline, and laboratory values have normalized.
—Patients should be referred for substance abuse treatment.

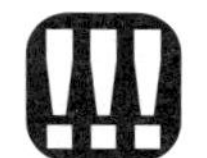

Pitfalls

DIAGNOSIS

• Mental status changes, hypertension, and hyperthermia should prompt evaluation for CNS bleed, infection, or infarct as well as infectious complications.
• The laboratory should be asked about substances that may cause a false-positive screen for amphetamines.

ICD-9-CM 969.7

Poisoning by psychotropic agents: psychostimulants.

See also: SECTION II, Hypotension, Seizures (Unexplained), and Ventricular Dysrhythmias chapters; SECTION III, Nitroprusside and Whole-Bowel Irrigation chapters; and SECTION IV, Methamphetamine and Methylphenidate chapters.

RECOMMENDED READING

Derlet RW, Rice P, Horowitz BZ, et al. Amphetamine toxicity: experience with 127 cases. *J Emerg Med* 1989;7:157–161.

Morgan JP. Amphetamine and methamphetamine during the 1990s. *Pediatr Rev* 1992;13:330–333.

Author: Katherine M. Hurlbut

Reviewer: Luke Yip

Amrinone

Basics

DESCRIPTION

Amrinone and milrinone are phosphodiesterase inhibitors that are used as inotropic agents.

FORMS AND USES

- Amrinone is an inotropic agent that is chemically distinct from catecholamines and cardiac glycosides.
- Milrinone is a less toxic derivative of amrinone that has 15 to 30 times the inotropic potency of amrinone.
- Therapeutic uses include the treatment of acute exacerbation of congestive heart failure refractory to standard therapy, pulmonary hypertension, heart failure following cardiac surgery, and hypotension refractory to standard therapy from poisoning with β-blockers, calcium channel blockers, or chloroquine.

TOXIC DOSE

- Doses of 450 mg/day orally are associated with thrombocytopenia.
- A toxic dose has not been well established. One case report describes death after infusion of 840 mg of amrinone over 3 days.

PATHOPHYSIOLOGY

- Amrinone and milrinone are selective phosphodiesterase 3 inhibitors.
- Phosphodiesterase inhibition causes an increase in intracellular cyclic AMP, which leads to increased intracellular calcium concentration and positive inotropy.
- These drugs augment cardiac performance by increasing contractility and causing peripheral vasodilatation with only a minor effect on the heart rate.

EPIDEMIOLOGY

- Poisoning is uncommon.
- Toxic effects following exposure are typically mild to moderate.

CAUSES

Poisoning is usually attributable to an inadvertant therapeutic overdose.

RISK FACTORS

- Hypersensitivity to bisulfites contraindicates the use of these drugs.
- Asthma is also a contraindication due to possible allergy to the sodium metabisulfite in the commercial product.

DRUG AND DISEASE INTERACTIONS

- These drugs may produce hypokalemia
- May exacerbate pulmonic and aortic stenosis or aortic outflow tract obstruction in idiopathic hypertrophic subaortic stenosis.
- Digoxin causes increased inotropic effects.
- Disopyramide can exacerbate hypotension.
- Furosemide causes precipitation of amrinone in solution.

PREGNANCY AND LACTATION

US FDA Pregnancy Category C. The drug exerts animal teratogenic or embryocidal effects, but there are no controlled studies in women, or no studies are available in either animals or women.

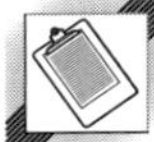

Diagnosis

DIFFERENTIAL DIAGNOSIS

Toxicologic causes of nausea, vomiting, and ventricular dysrhythmia include tricyclic antidepressants, chloroquine, and type 1a antidysrhythmic agents, among others.

SIGNS AND SYMPTOMS

Acute Overdose

- Cardiovascular. Hypotension and dysrhythmia (usually ventricular) are common.
- Gastrointestinal. Nausea, vomiting, diarrhea, and abdominal pain may occur (more common with oral therapy).

Chronic Therapy

- HEENT. Viral syndrome–like symptoms can occur.
- Hepatic. Hepatotoxicity is possible (more common with chronic oral therapy).
- Hematologic. Thrombocytopenia (dose-related) usually responds to dose reduction or discontinuation of treatment.

PROCEDURES AND LABORATORY TESTS

Essential Tests

No tests may be needed in asymptomatic patients.

Recommended Tests

- Acute ingestion

—ECG and cardiac monitoring to detect dysrhythmias.
—Serum electrolytes, BUN, creatinine, calcium, and magnesium in symptomatic patients to assess other potential causes of cardiac dysrhythmia.

- Chronic therapy. Complete blood count, liver enzymes, and serum electrolytes may be needed if patient develops symptoms.

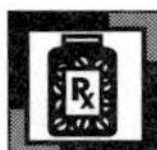

Treatment

- In the case of an acute intravenous overdose, amrinone administration should be discontinued and the patient placed on a cardiac monitor in an ICU.

DIRECTING PATIENT COURSE

The health-care professional should call the poison control center when:

- Severe or persistent effects develop.
- Coingestant, drug interaction, or underlying disease presents an unusual problem.

The patient should be referred to a health-care facility when:

- Toxic effects develop.
- Coingestant, drug interaction, or underlying disease presents an unusual problem.

Admission Considerations

Inpatient management in a monitored setting is warranted if the patient exhibits hypotension or dysrhythmia.

DECONTAMINATION

- Gastric lavage should be performed in pediatric (tube size 24–32 French) or adult (tube size 36–42 French) patients for large ingestions presenting within 1 hour of ingestion or if serious effects are present.
- One dose of activated charcoal (1–2 g/kg) should be administered without a cathartic if a substantial ingestion has occurred within the previous few hours.

ANTIDOTES

There is no specific antidote for amrinone poisoning.

ADJUNCTIVE TREATMENT

Hypotension

- Atropine should be used if hypotension is due to bradycardia.
- The patient should receive 10 to 20 ml/kg 0.9% saline intraveneously and be placed in the Trendelenburg position.
- Further fluid therapy should be guided by central pressure monitoring to avoid volume overload.
- A vasopressor may be added if needed.

Dysrhythmias

Standard advanced life support are used to treat dysrhythmias.

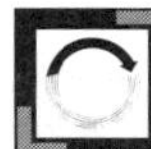

Follow-Up

PATIENT MONITORING

- Respiratory and hemodynamic function should be continuously monitored and supported.
- ECG should be obtained.

EXPECTED COURSE AND PROGNOSIS

- Acute ingestion usually causes toxicity within hours and resolves over days.
- Chronic toxicity often produces sequelae.

DISCHARGE CRITERIA/INSTRUCTIONS

Asymptomatic patients may be discharged after decontamination, 6 hours of observation, and psychiatric evaluation, if needed.

ICD-9-CM 972.9

Cardiac drugs.

See also: SECTION II, Hypotension and Ventricular Dysrhythmias chapters.

RECOMMENDED READING

Leboritz DJ, Lawless ST, Weise KL. Fatal amrinone overdose in a pediatric patient. *Crit Care Med* 1995;23:977–980.

Author: Edwin K. Kuffner

Reviewer: Gerald F. O'Malley

Angiotensin-Converting Enzyme Inhibitors

Basics

DESCRIPTION

Angiotensin-converting enzyme (ACE) inhibitors are common oral medications used in the treatment of hypertension.

FORMS AND USES

- Pharmaceutical preparations include benazepril (Lotensin), captopril (Capoten), enalapril (Vasotec), fosinopril (Monopril), lisinopril (Prinivil, Zestril), moexipril (Univasc), quinapril (Accupril), ramipril (Altace), and spirapril (Renormax).
- ACE inhibitors are used for the treatment of hypertension.

—Benazepril. 5-, 10-, 20-, or 40-mg tablets; adult dose 10 to 40 mg orally four times a day
—Captopril. 12.5-, 25-, 50-, or 100-mg tablets; adult dose 25 to 150 mg orally, divided twice or three times a day
—Enalapril. 2.5-, 5-, 10-, or 20-mg tablets; adult dose 10 to 40 mg orally four times a day
—Lisinopril. 2.5-, 5-, 10-, or 20-mg tablets; adult dose 10 to 40 mg orally four times a day

- Other uses for ACE inhibitors include the treatment of congestive heart failure, myocardial infarction, progressive renal impairment, and scleroderma renal crisis.

TOXIC DOSE

- Adults may ingest several hundred milligrams and develop minor hypotension that responds to crystalloid infusion.
- Children can ingest at least 100 mg without apparent toxicity.

PATHOPHYSIOLOGY

- ACE inhibitors prevent the conversion of angiotensin to angiotensin II, an extremely potent endogenous vasoconstrictor.
- Blockade of angiotensin II production produces orthostatic hypotension; however, frank hypotension is rare because of compensation by other bodily mechanisms.

EPIDEMIOLOGY

- Poisoning is uncommon.
- Hypotensive symptoms are usually not life threatening.
- Death occurs following massive ingestion or in the presence of coingestant or underlying disease state.

CAUSES

- Toxic ingestion is usually accidental.
- Child neglect or abuse should be considered if the patient is less than 1 year of age, suicide attempt if the patient is over 6 years of age.

RISK FACTORS

- Use in patients with renal failure may cause hyperkalemia.
- Both pediatric and geriatric patients are considered more sensitive to the hypotensive effect of ACE inhibitors.

DRUG AND DISEASE INTERACTIONS

Use with potassium supplements or potassium-sparing diuretics may cause severe hyperkalemia.

PREGNANCY AND LACTATION

- All agents included in this chapter are US FDA Pregnancy Category D. Evidence of human fetal risk exists, but benefits in certain situations (e.g., life-threatening situations or serious diseases) may make use of the drug acceptable despite its risks.
- Pregnancy testing should be conducted in all women of childbearing age prior to initiating ACE inhibitor therapy.

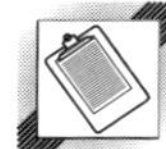

Diagnosis

DIFFERENTIAL DIAGNOSIS

- Toxicologic causes of hypotension include β-receptor or calcium channel blocker, various antidysrhythmics, tricyclic antidepressants, monoamine oxidase inhibitors, clonidine, imidazolines, α-methyldopa, nitrates, and α_1-receptor blocking agents, among others.
- Nontoxicologic causes include volume depletion, renal failure, adrenal insufficiency, autonomic dysfunction from diabetes, alcohol abuse, or other causes.

SIGNS AND SYMPTOMS

Hypotension may be acute and life threatening in massive overdose; overdose information is limited because of few reported cases.

HEENT

- Edema of the nose, throat, mouth, glottis, larynx, lips, and tongue (angioneurotic edema) may occur during therapeutic use or following overdose.
- Airway obstruction is possible.

Dermatologic

Dermatitis, exfoliative dermatitis, lichenoid eruptions, and lupus erythematosus-like reactions may occur during therapeutic use.

Cardiovascular

Hypotension may develop with either overdose or misuse.

Pulmonary

- Dyspnea, cough, and bronchospasm may occur during therapeutic use.
- Cough occurs in 5% to 20% of patients on chronic therapy, more commonly in women; cough will stop within days of discontinuing therapy.

Gastrointestinal

Alteration or loss of taste is possible (dysgeusia or ageusia).

Hepatic

- Liver enzyme abnormalities during chronic treatment are possible.
- Cholestatic-type hepatitis occurs rarely with therapeutic use.

Hematologic

- Blood loss secondary to gastrointestinal hemorrhage is possible.
- Disseminated intravascular coagulation is a rare complication.

Fluids and Electrolytes

Hyperkalemia may develop during therapy, particularly in patients with renal insufficiency.

Neurologic

Altered level of consciousness due to hypotension is possible in large overdose.

Genitourinary

- Proteinuria and glycosuria may occur during therapy.
- Nephrotic syndrome is possible, especially with preexisting decreased renal function.

PROCEDURES AND LABORATORY TESTS

Essential Tests

No tests may be needed in the asymptomatic patient.

Recommended Tests

- Serum electrolytes, BUN, and creatinine should be assayed to assess renal function and potassium level.
- Serum liver function and coagulation tests should be performed for symptomatic patients.
- ECG, serum acetaminophen, and aspirin levels should be tested in an overdose setting to detect occult ingestion.

Not Recommended Tests

There is no clinical benefit from obtaining ACE serum levels.

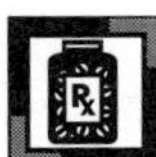

Treatment

- Treatment should focus on hemodynamic support.
- Dose and time of exposure should be determined for all substances involved.

DIRECTING PATIENT COURSE

The health-care professional should call the poison control center when:

- Respiratory symptoms, CNS depression, or other serious effects are present.
- Toxic effects are not consistent with ACE inhibitor toxicity.
- Coingestant, drug interaction, or underlying disease presents an unusual problem.

The patient should be referred to a health-care facility when:

- Angioneurotic edema or other toxic effects develop.
- Attempted suicide or homicide is possible.
- Patient or caregiver seems unreliable.
- Coingestant, drug interaction, or underlying disease presents an unusual problem.

Admission Considerations

Inpatient management is warranted if patient exhibits persistent hypotension or other serious effects including the potential for airway obstruction from angioedema.

DECONTAMINATION

Out of Hospital

Emesis should not be induced.

In Hospital

- Gastric lavage should be performed in pediatric (tube size 24–32 French) or adult (tube size 36–42 French) patients for large ingestion presenting within 1 hour of ingestion or if serious effects are present.
- One dose of activated charcoal (1–2 g/kg) should be administered if a substantial ingestion has occurred within the previous few hours.

ANTIDOTES

There is no specific antidote for ACE inhibitor poisoning.

ADJUNCTIVE TREATMENT

- Hypotension

—Atropine should be used to correct hypotension related to bradycardia.
—Hypotensive patients should receive fluid resuscitation with 0.9% saline in a 150- to 250-ml bolus (10–20 ml/kg in pediatrics) and be placed in the Trendelenberg position.
—Further fluid therapy should be guided by central pressure monitoring to avoid volume overload.
—Vasopressor may be added if needed. Dopamine is infused initially at 5 μg/kg/min and titrated to effect up to 20 μg/kg/min. If hypotension is unresponsive, norepinephrine may be added 0.1 to 0.2 μg/kg/min and titrated to effect. Caution: Tissue ischemia may result from high doses.

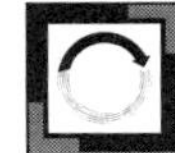

Follow-Up

PATIENT MONITORING

- Cardiac and respiratory function should be monitored continuously in symptomatic patients.
- Serum potassium should be followed closely in symptomatic patients.

EXPECTED COURSE AND PROGNOSIS

- Hypotension is common, usually develops early, but may persist for more than 24 hours.
- In severe cases, hyperkalemia or hypotension may develop.
- Angioneurotic edema may rarely produce airway obstruction.
- Recovery is usually complete unless complications of hypotension or hypoxia intercede.

DISCHARGE CRITERIA/INSTRUCTIONS

Asymptomatic patients with normal vital signs may be discharged from the emergency department or the hospital following gastric decontamination, observation for 4 to 6 hours, and a psychiatric evaluation, if needed.

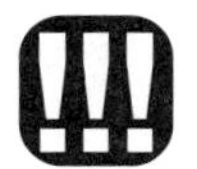

Pitfalls

DIAGNOSIS

Hyperkalemia may develop insidiously in patients with renal insufficiency or addition of diuretic, especially potassium-sparing types.

ICD-9-CM 972

Poisoning by agents primarily affecting the cardiovascular system.

See also: SECTION II, Hypotension chapter.

RECOMMENDED READING

Augenstein WL, Kulig KW, Rumack BH. Captopril overdose resulting in hypotension. *JAMA* 1988;259:3302–3305.

Trilli LE, Johnson KA. Lisinopril overdose and management with intravenous angiotensin II. *Ann Pharmacother* 1994;28:1165–1168.

Jackson EK, Garrison JC. Renin and angiotensin. In: Hardman JG, Gilman AG, Limbird LE, eds. *Goodman and Gilman's: the pharmacological basis of therapeutics, 9th ed.* New York: McGraw-Hill, 1996:733–758.

Author: Alvin C. Bronstein

Reviewer: Richard C. Dart

Anticholinergic Compounds

Basics

DESCRIPTION

- A wide variety of prescription and over-the-counter medications produce anticholinergic toxicity.
- The diagnosis is established based on physical signs; however, duration of effect is influenced by the half-life of the drug.

FORMS AND USES

Some anticholinergic medications include oxyphenomium (Antrenyl), benztropine (Cogentin), biperiden (Akineton), orphenadrine (Disipal, Marflex, Norflex), trihexyphenidyl, anisotropine (Valpin), butylscopolamine (Buscapina, Buscopan), clidinium (Librax, Quarzan), dicyclomine (Bentyl), glycopyrrolate (Robinul), isopropamide (Darbid), mepenzolate (Cantil), methantheline (Banthine), oxyphencyclimine (Daricon), propantheline (Pro-Banthine), trospium (Spasmex), flavoxate (Urispas), oxybutynin (Ditropan), cyclopentolate (Cyclogel), homatropine, tropicamide (Mydriacyl), belladonnna, atropine, *l*-hyoscyamine, Bellafoline, scopolamine, hyoscine, ipratropium (Atrovent), and diphenidol (Vontrol).

TOXIC DOSE

Toxicity may develop if more than three to four times the maximum daily dose is exceeded for an anticholinergic compound.

PATHOPHYSIOLOGY

Each compound competitively antagonizes acetylcholine, primarily at the muscarinic acetylcholine receptor.

EPIDEMIOLOGY

- Poisoning is common.
- Toxic effects are mild following accidental pediatric ingestion, but severe effects may develop following misuse or abuse.
- Death is rare and is usually attributable to trauma sustained during delirium.

CAUSES

- Ingestion by toddlers is usually accidental.
- Adolescent and adult cases usually involve misuse or abuse.
- Child neglect or abuse should be considered if the patient is less than 1 year of age, suicide attempt if the patient is over 6 years of age.

PREGNANCY AND LACTATION

- Dicyclomine and glycopyrrolate. US FDA Pregnancy Category B. Animal studies indicate no fetal risk and there are no controlled human studies, or animal studies show an adverse fetal effect but well-controlled studies in pregnant women do not.
- Most anticholinergic drugs. US FDA Pregnancy Category C. Studies have shown that the drug exerts animal teratogenic or embryocidal effects, but there are no controlled studies in women, or no studies are available in either animals or women.

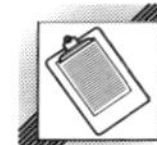

Diagnosis

DIFFERENTIAL DIAGNOSIS

Toxicologic causes include sympathomimetic agents; the presentation may be similar (tachycardia, mydriasis, and delirium), but sympathomimetic agents usually cause perspiration and bowel sounds are usually present.

SIGNS AND SYMPTOMS

- A large ingestion can result in florid anticholinergic syndrome: tachycardia, dilated pupils, a flushed appearance, decreased bowel sounds, urinary retention, and, occasionally, seizures.
- A patient may not exhibit all of the signs and symptoms of anticholinergic toxicity; it is common for patients to exhibit varying degrees of anticholinergic syndrome and for signs to fluctuate over time.

Vital Signs

- Sinus tachycardia is common; in its absence, the diagnosis of anticholinergic toxicity should be questioned.
- Mild hyperthermia is common.

HEENT

- Dry mucous membranes and mydriasis are common; mydriasis often produces blurred vision.
- Unilateral mydriasis and anisocoria have occurred after instillation of an ophthalmic cycloplegic agent or other anticholinergic drug into one eye.
- Ophthalmic administration of an anticholinergic agent can produce systemic anticholinergic toxicity.

Dermatologic

Warm, dry, and flushed skin is common.

Cardiovascular

Dysrhythmias have been reported, but are rare.

Gastrointestinal

Ileus and decreased bowel sounds are common.

Fluids and Electrolytes

Dehydration is common.

Musculoskeletal

Psychomotor agitation can produce rhabdomyolysis.

Neurologic

- Agitation with altered mental status is common; seizures may occur.
- Toxic psychosis with anxiety, paranoia, and hallucinations is well reported.
- CNS depression with drowsiness and lethargy progressing to coma is less common.
- Dystonic reactions and movement disorders have been reported.

Genitourinary/Renal

Urinary retention is common.

PROCEDURES AND LABORATORY TESTS

Essential Tests

Minimally symptomatic patients may not require laboratory testing.

Recommended Tests

- Serum electrolytes, BUN, and creatinine are measured to assess dehydration and potential renal injury from myoglobin.
- Creatine kinase may be elevated if rhabdomyolysis occurs.
- Urinalysis is ordered to assess dehydration or myoglobin-induced renal injury.
- ECG, serum acetaminophen, and aspirin levels are used to detect occult overdose.
  —Sinus tachycardia is common.
  —Malignant dysrhythmia is rare.

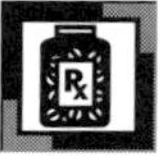

Treatment

- In the agitated patient, treatment focuses on control of agitation and protection from self-harm.
- In the patient with CNS depression, treatment focuses on airway management.
- The dose and time of exposure must be determined for all substances involved.

DIRECTING PATIENT COURSE

The health-care professional should call the poison control center when:

- Seizure, hyperthermia, rhabdomyolysis, or other severe effects are present.
- The use of physostigmine is considered.
- Toxic effects are not consistent with anticholinergic toxicity.
- A coingestant, drug interaction, or underlying disease presents an unusual problem.

The patient should be referred to a health-care facility when:

- Attempted suicide or homicide is possible.
- Patient or caregiver seems unreliable.
- Toxic effects develop.
- Coingestant, drug interaction, or underlying disease presents an unusual problem.

Admission Considerations

Inpatient management is warranted for patients in need of observation for persistent agitation, altered mental status, seizure, hyperthermia, or continued sedation.

DECONTAMINATION

Out of Hospital

Ipecac should be administered to induce emesis within 1 hour of ingestion for the alert patient who is too small to have effective gastric lavage.

In Hospital

- Ipecac should be administered to induce emesis within 1 hour of ingestion for the alert patient who is too small to have effective gastric lavage.
- Aspiration of gastric contents through a nasogastric tube may be helpful shortly after ingestion of a liquid preparation.
- Gastric lavage should be performed in pediatric (tube size 24–32 French) or adult (tube size 36–42 French) patients for large ingestions presenting within 1 hour of ingestion or if serious effects are present; lavage may be reasonable even 4 to 6 hours after ingestion due to gastrointestinal slowing.
- One dose of activated charcoal (1–2 g/kg) is administered without a cathartic if a substantial ingestion has occurred; one repeat dose of activated charcoal may be helpful 4 to 6 hours following the first dose due to slowed absorption.

ANTIDOTES

Physostigmine is an antidote used for the diagnosis of anticholinergic poisoning.

Indications

- Physostigmine is a diagnostic agent that distinguishes altered mental status due to anticholinergic toxicity from other causes of agitation and hallucination.
- Positive response to test may avoid CT and lumbar puncture for evaluation of altered mental status.

Contraindications

- Known allergy to cholinergic agonist or sulfites
- Overdose of tricyclic antidepressant, or ECG findings suggestive of it (QRS widening, R wave in the ECG lead aVR)
- History of asthma, heart disease, diabetes, seizure disorder, or inflammation of iris or ciliary body

Method of Administration

- Patient is connected to a cardiac monitor, and atropine is available at the bedside.
- Physostigmine is administered by slow intravenous push over 5 minutes; adults, 0.5 to 2.0 mg; pediatric, 0.02 mg/kg up to 2.0 mg; it may be repeated once after 5 to 10 minutes if the patient's mental status does not improve.

Potential Adverse Effects

- These are more common with larger doses and faster rates of administration.
- Muscarinic effects include nausea, vomiting, diarrhea, sweating, bronchorrhea, bradycardia, and hypotension; cardiac dysrhythmia may occur.
- Nicotinic effects (weakness, fasciculation) also may occur.
- Seizures may occur.

ADJUNCTIVE TREATMENT

Agitation or Hallucinosis

- A benzodiazepine with which the provider has experience is administered.

—Diazepam. Adult dose is 5 to 10 mg intravenously; pediatric dose is 0.2 to 0.5 mg/kg intravenously; dose is repeated at 10-minute intervals, titrating to effect
—Lorazepam is an alternative. Adult dose is 1 to 2 mg intravenously; pediatric dose is 0.05 mg/kg, repeated at 10-minute intervals, and titrated to effect; the airway should be monitored closely.

- Repeated doses of physostigmine are not recommended for behavior control, because although physostigmine reverses behavioral effects, the symptoms usually recur within 30 to 60 minutes.

Seizure

- A patent airway must be ensured.
- A benzodiazepine is administered for initial control. If seizures persist or recur, another anticonvulsant such as phenobarbital may be added.

Dysrhythmias or Conduction Abnormalities

- Standard ACLS guidelines for control of dysrhythmia should be followed.
- Seizures are to be controlled and acidemia corrected.
- If QRS widening or dysrhythmia persists, sodium bicarbonate is administered, 1 to 2 mEq/kg as an intravenous bolus, repeated as needed for widened QRS; the pH should not exceed 7.55.

Not Recommended Therapies

Physostigmine should not be used when the diagnosis of anticholinergic toxicity is already apparent.

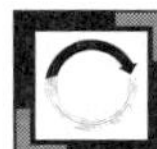

Follow-Up

PATIENT MONITORING

Vital signs, mental status, and fluid volume status should be followed until effects resolve.

EXPECTED COURSE AND PROGNOSIS

- Anticholinergic effects often persist for 24 to 48 hours; longer following a large exposure or continued gastrointestinal absorption due to anticholinergic effects.
- Hyperthermia and rhabdomyolysis can result from agitation that is improperly controlled, especially by the sole use of physical restraints.

DISCHARGE CRITERIA/INSTRUCTIONS

- From the emergency department. Patients who have not developed altered mental status, seizures, or dysrhythmia during 6 to 12 hours of observation (4 to 6 hours of observation following last dose of benzodiazapine) may be discharged following gastrointestinal decontamination and psychiatric evaluation, if needed.
- From the hospital. The patient may be discharged after resolution of toxic effects and psychiatric evaluation, if needed.

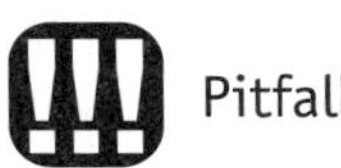

Pitfalls

DIAGNOSIS

- The health-care provider should consider other causes of altered mental status.
- A minor improvement in mental status should not be attributed to physostigmine; the beneficial effect of physostigmine is usually obvious.

TREATMENT

The health-care professional should not use physostigmine as a therapeutic agent instead of diagnostic agent or when the ECG suggests type 1a antidysrhythmic toxicity (e.g., tricyclic antidepressants).

ICD-9-CM 971.1

Poisoning by drugs primarily affecting the autonomic nervous system: parasympatholytics (anticholinergics and antimuscarinics) and spasmolytics.

See also: SECTION II, Seizures; SECTION III, Physostigmine chapter; and SECTION IV, Plants—Anticholinergic, Antihistamines—Nonsedating, Antihistamines—Over-the-Counter, Phenothiazines, and Antidepressants—Tricyclic chapters.

RECOMMENDED READING

Ellenhorn MJ. Antimuscarinic drugs. In: *Ellenhorn's medical toxicology,* 2nd ed. Baltimore: Williams & Wilkins, 1997:840–861.

Author: Edwin K. Kuffner

Reviewer: Richard C. Dart

Antidepressants—Bicyclic

Basics

DESCRIPTION

The bicyclic antidepressants are medications used orally in the treatment of depression and, in some cases, obsessive-compulsive disorder.

FORMS AND USES

- Venlafaxine hydrochloride (Effexor) is prescribed for depression at 75 mg/day orally, increasing to 225 to 375 mg/day over ensuing weeks.
- Venlafaxine is available in 25-mg, 37.5-mg, 50-mg, 75-mg, and 100-mg tablets.
- Viloxazine is an investigational bicyclic agent.
- Zimeldine was withdrawn from the worldwide market in 1983 because of association with Guillain-Barré syndrome.

TOXIC DOSE

The adult toxic dose is an ingestion of 4 g, which is associated with CNS depression.

PATHOPHYSIOLOGY

- Bicyclic antidepressants produce therapeutic effects by inhibiting the reuptake of serotonin and norepinephrine, thereby increasing synaptic concentrations.
- The drug is well absorbed from the gastrointestinal tract, with a large volume of distribution (6–7 L/kg).
- Metabolism occurs primarily through the cytochrome P450 system in the liver.

EPIDEMIOLOGY

- The incidence of poisoning is rising due to increased use and availability.
- Toxic effects following exposure are typically mild. Death has not yet been reported.

CAUSES

- Poisoning is usually the result of intentional ingestion.
- Child neglect should be considered if the patient is less than 1 year of age, suicide attempt if the patient is over 6 years of age.

Drug and Disease Interactions

- Blood levels of venlafaxine may increase if other drugs with similar induction of cytochrome P450 are discontinued.
- Combined ingestion of venlafaxine with a monoamine oxidase (MAO) inhibitor (isocarboxazid, phenelzine, tranylcypromine) may precipitate serotonin syndrome.
- CNS effects will be potentiated by sedative-hypnotic agents.
- Bicyclic antidepressants may potentiate the effects of sympathomimetic drugs.
- Due to cytochrome P450 induction, the dose should be decreased in the patient with hepatic or renal impairment.
- Older patients are more likely to be on polydrug regimens that could potentially contain drugs that interact with venlafaxine.

PREGNANCY AND LACTATION

- US FDA Pregnancy Category C. The drug exerts animal teratogenic or embryocidal effects, but there are no controlled studies in women, or no studies are available in either animals or women.
- No adverse maternal effects during pregnancy in humans have been reported.

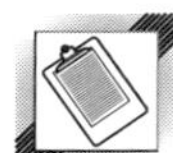

Diagnosis

DIFFERENTIAL DIAGNOSIS

- Toxicologic causes for CNS depression include, among others, anticonvulsants, alcohols, benzodiazepines, barbiturates, imidazolines, gammahydroxybutyrate (GHB), and narcotics.
- Nontoxicologic causes include metabolic abnormalities (hypoglycemia, hyponatremia, hypoxia), hypothermia, hypothyroidism, postictal states, infection or intracranial events (e.g., stroke or hemorrhage), and drug withdrawal.

SIGNS AND SYMPTOMS

The primary effect is mild CNS depression.

Vital Signs

- Tachycardia is common.
- Mild hypertension may occur.
- Hypothermia occurs rarely.
- Hyperthermia occurs if serotonin syndrome develops.

HEENT

Blurred vision and tinnitus may occur.

Dermatologic

Sweating may be present.

Cardiovascular

- Palpitations and hypertension develop initially.
- Conduction abnormalities such as prolonged QRS and QTc intervals occur rarely.
- Torsade de pointes have been reported with zimeldine.

Gastrointestinal

Nausea and vomiting, dry mouth, and constipation may occur.

Renal

Urinary retention may occur.

Fluids and Electrolytes

Syndrome of inappropriate antidiuretic hormone secretion may develop, although the mechanism is unclear.

Musculoskeletal

Tremor and myoclonus may develop.

Neurologic

- Headache may develop.
- Agitation may progress to confusion and mental status depression.
- Coma develops rarely and is not prolonged.
- Seizures have been reported rarely.

PROCEDURES AND LABORATORY TESTS

Essential Tests

No tests may be needed in minimally symptomatic patients.

Recommended Tests

- Serum electrolytes, BUN, and creatinine are measured to assess electrolyte abnormalities.
- Pulse oximetry is used to evaluate hypoxia as an etiology of altered mental status.
- ECG is used to evaluate the possibility of conduction abnormalities in massive ingestions.
- ECG, serum acetaminophen, and aspirin levels in an overdose setting are used to screen for occult ingestion.

Not Recommended Tests

Venlafaxine levels are not clinically useful.

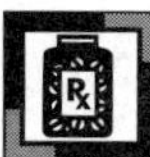

Treatment

- Treatment should focus on general supportive measures, treatment of seizures or hypotension, and monitoring for cardiac conduction abnormality.
- The dose and time of exposure should be determined for all substances involved.

DIRECTING PATIENT COURSE

The health-care professional should call the poison control center when:

- Cardiac, CNS, or other clinically significant effects are present.
- Toxic effects are not consistent with venlafaxine poisoning.
- Coingestant, drug interaction, or underlying disease present an unusual problem.

The patient should be referred to a health-care facility when:

- Attempted suicide or homicide is possible.
- Patient or caregiver seems unreliable.
- Cardiac, CNS, or other clinically significant effects are present.
- Toxic effects are not consistent with venlafaxine poisoning.
- Coingestant, drug interaction, or underlying disease presents an unusual problem.

Admission Considerations

Inpatient management is warranted for patients with seizure, cardiac conduction abnormality, or persistent sedation.

DECONTAMINATION

Out of Hospital

Decontamination is not recommended due to the potential for mental status depression.

In Hospital

- Gastric lavage should be performed in pediatric (tube size 24–32 French) or adult (tube size 36–42 French) patients for large ingestion presenting within 1 hour of ingestion or if serious effects are present.
- One dose of activated charcoal (1–2 g/kg) should be administered without a cathartic if a substantial ingestion has occurred within the previous few hours.

ANTIDOTES

There is no specific antidote for venlafaxine poisoning.

ADJUNCTIVE TREATMENT

- Physostigmine is contraindicated.
- Dysrhythmias or conduction abnormalities

—The standard advanced cardiac life support algorithms are used.
—Lidocaine is used for ventricular tachycardia or multifocal premature ventricular complexes. The adult dose is 50 to 100 mg intravenous bolus, followed by infusion of 2 to 4 mg/min titrated to desired effect. The pediatric dose is 1 mg/kg bolus, followed by infusion of 20 to 50 μg/kg/min titrated to effect. The bolus dose may be repeated in 10 to 15 minutes.
—Bretylium is administered at 5 mg/kg over 1 minute. If unsuccessful, the drug is administered at 10 mg/kg over 1 minute, repeated as necessary to a total dose of 30 mg/kg.

- Seizure

—A patent airway must be ensured.
—A benzodiazepine is administered for initial control. If seizures persist or recur, another anticonvulsant such as phenobarbital may be added.

- Hypotension. The patient should be treated with isotonic fluid infusion, Trendelenburg position, and, if needed, vasopressors. Dopamine is preferred and norepinephrine is added for refractory hypotension.
- Hemodialysis and hemoperfusion are not useful.

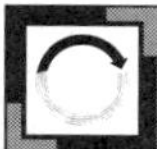

Follow-Up

PATIENT MONITORING

Cardiac and respiratory function should be monitored continuously until toxicity resolves.

EXPECTED COURSE AND PROGNOSIS

- Signs of toxicity usually develop within the first few hours after ingestion.
- Effects peak within 24 hours and resolve within 24 to 48 hours unless sequelae of seizures or hypotension intercede.
- Complications include:

—Hypoxic brain injury from prolonged seizures.
—Rhabdomyolysis with renal injury secondary to serotonin syndrome.

DISCHARGE CRITERIA/INSTRUCTIONS

The patient may be discharged from the emergency department or hospital when toxic effects resolve or stabilize, after decontamination, when ECG is normal for the patient, and after psychiatric evaluation, if needed.

PATIENT EDUCATION

Patients should be educated as to the hazards of combining bicyclic antidepressants with other medications, particularly MAO inhibitors or drugs that interfere with the cytochrome P450 system.

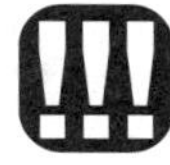

Pitfalls

DIAGNOSIS

- It is important to consider possible coingestants in suicidal attempts.
- All potential sources of altered mental status need to be evaluated.

TREATMENT

A potentially unprotected airway must be adequately controlled in an obtunded patient.

ICD-9-CM 969.0

Poisoning by psychotropic drugs: antidepressants.

See also: SECTION II, Serotonin Syndrome, Hypotension, and Seizure chapters.

RECOMMENDED READING

Ellenhorn MJ. Cyclic antidepressants. In: *Ellenhorn's medical toxicology: diagnosis and treatment of human poisoning,* 2nd ed. Baltimore: Williams & Wilkins, 1997:648–650.

Montgomery SA. Venlafaxine: a new dimension in antidepressant pharmacotherapy. *J Clin Psychiatry* 1993;54:119–126.

Author: Lada Kokan

Reviewer: Gerald F. O'Malley

Antidepressants—Tricyclic

Basics

DESCRIPTION

Tricyclic antidepressants (TCAs) are common oral medications used for the treatment of depression and several other medical disorders.

FORMS AND USES

- Pharmaceutical preparations include amitriptyline [Elavil, Etrafon (also contains perphenazine), Limbitrol (also contains chlordiazepoxide), Triavil (also contains perphenazine)], clomipramine (Anafranil), desipramine (Norpramin), doxepin (Adapin, Sinequan), dothiepin, imipramine (Tofranil), lofepramine, nortriptyline (Pamelor), protriptyline (Vivactil), and trimipramine (Surmontil).
- TCAs are used to treat depression, enuresis, headaches, chronic pain, and neuropathies, and are occasionally used for antihistamine effects.
- Representative doses for amitriptyline, desipramine, or imipramine are 75 to 300 mg/day in divided doses for adults; 50 to 100 mg/day for adolescents; and 1.0 to 1.5 mg/kg/day for children (9–12 years old).
- Representative doses for nortriptyline are 75 to 150 mg/day for adults; 30 to 50 mg/day in divided doses for adolescents.

TOXIC DOSE

Clinically significant toxicity has occurred in children at doses as low as 100 mg. Adults begin to develop toxic effects after ingesting two to three times the daily dose.

PATHOPHYSIOLOGY

- Cyclic antidepressants block the neuronal reuptake of norepinephrine, serotonin, and dopamine.
- Toxic effects are caused by myocardial sodium channel blockade as well as anticholinergic, adrenergic, and alpha-blocking effects.

EPIDEMIOLOGY

- Poisoning is common.
- Toxic effects following exposure are typically moderate.
- Severe toxicity or death may occur in large ingestions.

CAUSES

- Poisoning is usually a suicidal ingestion.
- Child neglect or abuse should be considered if the patient is less than 1 year of age, suicide attempt if the patient is over 6 years of age.

DRUG AND DISEASE INTERACTIONS

A concomitant overdose with a monoamine oxidase inhibitor may produce severe toxicity such as serotonin syndrome.

PREGNANCY AND LACTATION

- Clomipramine, desipramine, doxepin, and protriptyline. US FDA Pregnancy Category C. The drug exerts animal teratogenic or embryocidal effects, but there are no controlled studies in women, or no studies are available in either animals or women.
- Amitriptyline, dothiepin, imipramine, and nortriptyline. US FDA Pregnancy Category D. Evidence of human fetal risk exists, but benefits in certain situations (e.g., life-threatening situations or serious diseases) may make use of the drug acceptable.

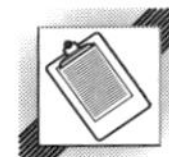

Diagnosis

DIFFERENTIAL DIAGNOSIS

- Other toxicologic causes of seizure include theophylline, isoniazid, and lindane.
- Other toxicologic causes of seizure that are especially associated with cardiac conduction abnormality include lidocaine, quinine, quinidine, encainide, cocaine, procainamide, and antihistamines.
- Nontoxicologic causes include status epilepticus from other causes (CNS tumor or bleed, meningitis, encephalitis, etc.).

SIGNS AND SYMPTOMS

Cardiac conduction abnormality, seizure, and CNS depression are characteristic and may be complicated by hyperthermia, acidosis, hypotension, rhabdomyolysis, and acute renal failure in serious cases.

Vital Signs

Tachycardia is common.

Cardiovascular

- Sinus tachycardia is common.
- Prolonged QRS and QT intervals and hypotension occur commonly and may deteriorate abruptly into ventricular dysrhythmia.

Pulmonary

- Respiratory depression or aspiration pneumonitis may develop.
- Adult respiratory distress syndrome has developed after severe overdose.

Renal

Acute renal failure may develop due to rhabdomyolysis.

Fluids and Electrolytes

Metabolic acidosis may develop due to seizures.

Neurologic

Altered mental status is common, ranging from drowsiness and confusion to seizures and coma.

PROCEDURES AND LABORATORY TESTS

Essential Tests

ECG with continuous cardiac monitoring is necessary.

- Sinus tachycardia is common.
- Limb lead QRS width greater than or equal to 0.1 seconds indicates toxicity.
- QRS width greater than or equal to 0.12 seconds is associated with an increased incidence of seizures; QRS width greater than or equal to 0.16 seconds is associated with an increased incidence of ventricular dysrhythmias.
- QRS complex with an R wave greater than or equal to 3 mm in lead aVR is associated with an increased risk of seizure or dysrhythmia.

Recommended Tests

- Arterial blood gases are measured because acidemia predisposes to more severe cardiac effects.
- Serum electrolytes, BUN, and creatinine levels are measured to assess other causes of hypotension, rhabdomyolysis, or dysrhythmia.
- Serum creatine kinase is assessed in patients with prolonged seizures or coma to assess rhabdomyolysis.
- Serum acetaminophen and aspirin levels in an overdose setting are used to detect occult ingestion.
- Head CT, lumbar puncture, bacterial cultures, and other tests are used to assess other causes of confusion, coma, or seizure.

Not Recommended Tests

Serum TCA levels are not clinically useful in overdose.

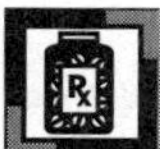

Treatment

• Treatment is focused on aggressive airway management, seizure control, support of cardiovascular function, and serum alkalinization in patients with dysrhythmia or QRS widening.
• The dose and time of exposure should be determined for all substances involved.

DIRECTING PATIENT COURSE

The health-care professional should call the poison control center when:

• Hypotension, dysrhythmia, QRS widening, seizure, or coma are present.
• Toxic effects are not consistent with TCA poisoning.
• Coingestant, drug interaction, or underlying disease presents an unusual problem.

The patient should be referred to a health-care facility when:

• Overdose effects are present (including persistent sinus tachycardia).
• Attempted suicide or homicide is possible.
• Patient or caregiver seems unreliable.
• Coingestant, drug interaction, or underlying disease presents an unusual problem.

Admission Considerations

Inpatient management in an intensive care setting is warranted for all patients with altered mental status, seizure, dysrhythmia (including persistent sinus tachycardia), or QRS widening.

DECONTAMINATION

Out of Hospital

Emesis should not be induced; coma or seizure may develop abruptly.

In the Hospital

• Gastric lavage should be performed in pediatric (tube size 24–32 French) or adult (tube size 36–42 French) patients for large ingestion presenting within 1 hour of ingestion or if serious effects are present.
• One dose of activated charcoal (1–2 g/kg) is administered without a cathartic if a substantial ingestion has occurred within the previous few hours.
• Due to anticholinergic effects, a second dose of activated charcoal (0.5–1.0 g/kg) may be worthwhile 2 to 4 hours after the first dose, but evidence does not support the use of further doses.

ANTIDOTES

There is no specific antidote for TCA poisoning.

ADJUNCTIVE TREATMENT

Recommended

Hypotension

• The patient should receive 10 to 20 ml/kg of 0.9% saline intravenously and be placed in the Trendelenburg position; further fluid therapy is guided by central pressure monitoring to avoid volume overload.
• If hypotension is unresponsive, a vasopressor is administered. The dose of dopamine is 2 to 5 μg/kg/min intravenously titrated to effect up to 20 μg/kg/min; rates above this are unlikely to provide further benefit. If hypotension continues to be unresponsive, norepinephrine may be added at 0.1 to 0.2 μg/kg/min and titrated to effect. Caution: A high rate of infusion may cause tissue ischemia.

Dysrhythmia or Conduction Abnormality

• Procainamide, quinidine, or other class IA antidysrhythmic agents should be avoided.
• Seizures must be controlled concurrently.
• If QRS widening or dysrhythmia develops, sodium bicarbonate is administered, 1 to 2 mEq/kg as an intravenous bolus, repeated as needed to the narrow QRS interval, but arterial pH should not exceed 7.55.
• Simultaneous hyperventilation and bicarbonate therapy must be administered with caution because the combination may cause severe alkalemia and clinical deterioration.
• Lidocaine may be added if sodium bicarbonate alone is not effective.

—Adult dosage is 50 to 100 mg by intravenous bolus, followed by an infusion of 2 to 4 mg/min, titrated to effect.
—Pediatric dosage is 1 mg/kg bolus up to 100 mg followed by infusion of 20 to 50 μg/kg/min, titrated to effect.
—The bolus dose may be repeated in 10 to 15 minutes.

Seizure

• A benzodiazepine is administered for initial control.

—Diazepam. Adult dose is 5 to 10 mg initially, repeated every 10 minutes or longer if needed; pediatric dose is 0.2 to 0.5 mg/kg, repeated every 10 minutes or longer if needed; airway should be monitored.
—Lorazepam. Adult dose is 2 to 4 mg by intravenous push over 2 to 5 minutes, repeated every 10 minutes or longer if needed; pediatric dose is 0.1 mg/kg by intravenous push over 2 to 5 minutes, not to exceed 4 mg per dose, and repeated every 10 minutes or longer if needed; airway should be monitored.

• If seizures persist or recur, another anticonvulsant such as phenobarbital or phenytoin should be added.

Not Recommended

• Continuous infusion of sodium bicarbonate is discouraged.
• The use of flumazenil in patients with ECG evidence of TCA overdose is contraindicated.

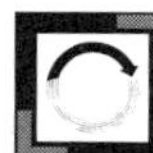

Follow-Up

PATIENT MONITORING

All patients should receive continuous respiratory and cardiac monitoring until discharge.

EXPECTED COURSE AND PROGNOSIS

• Most adverse effects develop early.
• Patients who survive this early period without sequelae usually recover completely.
• Possible complications include permanent neurologic injury from sustained hypotension, seizures, or hypoxia.

DISCHARGE CRITERIA/INSTRUCTIONS

• From the emergency department

—Patients who do not develop seizure, QRS widening, hypotension, or dysrhythmia (other than mild transient sinus tachycardia) during 6 hours of observation may be discharged after gastrointestinal decontamination and psychiatric evaluation, if needed.
—ECG criteria are less well defined in children, and most children should be admitted after significant TCA ingestion.

• From hospital. Patients may be discharged from the hospital after clinical effects have resolved and the ECG has been normal for 24 hours.

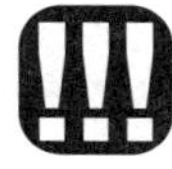

Pitfalls

DIAGNOSIS

Patients with TCA overdose generally do not have an overt anticholinergic syndrome.

TREATMENT

• Patients may deteriorate abruptly.
• Aggressive airway management and careful monitoring are critical.

ICD-9-CM 969.0

Poisoning by psychotropic agents: antidepressants.

See also: SECTION II, Hypotension, Neuroleptic Malignant Syndrome and Serotonin Syndrome, Seizure, and Ventricular Dysrhythmia; SECTION III, Sodium Bicarbonate chapters.

RECOMMENDED READING

Boehnert MT, Lovejoy FH. Value of the QRS duration versus the serum drug level in predicting seizures and ventricular arrhythmias after an acute overdose of tricyclic antidepressants. *N Engl J Med* 1985;313:474–479.

Callaham M, Kassel D. Epidemiology of fatal tricyclic antidepressant ingestion: implications for management. *Ann Emerg Med* 1985;14:1–9.

Author: Katherine M. Hurlbut

Reviewer: Richard C. Dart

Antidysrhythmic Agents—Class IA Quinidine and Disopyramide

Basics

DESCRIPTION

Quinidine and disopyramide are used for the treatment of life-threatening ventricular dysrhythmia.

FORMS AND USES

- Quinidine

—Quinidine gluconate 324 mg as sustained-release tablets (Quinaglute, Dura-Tabs); given orally, 324 to 972 mg every 8 to 12 hours.
—Quinidine sulfate 300 mg as sustained-release tablets (Quinidex, Extentabs) and 200 mg tablets as standard formulation; given orally, 200 to 400 mg every 4 to 6 hours.
—Quinidine polygalacturonate (Cardioquin) given orally, 275 mg two to three times daily.

- Disopyramide includes 100- and 150-mg tablets in standard (Norpace) and extended-release formulations (Norpace CR) and is given orally, 400 to 800 mg/day in divided doses.
- Procainamide is discussed in a separate chapter.

TOXIC DOSE

The precise toxic dose has not been established. However, toxic effects may develop just slightly above the therapeutic dose.

PATHOPHYSIOLOGY

- Antidysrhythmic class IA agents stabilize cardiac cell membranes by retarding the fast sodium channel, slowing phase zero of the action potential (depolarization), and depressing cardiac conduction velocity.
- Slowing of gastrointestinal motility following overdose due to anticholinergic effects of the drugs may result in delayed or prolonged toxicity.
- Diarrhea while on quinidine therapy is common and may potentiate ventricular dysrhythmias by producing hypokalemia.

EPIDEMIOLOGY

- Poisoning is uncommon.
- Toxic effects following exposure are typically mild to moderate.
- Death occurs rarely, primarily in patients who deteriorate before reaching medical care.

CAUSES

- Toxic ingestion is usually intentional.
- Child neglect or abuse should be considered if the patient is less than 1 year of age, suicide attempt if the patient is older than 6 years of age.

RISK FACTORS

A preexisting cardiac conduction defect predisposes the patient to adverse effects, even at therapeutic doses.

Drug and Disease Interactions

- Abrupt discontinuation of phenobarbital, phenytoin, or another cytochrome P450 inducer causes serum quinidine levels to increase.
- Quinidine potentiates other agents that prolong the QT interval.

PREGNANCY AND LACTATION

US FDA Pregnancy Category C. These drugs exert animal teratogenic or embryocidal effects, but there are no controlled studies in women, or no studies in either animals or women.

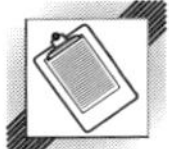

Diagnosis

DIFFERENTIAL DIAGNOSIS

- Toxicologic causes of CNS depression, seizure, and ECG conduction abnormality include class I antidysrhythmic agents, antihistamines, cocaine, β-receptors or calcium channel blockers, chloroquine, quinine, digoxin, phenothiazine, and cyclic antidepressants.
- Other causes of CNS depression and seizure include head trauma, elevated intracranial pressure, and electrolyte abnormalities.

SIGNS AND SYMPTOMS

- Primary effects are CNS depression, seizure, and ventricular dysrhythmia.
- Cinchona alkaloid toxicity (cinchonism) should be suspected in any patient describing sudden visual disturbance or tinnitus.

Vital Signs

Bradycardia and hypotension may accompany ventricular dysrhythmias.

HEENT

Cinchonism is a syndrome caused by quinidine-like drugs and is characterized by headache, fever, mydriasis, and tinnitus. Transient or permanent blindness may develop.

Cardiovascular

Severe depression of atrioventricular (AV) and ventricular conduction with ventricular tachycardia, ventricular fibrillation, and torsade de pointes may develop.

Pulmonary

Apnea and respiratory depression may occur in severe cases.

Gastrointestinal

Nausea, vomiting, and diarrhea are common.

Hematologic

Chronic quinidine use may produce immune disorders (e.g., hemolytic anemia, thrombocytopenia, a systemic lupus erythematosus-like syndrome, or sicca syndrome).

Neurologic

Coma and seizures may develop. A syncopal patient taking quinidine is considered to have suffered torsade de pointes until proven otherwise.

PROCEDURES AND LABORATORY TESTS

Essential Tests

- ECG with continuous monitoring is used to assess QRS widening, QTc prolongation, ST-T wave abnormalities. QTc prolongation greater than 50% indicates toxicity (more reliable indicator than spot drug levels).
- Serum electrolytes, calcium, magnesium, and phosphorus levels are measured to assess other causes of dysrhythmia.

Recommended Tests

- Plasma levels are available but unlikely to affect treatment of overdose. Quinidine may produce cinchonism with levels greater than 8 μg/ml and cardiac toxicity common with levels greater than 14 μg/ml.
- Serum acetaminophen and aspirin levels in an overdose setting should be measured to detect occult ingestion.

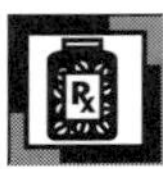

Treatment

- Treatment should focus on airway control and management of dysrhythmias.
- Dose and time of exposure should be determined for all substances ingested.

DIRECTING PATIENT COURSE

The health-care professional should call the poison control center when:

- Hypotension, dysrhythmia, or other severe effects are present.
- Toxic effects are not consistent with class IA antidysrhythmic poisoning.
- Coingestant, drug interaction, or underlying disease presents an unusual problem.

The patient should be referred to a health-care facility when:

- Attempted suicide or homicide is possible.
- Patient or caregiver seems unreliable.
- Toxic effects are present.
- Coingestant, drug interaction, or underlying disease presents an unusual problem.

Admission Considerations

Inpatient management is warranted for patients with cinchonism, patients who have cardiac, neurologic, or ocular effects, or those patients who have ingested a large amount of a sustained-release product.

DECONTAMINATION

Out of Hospital

Do not induce emesis; coma or seizure may develop abruptly.

In Hospital

- Gastric lavage is called for in pediatric (tube size 24–32 French) or adult (tube size 36–42 French) patients for large ingestion presenting within 1 hour of ingestion or if serious effects are present.
- One dose of activated charcoal (1–2 g/kg) should be administered without a cathartic if a substantial ingestion has occurred. Due to anticholinergic effects, a second dose of charcoal (0.5–1 g/kg) may be worthwhile 2 to 4 hours after the first dose.
- For patients who have ingested sustained-release preparations, whole-bowel irrigation should be considered.

ANTIDOTES

There is no specific antidote for class IA antidysrhythmic agents.

ADJUNCTIVE TREATMENT

- Cardiac pacing may be useful in patients with bradycardia or AV block not responsive to other measures.
- Hemodialysis is not useful for quinidine, but may be useful in severe disopyramide poisoning due to the small volume of distribution.
- Cardiac bypass may be used to maintain perfusion and to allow continued quinidine metabolism in patients with refractory dysrhythmia or hypotension.

Bradydysrhythmia

Standard agents, including atropine and isoproterenol, are usually ineffective. Early use of a pacemaker is recommended.

Ventricular Dysrhythmias

Sodium Bicarbonate

- $NaHCO_3$ 1 to 2 mEq/kg bolus intravenously is used to narrow the QRS complex. It may be repeated as needed to narrow the QRS complex, but arterial pH should not exceed 7.55. Simultaneous hyperventilation and bicarbonate therapy must be administered cautiously because it may cause severe alkalemia.
- Seizures need to be controlled concurrently.

Lidocaine

- Adult dose is 1.0 to 1.5 mg/kg intravenous push. Infusion should be titrated from 1 to 4 mg/min to maintain suppression. Boluses of 0.50 to 0.75 mg/kg are repeated and maintenance infusion increased every 5 to 10 minutes until ventricular tachycardia resolves or a total of 3 mg/kg has been given.
- Pediatric dose is 1 mg/kg intravenously, intraosseously, or endotracheally. The same dose may be repeated in 10 to 15 minutes. If a second dose is required, the infusion should be started at 20 to 50 μg/kg/min.
- The dose should be reduced in patients with hepatic insufficiency, congestive heart failure, or cardiogenic shock, or in patients over 70 years of age.

Phenytoin or Fosphenytoin

- Indications. Ventricular dysrhythmia that is unresponsive to other agents.
- Method of administration

—Phenytoin loading dose. Adult and pediatric dose is 15 to 20 mg/kg intravenously. The rate of infusion should not exceed 50 mg/min (adult) or 1.5 mg/kg/min (pediatric).
—Maintenance dose. Adult dose is 100 mg every 6 to 8 hours.
—ECG and blood pressure need monitoring during infusion; the infusion must be stopped if dysrhythmia or hypotension occurs.
—Fosphenytoin loading dose is 15 to 20 mg of phenytoin equivalents/kg given at a rate of 100 to 150 mg phenytoin equivalents/min.

- Bretylium should be avoided because β-blocking effects may worsen hypotension.
- Other class IA antidysrhythmic agents should be avoided because they may worsen dysrhythmias.

Torsade de Pointes

- If present, electrolyte abnormalities must be corrected.
- Procainamide, amiodarone, or bretylium should be avoided because they too prolong the QT interval.
- If patient is unresponsive, overdrive pacing may be used.

Magnesium Sulfate ($MgSO_4$)

- Adult dose is 1 to 2 g intravenous push; may be repeated in 10 to 15 minutes. Intravenous infusion is begun at 2 to 10 mg/min, titrated to antidysrhythmic effect.
- Pediatric dose is 25 to 50 mg/kg intravenously over 5 minutes.

Isoproterenol

- Adult dose is 2 to 4 μg/ml at an initial rate of 0.5 to 1.0 μg/min, titrated to effect.
- Pediatric dose is 0.1 μg/kg/min, titrated to effect.

Hypotension

- Primary treatment is correction of dysrhythmia.
- The patient should be administered 10 to 20 ml/kg 0.9% saline and, if needed, a vasopressor.

Seizures

- A patent airway must be ensured.
- Benzodiazepine is used for initial control. If seizures persist or recur, another anticonvulsant, such as phenobarbital, is added.

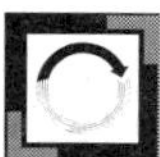

Follow-Up

PATIENT MONITORING

Patients require monitoring of electrolytes and cardiac rhythm throughout hospitalization.

EXPECTED COURSE AND PROGNOSIS

- After acute overdose, toxicity usually becomes apparent within hours.
- Survival is expected if patient receives appropriate aggressive care before anoxic injury intercedes.

DISCHARGE CRITERIA/INSTRUCTIONS

- From the emergency department. The asymptomatic patient with a normal ECG can be discharged after gastrointestinal decontamination, a 6-hour observation period (12 hours for sustained-release preparations), and psychiatric evaluation, if needed.
- From the hospital. The patient can be discharged after toxic effects have resolved and after psychiatric evaluation, if needed.

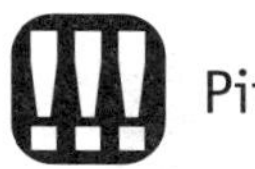

Pitfalls

DIAGNOSIS

It is important to recognize sustained-release preparations as the source of delayed or prolonged toxicity.

TREATMENT

The failure to correct diarrhea-induced hypokalemia may allow toxicity to develop at the therapeutic level of dosage.

ICD-9-CM 972.0

Poisoning by agents primarily affecting the cardiovascular system: cardiac rhythm regulators.

See also: SECTION II, Bradycardia, Hypotension, Seizures, and Ventricular Dysrhythmias chapters; and SECTION III, Procainamide chapter.

RECOMMENDED READING

Ellenhorn MJ. Antiarrhythmic drugs. In: *Medical toxicology. 2nd ed.* Baltimore: Williams & Wilkins, 1997:506–513.

Hruby K, Missliwetz J. Poisoning with oral antiarrhythmic drugs. *Int J Clin Pharmacol Ther Toxicol* 1985;23:253–257.

Authors: Gerald F. O'Malley and Katherine M. Hurlbut

Reviewer: Richard C. Dart

Antidysrhythmic Agents—Class IB

Basics

DESCRIPTION

The class IB antidysrhythmic agents include lidocaine, xylocaine, mexiletine, and tocainide.

FORMS AND USES

- Lidocaine HCL [EMLA cream (lidocaine 2.5%), viscous gel (2%–4% lidocaine)] is used as a topical anesthetic.
- Xylocaine for injection (50- or 100-mg prefilled syringes and ampules) is used for ventricular dysrhythmia as well as local anesthesia.
- Mexiletine HCL (Mexitil in 150-, 200-, or 250-mg capsules) is used for the treatment of life-threatening ventricular dysrhythmia. Dosage is 200 to 400 mg orally every 8 hours.
- Tocainide HCL (Tonocard in 100- or 600-mg tablets) is also used for the treatment of life-threatening ventricular dysrhythmia. Typical adult dosage is 1,200 to 1,800 mg/day in divided doses.
- Phenytoin HCL (Dilantin) is also used (see SECTION IV, Phenytoin chapter, for details).

TOXIC DOSE

Toxicity has occurred after ingestion of 5 to 10 mg/kg of lidocaine. The dose for tissue infiltration should not exceed 5 mg/kg (7 mg/kg for a lidocaine-epinephrine combination product).

PATHOPHYSIOLOGY

- Antidysrhythmic class IB agents depress phase IV depolarization of the cardiac action potential by producing a blockade of the fast inward sodium channel. This reduces spontaneous pacemaker activity and slows propagation of impulse conduction through myocardial tissue.
- These agents have a narrow therapeutic range, and toxicity may develop with therapeutic doses. Conduction delays and asystole may occur after a large intravenous dose of lidocaine.

EPIDEMIOLOGY

- Poisoning is uncommon.
- Toxic effects following an overdose are typically moderate, with death occurring in patients who deteriorate before reaching medical care or who receive a massive acute overdose.

CAUSES

- Toxicity from parenteral medication is often iatrogenic.
- An overdose from oral medications is usually an intentional ingestion
- Child neglect or abuse should be considered if the patient is less than 1 year of age, suicide attempt if the patient is over 6 years of age.

RISK FACTORS

A preexisting cardiac conduction defect predisposes the patient to adverse effects even at therapeutic doses.

DRUG AND DISEASE INTERACTIONS

- Theophylline enhances the toxicity of mexiletine.
- All antidysrhythmic class IB agents have an additive effect when combined with negative inotropic or chronotropic medications.

PREGNANCY AND LACTATION

All agents. US FDA Pregnancy Category C. The drug exerts animal teratogenic or embryocidal effects, but there are no controlled studies in women, or no studies are available in animals or women.

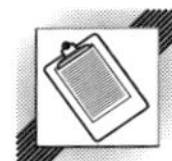

Diagnosis

DIFFERENTIAL DIAGNOSIS

- Toxicologic causes of CNS depression, seizure, and ECG conduction abnormalities include class I antidysrhythmics, antihistamines, cocaine, β-receptors or calcium channel blockers, quinine, chloroquine, digoxin, phenothiazine, and cyclic antidepressants, among others.
- Other causes of CNS depression and seizure include head trauma, elevated intracranial pressure, and electrolyte abnormalities.

SIGNS AND SYMPTOMS

Restlessness is often the first sign of toxicity. CNS effects typically develop before dysrhythmia. Toxicity of intravenous lidocaine is immediate.

Vital Signs

Bradycardia and hypotension are common after serious ingestion.

HEENT

- Diplopia and nystagmus have been reported with tocainide.
- Miosis and tinnitus have been reported with mexiletine and lidocaine at high doses.

Cardiovascular

Various dysrhythmias ranging from nodal bradycardia to third-degree atrioventricular (AV) block and asystole may occur.

Pulmonary

- Apnea and respiratory depression occur in a serious overdose.
- A diagnostic ECG effect has not been defined. Antidysrhythmic class IB agents do not typically affect the ECG in therapeutic doses, although the QT interval may be prolonged.

Gastrointestinal

Nausea, vomiting, and abdominal pain are common.

Hematologic

Methemoglobinemia may occur in lidocaine toxicity.

Neurologic

Neurologic effects occur early, ranging from restlessness, dizziness, and confusion to irritability, frank psychosis, seizure, and coma.

LABORATORY PROCEDURES AND TESTS

Essential Tests

- ECG with continuous monitoring is used to assess evidence of conduction delay, enhanced automaticity, or QTc prolongation. Should any of these be present, prompt aggressive treatment is needed.
- Serum levels may be available, but treatment should not be delayed for blood levels to confirm the diagnosis.
- Serum electrolytes, calcium, magnesium, BUN, creatinine, and glucose are measured to assess other causes of dysrhythmias.

Recommended Tests

- Arterial blood gas. Circumoral paresthesia and subtle mental status changes may be misidentified as anxiety or hyperventilation.
- Additional drug assays (lithium, opiates) should be performed as needed to assess other causes of mental status depression, seizures, or hypotension.
- Serum acetaminophen and aspirin levels should be measured in an overdose setting to detect occult ingestion.

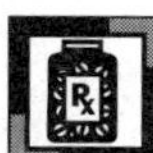

Treatment

- Treatment is focused on aggressive airway management, seizure control, and treatment of dysrhythmia.
- The dose and time of exposure should be determined for all substances involved.

DIRECTING PATIENT COURSE

The health-care professional should call the poison control center when:

- Altered mental status, bradycardia, or other severe effects are present.
- Toxic effects are not consistent with class IB antidysrhythmic poisoning.
- Coingestant, drug interaction, or underlying disease presents an unusual problem.

The patient should be referred to a health-care facility when:

- Attempted suicide or homicide is possible.
- Patient or caregiver seems unreliable.
- Toxic effects are present.
- Coingestant, drug interaction, or underlying disease presents an unusual problem.

Admission Considerations

Inpatient management is warranted for patients with apparent toxic effects of class IB antidysrhythmic agents.

DECONTAMINATION

Out of Hospital

Do not induce emesis; coma or seizures may develop abruptly.

In Hospital

- Gastric lavage should be performed in pediatric (tube size 24–32 French) or adult (tube size 36–42 French) patients for large ingestion presenting within 1 hour of ingestion or if serious effects are present.
- One dose of activated charcoal (1–2 g/kg) should be administered without a cathartic if a substantial ingestion has occurred within the previous few hours. However, this is not indicated for parenteral lidocaine exposure.

ANTIDOTES

There is no specific antidote for class IB antidysrhythmic agent poisoning.

ADJUNCTIVE TREATMENT

Bradydysrhythmia

- Atropine and isoproterenol are recommended, but usually ineffective. Early use of a pacemaker is recommended.
- Emergency cardiopulmonary bypass should be considered in life-threatening lidocaine toxicity because it can allow the liver to continue to metabolize lidocaine. Nontoxic levels may be reached within hours.

Ventricular Dysrhythmias

For stable patients, begin with drug therapy as described below. For unstable patients, use defibrillation followed by pharmacologic therapy.

- Sodium Bicarbonate. Administer $NaHCO_3$ 1 to 2 mEq/kg in an intravenous bolus and repeat as needed to suppress dysrhythmia, but do not exceed pH of 7.55. Simultaneous hyperventilation and bicarbonate therapy must be administered cautiously because it may cause severe alkalemia.
- Seizures should be controlled concurrently.
- Cardiac bypass may be used to maintain perfusion and allow continued quinidine or lidocaine metabolism in patients with refractory dysrhythmia or hypotension.
- Avoid bretylium because β-blocking effects may worsen hypotension. Avoid other class I antidysrhythmic agents because they may worsen the dysrhythmias.

Torsade de Pointes

- Correct electrolyte abnormalities if present.
- Avoid quinidine, disopyramide, procainamide, amiodarone, and bretylium, which also prolong the QT interval.
- Magnesium sulfate ($MgSO_4$)

—Adult dose is 1 to 2 g intravenous push, may be repeated in 10 to 15 minutes. Begin intravenous infusion at 2 to 10 mg/min, titrate upward to maintain antidysrhythmic effect.
—Pediatric dose is 25 to 50 mg/kg intravenously over 5 minutes.

- Isoproterenol

—Adult dose 2 to 4 μg/ml solution is infused intravenously at an initial rate of 0.5 to 1.0 μg/kg/min, titrated upward to effect.
—Pediatric dose is 0.1 μg/kg/min intravenous infusion, titrated to effect.
—If unresponsive, overdrive pacing may be used.

- Hypotension. The primary treatment is correction of the dysrhythmia. Also administer 10 to 20 ml/kg 0.9 saline, place patient in the Trendelenburg position, and administer a vasopressor, if needed. Dopamine is preferred, and norepinephrine is added for refractory hypotension.
- Seizures

—A patent airway must be ensured.
—A benzodiazepine is administered for initial control. If seizures persist or recur, another anticonvulsant such as phenobarbital may be added.

Cardiac Pacing

Cardiac pacing may be useful in patients with bradycardia or AV block who are not responsive to other measures.

- Not recommended. Hemodialysis, hemofiltration, hemoperfusion, forced diuresis, and urinary acidification are not recommended.

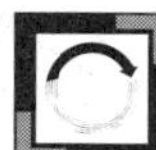

Follow-Up

PATIENT MONITORING

- Respiratory and cardiac function should be monitored continuously.
- Serial levels of mexiletine and tocainide should be monitored to assure they are decreasing.

EXPECTED COURSE AND PROGNOSIS

- The patient usually recovers unless sequelae of hypoxia intercede.
- Survival is expected if the patient receives appropriate aggressive care before anoxic injury intercedes.

DISCHARGE CRITERIA/INSTRUCTIONS

- From the emergency department. Discharge asymptomatic patients after gastrointestinal decontamination, a 6-hour observation period, and psychiatric evaluation, if needed.
- From the hospital. Discharge patients after toxic effects have resolved and after psychiatric evaluation, if needed.

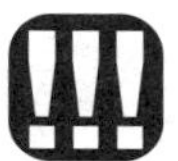

Pitfalls

DIAGNOSIS

- Failure to recognize subtle changes in mental status or neurological examination before seizures develop.
- An ECG alone should not be used to exclude antidysrhythmic class IB toxicity.

ICD-9-CM 968.5

Poisoning by other CNS depressants and anesthetics: surface (topical) and infiltration anesthetics.

See also: SECTION II, Hypotension and Seizure chapters; and SECTION III, Local Anesthetics and Phenytoin chapters.

RECOMMENDED READING

Brown DL, Skiendzielewski JJ. Lidocaine toxicity. *Ann Emerg Med* 1980;9:12;627–629.

Hruby K, Missliwetz J. Poisoning with oral antiarrhythmic drugs. *Int J Clin Pharmacol Ther Toxicol* 1985;23:253–257.

Author: Gerald F. O'Malley

Reviewer: Katherine M. Hurlbut

Antidysrhythmic Agents—Class IC

Basics

DESCRIPTION

The class IC antidysrhythmic agents include flecainide, propafenone, and moricizine.

FORMS AND USES

- Antidysrhythmic class IC agents are used in the treatment of life-threatening ventricular dysrhythmia.
- Flecainide (Tanbocor, in 50-, 100-, and 150-mg tablets). Adult dose is 100 to 200 mg twice daily. Pediatric dose is 100 to 200 $mg/m^2/day$ or 1 to 8 mg/kg/day in divided doses.
- Propafenone (Rhythmol, in 150- and 300-mg tablets). Adult dose is 600 to 900 mg/day orally. Pediatric dose is up to 600 $mg/m^2/24$ hours, or 8 to 10 mg/kg/day.
- Moricizine (Ethmozine, in 200-, 250-, and 300-mg tablets). Adult dose is 200 and 300 mg orally three times daily. Pediatric dose is not applicable because it is rarely needed in this group.
- Encainide, ajmaline, and prajmaline are used in Europe and the Middle East.

TOXIC DOSE

- Death has occurred after a flecainide ingestion of as little as three times the daily dose.
- Toxicity may develop at therapeutic drug levels in patients with underlying cardiac disease.

PATHOPHYSIOLOGY

- Antidysrhythmic class IC agents slow depolarization and conduction in normal cardiac tissue by inducing a blockade of the fast inward sodium channel during phase 0 (depolarization) of the action potential.
- Nonlinear kinetics are common for all agents; hence, a twofold increase in dosage may lead to a much greater elevation in the plasma level.

EPIDEMIOLOGY

- Poisoning is uncommon.
- Toxic effects are typically mild to moderate.
- Death occurs primarily in patients who collapse before medical care is received.

CAUSES

- Toxic ingestion is usually intentional.
- Child neglect or abuse should be considered if the patient is less than 1 year of age, suicide attempt if the patient is over 6 years of age.

RISK FACTORS

A preexisting cardiac conduction defect predisposes the patient to proarrhythmic effects even at therapeutic doses.

DRUG AND DISEASE INTERACTIONS

- Levels of antidysrhythmic class IC agents are increased by inhibitors of cytochrome P450: cimetidine, quinidine, ketoconazole, erythromycin, and birth control pills, among others.
- Class IC agents may cause lethal ventricular dysrhythmias when used to treat minimally symptomatic ventricular dysrhythmias after myocardial infarction.

PREGNANCY AND LACTATION

- Moricizine. US FDA Pregnancy Category B. Animal studies indicate no fetal risk, and there are no controlled human studies, or animal studies show an adverse fetal effect but well-controlled studies in women do not.
- Flecainide and propafenone. US FDA Pregnancy Category C. The drug exerts animal teratogenic or embryocidal effects, but there are no controlled studies in women, or no studies are available in animals or women.

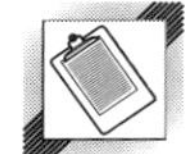

Diagnosis

DIFFERENTIAL DIAGNOSIS

- Toxicologic causes of CNS depression, seizure, and ECG conduction abnormality include class I antidysrhythmic agents, antihistamine, cocaine, β-receptor or calcium channel blockers, quinine, chloroquine, digoxin, phenothiazine, and cyclic antidepressants, among others.
- Other causes of CNS depression and seizure include head trauma, elevated intracranial pressure, and electrolyte abnormalities.

SIGNS AND SYMPTOMS

A large overdose that goes untreated often leads to severe cardiac dysrhythmia, depressed mentation, seizure, and cardiac arrest.

Vital Signs

Bradycardia and hypotension are common in a serious overdose.

Cardiovascular

- Conduction defects and wide-complex ventricular tachydysrhythmias are characteristic.
- Superventricular tachycardia with aberrant conduction also occurs.
- Atypical chest pain is reported in some patients in therapeutic doses.

Pulmonary

Propafenone may induce wheezing due to β-receptor blockade.

Gastrointestinal

Nausea and vomiting are common after an overdose.

Hepatic

An increase in liver transaminases may develop but is rarely severe.

Neurologic

- Visual hallucinations and dysarthria can occur in acute toxicity.
- Generalized depression of mental status, seizures may occur with serious overdose.

PROCEDURES AND LABORATORY TESTS

Essential Tests

- ECG with continuous monitoring is used to assess QRS widening, ST-T wave abnormalities, and QT prolongation. QT prolongation greater than 50% indicates toxicity. QRS widening or QT prolongation should prompt immediate intervention.
- Serum electrolytes, calcium, magnesium, BUN, and creatinine levels are measured to assess other causes of dysrhythmia.
- Arterial blood gas is measured in patients with clinical effects or receiving bicarbonate therapy.

Recommended Tests

- Serum acetaminophen and aspirin levels should be measured in an overdose setting to detect occult ingestion.
- Head CT, lumbar puncture, and bacterial cultures should be performed in patients with altered mental status of unknown etiology.

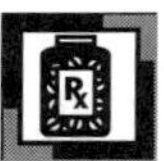

Treatment

- Treatment is focused on early airway management, seizure control and treatment of dysrhythmia.
- Dose and time of exposure should be determined for all substances involved.

DIRECTING PATIENT COURSE

The health-care professional should call the poison control center when:

- Altered mental status, cardiac toxicity, or other severe effects are present.
- Toxic effects are not consistent with class IC antidysrhythmic poisoning.
- Coingestant, drug interaction, or underlying disease presents an unusual problem.

The patient should be referred to a health-care facility when:

- Attempted suicide or homicide is possible.
- Patient or caregiver seems unreliable.
- Toxic effects are present.
- Coingestant, drug interaction, or underlying disease presents an unusual problem.

DECONTAMINATION

Out of Hospital

Do not induce emesis; coma or seizure may develop abruptly.

In Hospital

- Gastric lavage should be performed in pediatric (tube size 24–32 French) or adult (tube size 36–42 French) patients for large ingestion presenting within 1 hour of ingestion or if serious effects are present.
- One dose of activated charcoal (1–2 g/kg) should be administered without a cathartic if a substantial ingestion has occurred within the previous few hours.

Admission Consideration

Inpatient management is warranted for patients with apparent toxic effects or suspected suicidal ingestion of class IC antidysrhythmic agents.

ANTIDOTES

There is no specific antidote for class IC antidysrhythmic agent poisoning.

ADJUNCTIVE TREATMENT

Bradydysrhythmia

Standard agents including atropine and isoproterenol are usually ineffective. Early use of a pacemaker is recommended.

Ventricular Dysrhythmias

- For stable patients, begin with drug therapy as described below. For unstable patients use defibrillation followed by pharmacologic therapy as guided by the ACLS algorithm.
- Sodium bicarbonate. Administer $NaHCO_3$ 1 to 2 mEq/kg intravenous bolus and repeat as needed to narrow the QRS complex. Arterial pH should not exceed 7.55. Simultaneous hyperventilation and bicarbonate therapy must be administered cautiously because it may cause severe alkalemia. Control seizures concurrently.
- Lidocaine

—Adult dose is 1.0 to 1.5 mg/kg intravenous push. Titrate infusion from 1 to 4 mg/min to maintain suppression. Repeat with 0.5 to 0.75 mg/kg boluses and increase maintenance infusion every 5 to 10 minutes until ventricular tachycardia resolves or a total of 3 mg/kg has been given.
—Pediatric dose is 1 mg/kg intravenous push. May repeat same dose in 10 to 15 minutes. If a second dose is required, start infusion at 20 to 50 μg/kg/min.
—The dose should be reduced in patients with hepatic insufficiency, congestive heart failure, or cardiogenic shock, or in those over 70 years of age.

- Phenytoin or Fosphenytoin

—Phenytoin loading dose. Adults and pediatric dose is 15 to 20 mg/kg intravenous. The rate of infusion should not exceed 50 mg/min (adult) or 1.5 mg/kg/min (pediatric).
—Maintenance dose. Adult dose is 100 mg every 6 to 8 hours. Pediatric dose is 4 to 7 mg/kg/day in two divided doses.
—Monitor ECG and blood pressure during infusion; stop if dysrhythmia or hypotension occurs.
—Fosphenytoin loading dose is 15 to 20 or phenytoin equivalents/kg given at a rate of 100 to 150 phenytoin equivalents/min.

- Avoid bretylium because alpha blocking effects may worsen hypotension. Avoid class IA antidysrhythmic agents because they may worsen dysrhythmias.

Torsade de Pointes

- Correct electrolyte abnormalities if present.
- Avoid quinidine, disopyramide, procainamide, amiodarone or bretylium, which also prolong the QT interval.
- Magnesium sulfate ($MgSO_4$)

—Adult dose is 1 to 2 g intravenous push, and may be repeated in 10 to 15 minutes. Begin intravenous infusion at 2 to 10 mg/min, titrate to antidysrhythmic effect.
—Pediatric dose is 25 to 50 mg/kg intravenously over 5 minutes.

- Isoproterenol

—Adult dose is 2 to 4 μg/kg/min intravenous infusion, titrated to effect.
—Pediatric dose is 0.1 μg/kg/min intravenous infusion, titrated to effect.
—If unresponsive, overdrive pacing may be used.

Hypotension

The primary treatment is correction of the dysrhythmia. Also administer 10 to 20 ml/kg 0.9% saline, place patient in the Trendelenburg position, and administer a vasopressor, if needed. Dopamine is preferred and norepinephrine is added for refractory hypotension.

Seizures

- A patent airway must be ensured.
- A benzodiazepine is administered for initial control. If seizures persist or recur, another anticonvulsant such as phenobarbital may be added.

Cardiac Pacing

Cardiac pacing may be useful in patients with bradycardia or atrioventricular block not responsive to other measures.

Not Recommended

Hemodialysis, hemofiltration, hemoperfusion, forced diuresis, and urinary acidification are not recommended.

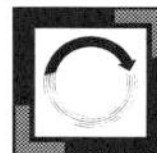

Follow-Up

PATIENT MONITORING

- Respiratory and cardiac function should be monitored continuously.
- Permanent neurologic injury may occur from hypotension, seizures, or hypoxia.

EXPECTED COURSE AND PROGNOSIS

- Most adverse effects develop soon after ingestion.
- Recovery is expected unless sequelae of hypoxia intercede.

DISCHARGE CRITERIA/INSTRUCTIONS

- From emergency department. There are no accepted criteria for discharge. Due to potential for delayed toxicity, most patients should be admitted if suicidal ingestion is possible.
- From the hospital. Discharge patient after toxic effects have resolved and after psychiatric evaluation, if needed.

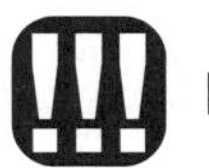

Pitfalls

DIAGNOSIS

Small increases in dosage may produce toxicity.

ICD-9-CM 968

Poisoning by other central nervous system depressants and anesthetics.

See also: SECTION II, Bradycardia, Hypotension, Seizure, and Ventricular Dysrhythmias chapters.

RECOMMENDED READING

Bigger JT, Hoffman BF. Antidysrhythmic drugs. In: Gilman et al., eds. *Pharmacologic basis of therapeutics.* New York: MacMillan, 1985:767–772.

Lewin NA, Osborn H. Antidysrhythmic agents. In: Goldfrank et al., eds. *Toxicologic emergencies,* 6th ed. Norwalk, CT: Appleton & Lange, 1998.

Author: Gerald F. O'Malley

Reviewer: Katherine M. Hurlbut

Antifungal Medications

Basics

DESCRIPTION

Antifungal medications include oral and parenteral medications active against an array of fungal infections.

FORMS AND USES

- Systemic preparations. Flucytosine (Ancobon), fluconazole (Diflucan), amphotericin B (Fungizone), clotrimazole (Lotrimin, Mycelex), nystatin (Mycostatin), ketoconazole (Nizoral), and itraconazole (Sporanox).
- Dermal preparations. Nystatin (Mycostatin, Mytrex, and Pedi-Dri).
- Vaginal preparations

—Butoconazole nitrate (Femstat), miconazole nitrate (Monistat 3), clotrimazole (Mycelex G, Lotrimin), terconazole (Terazol 3, Terazol 7), and tioconazole (Vagistat 1).
—See also SECTION IV, Griseofulvin chapter.

- Typical therapeutic dosages for systemic fungal infections

—Amphotericin B: 250 μg/kg/day with 1.0 mg/kg/day on alternate days, slow intravenous infusion over 4 to 6 hours
—Flucytosine 150 mg/kg/day orally in four divided doses
—Miconazole 1.8 to 3 g/day intravenously for 1 to 2 weeks (adults), or 20 to 40 mg/kg/day (children) in divided doses.
—Ketoconazole 200 to 400 mg/day orally
—Fluconazole 50 to 400 mg/day orally or intravenously
—Clotrimazole 10 mg to dissolve in the mouth every 4 hours
—Itraconazole 200 to 400 mg/day

- Therapeutic dosages for vaginal fungal infections

—Butoconazole 5 g vaginally every night for 3 days
—Miconazole 200 mg vaginally every night for 3 days
—Clotrimazole applied liberally to affected areas twice a day
—Terconazole 80 mg or 5 g vaginally every night for 3 days
—Tioconazole 4 to 6 g vaginally every night, one time dose

TOXIC DOSE

Toxic doses have not been established. Serious adverse effects may develop at therapeutic doses, particularly with amphotericin B.

PATHOPHYSIOLOGY

There are three antifungal categories:

- Polyene antifungals. The most important agent in this category is amphotericin B, which targets the kidney and the cardiovascular system.
- Synthetic nucleotide analogs. Flucytosine is the most important example. It interferes with DNA replication. Target organs are tissues that proliferate rapidly, such as bone marrow and gastrointestinal mucosal cells.
- Imidazole antifungals. Most are used topically to treat superficial fungal infections and exert their antifungal activity via alteration of fungal cell membranes and interference with the intracellular enzymes. Toxicity, when it occurs, is mild.

EPIDEMIOLOGY

- Poisoning is uncommon.
- Toxic effects following exposure are typically mild.
- In the case of amphotericin B, deaths have been reported after large intravenous overdose.
- Children, particularly neonates, may be at an increased risk for the development of cardiac toxicity from amphotericin.

CAUSES

- Overdose is usually attributable to accidental ingestion.
- Child neglect or abuse should be considered if the patient is less than 1 year of age, suicide attempt if the patient is over 6 years of age.

DRUG AND DISEASE INTERACTIONS

- Amphotericin B acts synergistically with any other drug that has nephrotoxic effects.
- The azole antifungals (e.g., ketoconazole) have increased plasma concentrations with digoxin, oral sulfonylurea, warfarin, and phenytoin.

PREGNANCY AND LACTATION

- Amphotericin B. US FDA Pregnancy Category B. Animal studies do not indicate a risk to the fetus, and there are no controlled human studies, or animal studies do show an adverse effect on the fetus but well-controlled studies in pregnant women have failed to demonstrate a risk to the fetus.
- Butoconazole, clotrimazole, flucytosine, fluconazole, itraconazole, ketoconazole, miconazole, nystatin, terconazole, and tioconazole. US FDA Pregnancy Category C. The drug exerts animal teratogenic or embryocidal effects, but there are no controlled studies in women, or no studies are available in either animals or women.
- All vaginal preparations are considered safe in pregnancy.
- Most of the azoles are secreted in breast milk in clinically significant amounts, and breastfeeding women should avoid their use.

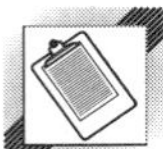

Diagnosis

DIFFERENTIAL DIAGNOSIS

Amphotericin B

Any toxicologic cause of acute renal failure, including heavy metals, ethylene glycol, herbal preparations, drugs of abuse (amphetamines, strychnine, cocaine, or pennyroyal oil), and over-the-counter drugs (aspirin or acetaminophen).

Flucytosine

- Any toxicologic or nontoxicologic cause of gastrointestinal distress, including gastroenteritis, heavy metals, nonsteroidal antiinflammatory drugs, salicylates, sulfasalazine, estrogen, ergotamine, and cathartics.
- Any toxicologic or nontoxicologic causes of bone marrow suppression, including neoplastic diseases, azathioprine, ganciclovir, and ticlopidine, among others.

SIGNS AND SYMPTOMS

- Polyene antifungals (e.g., amphotericin B). Nephrotoxicity occurs and may be associated with hyperkalemia, hypertension, ventricular dysrhythmia, and sudden death in overdose.
- Synthetic nucleotide analogs (e.g., flucytosine). Severe gastroenteritis and bone marrow depression may occur.
- Imidazole antifungals. Toxicity is limited to mild gastrointestinal effects.

Vital Signs

- Rapid infusion of amphotericin B may rarely result in cardiorespiratory arrest.
- Other agents may cause severe nausea and gastrointestinal fluid losses, which result in tachycardia and hypotension.
- Some of the azoles may cause fever as a side effect.

Dermatologic

- Amphotericin B can cause "red man" syndrome (rapid onset of erythema of hands, soles, face, and neck) during infusion.
- Fluconazole can cause Stevens-Johnson syndrome.

Cardiovascular

Amphotericin has rarely been associated with ventricular fibrillation, hypertension, and sudden cardiac death, probably due to hyperkalemia.

Pulmonary

Amphotericin B has been associated with pulmonary hypertension in therapeutic use.

Gastrointestinal

- Amphotericin B can cause nausea, vomiting, and diarrhea.
- Flucytosine can cause nausea and vomiting (universal), gastrointestinal hemorrhage, and sloughing.

Hepatic

- Amphotericin B can cause elevated liver function tests.
- All azoles may cause an asymptomatic elevation of transaminases.

Renal

Amphotericin B: azotemia in association with renal tubular acidosis is common.

Hematologic

- All three antifungal classes have been associated with rare cases of anemia, leukopenia, and thrombocytopenia.
- Amphotericin B has been associated with agranulocytosis, as well.

Fluids and Electrolytes

- Amphotericin B. Hypokalemia is common, but hyperkalemia seems involved when serious cardiac effects develop.
- Flucytosine. Hypokalemia with dehydration and loss of free body water may develop.

PROCEDURES AND LABORATORY TESTS

Essential Tests

- Amphotericin B or flucytosine

—ECG to detect cardiac rhythm disturbance
—Serum electrolytes, BUN, creatinine, and complete blood count (CBC) to detect hypokalemia, azotemia, and bone marrow suppression

Recommended Tests

- Amphotericin B

—Liver function test, PT/INR, PTT, calcium, magnesium, and phosphate may be abnormal following an overdose of certain of the azoles or amphotericin.
—CBC and platelet count should be monitored in the patient who is at risk for bone marrow depression.
—If gastrointestinal injury and sloughing is severe enough with flucytosine intoxication, endoscopy may allow quantification of mucosal damage.

Not Recommended Tests

Serum levels of any antifungal are not clinically useful.

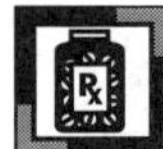

Treatment

- For all three classes, symptomatic and supportive care should be the focus of treatment.
- The dose and time of exposure should be determined for all substances involved.

DIRECTING PATIENT COURSE

The health-care provider should call the poison control center when:

- Cardiac arrest, severe hypertension, bone marrow suppression, or other severe effects are present.
- Toxic effects are not consistent with an antifungal agent.
- Coingestant, drug interaction, underlying disease presents an unusual problem.

The patient should be referred to a health-care facility when:

- Attempted suicide or homicide is possible.
- Patient or caregiver seems unreliable.
- Any toxic effects develop.
- Coingestant, drug interaction, or underlying disease presents an unusual problem.

Admission Considerations

Inpatient management is warranted for patients with cardiac dysrhythmia, persistent gastroenteritis, bone marrow depression, hepatitis, or coagulopathy.

DECONTAMINATION

Out of Hospital

- Amphotericin B. Emesis is not used because the drug is administered parenterally.
- Other agents. Ipecac should be administered to induce emesis within 1 hour of ingestion for alert pediatric or adult patients, if health-care evaluation will be delayed.

In Hospital

- Gastric lavage should be performed in pediatric (tube size 24–32 French) or adult (tube size 36–42 French) patients for large ingestion presenting within 1 hour of ingestion or if serious effects are present.
- One dose of activated charcoal (1–2 g/kg) should be administered without a cathartic if a substantial ingestion has occurred within the previous few hours.

ANTIDOTES

There is no specific antidote for antifungal poisoning.

ADJUNCTIVE TREATMENT

For hypotension, the patient is administered 10 to 20 ml/kg 0.9% saline and placed in the Trendelenburg position. If pressure is unresponsive, a vasopressor may be added. Dopamine is preferred, and norepinephrine is added for refractory hypotension.

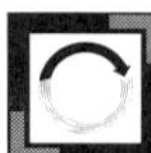

Follow-Up

PATIENT MONITORING

Patients with amphotericin B overdose should receive cardiac monitoring.

EXPECTED COURSE AND PROGNOSIS

Nearly all patients respond well to supportive therapy and recover.

DISCHARGE CRITERIA/INSTRUCTIONS

- From the emergency department. Asymptomatic patients may be discharged following decontamination, a 6-hour observation period, and a psychiatric evaluation, if needed.
- From the hospital. Patients may be discharged after stabilization or resolution of toxicity and, if needed, a psychiatric evaluation.

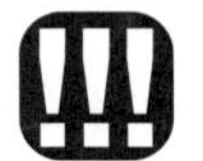

Pitfalls

DIAGNOSIS

The diagnosis of flucytosine- or azole-induced bone marrow suppression or gastrointestinal toxicity should be considered in patients that present with vague, nonspecific complaints.

ICD-9-CM 960.1

Poisoning by antibiotics: antifungal antibiotics.

See also: SECTION II, Hypotension chapter; and SECTION IV, Griseofulvin chapter.

RECOMMENDED READING

Como JA, Dismukes WE. Oral azole drugs as systemic antifungal therapy. *N Engl J Med* 1994;330:263–272.

Ellenhorn MJ, Schonwald S, Ordog G, Wasserberger J, eds. Antifungal drugs. In: *Ellenhorn's medical toxicology: diagnosis and treatment of human poisoning,* 2nd ed. Baltimore: Williams & Wilkins, 1997:270–284.

Author: Gerald F. O'Malley

Reviewer: Richard C. Dart

Antihistamines—Nonsedating

Basics

DESCRIPTION

The nonsedating antihistamines are prescription antihistamine medications that do not cause drowsiness.

FORMS AND USES

- Pharmaceutical preparations include acrivastine (Semprex-D, which also contains pseudoephedrine), astemizole (Hismanal), cetirizine (Zyrtec), fexofenadine (Allegra), and loratidine (Claritin; Claritin-D also contains pseudoephedrine).
- See also SECTION IV, Terfenadine chapter.
- These drugs are used in the treatment of seasonal allergic rhinitis, perennial allergic rhinitis, and chronic idiopathic urticaria.

—The recommended dose for astemizole is 10 mg daily for patients 12 years of age and older.
—The recommended dose for cetirizine is 5 to 10 mg daily for patients 12 years of age and older.
—The recommended dose for fexofenadine is 60 mg twice a day for patients 12 years of age and older.
—The recommended dose for loratidine is 10 mg daily for patients 12 years of age and older.

TOXIC DOSE

- Due to relatively recent availability, little information is available.
- Astemizole typically produces toxicity at therapeutic doses as a drug interaction that produces high plasma levels.
- Large doses of the other agents are usually needed to produce any toxicity.

PATHOPHYSIOLOGY

- Second-generation antihistamines are selective, peripheral H_1-receptor antagonists.
- Decreased occupancy of H_1-receptors in the brain is believed to be the mechanism of decreased drowsiness.
- These antihistamines are metabolized in the liver by the A3 family of cytochrome P450 enzymes, and drugs that interfere with metabolism may cause toxicity.

EPIDEMIOLOGY

- Poisoning is common.
- Toxic effects are typically mild with many of these products, but death has occurred with astemizole drug interaction or massive overdose of other agents.

CAUSES

- Toxic ingestion is usually suicidal.
- Toxic effects may occur when these antihistamines are taken in combination with other drugs.
- Child neglect or abuse should be considered if the patient is less than 1 year of age, suicide attempt if the patient is over 6 years of age.

RISK FACTORS

Toxicity is possible with therapeutic astemizole dose in patients with QT prolongation, kidney or liver dysfunction, or drug interaction.

DRUG AND DISEASE INTERACTIONS

- Drugs that inhibit the metabolism of astemizole may lead to severe dysrhythmia (ketoconazole, itraconazole, indinavir, fluvoxamine, clarithromycin, troleandomycin, and others).
- Drugs known to cause QT prolongation should be avoided (quinidine, disopyramide, procainamide, sotalol, ibutilide, pentamidine, propoxyphene, thioridazine, and others).

PREGNANCY AND LACTATION

- Acrivastine, cetirizine, loratidine. US FDA Pregnancy Category B. Animal studies indicate no fetal risk, and there are no controlled human studies, or animal studies show an adverse fetal effect but well-controlled studies in pregnant women do not.
- Astemizole, fexofenadine. US FDA Pregnancy Category C. The drug exerts animal teratogenic or embryocidal effects, but there are no controlled studies in women, or no studies are available in either animals or women.
- Loratidine and cetirizine appear in human breast milk and are generally not recommended for nursing mothers.

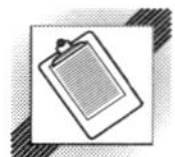

Diagnosis

DIFFERENTIAL DIAGNOSIS

- Toxicologic causes of syncope, QT prolongation, or torsade de pointes that may mimic astemizole toxicity include most antidysrhythmic drugs, thioridazine, and tricyclic antidepressants, among others.
- Nontoxicologic causes include severe hypomagnesemia, hypokalemia, ischemic heart disease, or any cause of ventricular dysrhythmia.

SIGNS AND SYMPTOMS

- Astemizole toxicity usually produces only mild symptoms such as dizziness; syncope, QT prolongation, torsade de pointes, and other conduction abnormalities may develop in severe cases.
- Acrivastine, cetirizine, loratidine, and fexofenadine produce mild effects, usually limited to nausea, headache, and sedation.

Vital Signs

Tachycardia may develop.

HEENT

Dry mouth and dizziness are common with each of the agents.

Dermatologic

Rash and urticaria occur rarely.

Cardiovascular

Astemizole may produce QT prolongation, torsade de pointes, ventricular dysrhythmia, hypotension, and cardiovascular collapse.

Gastrointestinal

Each of these agents cause nausea in overdose.

Hepatic

Hepatitis is reported rarely, after chronic use.

Neurologic

Anxiety, headache, somnolence, ataxia, tremors, and seizures may occur with large overdose.

PROCEDURES AND LABORATORY TESTS

Essential Tests

Asymptomatic patients may not require any laboratory studies.

Recommended Tests

- Serum electrolytes, BUN, and creatinine should be tested to assess other causes of cardiac dysrhythmia.
- Serum calcium and magnesium should be measured to assess their contribution to cardiac dysrhythmia.
- Serum acetaminophen and aspirin levels should be assayed to evaluate analgesic ingestion.
- Arterial blood gas, urine drug screen, and liver enzyme tests may be needed as indicated by clinical presentation.
- ECG and continuous cardiac monitoring are recommended; QT prolongation and ventricular dysrhythmias may occur, most likely after astemizole during drug interaction or overdose.

Not Recommended Tests

Serum drug levels are not readily available or useful.

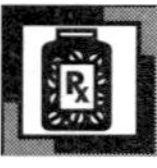

Treatment

- Treatment should focus on airway management and cardiac dysrhythmia.
- Dose and time of exposure should be determined for all substances involved.

DIRECTING PATIENT COURSE

The health-care professional should call the poison control center when:

- Altered mental status, seizure, cardiac dysrhythmia, or other severe effects are present.
- Toxic effects are not consistent with the reported poisoning.
- Coingestant, drug interaction, or underlying disease presents an unusual problem.

The patient should be referred to a health-care facility when:

- Attempted suicide or homicide is possible.
- Patient or caregiver seems unreliable.
- Symptoms develop.
- Coingestant, drug interaction, or underlying disease presents an unusual problem.

Admission Considerations

Inpatient management in a cardiac-monitored setting is warranted if:

- Patient is known to have astemizole overdose.
- Patient with ingestion of another nonsedating antihistamine has CNS complaint such as syncope or who develops CNS or cardiac toxicity.

DECONTAMINATION

Out of Hospital

Emesis should not be induced.

In Hospital

- Gastric lavage should be performed in pediatric (tube size 24–32 French) or adult (tube size 36–42 French) patients for large ingestion presenting within 1 hour of ingestion or if serious effects are present.
- One dose of activated charcoal (1–2 g/kg) should be administered without a cathartic if a substantial ingestion has occurred within the previous few hours.

ANTIDOTES

There is no specific antidote for nonsedating antihistamines.

ADJUNCTIVE TREATMENT

Torsade de Pointes

- Electrolyte abnormalities, if present, should be corrected.
- Administration of quinidine, disopyramide, procainimide, amiodarone, or bretylium should be avoided because these drugs also prolong the QT interval.
- Magnesium sulfate ($MgSO_4$) should be administered.

—Adult dose is 1 to 2 g by intravenous push; a continuous intravenous infusion should also be started at 2 to 4 g/h, titrated to antidysrhythmic effect. A repeat bolus of 1 to 2 g may be administered if dysrhythmia recurs.
—Pediatric dose is 25 to 50 mg/kg intravenously over 5 minutes.

- Isoproterenol (2–4 μg/ml) should be administered to adult patients at an initial rate of 0.5 to 1.0 μg/min, titrated to effect; pediatric dose is 0.1 μg/kg/min, titrated to effect.
- Torsade de pointes may require cardiac overdrive pacing.
- Ventricular dysrhythmias may require cardioversion.

Seizure

Seizures should be controlled with benzodiazepine followed by phenytoin or phenobarbital, if needed.

Hypotension

- Patient should receive 10 to 20 ml/kg 0.9% saline and be placed in the Trendelenburg position.
- Further fluid therapy should be guided by central pressure monitoring to avoid volume overload.
- If hypotension is unresponsive, a vasopressor should be administered.

—Dopamine: 2 to 5 μg/kg/min, titrated to effect; rates above 20 μg/kg/min are unlikely to provide further benefit.
—Norepinephrine infusion may be added at a rate of 0.1 to 0.2 μg/kg/min, titrated to effect if hypotension continues to be unresponsive.
—High rate of infusion may cause tissue ischemia.

- Hemodialysis and hemoperfusion are not recommended.

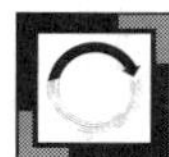

Follow-Up

PATIENT MONITORING

- Respiratory and cardiac function should be monitored continuously for at least 24 hours or as long as QTc is prolonged or dysrhythmias persist.
- Electrolytes and magnesium level should be monitored throughout the treatment course.

EXPECTED COURSE AND PROGNOSIS

- Most patients experience only sedation, which peaks and resolves during the first 24 hours.
- If ventricular dysrhythmia develops, sequelae are determined by occurrence of hypoxic injury.

DISCHARGE CRITERIA/INSTRUCTIONS

- From the emergency department. Asymptomatic patients who ingested cetirizine, loratidine, fexofenadine, or acrivastine may be discharged after decontamination, 6 hours of observation, and psychiatric evaluation, if needed.
- From the hospital

—Asymptomatic patients can be discharged after a 24-hour monitoring period and documentation of normal QTc and ECG.
—QT prolongation may persist for days; monitoring should continue until QTc is normal.

PATIENT EDUCATION

Patients taking astemizole should be made aware of potential drug interactions.

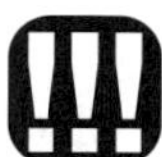

Pitfalls

DIAGNOSIS

- Signs and symptoms of overdose may initially be absent or nonspecific.
- Cardiac effects have been delayed up to 22 hours.
- QTc prolongation and torsade de pointes may be unrecognized.

TREATMENT

- Drugs that prolong QT interval should be avoided.
- Astemizole toxicity may require prolonged cardiac monitoring.

ICD-9-CM 963.0

Poisoning by antiallergic and antiemetic drugs.

See also: SECTION II, Hypotension, Seizure, and Ventricular Dysrhythmia chapters; and SECTION III, Terfenadine chapter.

RECOMMENDED READING

Nightingale SL. US Food and Drug Administration warnings issued on nonsedating antihistamines, terfenadine and astemizole. *JAMA* 1992;268:705.

Woosley RL. Cardiac actions of antihistamines. *Ann Rev Pharmacol Toxicol* 1996;36:233–252.

Author: Steven A. Seifert

Reviewer: Richard C. Dart

Antihistamines—Over-the-Counter

Basics

DESCRIPTION

Antihistamines include pharmaceuticals used in a wide range of products for over-the-counter (OTC) use.

FORMS AND USES

- OTC pharmaceutical preparations include antazoline, azatadine, bromodiphenhydramine, brompheniramine, buclizine, chlorcyclizine, chlorpheniramine, clemastine, cyclizine, cyproheptadine, dexbrompheniramine, dexchlorpheniramine, dimenhydrinate, diphenhydramine, diphenylpyraline, doxylamine, hydroxyzine, meclizine, methapyrilene, methdilazine, phenindamine, pheniramine, phenyltoloxamine, promethazine, pyrilamine, trimeprazine, tripelennamine, and triprolidine.
- These drugs are used in the treatment of allergic reactions and pruritus; in many combination products for the treatment of cold, cough, and allergy symptoms; as sleep aids; to treat motion sickness; and to treat dystonic reactions.

TOXIC DOSE

Toxic dose is variable; the estimation of dose is not clinically useful.

PATHOPHYSIOLOGY

- Therapeutic effects are due to competitive antagonism of the H_1-receptor.
- Toxicity is primarily due to anticholinergic (antimuscarinic) effects.

EPIDEMIOLOGY

- Poisoning is common.
- Toxic effects following exposure are typically mild to moderate.
- Death occurs in patients with large overdose.

CAUSES

- Toxic ingestion is usually suicidal or associated with recreational abuse.
- Child neglect or abuse should be considered if the patient is less than 1 year of age, suicide attempt if the patient is over 6 years of age.

RISK FACTORS

- Children may be more prone to CNS excitation and seizures.
- OTC antihistamines have abuse potential for psychedelic effects, particularly in adolescents.
- Elderly patients may be prone to CNS depression or hallucinosis at therapeutic doses and may be less tolerant of tachycardia.

DRUG AND DISEASE INTERACTIONS

- OTC antihistamines increase CNS depression when taken with other CNS depressants.
- Increased anticholinergic effect occurs when OTC antihistamines are taken with other anticholinergic agents.

PREGNANCY AND LACTATION

- Azatadine, chlorpheniramine, cyproheptadine dexchlorpheniramine, doxylamine, meclizine, and tripelennamine. US FDA Pregnancy Category B. Animal studies indicate no fetal risk and there are no controlled human studies, or animal studies show an adverse fetal effect but well-controlled studies in pregnant women do not.
- Antazoline, bromodiphenhydramine, brompheniramine, buclizine, chlorcyclizine, clemastine, cyclizine, dexbrompheniramine, dimenhydrinate, diphenhydramine, hydroxyzine, methdilazine, pheniramine, phenyltoloxamine, promethazine, pyrilamine, trimeprazine, and triprolidine. US FDA Pregnancy Category C. The drug exerts animal teratogenic or embryocidal effects, but there are no controlled studies in women, or no studies are available in either animals or women.

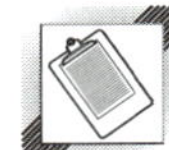

Diagnosis

DIFFERENTIAL DIAGNOSIS

- Toxicologic causes of anticholinergic effects include belladonna alkaloids, ophthalmic cycloplegics, antiparkinsonian drugs, antispasmodics, plants of the *Datura* genus (jimson weed), morning glory seeds, nutmeg, and several others.
- Other drugs that cause CNS depression or hallucinations and tachycardia include antidepressants, LSD, some mushrooms, cocaine, amphetamines, and phencyclidine.
- Nontoxicologic causes of altered mental status include conditions such as CNS infection, mass, or bleed; hyperthermia; and sepsis.

SIGNS AND SYMPTOMS

- Muscarinic anticholinergic effects predominate, including fever, tachycardia, mydriasis, flushed dry skin, CNS stimulation or depression, hallucinations, decreased bowel sounds, and urinary retention.
- Dysrhythmia, coma, seizures, and hypotension may develop in severe cases.

Vital Signs

- Tachycardia and mild hyperthermia are common.
- Mild hypertension may develop.
- Hypotension may develop with severe overdose.

HEENT

Mydriasis, blurred vision, and dry mucous membranes are common antimuscarinic effects.

Dermatologic

Skin is usually dry and flushed.

Cardiovascular

- Tachycardia and mild hypertension are common.
- QRS interval widening, ventricular dysrhythmias, QT prolongation, and hypotension may develop with severe overdose.

Gastrointestinal

Decrease in bowel sounds is common.

Hepatic

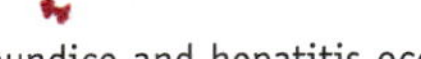

Cholestatic jaundice and hepatitis occur rarely.

Renal

- Urinary retention is common.
- Renal failure may occur rarely due to rhabdomyolysis or hypotension.

Fluids and Electrolytes

Metabolic acidosis may occur rarely due to hypotension or seizure.

Musculoskeletal

Rhabdomyolysis may occur rarely due to seizures or coma.

Neurologic

- CNS depression is common and may progress to coma.
- Paradoxically, CNS stimulation is also common and is characterized by agitation and hallucinations; in severe cases seizures may develop.
- Dystonia, chorea, parkinsonism, and dyskinesia have been reported with chronic use.

PROCEDURES AND LABORATORY TESTS

Essential Tests

No tests may be needed in minimally symptomatic patients with a clear history of nonsuicidal antihistamine ingestion.

Recommended Tests

- Complete blood count, blood cultures, and CSF should be assayed as needed to rule out other causes of altered mental status or hyperthermia.
- ECG, serum acetaminophen, and aspirin levels should be checked in an overdose setting to detect occult ingestion.
- Urine toxicology screen should be performed in patients with persistent tachycardia, QRS widening, prolonged QTc, or altered mental status of unclear etiology.
- Head CT is used as needed to determine cause of seizure or altered mental status.

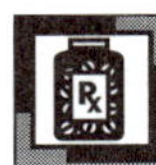

Treatment

- Dose and time of exposure should be determined for all substances involved.
- Treatment should focus on controlling agitation, maintaining the airway, reversing hyperthermia, and hemodynamic support.

DIRECTING PATIENT COURSE

The health-care professional should call the poison control center when:

- Coma, seizure, dysrhythmia, or other severe effects are present.
- The use of physostigmine is considered.
- Toxic effects are not consistent with antihistamine poisoning.
- Coingestant, drug interaction, or underlying disease presents an unusual problem.

The patient should be referred to a health-care facility when:

- A child has ingested more then three times the maximum daily dose of the medication. (Children who have ingested three times the maximum daily dose may be observed without gastric decontamination.)
- Attempted suicide or homicide is possible.
- Patient or caregiver seems unreliable.
- Toxic effects are present.
- Coingestant, drug interaction, or underlying disease presents an unusual problem.

Admission Considerations

Inpatient management is warranted if the patient exhibits altered mental status, seizure, persistently abnormal vital signs, or dysrhythmia.

DECONTAMINATION

Out of Hospital

Decontamination is not recommended.

In Hospital

- Gastric lavage should be performed in pediatric (tube size 24–32 French) or adult (tube size 36–42 French) patients for large ingestion presenting within 1 hour of ingestion or if serious effects are present.
- One dose of activated charcoal (1–2 g/kg) should be administered without a cathartic if a substantial ingestion has occurred within the previous few hours.

ANTIDOTES

Physostigmine is used for the diagnosis of antihistamine poisoning.

Indications

To distinguish altered mental status secondary to anticholinergic toxicity from other causes of agitation and hallucination.

Contraindications

- Known allergy to cholinergic agonist or sulfites
- Known or suspected tricyclic antidepressant overdose, or ECG findings suggestive of tricyclic antidepressant overdose (QRS interval widening, R wave in ECG lead aVR)
- Underlying health problems: asthma, heart disease, diabetes, inflammation of iris or ciliary body

Method of Administration

- Patient should be placed on cardiac monitor and have atropine available at the bedside.
- Adult dose is 1.0 to 2.0 mg, administered by slow intravenous push over 5 minutes; pediatric dose is 0.02 mg/kg up to 2.0 mg.
- Dose may be repeated once after 5 to 10 minutes if needed.
- Physostigmine will reverse behavioral effects, but symptoms will usually recur within 30 to 60 minutes.
- Repeated doses of physostigmine are not generally recommended for behavior control.

Adverse Effects

- Muscarinic effects may include nausea, vomiting, diarrhea, sweating, increased bronchial and salivary secretions, bradycardia, and hypotension; cardiac dysrhythmia may occur.
- Nicotinic symptoms (weakness, fasciculation) may also occur; seizures may occur.

ADJUNCTIVE TREATMENT

Agitation or Hallucinosis

A benzodiazepine may be used to control symptoms until resolution occurs.

- Diazepam. Adult dose is 5 to 10 mg (pediatric dose 0.2–0.5 mg/kg up to 5 mg) intravenously; doses may be repeated at 5-minute intervals, titrated to effect.
- Lorazepam. Adult dose is 2 to 4 mg (pediatric dose 0.05–0.1 mg/kg up to 2 mg) intravenously; doses may be repeated at 5-minute intervals, titrated to effect, while airway is monitored closely.

Hypotension

Hypotension should be treated in the standard manner, beginning with 10 to 20 ml/kg 0.9% saline intravenously.

Seizures

Seizures are treated in the standard manner, starting with a benzodiazepine.

Dysrhythmias or Conduction Abnormalities

- The initial effort should be to secure the airway, control seizures, and correct acidemia.
- If QRS widening or dysrhythmia persists, sodium bicarbonate should be administered as 1 to 2 mEq/kg intravenous bolus; this can be repeated as needed for widened QRS, but the pH should not be allowed to exceed 7.55.
- Lidocaine can be used for ventricular tachycardia or multifocal premature ventricular complexes.

—Adult dose is 50 to 100 mg intravenous bolus followed by infusion of 2 to 4 mg per minute, titrated to effect.
—Pediatric dose is 1 mg/kg bolus followed by infusion of 20 to 50 μg/kg/min, titrated to effect.
—Bolus dose may be repeated in 10 to 15 minutes.

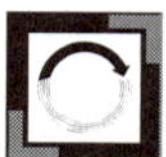

Follow-Up

PATIENT MONITORING

Electrolytes as well as respiration and cardiac function should be monitored throughout hospitalization.

EXPECTED COURSE AND PROGNOSIS

- Most patients recover uneventfully with supportive care.
- Sequelae of anoxia may develop if medical care is delayed.
- CNS effects may require several days to resolve.

DISCHARGE CRITERIA/INSTRUCTIONS

- From the emergency department. Patients who have not developed altered mental status, seizure, or dysrhythmia during 6 to 12 hours of observation may be discharged following gastrointestinal decontamination and psychiatric evaluation, if needed.
- From the hospital. A patient may be discharged after signs of toxicity have resolved for at least 12 hours.

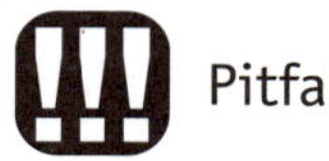

Pitfalls

DIAGNOSIS

A history of ingestion may be difficult to obtain due to recreational abuse.

TREATMENT

Anticholinergic effects generally recur 30 to 45 minutes after physostigmine administration.

ICD-9-CM 963.0

Poisoning by primarily systemic agents: antiallergic and antiemetic drugs.

See also: SECTION II, Hypotension, Seizure, and Ventricular Dysrhythmia chapters; and SECTION III, Physostigmine chapter.

RECOMMENDED READING

Koppel C, Tenczer J, Ibe K. Poisoning with over-the-counter doxylamine preparations: an evaluation of 109 cases. *Hum Toxicol* 1987;6:355–359.

Author: Katherine M. Hurlbut

Reviewer: Luke Yip

Basics

DESCRIPTION

Aminoglycosides are antimicrobial agents commonly used in the treatment of infections by gram-negative organisms.

FORMS AND USES

Aminoglycoside antimicrobials include amikacin (Amikin), gentamicin (Garamycin), kanamycin (Kanasig), netilmicin (Netromycin), neomycin (Neo-Myxin, Neocin), and tobramycin (Nebcin) and are used for the treatment of local or systemic infection, particularly infection with gram-negative bacterial organisms.

TOXIC DOSE

- A single overdose of any aminoglycoside rarely produces toxic effects.
- Gentamicin or tobramycin peak serum levels persistently above 12 μg/ml or trough levels greater than 2 μg/ml are associated with renal injury.
- Amikacin peak levels persistently above 20 μg/ml or trough levels greater than 8 μg/ml are associated with renal injury.

PATHOPHYSIOLOGY

An overdose of an aminoglycoside may result in nephrotoxicity and ototoxicity.

- Nephrotoxicity is the result of proximal tubular injury leading to acute tubular necrosis and subsequent oliguric renal failure.
- Ototoxicity manifests by cochlear and vestibular nerve dysfunction.
- Damage is dependent on dose, duration of therapy, preexisting renal disease or dysfunction, and concomitant use of other nephrotoxic or ototoxic drugs.

EPIDEMIOLOGY

- Intravenous overdose is usually the result of iatrogenic error.
- Oral overdoses are rare.
- Child neglect or abuse should be considered if patient is less than 1 year of age, suicide attempt if patient is over 6 years of age.

RISK FACTORS

- Nephrotoxicity is seen most frequently in the context of prolonged elevation of trough levels in elderly, dehydrated patients with underlying renal dysfunction or during treatment with other nephrotoxic drugs.
- Allergic sensitivity to antimicrobials is common. Patients with a history of sensitivity to other antimicrobial agents or sulfites are at increased risk.
- In the elderly, underlying renal disease may enhance the potential for toxicity.

DRUG AND DISEASE INTERACTIONS

- Aminoglycosides, when used with vancomycin, increase the incidence of nephrotoxicity and ototoxicity.
- When used with lincomycin, interstitial nephritis has occurred.
- Acute renal failure has resulted from the use of aminoglycosides with clindamycin.
- Ticarcillin may complex with either gentamicin or tobramycin, shortening its half-life. Therefore, the combination should not be used therapeutically.
- Aminoglycosides potentiate the effects of neuromuscular blockade (e.g., botulism).

PREGNANCY AND LACTATION

- Amikacin, gentamicin, and neomycin. US FDA Category C. The drug exerts animal teratogenic or embryocidal effects, but there are no controlled studies in women, or no studies are available in either animals or women.
- Kanamycin and tobramycin. US FDA Category D. Positive evidence of human fetal risk exists, but benefits in certain situations (e.g., life-threatening situations or serious diseases) may make use of the drug acceptable despite its risks.

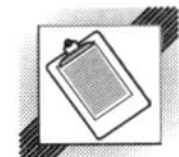

Diagnosis

DIFFERENTIAL DIAGNOSIS

- Toxicologic causes of renal injury include acetaminophen, chlorinated hydrocarbons, certain mushrooms, ethylene glycol, mercury, methemoglobinemia and rhabdomyolysis, among others.
- Other causes include hypotension, rhabdomyolysis, infection, and anatomical obstruction.

SIGNS AND SYMPTOMS

- The main toxicologic effects of aminoglycosides are nephrotoxicity and ototoxicity.
- Repeated inappropriately high doses are usually required to produce toxicity.

HEENT

- Partial or complete hearing loss may occur. Loss of high-frequency hearing may precede clinically apparent hearing loss.
- Vertigo occurs rarely.

Pulmonary

Apnea secondary to neuromuscular blockade may occur.

Renal

Especially if repeated, a high dosage may result in nephrotoxicity leading to renal failure.

Immunologic

Aminoglycosides have been reported to produce hypersensitivity reactions, including anaphylaxis.

PROCEDURES AND LABORATORY TESTS

Essential Tests

- Periodic trough and peak levels during therapy to maintain appropriate levels, serial levels following overdose.
- BUN, serum creatinine, and creatinine clearance to evaluate potential renal injury.

Recommended Tests

Audiology testing should be performed when toxicity is suspected or toxic levels are detected.

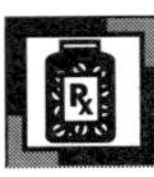

Treatment

- Treatment is focused on assessment of toxicity and general supportive renal care.
- Patients with normal renal function, who have received a single overdose, can usually be managed with conservative and supportive measures. Exceptions include aminoglycoside overdose in the presence of renal failure or the development of neuromuscular blockade.
- Dose and time of exposure should be determined for all substances involved.

DIRECTING PATIENT COURSE

- The health-care professional should call the poison control center when:
- Decreased hearing or other severe effects are present.
- Toxic effects are not consistent with aminoglycoside poisoning.
- Coingestant, drug interaction, or underlying disease presents an unusual problem.

The patient should be referred to a health-care facility when:

- Attempted suicide or homicide is possible.
- Patient or caregiver seems unreliable.
- Any toxic effects develop.
- Coingestant, drug interaction, or underlying disease presents an unusual problem.

Admission Considerations

Inpatient management is warranted for patients requiring electrolyte management or hemodialysis due to renal injury.

DECONTAMINATION

Out of Hospital

Induced emesis is not recommended due to rapid absorption and lack of toxicity following single acute overdose.

In Hospital

Gastric lavage should be performed in pediatric (tube size 24–32 French) or adult (tube size 36–42 French) patients for large ingestion presenting within 1 hour of ingestion or if serious effects are present.

ANTIDOTES

Treatment of Neuromuscular Blockade

- Physostigmine is a cholinergic agonist that that has been proposed to reverse neuromuscular blockade enhanced by the combination of aminoglycosides and neuromuscular blocking agents.
- It should not be used, however, if there is a significant possibility of cyclic antidepressant overdose.

ADJUNCTIVE TREATMENT

- The patient's urine output should be adequately maintained.
- Hypotension should be treated with isotonic fluid infusion, the Trendelenburg position, and vasopressors if needed. Dopamine is preferred; norepinephrine may be added for refractory hypotension.
- Due to high rates of elimination, dialysis is usually not necessary when renal function is adequate; however, it should be considered when renal failure is present.
- Physostigmine has been used to reverse neuromuscular blockade.
- Mechanical ventilation may rarely be required for prolonged respiratory depression, pulmonary edema, or prolonged neuromuscular blockade.

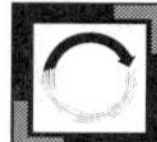

Follow-Up

PATIENT MONITORING

Renal function should be followed for 24 to 48 hours or until function stabilizes.

EXPECTED COURSE AND PROGNOSIS

- Nephrotoxicity is usually reversible if detected early and the specific medication is discontinued or removed by dialysis, but residual ototoxicity occurs occasionally.
- Immunocompromise secondary to marrow suppression (neomycin) may result in opportunistic infections. Antibiotic-associated bone marrow suppression usually reverses with discontinuation of the drug. However, permanent agranulocytosis has been reported.

DISCHARGE CRITERIA/INSTRUCTIONS

- From emergency department. Patients with normal renal and otic function may be discharged after gastrointestinal decontamination and psychiatric evaluation, if needed.
- From the hospital. Patients may be discharged after toxic effects resolve or stabilize and after psychiatric evaluation, if needed.

Pitfalls

Failure to monitor renal function and adjust dose appropriately may lead to renal injury.

ICD-9-CM 960

Poisoning by antibiotics.

See also: SECTION II, Hypotension chapter; and SECTION III, Physostigmine chapter.

RECOMMENDED READING

Butkus DE, de Torrente A, Terman DS. Renal failure following gentamicin in combination with clindamycin. *Nephron* 1976;17:307–313.

Green FJ, Lavelle KJ, Arnoff GR. Management of amikacin overdose. *Am J Kidney Dis* 1981;1:110–112.

Kacew S, Bergeron MG. Pathogenic factors in aminoglycoside-induced nephrotoxicity. *Toxicol Lett* 1990;51:237–239.

Koren G, Barzilay Z, Greenwald M. Tenfold errors in administration of drug doses: a neglected latrogenic disease in pediatrics. *Pediatrics* 1986;77:848–849.

Author: Steven A. Seifert

Reviewer: Richard C. Dart

Antimicrobials—Antituberculous Agents

Basics

DESCRIPTION

These medications are used for treatment of local or systemic infection with *Mycobacterium tuberculosis.*

FORMS AND USES

- Substances include aminosalicylic acid (Paser), capreomycin (Capastat), cycloserine (Seromycin), and ethambutol (Myambutol).
- See also SECTION IV, Isoniazid and Rifampin chapters.
- Cycloserine, capreomycin, and ethambutol are not recommended for pediatric use.

PATHOPHYSIOLOGY

Aminosalicylic Acid

- Aminosalicylic acid produces hypersensitivity or toxicity during therapeutic use through gastrointestinal, electrolyte, hepatic, and blood systems (i.e., blood dyscrasia).
- Overdosage has not been reported.

Capreomycin

- Exhibits renal, otic, and ophthalmic toxicity.
- Electrolyte and acid-base abnormalities, blood dyscrasia, and rashes may occur.
- Capreomycin is poorly absorbed from oral dosing.

Cycloserine

- Toxicity is manifested by CNS effects.
- Toxicity is closely related to serum levels and may result from chronic accumulation or acute overdose.
- Hypersensitivity reactions may occur.

EPIDEMIOLOGY

- Poisoning is uncommon.
- Toxic effects following exposure are typically mild to moderate, with death occurring only from coingestant or severe allergic reaction.

CAUSES

- Poisoning is usually the result of iatrogenic error.
- Child neglect should be considered if the patient is less than 1 year of age, suicide attempt if the patient is over 6 years of age.

PREGNANCY AND LACTATION

- Ethambutol. US FDA Pregnancy Category B. Animal studies indicate no fetal risk and there are no controlled human studies, or animal studies show an adverse fetal effect but well-controlled studies in pregnant women do not.
- Capreomycin and cycloserine. US FDA Pregnancy Category C. The drug exerts animal teratogenic or embryocidal effects, but there are no controlled studies in women, or no studies are available in either animals or women.

Diagnosis

DIFFERENTIAL DIAGNOSIS

- Renal failure. *Amanita phalloides* mushrooms, chlorinated hydrocarbons, *Cortinarius* species mushrooms, ethylene glycol, mercury, methemoglobinemia, rhabdomyolysis, and many others.
- Hepatotoxicity. Acetaminophen, *Amanita phalloides* mushrooms, anesthetic gases, aromatic or chlorinated hydrocarbons, arsenic, chronic ethanol, copper, chlorinated insecticides, iron, polychlorinated biphenyls, valproic acid, and many others.

SIGNS AND SYMPTOMS

- Aminosalicylic acid produces gastrointestinal symptoms, electrolyte abnormalities, hypersensitivity reactions, rashes, blood dyscrasia, hepatic injury, vasculitis, and encephalopathy.
- Capreomycin produces renal, otic, and ophthalmic toxicity, electrolyte and acid-base disturbances, blood dyscrasia, and skin rashes.
- Cycloserine effect is manifested primarily by CNS toxicity.
- Ethambutol toxicity primarily involves optic neuropathy.

Vital Signs

Aminosalicylic acid and ethambutol are associated with fever.

HEENT

- Capreomycin. Auditory and vestibular dysfunction with vertigo, tinnitus, hearing loss, and decreased visual acuity.
- Ethambutol. Optic neuropathy (chronic use), color vision disturbance, and blindness.

Dermatologic

Each agent can cause skin rash.

Cardiovascular

Cycloserine is associated with congestive heart failure.

Gastrointestinal

- Aminosalicylic acid. Nausea, vomiting, and abdominal pain.
- Ethambutol. Abdominal pain and nausea.

Hepatic

- Capreomycin or cycloserine. Hepatitis with elevated liver function tests.
- Ethambutol. Associated with cholestatic jaundice.

Renal

- Capreomycin poisoning commonly causes elevated creatinine and BUN and may be associated with tubular necrosis, metabolic alkalosis, hypokalemia, hyponatremia, hypochloremia, hypocalcemia, and hypomagnesemia.

Hematologic

- Aminosalicylic acid. Blood dyscrasia (agranulocytosis, neutropenia, thrombocytopenia, hemolytic anemia, mononucleosis-like or lymphoma-like disorders, hypoprothrombinemia).
- Capreomycin. Leukocytosis, leukopenia, eosinophilia (greater than 5% of patients on chronic therapy), and thrombocytopenia.
- Ethambutol. Thrombocytopenia and neutropenia.

Neurologic/Psychiatric

- Capreomycin. Neuromuscular block.
- Cycloserine. Drowsiness, headache, tremor, confusion, psychoses, paresis, paresthesia, seizures, and coma, as well as neuromuscular blockade.
- Ethambutol. Confusion, hallucinosis, and peripheral neuropathy (in chronic use).

Immunologic

- All agents. Reports of hypersensitivity reactions with anaphylaxis.
- Aminosalicylic acid. Hypersensitivity pneumonitis and vasculitis.

PROCEDURES AND LABORATORY TESTS

Essential Tests

- Capreomycin. Serum electrolytes, liver and renal function tests, complete blood count, and arterial blood gases.
- Cycloserine. Serum levels should be maintained below 30 μg/ml.

Recommended Tests

- ECG, serum acetaminophen, and aspirin levels in overdose setting to screen for occult ingestion.
- Aminosalicylic acid. Complete blood count (CBC) to assess for blood dyscrasia.
- Capreomycin. Liver function test to assess for injury; testing for auditory, vestibular, and ophthalmic function.
- Cycloserine. Liver function test to assess for injury.
- Ethambutol. CBC to assess for blood dyscrasia; liver function test and bilirubin levels to assess for injury; and ophthalmic evaluation.

Not Recommended Tests

Except for cycloserine, specific levels of agents are not helpful.

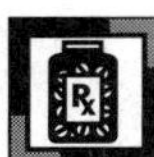

Treatment

- Treatment should be focused on airway management and supportive care.
- Specific therapy is generally not necessary; patients with normal renal function who have received an accidental overdose of these antimicrobials can usually be managed with conservative and supportive measures.
- Exceptions include the development or worsening of neuromuscular blockade, anaphylaxis, or severe symptoms from any toxicant.

DIRECTING PATIENT COURSE

The health-care professional should call the poison control center when:

- Toxic effects are not consistent with an antituberculous agent.
- Coingestant, drug interaction, or underlying disease presents an unusual problem.

The patient should be referred to a health-care facility when:

- Attempted suicide or homicide seems possible.
- Patient or caregiver seems unreliable.
- Any toxic effects develop.
- Coingestant, drug interaction, or underlying disease presents an unusual problem.

Admission Considerations

Inpatient management is warranted for patients who develop hypotension, respiratory or CNS depression, seizure, airway compromise, or dysrhythmia.

DECONTAMINATION

Decontamination is recommended if exposure is by the oral route.

Out of Hospital

Ipecac should be administered to induce emesis within 1 hour of ingestion for alert pediatric or adult patients if health-care evaluation will be delayed.

In Hospital

- Ipecac should be administered to induce emesis within 1 hour of ingestion for the alert patient who is too small to have effective gastric lavage.
- Gastric lavage should be performed in pediatric (tube size 24–32 French) or adult (tube size 36–42 French) patients for large ingestion presenting within 1 hour of ingestion or if serious effects are present.
- One dose of activated charcoal (1–2 g/kg) should be administered without a cathartic if a substantial ingestion has occurred within the previous few hours.

ANTIDOTES

Physostigmine is a cholinergic agonist that can be used to reverse neuromuscular blockade induced by cycloserine in combination with neuromuscular blocking agents.

ADJUNCTIVE TREATMENT

- Cycloserine toxicity should be treated with pyridoxine, 200 to 300 mg daily. Dialysis will remove cycloserine from the systemic circulation, but should be reserved for life-threatening complications.
- Hypotension. The patient should be treated with isotonic fluid infusion, Trendelenburg position, and, if needed, vasopressors. Dopamine is preferred and norepinephrine may be used for refractory hypotension.
- Seizures

—Patent airway must be assured.
—A benzodiazepine is administered for initial control.
—If seizures persist or recur, add another anticonvulsant, such as phenobarbital.

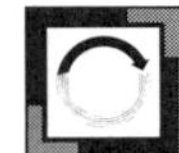

Follow-Up

PATIENT MONITORING

- Continuous ECG and pulse oximetry monitoring are used in patients with acute illness.
- For hepatotoxic agents (ethambutol), liver function tests should be followed daily until liver function is clearly improving.
- Renal dysfunction should be monitored daily until clearly improving.

EXPECTED COURSE AND PROGNOSIS

- Respiratory depression may result in hypoxia and related complications.
- Antibiotic renal and liver damage usually reverses with discontinuation of the drug.
- Immunocompromise secondary to bone marrow suppression (ethambutol) may result in opportunistic infections.
- Antibiotic-associated bone marrow suppression usually reverses with discontinuation of the drug; however, permanent agranulocytosis has been reported.
- Cycloserine. Recovery usually occurs with proper supportive care.
- Ethambutol. Permanent visual impairment may occur.

DISCHARGE CRITERIA/INSTRUCTIONS

- Discharge asymptomatic patients from the emergency department or hospital following 4 to 6 hours of observation and a psychiatric evaluation, if needed.
- Follow-up should be arranged for monitoring of liver or bone marrow function, as appropriate for the agent.

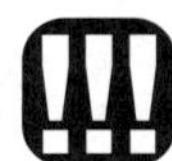

Pitfalls

DIAGNOSIS

Patient may not provide a history of self-medication with antibiotics.

ICD-9-CM 961.8

Poisoning by other antiinfectives, other antimycobacterial drugs.

See also: SECTION II, Hypotension and Seizure chapters; SECTION III, Physostigmine; and SECTION IV, Isoniazid, and Rifampin chapters.

RECOMMENDED READING

Darr M, Hamburger S, Ellerbeck E. Acid-base and electrolyte abnormalities due to capreomycin. *South Med J* 1982;75:627–628.

Gilman AG, Rall TW, Nies AS, et al., eds. *Goodman and Gilman's the pharmacological basis of therapeutics,* 8th ed. New York: Pergamon, 1990.

Author: Steven A. Seifert

Reviewer: Richard C. Dart

Antimicrobials—Macrolide

Basics

DESCRIPTION

The macrolide antimicrobials include erythromycin, azithromycin, clarithromycin, and other compounds with similar structure.

FORMS AND USES

- Macrolide antibiotics are used for the treatment of local or systemic infection with bacterial organisms.
- Macrolide antibiotics are available in a wide variety of forms, including azithromycin (Zithromax), erythromycin [base (E-Mycin), estolate, ethylsuccinate (EES), gluceptate, lactobionate, and stearate], clarithromycin (Biaxin), dirithromycin, and troleandomycin (Tao).

TOXIC DOSE

The macrolide antibiotics do not cause major toxicity in isolated acute overdose; they do, however, cause a number of adverse effects at therapeutic doses.

PATHOPHYSIOLOGY

- Toxic effects of the macrolides as a group include gastrointestinal irritation, cholestatic jaundice, ototoxicity, thrombophlebitis, and ventricular dysrhythmia; these effects are usually reversible upon discontinuation of the drug.
- Erythromycin may induce gastrointestinal symptoms, abdominal pain, thrombophlebitis, hearing loss, and exacerbation of weakness in myasthenia gravis.

DRUG AND DISEASE INTERACTIONS

Because they inhibit liver metabolism, macrolide antibiotics can increase the effects of benzodiazepines, calcium channel blockers, cyclic antidepressants, digoxin, ergotamine, estradiol, serotonin reuptake inhibitors, lovastatin (rhabdomyolysis), other macrolides, progesterone, theophylline, warfarin, and other agents.

EPIDEMIOLOGY

- Poisoning is uncommon.
- Toxic effects following exposure are typically mild.
- Death occurs only in conjunction with a coingestant.

CAUSES

- Macrolide antibiotic poisoning usually results from an accidental ingestion.
- Child neglect or abuse should be considered if the patient is less than 1 year of age, suicide attempt if the patient is over 6 years of age.

PREGNANCY AND LACTATION

- Azithromycin and erythromycin. US FDA Pregnancy Category B. Studies indicate no fetal risk and there are no controlled human studies, or animal studies show an adverse fetal effect but well-controlled studies in pregnant women do not.
- Clarithromycin. US FDA Pregnancy Category C. The drug exerts animal teratogenic or embryocidal effects, but there are no controlled studies in women, or no studies are available in either animals or women.

Diagnosis

DIFFERENTIAL DIAGNOSIS

Acute gastrointestinal effects can be caused by a wide variety of compounds, such as theophylline, salicylates, and caustic substances.

SIGNS AND SYMPTOMS

- Drug interactions are the primary cause of toxicity.
- Acute ingestion causes abdominal pain and other gastrointestinal effects.

HEENT

- Reversible ototoxicity characterized by a sensorineural hearing loss may occur.

Cardiovascular

- Ventricular dysrhythmias occur rarely in macrolide antibiotic toxicity.
- Erythromycin may produce thrombophlebitis.

Gastrointestinal

- Nausea, vomiting, abdominal pain, and diarrhea are common.
- Cholestatic jaundice, liver failure, and pseudomembranous colitis occur rarely.

Neurologic

- Erythromycin may exacerbate weakness in myasthenia gravis or cause sensorineural hearing loss.

PROCEDURES AND LABORATORY TESTS

Essential Tests

No test may be needed in minimally symptomatic patients.

Recommended Tests

- Serum electrolytes, BUN, and creatinine should be obtained in severe cases to assess volume depletion and electrolyte abnormalities.
- ECG, serum acetaminophen, and aspirin levels should be obtained in overdose settings to detect occult ingestion.
- Audiologic testing should be performed for hearing complaints.

Not Recommended Tests

Serum drug levels are not clinically helpful.

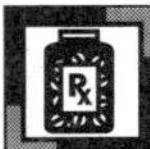

Treatment

- Treatment should focus on general supportive care and expectant care of adverse effects.
- Dose and time of exposure should be determined for all substances involved.

DIRECTING PATIENT COURSE

The health-care professional should call the poison control center when:

- Toxic effects develop.
- Coingestant, drug interaction, or underlying disease presents an unusual problem.

The patient should be referred to a health-care facility when:

- Attempted suicide or homicide is possible.
- The patient or caregiver seems unreliable.
- Toxic effects develop.
- Coingestant, drug interaction, or underlying disease presents an unusual problem.

Admission Considerations

Inpatient management is warranted for patients who develop persistent vomiting that is not controlled by antiemetic agents, or for other serious effects.

DECONTAMINATION

Out of Hospital

Emesis is not recommended because of the low toxic potential of macrolide antibiotics.

In Hospital

One dose of activated charcoal (1–2 g/kg) should be administered without a cathartic if a substantial ingestion has occurred within the previous few hours.

ANTIDOTES

There is no specific antidote available for macrolide antibiotic poisoning.

ADJUNCTIVE TREATMENT

- Hypotension is treated with isotonic fluid infusion, the Trendelenburg position, and vasopressors if needed; dopamine is preferred, and norepinephrine is used for refractory hypotension.
- Enhanced elimination by hemodialysis or hemoperfusion is not possible with macrolide antibiotics.

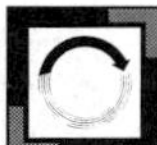

Follow-Up

PATIENT MONITORING

ECG and cardiac monitoring is recommended for patients with cardiac complaints.

EXPECTED COURSE AND PROGNOSIS

- Acute overdose is usually benign and managed with supportive and conservative care.
- Ototoxicity is usually reversible.

DISCHARGE CRITERIA/INSTRUCTIONS

Patients may be discharged from the emergency department or hospital when acute effects remit and following psychiatric evaluation, if needed.

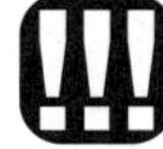

Pitfalls

DIAGNOSIS

- Macrolide antibiotic toxicity may be confused with ingestion of other agents or conditions that produce nonspecific CNS or respiratory depression, seizures, renal, bone marrow, or hepatic injury, or diarrheal illness.
- Patients often take over-the-counter medications and antibiotics on their own initiative, and occasionally fail to inform the health-care provider of these coingestants.

ICD-9-CM 960.3

Poisoning by antibiotics: erythromycin and other macrolides.

See also: SECTION II, Hypotension and Seizure chapters.

RECOMMENDED READING

Absher JR, Bale JF. Aggravation of myasthenia gravis by erythromycin. *J Pediatr* 1991;119:155–156.

Alcalay J, Halevy S, Theodor E, et al. Asymptomatic liver injury due to erythromycin stearate. *Drug Intell Clin Pharm* 1986;20:601–602.

Brandriss MW, Richardson WS, Barold SS. Erythromycin-induced QT prolongation and polymorphic ventricular tachycardia (torsades de pointes): case report and review. *Clin Infect Dis* 1994;18:995–998.

Author: Steven A. Seifert

Reviewer: Richard C. Dart

Basics

DESCRIPTION

These medications are used for the treatment of local or systemic infections.

FORMS AND USES

• Clindamycin (Cleocin) and lincomycin (Lincocin).
• Chloramphenicol (Cetina, Chloramphen, Chloromycetin, and Econochlor; also an ingredient of ophthalmic and veterinary products).
• The fluouroquinolones, which include ciprofloxin (Cipro), enoxacin (Penetrex), lomefloxacin (Maxaquin), norfloxacin (Norfloxil, Noroxin), ofloxacin (Oflox), pefloxacin, and vancomycin (Vancocin, Vancor).
• Fluoroquinolones should be avoided in patients 17 years of age and younger.

TOXIC DOSE

• Clindamycin and fluoroquinolones are expected to produce acute toxicity only after a large overdose.
• Death has occurred after a massive parenteral chloramphenicol overdose.

Pathophysiology

In contrast to their mechanism of action, the mechanism of toxicity is unclear for most antibiotics, perhaps due to their lack of serious toxicity in most cases.

Epidemiology

• Poisoning is uncommon.
• Toxic effects following exposure are typically mild, with death occurring only after massive overdose, usually involving parenteral administration.

CAUSES

• Poisoning is usually caused by iatrogenic error.
• Child neglect should be considered if the patient is less than 1 year of age, suicide attempt if the patient is over 6 years of age.

DRUG AND DISEASE INTERACTIONS

• Ciprofloxacin and enoxacin may increase levels of theophylline, caffeine, diphenhydramine, cyclosporine, and warfarin.
• Chloramphenicol clearance is decreased by cimetidine.

PREGNANCY AND LACTATION

• Clindamycin and lincomycin. US FDA Pregnancy Category B. Animal studies indicate no fetal risk and there are no controlled human studies, or animal studies show an adverse fetal effect but well-controlled studies in pregnant women do not.
• Ciprofloxacin, vancomycin, and chloramphenicol. US FDA Pregnancy Category C. The drug exerts animal teratogenic or embryocidal effects, but there are no controlled studies in women, or no studies are available in either animals or women.
• Gray baby syndrome may develop in a newborn infant with high serum levels of chloramphenicol.
• Fluoroquinolones are excreted in breast milk and should be avoided during breastfeeding.

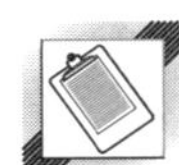

Diagnosis

DIFFERENTIAL DIAGNOSIS

Toxicologic causes of hepatotoxicity that may be complicated by renal injury include acetaminophen, anesthetic gases, aromatic or chlorinated hydrocarbons, arsenic, carbon tetrachloride, chronic ethanol, copper, chlorinated insecticides, iron, some species of mushrooms, thallium, and valproic acid.

SIGNS AND SYMPTOMS

• These products typically cause nausea and vomiting without other major effects after ingestion.
• Gray baby syndrome can occur after several doses of chloramphenicol. The term refers to rapid onset of vomiting, metabolic acidosis, cyanosis, irregular respiration, hypothermia, hypotension, and vasomotor collapse in neonates or toddlers who develop high plasma levels.

HEENT

• Chloramphenicol. Optic neuritis occurs rarely.
• Fluoroquinolones. Diplopia, color distortion occur rarely.
• Vancomycin. Auditory and vestibular eighth nerve injury may occur.

Dermatologic

• Chloramphenicol. Contact dermatitis, angioedema, and urticaria.
• Clindamycin and lincomycin. Stevens-Johnson syndrome and rash.
• Fluoroquinolones. Photosensitivity reactions and photoonycholysis.
• Vancomycin. Red man syndrome, referring to the rapid development of pruritus and erythema after infusion. Erythema multiforme and exfoliative dermatitis also have been reported.

Cardiovascular

• Clindamycin and lincomycin. Rapid intravenous administration may result in ventricular tachycardia or ventricular fibrillation, hypotension, or asystole.
• Vancomycin. Phlebitis, hypotension, and cardiac arrest may occur with rapid intravenous infusion.

Gastrointestinal

• Chloramphenicol. Nausea, vomiting, glossitis, stomatitis, diarrhea, and colitis may occur.
• Clindamycin and lincomycin. Diarrhea and colitis may occur.
• Fluoroquinolones may cause pseudomembranous colitis (rare) and hepatotoxicity, and liver enzyme elevation may occur.

Hepatic

• Clindamycin and lincomycin.
• Liver injury may occur.

Renal

• Clindamycin and lincomycin. Nephritis or acute renal failure.
• Fluoroquinolones. Hematuria, nephritis, and crystalluria.
• Vancomycin. Kidney injury.

Hematologic

• Chloramphenicol may cause bone marrow suppression. Dose-related suppression is acute and reversible. A second type, rare and non-dose-related, is late onset, progressive, nonreversible pancytopenia.
• Clindamycin and lincomycin. Sideroblastic anemia may result.
• Fluoroquinolones. Leukopenia or eosinophilia may occur.
• Vancomycin. Neutropenia and thrombocytopenia may occur.

Musculoskeletal

Fluoroquinolones. Joint tenderness and swelling.

Neurologic/Psychiatric

• Chloramphenicol. Headache, confusion, delirium, and peripheral neuritis.
• Fluoroquinolones. Headache, vomiting, abdominal pain, anxiety, paresthesia, cerebellar dysfunction, slurred speech, dizziness, drowsiness, seizures, hallucinations, and insomnia.

PROCEDURES AND LABORATORY TESTS

Essential Tests

No tests may be needed in asymptomatic patients.

Recommended Tests

• Chloramphenicol

—Arterial blood gases, serum electrolytes, BUN, and creatinine are used to assess metabolic acidosis.
—Complete blood count (CBC) is used to assess bone marrow effects.
—Serum drug level is used by some health professionals to ensure that drug levels do not exceed the therapeutic range. Levels greater than 50 μg/ml are associated with gray baby syndrome.

• Clindamycin or lincomycin

—If an acute large overdose occurs, ECG and continuous monitoring are needed to assess cardiovascular effects.

—CBC and platelet count are used to assess bone marrow effects.
—If treatment lasts more than 2 weeks, a serum liver function test is run to detect chemical hepatitis.
—Assays for stool occult blood and *Clostridium difficile* toxin are used to assess for pseudomembranous colitis.
—Proctosigmoidoscopy or barium-contrast enema is used to diagnose colitis.
—Fluoroquinolones. *Clostridium difficile* toxin assay in patients with diarrhea for suspected antibiotic-associated colitis.

Not Recommended Tests

Except for chloramphenicol, specific levels of antibiotic agents are not useful.

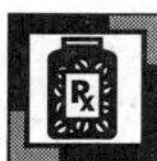

Treatment

Overdose with any of these antibiotics usually requires only supportive therapy.

DIRECTING PATIENT COURSE

The health-care professional should call the poison control center when:

- Severe or persistent effects develop.
- Toxic effects are not consistent with drug.
- Coingestant, drug interaction, or underlying disease presents an unusual problem.

The patient should be referred to a health-care facility when:

- Altered mental status, seizure, cardiac dysrhythmia, or other severe effects are present.
- Toxic effects develop.
- Coingestant, drug interaction, or underlying disease presents an unusual problem.

Admission Considerations

Inpatient management is warranted for patients who develop hypotension, respiratory or CNS depression, prolonged seizures, significant airway compromise, or persistent dysrhythmias.

DECONTAMINATION

Out of Hospital

Ipecac should be administered to induce emesis within 1 hour of ingestion for alert pediatric or adult patients if health-care evaluation will be delayed.

In Hospital

- Gastric lavage in pediatric (tube size 24–32 French) or adult (tube size 36–42 French) patients for large ingestion presenting within 1 hour of ingestion or if serious effects are present.
- One dose of activated charcoal (1–2 g/kg) should be administered without a cathartic if a substantial ingestion has occurred within the previous few hours.

ANTIDOTES

There are no specific antidotes available for these antimicrobials.

ADJUNCTIVE TREATMENT

- Antibiotic-associated pseudomembranous colitis is treated with replacement of fluids and electrolytes and with oral vancomycin.
- Antibiotic-associated colitis should not be treated with antidiarrheal agents.
- Optic neuritis secondary to chloramphenicol is treated with large doses of B vitamins.
- Hypothermia should be managed by slow passive or active rewarming, as indicated by core body temperature.
- Hypotension is treated with isotonic fluid infusion, the Trendelenburg position, and, if needed, vasopressors.
- Acute iatrogenic chloramphenicol overdose in neonates has been treated with exchange transfusion.
- Chloramphenicol clearance is moderately increased by hemodialysis in patients with impaired renal function.

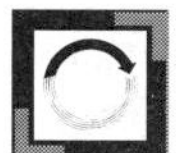

Follow-Up

PATIENT MONITORING

- Chloramphenicol

—Following a large overdose, patients should be observed for at least 12 hours.
—In gray baby syndrome, core body temperature, acid-base levels, and cardiovascular status must be monitored.
—CBC should be followed in chloramphenicol-treated patients for several weeks to months following discontinuation of long-term therapy.

- Clindamycin, lincomycin, and fluoroquinolones. In hepatic dysfunction, liver function tests should be followed daily until improvement is observed.

EXPECTED COURSE AND PROGNOSIS

- Rarely does renal or otic damage become permanent.
- Liver damage usually reverses with discontinuation of the drug.
- Chloramphenicol. Following an acute overdose, serious deterioration may be delayed for a few hours. Recovery is expected if cardiovascular support is given. Irreversible pancytopenia may result in associated complications such as infection.
- Clindamycin/lincomycin, fluoroquinolones, and vancomycin. These agents cause a mild course of illness with recovery expected.

DISCHARGE CRITERIA/INSTRUCTIONS

- From emergency department. Patients without bone marrow, liver, or renal toxicity may be discharged as symptoms resolve following gastrointestinal decontamination and psychiatric evaluation, if needed.
- From the hospital. Patients may be discharged when toxic effects resolve or stabilize and after psychiatric evaluation, if needed.

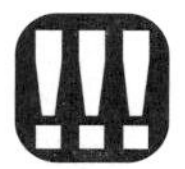

Pitfalls

DIAGNOSIS

Patient may not relate a history of self-medication with antibiotics.

ICD-9-CM 961

Poisoning by other antiinfectives.

See also: SECTION II, Hypotension chapter.

RECOMMENDED READING

Healy DP, Sahai JV, Fuller SH, et al. Vancomycin-induced histamine release and "red man syndrome": Comparison of 1- and 2-hour infusions. *Antimicrob Agents Chemother* 1990;34:550–554.

Nahata MC. Serum concentrations and adverse effects of chloramphenicol in pediatric patients. *Chemotherapy* 1987;33:322–327.

Author: Steven A. Seifert

Reviewer: Katherine M. Hurlbut

Antimicrobials—Penicillins and Cephalosporins

Basics

DESCRIPTION

Penicillins and cephalosporins are antibiotics used for the treatment of local or systemic infection with bacterial, rickettsial, mycoplasmal, and chlamydial organisms.

FORMS AND USES

- Penicillins. Penicillin-V or -G (Bicillin, Sycillin), amoxicillin (Amoxil, Augmentin, Unasyn), ampicillin, carbenicillin, cloxacillin, dicloxacillin, nafcillin (Nafcil, Unipen), methicillin, oxacillin, piperacillin, procaine penicillin, benzathine penicillin, and ticarcillin
- Cephalosporins. Cefaclor, cefadroxil (Duricef), cefamandole, cefazolin (Ancef), cefepime, cefixime (Suprax), cefmetazole, cefoperazone (Cefobid), cefotaxime (Claforan), cefotetan (Cefotan), cefoxitin (Mefoxin), cefprozil (Cefzil), ceftazidime, ceftriaxone (Rocephin), cefuroxime (Kefurox), cephalothin, cephradine, and cephalexin (Keflex)

TOXIC DOSE

- Toxic effects have occurred rarely after massive ingestion, but toxicity is unlikely with oral doses of less than 250 mg/kg.
- Allergic effects may occur at small doses.

PATHOPHYSIOLOGY

- Very large doses of amoxicillin or ampicillin may produce crystal formation in renal tubules.
- Cardiac conduction defects have occurred following rapid intravenous injection of potassium penicillin G.
- Some cephalosporins cause hypoprothrombinemia by inhibiting vitamin K-dependent microsomal carboxylase activity.

EPIDEMIOLOGY

- Ingestion is common.
- Toxic effects following exposure are typically mild.
- Death has not been reported after oral overdose.

CAUSES

- Toxic ingestion is usually accidental.
- Child abuse or neglect should be considered if the patient is less than 1 year of age, suicide attempt if the patient is over 6 years of age.
- Intravenous overdose usually results from iatrogenic error.

RISK FACTORS

- Patients allergic to other antimicrobials are at an increased risk for a hypersensitivity reaction.
- Patients with a true penicillin allergy have about a 10% incidence of hypersensitivity reactions to first-generation cephalosporins.

DRUG AND DISEASE INTERACTIONS

- A disulfiram-like reaction may occur with concurrent ingestion of cefoperazone, moxalactam, or cefamandole with ethanol.
- Underlying renal or hepatic dysfunction may predispose to adverse effects at therapeutic doses.

PREGNANCY AND LACTATION

- Cephalosporins and penicillins. US FDA Pregnancy Category B. Animal studies indicate no fetal risk, and there are no controlled human studies, or animal studies show an adverse fetal effect but well-controlled studies in pregnant women do not.
- Penicillins and cephalosporins cross into breast milk.

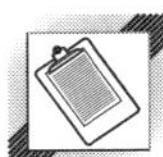

Diagnosis

DIFFERENTIAL DIAGNOSIS

- Toxicologic causes of renal failure and nephritis include nonsteroidal antiinflammatory drugs, ethylene glycol, mercury, and rhabdomyolysis.
- Other substances causing a disulfiram-like reaction are ethanol plus disulfiram or other substances that produce a similar reaction (carbon disulfide, metronidazole, chlorpropramide, glipizide, glyburide, and tolbutamide, among others).

SIGNS AND SYMPTOMS

Most ingestions of either a penicillin or a cephalosporin involve only nausea, vomiting, and abdominal pain; much larger doses may cause seizure and coma.

Vital Signs

Anaphylaxis may rarely develop, including hypotension, tachycardia, and increased respiratory rate.

Dermatologic

- Amoxicillin can cause Stevens-Johnson syndrome.
- Ampicillin can result in skin rash.
- Cefoperazone, moxalactam, or cefamandole with ethanol can cause flushing with a disulfiram-like reaction.

Cardiovascular

Penicillin-G can cause hyperkalemic cardiac arrest after rapid intravenous injection.

Pulmonary

Allergic reaction can cause wheezing and respiratory distress.

Gastrointestinal

Nausea, vomiting, diarrhea, and abdominal pain are common with both penicillins and cephalosporins.

Hepatic

- Cephalosporins cause impaired vitamin K1 production.
- Cefaclor can cause elevated hepatic enzymes.

Renal

Ampicillin and amoxicillin have caused hematuria and acute oliguric renal failure with large doses.

Hematologic

- Nafcillin. Leukopenia develops rarely.
- Cefamandole, cefazolin, cefmetazole, cefoperazone, and moxalactam. Prolonged prothrombin time rarely occurs.
- Cefaclor. Serum sickness, leukopenia, thrombocytopenia, and anemia have been observed.
- Ceftriaxone (intravenous). Hemolysis can occur.

Neurologic

- Penicillin (intravenous) can cause CNS depression, seizures, and coma.
- Procaine penicillin has been rarely associated with new onset of psychotic episodes (Hoigne syndrome), CNS excitation, and seizures.
- Cephalosporins may rarely cause encephalopathy, syncope, or seizure.

Immunologic

All penicillins and cephalosporins have been reported to produce hypersensitivity reactions and anaphylaxis.

PROCEDURES AND LABORATORY TESTS

Essential Tests

No test may be needed; asymptomatic patients require laboratory testing only after a large ingestion (e.g., tens of grams).

Recommended Tests

- Serum electrolytes, BUN, and creatinine are assessed in symptomatic patients; electrolyte abnormalities or renal insufficiency suggest significant exposure.
- CBC assesses anemia, thrombocytopenia, and leukopenia in symptomatic patients.
- ECG, serum acetaminophen, and aspirin in an overdose setting are used to detect occult ingestion.

Not Recommended Tests

- Specific levels of any penicillin or cephalosporin are not clinically useful.
- Serum creatinine measured by Jaffe's method: cefoxitin and cephalothin may result in false elevation.

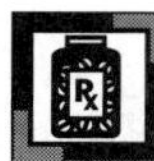

Treatment

- Treatment should focus on decontamination after large ingestion, airway management in severe cases, and supportive care.
- Dose and time of exposure should be determined for all substances involved.
- In most cases specific therapy will not be necessary.
- Patients with normal renal function can usually be managed with conservative supportive measures.

DIRECTING PATIENT COURSE

The health-care professional should call the poison control center when:

- Seizure or other severe effects are present.
- Toxic effects are not consistent with penicillin or cephalosporin poisoning.
- Coingestant, drug interaction, or underlying disease presents an unusual problem.

The patient should be referred to a health-care facility when:

- Attempted suicide or homicide is possible.
- Patient or caregiver seems unreliable.
- Serious toxic effects develop.
- Coingestant, drug interaction, or underlying disease presents an unusual problem.

Admission Considerations

Inpatient management is warranted if the patient develops hypotension, respiratory or CNS depression, seizures, airway compromise, or dysrhythmia, or has underlying medical conditions that warrant prolonged observation.

DECONTAMINATION

Out of Hospital

Emesis is not recommended due to the benign nature of most poisonings.

In Hospital

- Gastric lavage should be performed in pediatric (tube size 24–32 French) or adult (tube size 36–42 French) patients for massive ingestion presenting within 1 hour of ingestion or if serious effects are present.
- One dose of activated charcoal (1–2 g/kg) should be administered without a cathartic if a substantial ingestion has occurred within the previous few hours.

ANTIDOTES

There is no specific antidote for penicillin or cephalosporin toxicity.

ADJUNCTIVE TREATMENT

- Coagulopathy associated with cephalosporins can usually be managed by vitamin K1 administration at a dose of 10 mg orally or intramuscularly.
- If bleeding or thrombocytopenia have occurred, fresh-frozen plasma or platelet transfusion can be used.
- Hypotension. The patient should be treated with isotonic fluid infusion, the Trendelenburg position, and, if needed, vasopressors. Dopamine is preferred, and norepinephrine may be used for refractory hypotension.
- Seizures

—A patent airway must be ensured.
—A benzodiazepine is administered for initial control. If seizures persist or recur, another anticonvulsant such as phenobarbital may be added.

- Anaphylaxis

—Patent airway must be secured; 100% oxygen should be given.
 —If serious airway compromise is present, epinephrine should be administered immediately.
—Antihistamine can be used to block both H_1- and H_2-receptors.
 —Diphenhydramine. Adult dose is 25 to 50 mg intravenously every 6 to 8 hours; pediatric dose is 1 mg/kg intravenously up to 50 mg every 6 to 8 hours. Also administer Cimetidine. Adult dose is 300 mg intravenously every 6 hours; pediatric dose is 40 mg/kg/day intravenously divided into four doses (every 6 hours).
—Bronchospasm
 —Albuterol is administered, 0.15 mg/kg (maximum of 10 mg) in saline with humidified oxygen via nebulizer every 20 to 30 minutes.
 —Epinephrine 1:1,000. Adult dose is 0.3 to 0.5 ml subcutaneously; pediatric dose is 0.01 ml/kg up to 0.3 ml subcutaneously.

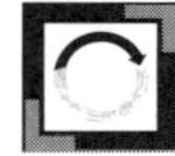

Follow-Up

PATIENT MONITORING

ECG and pulse oximetry should be monitored continuously in patients with anaphylaxis, seizure, dysrhythmias, or any other severe effects.

EXPECTED COURSE AND PROGNOSIS

- Most cases involve only gastrointestinal symptoms and resolve quickly.
- Allergic reactions are typically mild and self-limited.
- Severe anaphylaxis occurs rapidly and usually responds to medical management.

DISCHARGE CRITERIA/INSTRUCTIONS

- From the emergency department. Asymptomatic patients may be discharged after gastrointestinal decontamination and psychiatric evaluation, if needed.
- From the hospital. Patients may be discharged after toxic effects resolve or stabilize and after psychiatric evaluation, if needed.

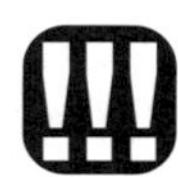

Pitfalls

DIAGNOSIS

It is important to ascertain whether other drugs or toxins were coingested.

TREATMENT

Excessive intervention should be avoided in mildly toxic exposures.

ICD-9-CM 960.0

Poisoning by antibiotics: penicillins.

See also: SECTION II, Hypotension and Seizure chapters.

RECOMMENDED READING

Alanis A, Weinstein AJ. Adverse reactions associated with the use of oral penicillins and cephalosporins. *Med Clin North Am* 1983;67:113–129.

Swanson-Biearman B, Dean BS, Lopez G, et al. The effects of penicillin and cephalosporin ingestions in children less than six years of age. *Vet Human Toxicol* 1988;30:66–67.

Author: Steven A. Seifert

Reviewer: Katherine M. Hurlbut

Antimicrobials—Sulfonamides

Basics

DESCRIPTION

- Sulfonamide antimicrobial agents are used for the treatment of local or systemic infection with bacterial, fungal, or parasitic agents.
- Sulfasalazine is used in ulcerative colitis.

FORMS AND USES

Sulfonamide antimicrobials include mafenide (Sulfamylon), silver sulfadiazine (Silvadene), sulfabenzamide (Sultrin), sulfacetamide (Bleph-10, Blephamide, Sulfacet-R, Sultrin), sulfadiazine, sulfadoxine (Fansidar), sulfamethizole (Urobiotic), sulfamethoxazole (Bactrim, Gantanol, Septra), sulfanilamide, sulfapyridine, sulfasalazine (Azulfidine), sulfathiazole (Sultrin), sulfinpyrazone (Anturane), and sulfisoxazole (Gantrisin, Pediazole).

TOXIC DOSE

Allergic reactions are the primary from of toxicity; any dose may induce reaction in a susceptible individual.

PATHOPHYSIOLOGY

- Dose-related hypersensitivity reactions are common. Acetylated metabolites are believed responsible for many of the toxic effects.
- Because sulfonamides are primarily excreted in the urine, renal failure increases the risk of adverse reactions.
- Stevens-Johnson syndrome is associated with the therapeutic use of either oral or ophthalmic preparations.

EPIDEMIOLOGY

- Allergic reactions are common, but poisoning is rare.
- Toxic effects following overdose are typically mild, with death occurring only from coingestant or severe allergic reaction.

CAUSES

- Ingestion is usually intentional, as part of a suicidal gesture.
- Child neglect or abuse should be considered if the patient is less than 1 year of age, suicide attempt if patients are over 6 years of age.

PREGNANCY AND LACTATION

- All agents. US FDA Pregnancy Category B. Animal studies indicate no fetal risk and there are no controlled human studies, or animal studies show an adverse fetal effect but well-controlled studies in pregnant women do not.
- All agents when used during near term pregnancies. US FDA Pregnancy Category D. Evidence of human fetal risk exists, but benefits in certain situations (e.g., life-threatening situations or serious diseases) may make use of the drug acceptable despite its risks.
- Sulfonamides in premature infants and neonates may cause kernicterus.
- Although excreted into breast milk, sulfonamides do not seem to pose a risk to otherwise healthy newborns [as opposed to those that are glucose-6-phosphate dehydrogenase (G-6-PD) deficient or have hyperbilirubinemia].

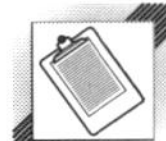

Diagnosis

DIFFERENTIAL DIAGNOSIS

The differential diagnosis includes any toxic cause of nausea and vomiting.

SIGNS AND SYMPTOMS

- Most common effects include nausea and vomiting, with possible hematologic effects.
- Kernicterus may present in premature newborns.
- Hypoglycemia may occur, especially in renal failure.

Vital Signs

- Fever may occur.
- Anaphylaxis-induced hypotension and tachycardia occur rarely.

HEENT

Conjunctivitis, myopia, glossitis, and optic neuritis may present as part of a hypersensitivity reaction.

Dermatologic

Hypersensitivity reactions may result in Stevens-Johnson syndrome, urticaria, maculopapular rashes, exfoliative rashes, and erythema nodosum.

Pulmonary

Hypersensitivity pneumonitis occurs rarely.

Gastrointestinal

Nausea and vomiting are frequent; diarrhea is rare.

Hepatic

Hepatitis, hepatocellular and/or cholestatic, may occur as part of a hypersensitivity reaction.

Renal

Acute tubular necrosis, oliguric renal failure, crystalluria, and hematuria may occur.

Hematologic

- Hemolytic anemia (G-6-PD deficiency predisposes), agranulocytosis, and thrombocytopenia may develop as part of a hypersensitivity reaction.
- Methemoglobinemia may develop rarely.

Neurologic/Psychiatric

Depression, headache, and hallucinosis occur rarely.

PROCEDURES AND LABORATORY TESTS

Essential Tests

No tests are usually needed in minimally symptomatic patients.

Recommended Tests

- Complete blood count is used to evaluate hematologic effects in symptomatic patients.
- Serum electrolytes, BUN, creatinine, and liver function tests to assess organ injury are indicated for symptomatic patients.
- Methemoglobin level is measured in symptomatic patients.
- ECG and serum acetaminophen and aspirin levels in overdose setting are used to detect occult ingestion.

Not Recommended

Specific levels of these agents are not useful.

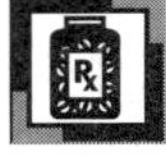

Treatment

- Treatment should be focused on airway management and general supportive measures, particularly if allergic response has occurred.
- The dose and time of exposure should be determined for all substances involved.

DIRECTING PATIENT COURSE

The health-care professional should call the poison control center when:

- Repetitive vomiting or other serious effects develop.
- Toxic effects are not consistent with sulfonamide poisoning.
- Coingestant, drug interaction, or underlying disease presents an unusual problem.

The patient should be referred to a health-care facility when:

- Attempted suicide or homicide is possible.
- Patient or caregiver seems unreliable.
- Toxic effects develop.
- Coingestant, drug interaction, or underlying disease presents an unusual problem.

Admission Considerations

Inpatient management is warranted for patients who develop any serious effects and who may have other sources of toxicity.

DECONTAMINATION

Out of Hospital

Induced emesis is not recommended due to low toxic potential.

In Hospital

- Gastric lavage should be performed in pediatric (tube size 24–32 French) or adult (tube size 36–42 French) patients for massive ingestion presenting within 1 hour of ingestion or if serious effects are present.

• One dose of activated charcoal (1–2 g/kg) should be administered without a cathartic if a substantial ingestion has occurred within the previous few hours.

ANTIDOTES

There is no specific antidote for sulfonamide poisoning.

ADJUNCTIVE TREATMENT

Methemoglobinemia

• The decision to treat methemoglobinemia is based primarily on evidence of CNS or cardiac ischemia.
• Supplemental oxygen needs to be administered.
• Methylene blue is the treatment. The dose is 1 to 2 mg/kg intravenously over 5 minutes.
• Clinical improvement should be apparent shortly after administration.
• Repeat the methemoglobin level after 30 minutes. If the level remains elevated and the patient is still symptomatic, a repeat dose of 1 to 2 mg/kg should be administered over 5 minutes.

Hypotension

The patient should be treated with isotonic fluid infusion, the Trendelenburg position, and, if needed, vasopressors. Dopamine is preferred, and norepinephrine may be used for refractory hypotension.

Seizures

• A patent airway must be ensured.
• A benzodiazepine is administered for initial control. If seizures persist or recur, another anticonvulsant such as phenobarbital followed by general anesthesia may be needed.

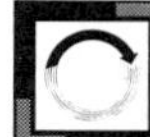

Follow-Up

PATIENT MONITORING

• Anaphylaxis. Respiratory and hemodynamic parameters need to be monitored continuously.
• Hepatotoxicity/renal impairment. Liver and/or kidney function tests should be monitored.

EXPECTED COURSE AND PROGNOSIS

• Most patients improve upon discontinuation of the medication(s) and provision of supportive care.
• Rarely is renal damage permanent.
• Liver damage from antibiotic-associated hepatotoxicity usually reverses with discontinuation of the drug.
• Antibiotic-associated bone marrow suppression usually reverses with discontinuation of the drug.

DISCHARGE CRITERIA/INSTRUCTIONS

Patients may be discharged from the emergency department or hospital when toxic effects resolve or stabilize and after psychiatric evaluation, if needed.

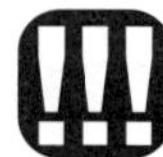

Pitfalls

DIAGNOSIS

• Toxicity may be confused with ingestion of other agents or with conditions that produce nonspecific gastrointestinal symptoms or renal, bone marrow, or hepatic injury.
• Patients often take antibiotics on their own, but may not relate that history.

TREATMENT

It is important to avoid excessive intervention in mildly toxic exposures.

ICD-9-CM 961.0

Poisoning by other antiinfectives: sulfonamides.

See also: SECTION II, Hypotension, Methemoglobinemia, and Seizure chapters.

RECOMMENDED READING

Carroll OM, Bryan PA, Robinson RJ. Stevens-Johnson syndrome associated with long-acting sulfonamides. *JAMA* 1966;195:691–693.

Carson JL, Strom BL, Duff A. Acute liver disease associated with erythromycins, sulfonamides, and tetracyclines. *Ann Intern Med* 1993;119:576–583.

Damergis JA, Stoker JM, Abadie JL. Methemoglobinemia after sulfamethoxazole and trimethoprim therapy. *JAMA* 1983;249:590–591.

Author: Steven A. Seifert

Reviewer: Katherine M. Hurlbut

Antineoplastic Medications

Basics

DESCRIPTION

- Antineoplastic agents are used in the treatment of various malignancies.
- Methotrexate also is used in the treatment of rheumatologic conditions.

FORMS AND USES

Antineoplastic agents include asparaginase (Elspar), bleomycin (Blenoxane), carboplatin (Paraplatin), carmustine (BCNU, BiCNU), chlorambucil (Leukeran), cisplatin (Platinol), cyclophosphamide (Cytoxan, NEOSAR), cytarabine (Cytosar U, Cytogam), dactinomycin (Cosmegen), daunorubicin citrate (DaunoXome), daunorubicin hydrochloride (Cerubidine), doxorubicin (Adriamycin, Rubex), ethylenimine, etoposide (VePesid), fluorouracil (Efudex cream and solution, Fluoroplex cream and solution, Fluothane), ifosfamide (Ifex), lomustine (CCNU, CeeNU), mechlorethamine (Mustargen), melphalan (Alkeran), methotrexate (Rheumatrex), mitomycin (mitomycin C, Mutamycin), nitrosureas, paclitaxel (Taxol), procarbazine (Matulane), streptozocin (Zanosar), vinblastine (Velban, Velsar), and vincristine (Oncovin, Vincasar).

PATHOPHYSIOLOGY

- Methotrexate. A structural analog of folate, it inhibits formation of nucleotides necessary for DNA and RNA synthesis.
- Pyrimidine analogs

—Cytarabine is a deoxycytidine analog, inhibiting DNA polymerase.
—5-Fluorouracil (5-FU) is a uracil analog, blocking thymidylate synthetase and incorporation into RNA and DNA.

- Vinca alkaloids (vincristine and vinblastine) bind tubulin and prevent polymerization into microtubules, interfering in cell replication.
- Etoposide affects DNA topoisomerase, causing DNA strand disruption.
- Taxol binds tubulin, preventing cell replication.
- Antibiotics (dactinomycin, daunorubicin, doxorubicin, bleomycin, and mitomycin) promote breakage and inhibit repair of DNA.
- Asparaginase depletes asparagine pools and inhibits protein synthesis.
- Carboplatin and cisplatin promote DNA cross-linking.
- Alkylating agents [nitrogen mustards (mechlorethamine, cyclophosphamide, ifosfamide, melphalan, and chlorambucil), ethylenimine, alkyl sulfonates, nitrosureas, and triazenes] form reactive intermediates that bind to nucleophilic moieties in DNA.

EPIDEMIOLOGY

- Overdose is uncommon, although adverse effects from therapeutic use are common.
- Toxic effects following exposure are typically moderate.
- Death occurs in patients with severe overdose or those receiving multiple agents with similar toxicities.
- Children are at greater risk for cardiotoxicity from doxorubicin and dactinomycin.
- The elderly are at greater risk for neurotoxicity from cytarabine, carboplatin, and mechlorethamine.

CAUSES

- Poisoning is usually an accidental iatrogenic incident.
- Child neglect or abuse should be considered if the patient is less than 1 year of age, suicide attempt if the patient is over 6 years of age.

RISK FACTORS

- Patients with underlying disease may be at increased risk.

—Cardiac (dactinomycin, doxorubicin, 5-FU, cisplatin, vinca alkaloids)
—Renal (cisplatin, streptozocin, nitrosureas, methotrexate, and mithramycin)
—Pulmonary (bleomycin)
—Neurologic (taxol, methotrexate, vincristine)

- Patients over 50 years of age or with renal insufficiency are at increased risk of toxicity from cytarabine.
- Risk factors for pulmonary fibrosis with bleomycin include a cumulative dose greater than 450 mg, a single dose greater than 25 mg/m^2, thoracic radiation, or oxygen administration.
- Mediastinal radiation, preexisting cardiac disease, concomitant use of cyclophosphamide, and use in the pediatric group increase risk of toxicity from doxorubicin and dactinomycin.

DRUG AND DISEASE INTERACTIONS

- Vincristine. Isoniazid and L-asparaginase may enhance neurotoxicity.
- Methotrexate. Nonsteroidal antiinflammatory drugs may increase the incidence of nephrotoxicity.

PREGNANCY AND LACTATION

- Most antineoplastics are known teratogens.
- Streptozocin, asparaginase, and dactinomycin. US FDA Pregnancy Category C. The drug exerts animal teratogenic or embryocidal effects, but there are no controlled studies in women, or no studies are available in animals or women.
- Antineoplastics. US FDA Pregnancy Category D. Positive evidence of human fetal risk exists, but benefits in certain situations (e.g., life-threatening situations or serious diseases) may make use of the drug acceptable despite its risks.
- Fluorouracil and methotrexate if used for rheumatoid arthritis or psoriasis. US FDA Pregnancy Category X. Studies in animals or humans have demonstrated fetal abnormalities or there is evidence of fetal risk based on human experience, or both, and the risk clearly outweighs any possible benefit.

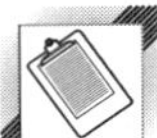

Diagnosis

DIFFERENTIAL DIAGNOSIS

Toxicologic causes of vomiting and diarrhea followed by bone marrow depression and possibly neurotoxicity include podophyllum, colchicine, arsenic, other heavy metal ingestion, and ricin.

SIGNS AND SYMPTOMS

Asparaginase

Hypersensitivity reactions (5%–20%), coagulopathy, pancreatitis, and decreased insulin production.

Bleomycin

Pulmonary fibrosis occurs in 5% of patients.

Carboplatin

- Nausea, vomiting and diarrhea are common.
- Myelosuppression is a dose-limiting effect.
- Hepatotoxicity occurs at high doses (greater than 1,500–2,000 mg/m^2). Fatal hepatotoxicity has occurred.
- Tinnitus and hearing loss occur at high doses.
- Peripheral neuropathy is more common in patients over 65 years of age.
- Renal insufficiency is associated with high dose (greater than 800–1,600 mg/m^2) and preexisting renal impairment.
- Hypomagnesemia, hypokalemia, hyponatremia, hypocalcemia, and anaphylaxis also have been reported.

Chlorambucil

Nausea, vomiting, bone marrow depression, seizures, ataxia, coma, irritability, and renal failure (rarely) have occurred.

Cisplatin

- Adverse effects include renal insufficiency (dose-limiting effect), tinnitus, high-frequency hearing loss, hypocalcemia, hypomagnesemia, hypophosphatemia, hypokalemia, anaphylactoid reactions, ataxia, sensory peripheral neuropathy, seizures, autonomic dysfunction, extrapyramidal effects, nausea, vomiting, and diarrhea, and increased liver enzyme levels.
- Neurotoxic effects are most often associated with a cumulative dose of 300 mg/m^2.
- Overdose effects include nausea, vomiting, diarrhea, hearing loss, respiratory failure, confusion, renal failure, increased liver enzyme levels, neurotoxicity, and myelosuppression.

Cyclophosphamide and Ifosfamide

- Hemorrhagic cystitis (5%–10%) is the most common adverse effect.
- Renal insufficiency, nausea, vomiting, diarrhea, stomatitis, syndrome of inappropriate secretion of antidiuretic hormone, hyperglycemia, and bone marrow suppression (leukopenia nadir at 7–12 days, thrombocytopenia at 10–15 days) may occur.

• High-dose ifosfamide may cause metabolic acidosis, mental status changes, cerebellar dysfunction, seizures, coma, and polyneuropathy.
• High-dose cyclophosphamide may cause cardiotoxicity, including decreased ECG voltage, and increased left ventricular mass at doses greater than 2.5 g/m^2/day.

Cytarabine

Cerebellar dysfunction, personality changes, parkinsonism, sensory peripheral neuropathy, and coma may develop.

Doxorubicin and Dactinomycin

• Overdose causes nausea, vomiting, diarrhea, stomatitis, and myelosuppression.
• Acute cardiotoxicity usually consists of ST changes and decreased ejection fraction and resolves within 24 hours.
• Acute myocarditis and pericarditis with conduction abnormalities are less common.
• Chronic cardiotoxicity is characterized by decreased ejection fraction and congestive heart failure and is related to the cumulative dose (greater than 20% incidence with total dose greater than 550 mg/m^2 doxorubicin or 950 mg/m^2 dactinomycin).
• Extravasation may cause significant local tissue destruction, swelling, pain, burning sensation, ulceration, and necrosis.

Etoposide

• Nausea, vomiting, and diarrhea are common.
• Myelosuppression is dose limiting; granulocyte nadir at 7 to 14 days, platelets at 9 to 16 days.
• Hepatic injury may develop at high doses (600–2,400 mg/m^2).
• Hypotension occurs with rapid intravenous infusion.
• Hypersensitivity reactions (bronchospasm and hypotension) and peripheral neuropathy also may occur.

Fluorouracil

• Vomiting, diarrhea, and lower gastrointestinal bleeding may occur.
• Lethargy, coma, ataxia, and upper motor neuron lesions with high intravenous doses or carotid arterial infusions may occur.
• ECG changes, myocardial ischemia, dilated cardiomyopathy, and cardiogenic shock may occur, usually in patients with preexisting cardiac disease.
• Bone marrow depression is dose limiting; granulocyte nadir occurs at 9 to 14 days, platelet nadir at 7 to 14 days.
• Extravasation causes local tissue irritation.

Mechlorethamine

• Eyes are irritated with splash contact.
• Ototoxicity, neurotoxicity (more common at high dose and older patients), CNS depression, nausea, vomiting, and bone marrow depression can occur.

Methotrexate

• Nausea and vomiting may begin within hours; mucositis, stomatitis, and diarrhea often develop within 7 to 14 days.
• Bone marrow suppression develops in 6 to 9 days and may last 2 weeks.
• Hepatic injury is associated with high or chronic dosing and usually resolves within 2 weeks of discontinuation.
• Acute tubular necrosis is reported with high intravenous doses.
• Increases in creatinine are associated with methotrexate levels greater than 4.5 μg/dl.
• Pulmonary effects may include infiltrates, dyspnea, cough, and tachypnea.
• Seizures, hemiparesis, behavioral changes, and reflex abnormalities have been associated with high intravenous doses.
• Intrathecal administration has been associated with chemical arachnoiditis (headache, neck stiffness, dizziness, fever, CSF pleocytosis), increased intracranial pressure and motor abnormalities (paresis, paraplegia, cranial nerve palsies, and ataxia).
• Necrotizing leukoencephalopathy includes cognitive disorders that can be delayed and is associated with intrathecal therapy or high intravenous doses given concurrently with cranial radiation.

Nitrosureas (Carmustine and Lomustine)

• Delayed bone marrow suppression (platelet nadir at 4 weeks, leukocytes at 5 weeks) may occur.
• Hypotension and tachycardia may occur with high-dose carmustine.
• Pulmonary fibrosis, CNS depression, nausea, vomiting, increased liver enzyme levels, and renal insufficiency can occur.
• Extravasation may cause serious local tissue destruction.

Paclitaxel (Taxol)

• Neutropenia is the dose-limiting effect.
• Other adverse effects include hypotension, dysrhythmias, congestive heart failure, headache, seizures, sensory neuropathy, coma, myalgias, pulmonary edema, anaphylaxis, autonomic neuropathy, mucositis, colonic perforation, increased liver function tests, renal insufficiency, optic neuritis, hypokalemia, nausea and vomiting, and ileus.
• Extravasation causes local tissue irritation.

Procarbazine

• A weak monoamine oxidase inhibitor, it may cause hypertension when administered with an indirect-acting sympathomimetic.
• Other effects include interstitial pneumonitis, paresthesia, neuropathy, hallucinations, seizures, coma, tremor, nausea, vomiting, diarrhea, and bone marrow suppression.

Vinblastine

• Myelosuppression is usually the dose-limiting effect; granulocyte nadir is at 7 to 14 days.
• Syndrome of inappropriate secretion of antidiuretic hormone, nausea, vomiting, myalgia, paresthesia, peripheral neuropathy, seizures and increased liver enzyme levels may occur.
• Extravasation may cause serious local tissue destruction.

Vincristine

• Symmetrical sensorimotor peripheral neuropathy (paresthesia, ataxia, decreased reflexes, and weakness) is generally the dose-limiting effect.
• Optic neuropathy, syndrome of inappropriate secretion of antidiuretic hormone, and bone marrow suppression also have been reported.
• In overdose, stomatitis, vomiting, diarrhea, fever, delirium, coma, seizures, and neuralgia may develop.
• Extravasation may cause significant local tissue destruction.

PROCEDURES AND LABORATORY TESTS

Essential Tests

• Complete blood count and platelet count. Myelosuppression is common at therapeutic doses of many antineoplastics; nadir counts usually develop after 7 to 14 days.
• Serum electrolytes, BUN, and creatinine tests are used to detect effects of prolonged vomiting and diarrhea. Nephrotoxicity may be caused by taxol, methotrexate, cyclophosphamide, cisplatin, and carboplatin.
• Ifosfamide may cause metabolic acidosis.

Recommended Tests

• Liver function tests (methotrexate, vinblastine, taxol, cisplatin, carboplatin, and etoposide). Hepatotoxicity may develop with therapeutic doses.
• ECG (doxorubicin, cyclophosphamide, dactinomycin, and fluorouracil). Cardiac toxicity may develop with therapeutic use.
• Methotrexate level is used to calculate an appropriate dose of leucovorin after methotrexate overdose.
• Urinalysis (cyclophosphamide and ifosfamide) is used to evaluate for hemorrhagic cystitis.
• Serum magnesium and phosphorus (carboplatin and cisplatin) are measured to detect hypomagnesemia and hypophosphatemia during therapeutic use.
• ECG, serum acetaminophen and aspirin levels are used in overdose setting to screen for occult ingestion.
• Audiometry may be useful after overdose of cisplatin and carboplatin, which cause hearing loss with therapeutic use.
• Electromyogram/nerve conduction velocity may be useful in patients with evidence of peripheral neuropathy after overdose of taxol, cisplatin, cytarabine, vincristine, vinblastine, carboplatin, etoposide, ifosfamide, and procarbazine.
• Echocardiography or radionuclide scan is used to detect doxorubicin cardiac toxicity.
• Chest radiograph may be useful after bleomycin overdose to detect pulmonary fibrosis.

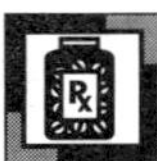

Treatment

- Treatment should focus on supporting cardiovascular function, detecting myelosuppression, and treating anemia, bleeding, and infection.
- Dose and time of exposure should be determined for all substances involved.

DIRECTING PATIENT COURSE

The health-care professional should call the poison control center when:

- Severe effects are present.
- Toxic effects are not consistent with antineoplastic poisoning.
- Coingestant, drug interaction, or underlying disease presents an unusual problem.

The patient should be referred to a health-care facility when:

- Attempted suicide or homicide is possible.
- Patient or caregiver seems unreliable.
- Any toxic effects develop.
- Coingestant, drug interaction, or underlying disease presents an unusual problem.

Admission Considerations

Inpatient management is warranted for patients with severe thrombocytopenia, anemia, or neutropenia; cardiac toxicity, suspected neutropenic sepsis, renal insufficiency, hepatotoxicity, mental status changes, seizures, or methotrexate toxicity requiring leucovorin therapy.

DECONTAMINATION

Out of Hospital

If acute ingestion has occurred, emesis should be induced with ipecac within 1 hour of ingestion for alert pediatric or adult patients if health-care evaluation will be delayed.

In Hospital

- If acute ingestion has occurred, gastric lavage should be performed in pediatric (tube size 24–32 French) or adult (tube size 36–42 French) patients for large ingestion presenting within 1 hour of ingestion or if serious effects are present.
- One dose of activated charcoal (1–2 g/kg) should be administered without a cathartic if a substantial ingestion has occurred within the previous few hours.

ANTIDOTES

Folic acid (Leucovorin) is a specific antidote for methotrexate poisoning.

- Indications

—Toxic methotrexate levels (1,000 μmol/L at 0 hours, 10 μmol/L at 24 hours, 0.5 μmol/L at 48 hours, or 0.05 μmol/L at 72 hours).
—Leucovorin should be administered at lower levels in patients with renal insufficiency or delayed methotrexate elimination.

- Contraindications. None.
- Method of administration

—Dose depends on levels, see nomogram or table in package insert.
—Range is 10 to 1,000 mg/m^2 every 6 hours orally, intramuscularly, or intravenously.

- Potential adverse effects. Anaphylactoid reactions.

ADJUNCTIVE TREATMENT

Amifostine

- Indications

—Protective against cisplatin-induced neurotoxicity and cyclophosphamide-induced myelosuppression
—Not studied in patients with overdoses but may have some utility

- Contraindications. Known hypersensitivity.
- Method of administration. 910 mg/m^2 intravenous infusion over 15 minutes.
- Adverse effects. Hypotension, dizziness, somnolence, hypocalcemia, hypomagnesemia, and flushing.

Dexrazoxane (Zinecard)

- Indications. Protection against doxorubicin-induced cardiac toxicity.
- Contraindications. Known allergy to dexrazoxane.
- Method of administration. 1,000 mg/m^2 intravenously or 10:1 dexrazoxane:doxorubicin ratio.
- Adverse effects. Nausea, vomiting, increased levels of liver function tests, myelosuppression, hypocalcemia, increased prothrombin time/partial thromboplastin time or international normalized ratio and increased amylase.

Granulocyte Colony-Stimulating Factor (GCSF)

- Indications. Neutropenia (absolute granulocyte count of less than 500/mm^3 or less than 1,000/mm^3 with fever or sepsis).
- Contraindications. Known hypersensitivity.
- Method of administration. 5 μg/kg/day subcutaneously or intravenously.

—Adverse effects. Hypotension, bone pain, and hypersensitivity reaction.

Sodium Bicarbonate

Urinary alkalinization may help prevent nephrotoxicity in methotrexate overdose; adult dose is a solution of 1 L D5W with 132 mEq sodium bicarbonate administered at two to three times maintenance fluid rates to maintain a urine pH of greater than 7.5; pediatric dose is 88 mEq sodium bicarbonate/L D5W.

Seizures

- A patent airway must be ensured.
- A benzodiazepine should be administered for initial control. If seizures persist or recur, another anticonvulsant such as phenobarbital should be added.
- Hypotension is treated with isotonic fluid infusion, the Trendelenburg position, and vasopressors if needed; dopamine is preferred, and norepinephrine is added for refractory hypotension.

Dysrhythmias or Conduction Abnormalities

- Seizures should be controlled and acidemia corrected.
- If QRS widening or dysrhythmias persist, sodium bicarbonate is administered at 1 to 2 mEq/kg intravenous bolus, repeated as needed to narrow QRS; arterial pH should not exceed 7.55.
- Lidocaine is used for ventricular tachycardia or multifocal premature ventricular complexes; adult dose is 50 to 100 mg intravenous bolus followed by infusion of 2 to 4 mg/min, titrated to desired effect; pediatric dose is 1 mg/kg bolus followed by infusion of 20 to 50 μg/kg/min, titrated to effect; bolus dose may be repeated in 10 to 15 minutes.
- If lidocaine is unsuccessful, bretylium is administered at 5 mg/kg over 1 minute; if unsuccessful, it is administered 10 mg/kg over 1 minute, repeated as necessary to total dose of 30 mg/kg.

Extravasation

• Infusion is stopped and as much infusate as possible is aspirated. The drug should then be diluted by injecting 10 to 15 ml 0.9% saline into the site.
• The limb is elevated and ice applied for 20 minutes four times a day.
• For vinca alkaloids or etoposide, warm compresses are applied or hyaluronidase (150 units hyaluronidase/L 0.9% saline) is infiltrated into the site to promote systemic uptake.
• Topical DMSO 100% every 6 hours has been used for extravasation caused by mitomycin-C, doxorubicin, or daunorubicin.
• Mechlorethamine. Infiltration with sodium thiosulfate 2% to 5% is used.
• Mitomycin-C extravasation is treated with topical DMSO 100% every 6 hours or subcutaneous infiltration with pyridoxine 100 mg/ml.
• Early surgical evaluation is needed for extravasation caused by doxorubicin, extravasation over a joint, or any case where tissue destruction is developing.
• Hydrocortisone infiltration (50 to 200 mg subcutaneously or intradermally) for doxorubicin and vinca alkaloids.

Glutamic Acid

May be used to prevent vincristine-induced neurotoxicity. A dose of 500 mg should be administered three times a day.

Hydration

Hydration reduces cisplatin nephrotoxicity and may reduce severity of hemorrhagic cystitis from cyclophosphamide and ifosfamide; adult dose is 5 to 6 L of an appropriate intravenous fluid per day. Furosemide is added at 10 mg every 8 to 12 hours or more as needed to maintain fluid balance.

Intrathecal Overdose

Intrathecal overdose or inadvertent intrathecal administration of an agent not designed for that use is initially treated with immediate removal of as much CSF as is clinically reasonable (usually 20 ml in an adult).

• Intrathecal methotrexate overdose has been treated with ventriculolumbar perfusion with warm normal saline or serial removal of 20-ml portions of CSF and replacement with equal volumes of warmed preservative-free normal saline (total volume exchanged 200–250 ml).
• Inadvertent intrathecal vincristine administration has been treated with CSF aspiration followed by ventriculolumbar perfusion with fresh frozen plasma.

Fluorouracil-induced Myelosuppression

This may be prevented with 300 mg allopurinol three times a day, but there has been no reported experience in its use in treating an overdose.

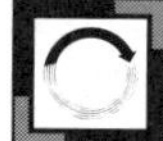

Follow-Up

PATIENT MONITORING

Patients who develop dysrhythmias, hemodynamic instability, chronic heart failure, bleeding, mental status changes, seizures, respiratory failure, or hepatic failure should be monitored in an ICU.

EXPECTED COURSE AND PROGNOSIS

• Most patients recover with supportive care.
• Permanent renal insufficiency and central or peripheral neurologic deficits may develop after overdose or therapeutic use.
• Patients with severe myelosuppression may succumb to neutropenic sepsis or uncontrolled bleeding.

DISCHARGE CRITERIA/INSTRUCTIONS

• From the emergency department

—Asymptomatic patients may be discharged if they have nontoxic methotrexate levels (if involved) and after gastrointestinal decontamination, 6 hours of observation, and psychiatric evaluation, if needed.
—Outpatient follow-up needs to be arranged prior to discharge for laboratory studies and neurologic evaluation as appropriate.

• From the hospital

—Patients may be discharged when able to tolerate oral feedings, mental status is improving, renal and hepatic function is stabilized, bleeding is controlled, and severe anemia or thrombocytopenia is improving.
—Outpatient follow-up needs to be arranged prior to discharge for laboratory studies and neurologic evaluation as appropriate.

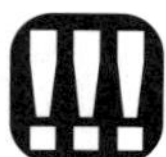

Pitfalls

FOLLOW-UP

Because some effects (e.g., myelosuppression), may not develop for more than a week after exposure, a follow-up appointment must be arranged prior to discharge.

ICD-9-CM 977

Poisoning by other and unspecified drugs and medicinal substances.

See also: SECTION II, Extravasation, Hypotension, and Seizures chapters; SECTION III, Folic Acid chapter.

RECOMMENDED READING

Wang RY, Calabresi P. Antineoplastic agents. In: Goldfrank LR, Flomenbaum NE, Lewin NA, et al., eds. *Goldfrank's toxicologic emergencies.* 6th ed. Norwalk, CT: Appleton & Lange, 1998.

Author: Katherine M. Hurlbut

Reviewer: Richard C. Dart

Antiparasitic Drugs

Basics

DESCRIPTION

The antiparasitic drugs include mebendazole, thiabendazole, and albendazole.

FORMS AND USES

Mebendazole (Vermox)

- Dosage applies to both adults and children.
- Enterobiasis. 100 mg once orally, consider repeat dose in 2 weeks.
- Ascariasis, trichuriasis, hookworm infection. 100 mg twice a day orally for 3 to 5 days.

Thiabendazole (Mintezol)

- Strongyloidiasis. 50 mg/kg in two doses for 2 days.
- Trichinosis. 50 mg/kg in two doses for 5 to 7 days.
- Cutaneous larva migrans. 25 mg/kg twice a day (a maximum of 3 g per day) for 2 to 5 days.

Albendazole (Albenza)

Typical dose for all patients over 2 years of age is 400 mg as a single oral dose; 200 mg for children 1 to 2 years of age.

PATHOPHYSIOLOGY

- Albendazole, mebendazole, and thiabendazole block the assembly of tubulin polymers. This causes depolymerization or complete breakdown of the microtubule and inhibition of protein secretion and glucose transport.
- These drugs are poorly absorbed and therefore affect primarily intestinal parasites and avoid systemic effects on the host.

EPIDEMIOLOGY

- Poisoning is becoming more common with the need to increase drug concentrations in an attempt to overcome drug resistance.
- Toxic effects following exposure are typically mild.

CAUSES

- Poisoning usually occurs by an accidental ingestion.
- Iatrogenic poisonings are due to drug interactions.
- Child neglect or abuse should be considered if the patient is less than 1 year of age, suicide attempt if the patient is over 6 years of age.

DRUG AND DISEASE INTERACTIONS

- Mebendazole. Cimetidine inhibits mebendazole metabolism and may increase plasma concentration.
- Thiabendazole. Inhibits metabolism of theophylline and may increase blood levels.
- Abendaxole. Dexamethadone and cimetidine may increase albudazole levels.

PREGNANCY AND LACTATION

- Mebendazole and thiabendazole. US FDA Pregnancy Category C. The drug exerts animal teratogenic or embryocidal effects, but there are no controlled studies in women, or no studies are available in either animals or women.
- Albendazole has not been assigned an FDA classification.
- Each of these drugs is relatively contraindicated in pregnancy.

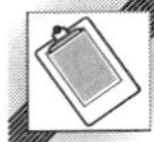

Diagnosis

DIFFERENTIAL DIAGNOSIS

Toxicologic causes that produce gastrointestinal upset and CNS depression include theophylline, salicylates, isopropanol, nonsteroidal antiinflammatory agents, and many others.

SIGNS AND SYMPTOMS

- Thiabendazole and related agents generally cause mild effects in an acute overdose.
- Thiabendazole appears to cause most adverse effects.

Vital Signs

Hypotension has occurred in a few severe poisonings.

HEENT

Tinnitus has been reported with thiabendazole.

Dermatologic

Each of these agents may cause rashes, urticaria and, rarely, Stevens-Johnson syndrome.

Gastrointestinal

- Anorexia, abdominal pain, nausea, vomiting, and diarrhea may develop.
- Elevated liver enzymes occur occasionally.

Renal

Hemolytic uremic syndrome may occur

Hematologic

Bone marrow depression has been associated with the use of mebendazole and albendazole.

Neurologic

- Dizziness, drowsiness, and headache have been reported.
- Seizure and Guillain-Barré syndrome have been associated with use, but the causal relationship is unclear.
- Hallucinations occur rarely.

PROCEDURES AND LABORATORY TESTS

Essential Tests

No tests may be needed in asymptomatic or minimally symptomatic patients.

Recommended Tests

- Liver function tests are used to monitor for hepatotoxicity.
- ECG and serum acetaminophen and aspirin levels are ordered to detect occult overdose.
- Serum levels are available in some places; however, they are used to confirm exposure, not to guide therapy.

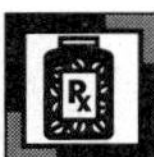

Treatment

- Treatment focuses on decontamination, supportive care, and identification of coingestants or complicating factors.
- The dose and time of exposure should be determined for all substances involved.

DIRECTING PATIENT COURSE

The health-care professional should call the poison control center when:

- CNS or other severe effects are present.
- Toxic effects are not consistent with mebendazole or thiabendazole.
- Coingestant, drug interaction, or underlying disease presents an unusual challenge.

The patient should be referred to a health-care facility when:

- Attempted suicide or homicide is possible.
- Patient or caregiver seems unreliable.
- Coingestant, drug interaction, or underlying disease presents an unusual challenge.

Admission Considerations

Inpatient management is warranted for patients with altered mental status.

DECONTAMINATION

Out of Hospital

Ipecac should be administered to induce emesis within 1 hour of ingestion for alert pediatric or adult patients if health-care evaluation will be delayed.

In Hospital

- Gastric lavage should be performed in pediatric (tube size 24–32 French) or adult (tube size 36–42 French) patients for large ingestion presenting within 1 hour of ingestion or if serious effects are present.
- One dose of activated charcoal (1–2 g/kg) should be administered without a cathartic if a substantial ingestion has occurred within the previous few hours.

ANTIDOTES

There is no specific antidote for poisoning by these agents.

ADJUNCTIVE TREATMENT

For seizures, a patent airway should be ensured and monitored closely, and a benzodiazepine should be administered for initial control.

- Diazepam

—The adult dose is 5 to 10 mg initially by intravenous push, repeated every 10 minutes as needed.
—The pediatric dose is 0.2 to 0.5 mg/kg, repeated every 10 minutes as needed.

- Lorazepam

—The adult dose is 2 to 4 mg initially by intravenous push, repeated every 10 minutes as needed.
—The pediatric dose is 0.1 mg/kg, repeated every 10 minutes as needed.
—Add another anticonvulsant, such as phenobarbital, if seizures persist or recur.

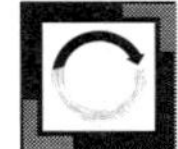

Follow-Up

PATIENT MONITORING

Cardiac monitoring is needed until the acute episode resolves.

EXPECTED COURSE AND PROGNOSIS

Toxic effects usually occur early, are not severe, and improve over 12 to 24 hours.

DISCHARGE CRITERIA/INSTRUCTIONS

- From the emergency department. Asymptomatic patients may be discharged after 8 hours of observation and after psychiatric evaluation, if needed.
- From the hospital. Patients may be discharged after sequelae have resolved.

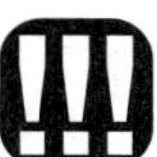

Pitfalls

DIAGNOSIS

Drug history is needed to identify drug interactions and coingestions.

ICD-9-CM 960.8

Poisoning by antibiotics: other specified antibiotics.

RECOMMENDED READING

Ellenhorn MJ. *Ellenhorn's medical toxicology: diagnosis and treatment of human poisoning,* 2nd ed. Baltimore: Williams & Wilkins, 1997.

Liu LX, Weller PF. Antiparasitic drugs. *N Engl J Med* 1996;334:1178–1184.

Author: Netti Riggs

Reviewer: Richard C. Dart

Antiprotozoal Medications

Basics

DESCRIPTION

Antiprotozoal medications include metronidazole (Flagyl, Protostat), chloroquine (Aralen), and hydroxychloroquine (Plaquenil).

FORMS AND USES

- Chloroquine

—For malaria, the adult dose is 160 to 200 mg intramuscularly, then 1 g orally, followed by 500 mg orally in 6 hours, and 500 mg orally daily for 2 days.
—For extraintestinal amebiasis, the adult loading dose is 1 g orally, followed by 500 mg daily for 2 to 3 weeks; the pediatric loading dose is 10 mg base/kg, orally, then 5 mg base/kg.
—Hydroxychloroquine. For malaria, the adult dose is 620 mg of the base initially, followed by 310 mg in 6 to 8 hours and 310 mg/day for 2 days.
—Metronidazole. For *Trichomonas* infection, intestinal amebiasis, and serious anaerobic infections, the adult dose is 375 to 1,000 mg, two to four times daily.

TOXIC DOSE

- Chloroquine has extreme potential toxicity; just three to four times the normal dose has caused death in either adults or children.
- Hydroxychloroquine may be fatal in an overdose above 10 g.
- Metronidazole. Although 2 to 3 g may cause mild symptoms, ingestion of 10 g rarely causes serious effects.

PATHOPHYSIOLOGY

Chloroquine is thought to act like class 1A antidysrhythmic agents by blocking the fast sodium channel, slowing phase zero of the action potential (depolarization), and depressing cardiac conduction velocity.

EPIDEMIOLOGY

- Poisoning by any of these agents is uncommon.
- Toxic effects are mild for metronidazole.

CAUSES

- A parenteral overdose is usually an iatrogenic error.
- An oral overdose is usually an intentional ingestion.
- Child neglect or abuse should be considered if the patient is less than 1 year of age, suicide attempt if the patient is over 6 years of age.

DRUG AND DISEASE INTERACTIONS

- Chloroquine and metronidazole levels are increased by cimetidine.
- Metronidazole potentiates the effect of oral anticoagulants.
- Phenytoin and phenobarbital increase clearance of metronidazole and result in reduced serum levels.
- Lithium levels may become toxic with use of metronidazole.

PREGNANCY AND LACTATION

- Metronidazole. US FDA Pregnancy Category B. Animal studies indicate no fetal risk and there are no controlled human studies, or animal studies show an adverse fetal effect but well-controlled studies in pregnant women do not.
- Chloroquine. US FDA Pregnancy Category D. Positive evidence of human fetal risk exists, but benefits in certain situations (e.g., life-threatening situations or serious diseases) may make use of the drug acceptable despite its risks.
- Metronidazole should be avoided in pregnant women.

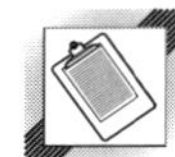

Diagnosis

DIFFERENTIAL DIAGNOSIS

- Chloroquine. Toxicologic causes of CNS depression, seizure, and ECG conduction abnormality include class I antidysrhythmic agents, antihistamines, cocaine, β-receptor or calcium channel blockers, quinine, digoxin, phenothiazine, and cyclic antidepressants.
- Metronidazole. Other causes of a disulfiram-like reaction include a combination of disulfiram and alcohol or other medications.

SIGNS AND SYMPTOMS

Chloroquine

Respiratory depression, cardiovascular collapse, seizures, and death occur in a serious overdose.

Hydroxychloroquine

- Neurotoxicity may occur with subacute myelooptic neuropathy, potentially leading to loss of vision.
- A delayed-onset, retrograde amnesia is reported following acute overdose.

Metronidazole

Nausea, vomiting, and ataxia occur in overdose; a disulfiram-like reaction occurs with ethanol.

Vital Signs

Chloroquine may cause tachycardia and hypotension.

HEENT

- Chloroquine and hydroxychloroquine. Tinnitus, sensorineural hearing loss, scotomas, blurred/clouded vision, and retinopathy (with chronic treatment) may occur.
- Hydroxychloroquine. Symptoms include retinopathy, decreased vision, scotoma and blurred vision, as well as corneal edema and opacities.

Dermatologic

- Chloroquine. Eruptions similar to lichen planus and pigmentary changes of skin and mucous membranes may occur.
- Hydroxychloroquine. Bleaching of hair, alopecia, pruritus, and skin eruptions (urticarial, lichenoid, exfoliative, and others) may occur.

Cardiovascular

Chloroquine may cause a widened QRS interval, inversion and depression of T-waves, and ventricular dysrhythmias, and cardiac arrest may occur suddenly after a large ingestion.

Pulmonary

Chloroquine may cause respiratory depression and arrest in severe cases.

Gastrointestinal

- Chloroquine and hydroxychloroquine. Anorexia, nausea, vomiting, diarrhea, and abdominal cramps may occur.
- Metronidazole. Nausea, vomiting, metallic taste, abdominal pain, and occasionally constipation may occur.

Hepatic

- Liver injury may occur in chloroquine-poisoned patients with glucose-6-phosphate dehydrogenase deficiency or alcoholic liver disease.
- Hydroxychloroquine has been associated with fulminant hepatic failure.

Renal

Metronidazole can cause dysuria, cystitis, polyuria, and dark urine.

Hematologic

- Chloroquine and hydroxychloroquine. Hemolytic anemia and methemoglobinemia have been reported.
- Metronidazole. Neutropenia and, rarely, thrombocytopenia may occur.

Neurologic/Psychiatric

- Chloroquine. Headache, neuropathy, visual disturbance, and agitation are followed by seizures and coma.
- Hydroxychloroquine. CNS irritability, psychosis, headache, nystagmus, ataxia, and seizures may occur.
- Metronidazole. Drowsiness, vertigo, seizures, and peripheral neuropathy may develop.

Immunologic

All of the drugs in this chapter have been reported to produce allergic reactions.

PROCEDURES AND LABORATORY TESTS

Essential Tests

- Chloroquine. ECG and cardiac monitoring to detect QRS and QTc widening which often precede ventricular dysrhythmia.
- Chloroquine or metronidazole. Complete blood count may detect neutropenia or thrombocytopenia, which is usually mild and reversible with cessation of the drug.

Recommended Tests

- Serum electrolytes, BUN, creatinine levels are ordered to evaluate altered mental status or cardiac dysrhythmia.
- Serum acetaminophen and aspirin levels in an overdose setting are used to detect occult overdose with analgesic medications.
- An ophthalmologic evaluation is ordered for any visual symptoms.

Not Recommended Tests

Specific drug levels are not clinically helpful.

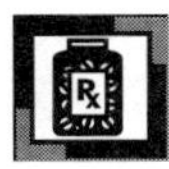

Treatment

- Chloroquine. Treatment focuses on airway management, supportive care, and administration of benzodiazepines and epinephrine in serious cases.
- Metronidazole. Treatment focuses on supportive care and management of hematologic abnormalities.
- The dose and time of exposure should be determined for all substances involved.

DIRECTING PATIENT COURSE

The health-care professional should call the poison control center when:

- Any toxic effects develop.
- Toxic effects are not consistent with expected toxicity.
- A coingestant, drug interaction, or underlying disease presents an unusual problem.

The patient should be referred to a health-care facility when:

- Attempted suicide or homicide is possible.
- Patient or caregiver seems unreliable.
- Any toxic effects develop.
- A coingestant, drug interaction, or underlying disease presents an unusual problem.

Admission Considerations

- Inpatient management is warranted for chloroquine- or hydroxychloroquine-poisoned patients who develop hypotension, respiratory or CNS depression, seizure, or dysrhythmia.
- For metronidazole, hospital admission is appropriate for patients with toxic effects that do not resolve promptly.

DECONTAMINATION

Out of Hospital

- Chloroquine and hydroxychloroquine. Do not induce emesis.
- Metronidazole. Ipecac should be administered to induce emesis within 1 hour of ingestion for alert pediatric or adult patients, if health-care evaluation will be delayed.

In Hospital

- Gastric lavage should be performed in pediatric (tube size 24–32 French) or adult (tube size 36–42 French) patients for large ingestion presenting within 1 hour of ingestion or if life-threatening effects are present.
- One dose of activated charcoal (1–2 g/kg) should be administered without a cathartic if a potentially toxic amount has been ingested.

ANTIDOTES

There is no specific antidote for overdose with any of these agents.

ADJUNCTIVE TREATMENT

- Chloroquine-induced dysrhythmia, hypotension, or seizure or history of ingestion of more than 5 g. Therapy should include early endotracheal intubation and administration of high doses of epinephrine and diazepam.

—Epinephrine. Infusion begins at 0.25 μg/kg/min, with the rate increased to maintain systolic blood pressure at greater than 100 mm Hg.
—Diazepam. The initial dose is 2 mg/kg infused over 30 minutes, followed by a continuous infusion of 1 to 2 mg/kg/day for 2 to 4 days depending on severity of toxicity; recurrence of cardiac dysrhythmia may respond to repeat diazepam bolus.

- Isolated seizures or altered mental status

—No data are available except for the treatment described above for chloroquine.
—Standard seizure management with more modest benzodiazepine doses may be used if these effects are isolated; however, it must be assured that the cardiac effects are absent.

- Not recommended therapies. No type of enhanced elimination is recommended.

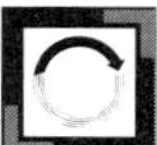

Follow-Up

PATIENT MONITORING

- Chloroquine and hydroxychloroquine. Respiratory and hemodynamic function should be monitored in an ICU.
- Metronidazole. Blood counts should be monitored as indicated by the initial laboratory results.

EXPECTED COURSE AND PROGNOSIS

- Acute overdoses with metronidazole usually peak in the first few hours and quickly resolve.
- A patient with chloroquine overdose typically deteriorates within a couple of hours, and death may occur abruptly; recovery may require days.
- Chloroquine may produce permanent hearing loss or sequelae of hypoxia, depending on whether complications occur.
- Retinopathy of chloroquine and hydroxychloroquine may persist or worsen despite treatment.

DISCHARGE CRITERIA/INSTRUCTIONS

- From the emergency department

—Chloroquine. It is unusual to discharge patients due to potentially lethal toxicity and narrow therapeutic ratio.
—Hydroxychloroquine. Patients without CNS or cardiac effects for 8 hours may be discharged after decontamination and psychiatric evaluation, if needed.
—Metronidazole. Patients may be discharged if toxicity does not develop over 2 to 4 hours, following gastrointestinal decontamination and psychiatric evaluation, if needed.

- From the hospital. Patients may be discharged after toxic effects have resolved or stabilized.

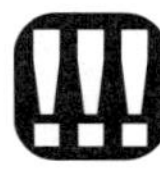

Pitfalls

DIAGNOSIS

Because chloroquine may produce rapid cardiovascular and CNS deterioration, the patient must be monitored very closely and receive early and aggressive care.

ICD-9-CM 961.7

Poisoning by other antiinfectives: antiviral drugs.

RECOMMENDED READING

Frytak S, Moertel CG, Childs DS, et al. Neurologic toxicity associated with high-dose metronidazole therapy. *Ann Intern Med* 1978;88:361–362.

Riou B, Barriot P, Rimailho A, et al. Treatment of severe chloroquine poisoning. *N Engl J Med* 1988;318:1–6.

Author: Steven A. Seifert

Reviewer: Luke Yip

Antivirals—Acyclovir Analogs, Amantadine, and Foscarnet

Basics

DESCRIPTION

These drugs are used in the treatment of herpes simplex and varicella zoster (acyclovir), cytomegalovirus (cidofovir and ganciclovir), herpes zoster (famciclovir and valacyclovir), or HIV infection (foscarnet and rimantadine).

FORMS AND USES

Antivirals discussed here include acyclovir (Zovirax), amantadine (Symmetrel), cidofovir (Vistide), famciclovir (Famvir), foscarnet (Foscavir), ganciclovir (Cytovene), ribavirin (Virazole), rimantadine (Flumadine), and valacyclovir (Valtrex).

PATHOPHYSIOLOGY

- Amantadine and rimantadine. The toxic mechanism includes anticholinergic effects. In addition, CNS and cardiac toxicity may develop similar to the tricyclic antidepressants.
- Cidofovir. The major toxicity is kidney proximal tubular cell injury.
- Ganciclovir. Toxicity is primarily manifested as bone marrow suppression and kidney injury.

EPIDEMIOLOGY

- Poisoning is uncommon.
- Toxic effects following exposure are typically mild to moderate.

CAUSES

- Acute toxicity is usually intentional.
- Child neglect should be considered if the patient is less than 1 year of age, suicide attempt if the patient is over 6 years of age.

DRUG AND DISEASE INTERACTIONS

Amantadine and Rimantadine

- Concomitant use of thioridazine may worsen tremor.
- Other anticholinergic agents may enhance toxicity.

Cidofovir

Administration with other nephrotoxic agents may increase the risk of kidney damage.

Foscarnet

- Use with pentamidine or other drugs that cause hypocalcemia may result in hypocalcemia.
- Concomitant use of drugs that may cause nephrotoxicity may produce kidney toxicity.
- Use with zidovudine and foscarnet may result in anemia.

Ganciclovir

- Neutropenia and anemia effects of didanosine and ganciclovir may be additive.
- Imipenem-cilastatin coadministered with ganciclovir has resulted in generalized seizures.
- Nephrotoxic drugs may have additive effects.

PREGNANCY AND LACTATION

- Famciclovir. US FDA Pregnancy Category B. Animal studies indicate no fetal risk and there are no controlled human studies, or animal studies show an adverse fetal effect but well-controlled studies in pregnant women do not.
- Acyclovir, amantadine/rimantadine, cidofovir, foscarnet, ganciclovir, and valacyclovir. US FDA Pregnancy Category C. The drug exerts animal teratogenic or embryocidal effects, but there are no controlled studies in women, or no studies are available in either animals or women.
- Ribavirin. US FDA Pregnancy Category X. Studies have demonstrated fetal abnormalities or there is evidence of fetal risk based on human experience, or both, and the risk clearly outweighs any possible benefit.

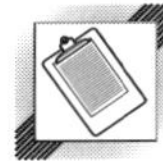

Diagnosis

DIFFERENTIAL DIAGNOSIS

- Renal failure. Aminoglycosides, chlorinated hydrocarbons, ethylene glycol, mercury, rhabdomyolysis, and other antiviral agents.
- Hepatotoxicity. Acetaminophen, anesthetic gases, aromatic hydrocarbons, arsenic, chronic ethanol, chlorinated insecticides, iron, polychorinated biphenyls, valproic acid, and other antiviral agents.

SIGNS AND SYMPTOMS

Acyclovir, Valacyclovir, and Famciclovir

Mild toxicity is manifested primarily by nausea, vomiting, and diarrhea.

Amantadine and Rimantadine

Amantadine and rimantadine have primarily anticholinergic effects, with CNS and cardiac toxicity.

Cidofovir

Overdose primarily results in renal insufficiency.

Foscarnet

The major toxicity is renal insufficiency.

Ganciclovir

Major toxicities are neutropenia, thrombocytopenia, anemia, and renal injury.

Ribavirin

The primary effect is anemia, followed by reticulocytosis.

Vital Signs

- Acyclovir and valacyclovir. Fever.
- Amantadine and rimantadine. Tachycardia, fever, and malignant hyperthermia.
- Ganciclovir. Fever.
- Ribavirin. Tachypnea, apnea, tachycardia, bradycardia.

HEENT

- Acyclovir and valacyclovir. Headache.
- Amantadine and rimantadine. Dry mouth and dilated pupils.
- Cidofovir. Low intraocular pressure.
- Ribavirin. Conjunctivitis.

Dermatologic

- Acyclovir and valacyclovir. Rash urticaria.
- Foscarnet. Rash and diaphoresis.
- Ribavirin. Rash.

Cardiovascular

- Amantadine and rimantadine. Tachycardia, ventricular ectopy (including torsade de pointes) and fibrillation, asystole, and chronic heart failure.
- Foscarnet. Dysrhythmia from electrolyte disturbance.
- Ribavirin

—Cardiac arrest, bradycardia, tachycardia, and ventricular ectopy may occur.
—Aerosol treatment of infants has resulted in death after massive exposure.

Pulmonary

- Amantadine and rimantadine. Adult respiratory distress syndrome.
- Foscarnet. Cough and dyspnea.
- Ribavirin. Dyspnea, bronchospasm, pneumothorax, and apnea.

Gastrointestinal

- Amantadine causes decreased gastrointestinal motility.
- All other agents produce nausea, vomiting, and diarrhea.

Hepatic

- Acyclovir and valacyclovir. Elevated levels on liver function test.
- Ribavirin. Elevated indirect bilirubin.

Renal

- Acyclovir and valacyclovir. Renal failure and obstructive nephropathy secondary to crystalluria.
- Cidofovir. Nephrotoxicity with proteinuria, glycosuria, and elevated serum creatinine.
- Foscarnet. Renal insufficiency.
- Ganciclovir. Renal insufficiency.

Hematologic

- Acyclovir and valacyclovir. Leukopenia and lymphadenopathy.
- Cidofovir. Neutropenia.
- Foscarnet. Anemia and granulocytopenia.
- Ganciclovir. Neutropenia, thrombocytopenia, and anemia.
- Ribavirin. Anemia and rebound reticulocytosis.

Musculoskeletal

Acyclovir and valacyclovir. Myalgia.

Neurologic/Psychiatric

- Acyclovir and valacyclovir. Lethargy, agitation, hallucinations, myoclonus, tremor, and coma.
- Amantadine and rimantadine. CNS depression, agitation, dystonias, confusion, hallucinations, and seizures; withdrawal of the drug is associated with neuroleptic malignant syndrome.
- Foscarnet. Seizures, headache, confusion, perioral tingling, and peripheral numbness.
- Ganciclovir. Seizures.

Endocrine

- Amantadine and rimantadine. Metabolic acidosis.
- Cidofovir. Metabolic acidosis and Fanconi's syndrome.
- Foscarnet. Hypokalemia, hypocalcemia, hypophosphatemia, hypomagnesemia, and hyperphosphatemia.

PROCEDURES AND LABORATORY TESTS

Essential Tests

- Acyclovir and valacyclovir. Liver and renal function tests.
- Cidofovir. Complete blood count (CBC), renal function tests, and levels of serum electrolytes and phosphate.
- Foscarnet. CBC, renal function tests, and levels of serum potassium, calcium, magnesium, and phosphate.
- Ganciclovir. CBC and liver and renal function tests.
- Ribavirin. CBC and liver function tests.

Recommended Tests

- Amantadine and rimantadine. Cardiac monitoring.
- Cidofovir. Periodic ocular function tests.
- Foscarnet. Cardiac monitoring.

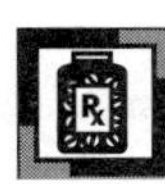

Treatment

- For each of these agents, patients with normal liver and renal function can usually be managed with conservative and supportive measures.
- Treatment should be focused on supportive care.
- Dose and time of exposure should be determined for all substances involved.

DIRECTING PATIENT COURSE

The health-care professional should call the poison control center when:

- Unexpected toxicity or other severe effects are present.
- Toxic effects are not consistent with antiviral toxicity.
- Coingestant, drug interaction, or underlying disease presents an unusual problem.

The patient should be referred to a health-care facility when:

- Attempted suicide or homicide is possible.
- Patient or caregiver seems unreliable.
- Unexpected toxic effects develop.
- Coingestant, drug interaction, or underlying disease presents an unusual problem.

Admission Considerations

Inpatient management is warranted for patients who develop hypotension, respiratory or CNS depression, seizures, significant airway compromise, or dysrhythmia.

DECONTAMINATION

Out of hospital

Ipecac-induced emesis is not recommended.

In Hospital

- Gastric lavage should be performed in pediatric (tube size 24–32 French) or adult (tube size 36–42 French) patients for large ingestion presenting within 1 hour of ingestion or if serious effects are present.
- One dose of activated charcoal (1–2 g/kg) should be administered without a cathartic if a substantial ingestion has occurred within the previous few hours.

ANTIDOTES

There are no specific antidotes available for the antiviral medications.

ADJUNCTIVE TREATMENT

- Amantadine and rimantadine

—Physostigmine should be considered for severe, anticholinergic effects unresponsive to supportive care.
—Plasma levels are reduced by hemodialysis.

- Cidofovir. Administration of probenecid may prevent or decrease nephrotoxicity in overdose.
- Acyclovir and valacyclovir. Hemodialysis may enhance removal of the drug in patients with renal failure.
- Foscarnet. Hemodialysis may increase body clearance, although its clinical usefulness has not been evaluated.
- Ganciclovir. Hemodialysis increases body clearance.
- Ribavirin. Hemodialysis is not effective.

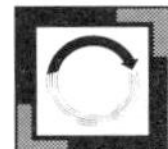

Follow-Up

PATIENT MONITORING

- Acyclovir and valacyclovir. Monitor CNS and renal function.
- Amantadine and rimantadine. Cardiac monitoring for 24 hours if signs of cardiac toxicity develop within 6 hours of ingestion.
- Cidofovir. Renal function should be monitored until stable.

EXPECTED COURSE AND PROGNOSIS

- Acyclovir and valacyclovir. Patients who have ingested up to 20 g have recovered uneventfully.
- Amantadine and rimantadine. Death from adult respiratory distress syndrome and cardiac dysrhythmia has occurred with 2 to 3 g in overdose.
- Cidofovir. Experience is limited in overdose. Recovery with some possible residual renal injury is expected.
- Foscarnet

—Recovery is expected with supportive care.
—Renal impairment may persist.
—Death from seizure has occurred.

- Ganciclovir. There is limited experience with the oral form of this drug. Recovery is likely.
- Ribavirin. Recovery is expected with supportive care.

DISCHARGE CRITERIA/INSTRUCTIONS

- From the emergency department. The asymptomatic patient can be discharged after an observation period of 4 to 6 hours and psychiatric evaluation, if needed.
- From the hospital

—Patients can be discharged when toxic effects have resolved or stabilized and after psychiatric evaluation, if needed.
—Patients with amantadine or rimantadine poisoning should be monitored for at least 24 hours.

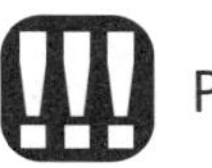

Pitfalls

TREATMENT

Class IA antidysrhythmic agents should be avoided for amantadine and rimantadine overdoses.

ICD-9-CM 961.7

Poisoning by other antiinfectives: antiviral drugs.

See also: SECTION II, Hyperthermia, Hypotension, Ventricular Dysrhythmias, and Seizure chapters; and SECTION III, Physostigmine chapter.

RECOMMENDED READING

Krieble BF, Rudy DW, Glick MR, et al. Case report: acyclovir/valacyclovir neurotoxicity and nephrotoxicity—the role for hemodialysis. *Am J Med Sci* 1993;305:36–39.

Pimentel L, Hughes B. Amantadine/rimantadine toxicity presenting with complex ventricular ectopy and hallucinations. *Pediatr Emerg Care* 1991;7:89–92.

Author: Steven A. Seifert

Reviewer: Richard C. Dart

Antivirals—Protease Inhibitors

Basics

DESCRIPTION

These substances are used for the treatment of local or systemic human immunodeficiency virus (HIV) infection.

FORMS AND USES

Indinavir (Crixivan), ritonavir (Norvir), and saquinavir (Invirase)

- Indinavir. 800 mg orally every 8 hours, 1 hour before or 2 hours after meals; dose is reduced to 600 mg every 8 hours with hepatic insufficiency.
- Ritonavir. 600 mg orally twice daily with food.
- Saquinavir. 600 mg orally within 2 hours of a meal.

PATHOPHYSIOLOGY

- Protease inhibitors are inhibitors of HIV proteases that cleave viral protein precursors necessary for viral replication.
- Major effects are gastrointestinal and peripheral neuropathies.
- Inhibitors also cause cytochrome P450 inhibition and increased activity of glucuronosyl transferases, resulting in numerous drug-to-drug interactions.
- Little information is available, but protease inhibitors are expected to have minimal toxicity following acute ingestion.

EPIDEMIOLOGY

- Poisoning is uncommon.
- Toxic effects are typically mild.
- Death occurs only rarely.

CAUSES

- Poisoning is usually an iatrogenic accident with intravenous medication.
- Child neglect should be considered if the patient is less than 1 year of age, suicide attempt if patient is over 6 years of age.

DRUG AND DISEASE INTERACTIONS

- Protease inhibitors may interact with other drugs metabolized by the liver. A partial list of drugs includes fentanyl, lidocaine, erythromycin, warfarin, carbamazepine, tricyclic antidepressants, selective serotonin reuptake inhibitors, and rifabutin.
- Increased protease inhibitor levels may develop when given with rifampin, quinine, β-blockers, calcium channel blockers, certain chemotherapeutic agents, corticosteroids, or other protease inhibitors.
- Ritonavir is formulated with alcohol and may produce a reaction when combined with disulfiram or drugs that produce a disulfiram-like reaction.
- Protease inhibitors and nucleoside or non-nucleoside reverse transcriptase inhibitors are often used in combination.

PREGNANCY AND LACTATION

US FDA Pregnancy Category B. Animal studies indicate no fetal risk and there are no controlled human studies, or animal studies show an adverse fetal effect but well-controlled studies in pregnant women do not.

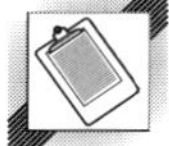

Diagnosis

DIFFERENTIAL DIAGNOSIS

- Renal failure. Acetaminophen, *Amanita phalloides* mushrooms, chlorinated hydrocarbons, *Cortinarius* species mushrooms, ethylene glycol, mercury poisoning, and rhabdomyolysis.
- Hepatotoxicity. Acetaminophen, aromatic hydrocarbons, arsenic, carbon tetrachloride, chronic ethanol, copper, chlorinated insecticides, iron, polychlorinated biphenyls, and valproic acid.

SIGNS AND SYMPTOMS

- Acute oral overdose is characterized by nausea, vomiting, and diarrhea.
- Adverse effects of chronic therapy include paresthesia and peripheral neuropathy.

Vital Signs

Tachycardia and hypoventilation occur rarely.

HEENT

Gingivitis may occur.

Cardiovascular

Hypotension, syncope, and palpitations occur rarely.

Pulmonary

Asthma, dyspnea, hypoventilation, pneumonia, pharyngitis, and rhinitis occur rarely.

Gastrointestinal

Nausea, vomiting, diarrhea, anorexia, pancreatitis, and gastrointestinal hemorrhage may occur after acute ingestion or during chronic therapy.

Hepatic

Liver function test abnormalities and increased enzyme levels may occur during therapy.

Renal

- Dysuria, hematuria, urinary tract infections, pyelonephritis, and renal failure occur rarely.
- Kidney stones have developed with ritonavir in 5% of patients.

Hematologic

Anemia, lymphadenopathy, lymphocytosis, leukopenia, and thrombocytopenia can occur.

Musculoskeletal

Arthralgia, muscle cramps, weakness, myositis, and muscle twitching can occur.

Neurologic/Psychiatric

- Headache is very common.
- Circumoral and peripheral paresthesia are common during therapy.
- Sensory and motor neuropathy, ataxia, confusion, seizures, tremor, urinary retention, and vertigo also may occur.

Endocrine

Diabetes mellitus, dehydration, edema, and gout can occur.

PROCEDURES AND LABORATORY TESTS

Essential Tests

No tests may be needed in minimally symptomatic patients after acute overdose.

Recommended Tests

- Complete blood count is used to assess bone marrow effects.
- Serum electrolytes, BUN, and creatinine are measured to assess renal effects in symptomatic patients.
- Liver enzymes, amylase, uric acid, and creatine kinase are measured to assess liver, pancreas, or muscle injury.
- ECG and serum acetaminophen and aspirin levels in overdose setting are used to detect occult ingestion.
- Chest radiography is often needed, but is usually related to underlying disease.

Not Recommended Tests

Specific levels are not clinically useful.

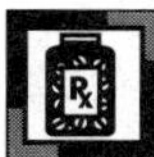

Treatment

- An overdose ingestion typically requires only symptomatic and supportive care. Treatment should be focused on airway management and support.
- Patients with normal liver function who have received an accidental overdose can usually be managed with conservative and supportive measures.
- Excessive intervention in mildly toxic exposures should be avoided.
- Dose and time of exposure should be determined for all substances involved.

DIRECTING PATIENT COURSE

The health-care professional should call the poison control center when:

- Seizure or other major effect develops.
- Toxic effects are not consistent with protease inhibitor poisoning.
- Coingestant, drug interaction, or underlying disease presents an unusual problem.

The patient should be referred to a health-care facility when:

- Attempted suicide or homicide is possible.
- Patient or caregiver seems unreliable.
- Any major toxic effect develops.
- Coingestant, drug interaction, or underlying disease presents an unusual problem.

Admission Considerations

Inpatient management is warranted for patients who develop any clinically significant toxic effect.

DECONTAMINATION

Out of Hospital

Induction of emesis is not recommended due to low potential for toxicity after acute ingestion.

In Hospital

- Gastric lavage should be performed in pediatric (tube size 24–32 French) or adult (tube size 36–42 French) patients for large ingestion presenting within 1 hour of ingestion or if serious effects are present.
- One dose of activated charcoal (1–2 g/kg) should be administered without a cathartic if a substantial ingestion has occurred within the previous few hours.

ANTIDOTES

There is no specific antidote for protease inhibitor poisoning.

ADJUNCTIVE TREATMENT

- Hypotension. The patient should be treated with isotonic fluid infusion, the Trendelenburg position, and, if needed, vasopressors. Dopamine is preferred and norepinephrine is added for refractory hypotension.
- Seizures

—A patent airway must be ensured.
—A benzodiazepine is administered for initial control. If seizures persist or recur, another anticonvulsant such as phenobarbital is added.

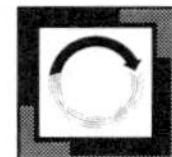

Follow-Up

PATIENT MONITORING

Patients should be observed until cardiovascular and neurologic functions are stable.

EXPECTED COURSE AND PROGNOSIS

- Following an acute overdose, the patient will exhibit mild symptoms with complete recovery expected unless complicated by underlying disease.
- CNS depression may lead to coma in severe cases.
- Respiratory depression may result in hypoxia and related complications.
- Associated conditions include local or systemic viral infection (HIV with or without clinical AIDS) and secondary opportunistic infections.

DISCHARGE CRITERIA/INSTRUCTIONS

Patient may be discharged from the emergency department or hospital when acute gastrointestinal effects are controlled and after completion of the psychiatric evaluation, if needed.

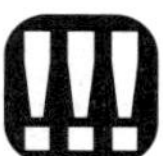

Pitfalls

DIAGNOSIS

Coingestants are often involved and require different therapy.

TREATMENT

Hemodialysis is not effective for protease inhibitor overdose.

ICD-9-CM 961.7

Poisoning by other antiinfectives: antiviral drugs.

See also: SECTION II, Hypotension and Seizure chapters.

RECOMMENDED READING

Danner SA, Carr A, Leonard JM, et al. A short-term study of the safety, pharmacokinetics, and efficacy of ritonavir, an inhibitor of HIV-1 protease. *N Engl J Med* 1995;333:1528–1533.

Author: Steven A. Seifert

Reviewer: Katherine M. Hurlbut

Antivirals—Reverse Transcriptase Inhibitors

Basics

DESCRIPTION

These antivirals are used to treat local or systemic infection by human immunodeficiency virus (HIV).

FORMS AND USES

- Non-nucleoside reverse transcriptase inhibitor. Nevirapine (Viramune).
- Nucleoside reverse transcriptase inhibitors. Didanosine (Videx), lamivudine (Epivir), stavudine (Zerit), zalcitabine (Hivid), and zidovudine (Retrovir).

PATHOPHYSIOLOGY

Nucleoside reverse transcriptase inhibitors are believed to produce altered mitochondrial function in nerve cells.

EPIDEMIOLOGY

- Poisoning is uncommon.
- Toxic effects following exposure are typically mild, with death occurring rarely.

CAUSES

- The cause of poisoning is usually an iatrogenic error or an intentional ingestion.
- Child neglect or abuse should be considered if the patient is less than 1 year of age, suicide attempt if the patient is over 6 years of age.

DRUG AND DISEASE INTERACTIONS

These drugs interact with one another and numerous other medications.

PREGNANCY

- Didanosine. US FDA Pregnancy Category B. Animal studies indicate no fetal risk and there are no controlled human studies, or animal studies show an adverse fetal effect but well-controlled studies in pregnant women do not.
- Nevirapine, lamivudine, stavudine, zalcitabine, and zidovudine. US FDA Pregnancy Category C. The drug exerts animal teratogenic or embryocidal effects, but there are no controlled studies in women, or no studies are available in either animals or women.

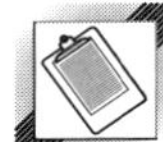

Diagnosis

DIFFERENTIAL DIAGNOSIS

- Renal failure. Acetaminophen, chlorinated hydrocarbons, ethylene glycol, heavy metals, methemoglobinemia, or rhabdomyolysis.
- Hepatotoxicity. Acetaminophen, anesthetic gases, aromatic hydrocarbons, arsenic, carbon tetrachloride, chronic ethanol, copper, chlorinated insecticides, iron, polychlorinated biphenyls, or valproic acid.

SIGNS AND SYMPTOMS

Nevirapine

There is limited experience in overdose. Minimal toxicity may occur, characterized by fatigue, headache, somnolence, and elevated liver function tests.

Didanosine

Possible effects of overdose include pancreatitis, seizures, peripheral neuropathy, diarrhea, hyperuricemia, hepatic dysfunction and lactic acidoses. It also may cause retinal depigmentation and optic neuritis in children.

Lamivudine

Overdose may produce fatigue, peripheral neuropathy, bone marrow suppression, nausea, vomiting, and diarrhea.

Stavudine

Overdose experience is limited. Peripheral neuropathy may occur.

Zalcitabine

Overdose experience is limited. Peripheral neuropathy, seizures, gastrointestinal effects, hepatitis, and pancreatitis may develop.

Zidovudine

Acute overdose may result in lethargy, bone marrow suppression, and, rarely, seizures.

HEENT

- Didanosine. Retinal depigmentation, optic neuritis, rhinitis, and epistaxis.
- Zalcitabine. Ototoxicity (hearing loss and tinnitus).
- Zidovudine. Tinnitus and nasal stuffiness.

Dermatologic

- Didanosine. Multiple rashes and Stevens-Johnson syndrome.
- Lamivudine. Rashes and alopecia.
- Zidovudine. Nail discoloration.

Cardiovascular

- Didanosine. Chronic heart failure, dysrhythmias, and thrombophlebitis.
- Zalcitabine. Dysrhythmia and palpitations.
- Gastrointestinal
- Didanosine. Pancreatitis (fatal) and diarrhea.
- Lamivudine. Anorexia, oral ulcerations, nausea, vomiting, and diarrhea.
- Zalcitabine. Esophageal ulcerations and pancreatitis (fatal).
- Zidovudine. Esophageal ulcerations, nausea, and pancreatitis (fatal).

Hepatic

- All agents may produce elevated liver function tests.
- Didanosine may result in fulminant liver failure.
- Zalcitabine may result in liver failure.

Hematologic

- Didanosine. Thrombocytopenia.
- Lamivudine. Thrombocytopenia and neutropenia.
- Zalcitabine. Thrombocytopenia, leukopenia, and neutropenia.
- Zidovudine. Granulocytopenia.

Musculoskeletal

- Didanosine. Myalgia, arthralgia, and weakness.
- Lamivudine. Myalgia and arthralgia.
- Stavudine. Elevation of creatine kinase levels.
- Zalcitabine. Arthralgia.
- Zidovudine. Myalgia and weakness.

Neurologic/Psychiatric

- Nucleoside analogs. Headache, painful peripheral neuropathy, seizures, and encephalopathy.
- Zidovudine. Mania.

Endocrine

- Nucleosides. Hypertriglyceridemia (possibly a marker for patients at risk for pancreatitis).
- Didanosine. Hypokalemia, hyperuricemia, and lactic acidosis, in association with liver failure.
- Zalcitabine. Lactic acidosis in association with liver failure.

Immunologic

Zalcitabine. Hypersensitivity reaction manifested by maculopapular rash, fever, eosinophilia, and exfoliation.

PROCEDURES AND LABORATORY TESTS

- Essential tests and procedures for nucleoside analogs include cardiac monitoring, liver function tests, complete blood count (CBC), and levels of electrolytes, platelets, creatine kinase, amylase, and uric acid.
- Underlying illness or complicating infections must be considered in interpreting results.

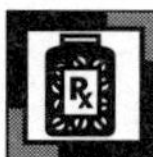

Treatment

- Patients with normal liver and renal function who have received an accidental overdose can usually be managed with conservative and supportive measures.
- Treatment should be focused on airway management and supportive care.
- The dose and time of exposure should be determined for all substances involved.

DIRECTING PATIENT COURSE

The health-care professional should call the poison control center when:

- Severe effects are present.
- Toxic effects are not consistent with antiviral poisoning.
- Coingestant, drug interaction, or underlying disease presents an unusual problem.

The patient should be referred to a health-care facility when:

- Attempted suicide or homicide is possible.
- Patient or caregiver seems unreliable.
- Toxic effects are not consistent with antiviral poisoning.
- Coingestant, drug interaction, or underlying disease presents an unusual problem.

Admission Considerations

Inpatient management is warranted when the patient develops hypotension, respiratory or CNS depression, prolonged seizures, significant airway compromise, or dysrhythmia.

DECONTAMINATION

Out of Hospital

Induction of emesis is not recommended.

In Hospital

- Gastric lavage should be performed in pediatric (tube size 24–32 French) or adult (tube size 36–42 French) patients for large ingestion presenting within 1 hour of ingestion or if serious effects are present.
- One dose of activated charcoal (1–2 g/kg) should be administered without a cathartic if a substantial ingestion has occurred within the previous few hours.

ANTIDOTES

There are no specific antidotes for antiviral agents.

ADJUNCTIVE TREATMENT

Didanosine. Hemodialysis may increase elimination.

Hypotension

The patient is treated with isotonic fluid infusion, the Trendelenburg position, and, if needed, vasopressors. Dopamine is preferred and norepinephrine is added for refractory hypotension.

Seizures

- A patent airway must be ensured.
- A benzodiazepine is administered for initial control. If seizures persist or recur, another anticonvulsant, such as phenobarbital, may be added.

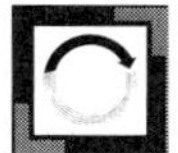

Follow-Up

PATIENT MONITORING

As indicated by clinical condition, CBC, electrolytes, and creatine kinase are monitored.

EXPECTED COURSE AND PROGNOSIS

- Overdose experience is limited for all agents.
- Didanosine

—Fulminant liver failure or pancreatitis may be fatal.
—Recovery is expected if liver failure or pancreatitis does not develop.

- Lamivudine. One patient who ingested 6 g developed no symptoms or laboratory abnormalities.
- Stavudine. In studies, 12 to 24 times the usual dosage produced no clinical effects.
- Zalcitabine. Recovery is expected.
- Zidovudine. Up to 50 g has been taken without fatality.

DISCHARGE CRITERIA/INSTRUCTIONS

- From the emergency department. The asymptomatic patient may be discharged following gastrointestinal decontamination and psychiatric evaluation, if needed.
- From the hospital. Patient may be discharged after toxic effects resolve or stabilize and after psychiatric evaluation, if needed.

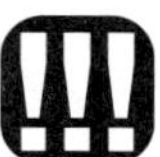

Pitfalls

DIAGNOSIS

Symptoms may be difficult to distinguish from underlying medical conditions as well as the effects of other medications.

ICD-9-CM 961.7

Poisoning by other antiinfectives: antiviral drugs.

See also: SECTION II, Hypotension and Seizure chapters.

RECOMMENDED READING

Fichtenbaum CJ, Clifford DB, Powderly WG. Risk factors for dideoxynucleoside-induced toxic neuropathy in patients with the human immunodeficiency virus infection. *J Acquir Immune Defic Syndr Hum Retrovirol* 1995;10:169–174.

Grob PM, Wu JC, Cohen KA, et al. Nonnucleoside inhibitors of HIV-1 reverse transcriptase: nevirapine as a prototype drug. *AIDS Res Hum Retrovir* 1992;8:145–152.

Author: Steven A. Seifert

Reviewer: Richard C. Dart

Arsenic

Basics

DESCRIPTION

Arsenic is a heavy metal used in a variety of household products and industrial processes; most household uses have been abandoned.

FORMS AND USES

- Included are arsenic acid; arsenious acid; arsenite; arsenous acid; arsenate; arsonic acid; and various arsenic, arsenous, and arsonic salts.
- See also SECTION IV, Arsine chapter.
- Arsenic is used to harden metals in glass manufacture; in the manufacture of pigments, insecticides, rodenticides, fungicides, wood preservatives; and as a dopant in semiconductors.
- It also has been a contaminant of well water, home-brewed alcohol ("moonshine"), opium, and wine.
- Arsenic is used in various homeopathic remedies and may be found in high concentrations in some folk remedies from China, India, Iran, Cambodia, and other areas of Southeast Asia.
- Arsenic is present in seafood, especially shellfish.

TOXIC DOSE

Lethal oral dose may range between 10 and 300 mg.

PATHOPHYSIOLOGY

- Toxicity is related to its inhibition of sulfhydryl enzymes and the uncoupling of oxidative phosphorylation.
- Cellular oxidative processes are disrupted, producing injury to multiple organs.

EPIDEMIOLOGY

- Arsenic poisoning is uncommon.
- Toxic effects are typically mild to moderate.
- Death occurs in severe or unrecognized cases.

CARCINOGENESIS

- Chronic ingestion of inorganic arsenic is associated with cancer of the skin, liver, bladder, kidney, and colon.
- Chronic inhalation is linked with lung cancer.

CAUSES

- Acute poisoning is usually an accidental ingestion.
- Chronic poisoning involves occupational or environmental exposure.
- Child neglect or abuse should be considered if the patient is less than 1 year of age, suicide attempt if the patient is over 6 years of age.

WORKPLACE STANDARDS

- ACGIH. TLV TWA is 0.2 mg/m^3 with no STEL.
- OSHA. PEL TWA is 0.5 mg/m^3 for organic; 0.01 mg/m^3 for inorganic.
- NIOSH. REL is 0.002 mg/m^3; IDLH is 5 mg/m^3.

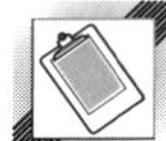

Diagnosis

DIFFERENTIAL DIAGNOSIS

- Toxicologic causes of acute gastrointestinal effects followed by neurologic toxicity include thallium, selenium, mercuric chloride, lead, salicylate, dinitrophenol, pentachlorophenol, and antineoplastics.
- Nontoxicologic causes include gastroenteritis and Landry–Guillain-Barré disease.

SIGNS AND SYMPTOMS

Acute Ingestion

- Severe hemorrhagic gastroenteritis develops within hours.
- Bone marrow depression, encephalopathy, cardiomyopathy, pulmonary edema, and cardiac dysrhythmia may occur over days.
- Peripheral neuropathy may develop in days to weeks.

Chronic Inhalation

Weakness, anorexia, hyperkeratosis, hyperpigmentation, hepatic injury, respiratory irritation, perforated nasal septum, tremor, or peripheral neuropathy may occur.

Vital Signs

Acute ingestion may be followed by tachycardia, hypotension, fever, or tachypnea.

HEENT

- Acute ingestion may be followed immediately by oral irritation and burning pain, metallic taste, and garlic odor.
- Alopecia may develop over several days.

Dermatologic

- Acute ingestion. Transverse white bands may appear on the nails (Aldrich-Mees lines) after 5 to 6 weeks.
- Chronic inhalation or ingestion. Patchy hypopigmentation and hyperpigmentation (eyelids, temples, axillae, neck, nipples, and groin) and hyperkeratosis (palms and soles) may develop; carcinoma in situ may develop over many years.

Cardiovascular

Acute ingestion may cause hypovolemic shock, and nonspecific ST-T changes; QTc prolongation and torsade de pointes have occurred.

Pulmonary

Patients with acute ingestion may develop noncardiogenic pulmonary edema or respiratory failure.

Gastrointestinal

Acute ingestion produces nausea, vomiting, abdominal pain, and diarrhea, and hemorrhagic gastroenteritis may develop.

Hepatic

Elevated liver function tests occur rarely after acute ingestion.

Renal

Acute ingestion causes acute tubular necrosis.

Hematologic

Acute or chronic exposure may cause anemia, agranulocytosis, thrombocytopenia, or aplastic anemia.

Fluids and Electrolytes

Severe gastroenteritis may cause fluid, electrolyte, and acid-base derangement.

Neurologic

- Acute ingestion
  - —Confusion, delirium, convulsions, encephalopathy, and coma may occur early in severe poisoning.
  - —A painful sensorimotor neuropathy in a "stocking-glove" distribution may begin weeks after exposure and may progress to respiratory failure.
- Chronic inhalation or ingestion. Tremor or peripheral neuropathy may be seen after several weeks or months.

PROCEDURES AND LABORATORY TESTS

Essential Tests

- Complete blood count with peripheral smear is used to assess bone marrow suppression.
  - —Pancytopenia may develop within days after acute poisoning; its nadir is at 7 to 14 days, and recovery occurs over 2 to 3 weeks.
  - —Chronic toxicity may cause anemia or aplastic anemia.
- Serum electrolytes, BUN, creatinine, and urinalysis are used to assess kidney injury.
- Blood and urine arsenic levels
  - —Whole blood arsenic (normal is less than 1 μg/dl) may be elevated early but declines rapidly.
  - —Urinary levels remain elevated for weeks (normal is less than 50 μg/l or less than 25 μg over 24 hours).

Recommended Tests

- ECG after acute exposure is used to detect dysrhythmia.
- Serum liver function tests, creatine kinase, and arterial blood gases are measured in patients with severe effects.
- Serum acetaminophen and aspirin levels are used in an overdose setting to screen for occult ingestion.
- Electromyelography/nerve conduction velocity is ordered if symptoms of peripheral neuropathy develop.
- Abdominal radiography may be useful following ingestion because arsenic compounds may be radiopaque.
- Head CT, lumbar puncture, and culture may be used to evaluate altered mental status.

Condition that May Alter Laboratory Results

Seafood produces elevation of the nontoxic form of arsenic in urine. Patients should abstain from eating seafood for 2 to 3 days prior to testing.

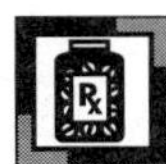

Treatment

- Treatment focuses on supporting hemodynamic function, managing the airway, treating dysrhythmias, and initiating chelation, if appropriate.
- The dose and time of exposure should be determined for all substances involved.
- Early consultation with a medical toxicologist is recommended.

DIRECTING PATIENT COURSE

The health-care professional should call the poison control center when:

- Toxic effects develop.
- Toxic effects are not consistent with arsenic poisoning.
- Coingestant, drug interaction, or underlying disease presents an unusual problem.

The patient should be referred to a health-care facility when:

- Any signs or symptoms or history of ingestion is present.
- Attempted suicide or homicide is possible.
- Patient or caregiver seems unreliable.
- Coingestant, drug interaction, or underlying disease presents an unusual problem.

Admission Considerations

Inpatient management is warranted for any symptomatic patient after acute exposure, any patient with unclear source of exposure, or a patient with major effects of chronic exposure (e.g., pancytopenia).

DECONTAMINATION

Out of Hospital

Ipecac should be administered to induce emesis within 1 hour of ingestion for alert pediatric or adult patients, if health-care evaluation will be delayed.

In Hospital

- Following large ingestions, gastric lavage should be performed in pediatric (tube size 24–38 French) or adult (tube size 36–42 French) patients presenting within 1 hour of ingestion or if serious effects are present.
- Gastric lavage should be considered if ingestion has occurred within 24 hours because some low-solubility arsenicals may be retained for prolonged periods. However, vomiting has often occurred spontaneously.
- One dose of activated charcoal (1–2 g/kg) should be administered without a cathartic if a substantial ingestion has occurred within the previous few hours.
- Whole-bowel irrigation may be useful if abdominal radiography reveals radiopaque material or if a poorly soluble arsenical was ingested.

ANTIDOTES

British Anti-Lewisite (BAL; Dimercaprol)

- Indications. BAL is used to treat a patient with severe poisoning (involving gastrointestinal bleeding, shock, dysrhythmias, or coma) or a patient unable to tolerate an oral agent (e.g., succimer).
- Contraindications

—Allergy to BAL or peanuts

- Method of administration

—A dose of 2.5 to 5 mg/kg is administered intramuscularly every 4 to 6 hours or 75 mg/m^2 intramuscularly every 4 hours.
—The dose is tapered over several days until an oral antidote can be tolerated.

- Adverse effects include headache, hypertension, tachycardia, fever, nausea, vomiting, and pain at the injection site.

—BAL may cause hemolysis in patients with glucose-6-phosphate dehydrogenase (G-6-PD) deficiency.

Succimer [Dimercaptosuccinic Acid (DMSA); Chemet]

- Indications

—Succimer is used in acute symptomatic arsenic poisoning.
—Use in chronic arsenic poisoning is occasionally recommended.
—Consultation with a medical toxicologist is recommended.

- Contraindications. Documented allergy to succimer precludes use.
- Method of administration. A dose of 10 mg/kg (or 350 mg/m^2) is administered by mouth three times a day for 5 days, followed by 10 mg/kg twice a day for 14 days.
- Adverse effects include nausea, vomiting, sulfur odor in bodily fluids, mild and transient elevation of transaminase levels, and a rash.

ADJUNCTIVE TREATMENT

- Hypotension. The patient should be treated with 10 to 20 ml/kg of 0.9 saline infusion, placed in the Trendelenburg position, and, if needed, treated with vasopressors. Dopamine is preferred, and norepinephrine is added for refractory hypotension.
- Ventricular dysrhythmias or conduction abnormalities occur rarely and are treated as indicated in the Ventricular Dysrhythmias chapter in SECTION II.

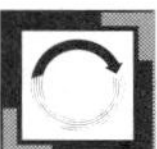

Follow-Up

PATIENT MONITORING

- Following acute ingestion, respiratory and cardiac function should be monitored continuously.
- Chelation should be continued until urinary arsenic excretion decreases to less than 25 μg/24 hours.

EXPECTED COURSE AND PROGNOSIS

- Toxicity develops rapidly after ingestion, but neuropathy and other injuries may require months to resolve and may leave residual injury.
- Possible complications include persistent polyneuropathy or CNS injury.

DISCHARGE CRITERIA/INSTRUCTIONS

- From the emergency department. An asymptomatic arsenic-exposed patient who is now in a clean environment and whose effects do not require hospitalization may be discharged following decontamination and psychiatric evaluation, if needed.
- From the hospital. The patient may be discharged to an arsenic-free environment when hemodynamic status, blood counts, and gastrointestinal tract allow outpatient management.

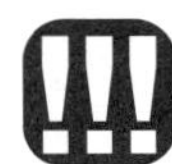

Pitfalls

DIAGNOSIS

Early manifestations may be confused with a primary gastrointestinal illness.

TREATMENT

The health-care professional must not delay chelation therapy in the symptomatic patient.

ICD-9-CM 985.1

Toxic effect of other metals: arsenic and its compounds.

See also: SECTION II, Hypotension and Ventricular Dysrhythmia chapters; and SECTION III, British Anti-Lewisite (Dimercaprol), Succimer, and Whole-Bowel Irrigation chapters.

RECOMMENDED READING

Gorby MS. Arsenic poisoning. *West J Med* 1988;149:308–315.

Kosnett M. Arsenic toxicity. In: Kreiss K, ed. *ATSDR case studies in environmental medicine #5*. Atlanta, GA: June, 1990.

Author: Luke Yip

Reviewer: Katherine M. Hurlbut

Arsine

Basics

DESCRIPTION

Arsine (AsH_3) is a colorless, nonirritating, inflammable gas with a garlicky odor.

FORMS AND USES

- Exposure to arsine usually occurs in the industrial/occupational setting when arsenic-containing products are exposed to strong acids or heated.
- Arsine may be produced during smelting and refining of metals and ores, galvanizing, soldering, etching, lead plating, metallurgy, burning fossil fuels, and the microelectronic/semiconductor industry (computer chips made of gallium arsenide are etched with strong acids).

TOXIC DOSE

Immediate death has occurred at 150 ppm.

PATHOPHYSIOLOGY

- Arsine rapidly enters red blood cells, depletes glutathione and produces rapid and severe Coombs' negative hemolytic anemia.
- Death may occur before the classic signs and symptoms of arsine poisoning develop.

EPIDEMIOLOGY

Poisoning is rare, but may be fatal.

CAUSES

Exposure usually occurs in the industrial/occupational setting.

RISK FACTORS

Exposure may go unnoticed because the odor is not noticeable during industrial use, and toxicity may develop with exposure below the odor threshold.

WORKPLACE STANDARDS

- ACGIH. TLV TWA is 0.05 ppm
- OSHA. PEL TWA is 0.05 ppm
- NIOSH. IDLH is 3 ppm

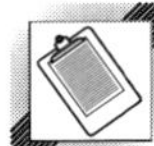

Diagnosis

SIGNS AND SYMPTOMS

- In cases where toxicity develops, there is usually a delay of 2 to 24 hours before toxicity becomes apparent.
- As hemolysis develops, symptoms of headache, weakness, chills, thirst, and abdominal pain develop.
- The triad of abdominal pain, hematuria, and bronze tint skin are characteristic of serious arsine poisoning.

HEENT

A garlic odor may be noticeable on the breath.

Dermatologic

Reddish staining of the conjunctiva and duskily bronzed skin (due to the presence of hemoglobin, not bilirubin) may develop within 12 to 36 hours.

Cardiovascular

- ECG changes include high-peaked T waves; T-wave changes are most pronounced 2 to 12 days after exposure.
- Ventricular dysrhythmia may develop.

Gastrointestinal

Nausea, vomiting, diarrhea, and abdominal pain.

Hematologic

Severe hemolysis may develop.

Urinary

- Dark red discoloration of the urine, hemoglobinuria, or hematuria frequently appears 4 to 12 hours after inhalation.
- Hemoglobinuria can cause acute tubular neurosis and renal failure.

PROCEDURES AND LABORATORY TESTS

Essential Tests

- Complete blood count with peripheral smear and serum haptoglobin should be obtained serially to evaluate for hemolysis.
- Serum electrolytes, BUN, and creatinine should be followed serially in symptomatic patients to assess toxicity.

Recommended Tests

- Blood and urine arsenic levels should be ascertained. Normal values are less than 20 μg/dl for blood, less than 50 μg/l in urine for occupational exposure.
- ECG to evaluate cardiac rhythym.

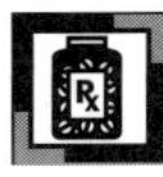

Treatment

- Treatment should focus on frequent monitoring of serum electrolytes and renal function, packed red blood cell transfusion, and aggressive supportive care to reduce further renal insult.
- Dose and time of exposure should be determined for all substances involved.

DIRECTING PATIENT COURSE

The health-care professional should call the poison control center when:

- Arsine exposure is suspected.
- Coingestant, drug interaction, or underlying disease presents an unusual problem.

The patient should be referred to a health-care facility when:

- History of arsine exposure is obtained.
- Coingestant, drug interaction, or underlying disease presents an unusual problem.

Admission Considerations

Inpatient management in an ICU is warranted for all patients with possible arsine poisoning.

DECONTAMINATION

Patient must be removed from the exposure and 100% oxygen should be administered.

ANTIDOTES

- There is no specific antidote for arsine poisoning.
- The use of British anti-Lewisite (BAL) in the treatment of acute arsine poisoning has been disappointing; it does not appear to prevent or reduce hemolysis.

ADJUNCTIVE TREATMENT

- Exchange transfusion has been advocated as the most efficient and effective management for acute, severe arsine poisoning.
- Intravenous fluids should be administered to the patient so that good urine output (1–2 ml/kg/h) is maintained.
- Exchange transfusion and hemodialysis may be required when renal insufficiency or failure develop.
- Diuretics, mannitol, and urinary alkalinization have been advocated, but supporting data are lacking.

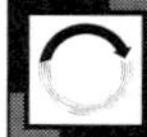

Follow-Up

EXPECTED COURSE AND PROGNOSIS

- Large exposures can cause death rapidly.
- Patients suffering from serious exposure often sustain multiple-organ injury.

DISCHARGE CRITERIA/INSTRUCTIONS

- Patients who are asymptomatic and hemodynamically stable for at least 24 hours after admission and show no evidence of hemolysis or worsening renal function may be discharged.
- Serum electrolytes, BUN, creatinine, and complete blood count should be repeated 1 to 2 days after discharge in patients who suffered toxic effects.

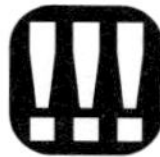

Pitfalls

DIAGNOSIS

Arsine poisoning may require 2 to 24 hours to develop symptoms.

TREATMENT

Failure to admit exposed patients to the ICU may allow injury to progress.

FOLLOW-UP

Premature discharge of the patient from the hospital can occur before onset of symptoms.

ICD-9-CM 987

Toxic effect of other gases, fumes, or vapors.

RECOMMENDED READING

Poisindex editorial staff: Arsine. In Rumack B, Reder PK, Gelman CR (eds.) Micromedex, Englewood Colorado (Edition expires August 31, 1998).

Author: Luke Yip

Reviewer: Kennon Heard

Asphyxiant Gases

Basics

DESCRIPTION

- This chapter covers gases that cause toxic effects by displacing oxygen from the atmosphere, thereby causing injury by hypoxia.
- Carbon monoxide poisoning and toxicity from pulmonary irritants are covered in separate chapters.

FORMS AND USES

Asphyxiant gases include acetylene, argon, butane, carbon dioxide, helium, hydrogen, inert gases, methane, natural gas, neon, nitrogen, and propane.

PATHOPHYSIOLOGY

- A simple asphyxiant displaces oxygen from the alveoli, thereby causing systemic hypoxia and finally tissue hypoxia.
- Toxic effects become noticeable when the ambient oxygen concentration drops below 15% and become severe when the concentration is below 10%.
- Due to their low vapor pressure, some of these agents cause frostbite if the agent comes in direct contact with tissue.

EPIDEMIOLOGY

- Poisoning is common.
- Toxic effects following exposure are typically mild and resolve quickly if the patient is removed before hypoxic tissue injury occurs.
- There are 10 to 20 deaths per year reported in the United States.
- Mass exposure has been reported after geologic events that release massive amounts of gas from natural underground stores.

CAUSES

- Minor exposures are usually accidental.
- Intentional abuse such as autoeroticism may result in severe exposure.
- Child neglect or abuse should be considered if the patient is less than 1 year of age, suicide attempt if the patient is over 6 years of age.

RISK FACTORS

- Intentional inhalational abuse of hydrocarbons increases the risk of hypoxic injury.
- A poorly ventilated area increases the risk of significant exposure to an asphyxiant gas.
- Patients with significant heart or lung disease may have symptoms at minimally decreased oxygen levels.
- The elderly are less tolerant of transient hypoxia.

DRUG DISEASE AND INTERACTIONS

Altitude potentiates the hypoxic effects.

PREGNANCY AND LACTATION

Severe maternal hypoxia may produce fetal hypoxia and distress.

WORKPLACE STANDARDS

- Butane

—ACGIH. TLV is 800 ppm (1900 mg/m^3).
—OSHA. Not listed.

- Carbon dioxide

—ACGIH. TLV TWA is 5,000 ppm (9,000 mg/m^3); STEL is 30,000 ppm (54,000 mg/m^3).
—OSHA. PEL TWA is 5,000 ppm (9,000 mg/m^3).
—ACGIH. TLV TWA is 2,500 ppm (4,500 mg/m^3).

- Propane

—OSHA. TLV is 1,000 ppm.

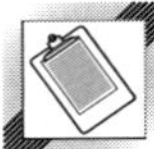

Diagnosis

DIFFERENTIAL DIAGNOSIS

- Toxicologic causes of hypoxia without other clinically apparent toxic effects include carbon monoxide, cyanide, hydrogen sulfide, methemoglobinemia.
- Nontoxicologic causes of hypoxia include pulmonary embolus, and other various hemoglobinopathies, among others.

SIGNS AND SYMPTOMS

Signs and symptoms of asphyxiants are directly related to the degree of hypoxia.

Vital Signs

Tachypnea and tachycardia are commonly initially followed by bradycardia, respiratory depression, and hypotension as death approaches.

HEENT

Mydriasis may occur as a preterminal effect.

Dermatologic

Diaphoresis and cyanosis may occur.

Cardiovascular

- Myocardial ischemia may complicate hypoxia.
- Tachycardia is superseded by various ventricular dysrhythmias and ending in idioventricular rhythm and asystole.

Pulmonary

Air hunger, tachypnea, and hyperpnea occur early, followed by respiratory depression as hypoxia worsens.

Neurologic

Headache and agitation are early signs, followed by lethargy and coma as hypoxia worsens.

PROCEDURES AND LABORATORY TESTS

Essential Tests

- Pulse oximetry or arterial blood gases are used to evaluate hypoxia.
- Carboxyhemoglobin or methemoglobin levels are measured if exposure is possible.
- Carboxyhemoglobin may cause inaccurate pulse oximetry results.

Recommended Tests

- Serum electrolytes, BUN, creatinine, and glucose levels are measured to assess other causes of altered mental status.
- ECG, serum acetaminophen and aspirin levels in overdose setting are used to detect an occult overdose.
- CT, lumbar puncture, and blood and CSF cultures are ordered as needed to evaluate the cause of altered mental status that persists despite oxygen therapy.

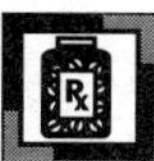

Treatment

- Focus treatment on oxygen therapy, airway management, and supportive care.
- The dose and time of exposure should be determined for all substances involved.

DIRECTING PATIENT COURSE

The health-care professional should call the poison control center when:

- The patient does not promptly improve with oxygen therapy.
- Toxic effects are not consistent with simple asphyxiants.
- A coingestant, drug interaction, or underlying disease presents an unusual problem.

The patient should be referred to a health-care facility when:

- Attempted suicide or homicide is possible.
- Patient or caregiver seems unreliable.
- Any toxic effects develop.
- Coingestant, drug interaction, or underlying disease presents an unusual problem.

Admission Considerations

Inpatient management is warranted for patients with persistent symptoms or hypoxia despite oxygen therapy.

DECONTAMINATION

Out of Hospital

The patient should be removed from exposure, and oxygen therapy should be initiated.

In Hospital

No decontamination is needed unless a coingestant is involved.

ANTIDOTES

High flow 100% oxygen should be administered.

ADJUNCTIVE TREATMENT

- Standard empiric therapy of altered mental status should be provided (naloxone, glucose determination, or D_{50} administration and thiamine) if the patient does not immediately respond to oxygen therapy.
- Seizures are a common manifestation of hypoxia. If they do not remit immediately with oxygen therapy, the patient should receive standard therapy beginning with benzodiazepine administration as described in SECTION II, Seizures chapter.

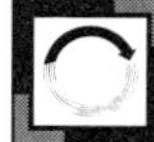

Follow-Up

PATIENT MONITORING

Patients with symptoms should be placed on a cardiac monitor and receive pulse oximetry.

EXPECTED COURSE AND PROGNOSIS

- Prognosis is directly related to the degree and duration of the hypoxic insult.
- Patients who are removed promptly from exposure should do well without long-term effects.
- Complications related to hypoxia may develop, such as myocardial ischemia or anoxic brain injury.

DISCHARGE CRITERIA/INSTRUCTIONS

- From the emergency department. Asymptomatic patients without other toxic exposure may be discharged after observation for 2 to 4 hours and after a psychiatric evaluation, if needed.
- From the hospital. Asymptomatic patients may be discharged after the resolution of the effects of hypoxia and after a psychiatric evaluation, if needed.

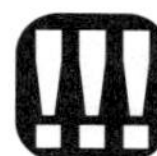

Pitfalls

DIAGNOSIS

- Failure to recognize concurrent toxicity, especially from carbon monoxide or pulmonary irritants, may result in morbidity from untreated poisoning.
- Frostbite may occur due to rapid evaporation of some of these agents.

TREATMENT

Unless precautions are taken, rescue attempts may cause injury to the rescuer as well as to the patient.

ICD-9-CM 987

Toxic effect of other gases, fumes, or vapors.

See also: SECTION II Seizures chapter; SECTION III, Carbon Monoxide chapter.

RECOMMENDED READING

Bresnitz EA. Simple asphyxiants and pulmonary irritants. In: Goldfrank LR, Flomenbuum, NE, Lewin NA, eds. *Goldfrank's toxicologic emergencies,* 6th ed. Norwalk, CT: Appleton & Lange, 1998.

Author: Kennon Heard

Reviewer: Katherine M. Hurlbut

Baclofen

Basics

DESCRIPTION

- Used to control muscle spasm and spasticity from multiple sclerosis, cerebral palsy, spinal cord injury, and other spinal cord diseases
- Baclofen (Lioresal) tablets (10 and 20 mg)
- Solutions for intrathecal injection (500 or 2,000 μg/ml)

FORMS AND USES

- Initial adult oral dose is 5 mg three times a day, titrated to a maximum of 20 mg four times a day.
- Initial adult and pediatric intrathecal dose is 50 μg, which may be increased to 100 μg in 25-μg increments. If a positive response is seen, a continuous intrathecal infusion is begun using 1.5 to 2 times the effective screening dose infused over 24 hours.

TOXIC DOSE

In adults, 300 to 1,000 mg orally has caused toxicity; more than 1.5 g may be fatal.

PATHOPHYSIOLOGY

Baclofen is a presynaptic gamma-aminobutyric acid (GABA) receptor agonist, reducing tonic activity of the spinal γ motor neurons.

EPIDEMIOLOGY

- Poisoning is uncommon.
- Toxic effects following exposure are typically mild to moderate.
- Death can occur in patients with large or multiple drug overdoses.

CAUSES

- Toxic ingestion is usually intentional.
- Child neglect or abuse should be considered if the patient is less than 1 year of age, suicide attempt if the patient is over 6 years of age.

DRUG AND DISEASE INTERACTIONS

- Renal insufficiency increases the risk of intoxication at normal doses.
- If ingested with other depressants, increased CNS depression may result.
- Decreased renal function in geriatric cases predisposes to toxicity at therapeutic doses.

PREGNANCY AND LACTATION

US FDA Pregnancy Category C. The drug exerts animal teratogenic or embryocidal effects, but there are no controlled studies in women, or no studies are available in either animals or women.

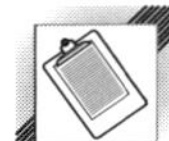

Diagnosis

DIFFERENTIAL DIAGNOSIS

- Toxicologic causes of CNS depression include ethanol, sedative or hypnotic agents, benzodiazepines, opioids, barbiturates, anticholinergics, and many others.
- Nontoxicologic causes of CNS depression include CNS disease such as infection, mass or bleed, seizures, withdrawal, or severe electrolyte abnormality.

SIGNS AND SYMPTOMS

Prominent effects are CNS depression, sometimes associated with seizures.

Vital Signs

- Bradycardia is common.
- Hypothermia, hypotension, and respiratory depression may develop in severe cases.

HEENT

Mydriasis is common.

Dermatologic

Skin bullae associated with prolonged coma may occur.

Cardiovascular

- Bradycardia is common; tachycardia occurs most often during recovery from overdose.
- Hypotension is common with severe overdose.
- Dysrhythmias, including atrioventricular block, premature ventricular contractions, and atrial fibrillation, occasionally develop after a large overdose.

Pulmonary

- Respiratory depression is common.
- Bronchospasm has been reported with therapeutic use in patients with reactive airways.

Gastrointestinal

Nausea and vomiting are common.

Hepatic

Elevated serum transaminase levels occasionally have been reported after overdose or during therapeutic use.

Renal

Incontinence and urinary retention may occur.

Musculoskeletal

Rhabdomyolysis may develop after prolonged seizures or coma.

Neurologic

- Confusion, agitation, and hallucinations may develop early and progress to coma, with hyporeflexia, flaccidity, and abnormal brain stem reflexes in severe cases.
- Myoclonus and seizures may occur.
- Dystonia, chorea, and tremor may develop with therapeutic use.
- Abrupt discontinuation after long-term use may cause withdrawal, accompanied by hallucinations, agitation, delirium, paranoia, and seizures.

Psychiatric

Depression, mania, and psychosis have been reported with therapeutic use.

PROCEDURES AND LABORATORY TESTS

Essential Tests

No tests may be needed in minimally symptomatic patients.

Recommended Tests

- ECG in symptomatic patients; bradycardia common
- Serum electrolytes, BUN, creatinine, and creatine kinase in patients with seizures, CNS depression, or coma; rhabdomyolysis may develop
- Arterial blood gases or pulse oximetry in patients with respiratory effects
- Serum acetaminophen and salicylate levels in overdose setting to detect occult ingestion
- Head CT, lumbar puncture, bacterial cultures as needed to rule out other causes of altered mental status

Not Recommended Tests

Serum baclofen levels are not clinically useful.

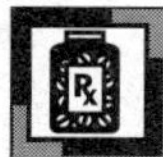

Treatment

- Treatment should focus on managing the airway, supporting cardiovascular function, and controlling seizures.
- Dose and time of exposure should be determined for all substances that could be involved.

DIRECTING PATIENT COURSE

The health-care professional should call the poison control center when:

- Hypotension, dysrhythmia, coma, seizures, or other serious effects are present.
- Toxic effects are not consistent with baclofen poisoning.
- Coingestant, drug interaction, or underlying disease presents an unusual problem.

The patient should be referred to a health-care facility when:

- Attempted suicide or homicide is possible.
- Patient or caregiver seems unreliable.
- Toxic effects develop.
- Coingestant, drug interaction, or underlying disease presents an unusual problem.

Admission Considerations

Inpatient management is warranted when CNS depression, seizure, dysrhythmias, or hypotension are present.

DECONTAMINATION

Out of Hospital

Emesis should not be induced; CNS depression may develop quickly.

In Hospital

- Gastric lavage should be performed in pediatric (tube size 24–32 French) or adult (tube size 36–42 French) patients presenting within 1 hour of a large ingestion or if serious effects are present.
- One dose of activated charcoal (1–2 g/kg) should be administered without a cathartic if a substantial ingestion has occurred within the previous few hours.
- Intrathecal overdose. If massive overdose occurs, immediately remove as much cerebrospinal fluid as is clinically reasonable (20–50 ml has been removed in adults).

ANTIDOTES

There is no specific antidote for baclofen poisoning.

ADJUNCTIVE TREATMENT

Hypotension

The patient should be treated with isotonic fluid infusion, the Trendelenburg position, and, if needed, vasopressors. Dopamine is preferred, and norepinephrine is added for refractory hypotension.

Seizure

- Adequate airway and oxygenation must be maintained.
- Benzodiazepines can be administered for initial control.

—Diazepam. Adult dose is 5 to 10 mg intravenously every 10 minutes or longer as needed; pediatric dose is 0.2 to 0.5 mg/kg intravenously every 10 minutes or longer as needed; need for intubation to be monitored closely.
—Lorazepam. Adult dose is 2 to 4 mg intravenous push over 2 to 5 minutes, repeated every 10 minutes or longer as needed; pediatric dose is 0.1 mg/kg intravenous push over 2 to 5 minutes, not to exceed 4 mg/dose, repeated every 10 minutes or longer as needed; need for intubation to be monitored closely.
—If seizures persist or recur, another anticonvulsant such as phenobarbital or phenytoin may be added.
—Other options for repeated seizures despite therapy include general anesthesia and neuromuscular blockade with EEG monitoring.

Withdrawal

- Benzodiazepines can be used for initial control. The dosing regimen is the same as for initial control of seizures.
- Resume baclofen therapy and taper dose gradually over days to weeks.

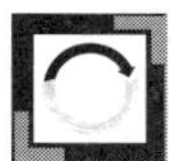

Follow-Up

PATIENT MONITORING

Cardiac and respiratory function must be monitored continuously.

EXPECTED COURSE AND PROGNOSIS

- Sequelae of prolonged seizures, hypoxia, or hypotension may occur.
- Coma may persist for several days, but most patients recover with supportive care unless sequelae of hypoxia intercede.

DISCHARGE CRITERIA/INSTRUCTIONS

- From the emergency department. Asymptomatic patients can be discharged following decontamination, 6 hours of observation, and psychiatric evaluation, if needed.
- From the hospital. The patient can be discharged after mental status returns to baseline and cardiovascular effects have resolved and after psychiatric evaluation, if needed.

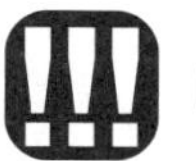

Pitfalls

DIAGNOSIS

Most patients on baclofen therapy have underlying neurologic disorders; changes in mental status may be difficult to detect.

TREATMENT

- Abrupt discontinuation of chronic baclofen use may precipitate withdrawal.
- Physostigmine has been used in some cases of baclofen overdose. In two cases, physostigmine use in baclofen overdose was associated with cardiac arrest; routine use is not recommended.
- Flumazenil also has been used, but its effectiveness has been erratic and seizures have occurred in the setting of mixed baclofen and benzodiazepine overdose; routine use is not recommended.
- Intrathecal overdose can be avoided by careful monitoring of mechanical pumps; two concentrations of intrathecal baclofen solution are available.

ICD-9-CM 968

Poisoning by other central nervous system depressants and anesthetics.

See also: SECTION II, Hypotension, Seizure, and Withdrawal—Depressants and Stimulants chapters.

RECOMMENDED READING

Delhaas EM, Brouwers JRBJ. Intrathecal baclofen overdose: report of 7 events in 5 patients and review of the literature. *Int J Clin Pharmacol Ther Toxicol* 1991;29:274–280.

Lee TH, Chess SS, Su SL, et al. Baclofen intoxication: report of 4 cases and review of the literature. *Clin Neuropharmacol* 1992;15:56–67.

Author: Katherine M. Hurlbut

Reviewer: Richard C. Dart

Barbiturates

Basics

DESCRIPTION

Barbiturates are a group of medications used primarily in the treatment of seizure and in some anesthesiology procedures.

FORMS AND USES

- Ultra short-acting barbiturates include methohexital (Brevital), thiamylal (Surital), and thiopental (Pentothal).
- Short-acting preparations include butabarbital (Buticaps, Butisol, Butalan), hexobarbital (Evipal), pentobarbital (Nembutal), and secobarbital (Seconal).
- Long-acting barbiturate preparations include mephobarbital (Mebaral), metharbital (Gemonil), phenobarbital (Arco-Lase, Bellatal belladonna with Phenobarbital Alkaloids, Donnatal, Luminal, Mudrane, Quadrinal, Rexatal, Solfoton), and primidone (Mysoline).
- Veterinary barbiturate products include phenobarbital (Beuthanasia, Euthanasia, Fatal, Lethal, Sleepaway, Succumb) and Secobarbital (Repose).
- Barbiturates can be used to control seizures.

—Phenobarbital. Adult dose is 60 mg two or three times per day; pediatric dose is 3 to 6 mg/kg/day.
—Primidone. Adult dose is 250 mg three or four times per day; maintenance dose for children under 8 years of age is 10 to 25 mg/kg/day.

- Barbiturates are also used for sedation.

—Butabarbital. Adult dose is 15 to 30 mg orally three or four times per day
—Secobarbital. 100 to 300 mg at bedtime

TOXIC DOSE

- To a naive user, toxicity may begin only slightly above the therapeutic dose.
- Tolerance develops rapidly, and regular abusers may tolerate huge doses.
- Death generally occurs from complications such as aspiration.

PATHOPHYSIOLOGY

- Barbiturates bind to a site that modulates the gamma-aminobutyric acid (GABA) receptor and increases the effects of GABA in the CNS.
- Primidone is metabolized to phenobarbital and phenylethylmalondiamid in the body.
- Phenylethylmalondiamid is biologically active and has effects similar to those of phenobarbital.

EPIDEMIOLOGY

- Poisoning is common.
- Toxic effects following exposure are typically mild to moderate.
- Death occurs rarely, most commonly in mixed ingestions or from complications such as aspiration.

CAUSES

- Toxic ingestion is usually suicidal.
- Child neglect or abuse should be considered if the patient is less than 1 year of age, suicide attempt if the patient is over 6 years of age.

RISK FACTORS

The elderly may be more sensitive to the sedative effects of barbiturates and have an increased risk of falling.

DRUG DISEASE AND INTERACTIONS

- CNS depression is increased by other depressants.
- Valproic acid and monoamine oxidase inhibitors may increase phenobarbital levels.
- Phenytoin and phenobarbital have variable interactions, either increasing or decreasing the level of one another.

PREGNANCY AND LACTATION

- US FDA Pregnancy Category D. Definite evidence of human fetal risk exists, but benefits in certain situations (e.g., life-threatening situations or serious diseases) may make use of the drug acceptable despite its risks.
- Phenobarbital is teratogenic.
- Barbiturates should be avoided in pregnancy.

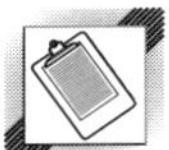

Diagnosis

DIFFERENTIAL DIAGNOSIS

- Toxicologic causes of mental status depression are numerous, including benzodiazepines, valproic acid, carbamazepine, ethanol, and opiates.
- Nontoxicologic causes include hypoglycemia, hypothermia, intracranial bleed or infection, hyponatremia or other electrolyte disorders, and hypoxia.

SIGNS AND SYMPTOMS

- The primary effect of intoxication is CNS depression.

Vital Signs

Hypotension, hypothermia, and apnea can occur.

HEENT

Nystagmus is common and may occur at therapeutic levels.

Dermatologic

Bullae may occur over pressure areas during coma.

Cardiovascular

- Hypotension is common with intravenous administration.
- Rapid infusion of phenobarbital may result in hypotension due to the propylene glycol diluent.

Pulmonary

Apnea occurs in a dose-related fashion.

Gastrointestinal

Idiosyncratic hepatitis has been reported.

Genitourinary

Massive crystalluria with proteinuria and hematuria has been reported with primidone ingestion.

Musculoskeletal

Rhabdomyolysis and compartment syndrome may occur from external pressure during coma.

Neurologic

- Ataxia, nystagmus, hyporeflexia, and somnolence occur initially and may occur at therapeutic levels.
- As levels of barbiturate increase, stupor and coma develop.

Endocrine

Hypoglycemia has been reported.

PROCEDURES AND LABORATORY TESTS

Essential Tests

Serum phenobarbital level should be checked if phenobarbital or primidone is the suspected toxicant.

Recommended Tests

- Pulse oximetry or arterial blood gases should be monitored to evaluate oxygenation in patients with CNS depression.
- Serum electrolytes, BUN, creatinine, and glucose should be assayed in patients with altered mental status.
- Serum creatine kinase should be checked to assess muscle injury in patients with prolonged coma.
- ECG, serum acetaminophen, and aspirin levels should be performed in an overdose setting to screen for occult ingestion.
- Head CT, lumbar puncture, bacterial cultures, and other tests should be performed in patients with altered mental status of unknown etiology.

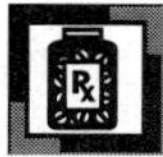

Treatment

- Treatment should focus on airway management, decontamination, and supportive care.
- Dose and time of exposure should be determined for all substances involved.

DIRECTING PATIENT COURSE

The health-care professional should call the poison control center when:

- Coma or other severe effects are present.
- Toxic effects are not consistent with barbiturate intoxication.
- Coingestant, drug interaction, or underlying disease presents an unusual problem.

The patient should be referred to a health-care facility when:

- Increased somnolence or other severe effects are present.
- Attempted suicide or homicide is possible.
- Patient or caregiver seems unreliable.
- Toxic effects are not consistent with barbiturate intoxication.
- Coingestant, drug interaction, or underlying disease presents an unusual problem.

Admission Considerations

Inpatient management is warranted if patients cannot care for themselves (e.g., ataxia, confusion) or have increasing phenobarbital levels following decontamination.

DECONTAMINATION

Out of Hospital

Emesis should not be induced.

In Hospital

- Gastric lavage should be performed in pediatric (tube size 24–32 French) or adult (tube size 36–42 French) patients for large ingestion presenting within 1 hour of ingestion or if serious effects are present.
- One dose of activated charcoal (1–2 g/kg) should be administered if a substantial ingestion has occurred within the previous few hours.

ANTIDOTES

There is no specific antidote for barbiturate poisoning.

ADJUNCTIVE TREATMENT

- Urinary alkalinization using sodium bicarbonate is sometimes employed in cases of phenobarbital intoxication.
- Urinary alkalinization increases phenobarbital clearance, but improved clinical outcomes (shortened duration of coma) have not been demonstrated; alkalinization does not increase clearance of other barbiturates.

Sodium Bicarbonate

- Adult

—Initial dose of sodium bicarbonate is one to two ampules (44 or 50 mEq per ampule) administered in an intravenous push.
—This should be followed by two to three ampules of sodium bicarbonate mixed in 1 L of D5W, infused at 200 ml/h.
—Urinary pH should be monitored hourly; the infusion rate should be increased within clinically reasonable boundaries to produce a urinary pH above 7.5.

- Pediatric

—Initial dose of sodium bicarbonate is 1 to 2 mEq/kg by intravenous push.
—This should be followed by one or two ampules of sodium bicarbonate (44 or 50 mEq per ampule) mixed in 1 L D5W, infused at a rate within clinically reasonable boundaries starting at 1.5 to 2.0 times the maintenance rate and adjusted to maintain the urinary pH above 7.5.

- The clinician should consider underlying medical conditions such as congestive heart failure, myocardial ischemia, and renal insufficiency when determining the infusion rate.
- Urinary alkalinization should continue until the patient has demonstrated clinical improvement.
- Supplemental potassium should be administered if the serum level is below 4.0 mEq/L.

Multiple-dose Activated Charcoal

- Phenobarbital clearance is increased by activated charcoal, but has not been shown to alter outcome; it does not increase clearance of other barbiturates.
- A typical treatment regimen is 25 to 50 g (0.5–1.0 g/kg) of activated charcoal orally every 2 to 4 hours.
- A cathartic can be administered with the first dose only.
- Activated charcoal should be discontinued if ileus or obstruction develops, if patient is not passing charcoal stools, or when phenobarbital level (in this instance of phenobarbital ingestion) falls below 45 μg/ml.

Hypotension

Hypotension following barbiturate poisoning should be treated in the standard manner, starting with rapid infusion of 10 to 20 ml/kg of 0.9% saline.

Charcoal Hemoperfusion or Hemodialysis

The clearance of phenobarbital is increased by these procedures, but because of the significant complication rate, these techniques are recommended only for persistent hypotension; in addition, they do not increase clearance of other barbiturates.

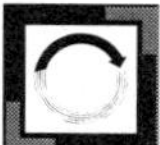

Follow-Up

PATIENT MONITORING

Patient should be monitored continuously for cardiac rhythm, oxygenation, and for complications of coma and aspiration.

EXPECTED COURSE AND PROGNOSIS

- Toxicity develops early; prolonged coma that resolves over several days may follow a large overdose.
- Sequelae of hypoxia, aspiration, and pressure necrosis of the skin and muscle may develop.

DISCHARGE CRITERIA/INSTRUCTIONS

- From the emergency department. Patients with improving symptoms and decreasing barbiturate levels may be discharged following gastrointestinal decontamination, a 4- to 6-hour observation period, and psychiatric evaluation, if needed.
- From the hospital. Patients with decreasing levels and good ambulation may be discharged with therapeutic antiseizure medications, if indicated.

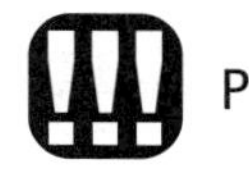

Pitfalls

DIAGNOSIS

Failure to evaluate other causes of altered mental status is a common error.

TREATMENT

Failure to provide early aggressive airway management can lead to increased risk of aspiration or respiratory failure.

FOLLOW-UP

Failure to demonstrate decreasing levels and good ambulation prior to discharge may allow a patient to be discharged prematurely.

ICD-9-CM 967.0

Poisoning by sedatives and hypnotics: barbiturates.

See also: SECTION II, Hypotension chapter; and SECTION III, Activated Charcoal and Sodium Bicarbonate chapters.

RECOMMENDED READING

Poisindex Editorial Staff. Long-acting barbiturates. In: Rumack BR, Sayers NK, Gelman CL, eds. *POISINDEX System.* Englewood, CO: Micromedex, Inc. (Edition expires November 30, 1997).

Author: Kennon Heard

Reviewer: Katherine M. Hurlbut

Barium

Basics

DESCRIPTION

Barium is a heavy metal used in commercial products.

FORMS AND USES

- Soluble forms of barium (i.e., barium carbonate, barium chloride, barium hydroxide) are highly toxic. Used in the past as rodenticides, they are no longer available in the United States for this use.
- Insoluble forms of barium (barium sulfate) used in radiographic procedures are not toxic.

TOXIC DOSE

- Toxicity varies by chemical form.
- Ingestion of 1 to 15 g (soluble forms) has caused death.

PATHOPHYSIOLOGY

- Absorption of barium from the gastrointestinal tract depends on the solubility of the compound. The solubility of barium salts, with the exception of barium sulfate, increases with decreasing pH.
- Inhaled barium is absorbed though the lung or directly from the basal membrane. Poorly soluble compounds may accumulate in the lungs.
- Barium plugs the potassium channel, allowing potassium efflux from the cell. Because influx is not affected, however, the level of extracellular potassium decreases, while that of intracellular potassium increases. Plasma potassium concentrations are thus lowered, with resultant profound hypokalemia and lowering of membrane potentials. Eventually muscles are unable to depolarize.
- Barium stimulates the release of acetylcholine and thereby stimulates smooth, striated, and cardiac muscle, resulting in violent peristalsis, arterial hypertension, muscle twitching, and disturbances in cardiac conduction.
- It also stimulates insulin secretion, resulting in hypoglycemia.

EPIDEMIOLOGY

Poisoning is uncommon.

CAUSES

Child neglect or abuse should be considered if the patient is less than 1 year of age, suicide attempt if the patient is over 6 years of age.

WORKPLACE STANDARDS

- ACGIH. TLV TWA is 0.5 mg/m^3
- OSHA. PEL TWA is 0.5 mg/m^3.
- NIOSH. IDLH is 250 mg/m^3.

Diagnosis

DIFFERENTIAL DIAGNOSIS

Barium toxicity is diagnosed based on history of exposure and multiorgan system signs and symptoms.

SIGNS AND SYMPTOMS

HEENT

Eye irritation, salivation, perioral paresthesia, and muscle twitching and paralysis, leading to difficulty speaking and swallowing.

Dermatologic

Irritation can occur, as can severe burns from metallic barium.

Cardiovascular

Hypertension, premature ventricular contractions, prolonged QT interval, ventricular tachycardia, ventricular fibrillation, and asystole.

Pulmonary

- Signs include respiratory muscle paralysis and respiratory failure.
- Inhalation can cause sore throat, bronchial irritation with coughing, shortness of breath, and pulmonary edema.
- Chronic exposure has resulted in baritosis with pulmonary nodules (benign pneumoconiosis).

Gastrointestinal

Nausea, vomiting, diarrhea, and severe abdominal pain may develop.

Renal

Acute renal failure may develop.

Musculoskeletal

- Weakness may progress to flaccid paralysis in serious cases.
- Stiffness, myoclonus, myalgia, rigidity, cramps, and rhabdomyolysis are also seen.

Neurologic

- Early central nervous system stimulation includes giddiness and anxiety followed by depression.
- Vertigo, tinnitus, mydriasis, headache, and seizures may develop.

Metabolic

Signs include profound hypokalemia and hypophosphatemia, as well as metabolic acidosis and hypoglycemia.

Endocrine

- Barium stimulates the adrenal gland, with resultant hyperadrenergic manifestations.
- Barium simulates insulin release, resulting in hypoglycemia.

PROCEDURES AND LABORATORY TESTS

Essential Tests

Blood chemistry. Studies should include assessment of electrolytes, determination of renal function, and hourly determination of blood glucose, serum potassium, calcium, phosphorus, and magnesium levels.

Recommended Tests

- Arterial blood gas or pulse oximetry should be performed to assess respiratory status.
- Urinalysis is used to detect renal injury.
- ECG and cardiac monitoring are used to detect dysrhythmias.
- Chest and abdominal radiography are used to assess for pulmonary infiltration.
- Measurement of barium in whole blood, plasma, and urine by atomic absorption. Five milliliters of blood should be collected, and urine should be collected in a metal-free, acid-washed container. Normal barium levels are less than 20 $\mu g/L$ in urine, less than 20 $\mu g/dl$ in plasma, and less than 40 $\mu g/dl$ in whole blood.

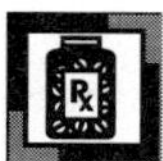

Treatment

Treatment should focus on aggressive supportive care and advanced cardiac life support (ACLS).

DIRECTING PATIENT COURSE

The health-care professional should call the poison control center when:

- Any symptoms develop.
- Coingestant, drug interaction, or underlying disease presents an unusual problem.

The patient should be referred to a health-care facility when:

- Toxic effects develop.
- Coingestant, drug interaction, or underlying disease presents an unusual problem.

Admission Considerations

Inpatient management is warranted when hypokalemia, severe muscle weakness, cardiac dysrhythmia, or other persistent effects develop.

DECONTAMINATION

Out of Hospital

Remove all clothing and jewelry and wash skin thoroughly.

In Hospital

- Remove all clothing and jewelry and wash skin thoroughly.
- Gastric lavage should be performed in pediatric (tube size 24–32 French) or adult (tube size 36–42 French) patients followed by administration of sodium sulfate (30 g in 250 ml of water) or magnesium sulfate to precipitate barium as the barium sulfate (insoluble) in the gastrointestinal tract.

ANTIDOTES

There is no specific antidote for barium poisoning.

ADJUNCTIVE TREATMENT

- Ventilatory support should be performed for respiratory failure and endotracheal intubation.
- Potassium should be administered for hypokalemia; large doses may be required.
- Administer nitroglycerin or nitroprusside for hypertension.
- Treat ventricular dysrhythmia using ACLS procedures. Procainamide has been used to control ventricular dysrhythmias. Ventricular fibrillation has been reported to be resistant to lidocaine.
- Diuresis induced by administration of furosemide has been associated with increased barium elimination.
- Hemodialysis may decrease the half-life of barium, but has not been studied clinically.
- Intravenous sodium sulfate (10 ml of 10% solution) every 15 minutes has been suggested to counteract the systemic effects of barium. However, it also has been implicated with acute renal failure caused by precipitation of barium sulfate in kidneys.

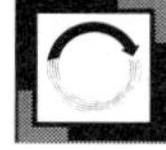

Follow-Up

PATIENT MONITORING

- Initially, chemistry profiles, including potassium, magnesium, calcium, and phosphate, should be determined at least hourly in serious cases.
- Respiratory and cardiac function should be monitored continuously in symptomatic patients.

EXPECTED COURSE AND PROGNOSIS

- Symptoms abate in most cases within 24 hours, although some patients may suffer muscle weakness and paralysis for more than 1 week.
- Acute poisoning may be fatal if not treated promptly.

DISCHARGE CRITERIA/INSTRUCTIONS

Asymptomatic patients may be discharged from the emergency department or hospital following decontamination, observation for at least 6 hours, and psychiatric evaluation, if needed.

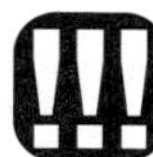

Pitfalls

Large parenteral doses of potassium (up to 420 mEq in 24 hours) may be necessary in the treatment of symptomatic barium poisoning; therefore, hourly monitoring of serum levels of potassium, as well as calcium, phosphorus, and magnesium, is necessary.

ICD-9-CM 985

Toxic effect of other metals.

RECOMMENDED READING

Roza O, Berman LB. The pathophysiology of barium: Hypokalemic and cardiovascular effects. *J Pharmacol Exp Ther* 1971;177:433–439.

Smith RP, Gosselin RE: Current concepts about the treatment of selected poisoning. *Ann Rev Pharmacol Toxicol* 1976;16:194–195.

Wetherill SF, Guarino MG, Cox RW. Acute renal failure associated with barium chloride poisoning. *Ann Intern Med* 1981;95:187–188.

Author: Luke Yip

Reviewer: Kennon Heard

Bee Sting

Basics

DESCRIPTION

Stings by the honey bee, the "killer bee," wasps, yellow jackets, and hornets are included in this chapter.

FORMS AND USES

Stings may be inflicted by:

- The European honey bee (*Apis mellifera*)
- The "Africanized bee" or "Brazilian killer bee" (*Apis mellifera scutellata* or *Apis mellifera adansoni*)

—Africanized or killer bees were introduced to South America from Africa and have spread northward, reaching the United States in 1990.
—Unless they adapt to climactic changes, the bees' range will remain limited to the southernmost United States.

- Stings by wasps, yellow jackets, and hornets are managed in the same manner.

TOXIC DOSE

- A single sting may cause anaphylaxis in susceptible individuals.
- Several hundred stings from either honey bees or killer bees are needed to produce serious systemic toxicity; fewer stings are needed to produce toxicity in children.
- Fewer stings from wasps are needed to produce toxicity.

PATHOPHYSIOLOGY

- Toxicity effects may be produced by two mechanisms.

—Anaphylaxis from immunoglobulin E (IgE)-mediated reaction. This effect is not related to the number of stings.
—Toxic reaction from multiple stings by swarming bees. Toxicity is due to direct toxic effect of venom, not from allergic response.

- Africanized or killer bees exhibit more aggressive behavior than honey bees, which makes the Africanized bees dangerous; however, their venom is not significantly different from that of domesticated European bees.
- Africanized bees swarm with minimal provocation, respond faster in greater numbers and aggressiveness, and have the capability to pursue victims over long distances (more than 20 km).

EPIDEMIOLOGY

- There have been approximately 350 fatal Africanized bee attacks worldwide, with 70 occurring in Venezuela in 1977 and 1978.
- Animal deaths have occurred from massive envenomation in the southwest United States.
- Due to smaller body mass, children are more at risk for systemic toxic reactions.

CAUSES

- Stings are nearly always accidental.
- Because Africanized bees attack with minimal provocation, any activity in the area of a hive can result in stings.

RISK FACTORS

- Patients allergic to any bee should be considered allergic to killer bees.
- Provoking bees is more likely to lead to their aggressive swarming behavior.

PREGNANCY AND LACTATION

- Supportive care of the mother following systemic illness is the best care for the fetus.
- Epinephrine causes placental vasoconstriction and should be used with caution; however, the benefit outweighs the risk in patients with anaphylaxis.

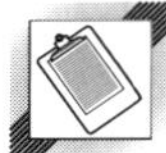

Diagnosis

A history of a single or multiple bee stings should be sought.

DIFFERENTIAL DIAGNOSIS

Other toxicologic causes of anaphylaxis include hymenoptera stings (e.g., wasps, hornets, fire ants, spiders, or marine envenomations) or bites (spiders or other insects).

SIGNS AND SYMPTOMS

The toxic effects of stings from hymenoptera species are similar.

- Direct effects of the venom include rapid onset of local pain as well as redness and swelling at the sting site.
- Allergic reactions include nausea, swelling of the involved extremity, urticaria, wheezing, and hypotension.

Vital Signs

- Tachycardia from pain or early anaphylaxis is common.
- Anaphylaxis can produce hypotension and bradycardia.

HEENT

Upper airway obstruction may occur in severe cases.

Dermatologic

- Toxic effects include wheal and flare at the sting site.
- Generalized urticaria can occur in isolation or as a part of anaphylaxis.

Cardiovascular

Tachycardia, hypotension, and shock can occur with anaphylaxis or with massive envenomation.

Pulmonary

- Direct effects of the venom include local swelling of the face or lips, which may cause airway obstruction.
- An allergic reaction may cause throat and chest tightness, stridor, airway edema, laryngospasm, and wheezing.

Gastrointestinal

Nausea, vomiting, and diarrhea can occur.

Renal

Direct effects of the venom can cause rhabdomyolysis and renal failure.

Neurologic

CNS depression and coma can occur.

PROCEDURES AND LABORATORY TESTS

Essential Tests

No specific tests are usually needed for stings without systemic effects.

Recommended Tests

- ECG, electrolyte levels, BUN, creatinine, arterial blood gases, and renal function tests may help to direct supportive treatment in symptomatic patients.
- Serum creatinine kinase should be measured in patients with systemic effects to assess rhabdomyolysis.

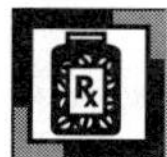

Treatment

Treatment should focus on managing the airway and supporting hemodynamic function.

DIRECTING PATIENT COURSE

The health-care professional should call the poison control center when:

- Systemic effects develop.
- Toxic effects are not consistent with bee envenomation.
- An underlying disease presents an unusual problem.

The patient should be referred to a health-care facility when:

- Anaphylaxis or other systemic effects develop.
- The estimated number of stings is over 50.
- The patient requires a tetanus shot.
- Toxic effects are not consistent with bee envenomation.
- An underlying disease presents an unusual problem.

Admission Considerations

Inpatient management is warranted for patients with cardiovascular instability, persistent or recurrent pulmonary symptoms, or systemic effects following a large number of stings.

DECONTAMINATION

Out of Hospital

- Stingers should be scraped rather than pulled out.
- Immobilization of severely stung limbs may decrease venom absorption.

In Hospital

Stingers should be scraped rather than pulled out.

ANTIDOTES

There is no specific antidote for hymenoptera venom.

ADJUNCTIVE TREATMENT

Urticaria or Local Itching

An antihistamine such as diphenhydramine is administered; adult dose is 25 to 50 mg intravenously or orally every 6 to 8 hours; pediatric dose is 1 mg/kg intravenously or orally up to 50 mg every 6 to 8 hours.

Local Pain or Swelling

- Ice packs wrapped in washcloths are applied to sting sites for 20 minutes of every hour.
- Nonsteroidal antiinflammatory drugs are given orally; for severe pain, a parenteral narcotic is given.

Bronchospasm

- Albuterol is administered 0.15 mg/kg (maximum of 10 mg) in saline with humidified oxygen via nebulizer every 20 to 30 minutes.
- Some clinicians also administer H_1- and H_2-receptor blocking drugs.

Anaphylaxis or Shock

- First, 100% oxygen is administered and the airway secured.
- Epinephrine should be administered immediately if the airway is compromised or hypotension is present. Hypertension is treated in the standard manner starting with rapid infusion of 0.9% saline 10 to 20 ml/kg.
- Antihistamines are administered to block both H_1- and H_2-receptors.

—Diphenhydramine. Adult dose is 25 to 50 mg intravenously every 6 to 8 hours; pediatric dose is 1 mg/kg intravenously up to 50 mg every 6 to 8 hours.
—Cimetidine is also administered; adult dose is 300 mg intravenously every 6 hours; pediatric dose is 40 mg/kg/day intravenously in divided doses every 6 hours.

- Epinephrine bolus is administered.

—The adult dose is 3 to 5 ml of 1:10,000 given as an intravenous push over 5 to 10 minutes; pediatric dose is 0.1 ml/kg given as an intravenous push over 5 to 10 minutes.
—The bolus should be followed with an infusion if necessary; 1 mg of 1:1,000 is diluted in 250 ml of D5W; dose should start at 1 μg/min, titrated to desired blood pressure.

- Epinephrine must be used with caution in the elderly.

Other

- Tetanus prophylaxis should be provided if patient is not up to date.
- Surgical removal of multiple stingers is rarely necessary.
- Severe facial or throat swelling may require surgical airway management.

Not Recommended Therapies

Locally applied meat tenderizer (papain) has not been proven effective.

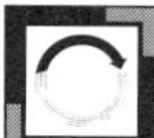

Follow-Up

PATIENT MONITORING

Continuous cardiac monitoring and pulse oximetry should be performed for patients with systemic effects or airway involvement.

EXPECTED COURSE AND PROGNOSIS

- Anaphylaxis can produce airway compromise, hypotension, and death within minutes of a sting.
- Direct venom effects appear to peak immediately; however, systemic effects (e.g., rhabdomyolysis) may worsen over a day or two.
- With aggressive supportive care, the prognosis is excellent if the patient is not moribund on arrival.

DISCHARGE CRITERIA/INSTRUCTIONS

- From the emergency department. Asymptomatic patients may be discharged after 4 hours of observation if no evidence of neurologic or cardiovascular toxicity develops.
- From the hospital. Patients may be discharged after toxic effects abate.

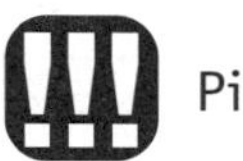

Pitfalls

DIAGNOSIS

The health-care professional must be able to recognize impending pulmonary or cardiovascular compromise.

TREATMENT

- The health-care professional must aggressively treat impending pulmonary or cardiovascular collapse.
- Mild symptoms should not be treated with epinephrine.

FOLLOW-UP

- Self-injectable epinephrine should be prescribed for sensitized individuals.
- If an allergic reaction has occurred, the patient should be evaluated by an allergist for desensitization.

ICD-9-CM 989

Toxic effect of other substances, chiefly nonmedicinal as to source.

See also: SECTION II, Hypotension chapter.

Author: Lada Kokan and Kennon Heard

Reviewer: Richard C. Dart

Benzene

Basics

DESCRIPTION

Benzene is a common aromatic hydrocarbon solvent found as a component of hundreds of commercial products.

FORMS AND USES

- It is primarily used as a chemical intermediate in the production of other chemical compounds such as styrene, cumene, cyclohexane, synthetic rubbers, gums, lubricants, lacquers, varnishes, dyes, pharmaceuticals, and agricultural chemicals.
- It is also used as a solvent in paints, thinners, inks, and adhesives.
- Safer alternatives have been substituted in many products, but benzene remains a low-level natural contaminant in many products such as gasoline (less than 2% benzene by volume).
- Benzene includes:

—Benzene (C_6H_6, benzol, coal or mineral naphtha)
—Cumene (isopropyl benzene)
—Styrene (vinyl benzene)
—Cyclohexane (benzene hexahydride)

TOXIC DOSE

PATHOPHYSIOLOGY

- Benzene is absorbed rapidly by inhalation and ingestion, and absorbed slowly through intact skin.
- It is metabolized in the liver and bone marrow by the cytochrome P450 mixed function oxidase system; phenol is the major metabolite.
- Benzene metabolites may form adducts with DNA and RNA, with carcinogenic effects.
- Bone marrow is the primary target organ of chronic exposure.
- Benzene metabolites are injurious to the renal, cardiac, and hepatic systems.
- Benzene is considered a group A carcinogen by the Environmental Protection Agency (there is no threshold for benzene's potential to cause leukemia).

EPIDEMIOLOGY

- Exposure is common and underreported, largely due to recreational "huffing" and inhalation of benzene-containing compounds.
- Toxic effects following exposure are typically related to the dose.
- Death is rare and generally secondary to acute high-dose exposure, resulting in profound CNS depression, asphyxiation, respiratory arrest, or cardiac dysrhythmia.

CAUSES

- Exposure typically occurs as a result of accidental occupational inhalation.
- Child neglect or abuse should be considered if the patient is less than 1 year of age, suicide attempt if the patient is over 6 years of age.

RISK FACTORS

Adolescents are at increased likelihood for inhaled benzene abuse.

DRUG AND DISEASE INTERACTIONS

Cytochrome P450 inducers such as phenobarbital, ethanol, chlordane, and parathion enhance benzene toxicity.

PREGNANCY AND LACTATION

Increased incidence of spontaneous abortion is possible following acute poisoning.

WORKPLACE STANDARDS

- ACGIH. TLV TWA is 0.5 ppm; STEL is 2.5 ppm.
- OSHA. PEL TWA is 10 ppm; PEL STEL is 5 ppm; ceiling is 25 ppm.
- NIOSH. REL TWA is 0.1 ppm

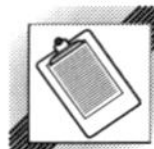

Diagnosis

DIFFERENTIAL DIAGNOSIS

- Toxicologic causes of depressed mental status include opioids, sedative or hypnotic agents, ethanol, gammahydroxybutyrate, rohypnol, clonidine, tricyclic antidepressants, methanol, anticonvulsants, and ethylene glycol, among others.
- Nontoxicologic causes of altered mental status include intracranial trauma or infection, hypoglycemia or other metabolic disturbances, and electrolyte abnormalities.
- Toxicologic and nontoxicologic causes of anemia and other bone marrow abnormalities include ionizing radiation, hematologic neoplasms, hemoglobinopathies, other chemical exposures (solvents, insecticides, and arsenic), smoking, and folic acid or B_{12} deficiency.

SIGNS AND SYMPTOMS

- Acute exposure may cause CNS depression and cardiac dysrhythmia.
- Chronic exposure may cause bone marrow depression, and malignancy may occur.

Vital Signs

Fever and tachycardia are common.

HEENT

- Splash contact (blepharospasm, corneal abrasion, chemical conjunctivitis, and lacrimation)
- Acute exposure: hoarseness, headache, mydriasis, ototoxicity, and tinnitus

Dermatologic

Prolonged skin exposure can cause dermatitis and, rarely, burns.

Cardiovascular

Sudden death after acute inhalation is believed to be related to ventricular dysrhythmia caused by myocardial sensitization to catecholamines and hypoxia induced by a simple asphyxiant effect.

Pulmonary

Cough; aspiration can cause a chemical pneumonitis.

Gastrointestinal

Vomiting, abdominal cramps, and gastrointestinal tract irritation can occur after ingestion.

Hepatic

Fatty liver and increased transaminases may occur.

Renal

Paroxysmal nocturnal hemoglobinuria may occur.

Hematologic

- Anemia, aplastic anemia, leukopenia, thrombocytopenia, and pancytopenia
- Acute myelomonocytic leukemia and chronic lymphocytic leukemia linked to chronic benzene exposure (latent period of 5–15 years)

Neurologic

- Initial transient CNS excitation: euphoria, nervousness, tremor, insomnia, nystagmus, headache ("benzol jag" is an acute occupational exposure characterized by confusion, euphoria, and ataxia)
- CNS depression: somnolence, confusion, vertigo, ataxia, seizures, and coma
- Chronic exposure associated with peripheral neuropathy, cognitive deficits, memory impairment, psychiatric disorders, encephalopathy, and emotional lability

PROCEDURES AND LABORATORY TESTS

Essential Tests

- Acute exposure. No tests needed in minimally symptomatic patients.
- Chronic exposure. Complete blood count (CBC) and reticulocyte count are needed.

Recommended Tests

- Acute exposure

—Serum electrolytes, BUN, and creatinine to assess CNS effects
—Arterial blood gases or pulse oximetry to assess oxygenation
—ECG and continuous cardiac monitoring to detect dysrhythmias
—Chest radiograph in patients with acute respiratory symptoms

- Chronic exposure

—CBC with differential to detect bone marrow effects
—Serum electrolytes, BUN, creatinine, and liver function tests to detect hepatic or renal injury
—Bone marrow evaluation in cases of chronic toxicity with hematologic abnormalities

Not Recommended

Levels of benzene and phenol (primary metabolite) are not clinically useful, except for workplace medical monitoring.

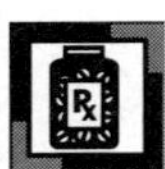

Treatment

DIRECTING PATIENT COURSE

- Focus treatment on airway management and hemodynamic support.
- Supportive care with appropriate airway management is vital; hemodynamic support may be required.
- Dose and time of exposure should be determined for all substances involved.

The health-care professional should call the poison control center when:

- Altered mental status or other serious effects are present.
- Toxic effects are not consistent with benzene poisoning.
- Coingestant, drug interaction, or underlying disease presents an unusual problem.

The patient should be referred to a health-care professional when:

- Attempted suicide or homicide is possible.
- Patient or caregiver seem unreliable.
- History of acute benzene exposure is obtained.
- Coingestant, drug interaction or underlying disease presents an unusual problem.

Admission Considerations

Inpatient management is warranted when cardiac dysrhythmia or persistent mental status depression is present.

DECONTAMINATION

Out of Hospital

- In cases of inhalation, patient should be removed from exposure and given supplemental oxygen.
- In cases of ingestion, emesis should not be induced due to rapid onset of CNS depression and risk of aspiration.

In Hospital

- Gastric lavage should be performed in pediatric (tube size 24–32 French) or adult (tube size 36–42 French) patients presenting within 1 hour of a large ingestion or if serious effects are present.
- One dose of activated charcoal (1–2 g/kg) should be administered without a cathartic if a substantial ingestion has occurred within the previous few hours.

ANTIDOTES

There is no specific antidote for benzene poisoning.

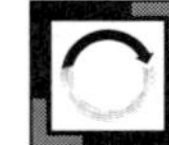

Follow-Up

PATIENT MONITORING

Respiratory and cardiac function should be monitored continuously in symptomatic patients.

EXPECTED COURSE AND PROGNOSIS

- Acute inhalation resolves quickly after termination of exposure.
- Sudden death can occur during acute exposure from cardiovascular catecholamine and dysrhythmia.
- Anemia, thrombocytopenia, or leukemia may occur in patients with chronic toxic exposure.

DISCHARGE CRITERIA/INSTRUCTIONS

- From the emergency department

—Following acute exposure, asymptomatic patients with normal neurologic examination results and without cardiac effects may be discharged after a 6-hour observation period and psychiatric evaluation, if needed.
—Patients suspected of abusing inhaled benzene require consideration for follow-up hematologic evaluation.

- From the hospital. Patients may be discharged after toxic effects resolve or stabilize and after psychiatric evaluation, if needed.

PATIENT EDUCATION

Appropriate counseling regarding the possible long-term hematologic effects is required for patients subject to chronic exposure.

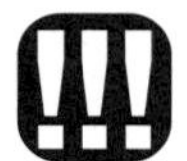

Pitfalls

DIAGNOSIS

- It is important to consider alternative diagnoses for alteration and depression in mental status.
- It is important to arrange for a hematologic workup in patients chronically exposed to benzene.

TREATMENT

Psychiatric evaluation should be ordered for chronic abusers of inhaled benzene.

ICD-9-CM 982.0

Toxic effect of solvents other than petroleum-based: benzene and homologues.

RECOMMENDED READING

Midzenski MA, McDiarmid MA, Rothman N, et al. Acute high dose exposure to benzene in shipyard workers. *Am J Ind Med* 1992;22:553–565.

U.S. Department of Health and Human Services. ATSDR case studies in environmental medicine: benzene toxicity. Monograph 11. Bethesda, MD: U.S. DHHS, October 1992.

Author: Alvin C. Bronstein

Reviewer: Gerald F. O'Malley

Benzocaine

Basics

DESCRIPTION

Benzocaine is a local anesthetic.

FORMS AND USES

- U.S. FDA-labeled indications for use include numerous indications involving mild to moderate localized pain or irritation.
- Benzocaine can be found in topical ointments, creams, gels, solutions, aerosols, and sprays.
- Formulations in which benzocaine is present include Tympagesic, Auralgan, Oragel, Benzodent, Orabase, Merocaine, Tyrozets, Americaine, Applicaine, BanSmoke, Burneze, Chigger-Tox, Dent's Toothache preparations, Dentispray, Dermoplast, Detane, Diet Ayds, Hurricaine, Lanacane, Numzident, Orajel, Orabase, SensoGARD, Slim Mint, Spec-T, Subcutin N, Teething Syrup, Topicaine, Trocaine, Unguentine, Vicks Children's Chloraseptic, Aerocaine, Aerotherm, Aezodent, Aidex, Allergen, Anbesol, Animine, Anocaine, Antibiotic Cold Sore Ointment, Antipyrine and Benzocaine Otic Solution, Anusept, Appedrine, and Auralgicin.
- Benzocaine is sometimes added to street drugs as an adulterant.

TOXIC DOSE

Ingestion of just 1 to 2 ml of 7.5% benzocaine gel can produce toxicity in infants.

PATHOPHYSIOLOGY

- Benzocaine is a local anesthetic that is metabolized to aniline and then further metabolized to phenylhydroxylamine and nitrobenzene.
- These potent agents (phenylhydroxylamine and nitrobenzene) are capable of oxidizing hemoglobin to methemoglobin, which results in methemoglobinemia.

—Methemoglobin is hemoglobin in the Fe^{3+} (oxidized) state instead of normal Fe^{2+} state.
—It is continuously produced in cells and reduced back to Fe^{2+} by the enzyme NADH (nicotinamide adenine dinucleotide, reduced form) methemoglobin reductase.

EPIDEMIOLOGY

- Poisoning is common due to the large number of over-the-counter products.
- Toxic effects following exposure are typically mild, and death occurs rarely.

CAUSES

- Toxicity usually occurs as a result of therapeutic misadventure.
- Child neglect or abuse should be considered if the patient is less than 1 year of age, suicide attempt if the patient is over 6 years of age.

RISK FACTORS

- Infants under the age of four months have greater susceptibility due to reduced NADH methemoglobin reductase activity.
- Topical use is not recommended in **children** less than 2 years of age.

PREGNANCY AND LACTATION

US FDA Pregnancy Category C. The drug exerts animal teratogenic or embryocidal effects, but there are no controlled studies in women, or no studies are available in either animals or women.

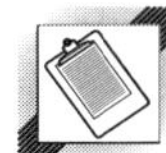

Diagnosis

DIFFERENTIAL DIAGNOSIS

- Toxicologic causes of methemoglobinemia include the use or ingestion of dapsone, nitrites, nitrates, chloroquine, primaquine, sulfonamide, aniline dyes, naphthalene, chlorates, phenacetin, mafenide acetate, phenazopyridine, resorcinol, aminobenzenes, and acetanilid.
- Nontoxicologic causes of methemoglobinemia primarily involve deficiency of NADH methemoglobin reductase.

SIGNS AND SYMPTOMS

- Toxic effects are caused by cellular hypoxia induced by decreased oxygen delivery to cells.

Vital Signs

Tachycardia, hypotension, and tachypnea are rare unless hemolysis or methemoglobinemia develop.

HEENT

Prolonged mucous membrane contact can result in irritation.

Dermatologic

- Cyanosis may develop due to methemoglobinemia.
- Rash is common with topical use.

Cardiovascular

Tachycardia and hypotension can result from methemoglobinemia.

Pulmonary

Dyspnea due to methemoglobin-induced hypoxia.

Gastrointestinal

Nausea and vomiting are common.

Hematologic

- Most cases of methemoglobinemia involve overdose.
- Idiosyncratic reactions have been reported following therapeutic doses.

Fluids and Electrolytes

Lactic acidosis due to relative hypoxia induced by methemoglobin.

Neurologic

- Altered mental status due to methemoglobin-induced hypoxia.
- Seizures occur in severe toxicity.

PROCEDURES AND LABORATORY TESTS

Essential Tests

- Methemoglobin level. Normal is less than 3%.
- If methemoglobin level is unavailable, a drop of the patient's blood can be placed upon a white sheet and compared with that of a normal control; blood with methemoglobinemia has a characteristic chocolate brown color.

Recommended Tests

- Arterial blood gases should be measured in symptomatic patients using a cooximeter because calculated oxygen saturations may be inaccurate in the presence of methemoglobin.
- Serum glucose-6-phosphate dehydrogenase (G-6-PD) determination should be made to determine etiology in patients with methemoglobinemia.
- Serum electrolytes, BUN, and creatinine can be used to assess for elevated anion gap acidosis.

Not Recommended Tests

Benzocaine in either plasma or urine can confirm exposure but qualitative levels are not clinically useful.

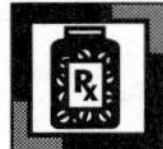

Treatment

- Treatment initially should focus on decontamination, supportive respiratory care, and administration of methylene blue, if indicated.
- Administration of 100% oxygen is critical in symptomatic patients.
- Dose and time of exposure should be determined for all substances involved.

DIRECTING PATIENT COURSE

The health-care professional should call the poison control center when:

- Cyanosis, acidosis, respiratory distress, or other severe effects are present.
- Toxic effects are not consistent with benzocaine poisoning.
- Coingestant, drug interaction, or underlying disease presents an unusual problem.

The patient should be referred to a health-care facility when:

- Attempted suicide or homicide is possible.
- Patient or caregiver seems unreliable.
- Coingestant, drug interaction, or underlying disease presents an unusual problem.

Admission Considerations

Inpatient management is warranted if the patient is symptomatic, exhibits an elevated methemoglobin level, or requires treatment with methylene blue.

DECONTAMINATION

Out of Hospital

- Emesis should be avoided due to potentially rapid onset of seizures and CNS depression.
- Exposed skin areas should be washed to limit further absorption.

In Hospital

- Ipecac-induced emesis is not recommended.
- Nasogastric aspiration using a nasogastric tube within the first 30 to 60 minutes following a large ingestion may be beneficial; however, because benzocaine is rapidly absorbed, gastric aspiration is useful only soon after ingestion.
- If there is concern of a coingestant, then gastric lavage with a large-bore orogastric tube may be indicated.
- One dose of activated charcoal (1–2 g/kg) should be administered without a cathartic if a substantial ingestion has occurred within the previous few hours.
- Exposed skin areas should be washed to limit further absorption.

ANTIDOTES

Methylene blue is used to reverse methemoglobinemia.

- Indications. The decision to treat methemoglobinemia is based primarily on the patient's clinical condition; any evidence of CNS or cardiac hypoxia (anxiety, confusion, hypotension, chest pain, etc.) indicates a need for treatment.
- Contraindications. Methylene blue is relatively contraindicated when patient has known NADH methemoglobin reductase deficiency or G-6-PD deficiency.
- Method of administration. 1 to 2 mg/kg should be given intravenously over 5 minutes.

—Clinical improvement should be apparent shortly after administration.
—Methemoglobin level should be repeated 30 minutes later.
—If the level remains elevated and the patient is still symptomatic, a repeat dose of 1 to 2 mg/kg intravenously over 5 minutes can be given.

- Potential adverse effects

—Hemolysis can occur in patients with G-6-PD deficiency.
—A paradoxical worsening of methemoglobinemia can occur with extremely large doses (unlikely with cumulative dose of less than 7 mg/kg).

ADJUNCTIVE TREATMENT

Exchange transfusion has been used rarely when life-threatening methemoglobinemia is refractory to methylene blue therapy or patient has severe G-6-PD deficiency.

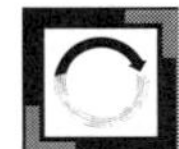

Follow-Up

PATIENT MONITORING

- Patient should be placed on continuous cardiac and hemodynamic monitoring.
- Serial methemoglobin levels should be checked until normal is approached and level does not recur after last dose of methylene blue.

EXPECTED COURSE AND PROGNOSIS

- Nearly all patients recover quickly if treatment is initiated before hypoxic injury occurs.
- Patients with hypoxic injury or G-6-PD deficiency may have prolonged course.

DISCHARGE CRITERIA/INSTRUCTIONS

- From the emergency room. Asymptomatic patients with a normal or decreasing methemoglobin level can be discharged after decontamination, a 4- to 6-hour period of observation, and psychiatric evaluation, if needed.
- From the hospital. Patient may be discharged when symptoms resolve and methemoglobin level is normal.

PATIENT EDUCATION

- Patient should return if fatigue, dyspnea, lightheadedness, shortness of breath, or cyanosis develop or recur.
- Patients with G-6-PD deficiency should be warned to avoid preparations containing benzocaine.

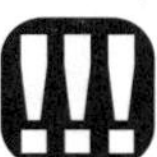

Pitfalls

DIAGNOSIS

- The pO_2 on the arterial blood gases reflects the partial pressure of oxygen dissolved in the blood and may be normal despite significant methemoglobinemia.
- A normal oxygen saturation by pulse oximetry does **not** rule out methemoglobinemia.
- Sulfhemoglobinemia produces effects indistinguishable from methemoglobinemia and should be suspected when methemoglobinemia fails to respond to methylene blue treatment.

TREATMENT

Methemoglobinemia may be recurrent despite treatment, especially in the face of continued gastrointestinal or dermal absorption of benzocaine.

ICD-9-CM 968.5

Poisoning by other central nervous system depressants and anesthetics: surface (topical) and infiltration anesthetics.

See also: SECTION II, Methemoglobinemia chapter; and SECTION III, Methylene Blue chapter.

RECOMMENDED READING

POISINDEX Editorial Staff. Benzocaine. In: Rumack BH, Hess AJ, Gelman CR, eds. *POISINDEX system*. Englewood, CO: Micromedex, Inc. (edition expires August 31, 1997).

Price D. Methemoglobinemia. In: Goldfrank LR, et al., eds. *Goldfrank's toxicologic emergencies*. 6th ed. Norwalk, CT: Appleton & Lange, 1998.

Author: Edwin K. Kuffner

Reviewer: Luke Yip

Benzodiazepines

Basics

DESCRIPTION

The benzodiazepines are used as sedatives, anxiolytics, and muscle relaxants, and include alprazolam (Xanax), brotizolam, chlordiazepoxide (Librium), chlorazepate (Tranxene), clobazam, clonazepam (Clonopin), diazepam (Valium), estazolam (Prosom), flurazepam (Dalmane), halazepam, lorazepam (Ativan), lormetazepam, medazepam, midazolam (Versed), nitrazepam, oxazepam (Serax), prazepam, temazepam (Restoril), triazolam (Halcion).

FORMS AND USES

- Anesthesia and sedation during procedures.
- Prescribed for their hypnotic, anxiolytic, anticonvulsant, and muscle-relaxant properties.

—Alprazolam. 0.25 to 0.5 mg orally three times per day.
—Chlordiazepoxide. For anxiety 5 to 25 mg orally four times per day; for alcohol withdrawal 25 to 100 mg intravenously or intramuscularly every 2 to 4 hours.
—Chlorazepate. 7.5 to 15 mg orally at night or twice per day.
—Diazepam. 2.5 to 5 mg increments intravenously up to 0.2 mg/kg; 2 to 10 mg orally three or four times per day.
—Flurazepam. 15 to 30 mg orally at night.
—Lorazepam. 0.5 to 2 mg intravenously, intramuscularly, or orally every 6 to 8 hours.
—Midazolam. 5 mg or 0.07 mg/kg intravenously.
—Oxazepam. 10 to 15 mg orally three or four times per day.
—Temazepam. 15 to 30 mg orally at bedtime.
—Triazolam. 0.125 to 0.5 mg orally at bedtime.

PATHOPHYSIOLOGY

- Benzodiazepines bind to the benzodiazepine receptor, augmenting the inhibitory neurotransmitter effect of gamma-aminobutyric acid (GABA).
- Hyperpolarization due to transmembrane chloride ion flux through a GABA-mediated channel produces decreased neuronal excitability.
- Toxic effects are typically mild to moderate.

EPIDEMIOLOGY

- Intentional ingestion is common.
- Death occurs rarely, usually involving coingestant such as ethanol, which accentuates respiratory depression.
- Young children are at increased risk of poisoning.
- The elderly are at risk, usually due to depressed renal and hepatic function.

CAUSES

- Toxic ingestion is usually intentional.
- Child neglect or abuse should be considered if the patient is less than 1 year of age, suicide attempt if the patient is over 6 years of age.

DRUG AND DISEASE INTERACTIONS

Toxic effects may be enhanced with coingestion of ethanol, barbiturates, or other CNS depressants.

PREGNANCY AND LACTATION

- Alprazolam, chlordiazepoxide, chlorazepate, diazepam, lorazepam, midazolam, and oxazepam. US FDA Pregnancy Category D. Evidence of human fetal risk exists, but benefits in certain situations (e.g., life-threatening situations or serious diseases) make use of the drug acceptable despite its risks.
- Flurazepam, temazepam, and triazolam. US FDA Pregnancy Category X. Studies demonstrate fetal abnormalities or there is evidence of fetal risk based on human experience, or both, and the risk clearly outweighs any possible benefit.
- Benzodiazepines are secreted in breast milk and can produce sedation in infants.

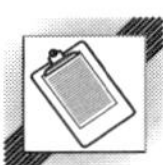

Diagnosis

DIFFERENTIAL DIAGNOSIS

- Toxicologic causes of respiratory and mental status depression include narcotics, ethanol, barbiturates, numerous sedative-hypnotic drugs, tricyclic antidepressants, and many others.
- Nontoxicologic causes include hypoxia, severe electrolyte abnormality, hypoglycemia, intracranial injury, meningitis, encephalitis, or postictal state, and many others.

SIGNS AND SYMPTOMS

The predominant effects are CNS depression with respiratory depression.

Vital Signs

Hypothermia and hypotension.

HEENT

Nystagmus, miosis, and diplopia.

Cardiovascular

Hypotension, bradycardia; tachycardia may develop as a response to hypotension.

Pulmonary

Respiratory depression; aspiration may occur.

Gastrointestinal

Nausea and vomiting, especially in children.

Musculoskeletal

Pressure injury may produce rhabdomyolysis or skin necrosis.

Neurologic

Impairment of speech and coordination, amnesia, ataxia, somnolence (rarely to the point of coma), confusion, depressed deep tendon reflexes, and dyskinesia.

PROCEDURES AND LABORATORY TESTS

Essential Tests

Testing may not be needed in asymptomatic patients.

Recommended Tests

- Serum electrolytes, BUN, and creatinine to assess causes of altered mental status.
- Pulse oximetry for assessment of altered mental status.
- Electrocardiogram, serum acetaminophen, aspirin, and ethanol levels in overdose setting to detect occult overdose.
- Urinalysis and serum creatine kinase if comatose to evaluate for rhabdomyolysis.
- Head CT, lumbar puncture, and chest radiographs as needed to evaluate respiratory complications and assess other causes of CNS depression.

Not Recommended Tests

Quantitative benzodiazepine levels are not clinically useful.

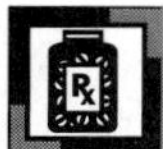

Treatment

DIRECTING PATIENT COURSE

- Treatment should focus on gastrointestinal decontamination and airway management.
- Supportive care with appropriate airway management is vital; endotracheal intubation may be needed to protect the airway.
- Dose and time of exposure should be determined for all substances involved.

The health-care professional should call the poison control center when:

- Significant CNS or respiratory depression, or other severe effects are present.
- Signs and symptoms are not consistent with benzodiazepine poisoning.
- Coingestant, drug interaction, or underlying disease presents an unusual problem.

The patient should be referred to a health-care facility when:

- Attempted suicide or CNS effects are present.
- Patient or caregiver seem unreliable.
- Any toxic effects develop.
- Coingestant, drug interaction, or underlying disease presents an unusual problem.

Admission Considerations

Inpatient management is warranted if persistent respiratory or CNS effects are present.

DECONTAMINATION

Out of Hospital

Emesis should not be induced due to potential for rapid deterioration.

In Hospital

- Emesis should not be induced.
- Gastric lavage should be performed in pediatric (tube size 24–32 French) or adult (tube size 36–42 French) patients for large ingestion presenting within 1 hour of ingestion or if serious effects are present.
- One dose of activated charcoal (1–2 g/kg) should be administered without a cathartic if a substantial ingestion has occurred within the previous few hours.

ANTIDOTES

Flumazenil (Romazicon) is a specific antidote for benzodiazepine intoxication.

- Indications. Reversal of benzodiazepine effects including profound sedation, respiratory depression, and coma.
- Contraindications. Seizures, known allergy to flumazenil, concurrent overdose of tricyclic antidepressant drugs, or use of cocaine or other seizure producing agents.
- Method of administration

—Adult dose is 0.1 to 0.2 mg intravenous push every 1 to 2 minutes until clinical effect or 1 to 2 mg given; if resedation occurs, may give 1 mg every 20 minutes to a maximum of 3 mg/h.
—Pediatric dose is 10 μg/kg intravenous push, titrated to effect.
—Caution: Resedation is possible 30 to 60 minutes after administration.

- Potential adverse effects. Agitation, vomiting, confusion, seizures, dysrhythmia, and flushing; may induce withdrawal.

ADJUNCTIVE TREATMENT

- Hemodialysis is not effective.
- Following decontamination, treatment is primarily supportive.
- Hypotension

—Patient should receive an intravenous infusion of 10 to 20 ml/kg 0.9% NaCl and be placed in the Trendelenburg position.
—Guide further fluid therapy by monitoring central pressure to avoid volume overload.

- If hypotension is unresponsive, a vasopressor should be administered.

—Dopamine. Patient should receive 2 to 5 μg/kg/min, titrated upward to desired effect; rates above 20 μg/kg/min are unlikely to provide further benefit.
—Norepinephrine. An infusion of 0.1 to 0.2 μg/kg/min intravenously, titrated to desired effect, should be given. High infusion rates may cause tissue ischemia.

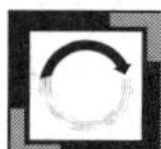

Follow-Up

PATIENT MONITORING

Patients should have continuous respiratory and hemodynamic monitoring.

EXPECTED COURSE AND PROGNOSIS

- Patients usually regain consciousness within 24 hours.
- Most patients recover completely unless hypoxia intercedes.
- In one study, only 5 of 702 poisoning patients died (a mortality rate of 0.007) and those cases were usually complicated by a coingestion.

DISCHARGE CRITERIA/INSTRUCTIONS

- From the emergency department. Asymptomatic patients may be discharged after decontamination, a 6-hour observation period, and psychiatric evaluation, if needed.
- From the hospital. Patients may be discharged when vital signs and mental status become normal and after psychiatric evaluation, if needed.

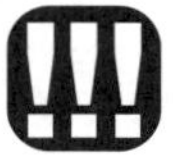

Pitfalls

DIAGNOSIS

Signs and symptoms of benzodiazepine overdose may closely resemble other conditions (both other ingestions and nontoxicologic conditions), resulting in misdiagnosis.

TREATMENT

Agents with long half-lives may require extended observation and care.

ICD-9-CM 969.4

Poisoning by psychotropic agents: benzodiazepine-based tranquilizers.

See also: SECTION II, Hypotension chapter; SECTION III, Flumazenil chapter; and SECTION IV, Sedative-Hypnotic Agents chapter.

RECOMMENDED READING

Buckley NA, Dawson AH, Whyte IM, O'Connell DL. Relative toxicity of benzodiazepines in overdose. *BMJ* 1995;310:219–221.

POISINDEX Editorial Staff. Benzodiazepines (management/treatment protocol). In: Rumack BH, Hess AJ, Gelman CR, eds. *POISINDEX system.* Englewood, CO: Micromedex, Inc. (edition expires August 31, 1997).

Author: Brian T. Williams

Reviewer: Richard C. Dart

Benzoyl Peroxide

Basics

DESCRIPTION

Benzoyl peroxide is a topical medication for the treatment of inflammatory acne, decubital or stasis ulcers, and pyoderma gangrenosum.

FORMS AND USES

Benzoyl peroxide is available as a 5% to 10% topical preparation.

TOXIC DOSE

- Acute oral toxicity has not been demonstrated.
- Inhalation may produce airway irritation.
- Moderation erythema and edema have occurred after exposure to 10% solutions.

PATHOPHYSIOLOGY

- Benzoyl peroxide has an antibacterial effect produced by slow release of active oxygen species as well as keratolytic, drying, and desquamative effects.
- It also may enhance aggregation of platelets.

EPIDEMIOLOGY

Minor skin effects are common. Other types of exposure are rare.

WORKPLACE STANDARDS

- OSHA. PEL TWA is 5 mg/m^3.
- NIOSH. IDLH is 1,000 mg/m^3.

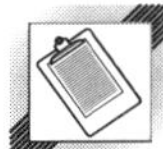

Diagnosis

SIGNS AND SYMPTOMS

- The primary effects are irritation of the eyes, nose, throat, and skin.

HEENT

- Inhalation produces irritation and inflammation of eyes, nose, and throat.
- Conjunctivitis and superficial corneal opacities have been noted.

Dermatologic

- Dermal application causes irritation of the skin.
- Erythema, peeling, drying, and itching of skin have been reported.
- Both primary irritant and sensitization dermatitis can occur.
- Cutaneous effects are greatest in the early weeks of treatment.
- Benzoyl peroxide can increase sebum excretion in the second month of treatment.

PROCEDURES AND LABORATORY TESTS

Essential Tests

No tests may be needed for asymptomatic or minimally symptomatic patients.

Recommended Tests

An ophthalmologic examination should be performed if irritation, pain, swelling, redness, or visual changes occur.

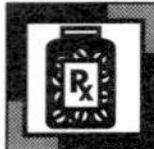

Treatment

DIRECTING PATIENT COURSE

Oral exposures in children and adults can be safely observed at home.

The health-care professional should call the poison control center when:

- Severe or persistent effects develop.
- Coingestant, drug interaction, or underlying disease presents an unusual problem.

The patient should be referred to a health-care facility when:

- There has been inhalation exposure.
- Irritation and pain persist after washing off a skin exposure.
- Coingestant, drug interaction, or underlying disease presents an unusual problem.

DECONTAMINATION

- Oral exposure. Immediate dilution with milk or water is recommended due to irritant effects.
- Gastric lavage should be performed in pediatric (tube size 24–32 French) or adult (tube size 36–42 French) patients for large ingestion presenting within 1 hour of ingestion or if serious effects are present.
- One dose of activated charcoal (1–2 g/kg) should be administered without a cathartic if a substantial ingestion has occurred within the previous few hours.

- Inhalation exposure

—Patients should be moved to fresh air.
—Humidified oxygen should be provided.

- Eye exposure. All eye exposures should be irrigated with water for at least 15 minutes.
- Skin exposure. Exposed areas should be washed thoroughly with soap and water.

ANTIDOTE

There is no specific antidote for benzoyl peroxide poisoning.

ADJUNCTIVE TREATMENT

Cool compresses may be applied, and topical steroids may be of benefit following skin exposure.

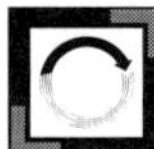

Follow-Up

PATIENT MONITORING

- Following dermatologic reactions, benzoyl peroxide treatment should be discontinued until reevaluation by a dermatologist.
- Corneal injuries should be treated with antibiotics and referred to an ophthalmologist.
- Inhalation exposures may be treated symptomatically after an initial period of airway observation.

DISCHARGE CRITERIA/INSTRUCTIONS

- From the emergency department. Patients with benzoyl peroxide toxicity may be discharged after symptoms resolve following decontamination and, if needed, psychiatric evaluation.
- From the hospital. Patients may be discharged after toxic effects resolve or stabilize and after psychiatric evaluation, if needed.

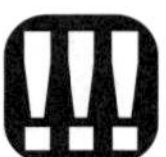

Pitfalls

Patch test reactions may be falsely negative in patients allergic to benzoyl peroxide.

ICD-9-CM 976

Poisoning by agents primarily affecting skin and mucous membrane, ophthalmologic, otorhinolaryngologic, and dental drugs.

RECOMMENDED READING

Jackson EM. Benzoyl peroxide: an old drug with new problems. *J Toxicol Cutan Ocular Toxicol* 1986;5:163–165.

Author: Michael Anderson

Reviewer: Richard C. Dart

Beryllium

Basics

DESCRIPTION

Beryllium is an element with unique physical characteristics that has led to varied technological uses.

FORMS AND USES

In addition to the mining industry, beryllium is used in atomic energy–related research; missile parts; tool and die manufacturing; dental laboratories; beryllium-copper alloy production; electronics; aerospace; and nuclear industries.

TOXIC DOSE

At lower air levels, the toxicity varies by duration and time of exposure. The air concentration considered immediately dangerous to health or life is 4 mg/m^3 of beryllium.

PATHOPHYSIOLOGY

- Beryllium poisoning is primarily an occupational disease.
- The principal source of toxicity is the inhalation of beryllium in the form of beryllium oxides (fumes), dusts of beryllium salts, metals, or alloys.

—Inhaled beryllium is transported from the airway to the interstitial lung space and regional lymph nodes, inducing a cellular immune response with activation of beryllium-specific T-lymphocytes.
—Inhalation of beryllium results in symptoms in a continuum from an acute chemical pneumonitis to a chronic, insidious granulomatous process.

- Cutaneous exposure by metal splinter or imbedded particles can cause dermatitis and sensitization to subsequent exposure.

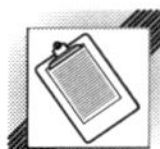

Diagnosis

Clinical diagnosis of chronic beryllium disease requires at least four of the following six features and at least one of the first two:

- Evidence of significant beryllium exposure
- Beryllium in lung tissue, lymph nodes, or urine
- Lower airway disease and consistent clinical course with this disease
- Radiographic evidence of interstitial disease
- Restrictive and or obstructive ventilatory abnormality or decreased diffusing capacity of carbon monoxide (D_{CO})
- Pathologic alterations consistent with beryllium disease in lung tissue or lymph nodes

DIFFERENTIAL DIAGNOSIS

Causes of chronic pulmonary disease include sarcoidosis, tuberculosis, and silicosis.

SIGNS AND SYMPTOMS

Acute Toxicity

- Acute symptomatic inhalation exposure is usually by high levels of beryllium and most likely is related to dose of exposure and solubility of the beryllium compound.
- Conjunctivitis and upper airway involvement may develop
- Epistaxis, facial pain, and nasopharyngitis occur.
- Edematous and hyperemic tissue in the nasal and pharyngeal regions may progress to ulceration, fissures, and perforation.
- Pulmonary. Chest pain, dry nonproductive cough, shortness of breath, rhonchi, tracheobronchitis, and chemical pneumonitis may occur.

Chronic Toxicity

- The primary chronic effect is granulomatous lung disease, although systemic involvement can occur.
- Latency period ranges from months to 30 years (average 6–10 years) from exposure to clinical illness.
- Incidence of lung cancer appears to be inversely related to the duration of exposure.
- Ulceration, noncaseating granulomas
- Impaired wound healing
- Right heart failure and cor pulmonale have occurred.
- Dyspnea on exertion has been accompanied by chest pain, cough, and weight loss.
- Bibasilar dry rales, cyanosis, clubbing, lymphadenopathy may occur.
- Noncaseating granulomas of the lung and involvement of other organs may be found.
- Nephrolithiasis has been observed.

PROCEDURES AND LABORATORY TESTS

Essential Tests

No tests are usually needed in asymptomatic patients.

Recommended Tests

- Chest radiographs range from normal to diffuse interstitial bilateral infiltrates with hilar adenopathy.
- Pulmonary function tests have revealed an obstructive pattern in approximately 33% of patients with berylliosis, restrictive in approximately 25%, and reduced carbon monoxide diffusing capacity in approximately 33%.
- Beryllium lymphocyte transformation test (preferably lymphocytes from bronchial lavage rather than blood) in conjunction with transbronchial biopsy will differentiate between chronic beryllium disease and sarcoidosis.
- A blood lymphocyte transformation test is useful in screening beryllium-exposed workers.

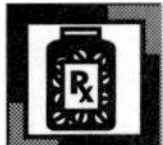

Treatment

DIRECTING PATIENT COURSE

The health-care professional should call the poison control center when:

- Toxic effects are not consistent with beryllium.
- Underlying disease presents an unusual problem.

The patient should be referred to a health-care facility when:

- Acute toxic effects develop.
- Underlying disease presents an unusual problem.

Admission Considerations

Inpatient management is warranted for hypoxic patients.

DECONTAMINATION

- Patient should be moved to fresh air for respiratory exposures.
- Skin should be irrigated copiously with water for dermal exposure.

ANTIDOTES

There is no antidote for beryllium toxicity.

ADJUNCTIVE THERAPY

- Skin disease

—Dermatitis usually resolves with cessation of exposure.
—Granulomas are treated by repetitive debridement or excision of the lesion.

- Chronic beryllium disease

—Corticosteroid therapy (prednisone 5–20 mg per day or four times per day) is associated with subjective and objective improvements.
—Exacerbation of symptoms may occur with withdrawal of steroids.

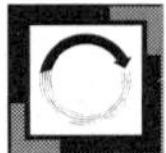

Follow-Up

EXPECTED COURSE AND PROGNOSIS

- Acute inhalation exposure

—Following termination of exposure, improvement typically occurs over 4 to 6 weeks.
—Bronchiectasis can be a long-term sequela of acute pneumonitis; approximately 17% of patients with acute exposure develop chronic beryllium lung disease.
—Acute disease may develop into a chronic form of berylliosis.

- There are no reports of long-term cures or evidence of remissions from chronic beryllium lung disease.
- Clinical progression is usually very gradual. Prolonged corticosteroid therapy is usually required.
- All cases should be reported to the Beryllium Case Registry.
- Referral to a physician experienced in the diagnosis and managment of beryllium disease is recommended.

ICD-9-CM 985.3

Toxic effect of other metals: beryllium and its compounds.

RECOMMENDED READING

Newman LS. Beryllium. In: Sullivan JB Jr, Krieger GR, eds. *Hazardous materials toxicology.* Baltimore: Williams & Wilkins, 1992:882–890.

Author: Luke Yip

Reviewer: Richard C. Dart

β-Receptor Blocking Drugs

Basics

DESCRIPTION

The β-receptor blocking drugs (β-blockers) are used in the treatment of hypertension, angina, myocardial infarction, cardiac dysrhythmia, cardiomyopathy, migraine headache, thyrotoxicosis, and topical use in glaucoma.

FORMS AND USES

- Pharmaceutical preparations of these substances include acebutolol, alprenolol, atenolol, betaxolol, Betoptic Ophthalmic, bisoprolol, Brevibloc, bucindolol, bufetolol, carteolol, Cartrol, esmolol, Inderal, Inderide (also contains hydrochlorothiazide), Kerlone, labetolol, Levatol, Lopressor, Lopressor HCT (also contains hydrochlorothiazide), Metipranolol, metoprolol, nadolol, oxprenolol, penbutolol, pindolol, practolol, propranolol, Sectral, Tenoretic (also contains chlorthalidone), Tenormin, Timolide (also contains hydrochlorothiazide), timolol, Timoptic, Toprol XL, Visken, Zebeta, and Ziac (also contains hydrochlorothiazide).
- Representative daily dosage

—Atenolol. Oral, 50 to 100 mg (200 mg maximum); intravenous, 5 to 10 mg.
—Betoptic Ophthalmic Solution. Ocular, 2 to 4 drops.
—Labetolol. Oral, 200 to 800 mg (2,400 mg maximum).
—Metoprolol. Oral, 100 to 400 mg.
—Propranolol. Oral, 40 to 320 mg; intravenous, 1 to 10 mg.
—Timolol. Oral, 10 to 60 mg.
—Timoptic. Ocular, 2 drops.

PATHOPHYSIOLOGY

- β-blocking agents are competitive antagonists at β_1, β_2, or both types of adrenergic receptors.
- Some agents also exhibit partial β-receptor agonist or antagonist activity.

EPIDEMIOLOGY

- Poisoning is uncommon.
- Toxic effects following exposure are typically mild to moderate, with death occurring in cases involving coingestants or large overdose.

CAUSES

- Toxic ingestion is usually intentional.
- Child neglect or abuse should be considered if the patient is less than 1 year of age, suicide attempt if the patient is over 6 years of age.

RISK FACTORS

- Patients with reactive airways disease may develop bronchospasm even at therapeutic doses.
- Elderly patients and those with underlying cardiovascular disease may be intolerant of even mild hypotension.
- Seizures and hypoglycemia are more common in children, particularly with propranolol.

DRUG AND DISEASE INTERACTIONS

- Coingestion of calcium channel blocker or digitalis may worsen bradycardia, dysrhythmias, and hypotension.
- Coingestion of other antihypertensives may worsen hypotension.

PREGNANCY AND LACTATION

- Acebutolol, metoprolol, and pindolol. US FDA Pregnancy Category B. Animal studies indicate no fetal risk and there are no controlled human studies, or animal studies show an adverse fetal effect but well-controlled studies in pregnant women do not.
- Atenolol, betaxolol, bisoprolol, carteolol, esmolol, labetolol, nadolol, penbutolol, propranolol, and timolol. US FDA Pregnancy Category C. The drug exerts animal teratogenic or embryocidal effects, but there are no controlled studies in women, or no studies are available in either animals or women.

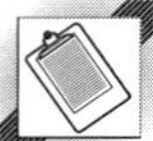

Diagnosis

DIFFERENTIAL DIAGNOSIS

- Toxicologic causes of bradycardia or heart block include calcium channel blockers, digitalis, class I antidysrhythmics, and clonidine.
- Nontoxicologic causes include ischemic heart disease and severe electrolyte abnormalities.

SIGNS AND SYMPTOMS

- Hypotension and bradycardia are common; life-threatening dysrhythmia may occur in severe cases.
- Bronchospasm, seizures, and hypoglycemia may occur.

Vital Signs

Bradycardia and hypotension are common.

Cardiovascular

May include severe bradycardia, atrioventricular blocks, intraventricular conduction delays, ventricular dysrhythmias, and congestive heart failure.

Pulmonary

- Bronchospasm is possible.
- Respiratory depression is possible in patients with hemodynamic instability.
- Pulmonary edema and acute respiratory distress syndrome may occur after a severe overdose.

Neurologic

- Seizures, most commonly after propranolol overdose
- CNS depression, coma (complicates profound hypotension)

Endocrine

Hypoglycemia, most commonly in children and diabetics after propranolol overdose.

PROCEDURES AND LABORATORY TESTS

Essential Tests

- ECG and continuous monitoring to detect dysrhythmia or ischemia
- Serum electrolytes, glucose, BUN, and creatinine to detect other causes of dysrhythmia or cause of drug accumulation

Recommended Tests

- Serum creatine kinase in patients with prolonged seizures or coma to detect rhabdomyolysis
- Serum acetaminophen and aspirin levels in an overdose setting to detect occult ingestion
- Lumbar puncture, bacterial cultures, and other tests in patients with altered mental status of unknown etiology
- Chest radiography in patients with pulmonary symptoms or coma

Not Recommended Tests

β-blocker levels are not clinically useful.

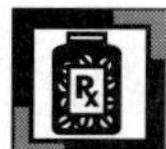

Treatment

DIRECTING PATIENT COURSE

- Treatment should focus on supportive care with appropriate airway management.
- Dose and time of exposure should be determined for all substances involved.

The health-care professional should call the poison control center when:

- Bradycardia, hypotension, altered mental status, or other severe effects are present.
- Toxic effects are not consistent with β-blocker poisoning.
- Coingestant, drug interaction, or underlying disease presents an unusual problem.

The patient should be referred to a health-care facility when:

- Attempted suicide or homicide is possible.
- Patient or caregiver seems unreliable.
- More than one daily dose of medication was ingested.
- Coingestant, drug interaction, or underlying disease presents an unusual problem.

Admission Considerations

Inpatient management is warranted if:

- Patient has ingested sustained-release preparation.
- Patient has toxic effects (hypotension, seizures, pulmonary edema, or dysrhythmia) other than mild bradycardia.

DECONTAMINATION

Out of Hospital

Emesis should not be induced; coma or seizures may develop abruptly.

In Hospital

- Gastric lavage in pediatric (tube size 24–32 French) or adult (tube size 36–42 French) patients presenting within 1 hour of substantial ingestion or if severe effects are present
- One dose of activated charcoal (1–2 g/kg) without a cathartic if a substantial ingestion has occurred within previous few hours
- Whole-bowel irrigation with a polyethylene glycol solution may be useful following ingestion of sustained-release preparation

ANTIDOTES

Glucagon

- Indications. Bradycardia and hypotension induced by β-receptor blocker; animal studies suggest that glucagon primarily affects heart rate without having a dramatic effect on blood pressure.
- Contraindication. Hypersensitivity to glucagon.
- Method of administration. Intravenous bolus of 50 to 150 μg/kg (5–10 mg in an adult) followed by an infusion of 2 to 10 mg/h, titrated to effect.
- Potential adverse effects. Frequent occurrence of vomiting and hyperglycemia. Acidosis may result from phenol diluent in some glucagon preparations. Check label and assure that saline is substituted for phenol diluent.

ADJUNCTIVE TREATMENT

- Hypotension

—Primary treatment is correction of dysrhythmia.
—If needed, patient may be infused with 10 to 20 ml/kg 0.9% saline and vasopressor such as dopamine.

- Intraaortic balloon pump has been used for hemodynamic support in overdoses unresponsive to drug therapy.
- Hemodialysis may increase elimination of acebutolol, atenolol, and nadolol, but is not expected to be useful for other β-blockers.

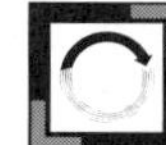

Follow-Up

PATIENT MONITORING

- Continuous cardiac and hemodynamic monitoring
- Serum glucose in diabetics and children
- Pulmonary status in patients with reactive airways disease

EXPECTED COURSE AND PROGNOSIS

- Most patients do well with gastrointestinal decontamination and supportive care. Factors producing greatest risk for complications include:

—Advanced age
—Underlying disease (especially cardiovascular)
—Coingestion of other myocardial depressant (calcium channel blockers, digitalis, clonidine, etc.)
—Massive ingestion of sustained release product

DISCHARGE CRITERIA/INSTRUCTIONS

- From the emergency department. Patients who have ingested an immediate-release formulation and are asymptomatic other than mild bradycardia may be discharged after gastric decontamination, a 6-hour observation period, and psychiatric evaluation, if needed.
- From the hospital. Patients may be discharged following gastrointestinal decontamination, resolution of cardiac effects, and psychiatric evaluation, if needed.

PATIENT EDUCATION

- Patients should be instructed carefully on the use and dosage of ophthalmic preparations.
- Patients should be warned to avoid simultaneous use of β-blockers and other agents with similar effects (calcium channel blocker, digitalis) when possible.

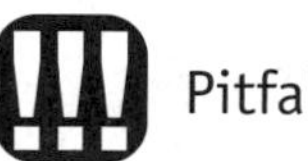

Pitfalls

DIAGNOSIS

- Ophthalmic drops can cause serious toxicity, particularly in the elderly.
- Sustained-release products may not produce toxic effects for several hours after overdose.

TREATMENT

Multiple modes of treatment (pressors, glucagon, isoproterenol, etc.) are often needed simultaneously in patients with severe effects.

ICD-9-CM 971.3

Poisoning by drugs primarily affecting the autonomic nervous system: sympatholytics (adrenergics).

See also: SECTION II, Hypotension chapter; SECTION III, Glucagon chapter.

RECOMMENDED READING

Love JN. Beta blocker toxicity: a clinical diagnosis. *Am J Emerg Med* 1994;12:356–375.

Taboulett P, Cariou A, Bordeaux A, et al. Pathophysiology and management of self-poisoning with beta blockers. *J Toxicol Clin Toxicol* 1993;31:531–551.

Author: Katherine M. Hurlbut

Reviewer: Richard C. Dart

β_2-Receptor Agonists

Basics

DESCRIPTION

β_2-receptor agonists are medications used to treat bronchospasm.

FORMS AND USES

- β_2-receptor agonists are used in the treatment of most types of asthma and chronic obstructive pulmonary disease. They are also used in the treatment of premature labor and hyperkalemia.
- Pharmaceutical preparations of the β_2-receptor agonists albuterol, terbutaline, isoetharine, metaproterenol, and ritodrine are variously available as solutions, aerosols, syrups, tablets, or sustained-release tablets.
- Common therapeutic doses of albuterol in the treatment of bronchospasms are as follows:

—Adult oral dose is up to 32 mg/day in divided doses three or four times daily.
—Pediatric oral dose for a child 2 to 6 years of age is 0.1 mg/kg per dose three times daily, up to 4 mg/day.
—Pediatric oral dose for a child 6 to 14 years of age is 2 mg three or four times daily.
—Adult dose of oral sustained-release formulation is 4 or 8 mg twice daily, up to 32 mg/day.
—Pediatric dose of oral sustained-release formulation for a child 6 to 12 years of age is 4 mg twice daily, up to 24 mg/day.

TOXIC DOSE

- Mild symptoms of toxicity begin when several times the usual dose is ingested.
- Death occurs only after massive ingestion or repeated, frequent inhalation overuse.

PATHOPHYSIOLOGY

- Binding to a β_2-adrenergic receptor activates the enzyme adenylate cyclase and thereby creates cyclic adenosine monophosphate (cAMP).
- Increased intracellular cAMP causes an influx of calcium and smooth muscle relaxation of the bronchi, gastrointestinal tract, and uterus.
- Increased cAMP also shifts potassium from extracellular to intracellular locations and lowers the serum potassium concentration.

EPIDEMIOLOGY

- Poisoning is common.
- Toxic effects following exposure are typically mild to moderate.
- Severe toxicity has resulted from dosing errors and intentional ingestion.
- Death is rare.

CAUSES

- Toxic ingestion is usually accidental or results from intentional overuse to control symptoms.
- Child neglect or abuse should be considered if the patient is less than 1 year of age, suicide attempt if the child is over 6 years of age.

DRUG AND DISEASE INTERACTIONS

Other sympathomimetic agents potentiate the sympathomimetic effects.

PREGNANCY AND LACTATION

- Ritodrine and terbutaline. US FDA Pregnancy Category B. Animal studies do not indicate a risk to the fetus and there are no controlled human studies, or animal studies do show an adverse effect on the fetus but well-controlled studies in pregnant women do not.
- Albuterol, isoetharine, and metaproterenol. US FDA Pregnancy Category C. The drug exerts animal teratogenic or embryocidal effects, but there are no controlled studies in women, or no studies are available in either animals or women.
- β_2-agonists inhibit uterine contractions and are used to prevent preterm labor.
- Fetal tachycardia may occur during therapeutic use in premature labor.

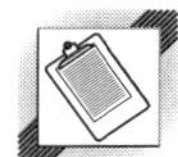

Diagnosis

DIFFERENTIAL DIAGNOSIS

- Other toxicologic causes of sympathomimetic toxicity include theophylline, cocaine, amphetamines, ephedrine, phenylpropanolamine, and many others.
- Nontoxicologic causes include hyperthyroidism, manic episode, alcohol or sedative-hypnotic withdrawal, and many others.

SIGNS AND SYMPTOMS

The patient is typically anxious with tachycardia, nausea, and vomiting; life-threatening cardiac effects are uncommon.

Vital Signs

Tachycardia is common.

HEENT

Moderately dilated pupils are common.

Dermatologic

Cool and clammy skin is common.

Cardiovascular

- Tachycardia and palpitations are common.
- Life-threatening dysrhythmias have been reported but are rare.

Pulmonary

- Paradoxical bronchospasm can occur rarely with therapeutic dosing.
- Pulmonary edema has occurred rarely with therapeutic dosing for premature labor.

Gastrointestinal

Nausea and vomiting are common.

Hematologic

- Thrombocytopenia has occurred after large overdose.
- Neutropenia and agranulocytosis have occurred during ritodrine therapy.

Fluids and Electrolytes

- Hyperglycemia and hypokalemia are common but rarely serious.
- Lactic acidosis and hypoglycemia may develop from prolonged hyperadrenergic state.

Musculoskeletal

Agitation can result in rhabdomyolysis.

Neurologic

- Mild intoxication can cause tremor, anxiety, restlessness, insomnia, and headaches.
- Severe intoxication can cause seizures.
- Syncope has been reported and may be secondary to hypotension.

Endocrine

Hyperglycemia and diabetic ketoacidosis may follow therapeutic dosing or overdose.

Psychiatric

Psychosis has occurred following therapeutic use or overdose.

PROCEDURES AND LABORATORY TESTS

Essential Tests

Serum electrolytes, glucose, BUN, and creatinine should be assayed to detect hypokalemia and hyperglycemia; acidosis and hypoglycemia may result from prolonged agitated state.

Recommended Tests

- Serum creatine kinase should be checked to detect rhabdomyolysis in patients with marked agitation.
- ECG and cardiac monitoring should be performed to detect dysrhythmias; sinus tachycardia is common, and other tachydysrhythmias or myocardial ischemia may develop.
- Serum acetaminophen and aspirin levels should be checked in overdose setting to detect occult ingestion.
- Head CT, lumbar puncture, and cultures may be needed in patients with altered mental status of undetermined origin.

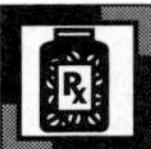

Treatment

• Treatment should focus on controlling tachycardia and agitation with the administration of benzodiazepines.
• Dose and time of exposure should be determined for all substances involved.

DIRECTING PATIENT COURSE

The health-care professional should call the poison control center when:

• Severe tachycardia, seizure, severe hypokalemia, or other severe effects develop.
• Toxic effects are not consistent with β_2-receptor agonist poisoning.
• Coingestant, drug interaction, or underlying disease presents an unusual problem.

The patient should be referred to a health-care facility when:

• Attempted suicide or homicide is possible.
• Patient or caregiver seems unreliable.
• Any toxic effects develop.
• Coingestant, drug interaction, or underlying disease presents an unusual problem.

Admission Considerations

Inpatient management is warranted if patient exhibits persistent tachycardia, agitation, or serious toxicity (hemodynamic instability, myocardial ischemia, or seizure).

DECONTAMINATION

Out of Hospital

Ipecac-induced emesis is not recommended.

In Hospital

• Gastric lavage should be performed in pediatric (tube size 24–32 French) or adult (tube size 36–42 French) patients for large ingestion presenting within 1 hour of ingestion or if serious effects are present. A smaller nasogastric tube may be used if a liquid preparation was ingested.
• One dose of activated charcoal (1–2 g/kg) should be administered without a cathartic if a substantial ingestion has occurred within the previous few hours.
• Whole-bowel irrigation may be used for a large ingestion involving a sustained-release preparation.

ANTIDOTES

There is no specific antidote for β_2-receptor agonist poisoning.

ADJUNCTIVE TREATMENT

• Multiple-dose activated charcoal. Multiple-dose activated charcoal increases clearance of β_2-agonists; following a large ingestion or in patients who have serious signs or symptoms, one to two extra doses of activated charcoal (0.5–1 g/kg) are indicated at 2- to 4-hour intervals are recommended.
• Persistent vomiting

—Suggested antiemetic adult regimens include metoclopramide 0.5 to 1.0 mg/kg plus diphenhydramine 25 to 50 mg, combined with prochlorperazine 10.0 mg or droperidol 2.5 mg intravenously.
—Ondansetron 8 mg intravenously infused over 15 minutes is an alternative.

• Seizure. A benzodiazepine with which the provider has experience should be administered.

—Diazepam. Adult dose is 5 to 10 mg intravenously; pediatric dose is 0.2 to 0.5 mg/kg intravenously; doses may be repeated at 10-minute intervals and titrated to effect.
—Lorazepam. Adult dose is 2 to 4 mg intravenously; pediatric dose is 0.05 mg/kg intravenously; doses may be repeated at 10-minute intervals and titrated to effect.
—Airway should be monitored closely.

• Hypertension. If hypertension does not respond to initial therapy or if end-organ damage develops (e.g., aortic dissection, CNS bleed, or myocardial infarction), a short-acting titratable agent such as nitroprusside should be administered.
• Tachydysrhythmia

—If extreme tachydysrhythmia, hypotension, or myocardial ischemia develops, esmolol should be administered in an intravenous bolus of 500 μg/kg infused over 1 minute, followed by an infusion of 50 μg/kg/min for 4 minutes.
—The loading dose may be repeated, followed by infusion at 100 μg/kg/min for 4 minutes.
—This titration may be repeated as needed until the heart rate is controlled or toxicity (hypotension) develops.

• Unopposed β-receptor stimulation is of theoretical concern during β-blockade; if heart rate or blood pressure increases dangerously during infusion, β-receptor stimulation may be the cause and should be discontinued.
• Hypotension

—The patient should receive 10 to 20 ml/kg 0.9% saline intravenously and be placed in the Trendelenburg position.
—Further fluid therapy should be guided by central pressure monitoring to avoid volume overload.
—A vasopressor may be added if needed. Dopamine is preferred and norepinephrine is added for refractory hypotension.

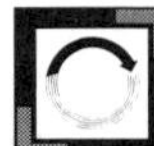

Follow-Up

PATIENT MONITORING

Symptomatic patients require continuous respiratory and cardiac monitoring until signs and symptoms of toxicity resolve.

EXPECTED COURSE AND PROGNOSIS

• Mild to moderate toxicity usually resolves over 4 to 6 hours.
• Severe toxicity may resolve within 24 hours unless a complication develops.
• Possible complications include tachycardia with rate-related myocardial ischemia and congestive heart failure, hypotension, hypertension, dysrhythmias, hypokalemia, and seizures.

DISCHARGE CRITERIA/INSTRUCTIONS

• From the emergency department. Asymptomatic patients can be discharged shortly after an inhalational exposure or 4 hours after ingestion; following gastrointestinal decontamination and psychiatric evaluation, if needed.
• From the hospital. Patient may be discharged when signs of toxicity have resolved and psychiatric evaluation, if needed.

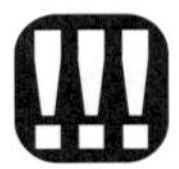

Pitfalls

TREATMENT

• Failing to administer sufficient benzodiazepine doses to effectively treat agitation and tachycardia may allow complications to develop.
• Failing to treat hypokalemia may facilitate dysrhythmia development.

ICD-9-CM 971

Poisoning by drugs primarily affecting the autonomic nervous system.

See also: SECTION II, Hypertension, Hypotension, Seizure, and Tachydysrhythmia (Unexplained) chapters; and SECTION III, Activated Charcoal, Nitroprusside, and Whole-Bowel Irrigation chapters.

RECOMMENDED READING

Katz VL, Seeds JW. Fetal and neonatal cardiovascular complications from β-sympathomimetic therapy for tocolysis. *Am J Obstet Gynecol* 1989;161:1–4.

Spitzer WO, Suissa S, Ernst P, et al. The use of β-agonists and the risk of death and near death from asthma. *N Engl J Med* 1992;326:501–506.

Author: Edwin K. Kuffner

Reviewer: Katherine M. Hurlbut

Bismuth

Basics

DESCRIPTION

Bismuth substances include bismuth subsalicylate (the primary form available in commercial products) as well as bismuth subcarbonate, bismuth oxycarbonate, bismuth subgallate, bismuth subnitrate, bismuth subchloride, bismuth triglycollamate, and bismuth sulfide.

FORMS AND USES

- Pharmaceutical preparations containing bismuth subsalicylate include Pepto-Bismol, Corrective Mixture, Infantol Pink, Pabizol with paregoric, and Pept-Aid Soothe.
- Bismuth subsalicylate is used as antibacterial against *Helicobacter pylori,* as a treatment for dyspepsia and diarrhea, and as a topical application for skin lesions.
- Typical dosages

—Bismuth subcitrate. 240 mg twice daily or 120 mg four times daily for 4 to 8 weeks (ulcer therapy).
—Bismuth subgallate. 0.6 to 2 g for gastrointestinal disturbances.
—Bismuth subsalicylate. 500 mg up to total 4 g/day for diarrhea therapy.

TOXIC DOSE

Toxicity from a single ingestion is unusual. It commonly develops from chronic exposure, particularly injections of bismuth.

PATHOPHYSIOLOGY

- Most medicinal bismuth products contain insoluble trivalent salts.
- Classification of bismuth compounds

—Group 1. Water-insoluble compounds, minimally absorbed, nontoxic (e.g., bismuth subcarbonate, bismuth subnitrate, bismuth subsalicylate).
—Group 2. Lipophilic compounds can produce hepatotoxicity and neurotoxicity (e.g., bismuth subgallate).
—Group 3. Absorbed and can lead to renal damage; includes water-soluble organic compounds (e.g., bismuth triglycollamate).
—Group 4. Minimal absorption, nontoxic, water-soluble compounds that hydrolyze to produce insoluble bismuth compounds (e.g., bismuth subchloride, bismuth sulfide).

- Excretion. Insoluble forms of bismuth are retained in the kidneys, bones, and gastric wall; slow elimination occurs by the kidneys. Soluble forms are quickly eliminated in urine and saliva.

EPIDEMIOLOGY

- Poisoning is uncommon.
- Toxic effects following exposure are typically mild, with death rarely occurring.

CAUSES

- Most common cause of poisoning is therapeutic misadventure.
- Child neglect or abuse should be considered if the patient is less than 1 year of age, suicide attempt if the patient is over 6 years of age.

RISK FACTORS

- Absorption of oral preparations increases in settings of altered intestinal mucosal integrity (e.g., Crohn's disease).
- Renal toxicity has occurred most frequently in patients with immature kidneys (particularly in children less than 3 years of age).

PREGNANCY AND LACTATION

- Bismuth subsalicylate. US FDA Pregnancy Category C. The drug exerts animal teratogenic or embryocidal effects, but there are no controlled studies in women, or no studies are available in either animals or women.
- Insoluble bismuth salts accumulate in the placenta; however, children born of mothers with bismuth encephalopathy appear normal at birth.

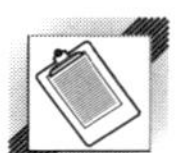

Diagnosis

DIFFERENTIAL DIAGNOSIS

Nontoxicologic causes of salivation, bluish discoloration of gums, loss of teeth, ulcerative stomatitis, and encephalopathy may include lead poisoning and mercury poisoning.

SIGNS AND SYMPTOMS

- Large or repeated exposures may produce increased salivation as an early effect, followed by encephalopathy and renal injury.

HEENT

Increased salivation, pyorrhea and ulcerative stomatitis may develop. A bluish line develops along gums due to bismuth deposition in fibrous tissues.

Dermatologic

A maculopapular rash ("erythema of the ninth day") may occur.

Cardiovascular

Myocardial injury has been reported after chronic exposure, although it rarely occurs.

Gastrointestinal

Nausea, vomiting, and diarrhea may occur in acute or chronic exposure.

Hepatic

Jaundice and fatty changes may develop in the liver with chronic exposure.

Renal

Proteinuria and microscopic hematuria occur early in the course of chronic exposure, whereas Fanconi syndrome, renal failure, and anuria may occur later.

Hematologic

Intestinal bacteria may reduce bismuth subnitrate to nitrate, which can cause methemoglobinemia and nitrate poisoning.

Musculoskeletal

Osteoarthropathy, osteoporosis, and osteomalacia may develop.

Neurologic

- Anorexia, headaches, malaise, confusion, tremors, and encephalopathy may occur.
- Encephalopathy may develop with chronic ingestion, starting with prodrome of malaise and lasting from weeks to months.
- Rapid deterioration may occur over 24 to 48 hours, including signs of confusion, dysarthria, gait disturbance, pseudotremor, and myoclonic jerks.

PROCEDURES AND LABORATORY TESTS

Essential Tests

- Results of liver function tests will be elevated if there is liver injury.
- Serum electrolytes, BUN, and creatinine levels are used to assess kidney injury.

Recommended Tests

- Salicylate levels are measured to check for salicylate toxicity.
- Bismuth levels are available from reference laboratories. Serum or blood bismuth levels less than 5 μg/dl are rarely toxic. However, levels do not correlate well with toxicity.

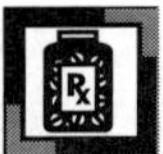

Treatment

- Treatment should be focused on termination of bismuth exposure.
- Treatment is primarily supportive once bismuth has been absorbed and deposited in the bones and other organs.
- Dose and time of exposure should be determined for all substances involved.

DIRECTING PATIENT COURSE

The health-care professional should call the poison control center when:

- Severe or persistent effects develop.
- Toxic effects are not consistent with bismuth poisoning.
- Coingestant, drug interaction, or underlying disease presents an unusual problem.

The patient should be referred to a health-care facility when:

- Attempted suicide or homicide is possible.
- Patient or caregiver seems unreliable.
- Toxic effects develop.
- Coingestant, drug interaction, or underlying disease presents an unusual problem.

Admission Considerations

Inpatient management is warranted if the patient exhibits altered mental status, renal dysfunction, or clinically significant effects.

DECONTAMINATION

Out of Hospital

Ipecac should be administered to induce emesis within 1 hour of an acute ingestion for the alert pediatric or adult patient if health-care evaluation will be delayed.

In Hospital

- Ipecac should be administered to induce emesis within 1 hour of acute ingestion for the alert patient who is too small to have effective gastric lavage.
- Gastric lavage should be performed in pediatric (tube size 24–32 French) or adult (tube size 36–42 French) patients presenting within 1 hour of a large ingestion.
- One dose of activated charcoal (1–2 g/kg) should be administered without a cathartic if a substantial ingestion has occurred within the previous few hours.

ANTIDOTES

d-*Penicillamine*

- Adult dose

—15 to 40 mg/kg/day orally, maximum 250 to 500 mg four times daily

- Pediatric dose

—20 to 30 mg/kg/day, once or twice daily

Dimercaprol

The dose for adult or pediatric patients is 3 mg/kg within 8 to 12 hours of bismuth ingestion.

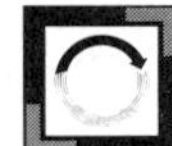

Follow-Up

PATIENT MONITORING

Specific monitoring is not necessary in uncomplicated cases.

EXPECTED COURSE AND PROGNOSIS

- Recovery is expected if encephalopathy and renal failure do not develop.
- Encephalopathy may take several weeks to resolve or may not improve.

DISCHARGE CRITERIA/INSTRUCTIONS

- From the emergency department. Patients may be discharged when clinical effects have stabilized and decontamination has been completed, and after psychiatric evaluation, if needed.
- From the hospital. Patients may be discharged after toxic effects resolve or stabilize and after psychiatric evaluation, if needed.

PATIENT EDUCATION

Use of bismuth subsalicylate preparations should be avoided in children under 16 years of age due to salicylate component.

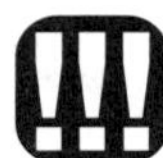

Pitfalls

DIAGNOSIS

Failure to consider bismuth exposure

FOLLOW-UP

- Bismuth subsalicylate-containing compounds can increase the risk of Reye syndrome in children due to salicylate.
- Avoid use of bismuth subsalicylate-containing compounds if using oral anticoagulants, probenecid, methotrexate, or other forms of salicylate.

ICD-9-CM 985.8

Toxic effects of specified metals (bismuth).

See also: SECTION II, British Anti-Lewisite and d-penicillamine chapters.

RECOMMENDED READINGS

Gryboski JD, Gotoff SP. Bismuth nephrotoxicity. *N Engl J Med* 1961;265:1289–1291.

Mendelowitz PC, Hoffman RS, Weber S. Bismuth absorption and myoclonic encephalopathy during bismuth subsalicylate therapy. *Ann Intern Med* 1990;112:140–141.

Pickering LK, Feldman S, Ericsson CD, Cleary TG. Absorption of salicylate and bismuth from bismuth subsalicylate-containing compound (Pepto-Bismol). *J Pediatr* 1981;99:654–656.

Author: Kathleen Graham

Reviewer: Luke Yip

Black Widow Spider

Basics

DESCRIPTION

Spiders of the genus *Latrodectus* include the following:

- *L. mactans*, the black widow, is found in the United States, South Africa, and South America.
- *L. hesperus* includes the brown widow, red widow, and other spiders, which are found in the United States.
- *L. hasseltii* is the red-back spider of Australia and New Zealand.
- *L. tredecimguttatus* is native to the Mediterranean, Eastern Europe, and Russia.
- *L. indistinctus* is the button spider of South Africa.

TOXIC DOSE

One bite is toxic.

PATHOPHYSIOLOGY

The venom acts at neuromuscular junctions to cause the release of acetylcholine and norepinephrine at postganglionic sympathetic synaptic sites. This produces uncontrolled muscle contraction.

EPIDEMIOLOGY

- Although poisoning is common, the toxic effects are typically mild to moderate; death is a rare event.
- Extremes of age and underlying cardiopulmonary disease increase the risk of death.

RISK FACTORS

Envenomation is usually an accidental incident and occurs through activities that place the victim in the spider habitat (e.g., putting hands in woodpiles and dark corners, harvesting grain by hand, or using an outhouse).

PREGNANCY AND LACTATION

Monitor pregnant patients for premature labor or spontaneous abortion; however, outcome is typically good.

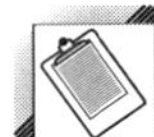

Diagnosis

DIFFERENTIAL DIAGNOSIS

Nontoxicologic causes of pain and cramping often accompanied by sweating include acute abdomen, myocardial infarction, or sickle cell crisis.

SIGNS AND SYMPTOMS

- Localized pain and cramping "migrating" from large muscle groups in the bitten extremity, to buttocks, abdomen, or chest over 30 to 120 minutes strongly suggests the diagnosis.
- Effects peak in the first few hours but may persist for days.

Vital Signs

Hypertension and tachycardia are common, but rarely require treatment.

HEENT

Although ptosis and eyelid edema may occur, these reactions are uncommon.

Dermatologic

- Diaphoresis is common.
- The bite site may show two small punctures with a small erythematous and diaphoretic area.

Cardiovascular

- Dysrhythmias and myocardial ischemia occur rarely.
- A bite to the arm or chest may produce pain that mimics myocardial ischemia.

Pulmonary

- Tachypnea and respiratory distress may develop.
- Respiratory failure has been reported but is rare.

Gastrointestinal

- Nausea and vomiting are common. Abdominal pain predominates.
- Boardlike rigidity of abdominal muscles may mimic acute abdomen.

Musculoskeletal

- Pain and spasm of large muscle groups develop within 30 minutes to 2 hours and resolve over 24 to 48 hours.
- Mild rhabdomyolysis has been reported.

Neurologic

- Weakness, hyperreflexia, headache, anxiety, and paresthesia are common and may persist for several days.
- Children may be irritable or drowsy.

Reproductive

- While there is concern that uterine muscle spasm could induce miscarriage or labor, pregnant women have had successful outcomes.
- Pregnant patients should be monitored for premature labor or spontaneous abortion.

PROCEDURES AND LABORATORY TESTS

Essential Tests

No tests may be needed in mildly symptomatic patients.

Recommended Tests

- ECG should be performed in patients with hypertension or chest pain. Effects of a bite to the arm may migrate to the chest, simulating myocardial ischemia.
- Creatine kinase is measured in patients with prolonged muscle spasm to rule out rhabdomyolysis.
- Arterial blood gas is used in patients with respiratory distress.
- Other tests may be needed to rule out acute abdomen (e.g., complete blood count, electrolytes, abdominal radiography, and computed tomography).

Treatment

Treatment should be focused on ensuring adequate ventilation and controlling muscle spasm and pain.

DIRECTING PATIENT COURSE

The health-care professional should call the poison control center when:

- Severe hypertension, myocardial ischemia, respiratory failure, intractable pain, or other severe effects are present.
- Signs and symptoms are not consistent with widow spider envenomation.
- Administration of antivenom is planned.
- Drug interaction or underlying disease presents an unusual problem.

The patient should be referred to a health-care facility when:

- The patient or caregiver seems unreliable.
- Toxic effects develop.
- Toxicity is not consistent with widow spider envenomation.
- An underlying disease presents an unusual problem.

Admission Considerations

Inpatient management is warranted in symptomatic pregnant patients or patients with persistent pain, respiratory distress, severe hypertension, or myocardial ischemia despite therapy.

ANTIDOTES

Black widow spider antivenom (*Lactrodectus mactans*) is available from Merck.

- Indications

—The primary indication is severe envenomation (marked hypertension, respiratory distress, myocardial ischemia, persistent pain despite parenteral opioids and muscle relaxants, or evidence of labor or miscarriage).
—Antivenom should be considered in patients with underlying cardiopulmonary disease.

- Contraindications include hypersensitivity to horse serum.
- Administration

—Antivenom should be administered in a monitored critical care setting, with preparation to manage the airway and treat anaphylaxis.
—The skin test involves injection of 0.02 ml of test solution (included with the antivenom) intradermally and observation for a wheal-and-flare reaction. A negative skin test does not rule out the possibility of a hypersensitivity reaction to antivenom.
—Antivenom is administered as one vial diluted in 50 to 100 ml of 0.9% saline administered intravenously over 20 to 30 minutes. Alternatively, one vial may be injected intramuscularly as described in the package insert.

- Adverse effects

—Acute allergic reactions, including anaphylaxis, may develop.
—Serum sickness (e.g., fever, rash, and myalgia) may occasionally develop 5 to 14 days after administration.

ADJUNCTIVE TREATMENT

The aggressive use of parenteral opioids and muscle relaxants provides the most effective pain relief short of antivenom. Frequent small bolus doses should be administered while monitoring respiratory and cardiac function.

Analgesics

- Morphine sulfate. Adult dose is 2 to 5 mg intravenously every 15 to 60 minutes as needed; pediatric dose is 0.05 mg/kg to 0.1 mg/kg up to 5 mg every 15 to 60 minutes intravenously as needed.
- Meperidine. Adult dose is 25 to 50 mg intravenously every 30 minutes to 4 hours as needed to a maximum dose of 300 mg. Pediatric dose is 1 to 2 mg/kg up to 50 mg intravenously or intramuscularly every 30 minutes to 4 hours.

Muscle Relaxants

- Diazepam. Adult dose is 2 to 10 mg intravenously every 1 to 4 hours. Pediatric dose is 0.04 to 0.3 mg/kg up to 10 mg intravenously every 1 to 4 hours as needed.
- Methocarbamol. Adult dose is 15 mg/kg intravenously over 5 minutes, followed by 15 mg/kg infusion over 4 hours. Pediatric dose is 15 mg/kg intravenously over 5 minutes every 6 hours.

Calcium Gluconate

- Calcium gluconate is used to relieve pain, although results are inconsistent. It is not as effective as opioids and muscle relaxants. Relapse of pain and cramping is common.
- Adult dose is 10 ml of 10% solution intravenously over 10 to 20 minutes, which may be repeated every 3 to 4 hours; pediatric dose is 50 mg/kg, up to 500 mg/kg/day.

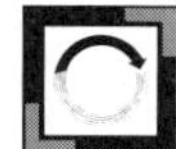

Follow-Up

PATIENT MONITORING

- Respiratory and cardiac function should be monitored continuously during acute episode and during treatment.
- Patients who receive antivenom may develop serum sickness (e.g., fever, rash, and arthralgia) 5 to 14 days later.

EXPECTED COURSE AND PROGNOSIS

- Toxic effects typically peak within hours and then improve over several days.
- Muscle pain, malaise, and weakness may persist for several days to weeks.
- No permanent sequelae are expected.

DISCHARGE CRITERIA/INSTRUCTIONS

- From the emergency department

—The patient may be discharged after 4 to 6 hours if pain control is achieved and severe complications do not develop.
—The patient should be discharged with an oral narcotic analgesic and muscle relaxant.

- From the hospital. The patient may be discharged when pain resolves.

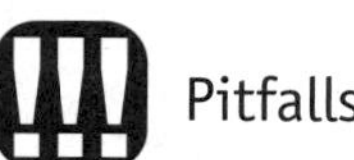

Pitfalls

DIAGNOSIS

- Widow spider bite may be confused with acute abdomen, particularly in young children and patients unaware of being bitten.
- Drug-seeking behavior should be considered in patients with recurrent presentations of widow spider bite.
- Widow spider bite of the upper extremity may mimic myocardial ischemia.

TREATMENT

- Aggressive use of parenteral narcotics and muscle relaxants may be needed for adequate pain control.
- *Latrodectus* antivenom should be considered in patients with persistent pain despite aggressive therapy.

ICD-9-CM 989.5

Toxic effect of venom.

See also: SECTION III, Black Widow Spider Antivenom chapter.

RECOMMENDED READING

Clark RF, Wethern-Kestner S, Vance MV, et al. Clinical presentation and treatment of black widow spider envenomation: a review of 163 cases. *Ann Emerg Med* 1992;21:782–787.

Moss HS, Binder LS. A retrospective review of black widow spider envenomation. *Ann Emerg Med* 1987;16:188–191.

Timms PK, Gibbons RB. Latrodectism—effects of the black widow spider bite. *West J Med* 1986;144:315–317.

Author: Katherine M. Hurlbut

Reviewer: Rivka S. Horowitz

Boric Acid and Borates

Basics

DESCRIPTION

- Boron is a natural component of many foods.
- Compounds containing boron are termed borates.
- Boric acid is colorless and odorless.

FORMS AND USES

- Boric acid is available as crystals, granules, and white powder.
- Borax is sodium borate and is widely used as a cleaning agent.
- Occupational sources include the manufacturing of glass, fire resistant materials, glazes, enamels, paints, paperboard, wood preservatives, cleaning compounds, insecticides, and herbicides.
- Household sources include medicated powders, topical astringents, antiseptic lotions, and insecticide for ants and roaches.
- In the past, it was also used as a topical home remedy for diaper rash and as an oral home remedy combined with honey for mucous membrane irritation in children.

TOXIC DOSE

- Boric acid ingestion of a few grams (1 teaspoon of 100% boric acid powder or granules) may be lethal in small children.
- Much larger doses are required in adults.

PATHOPHYSIOLOGY

- Dermal exposure is the most common route, but oral exposure results in greater toxicity.
- Severe toxicity in infants typically involves repeated exposure.
- The mechanism of toxicity is unknown.

EPIDEMIOLOGY

Death has occurred in some instances when boric acid was administered to infants orally as a home remedy.

WORKPLACE STANDARDS

- Sodium tetraborate anhydrous

—ACGIH. TLV TWA is 1 mg/m^3.
—OSHA. PEL TWA is 10 mg/m^3.

- Sodium tetraborate decahydrate

—ACGIH. TLV TWA is 5 mg/m^3.
—OSHA. PEL TWA is 10 mg/m^3.

- Sodium tetraborate pentahydrate

—ACGIH. TLV TWA is 1 mg/m^3.
—OSHA. PEL TWA is 10 mg/m^3.

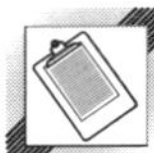

Diagnosis

DIFFERENT DIAGNOSIS

Other causes of nausea, vomiting, and diarrhea in combination with a skin rash primarily include infectious diseases.

SIGNS AND SYMPTOMS

Vital Signs

- Signs of dehydration are common.
- Fever is rare.

HEENT

- Mucous membrane involvement is common.
- Alopecia occurs rarely.

Dermatologic

- Localized erythema often progresses to diffuse erythema and then to generalized exfoliation.
- Exfoliation can be full thickness and indistinguishable from toxic epidermal necrolysis

Gastrointestinal

- Persistent nausea, vomiting, and diarrhea are very common.
- Vomitus and diarrhea may be bluish-green in color.
- Hematemesis and hematochezia are common.

Renal

Renal insufficiency with oliguria is common and may progress to anuric renal failure.

Fluids and Electrolytes

Dehydration with associated hypernatremia, hyperchloremia, and metabolic acidosis is common.

Neurologic

- Irritability, headache, abnormal movements, personality changes, and altered mental status are common.
- Symptoms may progress to seizures and coma.

PROCEDURES AND LABORATORY TESTS

Essential Tests

No test may be needed in asymptomatic patients.

Recommended Tests

- Serum electrolytes, BUN, and creatinine are used to assess severity and to guide supportive therapy.
- The normal serum boron concentration is less than 0.8 mg/dl. Elevated levels can confirm exposure, but do not correlate well with toxicity.
- ECG, serum acetaminophen and aspirin levels are used in overdose setting to detect occult ingestion.
- Head CT, lumbar puncture, and cultures should be performed as needed to evaluate altered mental status.

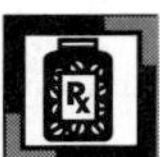

Treatment

Treatment should focus on general supportive care and correction of electrolyte abnormalities.

DECONTAMINATION

Out of Hospital

- Dermal

—If solid form, the crystals, granules, or powder are removed with a dry towel and the area is then irrigated copiously with water.
—If a solution containing boric acid is involved, irrigate the area copiously with water.

- Gastrointestinal

—Ipecac should be administered to induce emesis within 1 hour of ingestion for the alert pediatric or adult patient if health-care evaluation will be delayed.
—If vomiting has already occurred for an adult or pediatric patient, no further decontamination may be necessary.

In Hospital

- Dermal

—If solid form, the crystals, granules, or powder are removed with a dry towel and the area is then irrigated copiously with water.
—If a solution containing boric acid is involved, irrigate the area copiously with water.

- Gastrointestinal

—Ipecac should be administered to induce emesis within 1 hour of ingestion for the alert patient who is too small to have effective gastric lavage. If vomiting has already occurred, no further decontamination may be necessary.
—Gastric lavage should be performed in pediatric (tube size 24–32 French) or adult (tube size 36–42 French) patients for large ingestion presenting within 1 hour of ingestion or if serious effects are present.
—Activated charcoal is not recommended because it does not bind well with boric acid.

ANTIDOTES

There is no specific antidote to boric acid poisoning.

ADJUNCTIVE TREATMENT

- Urine output should be maintained at 1 to 2 ml/kg/h using isotonic intravenous fluid.
- Case reports suggest that hemodialysis, peritoneal dialysis, or exchange transfusion can remove borates and improve outcome.
- Sterile dressings should be applied to skin wounds.

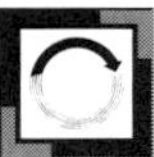

Follow-Up

PATIENT MONITORING

Fluid and electrolyte status, including renal function, should be monitored.

EXPECTED COURSE AND PROGNOSIS

- Following acute ingestion, toxicity may be delayed several hours; peak toxicity occurs in 1 to 2 days.
- Following chronic ingestion, recovery is slower and more likely incomplete.

ICD-9-CM 989

Toxic effect of other substances, chiefly nonmedicinal as to source.

RECOMMENDED READING

Baker MD, Bogeina SG. Ingestion of boric acid by infants. *Am J Emerg Med* 1986;4:358–361.

Author: Edwin K. Kuffner

Reviewer: Richard C. Dart

Botulism

Basics

DESCRIPTION

Botulism is a disease caused by botulinum toxin, which produces life-threatening muscle paralysis.

FORMS AND USES

- Pharmaceutical products. Purified botulinum toxin (BoTox, Oculinum) is used in the treatment of strabismus, blepharospasm, spasmodic dysphonia, hemifacial spasm, specific dystonia, and other movement disorders.
- Naturally occurring. *Clostridium botulinum* is a spore-forming, anaerobic, gram-positive bacillus. The spores contain one of eight strains of a potent neurotoxin A, B, C_{alpha}, C_{beta}, D, E, F, and G.

TOXIC DOSE

The toxin is extremely potent, with 0.05 μg (a taste of contaminated food) potentially fatal.

PATHOPHYSIOLOGY

- Botulism is caused by botulinum toxin, a neurotoxin produced by *C. botulinum*.
- The neurotoxin binds to presynaptic parasympathetic and sympathetic nerve terminals and to presynaptic motor nerve terminals at the end-plate, inhibiting the release of acetylcholine into the myoneurol synapse and thereby blocking muscle contraction.
- Spores germinate in an anaerobic environment with a pH greater than 4.6.
- There are four types of human botulism:

—Food-borne botulism, in which the toxin is formed before consumption. Common sources include home canned foods, fish without evisceration, and occasionally improperly prepared commercial products.
—Infant botulism, in which the toxin is produced by the organism in the immature gastrointestinal tract. Honey may contain botulinum spores and be the source of toxin.
—Infant-type botulism may occasionally occur in adults.
—Wound botulism in which traumatic wounds, often contaminated with soil, are the source.

- Eight serotypes of toxin are produced, with seven (A, B, C_{alpha}, C_{beta}, E, F, and G) reported to produce illness in humans.

EPIDEMIOLOGY

- The food-borne type often affects more than one victim, but rarely large numbers of victims.
- Toxic effects following exposure are typically moderate to severe.
- Death occurs, primarily in patients who do not receive adequate airway management.
- Children less than 6 months of age may develop infant botulism, in which the organism elaborates its toxin in the gastrointestinal tract.

CAUSES

- Food-borne botulism is caused by improper canning, processing, or storage of food, allowing spores to remain, germinate, and form toxin.
- Infant botulism has been associated with honey in the diet.

RISK FACTORS

- Adults with recent antibiotic use, achlorhydria, or prior intestinal surgery may be at risk for the adult form of infant-type botulism.
- Intravenous drug abuse is a risk factor for wound botulism.

DRUG AND DISEASE INTERACTIONS

Toxic effects are enhanced by drugs that cause neuromuscular blockade.

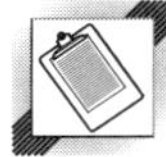

Diagnosis

A definite diagnosis of botulism is made when descending paralysis and at least one of the following are present:

- *C. botulinum* in culture
- Botulinum toxin in serum, stool, or implicated food source
- A compatible clinical illness in a person who is associated with a confirmed case

DIFFERENTIAL DIAGNOSIS

- Toxicologic causes of nausea, vomiting, and descending paralysis (which is initially subtle) include *Amanita muscaria* mushrooms, bacterial food poisoning, carbon monoxide, clostridium tetanus, diphtheria, organophosphate poisoning, paralytic shellfish poisoning, and tick paralysis, among others.
- Nontoxicologic causes of nausea, vomiting, and paralysis include Guillain-Barré syndrome, CNS vascular disease, dystonic reaction, Eaton-Lambert syndrome, myasthenia gravis, polio, postanesthetic paralysis, and primary muscular disorder, among others.

SIGNS AND SYMPTOMS

According to Type of Botulism

- Food-borne

—After the initial gastrointestinal symptoms of food poisoning, an incubation period of 18 to 36 hours (ranging from a few hours to several days) may occur.
—Early signs include dry mouth, difficulty in swallowing, and bulbar muscle weakness (e.g., blurred vision).
—Over several hours to days, descending extremity weakness develops and produces respiratory failure and death, if untreated.

- Infant

—Persistent hypotonia, constipation, tachycardia, difficulty in feeding, and a decreased gag reflex develop.
—Infant botulism most frequently occurs before 1 year of age.

- Wound

—Symptoms are similar to those of food-borne botulism except for a lack of gastrointestinal symptoms.
—It most commonly occurs in intravenous drug abusers and in patients with surgical wounds after an incubation period of 4 to 14 days.
—Examination of the wound is not diagnostic.

Vital signs

Tachypnea due to decreasing tidal volume may develop.

HEENT

- Bulbar muscle palsy and involvement of cranial nerves, especially abducens (VI) and oculomotor (III) nerves may occur.
- Fixed mydriasis may occur.

Cardiovascular

Cardiac arrest has occurred in patients on mechanical ventilation.

Pulmonary

- Respiratory muscle weakness and hypercarbia are late findings.
- Aspiration is common.

Gastrointestinal

Initial gastrointestinal distress, with nausea, vomiting, distention, and pain, are common but often not recognized as prodrome.

Neurologic

- Cranial nerve palsies and descending symmetric paralysis with intact mentation may occur.
- Deep tendon reflexes are diminished late.

PROCEDURES AND LABORATORY TESTS

Essential Tests

For patients with known exposure or in whom botulism is suspected clinically:

- Serum, stool, vomitus, gastric contents, wound, and suspect foods should be obtained for culture and toxin analysis. Antitoxin administration must not wait for confirmatory laboratory tests in symptomatic patients.
- Other tests should be performed as needed to evaluate for infectious or toxic causes.

Recommended Tests

- Serial assessment with pulse oximetry, arterial blood gases, and pulmonary function to monitor respiratory effects.
- Negative inspiratory force of less than 30% indicates the need for intubation.
- Electromyogram showing that repetitive nerve stimulation produces an incremental increase of small, compound muscle action potentials is diagnostic.
- A test using edrophonium chloride (Tensilon) may show mild improvement, but it is much less dramatic than with myasthenia gravis.

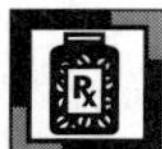

Treatment

- Treatment should focus on airway management and supportive care.
- Endotracheal intubation should be performed when the negative inspiratory force is less than 30% or any signs of respiratory failure or pulmonary aspiration develop.
- In food-borne cases, the dose and time of exposure for all possible exposures should be determined.
- The state health department should be notified immediately, and contact made with the Centers for Disease Control and Prevention (CDC).

DIRECTING PATIENT COURSE

The health-care professional should call the poison control center when:

- Botulism is suspected.
- Coingestant, drug interaction, or underlying disease presents an unusual problem.

Patients should be referred to a health-care facility when:

- Exposure to botulism is suspected.
- Diagnosis of botulism is entertained.

Admission Considerations

Inpatient treatment is warranted when botulism is suspected based on history or clinical signs.

DECONTAMINATION

- Gastric lavage should be performed in pediatric (tube size 24–32 French) or adult (tube size 36–42 French) patients who have ingested substantial quantities of food suspected to be contaminated and who present within 1 hour of ingestion or if their condition is serious.
- One dose of activated charcoal (1–2 g/kg) should be administered without a cathartic if a substantial ingestion has occurred within the previous few hours.
- Magnesium-containing cathartics should be avoided because they may depress neuromuscular conduction.
- Whole-bowel irrigation has been proposed by some to enhance elimination of the toxin in the gastrointestinal tract.

ANTIDOTES

- Antitoxins (mono-, bi-, or trivalent)

—Antitoxin is obtained by first calling CDC contact at your state health department.
—Antitoxins are available from the CDC: (404)639-3753 days, (404)639-2888 nights, weekends, and holidays.
—A specific antidote is available as a monovalent, bivalent (AB), and trivalent (ABE) antitoxin from the CDC.
—Trivalent is preferred if the specific type is unknown.

- Indications

—Food-borne botulism, confirmed or strongly suspected
—Wound botulism

- Contraindications. Known hypersensitivity to horse serum or to previous administration of antitoxin is a relative contraindication.
- Method of administration

—The initial dose is two vials administered intravenously.
—The dose should be repeated every 12 to 24 hours if condition worsens.

- Adverse effects

—Anaphylactic reaction to antitoxin occurs in approximately 2% of cases.
—The overall rate of adverse reactions is up to 17%.
—The likelihood of serum sickness in patients treated with antitoxin is 5% to 10%.

- Human botulism immune globulin

—This investigational drug is pentavalent (A, B, C, D, and E).
—It may be useful in infant botulism.

ADJUNCTIVE TREATMENT

- Food-borne botulism

—Treatment should be focused on initial decontamination and monitoring of respiratory function.
—Airway should be controlled and antitoxin administered.

- Infant botulism

—Respiratory and nutritional support should be administered.
—Antitoxin has not been proven to improve outcome.
—Human botulism immune globulin may be useful.
—The role of antibiotics has not been clearly demonstrated.

- Wound botulism

—Surgical debridement and respiratory support are primary.
—Antitoxin efficacy is not well established.
—The effectiveness of antibiotics is undecided.

- Not recommended therapies. Anticholinesterases such as edrophonium are not useful except as diagnostic agents.

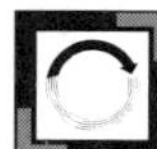

Follow-Up

EXPECTED COURSE AND PROGNOSIS

- If the patient is diagnosed early and treated with antitoxin and respiratory support, recovery over several months to a year is expected.
- Respiratory failure, when it occurs, usually develops within 12 hours of the onset of oculomotor (III) paralysis.
- Long-term neurologic symptoms of dysgeusia, exertional dyspnea, and easy fatigability occur rarely.
- Sequelae of hypoxia may develop in patients who present late or in whom airway is not controlled appropriately.

DISCHARGE CRITERIA/INSTRUCTIONS

- From the emergency department. All patients with suspected botulism should be admitted to the hospital.
- From the hospital. Patients with improving respiratory function may be discharged when their condition can be managed by a subacute care hospital.

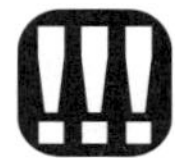

Pitfalls

DIAGNOSIS

- Diagnosis is often missed on initial presentation because of nonspecific initial gastrointestinal symptoms and the rarity of the disease.
- Impending respiratory failure may fail to be recognized.

TREATMENT

Early intubation and respiratory support are critical because the patient may die from complications of inadequate management.

FOLLOW-UP

Epidemiologic evaluation of source may fail to be performed.

ICD-9-CM 005.1

Other food poisoning (bacterial): botulism.

See also: SECTION III, Botulinum Antitoxin chapter.

RECOMMENDED READING

Davis LE. Botulinum toxin. From poison to medicine. *West J Med* 1993;158:25–29.

Hambleton P. *Clostridium botulinum* toxins. *J Neurol* 1992;239:16–20.

Hathaway CL. Botulism: the present status of the disease. *Curr Top Microbiol Immunol* 1995;195:55–57.

Author: Steven A. Seifert

Reviewer: Luke Yip

Brodifacoum and Long-Acting Anticoagulants

Basics

DESCRIPTION

Long-acting anticoagulants (super-warfarins) are warfarin derivatives used as rodenticides.

FORMS AND USES

This chapter discusses brodifacoum (Bromione, d-Con Mouse Prufe II, Havoc, Talon, Talon-G), difenacoum (Ratak), bromadiolone (Super-caid, Maki), chlorophacinone (Caid, Liphadione), diphacinone (Diphacin, Promar, Ramik), flocoumafen, pindone (Pival, Pivacin, Pivalyn, Tri-Ban), valone, and coumatetralyl.

TOXIC DOSE

- Mouthful amounts of rat bait have produced mild prothrombin time (PT) prolongation in children.
- Doses of 1 to 2 mg of brodifacoum may cause anticoagulation in adults.

PATHOPHYSIOLOGY

- Super-warfarins produce vitamin K deficiency by inhibiting the regeneration of active vitamin K, thereby inhibiting the formation of clotting factors II, VII, IX, and X.
- Anticoagulation is delayed until existing vitamin K stores are depleted.
- Half-lives of super-warfarins are long; a single ingestion may cause coagulopathy, which can last weeks to months.

EPIDEMIOLOGY

- Poisoning is common.
- Toxic effects following exposure occur rarely and are typically mild.
- Death is rare, usually due to hemorrhagic complications (especially intracranial) in adults with deliberate ingestion.

CAUSES

- Most cases involve accidental ingestion by children.
- Child neglect or abuse should be considered if the patient is less than 1 year of age, a suicide attempt if the patient is over 6 years of age.

DRUG AND DISEASE INTERACTIONS

Allopurinol, anabolic steroids, cephalosporins, chloral hydrate, cimetidine, clofibrate, cyclic antidepressants, erythromycin, ethanol, nonsteroidal antiinflammatory drugs, sulfonylureas, and thyroxine may potentiate anticoagulant effect.

PREGNANCY AND LACTATION

- Fetal intraventricular hemorrhage has been reported.
- Teratogenicity has been reported with other oral anticoagulants, such as coumadin.

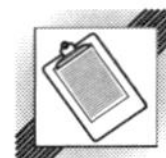

Diagnosis

DIFFERENTIAL DIAGNOSIS

- Toxicologic causes of anticoagulation include heparin, coumadin, and crotalid snake envenomation as well as hepatic failure from any cause (e.g., acetaminophen, *Amanita* species mushrooms).
- Nontoxicologic causes include hemophilia, vitamin K deficiency, or any cause of disseminated intravascular coagulation (sepsis or shock).

SIGNS AND SYMPTOMS

Accidental pediatric exposures usually cause minimal or no anticoagulation. However, intentional overdose may cause severe coagulopathy that may last weeks to months, often with bleeding (most common sites are gastrointestinal and genitourinary tracts).

Vital Signs

Hypotension and tachycardia may occur as a result of hemorrhage.

HEENT

Epistaxis or gingival bleeding may develop.

Dermatologic

Ecchymosis, hematoma, and occasionally necrosis (purple toe syndrome) may develop.

Cardiovascular

Pericardial tamponade may develop rarely.

Pulmonary

Hemothorax, hemoptysis, and alveolar hemorrhage are rare effects.

Gastrointestinal

- Hematemesis, hematochezia, or melena may occur.
- Gastroinestinal or retroperitoneal bleeding have been reported in adults with severe coagulopathy.

Renal

Hematuria may develop.

Hematologic

- PT, partial thromboplastin time (PTT), and international normalized ratio (INR) become prolonged.
- Platelet count and fibrinogen level remain unaffected, but fibrin split products may be elevated.

Musculoskeletal

Muscle hematoma, compartment syndrome, or hemarthroma develop rarely.

Neurologic

Intracranial hemorrhage is uncommon but is the most common cause of death.

Endocrine

Adrenal hemorrhage and insufficiency may occur rarely.

Genitourinary

Excessive vaginal bleeding and hematuria have been reported.

PROCEDURES AND LABORATORY TESTS

Essential Tests

- After accidental overdose, INR or PT should be measured in 24 to 48 hours.
- After deliberate ingestion, INR or PT levels should be obtained immediately and followed every 24 hours for 48 hours.
- Elevated INR or PT suggests significant exposure.

Recommended Tests

- PTT, fibrinogen, fibrin degradation products, complete blood count, platelets, guaic of stool, and type and crossmatch blood are ordered for patients with clinically significant prolongation of INR/PT.

—Thrombocytopenia or depressed fibrinogen suggests coagulopathy from another etiology.
—Anemia or guaiac-positive stool suggests significant toxicity.

- Levels of specific clotting factors are used to distinguish between an anticoagulant ingestion with liver dysfunction and a primary hematologic disorder.
- Serum levels of long-acting anticoagulants (from reference laboratories) are not useful in an acute setting, but they may confirm occult ingestion in child abuse or factitious disorder.
- Head CT followed by lumbar puncture is used in patients with altered mental status.
- Endoscopy may be useful if clinical evidence of gastrointestinal bleeding is present.

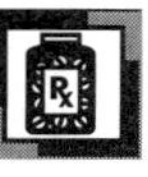

Treatment

- Treatment focuses on assessment and treatment of coagulopathy and control of bleeding.
- The dose and time of exposure should be determined for all substances involved.

DIRECTING PATIENT COURSE

The health-care professional should call the poison control center when:

- A history of anticoagulant ingestion is obtained.
- Toxic effects are not consistent with brodifacoum.
- Coingestant, drug interaction, or underlying disease presents an unusual problem.

The patient should be referred to a health-care facility when:

- Attempted suicide or homicide is possible.
- Patient or caregiver seems unreliable.
- Any toxic effects develop.
- Coingestant, drug interaction, or underlying disease presents an unusual problem.

Admission Considerations

Inpatient management is warranted for patients with frank bleeding or severe coagulopathy.

DECONTAMINATION

Out of Hospital

Ipecac should be administered to induce emesis within 1 hour of an acute single ingestion for an alert pediatric patient if health-care evaluation will be delayed.

In Hospital

- Ipecac should be administered to induce emesis within 1 hour of ingestion for the pediatric patient who is too small to have effective gastric lavage.
- Ipecac is not recommended in adults.
- Gastric lavage should be performed in pediatric (tube size 24–32 French) or adult (tube size 36–42 French) patients for large ingestion presenting within 1 hour of ingestion.
- One dose of activated charcoal (1–2 g/kg) should be administered without a cathartic if a substantial ingestion has occurred within the previous few hours.

ANTIDOTES

Vitamin K1 reverses the effect of brodifacoum on vitamin K regeneration.

Indications

- Marked prolongation of PT or INR without bleeding
- Severe prolongation of PT or INR and frank bleeding (may be used in conjunction with fresh or frozen plasma)

Method of Administration

- Marked prolongation of PT or INR without bleeding

—Vitamin K1 can be administered orally; adult initial dose is 50 to 100 mg/day initially in single or divided doses. Pediatric dose is not established; initial dose of 0.6 mg/kg or 10 to 15 mg is appropriate and will be titrated to effect in any case.
—INR and PT are repeated daily and dose is increased as needed to normalize INR or PT.
—Dosage may reach more than 200 mg/day.
—Daily dosing will be needed due to extremely long half-life.

- Severe prolongation of PT/INR and frank bleeding

—The initial dose of vitamin K1 for adults is 25 to 50 mg in D5W or 0.9% saline and infused intravenously at a rate not to exceed 1 mg/min. Pediatric dose is not established; initial dose of 0.6 mg/kg or 5 to 10 mg titrated to effect is reasonable starting dose.
—Dose is repeated two to four times daily until PT or INR normalize.
—Anaphylactoid reactions occur occasionally.
—Parenteral vitamin K1 doses as high as 400 mg have been used.
—Daily dosing will be needed due to extremely long half-life.

- Patients with prosthetic heart valves should not receive a high dose of vitamin K1 intravenously unless life-threatening bleeding is present.

Not Recommended Therapies

- No other form of vitamin K should be used (e.g., K2, menaquione, K3, menadione, K4, or menadiol).
- Phenobarbital may shorten the half-life of long-acting anticoagulants, but an improved outcome has not been demonstrated.

ADJUNCTIVE TREATMENT

- Patients with coagulopathy and active bleeding

—Fresh frozen plasma is administered; pediatric dose is 10 to 25 ml/kg; adult dose is 2 to 4 units intravenously.
—Based on serial INR and PT determinations, fresh frozen plasma is further administered as needed to return values toward normal.

- Bleeding and anemia. Packed red blood cells are administered as indicated.
- Both multiple-dose activated charcoal and cholestyramine have theoretical value because brodifacoum undergoes enterohepatic recirculation; however, they have not been demonstrated to alter outcome and are not routinely recommended.

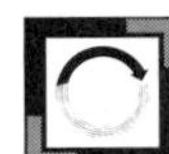

Follow-Up

PATIENT MONITORING

- Children with accidental ingestion should have PT and INR levels tested at 24 to 48 hours.
- In patients treated with vitamin K1, serial PT/INR will be needed until vitamin K therapy is no longer needed.

EXPECTED COURSE AND PROGNOSIS

- PT or INR becomes prolonged within 24 to 48 hours; peaks around 72 hours, and may persist for weeks or months in serious poisonings.
- Most patients will have no significant complications. Neurologic injury from intracranial bleeding or hypotension may occur in severe cases.

DISCHARGE CRITERIA/INSTRUCTIONS

- From the emergency department

—Asymptomatic children may be discharged after decontamination with follow-up PT or INR at 48 hours.
—Adults may be discharged if INR or PT is normal, after adequate decontamination and psychiatric evaluation, provided repeat PT or INR can be obtained 24 hours and 48 hours after ingestion.

- From the hospital

—Patient may be discharged when hemodynamically stable without active bleeding and normalizing INR/PT.
—Effective oral vitamin K1 dose must be established and regular follow-up ensured.

- A psychiatric evaluation should be obtained as indicated.

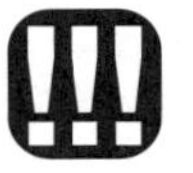

Pitfalls

DIAGNOSIS

Diagnosis can be elusive in adults with surreptitious ingestion.

TREATMENT

- Large oral or intravenous doses (greater than 200 mg) of vitamin K1 may be required for initial reversal of coagulopathy after intentional ingestion.
- Premature administration of vitamin K when coagulation is still normal is not recommended because it may instill a false sense of security by delaying the development of coagulopathy.

ICD-9-CM 964.2

Poisoning by agents primarily affecting blood constituents: anticoagulants.

See also: SECTION III, Vitamin K chapter; and SECTION IV, Coumadin chapter.

RECOMMENDED READING

Smolinske SC, Scherger DS, Kearns PS, et al. Superwarfarin poisoning in children: a prospective study. *Pediatrics* 1989;84:490–494.

Author: Luke Yip

Reviewer: Katherine M. Hurlbut

Bromides

Basics

DESCRIPTION

Bromide is a constituent in many drugs and chemicals, including some preparations of honatropine, halothane, neostigmine, pancuronium, pyridostigmine, quinine, scopolamine, and vecuronium. It is the active ingredient in ammonium bromide, bromvalerylurea, calcium bromide, carbromal, potassium bromide, and sodium bromide.

FORMS AND USES

- Bromides can be either organic or inorganic.

—Organic bromides include bromisoral, bromisoralum, bromocriptine, bromural, carbromal, and brompheniramine.
—Inorganic bromides include ammonium bromide, potassium bromide, sodium bromide, and calcium bromide.

- Dosage varies according to formulation.

TOXIC DOSE

- Acute ingestion of 10 g or more of carbromal may cause toxicity.
- Much smaller amounts produce toxicity with chronic ingestion.

PATHOPHYSIOLOGY

- The mechanism of toxicity may involve the substitution of bromide for chloride ions in extracellular and intracellular fluid.
- In bromide intoxication, the kidneys increase the elimination of chloride ions in an attempt to maintain a constant total halide concentration.

EPIDEMIOLOGY

- Poisoning is uncommon.
- Toxic effects following acute exposure are typically mild.
- Death occurs rarely, typically following at least 2 to 4 weeks of therapy in dehydrated, disabled patients.

CAUSES

- Most intoxications result from medicinal use. Occupational and environmental exposures do not cause intoxication.
- Poisoning is usually associated with intentional ingestion.
- Child neglect or abuse should be considered if the patient is less than 1 year of age, suicide attempt if the patient is over 6 years of age.

DRUG AND DISEASE INTERACTIONS

The elderly, dehydrated individuals, and patients with renal insufficiency are more susceptible to chronic intoxication.

PREGNANCY AND LACTATION

Bromide crosses the placenta. Case reports suggest that neonates born to intoxicated mothers have central nervous system depression and serum bromide levels higher than simultaneous maternal levels.

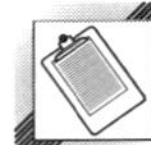

Diagnosis

DIFFERENTIAL DIAGNOSIS

- Toxicologic causes of confusion and CNS depression include, among many others, central nervous system depressants (e.g., barbiturates, benzodiazepines, sedative-hypnotics), lithium, phenytoin, and carbamazepine.
- Nontoxicologic causes include dementia, meningitis, cerebrovascular accident, central nervous system bleeding, and tumor.

SIGNS AND SYMPTOMS

- Acute intoxication is rare and may cause nausea and vomiting, CNS depression, coma, and, in severe cases, tachycardia, hypotension, and respiratory distress.
- Chronic intoxication is more common and is often characterized by gradual onset of confusion, behavioral changes, irritability, lethargy, slurred speech, weakness, abnormal reflexes, nystagmus, ataxia, toxic psychosis, anorexia, acneiform rash, an elevated serum chloride level, and a decreased anion gap.

Vital Signs

Fever occurs in about 25% of patients with chronic intoxication.

HEENT

Nystagmus and diplopia are common with chronic intoxication.

Dermatologic

An acneiform rash commonly develops with chronic intoxication and is termed *bromodera* (approximately 25% of all cases).

Cardiovascular

Tachycardia and hypotension are rare complications of severe acute intoxication.

Pulmonary

Acute respiratory distress syndrome is a rare complication of severe intoxication.

Gastrointestinal

Nausea and vomiting are common with acute or chronic intoxication.

Fluids and Electrolytes

- Spurious elevations in serum chloride and a decreased anion gap are common.
- Dehydration may predispose patients to chronic intoxication.

Neurologic

- Acute intoxication can cause central nervous system depression and coma.
- Chronic intoxication may cause lethargy, confusion, irritability, ataxia, dysarthria, nystagmus, tremor, abnormal reflexes, psychosis, hallucinations, weakness, and, rarely, abnormal cranial nerve findings. This symptom complex is termed *bromism*.

PROCEDURES AND LABORATORY TESTS

Essential Tests

- Serum electrolytes, BUN, and creatinine measurements. Elevated levels of serum chloride and a depressed anion gap suggest bromide intoxication (bromide is measured as chloride in many assays).
- Serum bromide level. A serum bromide level of 50 to 100 mg/dl may be associated with toxicity. A level greater than 200 mg/dl is generally associated with toxicity.

Recommended Tests

- Complete blood count, blood cultures, lithium levels, urine drug screen, cranial CT, and cerebral spinal fluid cultures may be necessary to rule out other causes of mental status changes.
- ECG, serum acetaminophen and aspirin levels should be checked in overdose setting to detect occult overdose.
- Imaging. Bromides may form bezoars and are often radiopaque. Visible tablets on abdominal radiographs suggest ongoing absorption.

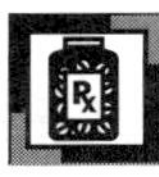

Treatment

- Treatment should focus on aggressive hydration and increasing urinary bromide excretion.
- The dose and time of exposure should be determined for all substances involved.

DIRECTING PATIENT COURSE

The health-care professional should call the poison control center when:

- Mental status changes, hypotension and other severe effects are present, or when the patient has underlying renal insufficiency.
- Signs and symptoms are not consistent with bromism.
- Coingestant, drug interaction, or underlying disease presents an unusual problem.

The patient should be referred to a health-care facility when:

- Attempted suicide or homicide is possible.
- Patient or caregiver seems unreliable.
- Symptoms are present.
- Coingestant, drug interaction, or underlying disease presents an unusual problem.

Admission Considerations

Inpatient managment is warranted when the patient's mental status changes or psychiatric effects, persistent dehydration or vomiting, renal insufficiency, or hypotension develop.

DECONTAMINATION

Out of Hospital

Ipecac should be administered to induce emesis within 1 hour of an acute single ingestion for alert pediatric or adult patients if healthcare evaluation will be delayed.

In Hospital

- Gastric lavage should be performed in pediatric (tube size 24–32 French) or adult (tube size 36–42 French) patients presenting within 1 hour of a large single ingestion.
- One dose of activated charcoal (1–2 g/kg) should be administered if a substantial ingestion has occurred within the previous few hours.

ANTIDOTES

There is no specific antidote for bromide poisoning.

ADJUNCTIVE TREATMENT

- Intravenous hydration. Infusion of 0.9% sodium chloride enhances urinary bromide excretion. An initial bolus of 10 to 20 ml/kg as clinically indicated should be administered followed by an infusion two to three times the maintenance fluid rate. Serum electrolyte and bromide levels should be monitored. Infusion should be discontinued when the symptoms have improved and the serum bromide level is less than 100 to 150 mg/dl.
- Diuresis. The addition of a diuretic (furosemide 10 mg intravenously every 6 to 12 hours) increases urinary bromide excretion beyond what is achieved with the administration of 0.9% sodium chloride alone. However, it is unknown whether diuresis improves clinical outcome, and dehydration is a potential complication if the fluid status is not carefully monitored.
- Hemodialysis can increase bromide clearance greatly. It is indicated in patients with underlying renal insufficiency and when attempts at intravenous chloride administration have been unsuccessful or are contraindicated.

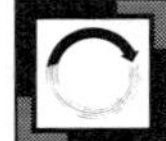

Follow-Up

EXPECTED COURSE AND PROGNOSIS

- Acute intoxication is rare, with clinical effects developing in hours and recovery occurring over 1 to 2 days.
- Patients with chronic intoxication develop symptoms over days to weeks and recover slowly with appropriate therapy.
- A syndrome involving sequelae of ataxia, dysarthria, tremor, and hyperreflexia with cerebellar atrophy has been described after chronic bromide intoxication.

DISCHARGE CRITERIA/INSTRUCTIONS

- From the emergency department. The patient may be discharged when serum electrolyte levels, vital signs, and mental status are normal after gastrointestinal decontamination, observation for 6 hours, and psychiatric evaluation, if needed.
- From the hospital. The patient may be discharged when mental status and neurologic examination results are normal or improving, psychiatric effects have resolved, electrolyte levels are normal, and the serum bromide level is less than 150 mg/dl. A psychiatric evaluation should be obtained prior to discharge as clinically appropriate.

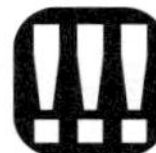

Pitfalls

- Bromide intoxication is different from bromine gas intoxication, which causes mainly pulmonary and dermatologic manifestations.
- Because clinical effects are nonspecific and bromide is rarely the main constituent of a drug, the possibility of bromide intoxication is rarely considered.

ICD-9-CM 967.3

Poisoning by sedatives and hypnotics: bromine compounds.

RECOMMENDED READING

Dax EC. Overdosage with bromides: a report on 59 cases. *BMJ* 1946;2:226–227.

Hanes FM, Yates A. Analysis of 400 instances of chronic bromide intoxication. *South Med J* 1938;31:667–671.

Harenko A. Neurologic findings in chronic bromisovalum poisoning. *Ann Med Int Fenn* 1967;57:181–188.

Maes V, Huyghens L, DeKeyser J, et al. Acute and chronic intoxication with carbromal preparations. *J Toxicol Clin Toxicol* 1985;23:341–346.

Author: Katherine M. Hurlbut

Reviewer: Richard C. Dart

Brown Recluse Spider Bite

Basics

- The brown recluse spider is one cause of necrotic arachnidism, a term applied to a syndrome that begins as a papule with initial local pain or itching. A small vesicle may form initially followed by a "bull's eye" or halo appearance (a central vesicle surrounded by erythema or ecchymosis). A pale, blanched ring may surround the discolored area. Over several days, a hard eschar may form in the center of the affected area. A full-thickness ulcer usually forms underneath it and often requires weeks to months to heal.
- The brown recluse is also known as the violin or fiddleback spider.

DESCRIPTION

- *Loxosceles reclusa* is the primary species known as brown recluse spider. Other species in the United States include *L. arizonica, L. deserta, L. laeta* (rare), and *L. unicolor.*
- Loxoscelism is a systemic syndrome resulting from the bite of the brown recluse spider. It is most likely to occur in children.
- Necrotic arachnidism has been reported following the bite of several different spider species worldwide, including chiracanthium (running spider), argiope (orb weaver), atrax (funnel web), phidippus (jumping spider), lycosa (wolf spider), and tegenaria (hobo spider).

TOXIC DOSE

One bite is toxic.

PATHOPHYSIOLOGY

- In the brown recluse spider, sphingomyelinase D appears to be the major venom component responsible for injury. It causes white blood cell infiltration, local tissue ischemia, and cell death, as well as red blood cell lysis. It also may injure endothelial cells, resulting in platelet activation and microvascular coagulation and obstruction.
- Fat cells appear more sensitive. More severe tissue necrosis may develop in areas of subcutaneous fat.

EPIDEMIOLOGY

- Envenomation is common.
- Toxic effects are typically mild to moderate, with death occurring rarely.
- The brown recluse spider and related species are found throughout South America and the southern United States; severe bites are most likely to occur in the southeastern United States.
- Children have an increased risk of a systemic reaction and hemolysis. Chronic circulation problems in older patients may impair healing.

RISK FACTORS

Bites are most likely to occur in the cool, dark environments where the spider is found.

PREGNANCY AND LACTATION

Both mother and fetus have generally done well despite the occurrence of maternal hemolysis. Pregnant patients should be managed as any other patient.

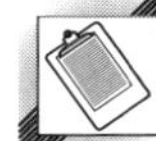

Diagnosis

DIFFERENTIAL DIAGNOSIS

- Any disease process that causes localized skin erythema and ulceration, especially if associated with constitutional symptoms (e.g., an infected insect bite or puncture wound, a venous stasis ulcer, vasculitis skin ulcer, and an ischemic or a diabetic skin ulcer).
- The bites of many other spiders found throughout the world reportedly cause necrotic arachnidism, as noted under the Description heading above.

SIGNS AND SYMPTOMS

- In local lesions, the initial bite usually occurs unnoticed. A few hours later, the patient notes a minimally painful and pruritic papule. Many cases resolve over the next few days. Some bites will enlarge over several days and then ulcerate. Healing may require weeks to months.
- The term *loxoscelism* refers to a systemic syndrome that is more common in children. Manifestations include fever, chills, arthralgia, coagulopathy and hemolysis, and may be complicated by seizures and coma.

Vital Signs

Fever and tachycardia are common if systemic effects develop.

Dermatologic

- Many patients develop only a papule and initial local pain or itching, which resolve over a few days.
- Necrotic arachnidism typically begins with a papule and initial local pain or itching. A small vesicle may form at the bite site. Over several hours, a bull's eye or halo appearance develops (a central vesicle surrounded by erythema or ecchymosis). A pale, blanched ring may surround the discolored area. Over several days, a hard eschar may form in the center of the affected area. A full-thickness ulcer often forms underneath it and often requires weeks to months to heal. In severe cases cutaneous necrosis may extend to involve subcutaneous fat and muscle.

Cardiovascular

Cardiovascular collapse occurs rarely, usually in patients with hemolysis and apparent systemic effects.

Renal

Renal failure has occurred in cases with severe hemolysis.

Hematologic

- Massive hemolysis may occur a day or so after envenomation, but it is rare and more common in children.
- Coagulation abnormalities are unusual; they may occur in severe cases.

Neurologic

- Lethargy, seizure, and coma may occur in severe cases.
- Transverse myelitis has been reported, but is rare.

PROCEDURES AND LABORATORY TESTS

Essential Tests

- There is no diagnostic test of envenomation by the brown recluse spider.
- No tests may be needed for minimally symptomatic patients.
- Complete blood count (CBC) is measured 48 to 72 hours after a bite in patients with systemic symptoms to rule out hemolysis.

Recommended Tests

- Serial CBC if hemolysis develops.
- Serum electrolytes, BUN, and creatinine levels are measured in patients with systemic symptoms to evaluate hemolysis and possible renal injury or hyperkalemia.
- In unusual cases, a bone scan may be needed if osteomyelitis from contiguous spread is suspected.

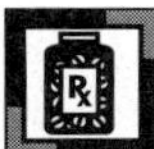

Treatment

• Many bites resolve spontaneously with simple wound care.
• No decontamination or first aid measures are recommended.
• Severe envenomation may require aggressive supportive care.
• No specific treatment has been shown to improve the size of a wound or the rate of healing.

DIRECTING PATIENT COURSE

The health-care professional should call the poison control center when:

• Systemic effects develop (e.g., altered mental status, hemolysis).
• Toxic effects are not consistent with necrotic arachnidism.
• A drug interaction or underlying disease presents an unusual problem.

The patient should be referred to a health-care facility when:

• The patient is very young.
• The patient or caregiver seems unreliable.
• Toxic effects are not consistent with necrotic arachnidism.
• Systemic effects or an underlying disease presents an unusual challenge.

ADMISSION CONSIDERATIONS

Inpatient management is warranted for patients with evidence of hemolysis or systemic effects; to administer fluid resuscitation and monitor blood count and renal function.

ANTIDOTES

There is no specific antidote for brown recluse spider venom.

ADJUNCTIVE TREATMENT

• The wound should be covered and standard local wound care provided, including tetanus toxoid, if needed.
• Surgical procedures. Surgical excision of a lesion is controversial. Early excision has been reported to produce a larger wound than supportive care. Some clinicians recommend excision (for cosmetic reasons) after several weeks, once the wound has stopped enlarging.
• Prophylactic antibiotics are not recommended.
• Infection occurs rarely and should be handled like an infected laceration. Remove necrotic material and administer antibiotic therapy.

Not Recommended

In the absence of an effective therapy, various speculative treatments have been recommended. Dapsone, electric shock, steroids, phentolamine, dextran, diphenhydramine, and hyperbaric oxygen have been proposed but not demonstrated to be effective.

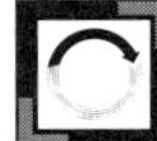

Follow-Up

PATIENT MONITORING

• Frequent wound checks for complications may be needed especially if original lesion was large.
• In patients with systemic effects, cardiac and respiratory function should be monitored continuously.

EXPECTED COURSE AND PROGNOSIS

• In mild cases, symptoms resolve after 1 to 2 days.
• Wounds may occasionally become infected.
• Necrotic lesions may require weeks to heal; large lesions may require skin grafts.
• Cases with a necrotic lesion may heal abnormally with thin, pigmented skin.
• Some clinicians recommend delayed excision (weeks after a bite) and primary closure (see Adjunctive Treatment).
• Fatal systemic reactions are rare.

DISCHARGE CRITERIA/INSTRUCTIONS

• From the emergency department. Discharge patients with no evidence of hemolysis or other systemic effects.
• From the hospital. Discharge patients whose systemic effects have resolved, and those with normal or improving renal function.

PATIENT EDUCATION

The patient should be advised that the wound may worsen over the first few days despite wound care.

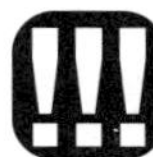

Pitfalls

DIAGNOSIS

• It is often difficult to identify an early lesion as a brown recluse bite.
• Necrotic arachnidism is frequently identified misleadingly as "brown recluse bite." Although the treatment is the same, most cases of necrotic arachnidism fail to manifest the severe effects that may be caused by true brown recluse spider bites.

TREATMENT

Dapsone is recommended by some practioners. However, the available data do not support its use, and it may produce methemoglobinemia.

ICD-9-CM 989.5

Toxic effect of other substances, chiefly nonmedicinal as to source: venom.

RECOMMENDED READING

Anderson PC. Loxosceles threatening pregnancy. *Am J Obstet Gynecol* 1991;165:1454–1456.

Phillips S, Kohn M, Baker J. Therapy of brown spider envenomation: a controlled trial of hyperbaric oxygen, dapsone and cyproheptadine. *Ann Emerg Med* 1995;25:363–369.

Wasserman GS, Anderson PC. Loxosceles and necrotic arachnidism. *J Toxicol Clin Toxicol* 1983–4;21:451–472.

Author: Kennon Heard

Reviewer: Richard C. Dart

Bupropion

Basics

DESCRIPTION

Bupropion (Wellbutrin, Zyban) is an oral monocyclic antidepressant medication.

FORMS AND USES

- Bupropion is used as an antidepressant and as an aid to smoking cessation.
- The usual starting dose is 100 mg twice a day, with a maximum dose of 450 mg/day.
- Sustained-release formulations are available.

TOXIC DOSE

Experience is limited; however, the mean dose in patients who had seizures during therapy was 8.3 mg/kg.

PATHOPHYSIOLOGY

- Bupropion is a monocyclic antidepressant structurally similar to amphetamine.
- It is a weak inhibitor of neuronal reuptake of dopamine, serotonin, and norepinephrine.
- The mechanism of its toxic effects is unknown.

EPIDEMIOLOGY

- Poisoning is uncommon.
- Toxic effects are typically mild.
- Death occurs rarely after a massive or mixed overdose.

CAUSES

- Toxic effects are usually due to intentional ingestion.
- Child neglect or abuse should be considered if the patient is less than 1 year of age, suicide attempt if the patient is over 6 years of age.

RISK FACTORS

- Seizures may occur at therapeutic doses, particularly in patients undergoing high-dose therapy (more than 600 mg/day), patients with bulimia, patients with head injury, patients taking drugs that decrease seizure threshold, or patients with a preexisting history of seizure disorder.
- Older patients may be less tolerant of orthostatic hypotension and tachycardia.

PREGNANCY AND LACTATION

US FDA Pregnancy Category B. Animal studies indicate no fetal risk and there are no controlled human studies, or animal studies show an adverse fetal effect but well-controlled studies in pregnant women do not.

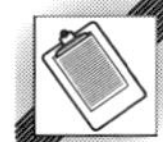

Diagnosis

DIFFERENTIAL DIAGNOSIS

- Toxicologic causes of altered mental status or seizures include sympathomimetic agents (e.g., amphetamines, cocaine, theophylline), lithium, isoniazid, and several others.
- Nontoxicologic causes of altered mental status or seizures include CNS infection or hemorrhage, thyrotoxicosis, underlying seizure disorder or noncompliance with seizure medications, and drug withdrawal.

SIGNS AND SYMPTOMS

- CNS depression or seizures are the most common effects.

Vital Signs

Tachycardia is common in overdose.

Cardiovascular

- Hypotension after overdose is rare, but orthostatic hypotension occurs with therapeutic use.
- Prolonged PR and QRS intervals have occurred in animal models of severe intoxication.

Gastrointestinal

Nausea and vomiting is common after overdose.

Neurologic

- Seizures may occur in some patients at therapeutic doses (see Risk Factors).
- Lethargy and confusion occur commonly; coma is rare.
- Tremors, hallucinations, paresthesia, and lightheadedness are also common.

PROCEDURES AND LABORATORY TESTS

Essential Tests

No tests may be needed for asymptomatic patients.

Recommended Tests

- Serum electrolytes, BUN, creatinine, and glucose should be measured in all patients with altered mental status.
- Oxygenation should be evaluated with pulse oximetry or arterial blood gases in patients with CNS depression.
- ECG, serum acetaminophen, and aspirin levels should be performed in an overdose setting to detect occult ingestion.
- Head CT, lumbar puncture, and cultures should be performed in patients with altered mental status of undetermined etiology.

Not Recommended Tests

Serum levels of bupropion are not clinically useful.

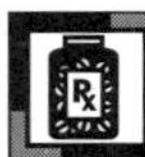

Treatment

- Treatment should focus on supportive care, including oxygen administration and appropriate airway management.
- Dose and time of exposure should be determined for all substances involved.

DIRECTING PATIENT COURSE

The health-care professional should call the poison control center when:

- Seizures or other severe effects are present.
- Toxic effects are not consistent with bupropion poisoning.
- Coingestant, drug interaction, or underlying disease presents an unusual problem.

The patient should be referred to a health-care facility when:

- Attempted suicide or homicide is possible.
- Patient or caregiver seems unreliable.
- Toxic effects develop.
- Coingestant, drug interaction, or underlying disease presents an unusual problem.

Admission Considerations

Inpatient management is warranted when the patient has seizures, altered mental status, or persistently abnormal vital signs.

DECONTAMINATION

Out of Hospital

Ipecac-induced emesis is not recommended because seizures may occur.

In Hospital

- Gastric lavage should be performed in pediatric (tube size 24–32 French) or adult (tube size 36–42 French) patients for large ingestion presenting within 1 hour of ingestion or if serious effects are present.
- One dose of activated charcoal (1–2 g/kg) should be administered without a cathartic if a substantial ingestion has occurred within the previous few hours.
- Whole-bowel irrigation with polyethylene glycol should be considered for the patient with ingestion of a sustained-release formulation.

ANTIDOTES

There is no specific antidote for bupropion poisoning.

ADJUNCTIVE TREATMENT

Seizure

- Adequate airway and oxygenation should be ensured.
- A benzodiazepine should be administered for initial control.

—Diazepam
—The adult dose is 5 to 10 mg initially, repeated every 5 to 10 minutes as needed.
—The pediatric dose is 0.2 to 0.5 mg/kg initially, repeated every 10 minutes as needed.
—The airway should be monitored closely.
—Lorazepam
—The adult dose is 2 to 4 mg administered by intravenous push over 2 to 5 minutes, repeated every 5 to 10 minutes as needed.
—The pediatric dose is 0.1 mg/kg administered by intravenous push over 2 to 5 minutes, not to exceed 4 mg per dose, and repeated every 5 to 10 minutes as needed.
—The airway should be monitored.

- If seizures persist or recur, another anticonvulsant such as phenobarbital or phenytoin should be added.

Hypotension

- The patient should be given 10 to 20 ml/kg 0.9% saline intravenously and placed in the Trendelenburg position.
- Further fluid therapy should be guided by central pressure monitoring to avoid volume overload.
- If hypotension does not respond to treatment, a vasopressor is administered.

—Dopamine
—The dose is 2 to 5 μg/kg/min, titrated to effect.
—Rates greater than 20 μg/kg/min are unlikely to provide further benefit.
—Norepinephrine
—The dose is 0.1 to 0.2 μg/kg/min, titrated to effect.

—High rates of infusion may cause tissue ischemia.

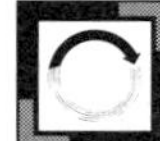

Follow-Up

PATIENT MONITORING

Cardiac and hemodynamic status should be monitored until effects resolve.

EXPECTED COURSE AND PROGNOSIS

Complete recovery usually occurs over 12 to 24 hours unless a coingestant is involved or sequelae of repeated seizures or hypoxia intercede.

DISCHARGE CRITERIA/INSTRUCTIONS

- From the emergency department

—An asymptomatic patient with normal vital signs may be discharged after gastrointestinal decontamination, 4 to 6 hours of observation, and psychiatric evaluation, if needed.
—Prolonged observation may be indicated for ingestion of a large amount of sustained-release formulation.

- From the hospital

—The patient may be discharged after seizures and tachycardia have resolved and mental status has returned to normal.
—The patient should be referred for psychiatric evaluation as appropriate.

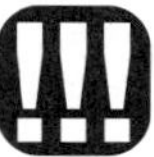

Pitfalls

DIAGNOSIS

Failure to consider ingestion of more life-threatening substances (e.g., tricyclic antidepressant) or nontoxicologic causes of altered mental status may result in the failure to treat a more life-threatening illness.

FOLLOW-UP

Failure to monitor ingestion of sustained-release formulation may result in missing delayed toxic effects.

ICD-9-CM 969.0

Poisoning by psychotropic agents: antidepressants.

See also SECTION II, Seizure (Unexplained) and Hypotension chapters; and SECTION III, Whole-Bowel Irrigation chapter.

RECOMMENDED READING

Davidson J. Seizures and bupropion: a review. *J Clin Psychiatry* 1989;50:256–261.

Spiller HA, Ramoska EA, Krenzelok EP, et al. Bupropion overdose: a 3-year multi-center retrospective analysis. *Am J Emerg Med* 1994;12:43–45.

Author: Kennon Heard

Reviewer: Katherine M. Hurlbut

Butorphanol

Basics

DESCRIPTION

Butorphanol (Stadol) is a synthetic opioid analgesic.

FORMS AND USES

- Butorphanol is available in injectable and nasal spray forms.
- The usual dose is 1 mg intravenously, 1 mg nasally (1 mg equals one spray), or 1 to 4 mg intramuscularly.

TOXIC DOSE

Some toxic effects (dysphoria) appear at therapeutic doses. Repeated administration probably produces tolerance; large doses may cause minimal effects.

PATHOPHYSIOLOGY

- Butorphanol is an agonist/antagonist at μ-receptors and an agonist at κ-receptors. Due to the κ stimulation, some patients experience dysphoria in addition to analgesia.
- Butorphanol is addictive for some patients.

EPIDEMIOLOGY

Poisoning is uncommon.

CAUSES

Child neglect or abuse should be considered if the patient is less than 1 year of age, suicide attempt if the patient is over 6 years of age.

DRUG AND DISEASE INTERACTIONS

Because of its antagonist activity at μ-receptors, butorphanol may precipitate withdrawal in opioid-addicted patients.

PREGNANCY AND LACTATION

- US FDA Pregnancy Category C. The drug causes animal teratogenic or embryocidal effects, but there are no controlled studies in women, or no studies are available in either animals or women.
- Very small amounts are passed in breast milk.
- Maternal overdose with butorphanol is well tolerated and treated as in nonpregnant patients.

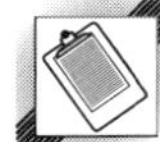

Diagnosis

DIFFERENTIAL DIAGNOSIS

Other toxicologic causes of CNS depression and small pupils include clonidine and all opioid agonists (e.g., codeine, meperidine, morphine, etc.).

SIGNS AND SYMPTOMS

HEENT

Miosis usually occurs with overdose.

Cardiovascular

- Bradycardia, hypotension, and vasodilatation may occur.
- Hypertension has been reported.

Pulmonary

- Respiratory depression occurs in a dose-related fashion.
- Pulmonary edema can occur with overdose.

Gastrointestinal

- Nausea and vomiting can occur.
- Constipation may occur in therapeutic doses.

Neurologic

Somnolence progressing to coma occurs with overdose.

PROCEDURES AND LABORATORY TESTS

Essential Tests

No tests may be needed in asymptomatic patients.

Recommended Tests

- Pulse oximeter or arterial blood gas levels are used to evaluate oxygenation.
- All patients with altered mental status should have blood glucose determined.
- Head CT, lumbar puncture, cultures, and other studies should be ordered as needed to evaluate other causes of altered mental status.
- Serum acetaminophen and aspirin levels are measured in overdose setting to detect occult ingestion.

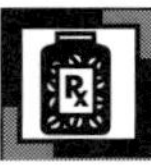

Treatment

DIRECTING PATIENT COURSE

The health-care professional should call the poison control center when:

- Severe or persistent effects develop.
- Coingestant, drug interaction, or underlying disease presents an unusual problem.

The patient should be referred to a health-care facility when:

- Toxic effects develop.
- Coingestant, drug interaction, or underlying disease presents an unusual problem.

DECONTAMINATION

Out of Hospital

Emesis should not be induced due to the possibility of mental status depression.

In Hospital

- Emesis should not be induced.
- One dose of activated charcoal (1–2 g/kg) should be administered without a cathartic if a substantial ingestion of nasal spray has occurred within the previous few hours.

ANTIDOTES

Naloxone is a specific antidote for opioid poisoning.

- Dose is 2 mg intravenously for respiratory depression
- This dose may be repeated up to 10 mg, but most patients will respond to 2 mg (see SECTION III, Naloxone and Nalmephene chapters for further details).

ADJUNCTIVE TREATMENT

Oxygen is to be administered and an intravenous line established.

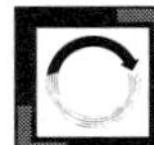

Follow-Up

PATIENT MONITORING

Continuous respiratory and cardiac monitoring should be performed.

EXPECTED COURSE AND PROGNOSIS

- Toxic effects occur soon after exposure.
- Complete recovery is expected unless sequelae of hypoxia intercede.

DISCHARGE CRITERIA/INSTRUCTIONS

- Following gastrointestinal decontamination, patients should be discharged when they are asymptomatic and have normal vital signs after a 4-hour observation period.
- Because butorphanol is increasingly recognized as a drug of abuse, referral to a substance abuse program should be considered.

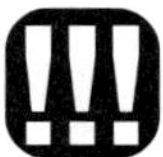

Pitfalls

DIAGNOSIS

Standard urine toxicology screens may not detect butorphanol.

ICD-9-CM 965.0

Poisoning by analgesics, antipyretics, and antirheumatics: opiates and related narcotics.

See also: SECTION III, Naloxone and Nalmephene chapter.

RECOMMENDED READING

Ellenhorn MG. Butorphanol. *Ellenhorn's medical toxicology,* 2nd ed. Baltimore: Williams & Wilkins, 1997:414–415.

Author: Kennon Heard

Reviewer: Richard C. Dart

Button or Disk Batteries

Basics

DESCRIPTION

- Button or disk batteries are used in a variety of electronic products (cameras, hearing aids, watches, calculators, toys, games, remote control devices). Typical sizes are 11.6 mm in diameter or smaller, but they may also be 15.6 mm (dime size) or 23.0 mm (quarter size) in diameter.
- The 23.0-mm batteries are most likely to lodge in the gastrointestinal tract and cause injury.
- Disk batteries contain metal salts bathed in a strong alkali; the metal contents may be lithium, magnesium, mercury, cadmium, zinc, silver, and nickel.

TOXIC DOSE

One battery is sufficient to cause gastrointestinal perforation.

PATHOPHYSIOLOGY

- Injury occurs when the battery becomes lodged in the gastrointestinal tract, usually the esophagus.
- Batteries also may be inserted in the nose or ear or lodge in the pharynx or airway.
- Injury may result from pressure necrosis, mechanical obstruction, or release of alkali if the battery leaks.
- Corrosive effects do not develop until the battery ruptures, usually several days or longer after ingestion.
- Release of mercury has resulted in elevated mercury levels, but toxicity has not been reported.

EPIDEMIOLOGY

- Disk battery ingestion is common.
- Toxic effects following exposure are typically mild; significant esophageal injuries occur rarely.

CAUSES

- Ingestion is usually accidental.
- Child neglect or abuse should be considered if the patient is less than 1 year of age, suicide attempt if the patient is over 6 years of age.

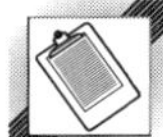

Diagnosis

DIFFERENTIAL DIAGNOSIS

- Toxicologic causes of isolated abdominal pain or gastrointestinal perforation include primarily ingestion of strong acid, base, or other caustic agent.
- Nontoxicologic causes of isolated abdominal pain include foreign body ingestion, ulcer disease, and gastrointestinal perforation from any cause.

SIGNS AND SYMPTOMS

Initial symptoms are minimal, but may involve effects of foreign body ingestion; later symptoms, if any develop, reflect gastrointestinal mucosal injury or perforation.

Vital Signs

- Fever or tachycardia suggests perforation.
- Tachypnea suggests aspiration.

HEENT

Drooling suggests esophageal or pharyngeal obstruction.

Pulmonary

- Stridor, cough, or dyspnea suggests aspiration; even an unimpressive, persistent cough may indicate bronchial battery location.
- Focal findings on pulmonary examination suggest bronchial location.
- If the battery is lodged in the esophagus, a tracheal-esophageal fistula may develop several days after ingestion.

Gastrointestinal

- Dysphagia, refusal to take fluids, or drooling suggests esophageal injury or obstruction.
- Regurgitation, vomiting, or abdominal pain suggests intestinal obstruction.
- Delayed dysphagia, pain, or fever may indicate perforation.
- Melena may indicate intestinal mucosal injury.

PROCEDURES AND LABORATORY TESTS

Essential Tests

- Plain abdominal and chest radiographs to locate the battery should be obtained on any patient with a potential ingestion.
- Posteroanterior and lateral radiographs should be performed to accurately locate the battery.
- If radiographic findings are negative, consider a lateral neck radiograph to see if the battery is located in the nasopharynx.
- Water-soluble radiocontrast studies may be needed if there is a possibility of perforation.

Recommended Tests

- If the recovered mercury or cadmium battery is not intact, mercury or cadmium levels should be determined.
- Complete blood count, serum electrolytes, BUN, and creatinine should be determined if obstruction or perforation is suspected.

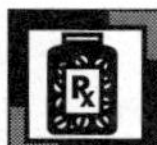

Treatment

• Supportive care with airway management is vital.
• The dose and time of exposure should be determined for all substances involved.

DIRECTING PATIENT COURSE

The health-care professional should call the poison control center when:

• Possible battery ingestion has occurred.
• Coingestant or underlying disease presents an unusual problem.

The patient should be referred to a health-care facility when possible battery ingestion has occurred.

Admission Considerations

Inpatient management is warranted if:

• Symptoms of perforation develop; immediate surgical consultation is warranted.
• Symptoms of esophageal injury or gastrointestinal obstruction are present.

DECONTAMINATION

Out of Hospital

Emesis should not be induced because it may cause the patient to aspirate the battery.

In Hospital

• No decontamination methods are needed acutely if the battery has passed into the stomach.
• If there is no progression of the battery through the intestine over several days, whole-bowel irrigation is recommended.

ANTIDOTES

There is no specific antidote for disk battery ingestion.

ADJUNCTIVE TREATMENT

• Glucagon, 1 mg intravenously, has been used to attempt to help the battery pass from the esophagus into the stomach; however, most patients will experience vomiting, and endoscopic removal is preferred.
• Patients with esophageal, pharyngeal, or tracheal location of batteries should undergo endoscopic removal of the battery; attempting to push the battery into the stomach with a nasogastric tube is not recommended.
• Metal detectors have been used to locate the battery, but their ability to ensure that the battery is past the esophagus has not been studied.

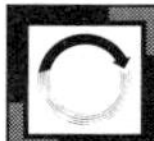

Follow-Up

PATIENT MONITORING

Stools should be strained in patients with batteries in the gastrointestinal tract; if the battery has not been found within 4 to 7 days, radiography should be repeated. Some authorities recommend more frequent radiography for large batteries (23.0 mm).

EXPECTED COURSE AND PROGNOSIS

• The battery typically passes in the stool within 3 days; however, passage occasionally takes up to 2 weeks.
• Gastrointestinal tract perforation or obstruction occurs rarely, usually after several days have passed.
• The patient may experience postobstructive pneumonia or develop a tracheal-esophageal fistula if the battery is aspirated.
• Mercury or cadmium toxicity from broken batteries is rare.

DISCHARGE CRITERIA/INSTRUCTIONS

• From the emergency department. Asymptomatic patients with batteries that have passed the lower esophageal sphincter may be discharged with instructions to return if they develop abdominal pain, fever, vomiting, or bloody stools; the patient's stools should be checked for the battery.
• From the hospital. Patients who can tolerate an oral diet and have passed the battery may be discharged.

PATIENT EDUCATION

Patients should be instructed to monitor their stools for the battery and contact their primary physician if they do not pass the battery within 4 to 7 days.

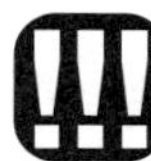

Pitfalls

DIAGNOSIS

• Patients with a battery lodged in the esophagus may be initially asymptomatic.
• If the battery is not located on chest and abdominal radiographs, a nasopharyngeal location should be ruled out with lateral neck radiography.
• Many battery ingestions are first misdiagnosed as viral gastroenteritis.

ICD-9-CM 985

Toxic effect of other metals.

See also: SECTION III, Whole-Bowel Irrigation chapter; and SECTION IV, Cadmium and Mercury chapters.

RECOMMENDED READING

Hoffman RS. Caustics and batteries. In: Goldfank LR, Flomenbaun NE, Lewin NA, et al. eds. *Goldfrank's toxicologic emergencies.* 6th ed. Norwalk, CT: Appleton & Lange, 1998.

Litovitz T, Schmitz BF. Ingestion of cylindrical and button batteries: an analysis of 2382 cases. *Pediat* 1992;89:747–757.

Author: Kennon Heard

Reviewer: Richard C. Dart

Cadmium

Basics

DESCRIPTION

Cadmium is a metal used in a variety of occupations (by jewelers, painters, and welders) and industries (battery manufacturing, paint and glaze manufacturing, electroplating, mining, and smelting, among others).

TOXIC DOSE

- Death has occurred following ingestion of solutions containing more than 25 mg/L; recovery has been reported after ingestion of liquid containing 16 mg/L cadmium.
- Cadmium is an International Agency for Research on Cancer I carcinogen.

PATHOPHYSIOLOGY

- Ingestion of cadmium may cause marked local gastrointestinal irritation and hemorrhage, with only a small amount of systemic absorption.
- Inhalation primarily causes irritation of respiratory system (see SECTION IV, Cadmium Fume Fever chapter).
- Kidney and liver injury may develop from substantial exposure by either oral or inhalational routes.
- Toxic effects following exposure are typically mild, with death occurring rarely following acute cadmium pneumonitis or chronic renal failure.

EPIDEMIOLOGY

- Poisoning is uncommon.
- Approximately 500,000 workers in the United States may be exposed to cadmium on the job.

CAUSES

Accidental occupational exposure is most frequent.

RISK FACTORS

- Impaired renal function or poor renal perfusion (as in congestive heart failure).
- Tobacco smoking increases cadmium levels.

PREGNANCY

- Possible decreased birth weight has been reported.
- Cadmium crosses the placenta; however, teratogenic effects have not been observed in humans.

WORKPLACE STANDARDS

- ACGIH. TLV TWA is 0.01 mg/m^3.
- OSHA. PEL: fume is 0.1 mg/m^3; dust is 0.2 mg/m^3.
- NIOSH. IDLH is 9 mg/m^2.

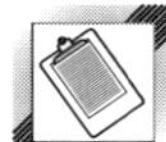

Diagnosis

DIFFERENTIAL DIAGNOSIS

- Toxicologic causes of renal failure include heavy metals, radiographic contrast media, and analgesic papillary necrosis.
- Nontoxicologic causes of chronic renal disease include infection, diabetes, hypertension, and Fanconi syndrome.

SIGNS AND SYMPTOMS

- Acute poisoning reflects the pathway of exposure.

—Acute life-threatening pneumonitis results from inhalation of cadmium fumes.
—Acute gastrointestinal effects result from ingestion.

- Chronic exposure results in renal insufficiency.

Vital Signs

- Acute

Tachycardia and hypotension may occur in severe cases.

- Chronic

Tachypnea and tachycardia may occur due to renal insufficiency.

HEENT

Chronic poisoning may result in yellow rings on the teeth; neck and facial edema, and salivation.

Dermatologic

Irritation may occur acutely.

Pulmonary

- Acute. Cadmium fume fever may occur.
- Chronic. Bronchitis, emphysema, or fibrosis may occur.

Cardiovascular

Development of hypertension during chronic exposure is a controversial topic; hypertension may be secondary to renal injury.

Gastrointestinal

- Acute. Salivation, vomiting, irritation of the mucosa, and increased bowel sounds and cramping may occur.
- Hemorrhagic gastroenteritis can occur in severe cases.

Hepatic

Liver enzyme elevation may occur.

Renal

- Acute. Flank pain and proximal tubular necrosis leading to acute tubular necrosis may occur in severe cases.
- Chronic. Proteinuria, aminoaciduria, glycosuria may occur.

Musculoskeletal

- Bone pain (Itai-Itai disease) and weakness may occur in chronic cases.
- Osteomalacia and osteoporosis may occur.

Neurologic

Headache, shivering, and nystagmus may occur.

PROCEDURES AND LABORATORY TESTS

Essential Tests

- Whole blood cadmium level

—Normal: 0.4 to 1 μg/L
—Smokers: 1 to 5 μg/L
—Toxicity: possible at $>$7 μg/L or serum cadmium $>$5 μg/L
—Level increases acutely; level does not reflect body burden until several months after acute exposure

- Urine cadmium level. Toxicity possible occurs at urine cadmium levels exceeding 3 μg/g creatinine.
- Serum electrolytes, BUN, creatinine, and urinalysis are advised for renal injury and volume changes after acute ingestion.

Recommended Tests

- Serum liver function tests for liver injury following serious acute ingestion
- Urine β_2-microglobulin, retinol binding protein, lysozyme, or *N*-acetyl-glucosaminidase; possible elevation in subclinical renal injury
- ECG, serum acetaminophen, and aspirin levels in overdose setting to detect occult ingestion
- Chest radiograph in patients with chronic toxicity to assess pulmonary fibrosis, presence of cancer
- Bone films to reveal osteomalacia, fractures in chronic cases

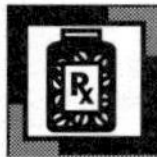

Treatment

- Treatment should focus on general supportive care, and management of renal failure in advanced cases.
- Dose and time of exposure should be determined for all substances involved.

DIRECTING PATIENT COURSE

The health-care professional should call the poison control center when:

- Cadmium toxicity is suspected.
- Coingestant, drug interaction, or underlying disease presents an unusual problem.

The patient should be referred to a health-care facility when:

- Patient or caregiver seem unreliable.
- Toxic effects develop.
- Coingestant, drug interaction, or underlying disease presents an unusual problem.

Admission Considerations

Inpatient management is warranted for patients with gastrointestinal toxicity following acute ingestion or renal failure following chronic exposure.

DECONTAMINATION

Out of Hospital

- Following inhalation, the patient should be moved to fresh air.
- The patient should also be removed from further exposure, including cigarettes.

In Hospital

- Gastric emptying is usually not warranted because of the chronic inhalation nature of most exposures.
- Decontamination of the skin or eyes with water should be considered following dust exposure.

ANTIDOTES

- There is no specific antidote for cadmium poisoning.
- Ethylenediaminetetraacetic acid ($CaNa_2$ EDTA) may increase urinary excretion if administered very soon after acute exposures; however, the role in humans is unclear (see SECTION III, EDTA chapter for dose), and consultation with a medical toxicologist is recommended.
- There is no evidence that chelation is effective in chronic cases.

ADJUNCTIVE TREATMENT

- Hypotension. The patient should be treated with isotonic fluid infusion, the Trendelenburg position, and, if needed, vasopressors. Dopamine is preferred, and norepinephrine is added for refractory hypotension.
- Hypertension should be treated if clinically indicated.
- Obstructive lung disease can be treated using inhaled bronchodilators and antiinflammatory agents.
- Osteomalacia and osteoporosis can be treated with calcium and vitamin D supplements to reduce bone pain.
- Reduced renal function. Nephrotoxic drugs should be avoided if possible.
- Hemodialysis is not useful unless needed for complications of renal failure (e.g., hyperkalemia).

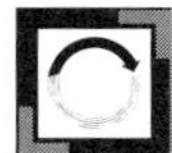

Follow-Up

PATIENT MONITORING

- Acute. Electrolytes, volume status, and complete blood counts may be needed to guide supportive care.
- Chronic. Electrolytes, BUN, creatinine.

EXPECTED COURSE AND PROGNOSIS

- Acute exposures

—Poisoning may be life threatening.
—Toxicity peaks within the first 24 hours, but corrosive, renal, or hepatic injury may require weeks to resolve, or may become permanent.

- Chronic exposures

—Renal insufficiency may progress, despite removal from exposure.
—Pulmonary injury is irreversible.
—Cadmium is an IARC I carcinogen; lung cancer is possibly related to exposure.

DISCHARGE CRITERIA/INSTRUCTIONS

- From the emergency department. Patients may be discharged after acute exposure if adverse effects do not develop within 4 to 6 hours. Perform decontamination and psychiatric evaluation, if needed.
- From the hospital. Patients may be discharged after renal and pulmonary injury have stabilized.

PATIENT EDUCATION

Patients who smoke should be strongly warned of the additive effects of cadmium in cigarettes on episodes of cadmium poisoning.

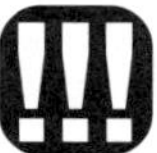

Pitfalls

DIAGNOSIS

Careful occupational history is needed to detect cadmium toxicity.

TREATMENT

It is important to avoid nephrotoxic drugs and therapies that decrease renal function.

ICD-9-CM 985.5

Toxic effect of other metals: cadmium and its compounds.

See also: SECTION II, Hypotension chapter; SECTION III, EDTA chapter; and SECTION IV, Cadmium Fume Fever chapter.

RECOMMENDED READING

Barnhart S, Rosenstock L. Cadmium chemical pneumonitis. *Chest* 1984;86:789–791.

Garry VF, Pohlman BL, Wick MR, Garvy JS, Zeisler R. Chronic cadmium intoxication: tissue response in an occupationally exposed patient. *Am J Indust Med* 1986;10:153–161.

Nogawa K, Kobayashi, Honda R. A study of the relationship between cadmium concentration in urine and renal effects of cadmium. *Environ Health Perspect* 1979;28:161–168.

Roels HA, Lauwerys RR, Buchet JP, Bernard AM, Vos A. Health significance of cadmium induced renal dysfunction: a five year follow up. *Br J Indust Med* 1989;46:755–764.

Author: Scott D. Phillips

Reviewer: Richard C. Dart

Cadmium Fume Fever/Pneumonitis

Basics

DESCRIPTION

- Cadmium fume fever is a transient febrile illness that occurs after inhalation of cadmium oxide fumes.
- Cadmium fume pneumonitis is a serious complication leading to hypoxia and occassionally death.
- Ingestion and inhalation of cadmium can produce other toxicity that is distinct from cadmium fume fever (see SECTION IV, Cadmium chapter).

FORMS AND USES

- Cadmium has broad industrial uses, ranging from the electroplating of steel, to antifriction bearings, to solder used in welding and brazing.
- Cadmium oxide is odorless. Poisoning can occur at concentrations too low to cause respiratory irritation.
- Cadmium oxide fumes result from burning cadmium in processes such as welding, heat-cutting, brazing, silver-soldering cadmium-plated or cadmium-containing metals, smelting, and refining.

TOXIC DOSE

Inhalation of cadmium oxide at a concentration of 40 mg/m^3 may be lethal.

PATHOPHYSIOLOGY

- Fumes of cadmium oxide cause direct injury to the lung.
- Symptoms typically develop over several hours as inflammation develops.

EPIDEMIOLOGY

- Poisoning is uncommon.
- Toxic effects following inhalation are typically mild to moderate, with death occurring in high-concentration exposures.

CAUSES

Toxicity usually results from occupational exposure.

WORKPLACE STANDARDS

NIOSH. IDLH is 9 mg/m^3.

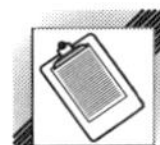

Diagnosis

Toxic causes of delayed pulmonary injury after inhalation exposure include phosgene, phosphine, other types of metal fume fever, oxides of nitrogen, and various types of metals.

SIGNS AND SYMPTOMS

- The physical examination may be initially unremarkable.
- The patient usually presents several hours after the initial inhalation exposure with flulike complaints such as upper airway irritation (cough, shortness of breath) headaches, nausea, chills, fever, and weakness.
- The onset of chest pain and dyspnea is often delayed for 24 to 36 hours.
- Severe cases. Within 72 hours and continuing up to 10 days, chest pain, dyspnea, cough, hemoptysis, wheezing, tracheobronchitis, pulmonary edema, and respiratory failure may occur. Approximately 20% of all cases are fatal.

Vital Signs

Tachycardia, tachypnea, and hypoxia may develop.

HEENT

Anosmia has been reported following chronic exposure.

Pulmonary

After an initial asymptomatic period, the effects range from mild sore throat irritation to severe dyspnea associated with hemorrhagic pulmonary edema that may be fatal.

PROCEDURES AND LABORATORY TESTS

Essential Tests

Arterial blood gases or pulse oximetry, chest radiograph, and pulmonary function tests should be performed in symptomatic patients.

Recommended Tests

- Analysis of the fumes or the material being used is the best method for determining the cause of the pneumonitis.
- Blood or urine cadmium levels above 5 $\mu g/L$ suggest excessive exposure.
- Urinary β_2-microglobulin levels may be elevated.

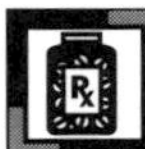

Treatment

Treatment should focus on supportive care with appropriate airway management.

DIRECTING PATIENT COURSE

The health-care professional should call the poison control center when:

- Severe or persistent effects develop.
- Drug interaction or underlying disease presents an unusual problem.

The patient should be referred to a health-care facility when:

- Patient or caregiver seems unreliable.
- Toxic effects develop.
- Drug interaction or underlying disease presents an unusual problem.

Admission Considerations

Inpatient management is warranted for any patient with a history of possible cadmium fume inhalation or who presents with dyspnea, cough, chest pain, hemoptysis, wheezing, tracheobronchitis, pulmonary edema, or respiratory distress.

DECONTAMINATION

- The patient should be moved to fresh air and 100% oxygen should be administered.
- Exposed skin and eyes should be copiously flushed with water.

ANTIDOTES

- There is no specific antidote available for cadmium poisoning.
- Chelation. There are no clear data to support the use of chelation therapy for acute inhalation of cadmium.
- Some investigators propose that immediate treatment with ethylenediaminetetraacetic acid (CaNa EDTA)may be effective.

—Adult dose is 75 mg/kg/day in 3 to 4 divided doses for 5 days, not to exceed 500 mg/kg. The course is repeated once after a drug-free period of 2 days.

ADJUNCTIVE TREATMENT

- If bronchospasm is evident, treatment with inhaled sympathomimetic agents should be considered.
- Aggressive pulmonary care for pneumonitis should be provided.
- Adequate ventilation and oxygenation should be maintained with close monitoring of arterial blood gases.
- Positive end-expiratory pressure in intubated patients or continuous positive airway pressure in nonintubated patients may be necessary.
- Based on anecdotal experience, some clinicians recommend early administration of methylprednisolone, 1 g intravenously as a single dose, in an attempt to prevent the later development of pulmonary edema.
- An antibiotic is indicated when there is evidence of infection.

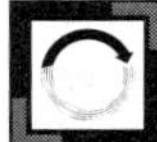

Follow-Up

PATIENT MONITORING

- Continuous cardiac and respiratory monitoring should be performed in symptomatic patients.
- Long-term follow-up including pulmonary function tests may be required.

EXPECTED COURSE AND PROGNOSIS

- If the patient survives the acute exposure, a restrictive ventilatory defect may persist.
- The restrictive impairment improves over time with the greatest improvement in the first 3 months.

DISCHARGE CRITERIA/INSTRUCTIONS

Asymptomatic patients may be discharged after a 12 hour observation period and documentation of normal or baseline pulmonary function.

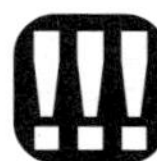

Pitfalls

DIAGNOSIS

- Following acute inhalation of cadmium fumes, there is little warning of impending pulmonary deterioration and there is a lag time of hours before ill effects become manifest.
- Unlike metal fume fever, which is self-limited and not life threatening, cadmium fume pneumonitis can be fatal.

ICD-9-CM 985.5

Toxic effect of other metals: cadmium and its compounds.

See also: SECTION III, Ethylenediaminetetraacetic Acid chapter; SECTION IV, Metal Fume Fever.

RECOMMENDED READING

Barnhart S, Rosenstoele L. Cadmium chemical pneumonitis. *Chest* 1984;86:789–791.

Author: Luke Yip

Reviewer: Ed Kuffner

Caffeine

Basics

DESCRIPTION

Caffeine is a methylxanthine medication most commonly used as a mild stimulant.

FORMS AND USES

- Caffeine, coffeinum, theobromine, and theophylline are methylxanthines.

—Caffeine is found in a wide variety of beverages
—Caffeine is a component in pharmaceutical preparations, including BC Remedy, Cafergot, Darvon Compound, DHC Plus, Esgic-Plus, Excedrin Asprin Free, Excedrin Extra Strength, Fioricet, Fiorinal, Goody's Headache Powders, Midol Maximum Strength, NoDoz, Norgesic Tablets, and Vanquish.

- Apnea of prematurity. Loading dose is 20 mg/kg caffeine citrate intravenously or orally, followed 2 to 3 days later by 5 to 10 mg/kg every 12 hours.
- Headache. Adult dose is 500 mg caffeine sodium benzoate intravenously for two doses.
- Prolongation of electroconvulsive seizures. Adult dose is 500 mg caffeine sodium benzoate 5 minutes before treatment.

TOXIC DOSE

- Adults may develop overt toxicity beginning at 1 g, with death reported at doses of 5 to 10 grams.
- Children have developed toxicity at doses of 36 mg/day.

PATHOPHYSIOLOGY

- Caffeine produces direct antagonism of adenosine receptors and inhibits phosphodiesterase, increasing intracellular cyclic adenosine monophosphate and calcium.
- In overdose, caffeine is associated with elevated levels of epinephrine and norepinephrine. These effects result in smooth muscle relaxation, vasodilation as well as cardiac and CNS stimulation.

EPIDEMIOLOGY

- Poisoning is common.
- Toxic effects are typically mild to moderate.
- Severe toxicity is rare, with death occurring only after massive ingestion or therapeutic dosing errors in infants.

CAUSES

- Poisoning is usually accidental in children or the result of therapeutic misuse in an adult.
- Child neglect or abuse should be considered if the patient is less than 1 year of age, suicide attempt if the patient is greater than 6 years of age.

RISK FACTORS

Patients at the extremes of age are more susceptible to the effects of caffeine.

DRUG AND DISEASE INTERACTIONS

Caffeine produces additive effects with sympathomimetic drugs.

PREGNANCY AND LACTATION

- US FDA pregnancy category B. Animal studies do not indicate fetal risk, and there are no controlled human studies, or animal studies do show an adverse effect but well-controlled human studies have failed to demonstrate fetal risk.
- Caffeine may potentiate the teratogenic effects of alcohol and tobacco.

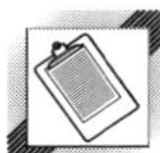

Diagnosis

- Caffeine is similar to theophylline.
- Severe caffeine toxicity causes nausea, vomiting, anxiety, tremors, seizures, dysrhythmia, hypotension, hypokalemia, and an increased anion gap metabolic acidosis.

DIFFERENTIAL DIAGNOSIS

- Toxicologic causes include intoxication with other sympathomimetic drugs (e.g., theophylline, cocaine, amphetamines, ephedrine, phenylpropanolamine) as well as lithium and monoamine oxidase inhibitors. The early stages of serotonin syndrome or neuroleptic malignant syndrome also may appear similar.
- Nontoxicologic causes include agitation from any cause (withdrawal, hypoglycemia, psychiatric disease, etc.).

SIGNS AND SYMPTOMS

Vital Signs

- Tachycardia is common, even with mild toxicity.
- Hypertension may be present early, but progresses to hypotension in more severe cases.
- Hyperthermia may develop in severe toxicity.

HEENT

Mydriasis is common as part of the sympathomimetic state.

Dermatologic

Diaphoresis may develop as part of the sympathomimetic state.

Cardiovascular

- Sinus tachycardia is common.
- A variety of either supraventricular or ventricular dysrhythmias may develop with severe toxicity.
- Hypotension may be heart rate related or a component of generalized cardiovascular collapse seen in severe toxicity.

Pulmonary

Respiratory failure develops rarely, following massive overdose.

Gastrointestinal

Nausea and vomiting are very common.

Fluids and Electrolytes

- Hypokalemia and hyperglycemia are common.
- Lactic acidosis may occur.

Musculoskeletal

Rhabdomyolysis may occur with psychomotor agitation.

Neurologic

- Anxiety, restlessness, insomnia, headache, and tremor are common following mild to moderate overdose.
- Tinnitus, altered mental status, hyperreflexia, clonus, photophobia, and seizures occur with severe intoxication.

Psychiatric

Delirium, psychosis, and hallucinations occur rarely.

PROCEDURES AND LABORATORY TESTS

Essential Tests

- Serum electrolytes, BUN, creatinine concentrations.

—The diuretic effect of caffeine may cause fluid and electrolyte abnormalities.
—An increased anion gap lactic acidosis may be associated with seizures, hypotension, or a hyperadrenergic state.

- ECG

—Sinus tachycardia is common.
—Various tachydysrhythmias may develop.
—Myocardial ischemia is possible.

Recommended Tests

- Serum creatine kinase concentration determination is recommended in symptomatic patients with agitation to detect rhabdomyolysis and guide fluid therapy.
- Urine or serum toxicology screen confirms exposure if history of exposure is absent.
- Serum theophylline level. Caffeine is metabolized to theophylline, and a nontoxic serum level of theophylline may be detected.

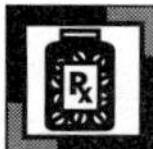

Treatment

- Focus treatment on decontamination, control of vomiting, support of hemodynamic function, and control of agitation.
- Dose and time of exposure should be determined for all substances involved.

DIRECTING PATIENT COURSE

The health-care professional should call the poison control center when:

- Persistent agitation, seizure, hypotension, or serious dysrhythmia is present.
- Signs and symptoms are not consistent with caffeine poisoning.
- Coingestant, drug interaction, or underlying disease presents an unusual problem.

The patient should be referred to a health-care facility when:

- Attempted suicide or homicide is possible.
- The patient or caregiver seems unreliable.
- Serious symptoms have developed.
- Coingestant, drug interaction, or underlying disease presents unusual challenge.

Admission Considerations

Inpatient management is warranted for patients with serious effects: cardiac dysrhythmia, seizures, hypotension, persistent vomiting or agitation, or electrolyte abnormalities.

DECONTAMINATION

Out of Hospital

Emesis should not be induced because of the risk of seizures and possibility of persistent emesis.

In Hospital

- Emesis should not be induced.
- Gastric lavage should be performed in pediatric (tube size 24–32 French) or adult (tube size 36–42 French) patients presenting within 1 hour of substantial ingestion or if serious effects are present. Gastric lavage is not indicated following repeated spontaneous vomiting.
- One dose of activated charcoal (1–2 g/kg) should be administered without a cathartic if substantial ingestion has occurred within the previous few hours.
- Following a large ingestion or in patients who have serious signs or symptoms, one to two extra doses of activated charcoal (0.5–1 g/kg) are recommended at 2- to 4-hour intervals.

ANTIDOTES

There is no specific antidote for caffeine poisoning.

ADJUNCTIVE TREATMENT

Persistent Vomiting Refractory to Initial Antiemetic

- Suggested antiemetic adult regimen is intravenous metoclopramide 0.5 to 1 mg/kg plus intravenous diphenhydramine 25 to 50 mg combined with intravenous prochlorperazine 10 mg or droperidol 2.5 mg.
- Intravenous ondansetron 8 mg infused over 15 minutes is an alternative in refractory cases.

Psychomotor Agitation

- A benzodiazepine familiar to the provider should be administered.

—Diazepam. Adult dose is 5 to 10 mg intravenously, pediatric dose is 0.2 to 0.5 mg/kg intravenously, repeated at 10-minute intervals, titrating to effect, or
—Lorazepam. Adult dose is 2 to 4 mg intravenously, pediatric dose is 0.05 mg/kg, intravenously, repeated at 10-minute intervals, titrating to effect.

- The airway should be monitored closely.

Tachydysrhythmia

- Overview. A variety of standard therapies for tachydysrhythmia have been used (esmolol, lidocaine, phenytoin, and procainamide), depending on rhythm.
- Esmolol. The loading dose is an intravenous bolus of 500 μg/kg infused over 1 minute followed by an infusion of 50 μg/kg/min for 4 minutes. If the response is inadequate, the loading dose is repeated and the infusion increased to 100 μg/kg/min for 4 minutes. Titration is continued until the heart rate is controlled or toxicity (hypotension) develops.
- Unopposed α-receptor stimulation is a theoretical concern during β-blockade. If heart rate or blood pressure increase precipitously during infusion, α-receptor stimulation may be the cause.
- Hypokalemia is common, and potassium should be replaced as needed.

Serious Complications of Intoxication

Hemodialysis is recommended when serious effects such as dysrhythmia, seizures, and hypotension complicate intoxication. It is rarely needed.

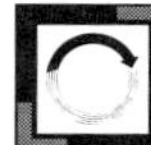

Follow-Up

PATIENT MONITORING

Symptomatic patients require continuous monitoring of respiratory and cardiac status and potassium levels until signs and symptoms of toxicity resolve.

EXPECTED COURSE AND PROGNOSIS

Signs and symptoms typically occur within 2 to 4 hours and peak within a few hours. If treated with appropriate supportive care, nearly all patients recover without sequelae.

DISCHARGE CRITERIA/INSTRUCTIONS

- From the emergency department. The asymptomatic patient can be discharged after gastrointestinal decontamination and 4- to 6-hour observation or after signs and symptoms have resolved, following psychiatric evaluation, if needed.
- From the hospital. The patient can be discharged after signs and symptoms of caffeine intoxication have resolved and following psychiatric evaluation, if needed.

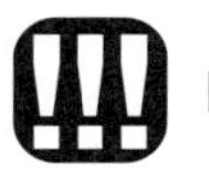

Pitfalls

DIAGNOSIS

- Waiting for the results of toxicologic screening should not delay instituting aggressive supportive care.
- Caffeine withdrawal symptoms may occur following chronic exposure, but would not be expected following an acute overdose.

TREATMENT

There should be no delay in consulting nephrology or transporting patients with life-threatening effects to a facility capable of performing hemodialysis

ICD-9-CM 969.7

Poisoning by psychotropic agents: psychostimulants.

See also: SECTION III, Activated Charcoal chapter.

RECOMMENDED READING

Aaronson LS, Macnee CL. Tobacco, alcohol, and caffeine use during pregnancy. *J Obstet Gynecol* 1989;18:279–287.

Benowitz NL, Osterloh J, Goldschlager N. Massive catecholamine release from caffeine poisoning. *JAMA* 1982;248:1097–1098.

Author: Edwin K. Kuffner

Reviewer: Katherine M. Hurlbut

Calcium Channel-Blocking Drugs

Basics

DESCRIPTION

Calcium channel-blocking drugs (CCBs) are commonly used to treat hypertension and certain cardiac dysrhythmias.

FORMS AND USES

- Typical pharmaceutical formulations include verapamil (Isoptin and Calan), diltiazem (Cardizem), nifedipine (Adalat and Procardia), amlodipine (Norvasc), bepridil (Vascor), isradipine (Dynacirc), nicardipine (Cardene), and nimodipine (Nimotop).
- Sustained-release products include verapamil (Calan SR, Isoptin SR, Covera-HS, and Verelan), diltiazem (Cardizem SR, Cardizem CD, and Dilacor XR), nifedipine (Procardia XL and Adalat CC), nicardipine (Cardene SR), felodipine (Plendil), and nisoldipine (Sular R).
- Treatment of hypertension.

—Typical adult dose of verapamil is 80 mg orally three times per day initially (maximum 360 mg/day); pediatric dose is 3 to 5 mg/kg/day orally in divided doses.
—Adult dose of nifedipine is 10 mg three times per day initially (maximum 120 mg/day); pediatric dose is 0.25 to 0.5 mg/kg.

TOXIC DOSE

- Ingestion of a gram or more of verapamil, nifedipine, or diltiazem can produce serious toxicity and possible death in an adult.
- The other medications in this class appear less toxic, but few data are available on overdose.

PATHOPHYSIOLOGY

- CCBs inhibit entry of extracellular calcium through voltage-dependent calcium channels, thereby reducing contraction of cardiac muscle.
- CCBs also relax arterial smooth muscle but have little effect on venous beds.

EPIDEMIOLOGY

- Poisoning is uncommon.
- Toxic effects following exposure are typically mild to moderate.
- Death occurs in cases involving coingestants or a massive overdose.

CAUSES

- Toxic ingestion is usually intentional.
- Child neglect or abuse should be considered if the patient is less than 1 year of age, suicide attempt if the patient is older than 6 years of age.

RISK FACTORS

Elderly patients and those with underlying cardiovascular disease may be intolerant of even mild hypotension.

DRUG AND DISEASE INTERACTIONS

- Hepatic disease decreases CCB elimination.
- Coingestion of β-blockers, digitalis, or class I antidysrhythmic agents may worsen bradycardia, dysrhythmias, and hypotension.
- Coingestion of other antihypertensives may worsen hypotension.

PREGNANCY AND LACTATION

- All CCBs. US FDA Pregnancy Category C. The drug exerts animal teratogenic or embryocidal effects, but there are no controlled studies in women, or no studies are available in either animals or women.
- Verapamil and nifedipine have been used as tocolytics.
- Verapamil administered to the mother may have cardiovascular effects on the fetus.
- Verapamil, diltiazem, nifedipine, and nicardiopine are excreted in human breast milk.

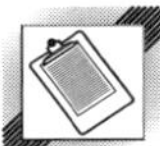

Diagnosis

DIFFERENTIAL DIAGNOSIS

- Toxicologic causes of bradycardia or heart block that resemble CCB overdose include β-receptor blocker, digitalis, class I antidysrhythmics, and clonidine, among others.
- Nontoxicologic causes include ischemic heart disease and severe electrolyte abnormalities such as hyperkalemia.

SIGNS AND SYMPTOMS

- CCBs suppress cardiac function to varying degrees in overdose.

—Verapamil and diltiazem are more effective than nifedipine at suppressing sinoatrial and atrioventricular nodal firing.
—Overdose with any of these agents may result in bradycardia and hypotension.

Vital Signs

Bradycardia and hypotension are common.

Cardiovascular

Effects may include severe bradycardia, atrioventricular block, intraventricular conduction delays, ventricular dysrhythmias, and congestive heart failure.

Pulmonary

- Respiratory depression may develop in patients with hemodynamic instability.
- Pulmonary edema and adult respiratory distress syndrome may develop after severe overdose.

Gastrointestinal

Nausea, vomiting, and ileus can occur.

Neurologic

- CNS depression and syncope can occur.
- Seizure occurs rarely.
- Coma may complicate profound hypotension.

Fluids and Electrolytes

Metabolic acidosis may develop in patients with hypotension.

PROCEDURES AND LABORATORY TESTS

Essential Tests

ECG and continuous monitoring should be performed to detect dysrhythmia or ischemia.

Recommended Tests

- Serum electrolytes, glucose, BUN, and creatinine should be assayed to detect other causes of dysrhythmia or origin of drug accumulation. Hyperglycemia resolves as CCB effects abate.
- Serum creatine kinase should be tested in patients with prolonged seizures or coma to detect rhabdomyolysis.
- Serum acetaminophen and aspirin levels should be measured in overdose setting to detect occult ingestion.
- Head CT, lumbar puncture, bacterial cultures, and other tests are used to assess altered mental status if etiology is unclear.
- Chest radiograph should be taken in a patient with pulmonary symptoms or coma.

Not Recommended Tests

CCB levels are neither easily attainable nor clinically useful.

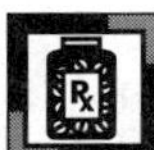

Treatment

- Treatment should focus on continuous ECG monitoring and treatment of dysrhythmia or hypotension.
- Dose and time of exposure should be determined for all substances involved.

DIRECTING PATIENT COURSE

The health-care provider should call the poison control center when:

- Bradycardia, hypotension, altered mental status, or other severe effects are present.
- Toxic effects are not consistent with CCB poisoning.
- Coingestant, drug interaction, or underlying disease presents an unusual problem.

The patient should be referred to a health-care facility when:

- Attempted suicide or homicide is possible.
- Patient or caregiver seems unreliable.
- Toxic effects develop.
- Coingestant, drug interaction, or underlying disease presents unusual problem, or more than one daily dose for age was ingested.

Admission Considerations

Inpatient management is warranted if patient is symptomatic or has ingested sustained release preparation.

DECONTAMINATION

Out of Hospital

Emesis should not be induced; coma or seizures may develop abruptly.

In Hospital

- Gastric lavage should be performed in pediatric (tube size 24–32 French) or adult (tube size 36–42 French) patients for large ingestion presenting within 1 hour of ingestion or if severe effects are present.
- One dose of activated charcoal (1–2 g/kg) should be administered without a cathartic if a substantial ingestion has occurred within the previous few hours.
- Whole-bowel irrigation with a polyethylene glycol solution should be considered following significant ingestion of sustained-release preparation.

ANTIDOTES

There is no specific antidote for CCB poisoning.

ADJUNCTIVE TREATMENT

- Hypotension

—The primary treatment is correction of dysrhythmia, if possible.
—Patient should receive 10 to 20 ml/kg 0.9% saline intravenously and be placed in the Trendelenburg position.
—Further fluid therapy should be guided by central pressure monitoring to avoid volume overload.
—A vasopressor may be added if needed. Dopamine initial dosage is 2 to 5 μg/kg/min titrated upward to effect. Dosages above 20 μg/kg/min are unlikely to have further effect. Norepinephrine may be added if hypotension is unresponsive to dopamine, 0.1 to 0.2 μg/kg/min, titrated to effect.

- If hypotension is unresponsive, or bradycardia, heart block, or signs of serious toxicity are present, calcium administration is recommended.

—Calcium chloride 10% is preferred over calcium gluconate.
—Initial dose for an adult is one ampule (10 ml of 10% solution) infused over 5 minutes; pediatric dose is 10 to 25 mg/kg, up to one ampule per dose.
—Dose may be repeated every 10 minutes as needed; however, if more than two additional treatments are needed, consultation with a poison center or medical toxicologist is recommended.
—Caution: Extravasation may cause skin necrosis.

- Bradycardia or hypotension that is refractory to standard interventions, including administration of atropine, calcium, and vasopressors is treated with glucagon.

—An intravenous bolus of 50 to 150 μg/kg (5–10 mg in an adult) of glucagon should be infused initially, followed by an infusion of 2 to 10 mg/h, titrated to effect.
—Vomiting and hyperglycemia occur frequently.
—If large doses are given, saline should be used to reconstitute the drug instead of the diluent included with the glucagon package.
—Hospital pharmacies often stock insufficient amounts of glucagon.

- Overdoses unresponsive to drug therapy. Intraaortic balloon pump has been used for hemodynamic support.

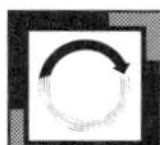

Follow-Up

PATIENT MONITORING

- Continuous respiratory, cardiac, and hemodynamic monitoring should be instituted.
- Serum glucose should be monitored in diabetics and children.

EXPECTED COURSE AND PROGNOSIS

- Most patients do well with gastrointestinal decontamination and supportive care.
- Course may be prolonged and complicated in patients with massive ingestion, advanced age, underlying cardiovascular disease, or coingestion of other myocardial depressant.
- Sequelae of prolonged hypotension may develop in severe cases.

DISCHARGE CRITERIA/INSTRUCTIONS

- From the emergency department. Asymptomatic patients may be discharged following gastric decontamination, 6 hours of observation, and psychiatric evaluation, if needed. Ingestion of a sustained-release product usually warrants 24-hour observation.
- From the hospital. Patients may be discharged following gastrointestinal decontamination, resolution of cardiac effects, and psychiatric evaluation. if needed.

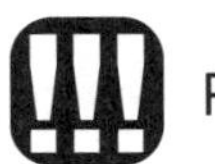

Pitfalls

DIAGNOSIS

Sustained-release products may not produce toxic effects for several hours after overdose.

TREATMENT

- Multiple modes of treatment (pressors, glucagon, isoproterenol, etc.) are often needed simultaneously in patients with severe effects.
- Elderly patients may be intolerant of even mild hypotension.

ICD-9-CM 972

Poisoning by agents primarily affecting the cardiovascular system.

See also: SECTION II, Hypotension chapter; SECTION III, Calcium Gluconate and Chloride and Glucagon chapters.

RECOMMENDED READING

Lewin N. Antihypertensive agents. In: Goldfrank LR, Flomenbaum NE, Lewin NA, et al., eds. *Goldfrank's toxicologic emergencies,* 6th ed. Norwalk, CT: Appleton & Lange, 1998.

Authors: Lada Kokan and Kennon Heard

Reviewer: Richard C. Dart

Camphor

Basics

DESCRIPTION

Camphor is a volatile organic compound with a distinctive odor that is used in many household products, usually at low concentrations.

FORMS AND USES

- The American Academy of Pediatrics Committee on Drugs concluded that camphor has no therapeutic role in medicine.
- Camphor is a colorless or white compound in the form of crystals, granules, or a translucent mass, with a pungent odor and taste.
- Camphor is available in hundreds of over-the-counter form spirits or liniments (Vicks Vaporub, Vicks Vaposteam, Camphophenique, Absorbent Rub, and others).
- Camphor has been used as an antipruritic and topical rubefacient, aphrodisiac, abortifacient, contraceptive, cold remedy, suppressor of lactation, and antiseptic.
- Camphor also has been used as a plasticizer, moth repellent, and preservative in pharmaceuticals and cosmetics; it is used in lacquers and varnishes, explosives, pyrotechnics, embalming fluid, camphorated parachlorophenol and paregoric.

TOXIC DOSE

- The lethal dose is reported to be 50 to 500 mg/kg (5 ml of 100% camphor for a 10-kg toddler).
- In adults, 2 g can produce toxicity.

PATHOPHYSIOLOGY

- Camphor is rapidly absorbed orally, but is also well absorbed via inhalation or skin.
- The precise mechanism of toxicity is unclear.
- Camphor acts as a local tissue irritant as well as a CNS stimulant.
- The most common route of exposure is ingestion, but other exposures have involved inhalation, dermal application, intranasal instillation, intraperitoneal injection, and mother-to-fetus by transplacental transfer.

EPIDEMIOLOGY

- Camphor poisoning is uncommon.
- Toxic effects following exposure are typically moderate to severe.
- Death occurs in a high proportion of cases.

CAUSES

- Toxicity usually results from accidental ingestion or misuse of product.
- Child neglect or abuse should be considered if the patient is less than 1 year of age, suicide attempt if the patient is over 6 years of age.

DRUG AND DISEASE INTERACTIONS

Patients with an underlying seizure disorder may be at increased risk for developing seizures.

PREGNANCY AND LACTATION

- US FDA Pregnancy Category C. The drug exerts animal teratogenic or embryocidal effects, but there are no controlled studies in women, or no studies are available in either animals or women.
- Camphor crosses the placenta and has been associated with one fetal death.
- The topical use of camphorated oil in pregnancy was not associated with teratogenic effects in one study.

WORKPLACE STANDARDS

- ACGIH (for synthetic camphor)

—TLV TWA is 2 ppm (12 mg/m^3).
—TLV STEL is 4 ppm (19 mg/m^3).

- NIOSH. IDLH is 200 mg/m^3.
- OSHA. PEL TWA is 2 mg/m^3.

Diagnosis

DIFFERENTIAL DIAGNOSIS

- Toxicologic causes of gastrointestinal effects and seizure include theophylline, caffeine, nicotine, carbamate or organophosphate pesticides, tricyclic antidepressants, stimulants (amphetamines, cocaine, and ephedrine), lindane, and strychnine.
- Nontoxicologic causes include Reye syndrome, intracranial mass, and porphyria.

SIGNS AND SYMPTOMS

Camphor rapidly produces gastrointestinal irritation and seizures following ingestion. The major manifestations are agitation and seizures associated with oral, throat, and gastric burning.

Vital Signs

Mild tachycardia is common.

HEENT

- Burning of the mouth and throat mucosa are common following ingestion.
- Mydriasis, flickering, darkening, or veiling of vision may occur.
- Ocular irritation, loss of the sense of smell, nasal irritation, and sore throat have occurred in workers exposed to approximately 2 ppm of camphor.
- The patient will often have the odor of camphor on the breath.

Dermatologic

Contact allergy and skin irritation have been reported.

Cardiovascular

- Mild tachycardia is common.
- Circulatory collapse is a rare effect that may develop with severe overdose.

Pulmonary

Postictal respiratory depression and apnea may occur.

Gastrointestinal

Oral and epigastric burning, nausea, and vomiting may develop.

Hepatic

- Mild intoxication may produce elevated liver function tests.
- Chronic ingestion may produce granulomatous hepatitis or fatty metamorphosis.

Neurologic

- Seizures are common; they may occur suddenly and without warning or may be preceded by fasciculation, mental confusion, and irritability.
- Confusion, agitation, delirium, irritability, and tremor also may be seen.

PROCEDURES AND LABORATORY TESTS

Essential Tests

No tests may be needed for asymptomatic patients.

Recommended Tests

- Serum electrolytes, BUN, creatinine, magnesium, and calcium levels should be assayed to evaluate altered mental status, cardiac dysrhythmia, or seizure.
- Serum liver function tests should be performed to detect hepatic injury.
- ECG, serum acetaminophen, and aspirin levels should be measured in an overdose setting to detect occult ingestion.

Not Recommended Tests

Camphor levels are not generally available.

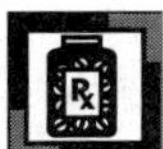

Treatment

- Treatment should focus on controlling seizures and airway management.
- Dose and time of exposure should be determined for all substances involved.

DIRECTING PATIENT COURSE

The health-care professional should call the poison control center when:

- Seizure or other serious effect develops.
- Toxic effects are not consistent with camphor poisoning.
- Coingestant, drug interaction, or underlying disease presents an unusual problem.

The patient should be referred to a health-care facility when:

- History of camphor ingestion greater than 10 mg/kg is obtained.
- Attempted suicide or homicide is possible.
- Patient or caregiver seems unreliable.
- Coingestant, drug interaction, or underlying disease presents an unusual problem.

Admission Considerations

Inpatient management is warranted for patients who develop any toxic effects of camphor exposure.

DECONTAMINATION

Out of Hospital

Emesis should not be induced; coma or seizures may develop abruptly.

In Hospital

- Gastric lavage should be performed in pediatric (tube size 24–32 French) or adult (tube size 36–42 French) patients for patients presenting within 1 hour of a large ingestion or if serious effects are present.
- One dose of activated charcoal (1–2 g/kg) should be administered without a cathartic if a substantial ingestion has occurred within the previous few hours.

ANTIDOTES

There is no specific antidote for camphor poisoning.

ADJUNCTIVE TREATMENT

- Seizure

—Adequate airway and oxygenation should be assured.
—A benzodiazepine familiar to the provider should be administered for initial control.
  —Diazepam. Adult dose is 5 to 10 mg intravenously initially, repeated every 10 minutes as needed; pediatric dose is 0.2 to 0.5 mg/kg intravenously every 10 minutes as needed.
  —Lorazepam. Adult dose is 2 to 4 mg intravenous push over 2 to 5 minutes, repeated every 10 minutes as needed; pediatric dose is 0.1 to 0.2 mg/kg intravenous push over 2 to 5 minutes (not to exceed 4 mg/dose), repeated every 10 minutes as needed.
  —Airway should be monitored closely.
—If seizures persist or recur, another anticonvulsant such as phenobarbital or phenytoin should be added.
—Other options for repeated seizures despite therapy include general anesthesia and neuromuscular blockade with EEG monitoring.

- Standard hemodialysis does not increase elimination of camphor.
- Case reports indicate that lipid hemodialysis or resin hemoperfusion may increase elimination of camphor; however, these techniques are not generally available, and indications for use are unknown.

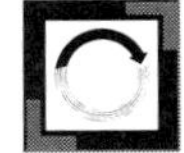

Follow-Up

PATIENT MONITORING

- Continuous respiratory and cardiac monitoring should be performed.
- The possibility of rhabdomyolysis should be monitored if repeated seizures occur.

EXPECTED COURSE AND PROGNOSIS

- Onset is rapid.
- Sequelae of seizures and hypoxia may develop in severe cases.
- Recovery is usually complete within 24 to 48 hours following ingestion unless sequelae of hypoxia intercede.

DISCHARGE CRITERIA/INSTRUCTIONS

- From the emergency department. Patients who remain asymptomatic during 6 to 8 hours of observation may be discharged following decontamination and psychiatric evaluation, if needed.
- From the hospital. Patient may be discharged when toxicity resolves or sequelae of toxicity are stable, following psychiatric evaluation, if needed.

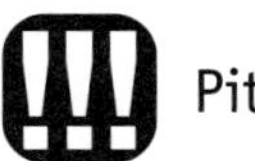

Pitfalls

DIAGNOSIS

Because of its hepatoneurotoxic effects, camphor toxicity may clinically mimic Reye syndrome.

ICD-9-CM 989

Toxic effect of other substances, chiefly nonmedicinal as to source.

See also: SECTION II, Seizure chapter.

RECOMMENDED READING

Cimenez JF, Brown AL, Arnold, et al. Chronic camphor ingestion mimicking Reye's syndrome. *Gastroenterology* 1983;84:394–398.

Ellenhorn MJ. Camphor. In: *Ellenhorn's medical toxicology: diagnosis and treatment of human poisoning,* 2nd ed. Baltimore: Williams & Wilkins, 1997:982–984.

Gibson DE, Moore GP, Pfaff JA. Camphor ingestion. *Am J Emerg Med* 1989;7:413.

Authors: Wei-Fong Kao and Jou-Fang Deng

Reviewer: Katherine M. Hurlbut

Cantharidin (Blister Beetle)

Basics

DESCRIPTION

- Cantharidin is a powder derived from crushed beetles of the order Coleoptera, Family Meloidae.
- Colorless, odorless, poorly soluble in water, cantharidin becomes biologically active and water soluble when reacted with alkali.

FORMS AND USES

- Pharmaceutical Preparations: 1% topical solution
- Animals: More than 2,000 species of blister beetles are known, primarily *Cantharis vesicatorea* (in Europe), *Epicauta vittata* (in the United States), and *Mylabris cichorii*. Cantharidin makes up 0.6% to 5% of the beetle's dry weight.
- Other: Black market powders, oils and solutions, generally marketed as an aphrodisiac (known as Spanish fly) and used in herbal medicine (predominantly in South Africa and China).
- Currently, cantharidin is used therapeutically only as a 1% topical solution for the treatment of warts.

TOXIC DOSE

Toxic effects are typically mild; however, an ingestion greater than 10 mg can be severe, with death occurring in patients ingesting greater than 60 mg.

PATHOPHYSIOLOGY

Cantharidin is a strong mucosal irritant and vesicant producing direct chemical irritation of mucosal tissue. This leads to vascular congestion and end-organ engorgement.

EPIDEMIOLOGY

- Poisoning is common. Most cases go unreported, however, particularly those following use as an aphrodisiac.
- Although the beetles inhabit the African and Asian continents, poisoning occurs in all countries due to transport and sale of the powder as an aphrodisiac.

CAUSES

- Poisonings have occurred via ingestion of a substance containing cantharidin, cutaneous exposure, or ingestion of the beetle itself.
- Most reported poisonings are the result of patients unknowingly ingesting a drink spiked with cantharidin by a hopeful suitor.

PREGNANCY AND LACTATION

Cantharidin is sometimes used as an abortifacient. Potential teratogenic effects are unknown.

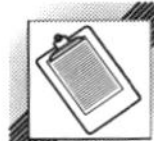

Diagnosis

The typical course is acute onset of gastroenteritis followed by oliguric renal failure in severe cases.

DIFFERENTIAL DIAGNOSIS

Other toxicologic causes of recurrent vomiting and systemic toxicity include arsenic, mercuric chloride, isopropanol, podophyllin, theophylline, colchicine, and many others.

SIGNS AND SYMPTOMS

Vital Signs

Initially normal except in serious cases in which systemic hemodynamic effects develop.

HEENT

- Mucosal edema, bullae, erosions, and bleeding of the oral mucosa may develop within hours of an ingestion.
- Severity seems to be proportional to concentration of preparation.

Dermatologic

- Symptoms may be delayed by several hours.
- Topical application may cause mild to severe blistering and ulceration if the preparation is not used properly.
- The severity of the effects appears to be proportional to the concentration of the preparation.

Cardiovascular

- Sinus tachycardia and nonspecific ECG changes may occur.
- Severe toxicity may terminate in ventricular tachycardia or fibrillation.

Pulmonary

The lungs are usually unaffected, although pulmonary edema, and hemorrhage have been reported.

Gastrointestinal

- Following ingestion, burning and blistering of mucosal surfaces with resultant dysphagia, vomiting, hematemesis, and crampy abdominal pain begin several hours after ingestion.
- Hematochezia or occult gastrointestinal bleeding may occur.

Renal

- Flank pain, polyuria, oliguria, dysuria, increased frequency, hematuria, and proteinuria may occur.
- Hematuria and proteinuria may persist for over 2 weeks.
- Acute renal failure may develop.

Hematologic

Mild disseminated intravascular coagulopathy has been reported.

Neurologic

Mental status depression, seizures, and coma may develop.

Genitourinary

Penile vascular engorgement leading to priapism may occur, as may petechiae, hemorrhagic bullae, and bleeding.

PROCEDURES AND LABORATORY TESTS

Essential Tests

- A complete blood count should be performed in symptomatic patients to evaluate hemorrhage, keeping in mind the lag in hemoglobin decrease in acute blood loss.
- Serum electrolytes, BUN, creatinine, and urinalysis should be performed in symptomatic patients to evaluate the effects of renal injury.
- Rectal examination for blood should be performed to assess gastrointestinal bleeding.
- Cardiac monitoring should be undertaken to assess ventricular dysrhythmias in symptomatic patients, which have been reported in some cases.

Recommended Tests

Coagulation studies should be performed in severe cases.

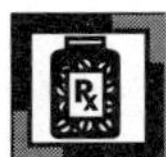

Treatment

- Focus treatment on supportive care of blood and fluid loss and detection of cardiac dysrhythmias.
- Dose and time of exposure should be determined for all substances involved.

DIRECTING PATIENT COURSE

The health-care professional should call the poison control center when:

- Severe or persistent effects develop.
- Signs and symptoms are not consistent with cantharidin poisoning.
- Coingestant, drug interaction, or underlying disease presents an unusual problem.

The patient should be referred to a health-care facility when:

- Attempted suicide or homicide is possible.
- Patient or caregiver seems unreliable.
- Signs and symptoms are not consistent with cantharidin toxicity.
- Toxic effects develop.
- Coingestant, drug interaction, or underlying disease presents an unusual problem.

Admission Considerations

Inpatient management is warranted for patients with evidence of cantharidin poisoning and should be admitted to a unit with cardiac monitoring for at least 24 hours.

DECONTAMINATION

Out of Hospital

Inducing emesis is not recommended due to strong gastrointestinal irritant effects.

In Hospital

- Gastric lavage should be performed in pediatric (tube size 24–32 French) or adult (tube size 36–42 French) patients for large ingestion presenting within 1 hour of ingestion or if serious effects are present, unless recurrent vomiting has occurred.
- One dose of activated charcoal (1–2 g/kg) should be administered without a cathartic if a substantial ingestion has occurred within the previous few hours.

ANTIDOTES

A specific antidote is not available for cantharidin poisoning.

ADJUNCTIVE TREATMENT

- Hypotension. The patient should be treated with isotonic fluid infusion, the Trendelenburg position, and, if needed, vasopressors. Dopamine is preferred, and norepinephrine is added for refractory hypotension.
- Consider transfusion of packed red blood cells if blood loss is substantial.
- Seizures

—A patent airway must be ensured.
—A benzodiazepine is administered for initial control. If seizures persist or recur, another anticonvulsant such as phenobarbital may be added.

- Bladder and ureteral irritation. Isotonic intravenous fluids should be administered to maintain a urine flow of greater than 4 L/day.
- Hemodialysis may be needed for renal failure, but does not increase excretion of toxin.

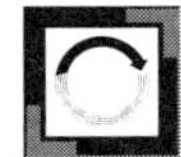

Follow-Up

PATIENT MONITORING

- Symptomatic patients should undergo continuous cardiac monitoring.
- Serial measurement of electrolyte and hematologic tests should be monitored in symptomatic patients.

EXPECTED COURSE AND PROGNOSIS

The effects of cantharidin poisoning are expected to peak within the first 24 hours and resolve over several days. Severe cases develop more rapidly.

DISCHARGE CRITERIA/INSTRUCTIONS

- From the emergency department. Asymptomatic patients may be discharged after gastrointestinal decontamination has been performed, a 6-hour observation period, and psychiatric evaluation, if needed.
- From the hospital. Patients with toxic affects may be discharged after 24 hours of cardiac monitoring or when cardiac and hematologic effects have resolved, and after psychiatric evaluation, if needed.

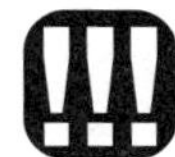

Pitfalls

DIAGNOSIS

Ingestion of a small amount of concentrated solution may result in lethal toxicity.

FOLLOW-UP

Renal injury in severe cases may require several days to resolve.

ICD-9-CM 976

Poisoning by agents primarily affecting skin and mucous membrane, ophthalmologic, otorhinolaryngologic, and dental drugs.

See also: SECTION II, Hypotension and Seizure chapters.

RECOMMENDED READING

Murphy MJ. Cantharidin. In: POISINDEX Editorial Staff, Rumack BH, Hess AJ, Gelman CR, eds. *POISINDEX system.* Englewood, CO: MICROMEDEX, Inc. (edition expires August 31, 1997).

Author: Jay Mullen

Reviewer: Rivka S. Horowitz

Capsaicin (Hunan-Hand Syndrome)

Basics

DESCRIPTION

Hunan-hand syndrome is a painful contact dermatitis resulting from the direct handling of chili peppers (*Capsicum annum*) or other plants containing the alkaloid capsaicin.

FORMS AND USES

- Capsaicin dermatitis is associated with preparation of Chinese or Mexican food because the peppers are commonly used as ingredients.
- Capsaicin is also a component of some incapacitating agents used by law enforcement agencies to subdue individuals.

TOXIC DOSE

- Toxic dose varies by content of capsaicin in the pepper and the duration of the exposure.
- Brief exposure usually produces no effects if the skin is thoroughly washed.

PATHOPHYSIOLOGY

- Capsaicin affects neuronal structures that contain substance P (the undecapeptide neurohumoral transmitter widely distributed in afferent sensory neurons), which is believed to be responsible for communication of pain and itching sensations from the periphery to the central nervous system.
- Stimulation of the cutaneous sensory neurons releases substance P and produces irritation, erythema, burning, or stinging pain without vesiculation.
- Symptoms are due to stimulation of nerve receptors, not local injury to the skin.

CAUSES

Direct handling of peppers without gloves in food preparation is the most common cause.

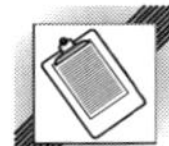

Diagnosis

DIFFERENTIAL DIAGNOSIS

Other toxicologic causes of burning and erythema of the hands include hydrogen fluoride, caustic exposure, contact with marine animals, and causes of peripheral neuropathy.

SIGNS AND SYMPTOMS

Diagnosis is based on a history of handling chili peppers combined with physical findings of irritation, erythema, and burning or stinging pain without vesiculation of areas that were in contact with the pepper or its juice.

HEENT

Ocular exposure may result in erythema, tearing, stinging, and burning pain.

Dermatologic

The exposed area may be erythematous. Vesiculation does not occur with a single exposure, but may with intense, prolonged, or chronic exposure.

Pulmonary

Inhalation of burning peppers or incapacitating spray may cause pulmonary irritation.

Gastrointestinal

Ingestion often causes gastrointestinal irritation, primarily diarrhea.

PROCEDURES AND LABORATORY TESTS

Essential Tests

No tests may be needed for asymptomatic patients.

Recommended Tests

- No tests are typically needed, except those needed to investigate differential diagnosis in unclear cases.
- Pulse oximetry and/or chest radiograph may be needed in patients with respiratory symptoms.

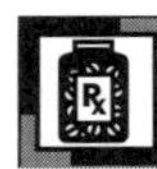

Treatment

Treatment is symptomatic and is challenging because of persistent pain.

DIRECTING PATIENT COURSE

- The health-care professional should call the poison control center when severe or persistent effects develop.
- The patient should be referred to a health-care facility when severe or persistent toxic effects develop.

Admission Considerations

Inpatient management is warranted for symptomatic patients with inhalation exposure.

DECONTAMINATION

- The exposed skin should be washed several times with warm soapy water.
- Alcohol wash may solubilize the remaining capsaicin. This may cause additional pain if the area has been abraded.
- Copious water irrigation is used for mucous membrane or ocular exposure.
- If exposure is respiratory, the patient should be moved to fresh air.

ANTIDOTES

There is no specific antidote for capsaicin poisoning.

ADJUNCTIVE TREATMENTS

- Cold water immersion may help, but seldom provides long-term pain relief.
- Application of lidocaine gel (2%) to the affected area has been reported to be the most consistent method of achieving pain relief.
- Irrigating or immersing the exposed area in vinegar water (5% glacial acetic acid) has been recommended and is continued for as long as the irritation recurs.
- Oral or parenteral analgesics may be required for pain relief.
- Respiratory support including supplemental oxygen may be needed for symptomatic patients following inhalation exposure.

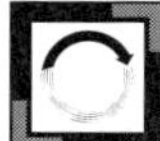

Follow-Up

PATIENT MONITORING

Symptomatic patients following inhalational exposure may need respiratory and cardiac monitoring.

EXPECTED COURSE AND PROGNOSIS

Although capsaicin-induced dermatitis may result in severe pain and discomfort, long-term sequelae have not been reported. Symptoms generally resolve over a period of 2 to 3 days.

DISCHARGE CRITERIA/INSTRUCTIONS

Patients may be discharged from the emergency department or hospital when toxic effects resolve and pain has been controlled.

PATIENT EDUCATION

Patients should be instructed to use gloves when working with hot or chili (jalapeno) peppers containing capsaicin in order to prevent dermal contact.

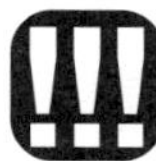

Pitfalls

DIAGNOSIS

Respiratory exposure may not be immediately apparent due to marked mucous membrane symptoms following inhalation.

ICD-9-CM 988

Toxic effect of noxious substances eaten as food.

RECOMMENDED READING

Anderson W. Relief of capsaicin contact dermatitis. *Ann Emerg Med* 1995;26:659.

Tominack RL, Spyker DA. Capsicum and capsaicin—a review: case report of the use of hot peppers in child abuse. *Clin Toxicol* 1987;25:591–601.

Williams SR, Clark RF, Dunford JV. Contact dermatitis associated with capsaicin: Hunan hand syndrome. *Ann Emerg Med* 1995;25:713–715.

Author: Luke Yip

Reviewer: Gerald F. O'Malley

Carbamate Insecticides

Basics

DESCRIPTION

Carbamate insecticides are relatively low toxicity chemicals used in many household, agricultural, and veterinary pest control products.

FORMS AND USES

- Carbamate insecticides are classified by their relative toxicity.
- Low-toxicity products include BPMC (Fenocarb), carbaryl (Sevin), isopocarb (Etrofolan and MIPC), MPMC (Meobal), MTMC (Meacrate and Tsumacide), and XMC (Cosban), and others.
- Moderate-toxicity products include bufencarb (Bux), carbosulfan, pirimicarb (Pirimor), promecarb and thiodicarb.
- High-toxicity products include aldicarb (Temik), aminocarb (Matacil), bendiocarb (Ficam), carbofuran (Furadan), dimetan (Dimetan), dimetilan (Snip), dioxacarb (Eleocron and Famid), formetanate (Carzol), methiocarb (Mesurol), methomyl (Lannate and Nudrin), oxamyl (Vydate), and propoxur (Baygon).

TOXIC DOSE

The toxic dosage of carbamate insecticides varies due to the wide range of products available.

PATHOPHYSIOLOGY

- Like organophosphate insecticides, carbamates inhibit acetylcholinesterase, resulting in the accumulation of acetylcholine and excessive stimulation of the acetylcholine receptor.
- Unlike organophosphates, however, the inhibition is reversible.
- Toxicity may manifest as nicotinic (muscle weakness, fasciculation, hypertension, and tachycardia) or muscarinic (diaphoresis, vomiting, diarrhea, etc.) effects.

EPIDEMIOLOGY

- Poisoning is common.
- Toxic effects are typically mild to moderate.
- Death is rare and usually occurs following a massive exposure or due to delayed treatment.

CAUSES

- Toxic ingestion is usually accidental.
- Dermal or inhalation exposure is usually occupational.
- Child neglect or abuse should be considered if the patient is less than 1 year of age, suicide attempt if the patient is over 6 years of age.

RISK FACTORS

- Agricultural workers, farmers, and gardeners who use pesticides are at increased risk of carbamate poisoning.
- Patients with congenitally low levels of acetylcholinesterase are at increased risk of toxicity from a given exposure.
- Patients with recent subtoxic exposure are at increased risk during reexposure.

DRUG AND DISEASE INTERACTIONS

- Carbamates prolong the activity of some paralytic agents.
- Gentamicin and other antibiotics may prolong carbamate toxicity.

PREGNANCY AND LACTATION

Carbamates cross the placenta; fetal death after ingestion has occurred.

WORKPLACE STANDARDS

- Carbaryl

—OSHA. PEL TWA is 5 mg/m^3.
—NIOSH. REL TWA is 5 mg/m^3.

- Aldicarb is not listed.
- Carbofuran. NIOSH. REL TWA is 0.1 mg/m^3.

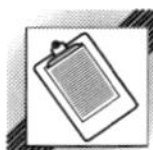

Diagnosis

DIFFERENTIAL DIAGNOSIS

- Other toxicologic causes of acute onset of acetylcholine effects include organophosphates, nicotine, carbachol, methacholine, arecoline, bethanechol, pilocarpine, and certain mushrooms, among others.
- Nontoxicologic causes include myasthenia gravis and Eaton-Lambert syndrome, among others.

SIGNS AND SYMPTOMS

- Muscarinic effects are manifested by the DUMBELS syndrome (**D**iaphoresis and diarrhea; **U**rination; **M**iosis; **B**radycardia, bronchospasm, and bronchorrhea; **E**mesis; excess **L**acrimation; and **S**alivation and seizures) and usually occur soon after exposure.

Vital Signs

Bradycardia, hypotension, and hypothermia may occur.

HEENT

Miosis, blurred vision, salivation, and lacrimation are common.

Dermatologic

Profuse diaphoresis is common.

Cardiovascular

- Hypotension and bradycardia are common with muscarinic agents.
- Cardiac depression and cardiovascular collapse may occur.
- Atrial fibrillation, atrioventricular blocks, and asystole may occur.

Pulmonary

- Bronchospasm and bronchorrhea are common.
- Pulmonary edema is common in severe cases.

Gastrointestinal

Nausea, vomiting, abdominal pain, and diarrhea are common; incontinence may occur.

Renal

Urinary incontinence is common, especially in severe cases.

Musculoskeletal

Fasciculation, weakness, paralysis, and respiratory failure may occur.

Neurologic

Confusion and seizures may occur.

PROCEDURES AND LABORATORY TESTS

Essential Tests

- Red blood cell cholinesterase level correlates roughly with effects; first sample should be drawn before treatment (plasma cholinesterase can be used if red blood cell cholinesterase is unavailable).

—Latent
  —No clinical manifestations are present.
  —Cholinesterase levels are 50% to 90% of baseline for patient.
—Mild
  —Patient is ambulatory and may experience nausea, vomiting, fatigue, headache, dizziness, sweating and salivation, tightness in the chest, and abdominal cramps or diarrhea.
  —Cholinesterase activity is 20% to 50% of baseline.
—Moderate
  —Patient cannot walk and experiences generalized weakness, difficulty in speaking, fasciculation, and miosis.
  —Cholinesterase activity is 10% to 20% of baseline.
—Severe
  —Patient is unconscious, with miosis, fasciculation, flaccid paralysis, increased secretions, moist rales, respiratory difficulty, and cyanosis.
  —Cholinesterase activity is less than 10% of baseline.

- Serum electrolytes, glucose, BUN, calcium, magnesium, phosphate, and creatinine should be assayed in symptomatic patients to detect other causes of dysrhythmia, weakness, or kidney injury.
- ECG and continuous cardiac monitoring should be performed to assess potential causes of hypotension and bradycardia.

Recommended Tests

- Serum acetaminophen and aspirin levels should be measured in an overdose setting to detect occult ingestion.
- Arterial blood gases should be measured if acidosis or hypoxia develop.
- Comprehensive urine drug screen should be performed if the source of intoxication is unknown (drugs abused may contain contaminants).

• Heat CT, lumbar puncture, bacterial cultures, and other tests as indicated should be performed in patients with altered mental status of unknown etiology.
• Negative inspiratory force should be followed to assess ventilatory capacity.
• Chest radiographs will assist evaluation of pulmonary edema.

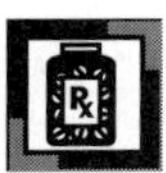

Treatment

• Treatment should focus on decontamination, airway management, and atropine administration
• Dose and time of exposure should be determined for all substances involved.

DIRECTING PATIENT COURSE

The health-care professional should call the poison control center when:

• Breathing difficulty, hypotension, or other severe effects are present.
• Toxic effects are not consistent with carbamate poisoning.
• Coingestant, drug interaction, or underlying disease presents an unusual problem.

The patient should be referred to a health-care facility when:

• Attempted suicide or homicide is possible.
• Patient or caregiver seems unreliable.
• Any toxic effects develop.
• Coingestant, drug interaction, or underlying disease presents an unusual problem.

Admission Considerations

Inpatient management is warranted if patient develops any toxic effects.

DECONTAMINATION

Out of Hospital

• Emesis should not be induced.
• Providers must wear protection to prevent contamination.
• All clothing should be removed from the patient and skin should be washed with soap and water.

In Hospital

• Health-care professionals should wear protective clothing.
• All clothing should be removed from the patient, and skin should be washed with soap and water.
• Gastric lavage should be performed in pediatric (tube size 24–32 French) or adult (tube size 36–42 French) patients for large ingestion presenting within 1 hour of ingestion or if serious effects are present.
• One dose of activated charcoal (1–2 g/kg) should be administered if a substantial ingestion has occurred within the previous few hours.

ANTIDOTES

Atropine and pralidoxime are antidotes for carbamate poisoning.

Atropine

• Indications. Control of bronchorrhea and other secretions
• Contraindication. Preexisting atropinization (dry airway, mydriatic pupils etc.)
• Method of administration

—Adult initial dose is 2 to 4 mg intravenously; dose may be repeated every 5 to 10 minutes as needed until lungs are clear to auscultation.
—Pediatric initial dose is 0.05 mg/kg intravenously; dose may be repeated every 5 to 10 minutes as needed until pulmonary secretions are controlled.
—In severe cases, rapid escalation of the dose may be needed.

• Adverse effects. Anticholinergic symptoms possible with excessive atropine.

Pralidoxime (2-PAM)

• Indications. Patients who require large doses of atropine or have serious signs of cholinergic toxicity.
• Contraindication. Ingestion of carbaryl is relative contraindication.
• Method of administration

—Adult dose is 1 to 2 g intravenously over 15 to 30 minutes or as a continuous intravenous infusion at 500 mg/h (preferred).
—Pediatric dose is 20 to 40 mg/kg intravenously over 15 to 30 minutes.

ADJUNCTIVE TREATMENT

Hypotension

• Atropine should be used if hypotension is due to bradycardia.
• Patient should receive 10 to 20 ml/kg 0.9% saline and be placed in the Trendelenburg position.
• Further fluid therapy should be guided by central pressure monitoring to avoid volume overload.
• A vasopressor may be added if needed. Dopamine is preferred, and norepinephrine is added for refractory hypotension.

Seizure

• Patent airway must be ensured.
• Benzodiazepine should be administered for initial control. If seizures persist or recur, another anticonvulsant such as phenobarbital may be added.

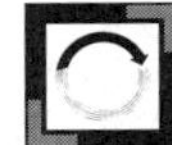

Follow-Up

PATIENT MONITORING

• Continuous respiratory and cardiac monitoring should be performed in symptomatic patients.
• In the case of occupational exposure, patients should not be allowed to work with organophosphate or carbamate pesticides until red blood cell cholinesterase levels have returned to 75% of known baseline.

EXPECTED COURSE AND PROGNOSIS

• Toxicity develops rapidly, peaks within hours, but may persist for days if patient does not receive antidotal treatment.
• Patients who receive early treatment usually recover without sequelae.

DISCHARGE CRITERIA/INSTRUCTIONS

• From the emergency department. Asymptomatic patients may be dishcarged after adequate decontamination, a 6-hour observation period, and psychiatric evaluation, if needed.
• From the hospital. Patients who have not required atropine for 24 hours may be discharged.

PATIENT EDUCATION

Patients should be warned not to return to work until cholinesterase levels of at least 75% of baseline have been documented.

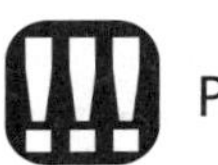

Pitfalls

DIAGNOSIS

Failure to adequately protect health-care providers may result in secondary exposures.

TREATMENT

Atropine should be administered until pulmonary secretions are improved; large doses may be required.

FOLLOW-UP

Patients should have demonstrated baseline or plateau of cholinesterase activity before handling pesticides again.

ICD-9-CM 989.3

Toxic effect of other substances, chiefly nonmedicinal as to source: organophosphate and carbamate.

See also: SECTION II, Cholinergic Syndrome, Hypotension, and Seizure chapters; SECTION III, Atropine and Pralidoxime chapters; and SECTION IV, Organophosphate Insecticides chapter.

RECOMMENDED READING

Rumack BH, Sayre NK, Gelman CR, eds. *POISINDEX system.* Englewood, CO: MICROMEDEX, Inc. (edition expires November 30, 1997).

Author: Kennon Heard

Reviewer: Luke Yip

Carbamazepine

Basics

DESCRIPTION

Carbamazepine is an oral antiseizure medication structurally similar to the tricyclic antidepressants.

FORMS AND USES

- Pharmaceutical preparations of carbamazepine include Tegretol, Epitol, and Atretol.
- Carbamazepine is used as an anticonvulsant, for trigeminal neuralgia, and for bipolar mood disorder.
- Typical doses are 200 mg orally twice a day, increased over a period of 2 weeks to a plateau therapeutic dose of 600 to 1,200 mg per day, divided three or four times daily (adult) or 20 to 70 mg/kg per day divided into three or four doses (child).

TOXIC DOSE

Ingestion of several grams by an adult (several hundred milligrams by a child) may cause ataxia and serious mental status depression.

PATHOPHYSIOLOGY

Carbamazepine selectively inhibits sodium channel recovery from inactivation, predominantly at epileptic foci; there is little effect on normal neuronal firing.

EPIDEMIOLOGY

- Poisoning is common.
- Toxic effects following exposure are typically mild or moderate.
- Death is rare unless coingestants are involved.

CAUSES

- Toxic ingestion is usually accidental.
- Child neglect or abuse should be considered if the patient is less than 1 year of age, suicide attempt if the patient is over 6 years of age.

RISK FACTORS

Geriatric patients are at increased risk of ataxia and falls.

DRUG AND DISEASE INTERACTIONS

- Ingestion of other CNS depressants produces additive CNS toxicity.
- Sodium valproate inhibits the metabolism of carbamazepine-10,11-epoxide, producing toxicity that is similar to carbamazepine toxicity.
- Macrolide antibiotics, propoxyphene, and azole antifungals or any inhibitor of the hepatic P450 enzymatic system may reduce metabolism and increase carbamazepine levels.

PREGNANCY AND LACTATION

US FDA Pregnancy Category C. The drug exerts animal teratogenic or embryocidal effects, but there are no controlled studies in women, or no studies are available in either animals or women.

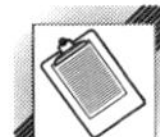

Diagnosis

DIFFERENTIAL DIAGNOSIS

- Toxicologic causes of generalized CNS depression are numerous and include other anticonvulsants, alcohols, benzodiazepines, barbiturates.
- Nontoxicologic causes include electrolyte abnormalities and CNS infection or bleed, among others.

SIGNS AND SYMPTOMS

- CNS depression, ranging from drowsiness to ataxia to coma, is the most common toxic effect.
- Cardiovascular conduction abnormalities have been reported, but are unusual.

Vital Signs

Tachycardia is common; bradycardia and hypotension occur occasionally.

HEENT

Nystagmus can occur at therapeutic doses or overdose.

Dermatologic

Allergic and nonspecific dermatitis, as well as eosinophilia, can occur.

Cardiovascular

- QT interval prolongation is common.
- Atrioventricular conduction delays are rare.

Pulmonary

Respiratory depression progressing to apnea may occur with severe overdose.

Gastrointestinal

Nausea and vomiting may occur.

Hematologic

Anemia and transient leukopenia are common; agranulocytosis and thrombocytopenia are rare. Aplastic anemia is also rare.

Hepatic

Transient elevation of liver enzymes may occur.

Renal

Acute tubular necrosis has been reported.

Fluids and Electrolytes

Water retention with hyponatremia may occur.

Musculoskeletal

Mild elevations of creatinine kinase have been reported, particularly after seizures.

Neurologic

- Drowsiness, ataxia, and slurred speech occur initially; coma may occur with severe overdose.
- Confusion and choreiform movements have been reported.
- Obtundation may wax and wane cyclically, perhaps due to cyclical absorption secondary to anticholinergic effects.

Endocrine

Mild hyperglycemia often develops.

PROCEDURES AND LABORATORY TESTS

Essential Tests

- Serum carbamazepine level should be assayed; ataxia and confusion may develop above the therapeutic level of 6 to 12 μg/dl.
- It is useful to document decreasing serum carbamazepine levels prior to discharge.

Recommended Tests

- ECG should be performed to evaluate for abnormal conduction or atrioventricular block.
- Serum electrolytes, BUN, and creatinine should be assayed in patients with altered mental status to evaluate for hyponatremia.
- CBC should be monitored for aplastic anemia with long-term therapy; leukopenia, anemia, and thrombocytopenia may occur.
- Liver function tests are used to monitor a patient for aminotransferase elevations with long-term therapy.
- Arterial blood gas or pulse oximetry is used to assess effects of CNS depression.
- Serum acetaminophen and aspirin levels are measured in overdose setting to detect occult ingestion.
- Head CT, lumbar puncture, and cultures should be ordered as needed to evaluate other potential causes of altered mental status.

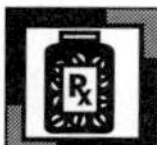

Treatment

- Treatment should focus on control of airway and dysrhythmia.
- Dose and time of exposure should be determined for all substances involved.

DIRECTING PATIENT COURSE

The health-care professional should call the poison control center when:

- Coma, dysrhythmia, hypotension or other serious effects are present.
- Toxic effects are not consistent with carbamazepine poisoning.
- Coingestant, drug interaction, or underlying disease presents an unusual problem.

The patient should be referred to a health-care facility when:

- Attempted suicide or homicide is possible.
- Patient or caregiver seems unreliable.
- Toxic effects develop.
- Coingestant, drug interaction, or underlying disease presents an unusual problem.

Admission Considerations

Inpatient management is warranted if patients exhibit altered mental status, cardiovascular toxicity, or other serious effects such as rising carbamazepine level.

DECONTAMINATION

Out of Hospital

Emesis should not be induced; CNS depression may develop.

In Hospital

- Gastric lavage should be performed in pediatric (tube size 24–32 French) or adult (tube size 36–42 French) patients for large ingestion presenting within 1 hour of ingestion or if serious effects are present.
- One dose of activated charcoal (1 to 2 g/kg) should be administered without a cathartic if a substantial ingestion has occurred within the previous few hours; due to anticholinergic effects and enterohepatic circulation, charcoal administration may be reasonable several hours after ingestion.

ANTIDOTES

There is no specific antidote for carbamazepine poisoning.

ADJUNCTIVE TREATMENT

- QRS widening or dysrhythmia

  —Sodium bicarbonate (1–2 mEq/kg) should be administered in an intravenous bolus and repeated as needed to narrow the QRS interval, but arterial pH should not exceed 7.45 to 7.55.
  —Simultaneous hyperventilation and bicarbonate therapy must be performed with caution because it may cause severe alkalemia and clinical deterioration.
  —Seizures must be controlled concurrently.

- Ventricular tachycardia or multifocal premature ventricular contractions not responding to bicarbonate therapy.

  —Lidocaine should be administered.
  —Adult dose is 50 to 100 mg in an intravenous bolus, followed by an infusion of 2 to 4 mg/min, titrated to effect.
  —Pediatric dose is 1 mg/kg bolus followed by infusion of 20 to 50 μg/kg/min, titrated to effect.
  —The bolus dose may be repeated in 10 to 15 minutes.

- Hypotension

—The primary treatment is correction of dysrhythmia.
—Patient should receive 10 to 20 ml/kg 0.9% saline and be placed in the Trendelenburg position.
—Further fluid therapy should be guided by central pressure monitoring to avoid volume overload.
—A vasopressor may be added if needed. Dopamine is preferred, and norepinephrine is added for refractory hypotension.

- Hemoperfusion decreases serum levels and should be considered for severe complications (seizures and dysrhythmias) not responding to standard therapy.
- Seizure

—A benzodiazepine is administered for initial control.
—Diazepam. Adult dose is 5 to 10 mg initially, repeated every 10 minutes or longer if needed; pediatric dose is 0.2 to 0.5 mg/kg, repeated every 10 minutes or longer if needed; airway should be monitored.
—Lorazepam. Adult dose is 2 to 4 mg by intravenous push over 2 to 5 minutes, repeated every 10 minutes or longer if needed; pediatric dose is 0.1 mg/kg by intravenous push over 2 to 5 minutes, not to exceed 4 mg per dose, and repeated every 10 minutes or longer if needed; airway should be monitored.
—If seizures persist or recur, another anticonvulsant such as phenobarbital or phenytoin should be added.

- Multiple-dose activated charcoal increases clearance but has not been shown to decrease morbidity or mortality.
- Physostigmine should not be used to treat anticholinergic symptoms.

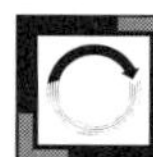

Follow-Up

PATIENT MONITORING

- For acute toxicity, cardiac, respiratory, and neurologic functions should be monitored.
- For chronic toxicity, complete blood count and liver function tests should be monitored.

EXPECTED COURSE AND PROGNOSIS

- Onset of effects after an acute ingestion occurs within hours.
- Most patients recover over a period of 24 hours, longer in cases with coma.

DISCHARGE CRITERIA/INSTRUCTIONS

- From the emergency department. Asymptomatic patients with normal ECG and falling carbamazepine levels during a 6-hour observation period may be discharged following gastrointestinal decontamination and psychiatric evaluation, if needed.
- From the hospital. Patient may be discharged after the resolution of neurologic and cardiac effects for 24 hours and psychiatric evaluation, if needed.

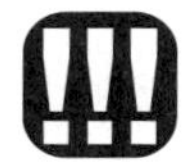

Pitfalls

DIAGNOSIS

Failure to consider other causes of altered mental status can lead to misdiagnosis.

TREATMENT

- Patients have exhibited "cyclical coma" after serious carbamazepine overdose, in which a patient's mental status improves initially but then deteriorates again due to periodic drug absorption.
- Formation of gastric pill concretions has been reported resulting in toxicity delayed up to 48 hours after presentation.
- Failure to assure declining carbamazepine levels may result in deterioration after discharge.

ICD-9-CM 966

Poisoning by anticonvulsants and anti-Parkinsonism drugs.

See also: SECTION II, Hypotension, Seizure, and Ventricular Dysrhythmia chapters.

RECOMMENDED READING

Ellenhorn MJ. Carbamazepine. In: *Medical toxicology: diagnosis and treatment of human poisoning*. Baltimore, MD: Williams & Wilkins 1997:597–599.

Seymour JF. Carbamazepine overdose: features of 33 cases. *Drug Safety* 1993;8:81–87.

Authors: Lada Kokan and Kennon Heard

Reviewer: Luke Yip

Carbon Disulfide

Basics

DESCRIPTION

Carbon disulfide is a sweet-smelling, colorless, and flammable liquid that is a vapor at room temperature.

FORMS AND USES

- Carbon disulfide is an industrial solvent used in the manufacture of adhesives, disinfectants, herbicides, rayon, and other synthetics.
- It is also used as a fumigant, metal treatment, and corrosion inhibitor.

TOXIC DOSE

- Inhalation of 4,800 ppm for an hour can be fatal; inhalation of 20 ppm may cause acute intoxication.
- Ingestion of 15 ml has been fatal.

PATHOPHYSIOLOGY

- Exposure may occur by either ingestion, inhalation, or skin contact.
- The precise mechanism of toxicity is unknown.
- Chronic exposure causes vascular endothelium damage, resulting in atherosclerosis.
- Carbon disulfide is not considered a carcinogenic substance.

EPIDEMIOLOGY

- Poisoning is rare.
- Toxic effects following exposure are typically mild, with death occurring only with massive exposure.

CAUSES

- Poisoning is usually an occupation-related accidental exposure involving inhalation.
- Child neglect or abuse should be considered if patient is less than 1 year of age, suicide attempt if the patient is over 6 years of age.

RISK FACTORS

Workers in factories producing adhesives, disinfectants, herbicides, rayon, and other synthetics are at increased risk of exposure.

PREGNANCY AND LACTATION

- Animal studies suggest an increased rate of spontaneous abortions.
- Human surveillance indicates an increased rate of birth defects.

WORKPLACE STANDARDS

- ACGIH. TLV TWA is 10 ppm.
- OSHA. PEL TWA is 20 ppm; ceiling is 30 ppm.
- NIOSH. REL TWA is 1 ppm; STEL is 10 ppm; IDLH is 500 ppm.

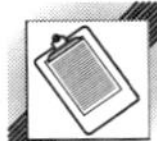

Diagnosis

DIFFERENTIAL DIAGNOSIS

- Toxicologic causes for acute mental status changes include carbon monoxide, hydrogen sulfide or cyanide, and asphyxiant gases.
- Peripheral neuropathy is also caused by acute exposure to mercury, lead, arsenic, manganese, and thallium.

SIGNS AND SYMPTOMS

- Acute exposure symptoms following inhalation include mucous membrane irritation (burning of lips, throat, and chest pain), appearance of intoxication and potentially severe CNS effects (seizure and coma).
- Chronic exposure results in CNS toxicity (cerebellar, atypical parkinsonism) and peripheral neuropathy.

Vital Signs

Tachypnea occurs with acute exposure.

HEENT

- Acute exposure causes lacrimation and mucous membrane irritation.
- Chronic exposure causes vascular disease in the retina.

Dermatologic

Acute exposure causes injury ranging from mild irritation to a full thickness burn.

Cardiovascular

- Acute exposure depresses myocardial function in animal models.
- Chronic exposure in humans increases the rate of atherosclerosis.

Pulmonary

Acute exposure causes dyspnea and transient decreases in oxygenation and vital capacity.

Gastrointestinal

Acute exposure results in nausea and vomiting.

Hepatic

Acute exposure decreases liver metabolism by the cytochrome P450 pathway in animal models.

Neurologic

- Acute exposure has resulted in CNS depression, seizures, and coma.
- With chronic exposure, peripheral polyneuropathy is most common, although brain atrophy, encephalopathy, and cerebellar effects also may occur.
- Atypical parkinsonism also has been reported.

Endocrine

Chronic inhalation exposure may lead to increased cholesterol and triglyceride production.

PROCEDURES AND LABORATORY TESTS

Essential Tests

No tests may be needed in asymptomatic patients.

Recommended Tests

- Patients with respiratory symptoms should undergo pulse oximetry or arterial blood gas analysis to assess oxygenation.
- Patients with chronic exposures may require screening of blood lipids to detect the presence of atherosclerotic heart disease.
- Head CT, lumbar puncture, bacterial cultures, and other tests should be administered as needed to assess altered mental status.
- Electromyography and nerve conduction velocity testing may show abnormalities in the patient with symptoms of neuropathy.
- CT scans of the brain may show cerebral atrophy.
- Urinary 2-Thiothiazdidine-4-carboxylic acid levels have been shown to correlate with exposure.

Not Recommended Tests

Blood and urine level tests are available, but data correlating levels with symptoms are lacking.

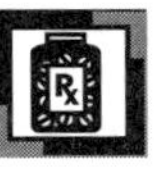

Treatment

- Treatment should focus on supportive care with appropriate airway management.
- The dose and time of exposure should be determined for all substances involved.

DIRECTING PATIENT COURSE

The health-care professional should call the poison control center when:

- CNS depression or other severe effects are present.
- Toxic effects are not consistent with carbon disulfide.
- Coingestion, drug interaction, or underlying disease presents an unusual problem.

Patients should be referred to a health-care professional when:

- Patient or caregiver seems unreliable.
- Attempted suicide or homicide is suspected.
- Toxic effects develop.
- Coingestant, drug interaction, or underlying disease presents an unusual problem.

Admission Considerations

Inpatient management is warranted for patients with CNS depression or signs of persistent irritation.

DECONTAMINATION

Out of Hospital

- Emesis should not be induced.
- Following inhalation, the patient should be moved to fresh air.
- Skin exposures should be irrigated with water for at least 15 minutes.

In Hospital

- Gastric aspiration with a nasogastric tube should be considered in patients presenting within 1 hour of a large ingestion or if serious effects are present.
- One dose of activated charcoal (1–2 g/kg) should be administered without a cathartic if a substantial ingestion has occurred within the previous few hours.
- Following inhalation exposure, oxygen is administered.
- Skin exposures should be irrigated with water for at least 15 minutes.

ANTIDOTES

There is no specific antidote for carbon disulfide poisoning.

ADJUNCTIVE TREATMENT

Seizures

- A patent airway must be ensured.
- A benzodiazepine is administered for initial control. If seizures persist or recur, another anticonvulsant such as phenobarbital may be added.

Bronchospasm

- Oxygen is administered, followed by albuterol 0.15 mg/kg (maximum of 10 mg) in saline with humidified oxygen via nebulizer every 20 to 30 minutes.
- If the peak expiratory flow is greater than 90% of predicted flow rate after initial dose, additional doses may not be needed.

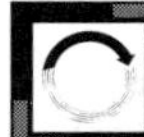

Follow-Up

PATIENT MONITORING

For acute inhalation exposure, follow the oxygen concentration and hemodynamic parameters.

EXPECTED COURSE AND PROGNOSIS

- Patients with acute exposures recover quickly if sequelae of hypoxia do not intercede.
- Chronic exposures can lead to permanent CNS toxicity, peripheral neuropathy, increased rates of cardiovascular disease and chronic gastritis.
- Neuropathy and encephalopathy do not appear to improve with termination of exposure.

DISCHARGE CRITERIA/INSTRUCTIONS

- From the emergency department. Asymptomatic patients may be discharged, following a 4- to 6-hour observation period and psychiatric evaluation, if needed.
- From the hospital. Patients may be discharged after acute effects resolve or stabilize.

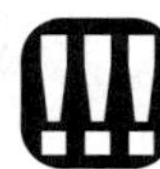

Pitfalls

DIAGNOSIS

In patients likely to have been exposed, carbon disulfide should be suspected when neuropathy occurs.

FOLLOW-UP

Patients with chronic exposure should have lipid profiles followed.

ICD-9-CM 987

Toxic effect of other gases, fumes, or vapors.

See also: SECTION II, Coma, Peripheral Neuropathy, and Seizures chapters.

RECOMMENDED READING

Abadin H, Liccione JJ. *Toxicologic profile for carbon disulfide.* Bethesda, MD: US Department of Health and Human Services, 1996.

Spyker DA, Gallanosa AG, Suratt PM. Health effects of acute carbon disulfide exposure. *J Toxicol Clin Toxicol* 1982;19:87–93.

Author: Kennon Heard

Reviewer: Richard C. Dart

Carbon Monoxide

Basics

DESCRIPTION

Carbon monoxide is a colorless and odorless gas generated by burning organic materials.

FORMS AND USES

- Common sources of exposure include the furnace, stove, water heater, gasoline power tools, automobile (or any internal combustion engine), especially if operated indoors.
- Carbon monoxide also may be produced by the metabolism of methylene chloride or nickel carbonyl.

TOXIC DOSE

- Most sources of carbon monoxide can produce sufficient amounts to rapidly produce life-threatening toxicity.
- Heavy cigarette smoking can produce a carboxyhemoglobin level of up to 12%.

PATHOPHYSIOLOGY

- Carbon monoxide binds to heme proteins, including hemoglobin and myoglobin. The term *carboxyhemoglobin* refers to hemoglobin to which carbon monoxide has bound. This displaces oxygen from hemoglobin and reduces the ability of hemoglobin to release oxygen to the tissues, thereby decreasing oxygen delivery and producing tissue hypoxia.
- Carbon monoxide also binds to mitochondrial proteins, resulting in microvascular dysfunction.

—This sets the stage for neutrophil infiltration of the endothelium and the release of proteases. Hypoxia causes the endothelial xanthine dehydrogenase to be converted to xanthine oxidase.
—This oxidase generates oxygen-free radicals and hydrogen peroxide, resulting in lipid peroxidation of the cell membrane.
—This may be the mechanism of delayed neuronal injury.

- Lack of sufficient oxygen produces anaerobic glycolysis and the production of lactic acidosis.

EPIDEMIOLOGY

- Carbon monoxide is a leading cause of poisoning death, with up to 8,000 deaths reported each year in the United States.
- Toxic effects following exposure are typically related to the dose (concentration × time).
- Death is common, and usually occurs before the patient reaches a health-care facility.

CAUSES

- The cause may be accidental or intentional.
- Child neglect or abuse should be considered if the patient is less than 1 year of age, suicide attempt if the patient is over 6 years of age.

RISK FACTORS

- Working in proximity to an internal combustion device such as a furnace or automobile engine increases the risk of carbon monoxide poisoning.
- Infants and children may be at higher risk of toxicity because their exposure is increased by high minute ventilation volume and high metabolic rate.
- Elderly patients are more susceptible to poisoning and may have a greater incidence of long-term sequelae.

PREGNANCY AND LACTATION

- Carbon monoxide may have teratogenic and embryotoxic potential when the exposure has been sufficient to cause maternal toxicity.
- Fetal carboxyhemoglobin is higher than that of the exposed mother. Exposure during pregnancy may lead to fetal CNS injury, death, and spontaneous abortion.

WORKPLACE STANDARDS

- ACGIH. TLV TWA is 25 ppm; TLV STEL is 400 ppm.
- NIOSH. REL TWA is 35 ppm; IDLH is 1,200 ppm.
- OSHA. PEL TWA is 50 ppm; PEL ceiling is 200 ppm.

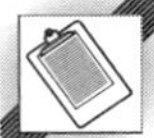

Diagnosis

DIFFERENTIAL DIAGNOSIS

- Toxicologic causes of altered mental status or coma combined with acidosis after an inhalation exposure include cyanide (smoke inhalation), hydrogen sulfide, and severe asphyxiant exposure.
- Other common causes of altered mental status include, among others, opioids, sedative-hypnotic agents, ethanol, gamma-hydroxybutyrate, rohypnol ("roofies"), α_2-receptor agonists (clonidine and tetrahydrozoline), tricyclic antidepressants, methanol, anticonvulsants, and ethylene glycol.
- Nontoxicologic causes include numerous intracranial events or electrolyte abnormalities.

SIGNS AND SYMPTOMS

The typical acute carbon monoxide poisoning initially produces headache, nausea, and vomiting, followed by progressive depression of mental status as the exposure continues. Organs with high oxygen utilization such as the brain and heart are the most affected.

Vital Signs

- Tachycardia, tachypnea, and mild hypertension are common.
- In severe cases, bradycardia and hypotension with respiratory depression may develop.
- Hypothermia is often present if coma has been prolonged.

HEENT

- Results of the funduscopic examination are usually normal, but in serious poisoning may reveal papilledema, optic atrophy, retinal hemorrhage, or vein engorgement.
- Visual field defects, including central scotomata, homonymous hemianopia, blindness, and retrobulbar neuritis have been reported.
- Sensorineural hearing loss has occurred rarely.

Dermatologic

- Bullae, vesicles, and erythematous patches that are not always associated with areas of direct pressure may occur.
- The classic cherry-red skin coloration is usually found only postmortem.

Cardiovascular

- Tachycardia, hypotension, peripheral vasodilation, cyanosis, shock, and cardiac arrest may develop.
- Ischemic chest pain may develop.

Pulmonary

- Dyspnea and pulmonary edema may occur.
- Aspiration pneumonia and adult respiratory distress syndrome often complicate severe exposure with coma.

Gastrointestinal

- Nausea and vomiting occur in both acute and subacute poisoning.
- Subacute and mild acute exposure may mimic gastrointestinal or viral illness.

Renal

- With significant poisonings, myoglobinuria and albuminuria have occurred.
- Both oliguric and nonoliguric renal failure have been reported.

Fluids and Electrolytes

- Lactic acidosis indicates serious poisoning.
- Volume depletion is common if coma has occurred.

Musculoskeletal

- Muscle necrosis may develop even in the absence of pressure injury, due to myocyte injury and death.
- Marked elevation in creatine kinase may occur.

Neurologic

- The CNS is the major target organ of carbon monoxide poisoning. In general, symptoms progress from headache, dizziness, disorientation and difficulty in thinking, to fainting, cerebral edema, coma, seizures, and death.
- In most cases, particularly those with mild effects, recovery is complete.
- Delayed neurologic sequelae (DNS) may occur following severe poisoning.

—The incidence ranges from 1% to 40%.
—DNS sequelae may include apathy, difficulty in speaking, visual loss, movement disorders, tremor, and parkinsonian syndrome.

Endocrine

Hyperglycemia following acute exposure has been reported.

PROCEDURES AND LABORATORY TESTS

Essential Tests

- Carboxyhemoglobin level from venous or arterial blood is measured to document exposure.

—Levels do not correlate well with toxicity, except at low levels.
—The half-life of carboxyhemoglobin is 4 to 6 hours while breathing room air, 40 to 90 minutes on 100% oxygen administered via a non-rebreathing face mask, and 30 to 40 minutes during treatment with hyperbaric oxygen.
—Smoking will produce carboxyhemoglobin levels of up to 12%.

- Serum electrolytes, BUN, and creatinine are measured to assess anion gap metabolic acidosis or renal injury.
- ECG and cardiac enzymes in symptomatic patients are used to assess potential myocardial ischemia (or cardiotoxic coingestant).

Recommended Tests

- Serum creatine kinase will become elevated if rhabdomyolysis occurs.
- Serum lactate should be measured in patients with metabolic acidosis. An elevated level indicates prolonged duration of carbon monoxide exposure.
- Serum liver function tests and coagulation tests are used in severe, comatose cases, where multiple organ failure may develop.
- Serum acetaminophen and salicylate levels in overdose setting are measured to evaluate occult ingestion.
- Serial mental status examinations, mini-mental status tests, or formal neuropsychiatric testing may be needed under certain conditions. Consultation with a medical toxicologist or other physician experienced in the application of these tests is recommended.
- Head CT or MRI with abnormalities within 6 hours of exposure indicate moderate to severe poisoning. Patients with gray matter changes (basal ganglion hypodensities on CT) may still have a good outcome. Those with white matter lesions often fare poorly.

Not Recommended Tests

Pulse oximetry will remain normal despite the presence of carboxyhemoglobin.

Carbon Monoxide

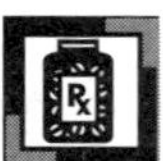

Treatment

• Treatment should focus on airway management, provision of supplemental oxygen, and hemodynamic support.
• Dose and time of exposure should be determined for all substances involved.

DIRECTING PATIENT COURSE

The health-care professional should call the poison control center when:

• Evidence of end-organ damage is present (altered mental status, acidosis, chest pain) or the patient's carboxyhemoglobin level is elevated.
• Patient is pregnant.
• Hyperbaric oxygen is being considered.
• Toxic effects are not consistent with carbon monoxide poisoning.
• Coingestant, drug interaction, or underlying disease presents an unusual problem.

The patient should be referred to a health-care facility when:

• History consistent with carbon monoxide poisoning is obtained.
• Attempted suicide or homicide is possible.
• Patient or caregiver seem unreliable.
• Coingestant, drug interaction, or underlying disease presents an unusual problem.

Admission Considerations

Inpatient management is warranted for pregnant patients, elderly patients, and all patients with serious exposure (neurologic signs or symptoms, chest pain, abnormal ECG, or acidosis).

DECONTAMINATION

Out of Hospital

The patient should be removed from exposure and administered supplemental oxygen.

In Hospital

Gastrointestinal decontamination should be performed if it is needed for coingestant.

ANTIDOTES

Oxygen at Normal Pressure

• Indications. All patients with possible carbon monoxide poisoning.
• Contraindications. None, possible CO_2 retention in patient with chronic obstructive pulmonary disease.
• Method of administration. 15 L/min via nonrebreather mask for 4 to 6 hours until patient becomes asymptomatic, carbon monoxide is excluded as cause, or hyperbaric oxygen is initiated.

Oxygen at Hyperbaric Pressure

• Consultation with a medical toxicologist or hyperbaric physician is recommended.
• Indications are not well defined, but include:

—Loss of consciousness
—Seizure
—Pregnant patient with carboxyhemoglobin level greater than 15%

• Contraindications

—Hemodynamically unstable patients
—Untreated pneumothorax

• Method of administration

—Hyperbaric medical service should be contacted.
—Typical hyperbaric regimen is 100% oxygen at 2.7 atmospheres absolute (ATA) for 30 minutes. The pressure is then decreased to 2.2 ATA for 90 min.
—Repeated treatments are sometimes provided until CNS is baseline. Often one additional treatment is performed.

• Potential adverse effects. Oxygen toxicity, barotrauma, pneumothorax, and seizures are all treated initially by discontinuation of hyperbaric treatment.

ADJUNCTIVE TREATMENT

• Hypotension. The patient should be treated with isotonic fluid infusion, the Trendelenburg position, and, if needed, vasopressors. Dopamine is preferred, and norepinephrine may be added for refractory hypotension.
• Myocardial ischemia is treated in the standard manner. The primary difficulty is the decision to perform hyperbaric therapy in a potentially unstable patient with myocardial ischemia. However, ischemia caused by carbon monoxide poisoning is often resistant to standard therapies.
• Seizures

—Patent airway must be ensured.
—A benzodiazepine is administered for initial control. If seizures persist or recur, another anticonvulsant such as phenobarbital may be added.
—In refractory cases consider general anesthesia with EEG monitoring.

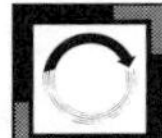

Follow-Up

PATIENT MONITORING

Respiratory and cardiac monitoring should be performed continuously in symptomatic patients.

EXPECTED COURSE AND PROGNOSIS

- Most patients with mild exposure do well with therapy of 100% oxygen by face mask.
- Toxic effects peak in the first few hours and often resolve over a few hours after discontinuation of exposure.
- Patients with more severe exposure may not recover completely. Sequelae may range from difficulty concentrating or personality changes to persistent vegetative state.
- In some cases, initial recovery is followed by persistent CNS injury or development of delayed neuropsychiatric sequelae.

DISCHARGE CRITERIA/INSTRUCTIONS

- From the emergency department. Asymptomatic or minimally symptomatic patients (without history of loss of consciousness) may be discharged after treatment with oxygen, when they become asymptomatic, and after psychiatric evaluation, if needed.
- From the hospital. Patients who meet the criteria for hyperbaric oxygen may be discharged after one or two treatments, if improved, and following psychiatric evaluation, if needed. Follow-up visits should be arranged for further therapy and serial evaluation.

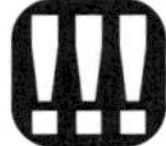

Pitfalls

DIAGNOSIS

Carbon monoxide poisoning should be considered in all patients with flulike symptoms, especially if multiple family members are affected.

TREATMENT

- It is important to consider hyperbaric oxygen for moderately or severely poisoned patients.
- It is vital to identify the source of exposure to prevent reexposure.
- A carboxyhemoglobin level drawn a few hours after end of exposure can be misleading because carbon monoxide has been eliminated. Therapy should be based on clinical manifestations.

FOLLOW-UP

It is necessary that the patient return if symptoms develop after the poisoning for evaluation of delayed neurologic sequelae.

ICD-9-CM 986

Toxic effect of carbon monoxide.

See also: SECTION II, Hypotension and Seizure chapters; SECTION III, Hyperbaric Oxygen chapter; and SECTION IV, Nickel Carbonyl chapter.

RECOMMENDED READING

Crocker PJ, Walker JS. Pediatric carbon monoxide toxicity. *J Emerg Med* 1985;3:443–448.

Ducasse JL, Celsis P, Marc-Vergnes JP. Noncomatose patients with acute carbon monoxide poisoning: hyperbaric or normobaric oxygenation? *Undersea Hyperbaric Med* 1995;22:9–15.

Gorman DF, Clayton D, Gilligan JE, et al. A longitudinal study of 100 consecutive admissions for carbon monoxide poisoning to The Royal Adelaide Hospital. *Anaesth Intens Care* 1992;20:311–316.

Koren G, Sharav T, Pastuszak A, et al. A multicenter, prospective study of fetal outcome following accidental carbon monoxide poisoning in pregnancy. *Reprod Toxicol* 1991;5:397–403.

Raphael JC, et al. Trial of normobaric and hyperbaric oxygen for acute carbon monoxide intoxication. *Lancet* 1989;19;414–418.

Thom SR, Taber RL, Mendiguren H, et al. Delayed neuropsychologic sequelae after carbon monoxide poisoning: prevention by treatment with hyperbaric oxygen. *Ann Emerg Med* 1995;25:474–480.

Author: Scott D. Phillips

Reviewer: Richard C. Dart

Carisoprodol

Basics

DESCRIPTION

Carisopradol is a centrally-acting oral skeletal muscle relaxant.

FORMS AND USES

- Pharmaceutical preparations include carisoprodol (Soma), carisoprodol in combination with salicylate (Soma Compound), and carisoprodol in combination with salicylate and codeine (Soma Compound with Codeine).
- Carisoprodol is a skeletal muscle relaxant for muscle spasm conditions.

—Adult dose is 350 mg orally, three times a day and at bedtime.
—This drug is not recommended for use by patients less than 12 years of age.

TOXIC DOSE

Ingestion of gram quantities may cause intoxication in an adult, death in a child.

PATHOPHYSIOLOGY

- Carisoprodol acts by blocking interneuronal activity in the descending reticular formation and spinal cord.
- Carisoprodol is metabolized to meprobamate in the liver and excreted by the kidney.
- This drug is frequently combined with aspirin and codeine; toxicity may result from these components in overdose.

EPIDEMIOLOGY

- Poisoning is uncommon.
- Toxic effects following exposure are typically mild.
- Death may occur from coingestant or in patients with inadequate airway management.

CAUSES

- Toxic ingestion is usually suicidal.
- Child abuse or neglect must be considered if the patient is less than 1 years of age, a suicide attempt should be considered if the child is older than 6 years of age.

RISK FACTORS

- Acute or chronic injury with muscle spasm
- Drug abuse or dependence

DRUG AND DISEASE INTERACTIONS

- Alcohol and other drugs that cause CNS depression may be additive to the effects of carisoprodol.
- Long-term use may lead to dependence and increased tolerance for narcotics.

PREGNANCY AND LACTATION

US FDA Pregnancy Category C. Studies have shown that the drug exerts animal teratogenic or embryocidal effects, but there are no controlled studies in women, or no studies are available in either animals or women.

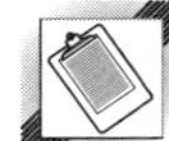

Diagnosis

DIFFERENTIAL DIAGNOSIS

Carisoprodol overdose causes nonspecific CNS depression and may be difficult to distinguish from the numerous other drugs that produce similar nonspecific signs (ethanol, benzodiazepines, and other muscle relaxants, among others).

SIGNS AND SYMPTOMS

- The primary effect of overdose is CNS depression leading to respiratory depression, coma, and death (in cases with inadequate airway management).

Vital Signs

Mild tachycardia and postural hypotension can occur.

Dermatologic

Erythema multiforme, pruritic rash, facial flush, and fixed drug eruption occur rarely.

Cardiovascular

Tachycardia and postural hypotension are common.

Gastrointestinal

Nausea, vomiting, and epigastric distress may occur.

Hematologic

Leukopenia occurs during chronic therapy, rarely.

Musculoskeletal

Transient idiosyncratic reaction manifested by extreme weakness and transient quadriplegia rarely occurs during chronic therapy.

Neurologic

- Mild CNS depression is common and may become severe.
- Transient idiosyncratic reaction manifested by ataxia, loss of vision, diplopia, mydriasis, dysarthria, agitation, and confusion occurs rarely.

PROCEDURES AND LABORATORY TESTS

Essential Tests

No tests may be needed because most cases involve only mild CNS effects.

Recommended Tests

- Arterial blood gas, pulse oximetry, serum electrolytes, BUN, and creatinine should be monitored in patients with alteration in mental status or cardiovascular effects.
- ECG, serum acetaminophen, and aspirin levels should be obtained in patients with intentional overdose to detect occult ingestion.

Not Recommended Tests

Carisoprodol levels are not clinically useful.

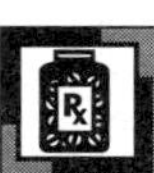

Treatment

- Treatment should focus on airway management and hemodynamic support.
- Dose and time of exposure should be determined for all substances involved.
- Mechanical ventilation may be needed for respiratory depression.

DIRECTING PATIENT COURSE

The health-care professional should call the poison control center when:

- Altered mental status or hemodynamic effects occur.
- Signs and symptoms are not consistent with carisoprodol toxicity.
- Coingestant, drug interaction, or underlying disease presents an unusual problem.

The patient should be referred to a health-care facility when:

- Any clinical effects become apparent.
- Coingestant, drug interaction, or underlying disease presents an unusual problem.

Admission Considerations

Inpatient management is warranted if patients develop profound weakness, hypotension, respiratory or CNS depression, seizure, significant airway compromise, persistent or life-threatening dysrhythmia, or have underlying medical conditions that warrant prolonged observation.

DECONTAMINATION

Out of Hospital

Emesis should not be induced because of the possibility of CNS or respiratory depression.

In Hospital

- Gastric lavage should be performed in pediatric (tube size 24–32 French) or adult (tube size 36–42 French) patients for large ingestion presenting within 1 hour of ingestion or if serious effects are present.
- One dose of activated charcoal (1–2 g/kg) should be administered without a cathartic if a substantial ingestion has occurred within the previous few hours.

ANTIDOTES

There is no specific antidote for carisoprodol poisoning.

ADJUNCTIVE TREATMENT

Hypotension

- Patient should receive 10 to 20 ml/kg 0.9% saline and be placed in the Trendelenburg position.
- Further fluid therapy should be guided by central monitoring or right heart catheter to avoid volume overload.
- If hypotension is unresponsive, a vasopressor should be administered.

—Dopamine. Dosage for adult or pediatric patient is 2 to 5 μg/kg/min, titrated to desired effect; rates above 20 μg/kg/min are unlikely to provide further benefit.
—Norepinephrine. If hypotension is unresponsive, 0.1 to 0.2 μg/kg/min should be added and titrated to desired effect.

- Other options include phenylephrine and levarterenol.
- A high rate of infusion may cause tissue ischemia.

Seizure

- A benzodiazepine should be administered for initial control.

—Diazepam. Adult dose is 5 to 10 mg intravenously, repeated every 10 minutes, if needed; pediatric dose is 0.2 to 0.5 mg/kg, repeated every 10 minutes, if needed.
—Lorazepam. Adult dose is 2 to 4 mg intravenous push over 2 to 5 minutes, repeated every 10 minutes, if needed; pediatric dose is 0.1 mg/kg intravenous push over 2 to 5 minutes, not to exceed 4 mg/dose, repeated every 10 minutes or longer, if needed.

- The need for intubation should be monitored closely.
- If seizures persist or recur, another anticonvulsant such as phenobarbital or phenytoin may be added.

Not Recommended

Diuresis is not useful in enhancing elimination.

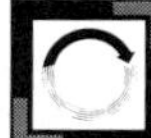

Follow-Up

PATIENT MONITORING

Respiratory status and cardiac rhythm should be monitored continuously until dysrhythmias resolve and patient is stable.

EXPECTED COURSE AND PROGNOSIS

- Most cases have minimal effects and resolve within hours.
- Recovery is the rule in cases with mental status depression or respiratory depression, unless adequate airway could not be provided.
- Sequelae of hypoxia are possible complications.

DISCHARGE CRITERIA/INSTRUCTIONS

- From the emergency department. Patients who develop no signs or transient CNS or respiratory depression that resolves within 6 hours after ingestion may be discharged after decontamination and psychiatric evaluation, if needed.
- From the hospital. Patients may be discharged upon resolution of CNS or respiratory depression, hypotension, and psychiatric evaluation, if needed.

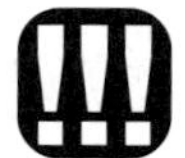

Pitfalls

DIAGNOSIS

- Carisoprodol toxicity may be confused with that of other agents that produce nonspecific CNS or respiratory depression.
- Idiosyncratic reaction is uncommon and may be mistaken for conditions that produce cranial nerve palsy.
- Failure to screen for common combination drugs of salicylate and narcotics can lead to misdiagnosis.

ICD-9-CM 968.0

Poisoning by central nervous system muscle tone depressants (Carisoprodol).

See also: SECTION II, Hypotension and Seizure chapters.

RECOMMENDED READING

Littrell RA, Hayes LR, Stillner V. Carisoprodol (Soma): a new and cautious perspective of an old agent. *South Med J* 1993;86:754–756.

Littrell RA, Sage T, Miller W. Case report: meprobamate dependence secondary to carisoprodol (Soma) use. *Am J Drug Alcohol Abuse* 1993;19:133–134.

Olsen H, Koppang E, Alvan G, et al. Carisoprodol elimination in humans. *Ther Drug Monit* 1994;16:337–340.

Author: Steven A. Seifert

Reviewer: Richard C. Dart

Caustics—Acidic

Basics

DESCRIPTION

Acids are caustic substances with a pH of less than 7.

FORMS AND USES

- Acidic caustic substances include phosphoric acid, sulfuric acid, oxalic acid, acetic acid, hydrochloric acid, formic acid, and nitric acid. Hydrofluoric acid, boric acid, chromic acid, selenious acids are included in separate chapters.
- Acids are used in a variety of household products: toilet bowl cleaners, descalers, metal cleaners, antirust compounds, battery fluid, and pool sanitizers.
- Industrial uses of concentrated acids include plating, photography, cement manufacturing, leather tanning, bleaching, metal refining, plumbing, engraving, metal cleaning, rustproofing, chemicals, munitions and fertilizer manufacturing, hat making, printing, dyeing, rayon manufacturing, hair-wave neutralizing, airplane glue manufacturing, blueprint paper production, cellulose formate manufacturing, and many other areas of production.

TOXIC DOSE

The toxic dose varies tremendously by type and concentration of acid.

PATHOPHYSIOLOGY

- Acids cause coagulation necrosis on contact with mucosal surfaces, destroying submucosal structures.
- Fumes may cause airway irritation, bronchospasm, and adult respiratory distress syndrome in severe cases.

EPIDEMIOLOGY

- Poisoning is common.
- Toxic effects following exposure are typically mild.
- Death occurs after ingestion of a large amount of dilute solution or a smaller amount of concentrated, highly acidic compounds.
- Occupational exposure to acid mists is associated with laryngeal cancer.

CAUSES

- Toxic ingestion is usually accidental in children.
- Adult toxicity is most likely to result from suicidal or occupational exposure.
- Child neglect or abuse should be considered if the patient is less than 1 year of age, suicide attempt if the patient is older than 6 years of age.

WORKPLACE STANDARDS

Hydrochloric Acid

- ACGIH. TLV ceiling is 5 ppm (7 mg/m^3).
- OSHA. PEL ceiling is 5 ppm (7 mg/m^3).
- NIOSH

—REL ceiling is 5 ppm (7mg/m^3).
—IDLH is 50 ppm.

Nitric Acid

- OSHA

—PEL TWA is 2 ppm (5 mg/m^3).
—STEL is 4 ppm (10 mg/m^3).

- NIOSH. IDLH is 25 ppm.

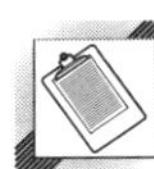

Diagnosis

DIFFERENTIAL DIAGNOSIS

- Other toxicologic causes of gastrointestinal injury include ingestion of alkaline caustic agents or massive ingestion of hypochlorite or other gastrointestinal irritant.
- Nontoxicologic causes of acute gastrointestinal pain and bleeding include peptic ulcer disease and perforated viscus.

SIGNS AND SYMPTOMS

- Ingestion may produce gastrointestinal burns, most commonly in the stomach, but oral and esophageal burns may occur as well; perforation is a rare complication.
- Metabolic acidosis, shock, gastrointestinal hemorrhage, and renal failure are rare complications of serious ingestion.

Vital Signs

Tachypnea is common after inhalation.

HEENT

- Ocular exposure effects range from corneal burns to opacification, blindness, and perforated globe.
- Oral burns may develop.

Dermatologic

Dermal toxicity ranges from irritation to full-thickness burns.

Cardiovascular

Cardiovascular collapse is a rare complication of severe exposure.

Pulmonary

- Bronchospasm may occur after inhalation.
- In severe cases adult respiratory distress syndrome may develop.
- Upper airway edema may develop after inhalation or aspiration.

Gastrointestinal

- Injuries are more common after deliberate ingestion of strong acids.
- Esophageal injury is usually maximal in the middle and lower thirds of the esophagus; gastric burns are more common.
- Gastrointestinal bleeding or perforation may occur acutely after grade III (full-thickness) injury.

Renal

Acute renal failure occurs rarely, generally caused by hypotension.

Hematologic

- Hemolysis has occurred after severe formic, acetic, or sulfuric acid exposure.
- Disseminated intravascular coagulation is a rare complication in severe cases.

Fluids and Electrolytes

- Metabolic acidosis may develop in cases complicated by shock.
- Extensive gastrointestinal injury may result in massive fluid loss.
- Hyperkalemia may develop secondary to hemolysis.
- Hyperphosphatemia has occurred after phosphoric acid ingestion.

PROCEDURES AND LABORATORY TESTS

Essential Tests

- Complete blood count should be obtained to detect hemolysis or gastrointestinal bleeding.
- Electrolytes, BUN, and creatinine should be obtained to evaluate for metabolic acidosis or renal failure associated with severe injury and shock.

Recommended Tests

- Coagulation studies (prothrombin time/partial thromboplastin time or international normalized ratio, fibrinogen, fibrin degradation products) should be obtained in patients with severe effects.
- Chest radiograph should be obtained for pulmonary symptoms or if gastrointestinal perforation is expected.
- A barium swallow and small-bowel follow-through should be obtained several weeks after ingestion to assess delayed gastrointestinal complications, such as strictures, that may develop after grade II or III injury (burn extends deeper than mucosa of gastrointestinal tract).
- Endoscopy is recommended after deliberate or large ingestion and in patients who are symptomatic or have oral burns; the likelihood of complications (strictures, obstruction, bleeding, and perforation) is related to the severity of the injury.

—Grade I. Mucosal hyperemia and superficial epithelial desquamation with intact mucous membranes.
—Grade II. Superficial blisters, ulcers, and hyperemia; patchy membranous mucosal exudates.
—Grade III. Necrosis and total loss of esophageal epithelium.

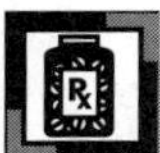

Treatment

- Treatment should focus on hemodynamic support and evaluating the injury.
- Aggressive airway management after aspiration or inhalation exposure is indicated because airway edema may develop rapidly.
- Dose and time of exposure should be determined for all substances involved.

DIRECTING PATIENT COURSE

- Emergency surgical evaluation is needed for patients with signs of perforation.
- Laparoscopic evaluation should be considered in patients with third-degree injury because transmucosal gastric burns or perforation may be present.

The health-care professional should call the poison control center when:

- Hypotension, gastrointestinal bleeding, perforation, metabolic acidosis, or other severe effects are present.
- Toxic effects are not consistent with acid exposure.
- Coingestant, drug interaction, or underlying disease presents an unusual problem.

The patient should be referred to a health-care facility when:

- Attempted suicide or homicide is possible.
- Patient or caregiver seems unreliable.
- Any symptoms develop.
- Coingestant, drug interaction, or underlying disease presents an unusual problem.

Admission Considerations

Inpatient management is warranted if:

- Patients have oral burns or symptoms (drooling, dysphagia, and stridor), unless endoscopy is immediately available and excludes grade II or III injury.
- Patients have grade II or III gastrointestinal injury noted on endoscopy.
- Patients exhibit dyspnea, wheezing, stridor, upper airway edema or burns, or any degree of respiratory distress.

DECONTAMINATION

Out of Hospital

- Emesis should not be induced.
- Neutralization with a basic solution should not be attempted because it may cause thermal injury.
- Ingestion should be diluted with 4 to 8 ounces of milk or water.
- Exposed mouth, skin, and eyes should be irrigated copiously with water.
- Patients with inhalation injury should be removed from further exposure.

In Hospital

- Oxygen should be administered to all patients with pulmonary symptoms.
- Following an ingestion, gastric lavage should not be performed because of the potential for perforation.
- Ingestion that occurred within the preceding 30 minutes should be diluted with 4 to 8 ounces of milk or water; neutralization with an alkaline solution is not recommended.
- Activated charcoal should not be administered unless a toxic coingestant is involved.
- Exposed eyes should be irrigated with sterile water or saline for at least 20 minutes; irrigation should continue until the pH of the cul de sac has returned to normal.
- Exposed skin should be irrigated with copious amounts of water.

ANTIDOTES

There is no specific antidote for caustic acid poisoning.

ADJUNCTIVE TREATMENT

- Intravenous crystalloid (10 to 20 ml/kg) should be administered for hypotension.
- Steroids should be considered for patients showing second-degree burns under endoscopy. The decision to administer steroids should involve a toxicologist, gastroenterologist, or surgeon experienced in managing these injuries.

—Steroids are not indicated for first-degree burns because stricture formation is unlikely.
—They are generally not indicated for third-degree burns because steroids increase the risk of perforation.

- Antibiotics are used only for suspected infection or perforation.
- Packed red blood cells and fresh frozen plasma may be needed if severe hemorrhage or hemolysis develops.

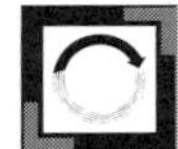

Follow-Up

PATIENT MONITORING

Patients with grade II or III gastrointestinal injury, those awaiting endoscopic evaluation, and those with significant inhalation exposure should be monitored in an intensive care setting.

EXPECTED COURSE AND PROGNOSIS

- Patients with first-degree injuries generally recover uneventfully.
- Patients with second-degree injuries may develop fistulas, strictures, or gastric outlet obstruction, but generally survive.
- Acute third-degree injuries are often complicated by gastrointestinal bleeding, shock, perforation, stricture, renal failure, and high mortality rate.

DISCHARGE CRITERIA/INSTRUCTIONS

- From the emergency department. Patients who are asymptomatic after taste ingestion and patients with no visible gastrointestinal injury or those with documented grade I gastrointestinal injury and tolerating oral intake may be discharged after a 6-hour observation period and psychiatric evaluation, if needed.
- From the hospital.

—Patients with documented grade II injuries may be discharged when they are tolerating a soft diet, with follow-up endoscopy or upper gastrointestinal series to detect sequelae.
—Patients with grade III injuries may be discharged when complications have resolved and adequate nutrition (enteral or parenteral) is achieved.

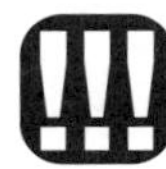

Pitfalls

DIAGNOSIS

- Oral burns may not adequately reflect the severity of distal gastrointestinal injury.
- Upper airway edema may develop abruptly after inhalation or aspiration.

FOLLOW-UP

Patients with grade II esophageal injury are at risk for stricture formation, gastric outlet obstruction, and possibly carcinoma; periodic follow-up and possibly dilation or surgery may be required.

ICD-9-CM 983.1

Toxic effect of acids.

See also: SECTION II, Hypotension chapter; SECTION IV, Ammonia, Boric Acid and Borates, Caustics—Basic, Chromium, Hydrofluoric Acid, and Selenium chapters.

RECOMMENDED READING

Dilawari JB, Singh S, Rao PN, et al. Corrosive acid ingestion in man: a clinical and endoscopic study. *Gut* 1984;25:183–187.

Wu M, Lai W. Surgical management of extensive corrosive injuries of the alimentary tract. *Surg Gynecol Obstet* 1993;177:12–16.

Zarger SA, Kochhar R, Nagi B, et al. Ingestion of corrosive acids: spectrum of injury to upper gastrointestinal tract and natural history. *Gastroenterol* 1989;97:702–707.

Author: Katherine M. Hurlbut

Reviewer: Richard C. Dart

Caustics—Basic

Basics

DESCRIPTION

Caustic alkaline chemicals are typically used in a wide array of cleaning products.

FORMS AND USES

- Caustic alkaline (basic) substances include ammonia, borax, calcium carbide, calcium hydroxide, calcium oxide, caustic potash, caustic soda, Clinitest tablets, diethanolamine, diethylenetriamine, isopropylamine, isopropyl aminoethanol, lime, lye, Portland cement, potassium carbonate, potassium hydroxide, potassium nitrate, potassium oxide, sodium carbonate, sodium hydroxide, sodium metasilicate, sodium oxide, sodium silicate, sodium tripolyphosphate, tetraethylenepentamine, triethylenetetramine, and trisodium phosphate.
- Corrosive alkaline chemicals are used in drain and pipeline cleaners; oven cleaners; denture cleaners; bathroom, household, and industrial cleaners; hair relaxers; electric dishwasher soaps and low-phosphate detergents; fertilizers; Portland cement; automobile air bags; and Clinitest tablets.

TOXIC DOSE

Just a few milliliters of highly caustic alkali (e.g., sodium hydroxide) can cause severe injury.

PATHOPHYSIOLOGY

- Alkaline corrosives saponify the fat in cell membranes, destroying the cell and causing liquefaction necrosis.
- These substances may be simply irritating or truly corrosive, depending on the molarity, concentration, amount ingested, and other factors.
- In general, significant gastrointestinal injury is not associated with alkaline products with a pH of less than 11.5.

EPIDEMIOLOGY

- Poisoning is common.
- Toxic effects following exposure are typically mild after inadvertent "taste" exposures of a household product in children.
- Severe injury or death occur more often after suicidal ingestion or industrial accidents.

CAUSES

- Toxic ingestion is usually accidental.
- Child neglect or abuse should be considered if the patient is less than 1 year of age, suicide attempt if the patient is over 6 years of age.

RISK FACTORS

Underlying pulmonary disease confers greater risk after inhalation.

WORKPLACE STANDARDS

Sodium hydroxide

- ACGIH. TLV TWA is 2 mg/m^3.
- OSHA. PEL TWA is 2 mg/m^3.
- NIOSH. IDLH is 10 mg/m^3.

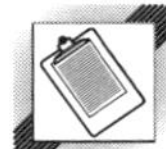

Diagnosis

DIFFERENTIAL DIAGNOSIS

- Toxicologic causes of caustic injury include ingestion of iron, acids, button batteries, phenol, copper sulfate, hydrogen peroxide, silver nitrate, zinc chloride, ethylene dichloride, mercuric chloride, formaldehyde, and other compounds.
- Nontoxicologic causes of caustic injury depend on the route of injury.

—After ingestion, caustic injury should be differentiated from esophagitis, gastritis, peptic or duodenal ulcers, or perforated ulcer.
—After inhalation exposure, caustic injury should be differentiated from reactive airway disease, epiglottitis, adult respiratory distress syndrome, pulmonary edema, and upper airway edema of other etiologies.

SIGNS AND SYMPTOMS

- Caustic burns of the mouth and esophagus are most common, but gastric or intestinal burns may occur with large ingestion; the presence or absence of oral burns does not correlate with the presence of esophageal burns.
- Inhalation exposure can cause wheezing, upper airway edema, and, in severe cases, pulmonary edema.
- Shock, metabolic acidosis, and renal failure are rare complications seen with severe gastrointestinal burns.

Vital Signs

Tachycardia is common; hypotension may develop in severe cases.

HEENT

- Ocular exposure may result in corneal burns, opacification, visual loss, and/or perforated globe.
- Oropharyngeal burns may develop.

Dermatologic

Dermal contact may cause irritation or chemical burns.

Pulmonary

- Inhalation may cause bronchospasm, upper airway edema or obstruction, laryngospasm, or adult respiratory distress syndrome.
- Young children are at greater risk of severe upper airway edema after ingestion.

Gastrointestinal

- Gastrointestinal burns may develop after ingestion.
- Esophageal burns are most common, occurring in 5% to 35% of patients.
- Gastric burns are less common, and intestinal burns are unusual except after large ingestions.
- Most patients with significant gastrointestinal burns develop vomiting, drooling, and stridor.
- Peritoneal signs may be present if perforation occurs.

Renal

Renal failure is a rare complication of severe burns, accompanied by shock and gastrointestinal bleeding.

Fluids and Electrolytes

Metabolic acidosis may develop in patients with severe gastrointestinal bleeding or massive tissue necrosis after corrosive ingestion.

PROCEDURES AND LABORATORY TESTS

Essential Tests

No tests may be needed after a minor "sip" ingestion of a household product.

Recommended Tests

- Complete blood count, serum electrolytes, BUN, and creatinine should be assayed in patients with gastrointestinal symptoms; anemia, metabolic acidosis, and renal failure are usually the result of complications (bleeding, shock, and massive tissue necrosis) and are associated with a poorer prognosis.
- Arterial blood gases should be measured in patients with pulmonary symptoms; hypoxia generally occurs only after severe inhalation exposure.
- Chest radiography should be undertaken in patients with pulmonary symptoms; upright chest and abdominal radiographs should be taken when perforation is suspected.
- Barium swallow imaging may be needed to detect gastrointestinal strictures and obstruction in the weeks after ingestion.
- Gastrointestinal endoscopy should be performed within 24 hours of ingestion in patients at risk for significant burns; indications include stridor, drooling, or vomiting, and adults with suicidal or large ingestions (the absence of oropharyngeal burns does not reliably exclude esophageal or gastric burns).

—Grade I. Mucosal hyperemia AND superficial epithelial desquamation with intact mucous membranes
—Grade II. Superficial blisters, ulcers, and hyperemia; patchy membranous mucosal exudates.
—Grade III. Necrosis and total loss of esophageal epithelium.

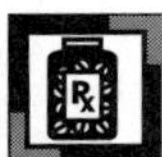

Treatment

- Treatment should focus on airway control, support of hemodynamic function, and assessment of burn severity.
- Intubation can be extremely difficult; cricothyrotomy or tracheostomy may be necessary.
- Dose and time of exposure should be determined for all substances involved.
- Surgical evaluation must be considered for any patient with Grade III esophageal injury to assess the extent of gastric or duodenal burns.
- Any patient with a suspected perforation is a surgical emergency; the absence of free air on abdominal or chest radiographs does not reliably exclude perforation.

DIRECTING PATIENT COURSE

The health-care professional should call the poison control center when:

- Serious effects (Grade I or Grade II burns or complications of hypotension, acidosis, hypoxia, gastrointestinal bleeding, or perforation) are present.
- Toxic effects are not consistent with alkaline corrosive poisoning.
- Coingestant or underlying disease presents an unusual problem.

The patient should be referred to a health-care facility when:

- Attempted suicide or homicide is possible.
- Patient or caregiver seems unreliable.
- Toxic effects are present.
- Coingestant or underlying disease presents an unusual problem.

Admission Considerations

Inpatient management is warranted if the patient exhibits Grade II or III burns, bleeding, hypotension, respiratory distress, wheezing, hypoxia, of upper airway injury, or if endoscopy is needed.

DECONTAMINATION

- Decontamination is not recommended after caustic ingestion.
- Emesis should not be induced with ipecac.
- Neutralization with an acidic solution should not be attempted because it may cause thermal burns.
- Ingestion may be diluted with a small amount (4 ounces) of milk or water; nothing else should be taken orally until injury is evaluated.
- Gastric lavage should not be performed because this may worsen gastrointestinal injury.
- Activated charcoal should not be administered unless a coingestant is suspected because it may induce vomiting and obscure endoscopy findings.
- Exposed eyes should be irrigated with sterile water or saline for at least 20 minutes; irrigation should continue until the pH of the cul de sac has returned to normal.

ANTIDOTES

There is no specific antidote for alkaline corrosive poisoning.

ADJUNCTIVE TREATMENT

- Steroid administration is recommended in certain cases to reduce stricture formation after alkaline-induced esophageal burns.

—Steroids should be considered in patients with Grade II burns.
—They are not indicated with Grade I burns because strictures are unlikely to develop.
—Steroids also should be avoided with Grade III burns because the risk of perforation is greater and strictures often form regardless of therapy.
—The adult or pediatric dose is 0.1 mg/kg of dexamethasone or prednisone 1 to 2.5 mg/kg for 3 weeks then taper off.

- Prophylactic use of antibiotics has not shown any benefit.
- Hypotension is treated in the standard manner, beginning with infusion of 0.9% saline, 10 to 20 ml/kg. Further management is described in SECTION II, Hypotension chapter.

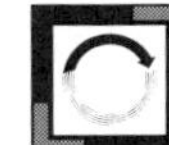

Follow-Up

PATIENT MONITORING

- Airway must be monitored carefully in patients with inhalation or significant oral exposure.
- Blood pressure and temperature should be monitored, and serial abdominal examinations should be performed in patients with Grade III burns.

EXPECTED COURSE AND PROGNOSIS

- Children generally do well after taste ingestion.
- Adults with deliberate ingestion or industrial exposures are most likely to sustain complications or death.
- Delayed sequelae of gastrointestinal burns may include stricture formation, gastrointestinal bleeding, pyloric stenosis, perforation, and tracheoesophageal or aortotracheal fistula formation.
- Patients who develop esophageal burns and stricture are at increased risk for esophageal cancer (1,000-fold increase in risk; latency 12–40 years).

DISCHARGE CRITERIA/INSTRUCTIONS

- From the emergency department. Patients who are asymptomatic after taste ingestion and patients with Grade I burns or documented absence of gastrointestinal burns who are tolerating oral intake may be discharged after 6 hours of observation and psychiatric evaluation, if needed.
- From the hospital. Patients with documented Grade II or III burns may be discharged when they are tolerating a soft diet (or parenteral nutrition), with follow-up endoscopy or upper gastrointestinal series to detect stricture formation.

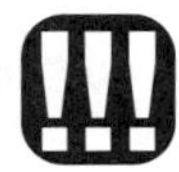

Pitfalls

DIAGNOSIS

The absence of oropharyngeal burns does not reliably exclude esophageal or gastric burns.

TREATMENT

Children less than 1 year of age are at increased risk for developing upper airway edema requiring intubation after minor alkaline corrosive ingestion.

FOLLOW-UP

Patients with stricture formation require periodic evaluation for esophageal carcinoma.

ICD-9-CM 983.9

Toxic effect of corrosive aromatics, acids, and caustic alkalis: caustic alkalis.

See also: SECTION II, Hypotension chapter.

RECOMMENDED READING

Hoffman RS. Caustics and batteries. In: Goldfrank LR, Flomenbaum NE, Lewin NA, et al., eds. *Goldfrank's toxicologic emergencies,* 6th ed. Norwalk, CT: Appleton & Lange, 1998.

Author: Katherine M. Hurlbut

Reviewer: Richard C. Dart

Chloral Hydrate

Basics

DESCRIPTION

Chloral hydrate is an oral sedative-hypnotic agent.

FORMS AND USES

- Chloral hydrate is used for sedation and hypnosis, treatment of insomnia, adjunct to perioperative anesthesia and analgesia, and the treatment of alcohol withdrawal.
- Chloral hydrate is available as syrup (250 mg/5 ml, 500 mg/5 ml), tablet (250 and 500 mg), or suppository (325, 500, and 650 mg).
- Typical adult therapeutic dose for sedation and hypnosis is 0.5 to 1 g orally; pediatric, 25 to 50 mg/kg/day orally up to 1 g in three or four divided doses.

TOXIC DOSE

- Range of toxicity varies widely as for most sedative-hypnotic agents.
- Ingestion of more than the therapeutic dose may cause CNS depression.

PATHOPHYSIOLOGY

- Chloral hydrate is metabolized to trichloroethanol (TCE), which is largely responsible for its action and has a half-life of 4 to 12 hours.
- TCE is then metabolized to trichloroacetic acid (TCA), which is highly protein-bound and displaces other drugs (e.g., warfarin) from protein binding sites.
- Concurrent ethanol ingestion potentiates formation of TCE, producing greater toxicity.
- Withdrawal syndrome after cessation of prolonged abuse has been reported.

EPIDEMIOLOGY

- Poisoning is uncommon.
- Toxicity is usually mild.
- Death is rare, occurring in patients in whom the airway is not controlled.

CAUSES

- Toxicity usually results from pediatric accidental ingestion or adult abuse.
- Child neglect or abuse should be considered if the patient is less than 1 year of age, suicide attempt if the patient is over 6 years of age.

DRUG AND DISEASE INTERACTIONS

- Administration with other sedative-hypnotics will produce additive effect.
- Disulfiram-like reaction may occur when ingested with ethanol.

PREGNANCY AND LACTATION

- FDA Pregnancy Category C. The drug exerts animal teratogenic or embryocidal effects, but there are no controlled studies in women, or no studies are available in animals or women.
- Excretion in breast milk has been reported.

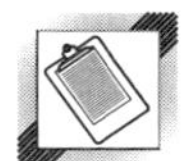

Diagnosis

DIFFERENTIAL DIAGNOSIS

Other toxicologic causes of CNS depression are numerous, including all sedative-hypnotic agents, narcotics, alcohols, barbiturates, tricyclic antidepressants, and many others.

SIGNS AND SYMPTOMS

Vital Signs

Bradypnea, hypotension, and hypothermia may occur in severe cases.

HEENT

Symptoms may include miosis, a peculiar and acrid pearlike odor on the breath, mucous membrane irritation, and laryngospasm.

Cardiovascular

Supraventricular and ventricular dysrhythmias, hypotension, and depression of myocardial contractility may occur in severe cases.

Pulmonary

Bradypnea may develop.

Gastrointestinal

Nausea, vomiting, esophageal and abdominal pain are common.

Neurologic

Lightheadedness, headache, ataxia, altered mental status, coma, and decreased deep tendon reflexes may occur.

PROCEDURES AND LABORATORY TESTS

Essential Tests

No tests may be needed in asymptomatic patients.

Recommended Tests

- Serum electrolytes, BUN, and creatinine are used to assess other causes of CNS depression.
- ECG is used to detect dysrhythmia.
- Pulse oximetry is used to assess oxygenation.
- Serum acetaminophen and aspirin levels should be obtained in an overdose setting to detect occult overdose.
- Trichloroethanol and urochloralic acid (metabolite of TCA) levels may help to confirm exposure but are not available rapidly for clinical use.
- Chloral hydrate is radiopaque and may be visible on an abdominal x-ray; however, the absence of radiopacities does not rule out an ingestion.

Not Recommended Tests

Measuring the serum chloral hydrate level is not useful.

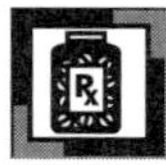

Treatment

Supportive care and airway management are mainstays of therapy.

DIRECTING PATIENT COURSE

The health-care professional should call the poison control center when:

- Severe or persistent effects develop.
- Coingestant, drug interaction, or underlying disease presents an unusual problem.

The patient should be referred to a health-care facility when:

- Toxic effects develop.
- Coingestant, drug interaction, or underlying disease presents an unusual problem.

Admission Considerations

Inpatient management is warranted for patients with CNS depression, hypotension, or cardiac dysrhythmia.

DECONTAMINATION

Out of Hospital

Ipecac should not be administered because of the potential for CNS depression.

In Hospital

- Emesis should not be induced because of the potential for rapid deterioration.
- Gastric lavage should be performed in pediatric (tube size 24–32 French) or adult (tube size 36–42 French) patients for large ingestion presenting within 1 hour of ingestion or if serious effects are present.
- One dose of activated charcoal (1–2 g/kg) should be administered without a cathartic if a substantial ingestion has occurred within the previous few hours.

ANTIDOTES

There is no specific antidote for chloral hydrate poisoning.

ADJUNCTIVE TREATMENT

- Cardiac dysrhythmias should be treated according to standard Advanced Cardiac Life Support System protocols.
- Case reports suggest that hemodialysis and charcoal hemoperfusion can improve outcome by removing chloral hydrate and trichloroethanol.

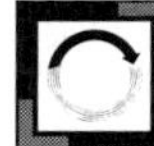

Follow-Up

PATIENT MONITORING

ECG should be obtained and respiratory, cardiac, and hemodynamic status monitored continuously.

EXPECTED COURSE AND PROGNOSIS

Toxic effects begin within minutes; recovery occurs over hours unless sequelae of hypoxia intercede.

DISCHARGE CRITERIA/INSTRUCTIONS

- From the emergency department. Asymptomatic patients may be discharged after decontamination, observation for 4 to 6 hours, and psychiatric evaluation, if needed.
- From the hospital. Patients may be discharged when toxic effects have resolved, and following decontamination and psychiatric evaluation, if needed.

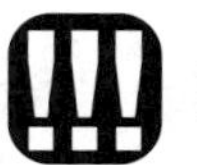

Pitfalls

DIAGNOSIS

Clinician should consider all the potential causes of CNS depression, toxicologic and nontoxicologic.

ICD-9-CM 967.1

Poisoning by chloral hydrate group.

See also: SECTION II, Ventricular Dysrhythmia chapter.

RECOMMENDED READING

Ellenhorn MJ. *Medical toxicology,* 2nd ed. Baltimore: Williams & Wilkins, 1997:695.

Author: Edwin K. Kuffner

Reviewer: Richard C. Dart

Chloride

Basics

DESCRIPTION

- Chlorine gas is a greenish-yellow, heavier-than-air gas with a pungent irritating odor.
- Under pressure or in combination with other chemicals, chlorine can exist as a liquid, a solid, or a gas.

FORMS AND USES

- Chlorine liquid is used to produce chlorine gas for use as an industrial disinfectant.
- Occupational exposures may occur during manufacturing of rubber and plastics, the bleaching of fabrics, the production of hydrochloric acid, and in the course of water and sewage purification.
- Other commonly used chemicals containing chlorine include household products such as bleach (e.g., Clorox) and other products containing sodium hypochlorite.

TOXIC DOSE

- Inhalation toxicity depends on concentration of gas and duration of exposure. Just one or two breaths of concentrated chlorine gas can produce serious injury.
- Ingestion of household bleach (5% sodium hypochlorite) is generally nontoxic; ingestion of more concentrated solutions may cause caustic injury.

PATHOPHYSIOLOGY

- Chlorine combines with water and liberates hypochlorous acid, hydrochloric acid, and oxygen free radicals, which are cytotoxic.
- Mixture of household bleach (hypochlorite) with ammonia-containing compounds may produce chloramine, a volatile irritant gas that produces effects similar to chlorine.
- Mixture of bleach with an acid may produce chlorine gas.

EPIDEMIOLOGY

- Poisoning is common and often occurs in the home.
- Toxic effects following inhalation exposure are typically mild to moderate, with death occurring in high-concentration exposures.

CAUSES

- Toxicity usually results from a household or occupational accident.
- Child neglect or abuse should be considered if the patient is less than 1 year of age, suicide attempt if the patient is over 6 years of age.

RISK FACTORS

Children may be more severely affected by chlorine gas because it is heavier than air and concentrates closer to the ground.

DRUG AND DISEASE INTERACTIONS

Patients with preexisting pulmonary disease are more susceptible to injury.

PREGNANCY AND LACTATION

High concentrations of hypochlorite are teratogenic in animal studies.

WORKPLACE STANDARDS

- Chlorine

—OSHA. PEL TWA is 0.5 ppm; PEL STEL is 1 ppm.
—NIOSH. IDLH is 25 ppm.

- Chlorine dioxide. OSHA. PEL TWA is 0.1 ppm (0.3 mg/m^3).
- Chlorine trifluoride. ACGIH. TLV (ceiling limit) is 0.1 ppm (0.4 mg/m^3).
- Odor detectable at concentrations of 0.5 ppm.

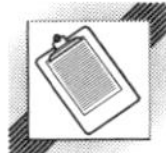

Diagnosis

DIFFERENTIAL DIAGNOSIS

Toxicologic causes of acute pulmonary injury include acrolein, ammonia, bromine, smoke inhalation, and phosgene, among others.

SIGNS AND SYMPTOMS

- Most serious exposures occur by inhalation and rapidly produce upper airway irritation and cough.
- Acute worsening may occur hours after inhalation exposure.

Vital Signs

- Tachycardia, tachypnea, and hypoxia are common following inhalation.
- Fever may develop if chemical pneumonitis and pulmonary edema occur.

HEENT

- Mucous membrane irritation (rhinorrhea and blepharospasm) is common.
- Upper airway obstruction may occur after high-concentration inhalation exposure.
- Conjunctivitis or corneal burns may occur from splash or high concentration exposure.

Dermatologic

Erythema and dermatitis are common following dermal exposure and related to concentration and duration of exposure.

Pulmonary

- Cough, chest pain, dyspnea, and bronchospasm are common following low-level exposures; wheezing, rhonchi, and rales also occur.
- Noncardiogenic pulmonary edema may occur following high-level inhalation exposure, but may be delayed for several hours.
- Reactive airway disease may develop after either severe acute or chronic inhalation exposure.

Gastrointestinal

- Nausea and vomiting are common following either ingestion or inhalation.
- Caustic gastrointestinal injury may follow ingestion of a large amount or a high-concentration solution.

Neurologic

- Headache and lightheadedness are common following low-level inhalation exposure.
- Syncope has occurred following high-level inhalation exposure.

PROCEDURES AND LABORATORY TESTS

Essential Tests

No specific tests are required following many mild exposures, especially ingestion of low-concentration solutions.

Recommended Tests

- Arterial blood gas and pulse oximetry should be monitored in symptomatic patients; hypoxia indicates severe injury or bronchospasm.
- Serum electrolytes, BUN, and creatinine should be assayed after serious inhalation or large-ingestion exposures; hyperchloremia or acidosis may occur.
- ECG, serum acetaminophen, and aspirin levels should be measured in an overdose setting to detect occult overdose.
- Chest radiography may reveal infiltrates in symptomatic patients, but normal chest radiographs obtained shortly after exposure do not preclude the development of delayed pulmonary effects.
- Pulmonary peak flows should be monitored to follow progress of bronchospasm.
- Bronchoscopy may be needed for severe pulmonary effects.
- Endoscopy should be considered for persistent gastrointestinal complaints following ingestion.

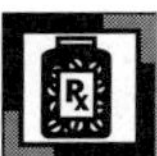

Treatment

- Supportive care with appropriate airway management is vital, with endotracheal intubation considered in serious exposures.
- Dose and time of exposure should be determined for all substances involved.
- Patients with dermal or ocular exposures should be checked for burns following irrigation procedures.

DIRECTING PATIENT COURSE

The health-care professional should call the poison control center when:

- Bronchospasm, airway obstruction, pulmonary edema, gastrointestinal, dermal injury, or other severe effects are present.
- Signs and symptoms are not consistent with chlorine poisoning.
- Coingestant, drug interaction, or underlying disease presents an unusual problem.

The patient should be referred to a health-care facility when:

- Attempted suicide or homicide is possible.
- Patient or caregiver seems unreliable.
- Symptoms more than a mild cough are present.
- Coingestant, drug interaction, or underlying disease presents an unusual problem.

Admission Considerations

Inpatient management is warranted if:

- Patient has experienced a high-concentration inhalation exposure.
- Patient exhibits upper airway edema, second- or third-degree burns, hypoxia, persistent respiratory symptoms, or caustic gastrointestinal injury.

DECONTAMINATION

Out of Hospital

- Inhalation. Patient should be removed from source of exposure.
- Ingestion. Emesis should not be induced.
- Dermal or ocular exposure. Affected area should be irrigated copiously with water.

In Hospital

- Ingestion

—Ipecac induced emesis is not recommended.
—Gastric contents should be aspirated gently with a nasogastric tube in patients presenting within 1 hour of a large ingestion; a large-bore orogastric tube is not recommended.
—Dermal. Affected area should be irrigated copiously with water or 0.9% saline.
—Ocular. Eyes should be irrigated copiously with 0.9% saline.

ANTIDOTES

There is no specific antidote for chlorine poisoning.

ADJUNCTIVE TREATMENT

Bronchospasm

- Oxygen should be administered, followed by albuterol 0.15 mg/kg (maximum of 10 mg) in saline with humidified oxygen via nebulizer every 20 to 30 minutes.

—If the peak expiratory flow rate (PEFR) is greater than 90% of predicted after initial dose, additional doses may not be needed.
—Patient should be monitored continually for response.

- Methylprednisolone and prednisone are used in the same manner as for asthma.

—Adult dose of methylprednisolone is 60 to 125 mg (1–1.5 mg/kg) given intravenously (pediatric, 1–2 mg/kg) every 6 to 8 hours.
—This may be decreased to a single daily dose and tapered.

- Prednisone, 2 mg/kg orally for several days, should be considered for cough or bronchospasm following inhalation exposure.
- Nebulized sodium bicarbonate has been recommended, but recent evidence indicates it is ineffective, and animal evidence suggests that it may cause a chemical pneumonitis.

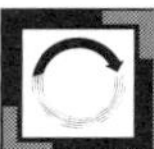

Follow-Up

PATIENT MONITORING

- In an acute episode, continuous cardiac and respiratory monitoring should be performed.
- Long-term monitoring of pulmonary complications with pulmonary function tests is often needed.

EXPECTED COURSE AND PROGNOSIS

- Patients with low-level inhalation usually recover without sequelae.
- High-concentration or prolonged exposure may result in severe symptoms and permanent sequelae.
- Interstitial lung disease, pulmonary fibrosis, and reactive airway disease may occur following either severe acute or chronic inhalation exposure.

DISCHARGE CRITERIA/INSTRUCTIONS

- From the emergency department. A patient with hypochlorite solution ingestion or asymptomatic minor inhalation exposure may be discharged after symptoms have resolved.
- From the hospital. Patient may be discharged when respiratory symptoms and other effects are improving.

PATIENT EDUCATION

Patients should be instructed to return if they develop persistent coughing, difficulty in breathing, or chest pain.

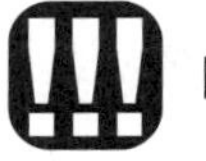

Pitfalls

DIAGNOSIS

Chest radiograph may be normal shortly after exposure and does not preclude subsequent pulmonary edema.

ICD-9-CM 983.9

Toxic effects of corrosive aromatics, acids, and caustic alkalis.

See also: SECTION IV, Caustics–Acidic chapter.

RECOMMENDED READING

Courteau JP, Cushman R, Bouchard F, et al. Survey of construction workers repeatedly exposed to chlorine over a three- to six-month period in a pulpmill. 1. Exposure and symptomatology. *Occup Environ Med* 1994;51:219–224.

Schonhofer B, Voshaar T, Kohler D. Long-term lung sequelae following accidental chlorine gas exposure. *Respiration* 1996;63:155–159.

Author: Edwin K. Kuffner

Reviewer: Katherine M. Hurlbut

Cholinergic Agonist Medications

Basics

DESCRIPTION

Cholinergic agonism is caused by a wide variety of drugs, chemicals, and naturally occurring substances. Cholinergic agonists mimic the action of acetylcholine, a naturally occurring neurotransmitter found in various organs and tissues.

FORMS AND USES

Pharmaceutical preparations include acetylcholine (Miochol), bethanechol (Urecholine, Duvoid, and Myotonachol), carbachol (Isoptocarbachol and Carboptic), methacholine (Provocholine), and pilocarpine (Isoptocarpine, Pilocar, PilostatV, Adsorbocarpine, and Akarpine).

- Acetylcholine. One-half to 2 ml of a 1% solution is used as a miotic.
- Bethanechol

—The oral dose is 10 to 50 mg three to four times a day, and the subcutaneous dose is 5 mg three to four times a day.
—It is used to treat acute postoperative and postpartum nonobstructive urinary retention and neurogenic atony of the urinary bladder with retention.

- Carbachol

—Up to 0.5 ml intraocularly is used to produce miosis during surgery.
—To relieve intraocular pressure of glaucoma, two drops up to three times daily of a 1.5%, 2.25%, or 3% solution can be used.

- Methacholine. Methacholine is a bronchoconstricting agent used in the diagnosis of hyperreactive airway disorders. It is not meant to be used therapeutically.
- Pilocarpine

—Pilocarpine is available in 4% gel; ophthalmic solutions of 0.25%, 0.5%, 1%, 2%, 3%, 4%, 5%, 6%, 8%, and 10%; and a controlled-release ocular insert providing 20 and 40 μg/h for 7 days.
—It is used for the treatment of primary open-angle glaucoma and xerostomia.

- Natural products containing arecoline include *Pilocarpus* plants, seeds of *Areca catechu*, and the leaves of the Piper betel (betel leaf). Fungi (mushrooms) from the *Boletus, Inocybe*, and *Clitocybe* genera contain muscarine.

TOXIC DOSE

Two or three times the daily dose will provide cholinergic effects in many patients.

PATHOPHYSIOLOGY

- Cholinergic agonists directly excite postganglionic cholinergic receptors and are selective for various muscarinic and nicotinic receptor sites.
- Acetylcholine, methacholine, bethanechol, and pilocarpine primarily affect muscarinic receptors, activating urinary, gastrointestinal, cardiac, uterine, bronchial, exocrine, CNS cortex, vascular, and brainstem receptors.
- Carbachol directly excites muscarinic sites but also causes the release of acetylcholine at the nicotinic receptors in the postganglionic autonomic nervous system, neuromuscular skeletal muscle junction, and adrenal medulla.

EPIDEMIOLOGY

- Poisoning is uncommon.
- Toxic effects following exposure are typically moderate; death occurs rarely.

CAUSES

- Toxic ingestion is usually suicidal.
- Child neglect or abuse should be considered if the patient is less than 1 year of age, suicide attempt if the patient is older than 6 years of age.

DRUG AND DISEASE INTERACTIONS

- Acetylcholine in combination with metoprolol may cause bronchospasm.
- Bethanechol taken with donepezil or tacrine causes synergistic cholinergic effects, which can result in cholinergic toxicity.
- Pilocarpine and sulfacetamide may cause precipitation when instilled in the same eye unless administration is separated by 15 to 20 minutes.

PREGNANCY AND LACTATION

Acetylcholine, bethanechol, carbachol, and pilocarpine. US FDA Pregnancy Category C. The drug exerts animal teratogenic or embryocidal effects, but there are no controlled studies in women, or no studies are available in either animals or women.

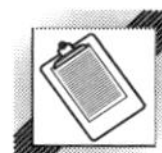

Diagnosis

DIFFERENTIAL DIAGNOSIS

Toxicologic causes of muscarinic symptoms include organophosphate or carbamate insecticides and therapeutic cholinesterase inhibitors like donepezil and tacrine.

SIGNS AND SYMPTOMS

- A mnemonic for cholinergic effects is DUMBELS: **D**iaphoresis and **D**iarrhea; **U**rination; **M**iosis; **B**radycardia and **B**ronchospasm; **E**mesis; excess **L**acrimation; and **S**alivation and **S**eizures.
- Nicotinic effects such as weakness, muscle cramps, paralysis, hypertension, and tachycardia may occur with carbachol, methacholine, and arecoline.
- Therapeutic doses of bethanechol given intravenously can cause shock or sudden cardiac arrest.

Vital Signs

- Tachypnea and hypothermia may develop.
- Muscarinic compounds may cause hypotension and bradycardia.
- Nicotinic compounds (carbachol, methacholine, arecoline) may cause hypertension and tachycardia.

HEENT

- Systemic exposure causes salivation, lacrimation, and miosis.
- Topical exposure to the eye may cause miosis, pain, eyelid twitching, and blurred vision.

Dermatologic

Profuse sweating can occur.

Cardiovascular

- Hypotension with reflex tachycardia occurs with low doses, whereas high doses cause bradycardia.
- Decreased cardiac contractility, shock, atrial fibrillation, cardiac arrest, and heart block can occur.

Pulmonary

- Bronchospasm, tachypnea, dyspnea, increase in pulmonary secretion, and pulmonary edema may develop.
- Asthmatic patients are especially susceptible.

Gastrointestinal

Nausea, vomiting, diarrhea, and abdominal pain may be present.

Renal

Urinary incontinence is possible.

Fluids and Electrolytes

Fluid depletion and electrolyte imbalances may occur.

Musculoskeletal

Compounds with greater nicotinic activity (carbachol, methacholine) may cause muscle cramps, muscle weakness, and fasciculation.

Neurologic

- Vertigo, tremors, seizures, and coma may occur.
- Pilocarpine has caused frontal headaches.
- Compounds with greater nicotinic activity may cause weakness and paralysis.

PROCEDURES AND LABORATORY TESTS

Essential Tests

No tests may be needed in minimally symptomatic patients.

Recommended Tests

- ECG should be obtained and continuous cardiac monitoring initiated in symptomatic pa-

tients; various dysrhythmias and heart block may occur.
- Arterial blood gases should be measured in the event of prolonged seizures.
- Serum electrolytes, BUN, and creatinine should be measured to assess effects of fluid loss, seizure, or cardiac effects.
- Serum creatine kinase can be used to assess muscle injury if repeated seizures occur.
- Serum acetaminophen and aspirin levels should be screened in an overdose setting to detect occult ingestion.
- Peak flow or pulmonary function monitoring should be instituted for patients with bronchospasm or dyspnea.
- Chest radiography can be used to assess causes of hypoxia (bronchospasm versus pulmonary edema).
- Head CT should be obtained as needed to rule out other causes of coma and seizures.

Not Recommended Tests

Serum levels of cholinergic agents are not clinically useful.

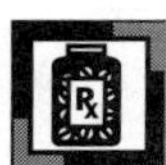

Treatment

- Treatment should focus on airway management, seizure control, and administration of atropine.
- Dose and time of exposure should be determined for all substances involved.

DIRECTING PATIENT COURSE

The health-care professional should call the poison control center when:

- Seizures, coma, dysrhythmia, hypotension, acidemia, bronchospasm, or other serious effects are present.
- Toxic effects are not consistent with cholinergic poisoning.
- Coingestant, drug interaction, or underlying disease presents an unusual problem.

The patient should be referred to a health-care facility when:

- Attempted suicide or homicide is possible.
- Patient or caregiver seems unreliable.
- Any toxic effects develop.
- Coingestant, drug interaction, or underlying disease presents an unusual problem.

Admission Considerations

Inpatient management in an intensive care unit is warranted if patient develops apparent cholinergic effects.

DECONTAMINATION

Out of Hospital

Emesis should not be induced; spontaneous emesis or seizures may develop abruptly.

In Hospital

- Gastric lavage should be performed in pediatric (tube size 24–32 French) or adult (tube size 36–42 French) patients for large ingestion presenting within 1 hour of ingestion or if serious effects are present.
- One dose of activated charcoal (1–2 g/kg) should be administered without a cathartic if a substantial ingestion has occurred within the previous few hours.

ANTIDOTES

Atropine

- Indication is control bronchorrhea and other secretions.
- Method of administration

—The adult dose is 2 mg intravenously initially; subsequent doses in 2 mg increments are administered every 5 to 10 minutes as necessary until pulmonary secretions are controlled.
—The pediatric dose is 0.05 mg/kg intravenously initially; subsequent doses in 2 mg increments are administered every 5 to 10 minutes as necessary until pulmonary secretions are controlled.
—Endpoint of atropine therapy is adequate oxygenation and resolution of pulmonary secretions and edema.

ADJUNCTIVE TREATMENT

Hypotension

- Atropine can correct hypotension related to bradycardia.
- Patient should receive 10 to 20 ml/kg 0.9% saline intravenously and be placed in the Trendelenburg position.
- Further fluid therapy can be guided by central pressure monitoring to avoid volume overload.
- Vasopressor can be added if needed.

Seizures

- A patent airway must be ensured.
- A benzodiazepine is administered for initial control. If seizures persist or recur, another anticonvulsant such as phenobarbital may be added.

Bronchospasm

- Albuterol 0.15 mg/kg (maximum of 10 mg) can be given in saline with humidified oxygen via nebulizer every 20 to 30 minutes; if the peak expiratory flow rate is greater than 90% predicted after initial dose, additional doses may not be needed.
- Response should be monitored; the use of steroids should be considered if symptoms persist.

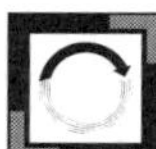

Follow-Up

PATIENT MONITORING

Respiratory and cardiac parameters should be monitored continuously on all symptomatic patients.

EXPECTED COURSE AND PROGNOSIS

- Onset of toxicity peaks within 6 to 12 hours of exposure, but may require several days for complete recovery.
- If complications of seizures or prolonged hypoxia develop, recovery may be prolonged.

DISCHARGE CRITERIA/INSTRUCTIONS

- From the emergency department. Asymptomatic patients may be discharged following decontamination, a 4- to 6-hour observation period, and psychiatric evaluation, if needed.
- From the hospital. Patients may be discharged after toxic effects have resolved or stabilized and psychiatric evaluation has been completed, if needed.

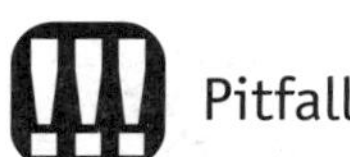

Pitfalls

TREATMENT

- Prompt seizure control is critical; general anesthesia or neuromuscular paralysis and EEG monitoring may be required.
- Excessive atropine in a mild poisoning may cause anticholinergic symptoms.

FOLLOW-UP

Renal failure and CNS injury secondary to prolonged seizures occur rarely.

ICD-9-CM 971.0

Poisoning by drugs primarily affecting the autonomic nervous system: parasympathomimetics (cholinergics).

See also: SECTION II, Hypotension and Seizures chapters; SECTION III, Atropine chapter.

RECOMMENDED READING

Hardman JG, Limbird LE, Molinoff PB, et al., eds. *Goodman & Gilman's the pharmacological basis of therapeutics*, 9th ed. New York: McGraw-Hill, 1996.

Author: Robin Millin

Reviewer: Richard C. Dart

Chromium

Basics

DESCRIPTION

Chromium is widely used in the metallurgical, refractory, and chemical industries as well as the tanning industry, pigment production, graphics, and many others.

FORMS AND USES

- Chromium compounds exist in a variety of valence states. Cr II (bivalent and basic), Cr III (trivalent and amphoteric), and Cr VI (hexavalent and acidic) are the commercially important forms.
- Compounds containing hexavalent chromium include chromic acid, potassium chromate, potassium dichromate, and sodium dichromate.

TOXIC DOSE

The lethal oral adult dose of has been estimated to be between 0.5 and 1.0 g of hexavalent chromium.

PATHOPHYSIOLOGY

- There is little conclusive evidence of toxic effects of divalent and trivalent chromium.
- The chromium in biological materials is usually trivalent.

EPIDEMIOLOGY

- Chromium may cause bronchogenic lung cancer in humans, the risk of which is increased by cigarette smoking.
- Chrome ulcers are common in tannery workers.
- Acute irritative dermatitis and allergic eczematous dermatitis are widespread in housewives, woodworkers, cement workers, limestone workers, radio factory workers, painters, and furniture polishers.
- Allergy to metals containing chromium, such as in acupuncture needles or military uniforms, is commonly reported.

CAUSES

- Most exposures are occupational.
- Child neglect or abuse should be considered if the patient is less than 1 year of age, suicide attempt if the patient is over 6 years of age.

WORKPLACE STANDARDS

For hexavalent chromium, expressed as chromium:

- ACGIH. TLV TWA (chromate) is 0.05 mg/m^3.
- OSHA. PEL TWA is 0.1 ppm (0.25 mg/m^3).
- NIOSH. IDLH is 15 mg/m^3.

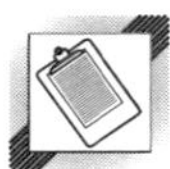

Diagnosis

DIFFERENTIAL DIAGNOSIS

Other causes of caustic skin or gastrointestinal injury include acidic or basic corrosives.

SIGNS AND SYMPTOMS

Systemic effects resulting from acute ingestion include circulatory collapse, shock, and death.

Dermatologic

- Chrome ulcers are usually painless and occur most commonly on the fingers and hands.
- Acute irritative dermatitis and allergic eczematous dermatitis can occur and may be associated with yellow or orange skin discoloration.

Pulmonary

- High concentrations have been found in lung tissue after inhalation, which causes a pneumoconiosis that can be seen on chest radiograph.
- Both bronchial asthma and anaphylaxis have been reported after inhalation of chromium-containing dust.
- A corrosive reaction from chromium-containing mist commonly leads to ulceration and perforation of the nasal septum, particularly in welders.
- Systemic effects resulting from acute ingestion include pulmonary edema.

Gastrointestinal

Following ingestion, oral and gastrointestinal burns with hemorrhage are common.

Hepatic

Systemic effects resulting from acute ingestion include acute hepatitis.

Renal

Systemic effects resulting from acute ingestion include renal failure.

Hematologic

Systemic effects resulting from acute ingestion include thrombocytopenia and anemia.

Neurologic

Systemic effects resulting from acute ingestion include encephalopathy.

PROCEDURES AND LABORATORY TESTS

Essential Tests

No tests may be needed in asymptomatic patients.

Recommended Tests

- CBC, serum electrolytes, BUN, creatinine, liver function tests, and coagulation studies should be followed, as indicated by clinical condition.
- CT or MRI scanning from the nose to the abdomen must be considered in the first few days as a guide, due to the late development of abscess.

Not Recommended Tests

Blood or serum levels have not been found to be clinically useful.

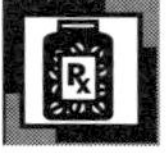

Treatment

Treatment should focus on general supportive care and decontamination.

DIRECTING PATIENT COURSE

The health-care professional should call the poison control center when:

- History of ingestion of hexavalent chromium is obtained.
- Toxic effects are not consistent with chromium poisoning.
- Coingestant or underlying disease presents an unusual problem.

Patients should be referred to a health-care facility when:

- History of ingestion of hexavalent chromium is obtained.
- Attempted suicide or homicide is possible.
- Coingestant or underlying disease presents an unusual problem.

Admission Considerations

Inpatient management in an intensive care setting is warranted for symptomatic patients after ingestion.

DECONTAMINATION

Ingestion

- Overall management is similar to acidic caustic agents
- Dilution with water or milk can be administered in the outpatient setting. Emesis should not be induced.
- Ascorbic acid, which reacts with hexavalent chromium to form the less toxic trivalent form, can be administered at 1 g per 0.135 g elemental chromium ingested.
- Activated charcoal is of questionable benefit.

Dermal

The skin should be washed copiously with tepid water and soaked in a 10% to 20% solution of ascorbic acid for 15 minutes.

ANTIDOTES

Dimercaprol (British anti-Lewisite), a heavy metal chelator, has been used successfully in some cases.

ADJUNCTIVE TREATMENT

- Ingestion. If significant gastrointestinal injury has occurred following ingestion, parenteral nutrition should be considered.
- Dermal. Wound care should include appropriate topical or systemic antibiotics, vitamin C, and tetanus prophylaxis.
- Inhalation

—If dust inhalation is a possibility, the inside of the nose should be washed daily and the nasal septum covered with zinc or barium ointment.
—Asthma attacks or anaphylaxis should be treated as usual.

- Hemodialysis has not been shown to have greater clearance rates than inherent renal clearance.

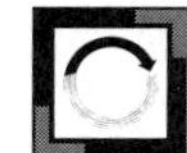

Follow-Up

PATIENT MONITORING

Respiratory and cardiac monitoring should be performed continuously in symptomatic patients.

EXPECTED COURSE AND PROGNOSIS

- After acute ingestion, toxic effects usually peak within 24 hours, but caustic injury may require weeks to heal.
- Chronic inhalation may produce persistent pulmonary disease.

DISCHARGE CRITERIA/INSTRUCTIONS

- From the emergency department. Asymptomatic patients may be discharged after decontamination.
- From the hospital. Patient may be discharged when toxic effects resolve or stabilize.

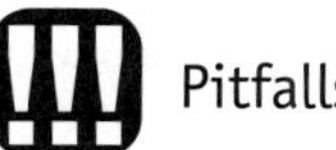

Pitfalls

FOLLOW-UP

Grade II or III esophageal burns need follow-up gastrointestinal series to detect strictures.

ICD-9-CM 985.6

Toxic effect of other metals: chromium.

See also: SECTION III, British Anti-Lewisite (dimercaprol); SECTION IV, Caustics—Acidic.

RECOMMENDED READING

Deng JF, Fleeger AK, Sinks T. An outbreak of chromium ulcer in a manufacturing plant. *Vet Human Tox* 1990;32:142–146.

Authors: Scott D. Phillips and Melanie A. Wells

Reviewer: Richard C. Dart

Ciguatera Fish Poisoning

Basics

DESCRIPTION

• Ciguatera fish poisoning is the common name for the toxic effects caused by eating tropical reef fish that themselves have ingested quantities of a toxic dinoflagellate (*Gambierdiscus toxicus*).
• *G. toxicus* produces toxins including ciguatoxin, maitotoxin, and scaritoxin.
• Fish that are most commonly ciguatoxic include amberjack, barracuda, cinnamon, dolphin, eel, emperor, grouper, kingfish, paddletail, parrot fish, red snapper, sea bass, Spanish mackerel, and surgeon fish.

TOXIC DOSE

Toxicity is related to the amount of fish ingested; large fish and viscera contain more toxin.

PATHOPHYSIOLOGY

• Ciguatoxin causes gastrointestinal distress within minutes to hours after ingestion.
• Ciguatoxin also causes a variety of neurologic symptoms, including paresthesias and hot-cold sensory reversal.
• Ciguatoxin does not harm the fish but is stored in its tissues.

EPIDEMIOLOGY

• Poisoning is common.
• Toxic effects following exposure are typically mild to moderate; death occurs rarely.
• Although endemic in the tropics and subtropics, poisoning has been reported in nontropical areas as the result of tourism and importation of fish; most outbreaks in the United States begin in the Caribbean, Hawaii, or Florida.

CAUSES

Ciguatera poisoning can occur following the ingestion of tropical reef-dwelling fish whose diet includes the dinoflagellate *G. toxicus*.

PREGNANCY AND LACTATION

• An infant delivered 2 days after maternal ciguatoxin poisoning had facial palsy, myotonia of hand muscles, respiratory distress syndrome, and meconium aspiration; however, normal birth after severe maternal poisoning also has been reported.
• Premature labor and spontaneous abortion have been reported.
• Breastfeeding should be avoided after eating ciguatoxic fish.

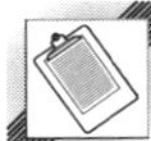

Diagnosis

DIFFERENTIAL DIAGNOSIS

• Toxicologic causes of gastroenteritis include food poisoning (scombroid, neurotoxic shellfish, and bacterial), organophosphate or carbamate insecticide poisoning, botulism, monosodium glutamate, and many others.
• Common nontoxicologic causes include viral gastroenteritis.

SIGNS AND SYMPTOMS

• Paresthesias are the hallmark of ciguatera poisoning.
• The first episodes of ciguatera poisoning are more likely to involve cardiovascular and gastrointestinal manifestations; subsequent episodes are more severe and commonly include chills, arthralgia, and neurologic findings.

Vital Signs

• Hypotension, hyperthermia, bradycardia, and respiratory depression occur in severe cases.
• Hypothermia occurs rarely.

HEENT

• Facial flushing, numbness, and oral paresthesia; metallic taste
• Curious sensation of looseness and pain in the teeth
• Extraocular paresis, blurred vision, dilated pupils, photophobia, lacrimation, and transient blindness
• Dysphonia and hypersalivation possible

Dermatologic

• Diaphoresis is common.
• Pruritus may be followed by cellulitis.
• Urticaria, acne, alopecia, and nail loss occur rarely.

Cardiovascular

• Sinus bradycardia and hypotension
• Extrasystoles, T-wave changes, and dysrhythmia

Pulmonary

• Respiratory depression, dyspnea, and bronchospasm
• In severe cases, respiratory paralysis

Gastrointestinal

• Nausea, vomiting, abdominal pain, and diarrhea that is watery and nonbloody
• Incapacitating hiccoughs possible

Fluids and Electrolytes

Hyperkalemia and dehydration are possible.

Musculoskeletal

• Arthralgia, myalgia, and neck stiffness
• Muscle paralysis of the limb and facial muscles
• Muscle breakdown with increased creatine kinase possible

Neurologic

• Numbness or tingling of the extremities are the most common presentation.
• Headaches are also common.
• Hot-cold temperature sensory reversal usually occurs 2 to 5 days after ingestion. It is frequently localized to the palms of the hands, soles of the feet, lips and mucous membranes of the mouth, and a painful burning sensation upon contact with cold objects.
• Extremity tremor and weakness, vertigo, ataxia, and cranial nerve palsy may occur.
• Drowsiness, fatigue, malaise, tremors, and visual hallucinations may occur.
• Delirium and coma are possible in severe cases.

Genitourinary

• Dysuria and urethritis
• Painful ejaculation and dyspareunia in the sexual partner occasionally reported

PROCEDURES AND LABORATORY TESTS

Essential Tests

• Serum electrolytes, BUN, creatinine, calcium, and magnesium assays to assess electrolyte abnormality as cause of illness
• Serum creatine kinase assay to assess possible muscle injury
• ECG and cardiac monitoring
• Pulse oximetry to assess hypoxia

Recommended Tests

• Head CT, lumbar puncture, and bacterial cultures as clinically indicated to evaluate altered mental status
• Red blood cell and serum cholinesterase assays if insecticide exposure possible

Not Recommended Tests

EMG is not recommended because results have been normal in all patients studied.

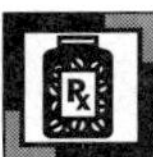

Treatment

Treatment should focus on early administration of mannitol and supportive care of respiratory and cardiovascular function.

DIRECTING PATIENT COURSE

The health-care professional should call the poison control center when:

- Severe poisoning occurs.
- Toxic effects are not consistent with ciguatera fish poisoning.
- Coingestant, drug interaction, or underlying disease presents an unusual problem.

The patient should be referred to a health-care facility when:

- Attempted suicide or homicide is possible.
- Patient or caregiver seems unreliable.
- Toxic effects develop.
- Coingestant, drug interaction, or underlying disease presents an unusual problem.

Admission Considerations

Inpatient management is warranted if any symptoms are present because toxicity may worsen.

DECONTAMINATION

Out of Hospital

Ipecac should be considered to induce emesis within 1 hour of ingestion for the alert pediatric or adult patient if health-care evaluation will be delayed.

In Hospital

- Ipecac should be considered to induce emesis within 1 hour of ingestion for the alert patient who is too small to undergo effective gastric lavage.
- Gastric lavage should be performed in pediatric (tube size 24–32 French) or adult (tube size 36–42 French) patients who present within 1 hour of a large ingestion or if serious effects are present.
- One dose of activated charcoal (1–2 g/kg) should be administered without a cathartic if a substantial ingestion has occurred within the previous few hours.

ANTIDOTES

There is no specific antidote for ciguatera poisoning.

ADJUNCTIVE TREATMENT

- Mannitol can be administered to a patient with neurologic symptoms from ciguatera fish poisoning.

—Dehydration should be corrected prior to administration of mannitol.
—The dosage for adult or pediatric cases is 1 g/kg intravenously over 30 to 60 minutes; a second dose may be indicated.
—The maximum dosage is 1 g/kg at a rate of 500 ml/h.
—Treatment within 24 hours of symptom onset is associated with higher success rate.

- Antiemetic or antidiarrheal preparations may be administered as clinically indicated.
- Seizure

—Adequate airway must be maintained.
—Benzodiazepine can be given for initial control; if seizures persist or recur, another anticonvulsant such as phenobarbital may be added.

- Hypotension

—The patient should be treated with isotonic fluid infusion, the Trendelenburg position, and, if needed, vasopressors. Dopamine is preferred, and norepinephrine is added for refractory hypotension.

- Bradycardia

—Atropine should be administered if bradycardia causes hypotension.
—Adult dose is 0.5 to 1 mg intravenously, repeated in 5 minutes as needed up to 2 mg.
—Pediatric dose is 0.02 mg/kg intravenously, repeated every 5 minutes as needed up to 1 mg
—If bradycardia and hypotension are unresponsive to atropine, isoproterenol can be considered.

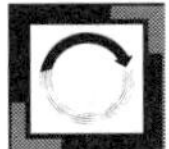

Follow-Up

PATIENT MONITORING

Electrolytes, urinary output, cardiac rhythm, and neurologic effects should be monitored throughout the acute phase of ciguatera poisoning.

EXPECTED COURSE AND PROGNOSIS

- Onset of illness may occur within minutes to 30 hours after ingestion.
- Gastrointestinal symptoms and myalgia typically begin within 6 hours following ingestion and usually resolve within 3 days.
- Pruritus often develops more than 30 hours from the time of ingestion and may persist for weeks.
- Weakness, sensory disturbances, vertigo, and ataxia last 12 hours to 10 days but may persist for months or years in severe cases.
- Early treatment may attenuate or prevent development of chronic neurologic symptoms.
- Toxicity may be more severe with subsequent poisoning.

DISCHARGE CRITERIA/INSTRUCTIONS

- From the emergency department. Asymptomatic or minimally symptomatic patients can be discharged following gastrointestinal decontamination and observation for at least 6 hours.
- From the hospital. Patient can be discharged when oral intake is adequate and neurologic effects have stabilized.

PATIENT EDUCATION

- Patients should avoid further seafood ingestion, alcohol, marijuana, opiates, barbiturates, solvents, herbicides, insecticides, glues, epoxies, ethers, resins, cosmetics, and nuts and grains because these substances may aggravate symptoms or slow recovery. These restrictions should be maintained 3 to 6 months after resolution of symptoms, 12 months in patients who were severely affected.
- Patients should avoid eating fish weighing more than about 3 pounds.

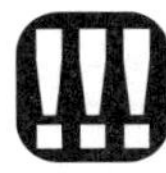

Pitfalls

DIAGNOSIS

Patients may not present until hours to days after the onset of symptoms; history regarding travel and foods may be the only clues.

TREATMENT

- If mannitol is administered, hyponatremic dehydration may occur, especially in children.
- Neurologic symptoms may not respond to pharmacologic treatment.

ICD-9-CM 988.0

Toxic effect of noxious substances eaten as food: fish and shellfish.

See also: SECTION II, Bradycardia, Hypotension, and Seizure chapters.

RECOMMENDED READING

Pern JH, Lewis RJ, Ruff T, et al. Ciguatera and mannitol: experience with a new treatment regimen. *Med J Aust* 1989;151:77–80.

Swift AEB, Swift TR. Ciguatera. *Clin Toxicol* 1993;31:1–29.

Williams RK, Palafox NA. Treatment of pediatric ciguatera fish poisoning. *Am J Dis Child* 1990;144:747–748.

Author: Luke Yip

Reviewer: Katherine M. Hurlbut

Cisapride

Basics

DESCRIPTION

- Cisapride is an oral medication used in the treatment of gastroesophageal reflux disease.
- Cisapride, found in pharmaceutical preparations, including Propulsid, Risamol, and Alimix.

FORMS AND USES

- Cisapride is used to treat gastroesophageal reflux disease and gastrointestinal dysmotility.
- Adult dose is up to 20 mg, four times a day orally.
- Pediatric starting dose is 0.2 mg/kg/day orally divided four times a day.
- The safety and efficacy of cisapride have not been established in children.

TOXIC DOSE

Ingestion of several times the daily dose may produce toxicity.

PATHOPHYSIOLOGY

- Cisapride increases gastrointestinal motility by stimulating the release of acetylcholine.
- The parent drug is responsible for toxicity.

EPIDEMIOLOGY

- Poisoning is rare, and toxic effects following exposure are mild.
- Death may occur in patients with massive overdose who develop cardiac dysrhythmia or during concurrent treatment with cisapride and a drug that inhibits cytochrome P450.

CAUSES

- Poisoning is usually intentional.
- Child neglect or abuse should be considered if the patient is less than 1 year of age, suicide attempt if the patient is over 6 years of age.

RISK FACTORS

- Renal insufficiency allows drug accumulation.
- History of coronary artery disease or previous cardiac dysrhythmia, especially atrial fibrillation, increases the risk of toxic effects.
- Cisapride has an increased half-life in elderly patients.

DRUG AND DISEASE INTERACTIONS

- Cisapride interacts with drugs that inhibit cytochrome P450 3A4, including ketoconazole, itraconazole, miconazole, fluconazole, clarithromycin, erythromycin, and troleandomycin.
- Cimetidine increases plasma concentrations of cisapride.
- Coingestion of drugs that prolong the QT interval or are arrhythmogenic is a risk factor.

PREGNANCY AND LACTATION

- US FDA Pregnancy Class C. The drug exerts animal teratogenic or embryocidal effects, but there are no controlled studies in women, or no studies are available in either animals or women.
- Cisapride distributes poorly into breast milk.

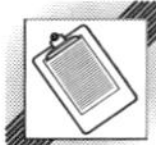

Diagnosis

DIFFERENTIAL DIAGNOSIS

- Other toxicologic causes of prolonged QT interval and cardiac dysrhythmia include tricyclic antidepressants, phenothiazines, chloroquine, astemizole, class I antidysrhythmic drugs, and several others.
- Nontoxicologic causes include hypocalcemia, hypokalemia, ischemic heart disease, torsade de pointes, congenital prolonged QT, and several others.

SIGNS AND SYMPTOMS

- The patient is usually asymptomatic.
- Severe cases may present with syncope or cardiac dysrhythmia manifested initially by prolonged QT interval.

Cardiovascular

Potentially fatal cardiac dysrhythmias include QT prolongation, ventricular tachycardia, ventricular fibrillation, and torsade de pointes.

Gastrointestinal

Diarrhea and abdominal pain are common adverse events.

Neurologic

The multiple effects (confusion, syncope) are all related to decreased CNS perfusion in severe cases.

PROCEDURES AND LABORATORY TESTS

Essential Tests

ECG and cardiac monitoring are performed to detect prolonged QT interval.

Recommended Tests

- Serum electrolytes, BUN, creatinine, calcium, magnesium are assessed in patients with ECG abnormalities or altered mental status.
- Serum acetaminophen and aspirin levels are measured in overdose setting to detect occult ingestion.

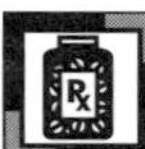

Treatment

- Treatment should focus on detection and therapy of cardiac dysrhythmia.
- The dose and time of exposure should be determined for all substances involved.

DIRECTING PATIENT COURSE

The health-care professional should call the poison control center when:

- Severe or persistent effects develop.
- The signs and symptoms are not consistent with cisapride overdose.
- Coingestant, drug interaction, or underlying disease presents an unusual problem.

The patient should be referred to a health-care facility when:

- Attempted suicide or homicide is possible.
- Patient or caregiver seems unreliable.
- Any symptoms are present.
- Coingestant, drug interaction, or underlying disease presents an unusual problem.

Admission Considerations

Inpatient management is warranted when patients develop cardiac or neurologic manifestations.

DECONTAMINATION

Out of Hospital

Ipecac should be administered to induce emesis within 1 hour of ingestion for the alert pediatric or adult patient if health-care evaluation will be delayed.

In Hospital

- Ipecac-induced emesis within 1 hour of ingestion should be administered to the pediatric patient who is too small to have effective gastric lavage due to orogastric tube size constraints.
- Gastric lavage should be performed in pediatric (tube size 24–32 French) or adult (tube size 36–42 French) patients for substantial ingestion presenting within 1 hour of ingestion or if serious effects are present.
- One dose of activated charcoal (1–2 g/kg) should be administered without a cathartic if a substantial ingestion has occurred within the previous few hours.

ANTIDOTES

There is no specific antidote for cisapride poisoning.

ADJUNCTIVE TREATMENT

Dysrhythmia or Conduction Abnormality

- Seizures must be controlled and acidemia corrected.
- If QRS widening or dysrhythmias persist, sodium bicarbonate 1 to 2 mEq/kg bolus should be administered intravenously, repeated as needed to suppress dysrhythmia while maintaining arterial pH less than 7.55.
- Lidocaine is used for ventricular tachycardia or multifocal premature ventricular complexes.

—Adult dose is 50 to 100 mg intravenous bolus followed by an infusion of 2 to 4 mg/min titrated to desired effect.
—Pediatric dose is 1 mg/kg bolus intravenously, followed by infusion of 20 to 50 μg/kg/min titrated to effect.
—The bolus dose may be repeated in 10 to 15 minutes for both pediatric and adult.

- Bretylium is administered at 5 mg/kg over 1 minute. If unsuccessful, a dose of 10 mg/kg is administered over 1 minute, repeated as necessary to total dose of 30 mg/kg.

Torsade de Pointes

- Electrolyte abnormalities are to be corrected if present.
- The adult dose of magnesium sulfate ($MgSO_4$) is 1 to 2 g intravenous push, which may be repeated in 10 to 15 minutes. The intravenous infusion begins at 2 to 10 mg/min, titrated upward to sustain antidysrhythmic effect. The pediatric dose is 25 to 50 mg/kg intravenously over 5 minutes.
- Isoproterenol and sequential overdrive cardiac pacing should be administered if there is no response.
- Verapamil, quinidine, disopyramide, procainamide, and sotalol should be avoided.

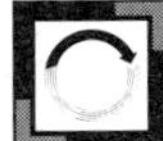

Follow-Up

PATIENT MONITORING

Continuous respiratory and cardiac monitoring in an intensive care unit should be performed in symptomatic patients or following large ingestion.

EXPECTED COURSE AND PROGNOSIS

- Most patients manifest few effects and suffer no permanent effects.
- Cardiac dysrhythmia is usually responsive to treatment.
- Death occurs rarely, when malignant dysrhythmia occurs outside the hospital.

DISCHARGE CRITERIA/INSTRUCTIONS

- From the emergency department. Patients asymptomatic for 6 hours after overdose and who have undergone gastrointestinal decontamination may be discharged following psychiatric evaluation as appropriate.
- From the hospital. Patients may be discharged after mental status, ECG, and vital signs have returned to normal, and psychiatric evaluation is complete.

PATIENT EDUCATION

Patients should be warned about concurrent use with contraindicated medications.

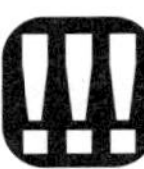

Pitfalls

DIAGNOSIS

The use of cisapride must be avoided when increased GI motility could be harmful: gastrointestinal hemorrhage, bowel perforation, or mechanical obstruction.

ICD-9-CM 973.4

Poisoning by digestants.

See also: SECTION II, Hypotension and Ventricular Dysrhythmia chapters; SECTION III, Magnesium Sulfate chapter.

RECOMMENDED READING

Bran S, Murray WA, Hirsch IB, Palmer JP. Long QT syndrome during high-dose cisapride. *Arch Intern Med* 1995;155:765–768.

Wysowski DK, Bacsanyi J. Cisapride and fatal arrhythmia. *N Engl J Med* 1996;335:290–229.

Author: Kathleen Graham

Reviewer: Richard C. Dart

Clonidine

Basics

DESCRIPTION

Clonidine, an α_2-receptor agonist, is available as Catapres (0.1-, 0.2-, and 0.3-mg tablets); Catapres-TTS (2.5-, 5.0-, and 7.5-mg transdermal patches); and Combipres (0.1-, 0.2-, and 0.3-mg tablets).

FORMS AND USES

- Hypertension. 0.1 mg by mouth twice a day to a maximum of 2.4 mg/day; clonidine transdermal 1 patch/wk; 0.1 to 0.3 mg/day.
- Opiate and nicotine withdrawal. As much as 25 μg/kg/day in divided doses.
- Also used for prophylaxis of migraine headache, and the flushing associated with menopause and dysmenorrhea.

TOXIC DOSE

- Adults have survived doses greater than 10 mg.
- Children have become symptomatic after ingestion of 1 tablet (0.1 mg) clonidine.
- Deaths have been reported from children sucking on discarded clonidine patches.

PATHOPHYSIOLOGY

- Clonidine is an α_2-receptor agonist that inhibits sympathetic outflow by presynaptic α_2 stimulation in the brainstem and medulla; it causes peripheral α-receptor stimulation as well.
- The precise mechanisms of action or toxicity are unknown.

EPIDEMIOLOGY

- Poisoning is uncommon.
- Toxic effects following exposure are typically mild to moderate, with death occurring in cases of large overdose where medical intervention is not immediately available.

CAUSES

- Toxic ingestion is usually intentional.
- Child neglect or abuse should be considered if the patient is less than 1 year of age, suicide attempt if the patient is over 6 years of age.

DRUG AND DISEASE INTERACTIONS

Sedating agents may enhance CNS depression caused by clonidine; other antihypertensive agents may increase the hypotensive effect.

PREGNANCY AND LACTATION

- US FDA Pregnancy Category C. The drug exerts animal teratogenic or embryocidal effects, but there are no controlled studies in women, or no studies are available in either animals or women.
- Clonidine is secreted in breast milk in clinically significant amounts.

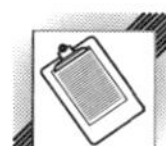

Diagnosis

DIFFERENTIAL DIAGNOSIS

- Toxicologic causes of CNS depression include anticonvulsants, alcohols, benzodiazepines, barbiturates, narcotics, other imidazolines, gamma-hydroxybutrate and many others.
- Nontoxicologic causes of CNS depression include metabolic changes such as hypoglycemia, hyponatremia, hypoxia, hypothermia, hypothyroidism, and postictal states; infectious causes such as meningitis or sepsis; space-occupying lesions; trauma; and tumors.

SIGNS AND SYMPTOMS

Sedation, apnea, hypotension, bradycardia, and miosis are characteristic. The toxic effects of clonidine are often mistaken for a narcotic overdose.

Vital Signs

- Initial transient hypertension (usually occurs before reaching health care) can be followed by hypotension, bradycardia, hypothermia, and hypoventilation.
- Apnea may develop; patients will respond to stimulation (such as stroking foot) by resuming normal breathing pattern but revert to hypoventilation or even apnea when not touched or otherwise stimulated.

HEENT

Miosis and dry mucous membranes are characteristic.

Dermatologic

Pallor is common.

Cardiovascular

- Bradycardia is common; atrioventricular nodal blocks occur rarely.
- Cardiac ischemia may develop in hypotensive patients.

Pulmonary

Respiratory depression may progress to apnea.

Neurologic

- CNS depression ranges from lethargy to coma; ataxia, hyporeflexia, and hypotonia may occur.
- Seizures occur rarely.

Endocrine

Weight gain, gynecomastia, and interference with the renin-angiotensin-aldosterone system are infrequent physiologic effects.

PROCEDURES AND LABORATORY TESTS

Essential Tests

No tests are usually needed in asymptomatic patients

Recommended Tests

- ECG and cardiac monitoring should be performed to assess bradycardia and atrioventricular nodal blocks. Cardiac ischemia may develop in hypotensive patients.
- Serum electrolytes, BUN, and creatinine are assayed to assess electrolyte causes of altered mental status or hypotension.
- Arterial blood gas or pulse oximetry is performed for assessment of altered mental status.
- Head CT, lumbar puncture, bacterial cultures are obtained to assess altered mental status.
- Serum acetaminophen and aspirin levels are determined in an overdose setting to assess occult ingestion.

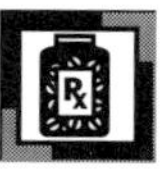

Treatment

- Treatment should focus on airway management and general supportive care.
- The dose and time of exposure should be determined for all substances involved.

DIRECTING PATIENT COURSE

The health-care professional should call the poison control center when:

- Hypotension or altered mental status develops.
- Toxic effects are not consistent with clonidine.
- Coingestant, drug interaction, or underlying disease presents an unusual problem.

The patient should be referred to a health-care facility when:

- Attempted suicide or homicide is possible.
- Patient or caregiver seems unreliable.
- Toxic effects develop.
- Coingestant, drug interaction, or underlying disease presents an unusual problem.

Admission Considerations

Inpatient management is warranted for:

- Small children with a history of clonidine ingestion
- Adults who develop toxic effects

DECONTAMINATION

Out of Hospital

Emesis should not be induced because CNS depression may develop quickly.

In Hospital

- Gastric lavage should be performed in pediatric (tube size 24–32 French) or adult (tube size 36–42 French) patients for large ingestion presenting within 1 hour of ingestion or if serious effects are present.
- One dose of activated charcoal (1–2 g/kg) should be administered without a cathartic if a substantial ingestion has occurred within the previous few hours.
- In cases of suspected ingestion of clonidine patches, whole-bowel irrigation is recommended.

ANTIDOTES

- There is no specific antidote for clonidine poisoning.
- Naloxone is typically used to treat patients with depressed mental status of unknown etiology; however, its role in clonidine overdose is unclear (some studies suggest efficacy in reversing opioid-like effects and cardiovascular depression, but it is likely that body stimulation is responsible).

—Patients with coma and respiratory depression are treated with 2 mg intravenously initially and observed for clinical improvement.
—Dose may be doubled to 4 mg intravenously; if no improvement is seen, more naloxone is unlikely to have an effect

ADJUNCTIVE TREATMENT

- Hypotension. The patient should be treated with isotonic fluid infusion, the Trendelenburg position, and, if needed, vasopressors. Dopamine is preferred, and norepinephrine is added for refractory hypotension.
- Hypertension. If end-organ damage develops (rare), treatment with a titratable antihypertensive such as nitroprusside should be initiated.
- Bradycardia should be treated initially according to Advanced Cardiac Life Support guidelines; but if bradycardia persists, **cardiac pacing** could be effective.
- Hemodialysis, multiple-dose activated charcoal, and urinary alkalinization have not been demonstrated to be effective.

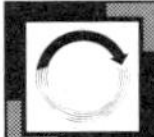

Follow-Up

PATIENT MONITORING

Respiratory function and cardiac rhythm should be monitored continuously.

EXPECTED COURSE AND PROGNOSIS

- Toxic effects typically peak soon after ingestion of tablets, but may be delayed after ingestion of a patch.
- Complete recovery occurs if adequate airway management is maintained.
- Bradycardia, hypotension, and apnea may persist for more than 24 hours following severe overdose.

DISCHARGE CRITERIA/INSTRUCTIONS

- From the emergency department. Asymptomatic patients may be discharged following cardiac monitoring during a minimum 4- to 6-hour observation period and after psychiatric evaluation, if needed.
- From the hospital. Patients may be discharged when CNS, respiratory, and cardiovascular effects have resolved or stabilized, and after psychiatric evaluation, if needed.

PATIENT EDUCATION

- Adults should be instructed to keep clonidine pills and patches out of reach of children.
- Clonidine patches should be disposed of in childproof containers; when discarded, patches may contain up to 75% of their original content.

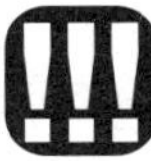

Pitfalls

DIAGNOSIS

The toxic effects of clonidine are often mistaken for a narcotic overdose.

TREATMENT

- Treatment of the initial transient hypertensive event with a long-acting antihypertensive may complicate management of subsequent clonidine-induced hypotension.
- Sequelae of hypoxia may occur if airway control is not achieved early.

ICD-9-CM 972.6

Poisoning by agents primarily affecting the cardiovascular system: other antihypertensive agents.

See also: SECTION II, Hypertension and Hypotension chapters; and Section III, Naloxone and Nalmephene chapter.

RECOMMENDED READING

Anderson RJ, Hart GR. Clonidine overdose. *Ann Emerg Med* 1981;10:107–112.

Caravati EM. Clonidine. In: Tintinalli JE, et al., eds. *Emergency medicine: a comprehensive study guide,* 4th ed. New York: McGraw-Hill, 1996:805–807.

Wiley JF, Wiley CC, Torrey SB, et al. Clonidine poisoning in young children. *J Pediatr* 1990;116:654.

Authors: Lada Kokan and Gerald F. O'Malley

Reviewer: Richard C. Dart

Cobalt

Basics

DESCRIPTION

Cobalt is an essential trace element (cyanocobolamine is vitamin B12).

FORMS AND USES

- Cobalt is a component of high-speed steel superalloys, jet engines, magnets, and cutting tools; cement (with chromium and nickel); and hard metal, a mixture of tungsten carbide (70%–95%), cobalt (5%–25%), and other trace metals (<5%).
- Cobalt blue is a pigment used in glass, china, and paint.
- Cobalt is used as a catalyst in the oil and chemistry industry and is used to blend tungsten and carbon by powdered metallurgy.

TOXIC DOSE

- Acute inhalation of 20 mg/m^3 is potentially lethal.
- Chronic inhalation of 1 to 2 mg/m^3 is associated with fatal pulmonary disease.

PATHOPHYSIOLOGY

The mechanism of cobalt toxicity is not well described.

- Induction of pulmonary fibrosis may be related to cobalt's high protein solubility.
- Cobalt may contribute to allergic dermatitis and reactive airway disease by acting as a hapten with endogenous proteins.

EPIDEMIOLOGY

- Cobalt poisoning is uncommon.
- Toxic effects following exposure are typically mild.
- Death occurs rarely and only from chronic exposure.

CAUSES

Cobalt toxicity is usually an occupational hazard associated with long-term exposure.

RISK FACTORS

Cobalt toxicity is an occupational hazard for construction workers, masons (from contact with cement), workers in the electroplating industry, diamond polishers, cobalt refining, and hard metal production, among many others.

WORKPLACE STANDARDS

- OSHA. PEL TWA is 0.1 mg/m^3.
- NIOSH. REL TWA is 0.05 mg/m^3; IDLH is 20 mg/m^3.

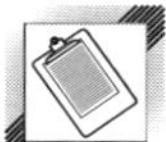

Diagnosis

The diagnosis of cobalt poisoning is established by a history of occupational exposure accompanied by skin sensitization or pulmonary disease.

DIFFERENTIAL DIAGNOSIS

- Other toxicologic causes of skin sensitization include nickel and chromium.
- Nontoxicologic causes that produce similar pulmonary symptoms include chronic obstructive pulmonary disease from any cause, as well as chronic recurrent bronchospasm, infectious pneumoconioses, and reactive airway diseases.

SIGNS AND SYMPTOMS

Vital Signs

Tachycardia, tachypnea, and decreased pulse oximetry are common following chronic cobalt inhalation.

HEENT

Mucous membrane irritation may occur following cobalt dust exposure.

Dermatologic

- Skin sensitization and dermatitis are common; cross-sensitization may occur with chromium and nickel.
- "Cement worker's eczema" may be due to cobalt.
- A red, often pruritic, papular rash known as cobalt itch may develop.
- Facial flushing has been reported following ingestion.

Cardiovascular

Cardiomyopathy has occurred in the past due to the addition of cobalt in beer, but is no longer seen due to food regulations.

Pulmonary

- Lung toxicity usually requires chronic exposure to cobalt.
- Nonproductive cough and dyspnea are common among workers exposed to dusts containing cobalt.
- Obstructive lung disease, interstitial fibrosis (hard metal lung disease), and reactive airway disease may develop with chronic exposure.
- Interstitial pneumonitis may develop following acute inhalation, but is rare.

Gastrointestinal

Nausea, vomiting, diarrhea, and abdominal pain occur following ingestion but also have been reported following inhalation.

Renal

Glomerulonephritis may occur following chronic exposure, but is rare.

Hematologic

Cobalt chloride boosts red cell production, causing polycythemia.

Endocrine

Hypothyroidism and thyroid hyperplasia (goiter) were also noted in patients that developed cardiomyopathy following cobalt addition to beer.

PROCEDURES AND LABORATORY TESTS

Essential Tests

- For acute inhalation or ingestion, no tests are essential.
- For symptomatic patients with chronic exposure, complete blood count, serum electrolytes, creatinine, urinalysis and thyroid function, pulmonary function tests may be ordered. Findings may indicate polycythemia, glomerulonephritis, or hypothyroidism.

Recommended Tests

- Arterial blood gas (ABG) analysis to evaluate pulmonary gas exchange should be performed for patients with persistent pulmonary effects of cobalt exposure.
- Urinary cobalt level may be used to confirm exposure.

—Normal level of urinary cobalt is 0.1 to 0.2 $\mu g/L$.
—Serum levels are not clinically useful for acute or chronic toxicity.

- Chest radiography may be helpful in evaluating pulmonary effects.

—It is especially useful in patients who have persistent pulmonary complaints, hypoxia, or abnormal ABG analysis results.
—Findings consistent with interstitial lung disease of chronic cobalt exposure include small nodular densities and infiltrates.

- Pulmonary function test results are usually abnormal in patients who have symptomatic interstitial fibrosis, reactive airway disease, or chronic obstructive pulmonary disease.
- Dermal patch testing may be useful in diagnosis of cobalt-induced allergic dermatitis.

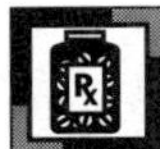

Treatment

- Discontinuation of exposure is the mainstay of therapy.
- Patients should be placed on supplemental oxygen and treated initially for wheezing with nebulized β_2-agonists.
- Dose, time, and duration of exposure should be determined for all substances involved.
- The need for consultation with a pulmonologist should be assessed.

DIRECTING PATIENT COURSE

The health-care professional should call a poison control center when:

- Signs and symptoms are not consistent with cobalt poisoning.
- Coingestant, drug interaction, or underlying disease presents an unusual problem.

The patient should be referred to a health-care facility when:

- Rash, respiratory distress, or other toxic effects are present.
- Coingestant, drug interaction, or underlying disease presents an unusual problem.

Admission Considerations

Inpatient management is warranted if the patient exhibits respiratory distress, evidence of upper airway edema, hypoxia, or persistent recalcitrant wheezing.

DECONTAMINATION

Out of Hospital

- Ingestion. Ipecac should be administered within 1 hour of large ingestion for the alert pediatric or adult patient if health-care evaluation will be delayed.
- Inhalation. The patient should be removed from source of exposure, and oxygen should be administered if available.
- Dermal exposure. The exposed area should be washed thoroughly with soap and water.

In Hospital

- Ipecac should be administered to induce emesis within 1 hour of ingestion for the alert patient who is too small to undergo effective gastric lavage.
- Gastric lavage should be performed in pediatric (tube size 24–32 French) or adult (tube size 36–42 French) patients presenting within 1 hour of a large ingestion or if serious effects are present.
- One dose of activated charcoal (1–2 g/kg) should be administered without a cathartic if a large ingestion has occurred within the preceding few hours.

ANTIDOTES

- There is no specific antidote for cobalt poisoning.
- British anti-Lewisite and calcium ethylenediaminetetraacetic acid increase cobalt excretion in animal models, but their use in human overdose is unclear, so neither is routinely recommended.

ADJUNCTIVE TREATMENT

- For bronchospasm:

—Oxygen, followed by albuterol 0.15 mg/kg (maximum of 10 mg) in saline with humidified oxygen, should be administered via nebulizer every 20 to 30 minutes, and the patient should be monitored for response; if the peak expiratory flow rate is greater than 90% predicted after initial dose, additional doses may not be needed.
—Methylprednisolone 60 to 125 mg (1.0–1.5 mg/kg) given intravenously (children 1–2 mg/kg) every 6 to 8 hours; this dosage may be decreased to a single daily dose and tapered.
—The methylprednisolone dose may be converted to prednisone, 2 mg/kg orally for several days.
—Case reports suggest that corticosteroids and cytotoxic agents may be beneficial in managing pulmonary interstitial fibrosis, but there are no well-designed human studies demonstrating efficacy.

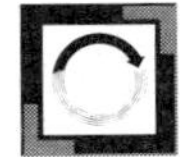

Follow-Up

PATIENT MONITORING

- Patients should be observed in a monitored setting until respiratory symptoms resolve.

EXPECTED COURSE AND PROGNOSIS

- Most patients with low-level acute inhalation exposure need not be evaluated in a health-care facility.
- Patients suffering high-level inhalation exposures resulting in severe pulmonary symptoms may have a protracted hospital course.
- Skin sensitization may develop from chronic cobalt exposure and is usually permanent.
- Chronic obstructive lung disease may develop with chronic cobalt exposure.

DISCHARGE CRITERIA/INSTRUCTIONS

- From the emergency department. Asymptomatic patients or patients in whom symptoms resolve quickly may be discharged immediately after evaluation. Follow-up should be provided for patients with substantial inhalation exposures.
- From the hospital. Patients may be discharged when pulmonary or cardiovascular complaints have resolved or become stable.
- An industrial hygienist should be consulted for workplace evaluation, and the patient's need for work restriction or removal from the workplace should be evaluated.

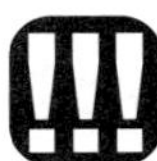

Pitfalls

TREATMENT

Workers with either dermatologic or pulmonary signs or symptoms of cobalt toxicity should be removed from the source of exposure until evaluation has been completed.

FOLLOW-UP

- Patients with abnormal pulmonary function tests should be followed closely, even after removal from the source of exposure.
- Workers with documented hypersensitivity reactions (contact dermatitis or respiratory symptoms) should be removed from the workplace.

ICD-9-CM 985

Toxic effect of other metals.

RECOMMENDED READING

Shirakawa T, Kusaka Y, Fujimura N, et al. Occupational asthma from cobalt sensitivity in workers exposed to hard metal dust. *Chest* 1989;95:29–37.

Templeton DM. Cobalt. In: Sullivan JB Jr, Krieger GR, eds. *Hazardous materials toxicology.* Baltimore: Williams & Wilkins, 1992:853–859.

Author: Edwin K. Kuffner

Reviewer: Richard C. Dart

Cocaine

Basics

DESCRIPTION

Cocaine is a widespread drug of abuse as well as a pharmaceutical product used to produce vasoconstriction of the nasal mucosa.

FORMS AND USES

- Pharmaceutical cocaine is available in aqueous solutions of 4% to 10% for use as a topical anesthetic and vasoconstrictor and is often combined with tetracaine and adrenaline to form Tetracaine Adrenaline Cocaine (TAC), a topical anesthetic.
- The coca plant, *Erythroxylan coca,* is the source of cocaine. Dried coca leaves contain approximately 2% cocaine
- "Crack" cocaine is the crystalline base form of cocaine that is heat stable and may be smoked.
- Slang terms include coke, crack, snow, rock, and white girl, among many others.

TOXIC DOSE

Individual toxic response to cocaine varies widely; in patients who are not chronic users, nasal application of 25 mg (less than 1 ml of 4% solution) has resulted in death.

PATHOPHYSIOLOGY

Cocaine increases the concentration of norepinephrine in the synapse by increasing release of norepinephrine from neurons in both the CNS and peripheral nervous systems and blocking its reuptake at the presynaptic membranes of the sympathetic nervous system.

EPIDEMIOLOGY

- Cocaine is one of the most frequently used illicit drugs, and poisoning is common.
- Death occurs in patients with severe toxic effects, such as seizure, dysrhythmia, or hyperthermia.

CAUSES

- Cocaine poisoning usually results from recreational cocaine abuse.
- Severe toxicity may develop in "body-packers" or "body-stuffers."
- Child neglect should be considered in pediatric patients.

DRUG AND DISEASE INTERACTIONS

- Cocaine has a synergistic effect with other sympathomimetic agents (e.g., amphetamines).
- Cocaine may interact with monoamine oxidase inhibitor antidepressants (e.g., phenelzine or tranylcypromine) to cause severe hypertension, hyperthermia, and death.

PREGNANCY AND LACTACTION

- US FDA Pregnancy Classification X. Studies in animals or humans have demonstrated fetal abnormalities, or there is evidence of fetal risk based on human experience, or both, and the risk clearly outweighs any possible benefit.
- Maternal cocaine use during pregnancy is associated with spontaneous abortion, placenta previa, abruptio placentae, fetal prematurity, low birth weight, multiple intestinal atresia, and necrotizing enterocolitis.

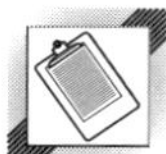

Diagnosis

DIFFERENTIAL DIAGNOSIS

- Other toxicologic causes of adrenergic excess include other sympathomimetic agents (e.g., amphetamine, methamphetamine), neuroleptic malignant syndrome, and serotonin syndrome.
- Nontoxicologic causes of adrenergic excess include hyperthyroidism, manic episode, alcohol or sedative withdrawal, and pheochromocytoma.

SIGNS AND SYMPTOMS

Vital Signs

- Hypertension, tachycardia, and mild hyperthermia are common.
- Severe hyperthermia and hypotension may develop in overdose.
- Shock may result from severe overdose.

HEENT

Mydriasis may occur, along with nasal mucosal ischemia or septal perforation (with chronic abuse)

Dermatologic

Pallor and diaphoresis are common.

Cardiovascular

- Acute toxic effects may include myocardial ischemia and infarction, aortic dissection, cardiac sudden death, and dysrhythmias.
- Chronic cocaine abuse may cause myocarditis and cardiomyopathy.

Pulmonary

- Pneumomediastinum, pneumothorax, and pulmonary hemorrhage may be seen in freebase and crack cocaine smokers.
- Pulmonary hypertension and pulmonary edema may develop.

Gastrointestinal

- Bowel ischemia and infarction due to splanchnic vasospasm may occur in patients of all ages.
- Necrotizing enterocolitis may occur in neonates.

Hepatic

Hepatic necrosis may develop in patients with severe hyperthermia.

Renal

Acute renal failure may occur as a complication of rhabdomyolysis.

Fluids and Electrolytes

Lactic acidosis may occur.

Musculoskeletal

Rhabdomyolysis may occur due to hyperthermia, agitation, and seizures.

Neurologic

- Agitation and seizures are common.
- Intracranial hemorrhage, ischemic infarcts, and cerebral vasculitis occur in rare cases.

Vascular

Peripheral ischemia may follow intraarterial injection.

Psychiatric

Psychosis, paranoid delusions, and mania are common.

PROCEDURES AND LABORATORY TESTS

Essential Tests

Laboratory testing may not be needed in asymptomatic or minimally symptomatic patients.

Recommended Tests

- ECG and cardiac monitoring should be performed in symptomatic patients.
  - —Sinus tachycardia is common; other dysrhythmias (supraventricular and ventricular) suggest severe toxicity.
  - —Acute ischemia and infarction may occur.
- Serum electrolytes, BUN, creatinine, glucose, and urinalysis should be obtained to assess renal injury and effects.
- Complete blood count, liver function tests, coagulation studies, and serum creatine kinase should be obtained in patients with hyperthermia or marked agitation.
- Serum acetaminophen and aspirin levels in an overdose setting may detect occult ingestion; the urinary cocaine screen may detect cocaine metabolites several days after exposure.
- Head CT, lumbar puncture, pulse oximetry, and toxicology studies are used to evaluate other causes of seizure and altered mental status.
- Chest radiography should be performed in patients with chest pain, pulmonary symptoms, or hypoxia.
- Abdominal radiographs should be performed in patients suspected of ingesting packets of cocaine.

Not Recommended Tests

Serum cocaine levels are not clinically useful.

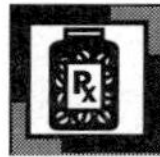

Treatment

- Initial treatment should focus on controlling agitation, seizures, and hyperthermia, and supporting hemodynamic function.
- Dose and time of exposure should be determined for all substances involved.

DIRECTING PATIENT COURSE

The health-care professional should call the poison control center when:

- Signs and symptoms are not consistent with cocaine poisoning.
- Severe effects such as altered mental status, seizure, cardiac dysrhythmia or ischemia, hyperthermia, or other end-organ damage are present.
- Coingestant, drug interaction, or underlying disease presents an unusual problem.

The patient should be referred to a health-care facility when:

- Attempted suicide or homicide is possible.
- The patient or caregiver seems unreliable.
- Any toxic effects develop.
- Coingestant, drug interaction, or underlying disease presents an unusual problem.

Admission Considerations

Inpatient management is warranted when minor toxic effects do not resolve quickly or with ischemic chest pain, hyperthermia, or other end-organ injury.

DECONTAMINATION

Out of Hospital

Emesis should not be induced because of its potential for causing seizures.

In Hospital

- Gastric lavage is generally not indicated in cocaine poisoning because cocaine ingestion is uncommon.
- If ingestion has occurred, one dose of activated charcoal (1–2 g/kg) should be administered if the ingestion is substantial and has occurred within the previous few hours.
- Whole-bowel irrigation should be considered for patients suspected of ingesting packets of cocaine

ANTIDOTES

There is no specific antidote for cocaine poisoning.

ADJUNCTIVE TREATMENT

- Control of agitation. A benzodiazepine familiar to the provider should be administered.

—Diazepam. Adult dose is 5 to 10 mg intravenously. Pediatric dose is 0.2 to 0.5 mg/kg intravenously, doses repeated at 10-minute intervals, titrating to effect.
—Airway should be monitored closely.
—Haloperidol should be avoided in treating cocaine toxicity because it may interact with cocaine to cause hyperthermia.

- Hypertension. If hypertension is not responsive to benzodiazepines, or end-organ damage develops (aortic dissection, CNS bleed, myocardial infarction), a short-acting, titratable antihypertensive agent, such as nitroprusside, should be administered.
- Hypotension. The patient should be treated with isotonic fluid infusion, the Trendelenburg position, and, if needed, vasopressors. Dopamine is preferred, and norepinephrine is added for refractory hypotension.
- Seizures

—A patent airway must be ensured.
—A benzodiazepine is administered for initial control. If seizures persist or recur, another anticonvulsant such as phenobarbital may be added.

- Ventricular dysrhythmia or conduction abnormality

—The health-care provider must first control seizures and correct acidemia.
—If QRS widening or dysrhythmia persists, sodium bicarbonate may be administered: 1 to 2 mEq/kg intravenous bolus, repeated as needed to narrow the QRS interval, but not to exceed an arterial pH of 7.55.
—Bretylium. 5 mg/kg over 1 minute; if unsuccessful, 10 mg/kg over 1 minute is administered, repeated as necessary to total dose of 30 mg/kg.

- Rhabdomyolysis. Acidemia and hyperkalemia should be corrected, and adequate hydration and urine output (1–2 ml/kg/h) should be ensured.

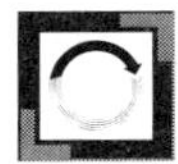

Follow-Up

PATIENT MONITORING

Symptomatic patients require continuous cardiac and hemodynamic monitoring and frequent temperature measurement.

EXPECTED COURSE AND PROGNOSIS

- Patients generally recover within hours from mild or moderate intoxication.
- Health-care providers must also be alert for signs and symptoms of complications of cocaine poisoning:

—End-organ injury from hypertension
—Cerebral injury from uncontrolled seizures, cerebrovascular accident, or cerebral vasculitis or hemorrhage
—Acute renal failure due to rhabdomyolysis or hypotension
—Cardiac dysfunction due to ischemia, cardiomyopathy, valvular disease, or aortic dissection
—Peripheral vasculitis and cardiac valvular disease due to chronic intravenous abuse
—Complications and long-term sequelae are more common in massive, or chronic, intravenous or inhalational abuse

DISCHARGE CRITERIA/INSTRUCTIONS

- From emergency department. Patients may be discharged after cocaine effects have resolved, vital signs and mental status have returned to baseline, and myocardial ischemia has been ruled out.
- From hospital. Patients may be discharged after cocaine effects have resolved or stabilized, vital signs and mental status have returned to baseline, and laboratory values have normalized.
- Refer patients for substance abuse treatment.

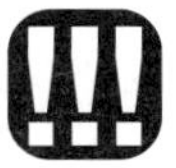

Pitfalls

DIAGNOSIS

- Mental status changes, seizures, hypertension, and hyperthermia should prompt evaluation for CNS bleed or infarction and infection.
- Chest pain should prompt evaluation for myocardial infarction, aortic dissection, or pneumomediastinum.

TREATMENT

- Hyperthermia requires early and aggressive treatment.
- Intravenous abusers are at risk for complications of intravenous drug abuse.

ICD-9-CM 968.5

Poisoning by other central nervous system depressants and anesthetics: surface (topical) and infiltration anesthetics.

See also: SECTION II, Body Packer/Body Stuffer, Coma, Hypertension, Hypotension, Seizures, Ventricular Dysrhythmias chapters; and SECTION III, Nitroprusside and Whole-Bowel Irrigation chapters.

RECOMMENDED READING

Cregler LL, Mark H. Medical complications of cocaine abuse. *N Engl J Med* 1986;315:1495–1500.

Goldfrank LR, Hoffman RS. The cardiovascular effects of cocaine. *Ann Emerg Med* 1991;20:165–175.

Hollander JE. The management of cocaine-associated myocardial ischemia. *N Engl J Med* 1995;333:1267–1272.

Author: Edward W. Cetaruk

Reviewer: Luke Yip

Cocaine "Washed-Out" Syndrome

Basics

DESCRIPTION

• Cocaine washed-out syndrome involves depressed mental status, ranging from lethargy to deep coma, following binge use of cocaine or another stimulant.
• Other causes of altered mental status must be excluded.

TOXIC DOSE

Repeated use over days (binge use) is required to produce the syndrome.

PATHOPHYSIOLOGY

• The syndrome is possibly related to depletion of CNS catecholamines by repeated cocaine abuse.
• Similar cases have been noted after binge use of other stimulants such as methamphetamines.

EPIDEMIOLOGY

The syndrome occurs in 0.2% to 11.6% of patients presenting to the emergency department with illness related to recent cocaine use.

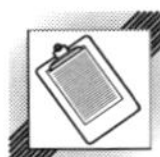

Diagnosis

DIFFERENTIAL DIAGNOSIS

• This is a diagnosis of exclusion.
• Other causes of depressed mental status should be investigated: poisoning by other agents, hypoxia, hypoglycemia, electrolyte abnormality or intracranial infection, bleeding, or ischemia.

SIGNS AND SYMPTOMS

No pathognomonic signs develop. The patient is in a deep coma without apparent cause unless history of binge use of cocaine is obtained.

Vital Signs

Vital signs are typically normal despite presence of coma.

HEENT

Pupils are typically mid-position.

Dermatologic

Stigmata of intravenous drug use may be present.

Neurologic

• Depressed mental status may range from mild lethargy to deep coma.
• No localizing neurological signs should be present.

PROCEDURES AND LABORATORY TESTS

Essential Tests

• Serum electrolytes, BUN, creatinine, liver function tests to determine other causes of coma
• Arterial blood gases to detect hypoxia or methemoglobinemia
• ECG, serum acetaminophen and aspirin levels are measured in overdose setting to detect occult ingestion
• Head CT, lumbar puncture, and cultures to assess other causes of coma

Recommended Tests

In unusual cases, tests to detect hypoadrenal or hypothyroid function may be appropriate.

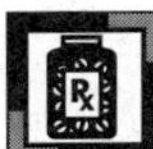

Treatment

Therapy should focus on supportive care and management of airway.

DIRECTING PATIENT COURSE

The health-care professional should call the poison control center when:

- Persistent CNS depression is present.
- Coingestant, drug interaction, or underlying disease presents an unusual problem.

The patient should be referred to a health-care facility when:

- All patients with CNS depression should be examined in a health-care facility.

ADMISSION CONSIDERATIONS

All patients should be admitted.

Out of Hospital

Emesis should not be induced.

In Hospital

- Emesis and gastric lavage are not recommended.
- One dose of activated charcoal (1–2 g/kg) should be administered without a cathartic if a substantial ingestion has occurred within the previous few hours.

ANTIDOTES

No specific treatment or antidote is available.

ADJUNCTIVE TREATMENT

Supportive care should be provided in a monitored setting.

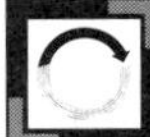

Follow-Up

PATIENT MONITORING

Respiratory and cardiac function should be monitored continuously.

EXPECTED COURSE AND PROGNOSIS

- Patient's mental status should begin to improve within several hours, occasionally requiring as much as 24 hours.
- Complete recovery usually occurs unless complications such as aspiration develop.

DISCHARGE CRITERIA/INSTRUCTIONS

The patient may be discharged when mental status returns to normal.

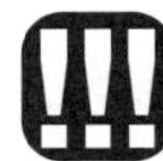

Pitfalls

DIAGNOSIS

- It is important to investigate diagnoses of electrolyte abnormality, intracranial lesion, or infection.
- Prolonged coma prior to treatment may allow development of compartment syndrome.

ICD-9-CM 304.0

Poisoning by psychotropic agents: drug dependence.

See also: SECTION II, Coma.

RECOMMENDED READING

Sporer KA, Lesser SH. Cocaine washed out syndrome. *Ann Emerg Med* 1992;21:112.

Author: Richard C. Dart

Reviewer: Katherine M. Hurlbut

Colchicine

Basics

DESCRIPTION

Colchicine is a medication used in the treatment of gout and is present in some plants.

FORMS AND USES

- USP colchicine is available as 0.5- and 0.6-mg tablets and as solution (0.5 mg/ml) for injection.
- For chronic gouty arthritis, the adult dose is 0.6 mg hourly by mouth until improvement is noted or diarrhea develops, to a maximum of 6 mg.
- Colchicine is also used for familial Mediterranean fever.
- Plants include *Colchicum autumnale* (autumn crocus, wild or meadow saffron), and *Gloriosa superba* (glory lily, naked lady, naked boy, son-before-the-father).
- All parts of the plants are poisonous, but the highest colchicine concentration is in the bulb.

TOXIC DOSE

Reported fatal doses range from 7 to 60 mg (usually more than 0.8 mg/kg).

PATHOPHYSIOLOGY

- Colchicine binds selectively and reversibly to microtubules, causing metaphase arrest and preventing many cell functions.
- Rapidly dividing cells are the most sensitive to colchicine.

EPIDEMIOLOGY

- Poisoning is uncommon.
- Toxic effects following exposure are typically moderate to severe.
- Ingestion of more than 0.8 mg/kg is often fatal.

CAUSES

- Poisoning is usually intentional.
- Child neglect should be considered if the patient is less than 1 year of age.
- A suicide attempt should be considered in patients over 6 years of age.

DRUG AND DISEASE INTERACTIONS

Administration of drugs that inhibit cytochrome P450 (cimetidine, tolbutamine, and erythromycin) may increase toxicity by reducing clearance.

PREGNANCY AND LACTATION

US FDA Pregnancy Category D. Positive evidence of human fetal risk exists, but benefits in certain situations (e.g., life-threatening situations or serious diseases) may make use of the drug acceptable despite its risks.

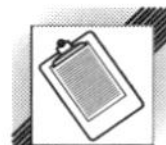

Diagnosis

DIFFERENTIAL DIAGNOSIS

- Toxic agents that produce severe vomiting and diarrhea followed by metabolic acidosis and systemic deterioration include iron, organophosphates, salicylate, podophyllin, and antineoplastics.
- Nontoxic causes may include infectious gastroenteritis, hyperthyroidism, early diabetic ketoacidosis, alcohol withdrawal, and various endocrine abnormalities, among others.

SIGNS AND SYMPTOMS

- Latent period (2–12 hours). Before symptoms develop.
- Phase 1 (2–24 hours). Nausea, vomiting, diarrhea, gastrointestinal hemorrhage, hypotension, and leukocytosis.
- Phase 2 (1–7 days). Delirium, seizures, coma, ascending peripheral neuropathy, myocardial depression, hypotension, adult respiratory distress syndrome, dysrhythmias, respiratory failure, renal and hepatic failure, coagulopathy, and myelosuppression (nadir at 4–7 days).
- Phase 3 (7–10 days). Rebound leukocytosis, alopecia, and persistent neuropathy and myopathy.
- Toxicity after plant ingestion is usually less severe.

Vital Signs

- Hypotension and tachycardia may occur early from volume loss or during phase 2 secondary to myocardial injury.
- Fever is common and needs to be distinguished from sepsis if neutropenic.

HEENT

- Oral pain and stomatitis may develop.
- Colchicine is a severe eye irritant.

Dermatologic

Alopecia is common 7 days or more after exposure.

Cardiovascular

Myocardial injury with ST elevation and decreased cardiac contractility has been reported.

Pulmonary

- Respiratory failure may develop secondary to peripheral neuropathy and myopathy in severe cases.
- Adult respiratory distress syndrome is common in severe cases.

Gastrointestinal

Nausea, vomiting, severe abdominal pain, diarrhea, and hemorrhagic gastroenteritis are common early after ingestion.

Hepatic

Elevated liver enzymes and prolonged international normalized ratio (INR) have been reported.

Renal

- Azotemia, proteinuria, hematuria, and myoglobinuria may occur.
- Oliguria and renal failure may develop in severe cases.

Hematologic

- Peripheral leukocytosis occurs in phase 1 and on recovery.
- Leukopenia and thrombocytopenia reach a nadir after 4 to 7 days.
- Disseminated intravascular coagulopathy may develop with severe poisoning.

Fluids and Electrolytes

Dehydration and electrolyte disturbances from gastrointestinal losses may occur.

Musculoskeletal

- Myopathy with rhabdomyolysis and myoglobinuria may occur.
- Weakness may last several weeks.

Neurologic

Confusion, coma, loss of deep tendon reflexes, seizures and ascending paralysis have been reported with severe intoxication.

Reproductive

Down syndrome and trisomy 23 associated with *in utero* exposure.

PROCEDURES AND LABORATORY TESTS

Essential Tests

- Serum electrolytes, BUN, and creatinine. Dehydration and electrolyte abnormalities in first 24 hours or renal failure in phase 2 suggest severe poisoning.
- Complete blood count, platelets, and prothrombin time/INR. Initial leukocytosis followed by leukopenia, thrombocytopenia, and coagulopathy suggest severe poisoning.
- Liver function test. Hepatic injury suggests moderate to severe poisoning.

Recommended Tests

- ECG, serum acetaminophen and aspirin levels are measured in an overdose setting to detect occult overdose.
- Blood, urine, and spinal fluid cultures and a urine toxicology screen are ordered as needed to evaluate other causes.

Not Recommended Tests

Colchicine levels are not clinically useful.

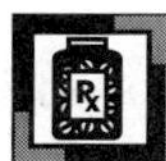

Treatment

- Treatment should focus on aggressive supportive care of volume depletion, hypotension, and potential complications such as adult respiratory distress syndrome.
- The dose and time of exposure must be determined for all substances.

DIRECTING PATIENT COURSE

The health-care provider should call the poison control center when:

- Severe gastroenteritis, hypotension, or mental status changes are present.
- Signs and symptoms are not consistent with colchicine.
- Coingestant, drug interaction, or underlying disease presents an unusual problem.

The patient should be referred to a health-care facility when:

- Attempted suicide or homicide is possible.
- Patient or caregiver seems unreliable.
- Signs or symptoms develop.
- Coingestant, drug interaction, or underlying disease presents an unusual problem.

Admission Considerations

Inpatient management is warranted for all patients with symptoms.

DECONTAMINATION

Out of Hospital

- The patient is often already vomiting.
- Emesis can be induced with ipecac for either pediatric or adult patients, if this can be performed within 30 minutes of ingestion.

In Hospital

- Gastric lavage should be performed in pediatric (tube size 24–32 French) or adult patients (tube size 36–42 French) presenting within 1 hour of a large ingestion or if serious effects are present.
- One dose of activated charcoal (1–2 g/kg) should be administered without a cathartic if a substantial ingestion has occurred within the previous few hours.
- Because colchicine undergoes enterohepatic recirculation, multiple-dose charcoal is theoretically of value but has not been proven (see SECTION III, Activated Charcoal chapter).

ANTIDOTES

There is no antidote for colchicine poisoning.

ADJUNCTIVE TREATMENT

Hypotension

- Patient should be administered 10 to 20 ml/kg 0.9% saline and placed in the Trendelenburg position.
- Further fluid therapy should be guided by central monitoring or right heart catheter to avoid volume overload.
- If hypotension persists, a vasopressor should be administered.

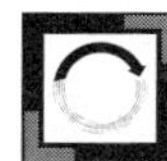

Follow-Up

PATIENT MONITORING

- Cardiac and respiratory function should be monitored continuously.
- Serial complete blood counts, renal function, and coagulation studies are used to follow toxicity.

EXPECTED COURSE AND PROGNOSIS

- The early course is volatile.
- Patients who survive the first several days generally recover, although death from neutropenic sepsis may occur at 4 to 7 days.
- **Possible complications** include prolonged neuropathy and renal failure.

DISCHARGE CRITERIA/INSTRUCTIONS

- From the emergency department. Patients who remain asymptomatic during 24 hours of observation after appropriate decontamination may be discharged.
- From the hospital. Patients may be discharged after hemodynamic, hematologic, pulmonary, hepatic, and neurologic effects have stabilized.

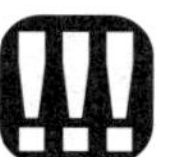

Pitfalls

DIAGNOSIS

The early presentation of colchicine poisoning may be confused with sepsis or meningitis.

TREATMENT

Presumptive antibiotic therapy should be provided to neutropenic patients who may develop sepsis during the phase 2.

ICD-9-CM 989

Toxic effect of other substances, chiefly nonmedicinal as to source

See also: SECTION II, Hypotension chapter; and SECTION III, Activated Charcoal chapter.

RECOMMENDED READING

Folpini A, Furfori P. Colchicine toxicity: clinical features and treatment. *Clin Toxicol* 1995;33:71–77.

Authors: Wei-Fong Kao and Jou-Fang Deng

Reviewer: Katherine M. Hurlbut

Cone Snail

Basics

DESCRIPTION

- There are 300 to 500 species of cone snails (genus *Conus*) that inhabit coral reefs throughout the world, especially in the Indo-Pacific area.
- Cone snails are nocturnal predators that burrow under sand and coral during the day and crawl on the sandy floor at night in search of annelid worms, small fish, and other mollusks for food.

FORMS AND USES

- *Conus geographus* has been responsible for most human fatalities (probably because of its larger size, up to 6 inches in length).
- *C. tulipa, C. magus, C. purascens,* and others also have been implicated.
- *C. tulipa* has the most toxic venom but reaches a size of only 3 inches.

TOXIC DOSE

A single sting from *C. geographus* is potentially lethal; over 20 fatalities have been reported due to accidental stings.

PATHOPHYSIOLOGY

- The venom, known as conotoxin, is synthesized in a venom duct that leads to the radula tooth. At close range, the snail fires the radula tooth into the prey. Venom is delivered by contraction of a muscular venom bulb. The snail then ingests the prey.
- Each tooth is used only once; others are available and stored in the radula sac.
- Conotoxins are neurotoxic peptides.

—α-conotoxins are postsynaptic neurotoxins that inhibit the nicotinic acetylcholine receptor and bind to similar sites as curare, cobra venom toxins, or α-bungarotoxin.
—Ω-conotoxins inhibit neuronal calcium channels and block neuromuscular synapses.
—Virgotoxin is a cardiotoxic protein that has direct action on vertebrate cardiac muscle.
—μ-conotoxin inhibits voltage-sensitive sodium channels and blocks propagation of action potentials in vertebrate muscle membranes.
—κ-conotoxins target potassium channels.

EPIDEMIOLOGY

- Poisoning is rare.
- Humans have typically been stung while handling the snails or collecting shells on the beach or on coral reefs.
- Toxic effects following exposure are typically moderate to severe.
- Death occurs rarely.

CAUSES

Poisoning is usually caused by handling a snail.

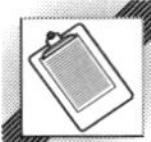

Diagnosis

Diagnosis is made on the history of handling a cone shell and the onset of localized pain.

DIFFERENTIAL DIAGNOSIS

Other conditions that produce localized acute pain in the body part affected should be considered (e.g., infection or trauma).

SIGNS AND SYMPTOMS

- Initial signs and symptoms may include local stinging, burning, numbness, and cyanosis or ischemia at the puncture site.
- Numbness and tingling may remain localized but may spread rapidly to involve the entire body, with the lips and mouth particularly affected.
- The symptoms increase in severity for 3 to 6 hours, and recovery occurs over 24 hours, although a localized reaction may last for several weeks.

Vital Signs

Tachycardia is often present.

Dermatologic

- Local stinging, burning, numbness, and cyanosis or ischemia at the puncture site develop early.
- A localized reaction may last for several weeks.

Pulmonary

- Dyspnea is sometimes noted.
- In animals, death is from respiratory depression; however, this has not been reported in humans.

Neurologic

In severe cases, muscle incoordination, dysphagia, paralysis, and coma may ensue.

PROCEDURES AND LABORATORY TESTS

Essential Tests

No tests may be needed if toxic effects fail to develop during an observation period of 4 to 6 hours.

Recommended Tests

In symptomatic cases:

- ECG is used to detect cardiac dysrhythmia if hypoxia develops.
- Arterial blood gases or pulse oximetry is ordered to detect hypercapnia or hypoxia.
- Pulmonary function testing may be appropriate to detect pulmonary involvement.

Not Recommended Tests

Conotoxin levels are not available.

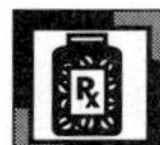

Treatment

Treatment focuses on pain control, the monitoring of respiratory status in severe cases, and tetanus prophylaxis, if needed.

DIRECTING PATIENT COURSE

The health-care professional should call the poison control center when:

- Paralysis or other severe effects are present.
- Toxic effects are not consistent with cone snail poisoning.
- An underlying disease presents an unusual challenge.

The patient should be referred to a health-care facility when:

- Attempted suicide or homicide is possible.
- Patient or caregiver seems unreliable.
- Symptoms develop.
- An underlying disease presents an unusual challenge.

Admission Considerations

Inpatient management is warranted for patients with pain requiring parenteral pain medication or with systemic effects of envenomation.

DECONTAMINATION

The wound should be immersed in hot water (105°F) for short periods to inactive the toxin.

ANTIDOTES

There is no specific antidote for cone snail envenomation.

ADJUNCTIVE TREATMENT

- The initial treatment is similar to early snakebite treatment; the extremity should be immobilized, the patient kept at rest, and reassurance provided.
- Tetanus prophylaxis is indicated as with all other bites and stings.
- Immersion in hot water for 30 to 60 minutes may provide pain relief. Parenteral opioid administration may be necessary for control of pain.
- Life support includes respiratory and cardiovascular support as needed.

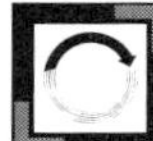

Follow-Up

PATIENT MONITORING

Continuous cardiac and respiratory monitoring should be performed until systemic venom effects resolve.

EXPECTED COURSE AND PROGNOSIS

- Numbness and tingling may rapidly spread to involve the entire body, with the lips and mouth particularly affected.
- Symptoms increase in severity for 3 to 6 hours: recovery occurs over 24 hours.
- A localized reaction at the sting site may last for several weeks.

DISCHARGE CRITERIA/INSTRUCTIONS

Asymptomatic patients may be discharged from the emergency department or hospital when their local effects are resolving, they develop no systemic effects, or the effects resolve during observation for several hours.

PATIENT EDUCATION

- Patients should be warned not to pick up patterned snails without wearing leather gloves.
- Fatal stings have occurred through clothing.

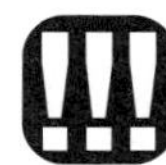

Pitfalls

TREATMENT

Hot water immersion is not always effective.

ICD-9-CM 989

Toxic effect of other substances, chiefly nonmedicinal as to source.

RECOMMENDED READING

POISINDEX Editorial Staff: Conotoxin. In: Rumack BH, Hess AJ, Gelman CR, eds. *POISINDEX system*. Englewood, CO: MICROMEDEX, Inc. (edition expires May 31, 1998).

Author: Melanie A. Wells

Reviewer: Richard C. Dart

Copper

Basics

DESCRIPTION

Copper is a reddish-brown metal. Copper sulfate is caustic salt composed of blue crystals or liquid.

FORMS AND USES

- Substances covered in this chapter include metallic copper, copper sulfate (cupric sulfate), cupric oxide, cuprous oxide, cupric acetate, cupric acetoarsenate, cupric arsenite, cupric carbonate, cupric chloride, cupric chromate, cuprous cyanide, cupric tungstate, cupric hydroxide, cupric nitrate, and cupric selenide.
- Copper is used in battery work, electroplating, fungicides and insecticides, plumbing, soldering, welding, ceramics, paints, pigments, pyrotechnics, photography, water purification, animal foods, petroleum distillation, and pharmaceuticals.
- Copper sulfate may be found in children's chemistry sets and crystal gardens and in Clinitest tablets.

TOXIC DOSE

- Copper sulfate is the most toxic form. Renal failure and death have been reported after ingestion of 1 g of copper sulfate.
- Death has occurred after a few swallows of water (29 μg/ml copper sulfate) from a crystal garden.

PATHOPHYSIOLOGY

- Chronic exposure to copper sulfate during spraying has been associated with interstitial pulmonary granulomas and fibrohyaline scars that contain large amounts of copper.
- Copper sulfate has caused alkaline corrosive mucosal injury after ingestion.
- Copper inhibits sulfhydryl enzymes, allowing production of free radicals and increasing susceptibility to lipid peroxidation, thereby causing hemolysis, hepatotoxicity, and nephrotoxicity.

EPIDEMIOLOGY

- Poisoning is uncommon.
- Toxic effects during chronic exposure are mild.
- Death may occur after ingestion of copper sulfate in high concentration.
- Carcinogenesis. The risk of adenocarcinoma is increased after chronic exposure to copper sulfate spray, believed to be due to arsenite contaminant.

CAUSES

- Chronic exposure is usually occupational.
- Acute exposure is usually from accidental ingestion.
- Child neglect or abuse should be considered if the patient is less than 1 year of age, suicide attempt if the patient is over 6 years of age.

WORKPLACE STANDARDS

Metallic copper

- ACGIH. TLV TWA is 0.2 mg/m^3 (fumes).
- OSHA. PEL TWA is 0.1 mg/m^3 (fumes); 1 mg/m^3 (dusts and mists).
- NIOSH.

—REL TWA is 0.2 mg/m^3 (fumes); 1 mg/m^3 (dusts and mists).
—IDLH is 100 mg/m^3.

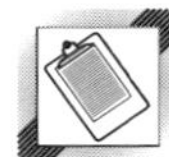

Diagnosis

DIFFERENTIAL DIAGNOSIS

- Toxicologic causes of acute gastrointestinal caustic effect include alkaline or acid solutions, phenol, several of the inorganic metal salts, and hydrogen peroxide, among others.
- Toxicologic causes of hepatic necrosis and renal failure include *Amanita phalloides* mushroom, acetaminophen, and carbon tetrachloride, among others.
- Toxicologic causes of interstitial lung disease include chronic exposure to beryllium, cobalt, coal mining, or multiple allergens (e.g., farmer's lung).
- Other causes of gastrointestinal effects include esophagitis, gastritis, peptic or duodenal ulcers, and perforated ulcer.

SIGNS AND SYMPTOMS

- Copper sulfate ingestion causes initial vomiting, diarrhea, abdominal pain, and corrosive injury leading to bleeding, perforation, shock, hemolysis, and renal and hepatic failure in severe cases.
- Chronic occupational exposure rarely causes serious illness.
- Metal fume fever may develop with exposure to copper fumes.

Vital Signs

Hypotension and tachycardia occur after copper sulfate ingestion.

HEENT

- Copper sulfate crystals have caused severe corneal injury.
- Oral burns may develop after copper sulfate ingestion.

Dermatologic

- Copper sulfate can cause dermal irritation.
- Chronic copper exposure can cause blue-green discoloration of skin and hair.

Cardiovascular

Cardiovascular collapse and ventricular dysrhythmias may develop after severe copper sulfate ingestion.

Pulmonary

- Chronic exposure to copper sulfate spray is associated with interstitial disease with granulomas and fibrohyaline scars.
- Some patients progress to pulmonary fibrosis.

Gastrointestinal

Early effects of copper sulfate ingestion include vomiting, diarrhea (may be blue-green), and abdominal pain, with corrosive gastrointestinal injury, hemorrhage, and perforation in severe cases.

Hepatic

Copper sulfate may cause centrilobular hepatic necrosis with elevated liver function tests and jaundice after 2 to 3 days, which may progress to hepatic failure.

Renal

- Copper sulfate may cause hematuria or hemoglobinuria from hemolysis.
- Acute renal failure may occur after severe poisoning.

Fluids and Electrolytes

Fluid and electrolyte disturbances and metabolic acidosis from severe vomiting and diarrhea may occur after copper sulfate ingestion.

Musculoskeletal

Rhabdomyolysis develops rarely after copper sulfate ingestion.

Neurologic

Coma and hepatic encephalopathy may occur after severe ingestion.

PROCEDURES AND LABORATORY TESTS

Essential Tests

No tests may be needed in asymptomatic patients.

Recommended Tests

- Complete blood count with peripheral smear may be performed to assess hemolysis.
- Serum electrolytes, BUN, and creatinine are measured in symptomatic patients to assess electrolyte disturbance or metabolic acidosis.
- Prothrombin time and liver function tests may be elevated in acute liver injury.
- Serum copper levels may be measured in symptomatic patients.

—Normal serum copper is 1 μg/ml.
—Greater than 5 μg/ml is considered toxic.

- ECG, serum acetaminophen, and aspirin levels may be performed in an overdose setting to detect occult overdose.
- Chest radiograph may be performed in symptomatic patients; copper salts may be radiopaque.
- Abdominal radiography may be useful to assess adequacy of decontamination.

• Gastrointestinal endoscopy is performed within 24 hours of ingestion of corrosive copper salt for patients with stridor, drooling, or vomiting or for adults with suicidal or large ingestions to assess extent of mucosal injury.

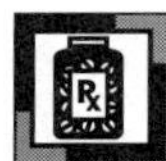

Treatment

• Treatment should focus on replacing gastrointestinal losses of fluid and blood, assessing gastrointestinal burns, and evaluating hemolysis, renal, and hepatic injury.
• Dose and time of exposure should be determined for all substances involved.
• Consultation with a medical toxicologist and other specialists, such as a gastroenterologist, is highly recommended.
• Patients with corneal burns should immediately be referred to an ophthalmologist.

DIRECTING PATIENT COURSE

The health-care professional should call the poison control center when:

• History of ingestion of copper sulfate is obtained.
• Toxic effects are not consistent with copper poisoning.
• Coingestant, drug interaction, or underlying disease presents an unusual problem.

Patients should be referred to a health-care facility when:

• History of ingestion of copper sulfate is obtained.
• Attempted suicide or homicide is possible.
• Patient or caregiver seems unreliable.
• Coingestant, drug interaction, or underlying disease presents an unusual problem.

Admission Considerations

Inpatient management in an intensive care setting is warranted when the patient has symptoms after ingestion of corrosive copper salt.

DECONTAMINATION

Out of Hospital

• Emesis should not be induced.
• Stomach contents should be diluted (by encouraging the patient to drink) with a small amount (4 ounces) of milk or water.
• Exposed eyes and skin should be irrigated with water.

In Hospital

• Stomach contents should be diluted (by encouraging the patient to drink) with a small amount (4 ounces) of milk or water.
• Gastric aspiration with a flexible tube should be performed in patients who have not already had repeated emesis within 1 hour of ingestion of a corrosive copper salt.
• Gastric lavage is not recommended because there is some risk of perforation during lavage after corrosive ingestion.
• Copper will adhere somewhat to activated charcoal, and if a noncorrosive form of copper is ingested, then one dose of activated charcoal (1–2 g/kg) should be administered without a cathartic.
• Exposed eyes should be irrigated with copious amounts of water, and a slit-lamp examination should be performed.
• Exposed skin should be irrigated with copious amounts of water and washed with soap.

ANTIDOTES

• Copper is bound to metal chelators, but there is little experience with chelation after acute copper intoxication.
• It is generally used for serious exposures, but the efficacy of this practice is unknown.
• Consultation with a medical toxicologist is advised.
• D-penicillamine

—Indication. Symptomatic, acute copper sulfate ingestion or chronic intoxication (Wilson's disease).
—Contraindications. Allergy to penicillin or penicillamine.
—Dose. 20 to 30 mg/kg orally, divided into four doses daily.
—Potential adverse effects
  —Rash, fever, leukopenia, thrombocytopenia, eosinophilia, and hemolytic anemia may occur.
  —The antidote may be difficult to administer due to vomiting.
—Other chelating agents. Ethylenediaminetetraacetic acid (EDTA) and British anti-Lewisite (dimercaprol) also have been used for copper intoxication.

ADJUNCTIVE TREATMENT

Hypotension

• The patient should be given 10 to 20 ml/kg 0.9% saline intravenously and placed in the Trendelenburg position.
• Further fluid therapy should be guided by central pressure monitoring to avoid volume overload.
• If hypotension is unresponsive, a vasopressor should be administered. Dopamine is preferred, and norepinephrine is added for refractory hypotension.

Steroids

• Studies suggest that steroids reduce stricture formation after alkaline-induced esophageal burns, but no data are available for copper sulfate burns.
• Steroids should be considered for patients with grade 2 burns.

Surgery

If the patient has Grade III esophageal injury or perforation, consider surgical consultation to assess the extent of gastric or duodenal burns.

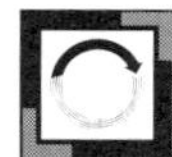

Follow-Up

PATIENT MONITORING

Patients who are symptomatic after ingestion of copper salt should be monitored in an intensive care unit.

EXPECTED COURSE AND PROGNOSIS

• Patients who survive the first 24 hours after copper sulfate ingestion generally recover.
• Renal insufficiency, sequelae of prolonged hypotension, and esophageal strictures may persist.

DISCHARGE CRITERIA/INSTRUCTIONS

• From the emergency department. Asymptomatic patients may be discharged after 6 hours of observation, gastrointestinal decontamination, and psychiatric evaluation, if needed.
• From the hospital. Patients may be discharged when hemolysis and gastrointestinal bleeding are controlled, renal function is stable, hepatic function is improving, and adequate nutrition has been established.

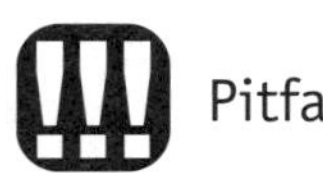

Pitfalls

FOLLOW-UP

Grade II or III esophageal burns require a follow-up upper gastrointestinal series to detect strictures.

ICD-9-CM 985.8

Toxic effect of other metals: other specified metals.

See also: SECTION II, Hypotension and Metal Fume Fever chapters; SECTION III, British Anti-Lewisite, Ethylenediaminetetraacetic Acid (EDTA), and Penicillamine chapters; and SECTION IV, Caustics—Basic chapter.

RECOMMENDED READING

Jantsch W, Kulig K, Rumack BH. Massive copper sulfate ingestion resulting in hepatotoxicity. *J Toxicol Clin Toxicol* 1984;22:585–588.

Schwartz E, Schmidt E. Refractory shock secondary to copper sulfate ingestion. *Ann Emerg Med* 1986;15:952–954.

Author: Scott D. Phillips

Reviewer: Katherine M. Hurlbut

Coumadin and Warfarin

Basics

DESCRIPTION

Coumadin and warfarin are oral anticoagulant medications.

FORMS AND USES

- Coumadin and the short-acting coumarin-type anticoagulants are pharmaceutical preparations of warfarin.
- Coumadin is used in the prophylaxis and treatment of venous thrombosis, pulmonary embolism, and valvular thrombi; for prophylaxis of thrombus formation in atrial fibrillation; and as an adjunct in the treatment of coronary occlusion.
- Dose is titrated to maintain a prothrombin time (PT) of 1.5 to 2.5 times control, or international normalized ratio (INR) of 2.0 to 4.5, typically requiring 2.5 to 7.5 mg/day.
- Warfarin is still used occasionally as a rodenticide in lacing baits for mouse and rat control.

TOXIC DOSE

- Repeated ingestion over 2 to 3 days is needed to produce anticoagulation.
- A single ingestion does not produce anticoagulation unless a massive amount is ingested.

PATHOPHYSIOLOGY

- Warfarin induces vitamin K deficiency by inhibiting the regeneration of active vitamin K and thereby the activation of clotting factors II, VII, IX, and X.
- Anticoagulation is delayed until coagulation factors are depleted.
- Due to its relatively short half-life, a single ingestion of coumadin or warfarin cannot inhibit synthesis of clotting factors long enough to produce anticoagulation.

EPIDEMIOLOGY

- Poisoning is uncommon.
- Toxic effects following exposure are typically mild to moderate.
- Death occurs in chronic ingestion leading to hemorrhage.

CAUSES

- Toxic ingestion is usually accidental, by a child.
- Child neglect or abuse should be considered if the patient is less than 1 year of age, suicide attempt if the patient is over 6 years of age.

RISK FACTORS

Health-care workers have been reported to use coumadin to induce factitious coagulopathy.

DRUG AND DISEASE INTERACTIONS

- Drugs potentiate anticoagulant effect of coumadin and warfarin include: allopurinol, anabolic steroids, cephalosporin, chloral hydrate, cimetidine, clofibrate, cyclic antidepressants, erythromycin, ethanol, nonsteroidal antiinflammatory drugs, sulfonylureas, thyroxine, and many others.
- Coumadin and warfarin may produce bleeding at lower levels in patients with preexisting coagulation abnormality.

PREGNANCY AND LACTATION

- US FDA Pregnancy Category D. Positive evidence of human fetal risk exists, but benefits in certain situations (e.g., life-threatening situations or serious diseases) make use of the drug acceptable despite its risks.
- Warfarin is a known teratogen.
- Breastfeeding is acceptable during coumadin therapy.

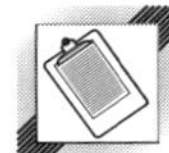

Diagnosis

DIFFERENTIAL DIAGNOSIS

- Toxicologic causes of anticoagulation include ingestion of brodifacoum, parenteral heparin overdose, crotalid snake bite, thrombolytic administration, or any poison that produces hepatic failure.
- Nontoxicologic causes include hemophilia, sepsis, and other causes of disseminated intravascular coagulation, and vitamin K deficiency.

SIGNS AND SYMPTOMS

Unexpected bleeding or bruising is the hallmark of warfarin toxicity.

Vital Signs

Hypotension and tachycardia may occur as a result of hemorrhage.

HEENT

Epistaxis and gingival bleeding may occur.

Dermatologic

- Bruising and petechiae may develop.
- Purple toe syndrome (discoloration of feet and toes) occurs rarely during therapeutic use.
- Idiopathic skin necrosis is another complication of therapeutic use.

Pulmonary

- Upper airway bleeding may occur.
- Alveolar hemorrhage occurs rarely.

Gastrointestinal

Abdominal pain, hematemesis, and hematochezia may occur.

Renal

Hematuria may occur.

Musculoskeletal

Compartment syndrome, carpal tunnel syndrome, and hemarthrosis occur rarely.

Neurologic

- Intracranial hemorrhage is rare but catastrophic.
- Spontaneous epidural hemorrhage has been reported; symptoms include paresis, back pain, and urinary incontinence.

Reproductive

Menorrhagia may be a sign of anticoagulation.

PROCEDURES AND LABORATORY TESTS

Essential Tests

No tests are usually needed following a single accidental ingestion.

Recommended Tests

If the patient is symptomatic or chronic ingestion is suspected:

- INR or PT should be measured 12 to 24 hours postingestion to assess coagulation effect; if normal, no further evaluation is needed for warfarin ingestion.
- Partial thromboplastin time, fibrinogen, fibrin degradation products, complete blood count, platelets, stool test for blood, and blood type and crossmatch should be performed in patients with clinically significant prolongation of INR/PT or bleeding.

—Thrombocytopenia or depressed fibrinogen suggests coagulopathy from another etiology.
—Anemia or guaiac-positive stools suggest significant warfarin toxicity.

- Head CT followed by lumbar puncture should be performed in patients with altered mental status; coagulopathy may need to be reversed before lumbar puncture.
- Endoscopy may be useful if clinical evidence of gastrointestinal bleeding is present.

Not Recommended Tests

Serum levels of warfarin are not clinically helpful.

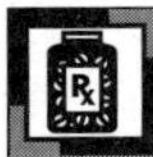

Treatment

- Treatment should focus on assessment and treatment of coagulopathy and control of bleeding.
- Dose and time of exposure should be determined for all substances involved.

DIRECTING PATIENT COURSE

The health-care professional should call the poison control center when:

- Hemorrhage is present.
- Toxic effects are not consistent with warfarin.
- Coingestant, drug interaction, or underlying disease presents an unusual problem.

The patient should be referred to a health-care facility when:

- Repeated ingestion of warfarin or coumadin is possible.
- Attempted suicide or homicide is possible.
- Patient or caregiver seems unreliable.
- Any toxic effects develop.
- Coingestant, drug interaction, or underlying disease presents an unusual problem.

Admission Considerations

Inpatient management is warranted if patient exhibits frank bleeding, severe coagulopathy, or marked anemia.

DECONTAMINATION

Out of Hospital

Decontamination is not needed for ingestion of a few tablets of coumadin or a handful of rodent bait.

In Hospital

- Decontamination is not needed for ingestion of a few tablets of coumadin or a handful of rodent bait.
- If the amount potentially ingested was large, gastric lavage should be considered in pediatric (tube size 24–32 French) or adult patients (tube size 36–42 French) presenting within 1 hour of ingestion; not recommended if bleeding is already present.
- One dose of activated charcoal (1–2 g/kg) should be administered without a cathartic if a substantial ingestion has occurred within the previous few hours.

ANTIDOTES

Vitamin K1

- Indication. Marked prolongation of PT or INR without bleeding.
- Method of administration. Vitamin K1 should be administered orally.

—Adult dose is 50 to 100 mg/day initially in single or divided doses.
—Pediatric dose is 0.6 mg/kg/day initially in single or divided doses.

- INR or PT should be repeated daily, and dose increased as needed to normalize INR or PT.
- Dosage may reach more than 200 mg/day in severe cases.
- Caution: Complete reversal may not be desired in patients with medical need for therapeutic anticoagulation.
- Indication. Severe prolongation of PT or INR and frank bleeding (the patient should first receive fresh frozen plasma as described below in ADJUNCTIVE THERAPY).
- Method of administration. Vitamin K1 should be administered intravenously.

—Vitamin K1 (25–50 mg) should be diluted with D5W or 0.9% saline and infused slowly at a rate not to exceed 1 mg/min. Dose is not well established in children; initial dose of 0.6 mg/kg or 5 to 10 mg, titrated to response, is a reasonable starting dose.
—Dose should be repeated two to four times daily; clinician should be prepared to treat anaphylactoid reactions.
—Parenteral vitamin K1 in doses as high as 400 mg per day have been used.

- Adverse effects and precautions

—Anaphylactoid reactions and even death have occurred during intravenous use of vitamin K1.
—In a patient who is anticoagulated for prosthetic valve, vitamin K1 should not be given unless anticoagulation is life-threatening.
—No other form of vitamin K should be used (e.g., K2, K3, menadione, K4, or menadiol).

ADJUNCTIVE TREATMENT

- Marked coagulopathy and active bleeding

—Fresh-frozen plasma should be administered intravenously; the pediatric dose is 15 to 25 ml/kg, and the adult dose is 2 to 4 units.
—On the basis of serial INR and PT determinations, further fresh-frozen plasma may be needed.

- Bleeding with anemia. Packed red blood cells should be administered as indicated.

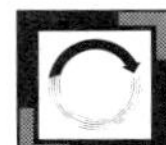

Follow-Up

PATIENT MONITORING

Serial INR or PT monitoring is used to guide therapy of patients with coagulopathy.

EXPECTED COURSE AND PROGNOSIS

- Complications of hypotension from hemorrhage or intracranial bleeding occur rarely.
- If vitamin K therapy is instituted before bleeding complications cause injury, a complete recovery is expected.

DISCHARGE CRITERIA/INSTRUCTIONS

- From the emergency department. Asymptomatic patients with acute single ingestion that is not massive may be discharged after gastrointestinal decontamination and psychiatric evaluation, if needed.
- From the hospital.

—Patients may be discharged when hemodynamically stable without active bleeding and when INR or PT is normalizing.
—Effective oral vitamin K1 dose must be established and regular follow-up assured; psychiatric evaluation should be obtained as indicated.

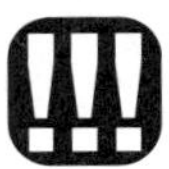

Pitfalls

DIAGNOSIS

Measuring PT/INR too soon following ingestion may result in a false sense of security. At least 12 to 24 hours should elapse prior to measuring INR or PT.

TREATMENT

- Large doses of vitamin K may be required; undertreatment is common.
- Severe warfarin overdose in patients requiring therapeutic anticoagulation, e.g., patients with prosthetic heart valves, may require slow partial reversal of anticoagulation; PT should be monitored several times daily to assist in determining quantity and times of fresh-frozen plasma therapy.

ICD-9-CM 964.2

Poisoning by agents primarily affecting blood constituents: anticoagulants.

See also: SECTION III, Vitamin K chapter.

RECOMMENDED READING

Hirsh J. Oral anticoagulant drugs. *N Engl J Med* 1991;324:1865–1875.

Author: Luke Yip

Reviewer: Katherine M. Hurlbut

Cyanide

Basics

DESCRIPTION

Cyanide is a chemical present in many industrial and household products and used in chemical processes. It is also present in some plants.

FORMS AND USES

- Industrial sources of cyanide include alkaline cyanide salts (HCN, KCN, CaCN), hydrocyanic acid, cyanogen (cyanogen bromide, chloride, and iodide), metal cyanides (iron and mercury), aliphatic thiocyanates [isobornyl thiocyanoacetate (Thanite), Lethane 60, or 384], nitriles, nitroprusside, and inhaled smoke, especially from burning plastic materials.
- Plant sources of cyanide include amygdalin cyanogenic glycosides (apple, peach, apricot, plum, cherry, and almond seeds), Laetrile tablets, bitter cassava, lima bean, sorghum, and bamboo.

TOXIC DOSE

- Cyanide gas. Inhalation of 90 ppm exposure for 30 minutes may be lethal.
- Cyanide salts. Ingestion of 200 mg may be lethal to adult.

PATHOPHYSIOLOGY

- Cyanide binds to heme iron in the cytochrome a-a_3 complex, inhibiting the final step of oxidative phosphorylation and preventing adenosine triphosphate production.
- This forces the organism to convert from anaerobic metabolism with a shift from pyruvate to lactate production and accumulation of lactic acid.
- Many metalloenzyme systems are affected by cyanide.

EPIDEMIOLOGY

- Poisoning is rare.
- Toxic effects following exposure are typically severe.
- Death occurs most frequently after acute inhalation exposure.

CAUSES

- Exposure is usually accidental in industrial employees.
- Child neglect or abuse should be considered if the patient is less than 1 year of age, suicide attempt if the patient is over 6 years of age.

RISK FACTORS

Geriatric patients with cardiovascular disease may be more prone to the development of cerebral and cardiac injury.

PREGNANCY AND LACTATION

- Chronic maternal cyanide poisoning is associated with low birth weight.
- Animal studies indicate teratogenic effects.

WORKPLACE STANDARDS

- Cyanide salts

—ACGIH. TLV (ceiling) is 5 mg/m^3.
—OSHA. PEL (ceiling limit) is 5 mg/m^3.

- Cyanogen

—ACGIH. TLV is 21 mg/m^3.
—OSHA. PEL (ceiling limit) is none.

- Cyanogen chloride

—ACGIH. TLV is 0.6 mg/m^3.
—OSHA. PEL (ceiling limit) is none.

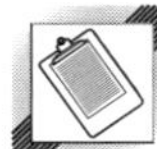

Diagnosis

DIFFERENTIAL DIAGNOSIS

- Toxicologic causes of abrupt onset of headache, dyspnea, confusion, and circulatory collapse include hydrogen sulfide, carbon monoxide, large inhalation of irritant, or asphyxiant gas.
- Other causes of metabolic acidosis include iron, toxic alcohols, renal failure, diabetic or alcoholic ketoacidosis, isoniazid, lactic acidosis, and salicylates.

SIGNS AND SYMPTOMS

- Inhalation often causes rapidly progressive headache, vomiting, dyspnea, fatigue, confusion, seizures, and coma.
- Circulatory collapse and death may occur within minutes.
- After ingestion, onset of effects may be delayed and progression is usually slower.

Vital Signs

Tachycardia and tachypnea occur early, followed by bradycardia and apnea in severe cases.

HEENT

- Mydriasis is common.
- Retinal arteries and veins appear similarly red.
- Blindness or optic neuritis may occur in chronic exposure.

Dermatologic

- Irritation and pruritus may occur with skin exposure.
- Moist sodium cyanide may cause burns.

Cardiovascular

Tachycardia and hypertension are early signs that give way to bradycardia and hypotension in later phases of toxicity (progression may be very rapid).

Pulmonary

- Respiratory tract irritation and noncardiogenic pulmonary edema may occur.
- Cyanosis is a late finding.

Gastrointestinal

Nausea, vomiting, and abdominal pain may occur following either ingestion or inhalation.

Fluids and Electrolytes

Metabolic acidosis and elevated serum lactate are common in significant poisoning.

Neurologic

- Headache and CNS stimulation with agitation may occur.
- Seizures and coma are a late finding or indicative of serious poisoning.

PROCEDURES AND LABORATORY TESTS

Essential Tests

- Arterial blood gases. Metabolic acidosis indicates poisoning.
- Serum electrolytes and lactate. Elevated anion gap metabolic acidosis is common.
- Blood cyanide levels following acute exposure

—Asymptomatic. Less than 0.2 μg/ml (mg/L)
—Tachycardia. 0.5 to 1.0 μg/ml (mg/L)
—Obtundation. 1.0 to 2.5 μg/ml (mg/L)
—Coma. 2.5 to 3.0 μg/ml (mg/L)
—Death. Greater than 3.0 μg/ml (mg/L).
—Caution should be exercised in interpretation; results are unreliable in many laboratories and levels alone should not guide therapy.

Recommended Tests

ECG and serum acetaminophen and aspirin levels should be determined to detect myocardial ischemia and, in an overdose setting, to detect occult overdose.

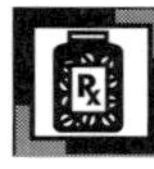

Treatment

- Treatment should focus on aggressive supportive care with appropriate airway management.
- Patients often survive with good supportive care alone.
- Dose and time of exposure should be determined for all substances involved.
- Consultation with a medical toxicologist is recommended.

DIRECTING PATIENT COURSE

The health-care professional should call the poison control center when:

- Any known cyanide exposure has occurred.
- Patient has unexplained increased anion gap metabolic acidosis.
- Coingestant or underlying disease presents an unusual problem.

The patient should be referred to a health-care facility when:

- Any known cyanide exposure occurs.
- Patient or caregiver seems unreliable.

• Coingestant or underlying disease presents an unusual problem.

Admission Considerations

Inpatient management is warranted for symptomatic patients or those with probable ingestion (delayed effects possible).

DECONTAMINATION

Out of Hospital

• Emesis should not be induced.
• The patient should be removed from exposure, the airway assured, and supplemental oxygen provided.
• If skin exposure occurs, exposed areas should be washed and clothing removed.

In Hospital

• Emesis should not be induced.
• Gastric lavage should be performed in pediatric (tube size 24–32 French) or adult (tube size 36–42 French) patients presenting within 1 hour of ingestion or if serious effects are present.
• One dose of activated charcoal (1–2 g/kg) should be administered without a cathartic if a substantial ingestion has occurred within the previous few hours.

ANTIDOTES

The cyanide antidote package contains a specific antidote for cyanide poisoning. See SECTION III, Cyanide Antidote Package chapter, for details of use.

Indications for Cyanide Antidote Package

• A patient with known cyanide poisoning and serious clinical effects (hypotension, metabolic acidosis, altered mental status, etc.) should receive treatment.
• For a patient with known cyanide exposure but without clinical effects, treatment with sodium thiosulfate component alone should be considered.
• For a patient with suspected cyanide poisoning (e.g., altered mental status and acidosis in a smoke inhalation victim), treatment with sodium thiosulfate component alone should be considered.
• For prevention and treatment of cyanide toxicity associated with nitroprusside infusion, concurrent infusion of sodium thiosulfate with nitroprusside has been used to prevent cyanide accumulation.

ADJUNCTIVE TREATMENT

Hypotension

• The patient should be given 10 to 20 ml/kg 0.9% saline and placed in the Trendelenburg position.
• Further fluid therapy should be guided by central pressure monitoring to avoid volume overload.
• If hypotension is unresponsive, a vasopressor should be administered.

—Dopamine
—The dose is 2 to 5 μg/kg/min intravenously, titrated upward to effect.
—Rates greater than 20 μg/kg/min are unlikely to provide further benefit.
—Norepinephrine
—The rate is 0.1 to 0.2 μg/kg/min intravenously, titrated to effect.
—A high rate of infusion may cause tissue ischemia.

Sodium Bicarbonate

Sodium bicarbonate may be considered if arterial pH falls below 7.20, but its use is controversial.

Hyperbaric Oxygen

• Hyperbaric oxygen is a potential therapy to prevent delayed neurologic sequelae.
• Its use should not delay administration of the antidote package.

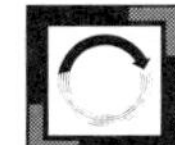

Follow-Up

PATIENT MONITORING

• Continuous respiratory and cardiac monitoring should be performed in all patients. Acid-base status should be followed frequently in symptomatic patients.
• During recovery, the patient should be followed for delayed neurologic sequelae.

EXPECTED COURSE AND PROGNOSIS

• Many patients survive with aggressive supportive care.
• Severely symptomatic patients often suffer sequelae of hypoxia.
• Possible complications include delayed neurologic sequelae similar to those of carbon monoxide poisoning: chronic headache, personality change, memory deficits, extrapyramidal sequelae, optic neuropathy, and parkinsonian syndrome.

DISCHARGE CRITERIA/INSTRUCTIONS

• From the emergency department.

—A patient with a minor exposure who has not developed symptoms may be discharged after 8 hours of observation, decontamination, and psychiatric evaluation, if needed.
—Oral cyanide ingestion and nitriles may have a delayed onset of symptoms.

• From the hospital. The patient may be discharged when all signs, symptoms, and laboratory abnormalities have resolved and medical and psychiatric follow-up has been arranged.

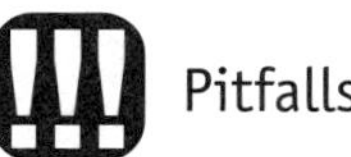

Pitfalls

DIAGNOSIS

• Symptoms may be delayed after nitrile exposure or oral cyanide ingestion.
• Cyanide may fail to be recognized as a cause of metabolic acidosis.
• Cyanide or nitriles may fail to be recognized from a worksite or job description.
• Associated conditions are smoke inhalation and carbon monoxide or hydrogen sulfide poisoning.

TREATMENT

• Dosing of sodium nitrite and sodium thiosulfate may be inadequate.
• Skin or gastrointestinal exposures may fail to be decontaminated.
• In the presence of renal failure, thiocyanate may accumulate and result in nausea, vomiting, and muscle cramps.

ICD-9-CM 989.0

Cyanide (compounds) (hydrogen) (potassium) (sodium).
987.7 Cyanide dust or gas (inhalation).
989.0 Cyanide fumigant.
989.0 Cyanide pesticide (dust) (fumes).

See also SECTION II, Anion Gap Metabolic Acidosis (Unexplained) and Hypotension chapters; SECTION III, Cyanide Antidote Package, Hyperbaric Oxygen, and Nitroprusside chapters.

RECOMMENDED READING

Agency for Toxic Substances and Disease Registry. Toxicological profile for cyanide. Atlanta: US Department of Health and Human Services, Public Health Service, 1989. DHHS report no. ATSDR/TP-89/12; NTIS report no. PB/90/162058/AS.

Hall AH, Rumack BH. Clinical toxicology of cyanide. *Ann Emerg Med* 1986;15:1067–1074.

Kulig K. Cyanide antidotes and fire toxicology. *N Engl J Med* 1991;325:1801–1802.

Author: Scott D. Phillips

Reviewer: Luke Yip

Cyclobenzaprine

Basics

DESCRIPTION

Cyclobenzaprine hydrochloride (Flexeril) is an oral muscle relaxant.

FORMS AND USES

- Cyclobenzaprine is commonly prescribed as a relaxant for the skeletal muscles.
- The usual dose is 10 mg orally three times a day.

TOXIC DOSE

The toxic dose is poorly characterized, but several hundred milligrams may cause death.

PATHOPHYSIOLOGY

- Cyclobenzaprine has anticholinergic, antihistaminic, and sedative properties.
- Anticholinergic side effects are frequent at therapeutic doses.
- Deaths from this drug are primarily caused by CNS depression, not by cardiac toxicity.

DRUG AND DISEASE INTERACTIONS

Cyclobenzaprine potentiates CNS depression caused by other sedating drugs.

PREGNANCY AND LACTATION

US FDA Pregnancy Category B. Animal studies indicate no fetal risk and there are no controlled human studies, or animal studies show an adverse fetal effect, but well-controlled studies in pregnant women do not.

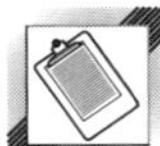

Diagnosis

DIFFERENTIAL DIAGNOSIS

Toxicologic causes of CNS depression include tricyclic antidepressants, ethanol, barbiturates, sedative-hypnotic drugs, and many others.

SIGNS AND SYMPTOMS

Typical overdose presentation. Tachycardia, tachypnea, confusion, and agitation, progressing to delirium, respiratory depression, and coma in severe cases.

HEENT

Mydriasis, dry mouth, blurred vision, hyperthermia.

Dermatologic

Warm, flushed, dry skin.

Cardiovascular

Sinus tachycardia; ventricular dysrhythmia occurs rarely.

Gastrointestinal

Decreased or absent bowel sounds.

Musculoskeletal

Rhabdomyolysis, rarely.

Renal

Urinary retention, renal failure secondary to dehydration, and rhabdomyolysis.

Neurologic

Drowsiness, dizziness, fatigue, confusion, agitation, somnolence, hallucinations, seizures

PROCEDURES AND LABORATORY TESTS

Essential Tests

No tests are usually needed for asymptomatic patients.

Recommended Tests

- Pulse oximetry, serum electrolytes, BUN, creatinine, and blood glucose should be measured to assess altered mental status.
- ECG, acetaminophen and aspirin level should be assayed to evaluate occult ingestion in an overdose setting.
- Serum creatine phosphokinase should be performed for patients with prolonged periods of unconsciousness.
- Despite the lack of clinical evidence of serious cardiac toxicity, continuous cardiac monitoring has been advocated in cyclobenzaprine overdose situations because of its structural similarity to tricyclic antidepressants.
- Judicious use of physostigmine 1 to 2 mg intravenously over 2 to 3 minutes may be used to diagnose anticholinergic syndrome; clinical response should be evident within a few minutes.

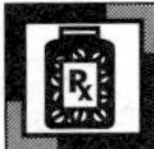

Treatment

- Therapy should focus on empiric therapy of altered mental status (e.g., oxygen, naloxone, glucose, and thiamine) and maintenance of airway.
- Dose and time of exposure should be determined for all substances involved.
- Other causes of altered mental status (infection, trauma, etc.) should be considered.

DIRECTING PATIENT COURSE

The health-care professional should call the poison control center when:

- CNS depression or other toxic effects develop.
- Toxic effects are not consistent with cyclobenzaprine.
- Coingestant, drug interaction, or underlying disease presents an unusual problem.

The patient should be referred to a health-care facility when:

- Attempted suicide or homicide is possible.
- Patient or caregiver seems unreliable.
- Coingestant, drug interaction, or underlying disease presents an unusual problem.

Admission Considerations

Inpatient management is warranted for patients with an altered level of consciousness or hemodynamic instability following 6 hours of observation.

DECONTAMINATION

Out of Hospital

Do not induce emesis.

In Hospital

- Gastric lavage should be performed in pediatric (tube size 24–32 French) or adult (tube size 36–42 French) patients presenting within 1 hour of a large ingestion or if serious effects are present.
- One dose of activated charcoal (1–2 g/kg) should be administered without a cathartic if a substantial ingestion has occurred within the previous few hours.

ANTIDOTES

There is no specific antidote for cyclobenzaprine poisoning.

ADJUNCTIVE TREATMENT

Hypotension

- Saline (10–20 ml/kg 0.9%) should be administered and the patient placed in the Trendelenburg position.
- Further fluid therapy should be guided by central pressure monitoring to avoid volume overload.
- A vasopressor may be added if needed. Dopamine is preferred and norepinephrine is added for refractory hypotension.

Anticholinergic Syndrome

Reversal of anticholinergic toxicity by physostigmine is used to determine whether altered mental status is due to anticholinergic effects. (See SECTION III, Physostigmine.)

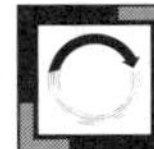

Follow-Up

PATIENT MONITORING

Respiratory and cardiac function should be monitored continuously in symptomatic patients.

EXPECTED COURSE AND PROGNOSIS

- Toxicity usually develops within hours, but may be delayed due to anticholinergic effects.
- Complete recovery over 1 to 2 days is expected unless sequelae of hypoxia or hypotension intercede.

DISCHARGE CRITERIA/INSTRUCTIONS

Asymptomatic patients may be discharged after 6 hours of observation and a psychiatric evaluation, if needed.

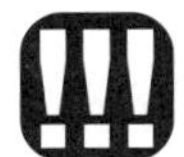

Pitfalls

DIAGNOSIS

Failure to consider other causes of altered mental status may result in missing life-threatening problems.

ICD-9-CM 968

Poisoning by other central nervous system depressants and anesthetics.

See also: SECTION II, Anticholinergic Syndrome and Hypotension chapters; and SECTION III, Physostigmine chapter.

RECOMMENDED READING

Ellenhorn MJ. Muscle relaxants. In: *Medical toxicology: diagnosis and treatment of human poisoning.* Baltimore: Williams & Wilkins, 1997:937–953.

Author: Luke Yip

Reviewer: Kennon Heard

Cyclosporine

Basics

DESCRIPTION

Cyclosporine (Sandimmune, Neoral) is used for immunosuppression following organ transplantation and for treatment of autoimmune disorders.

FORMS AND USES

Cyclosporine formulations are available for oral, rectal, ophthalmic, or pulmonary aerosol administration.

TOXIC DOSE

- Acute single ingestion of several grams or more has not been reported to produce toxicity.
- Repeated therapeutic ingestion may produce toxicity when trough serum levels exceed 500 mg/ml.

PATHOPHYSIOLOGY

Cyclosporine causes immunosuppression by suppressing helper T-lymphocyte release of lymphokines.

DRUG AND DISEASE INTERACTIONS

- Drugs or conditions that increase cyclosporine levels.

—Erythromycin, metoclopramide, and grapefruit juice increase absorption of cyclosporine.
—Acetazolamide, allopurinol, carvedilol, cimetidine, ciprofloxacin, cisapride, clarithromycin, erythromycin, fluconazole, ketoconazole, diltiazem, glipizide, glyburide, levofloxacin, methylprednisolone, metoclopramide, verapamil, nonsteroidal anti-inflammatory agents, oral contraceptives, prednisone, and many other drugs decrease clearance from the blood.
—Erythromycin decreases biliary excretion.
—Amiodarone, chloroquine, doxycycline, and nifedipine increase cyclosporine levels by an unknown mechanism.

- Other interactions

—Aminogylcosides, amphotericin B, ganciclovir, diclofenac, and melphalan, among other drugs, enhance nephrotoxicity, as well as increase the incidence of lovastatin-induced myalgia, myositis, rhabdomyolysis, and acute renal failure.
—Nifedipine increases the incidence of gingival hyperplasia.
—High-dose methylprednisolone increases the incidence of seizures.

PREGNANCY AND LACTATION

US FDA Pregnancy Category C. The drug exerts animal teratogenic or embryocidal effects, but there are no controlled studies in women, or no studies are available in animals or women.

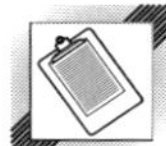

Diagnosis

DIFFERENTIAL DIAGNOSIS

- Cyclosprine may cause elevated hemacrit, decreased white blood cell count, decreased platelet count, thromboembolism, hypertension, several forms of CNS dysfunction, hyperglycemia, and progressive renal insufficiency.
- Cyclosporine should be considered the likely cause, but other common causes also should be evaluated in patients receiving cyclosporine therapeutically.

SIGNS AND SYMPTOMS

Vital Signs

Hypertension is common during chronic therapy and has been reported following a single acute overdose.

HEENT

- Facial flushing and abnormal taste perception can occur.
- Gingival hyperplasia may develop during chronic therapy.

Gastrointestinal

After acute ingestion, nausea and vomiting are common.

Hepatic

Hyperbilirubinemia may develop during chronic therapy.

Renal

Renal insufficiency, hyperkalemia, and hypomagnesemia are common during chronic therapy

Fluids and Electrolytes

Following an acute ingestion, minimal elevation of serum creatinine has occurred.

Neurologic

- Following acute ingestion, headache and CNS depression are common.
- During chronic therapy, less common effects include tremors, CNS depression, seizures, visual hallucinations, and cortical blindness.

Hormonal

Hypoglycemia may develop during chronic therapy.

PROCEDURES AND LABORATORY TESTS

Essential Tests

No tests may be needed in asymptomatic patients.

Recommended Tests

- In patients treated chronically, complete blood count, serum electrolytes, BUN, creatinine, and bilirubin are used to evaluate primary adverse effects of cyclosporine.
- Head CT, lumbar puncture, and cultures are ordered to evaluate other causes of altered mental status.
- Plasma levels are useful for confirming an acute overdose. Monitoring of plasma levels is important for patients on chronic therapy both to prevent cyclosporine toxicity and to ensure adequate immunosuppression. Therapeutic trough plasma concentrations are 50 to 300 mg/ml and whole blood levels have been reported in the range of 100 to 500 mg/ml.

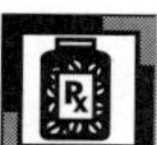

Treatment

Treatment should focus on general symptomatic and supportive care.

DIRECTING PATIENT COURSE

The health-care professional should call the poison control center when:

- Severe or persistent effects develop.
- Coingestant, drug interaction, or underlying disease presents an unusual problem.

The patient should be referred to a health-care facility when:

- Attempted suicide or homicide is possible.
- Patient or caregiver seems unreliable.
- Toxic effects develop.
- Coingestant, drug interaction, or underlying disease presents an unusual problem.

DECONTAMINATION

Out of Hospital

Ipecac should be avoided due to the low toxicity associated with acute ingestions.

In Hospital

- Ipecac should be avoided due to the low toxic potential.
- Gastric lavage is rarely indicated due to the limited toxicity following acute overdose. When it is indicated (e.g., toxic coingestants), it should be performed in pediatric (tube size 24–32 French) or adult (tube size 36–42 French) patients presenting within 1 hour of ingestion or if serious effects are present.
- One dose of activated charcoal (1–2 g/kg) should be administered without a cathartic if a substantial ingestion has occurred within the previous few hours.

Admission Considerations

Inpatient management may be warranted for patients who have documented CNS depression or evidence of acute renal insufficiency.

ANTIDOTES

There is no specific antidote for cyclosporine poisoning.

ADJUNCTIVE TREATMENT

- Nifedipine is useful for treating hypertension associated with chronic therapy because it may confer a renal protective effect.
- Hemodialysis does not appear to be clinically useful.

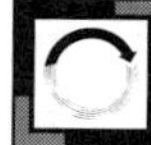

Follow-Up

PATIENT MONITORING

- Following an acute overdose, renal function and cyclosporine levels must be reevaluated within a day or two.
- During chronic therapy, renal function, bilirubin, and plasma levels are monitored regularly.

EXPECTED COURSE AND PROGNOSIS

Experience with acute overdose is limited but has not produced significant toxicity in either adults or children.

DISCHARGE CRITERIA/INSTRUCTIONS

Patients may be discharged from the emergency department or hospital when toxic effects resolve or stabilize and after psychiatric evaluation, if needed.

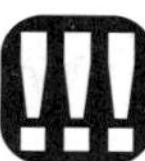

Pitfalls

Failure to monitor cyclosporine levels, renal function, and liver function during chronic therapy may allow severe toxicity to develop.

ICD-9-CM 963.1

Poisoning by antineoplastic and immunosuppressive drugs.

RECOMMENDED READING

Ellenhorn MJ. Immunotoxicology. *Cyclosporine.* Baltimore: Williams & Wilkins, 1997:779–783.

Author: Edwin K. Kuffner

Reviewer: Richard C. Dart

Dapsone

Basics

DESCRIPTION

Dapsone is an oral antimicrobial medication that is also used for some skin disorders.

FORMS AND USES

- Dapsone (Avlosulfon and Sulfona) is available in 25- and 100-mg tablets.
- Dermatitis herpetiformis is typically treated with an adult initial dose of 50 mg/day with individual variation ranging from 50 to 300 mg/day.
- Leprosy is treated with an adult dose of 100 mg/day; pediatric dose is 1 to 2 mg/kg/day up to 100 mg/day.
- Other uses have included AIDS-related infections, necrotic arachnidism, leishmaniasis, dermatoses and immune-mediated conditions, rheumatoid arthritis, vasculitis, *Pneumocystis carinii* pneumonia, and chloroquine-resistant malaria.

TOXIC DOSE

In adults, 1 g can cause toxicity, and 3 to 5 g or more can result in death.

PATHOPHYSIOLOGY

Mechanism of toxicity is primarily production of methemoglobinemia by a metabolite, monoacetyldapsone.

EPIDEMIOLOGY

- Poisoning has become common owing to its increased use in the treatment of AIDS-related infections.
- Toxic effects are usually mild but can be life threatening.
- Deaths have been reported from hemolytic and aplastic anemia, erythema multiforme, and the sulfone syndrome.
- Neonates are at increased risk for both methemoglobinemia and hemolytic anemia because of their immature glucose-6-phosphate dehydrogenase (G-6-PD) enzyme system.

CAUSES

- Toxicity is usually caused by therapeutic overuse.
- Child neglect or abuse should be considered if the patient is less than 1 year of age, suicide attempt if the patient is over 6 years of age.

RISK FACTORS

- G-6-PD deficiency is a relative contraindication for the use of dapsone; methemoglobinemia occurs at a lower exposure level and is more severe than in normal individuals.
- Methemoglobin reductase deficiency or the presence of hemoglobin M is a risk factor.

DRUG AND DISEASE INTERACTIONS

- Trimethoprim increases dapsone levels.
- Pyrimethamine increases incidence of hemolysis and methemoglobinemia.
- Concurrent use of rifampin decreases dapsone levels.

PREGNANCY AND LACTATION

- FDA Pregnancy Category C. The drug exerts animal teratogenic or embryocidal effects, but there are no controlled studies in women, or no studies are available in either animals or women.
- Breastfed infants can develop dapsone toxicity from the treated mother.

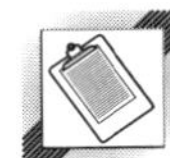

Diagnosis

DIFFERENTIAL DIAGNOSIS

- Toxicologic causes of methemoglobinemia or hemolysis include arsine, alpha methyldopa, naphthalene, quinidine, penicillin, nitrites and nitrates, local anesthetics, chloroquine, primaquine, sulfonamides, aniline dyes, and phenacetin.
- Nontoxicologic causes include neonatal diarrheal syndromes and methemoglobin reductase deficiency.

SIGNS AND SYMPTOMS

- Toxicity is usually caused by chronic therapeutic administration and includes rash, hemolysis, and methemoglobinemia.
- Acute overdose rarely causes hemolysis, but often causes methemoglobinemia.

Vital Signs

- Tachycardia, hypotension, and tachypnea occur if hemolysis or methemoglobinemia develops.
- Fever occurs occasionally during chronic therapy.

HEENT

- Blurred vision, conjunctivitis, stomatitis, and tinnitus have been reported.
- Optic atrophy during chronic therapy occurs rarely.

Dermatologic

- Cyanosis from methemoglobinemia may occur.
- Multiple types of rash have been reported.

Cardiovascular

Tachycardia and hypotension can result from methemoglobinemia.

Pulmonary

- Dyspnea may occur.
- Pulmonary eosinophilia has been reported during chronic therapy.

Gastrointestinal

- Nausea, vomiting, and abdominal pain are common following acute overdose.
- Pancreatitis and porphyria occur rarely.

Hepatic

Hepatitis and cholestatic jaundice occur rarely, following either acute overdose or chronic therapy.

Renal

- Acute renal failure and acute tubular necrosis may develop after acute hemolysis.
- Nephrotic syndrome with hypoalbuminemia has been reported.
- Acute porphyria occurs rarely.

Hematologic

- Methemoglobinemia may occur with either acute overdose or chronic therapy.
- Symptoms may not develop for hours to days following an acute exposure.
- Sulfhemoglobinemia may occur following acute overdose or during chronic therapy.
- Thrombocytopenia, agranulocytosis, and aplastic anemia occur rarely and are usually reversible.

Fluids and Electrolytes

Metabolic acidosis from elevated lactate may occur.

Neurologic

- Dose-related peripheral motor neuropathy occurs rarely; most commonly with chronic therapy but also following massive acute ingestion.
- Concurrent sensory involvement has also been reported.
- Headache, dizziness, insomnia, psychosis, and altered mental status have been reported with chronic therapy.

Immunologic

- Hypersensitivity reactions, usually rash alone, are common.
- Sulfone syndrome (fever, exfoliative dermatitis, hepatotoxicity with jaundice, lymphadenopathy, hemolysis, and methemoglobinemia associated with chronic therapy) occurs rarely.

PROCEDURES AND LABORATORY TESTS

Essential Tests

The asymptomatic patient may need no laboratory testing.

Recommended Tests

- Complete blood count may be performed to evaluate for the presence of hemolysis.
- Arterial blood gases and methemoglobin level may be determined.

—If methemoglobin level is 1% to 5%, then there are no expected signs and symptoms.
—If methemoglobin level is 5% to 20%, asymptomatic cyanosis is expected.

—If methemoglobin level is 20% to 50%, symptoms of hypoxia—dyspnea, headache, and fatigue—are expected.
—If methemoglobin level is 50% to 70%, life-threatening signs of hypoxia occur, including altered mental status, chest pain, and metabolic acidosis.

- Serum bilirubin, lactate dehydrogenase, and serum haptoglobin may be measured to evaluate hemolysis.
- Direct and indirect Coombs test may be performed to evaluate hemolysis.
- Sulfhemoglobin level may be determined; effects of sulfhemoglobinemia are similar to those of methemoglobinemia and should be suspected when apparent methemoglobinemia fails to respond to methylene blue treatment.
- ECG, serum acetaminophen and aspirin levels should be performed in an overdose setting to detect occult ingestion.

Not Recommended Tests

Dapsone serum levels are not clinically useful.

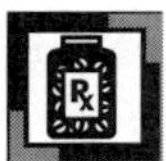

Treatment

- Treatment should focus on decontamination, general supportive care, and treatment of methemoglobinemia.
- Dose and time of exposure should be determined for all substances involved.

DIRECTING PATIENT COURSE

The health-care professional should call the poison control center when:

- Cyanosis, acidosis, hemolysis, or other severe effects are present.
- Toxic effects are not consistent with dapsone poisoning.
- Coingestant, drug interaction, or underlying disease presents an unusual problem.

The patient should be referred to a health-care facility when:

- Attempted suicide or homicide is possible.
- Patient or caregiver seems unreliable.
- Any toxic effects develop.
- Coingestant, drug interaction, or underlying disease presents an unusual problem.

Admission Considerations

Inpatient treatment is warranted when patient has signs of hemolytic anemia, agranulocytosis, or methemoglobinemia resistant to therapy.

DECONTAMINATION

Out of Hospital

Emesis should be induced with ipecac within 1 hour of ingestion for the alert pediatric or adult patient if health-care evaluation will be delayed, especially if the patient is G-6-PD deficient.

In Hospital

- Gastric lavage should be performed in pediatric (tube size 24–32 French) or adult (tube size 36–42 French) patients for large ingestion presenting within 1 hour of ingestion or if serious effects are present.
- One dose of activated charcoal (1–2 g/kg) should be administered without a cathartic if a substantial ingestion has occurred within the previous few hours.
- Administration of one or two repeat doses of activated charcoal (0.5 g/kg) without a cathartic should be considered after large ingestions, especially in patients who have serious effects.

ANTIDOTES

There is no specific antidote for dapsone. Methylene blue is used for treatment of methemoglobinemia.

Methylene Blue

- Indication. Symptoms of hypoxia attributable to methemoglobinemia.
- Contraindications. Known NADH methemoglobin reductase deficiency or 100% G-6-PD deficiency
- Method of administration

—The dose is 1 to 2 mg/kg administered intravenously over 5 minutes.
—Methemoglobin level should be determined again 30 minutes after the initial dose.
—If methemoglobin level remains elevated and the patient is still symptomatic, a repeat dose of 1 to 2 mg/kg should be administered.

- Adverse effects

—Hemolysis in patients with G-6-PD deficiency
—Paradoxical worsening of methemoglobinemia with large doses (>7 mg/kg of methylene blue)

ADJUNCTIVE TREATMENT

Exchange transfusion may be indicated rarely for methemoglobinemia unresponsive to methylene blue therapy in patients with known NADH methemoglobin reductase deficiency or 100% G-6-PD deficiency and life-threatening hypoxia; a hematologist should be consulted.

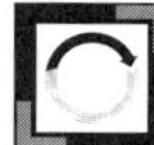

Follow-Up

PATIENT MONITORING

- Depending on toxic effects, the patient should be monitored for hemodynamic instability, hypoxia, hemolytic anemia, and serial methemoglobin levels.
- Prior to initiation of chronic dapsone therapy, patients should have G-6-PD status, complete blood count, BUN, creatinine, liver function tests, and urinalysis performed.

EXPECTED COURSE AND PROGNOSIS

- Methemoglobinemia or hemolysis peaks in the first day and then resolves over 1 to 2 days with appropriate therapy.
- Patients with neuropathy and sulfone syndrome usually recover completely after discontinuation of therapy.

DISCHARGE CRITERIA/INSTRUCTIONS

- From the emergency department. Asymptomatic patients who have had an acute overdose may be discharged after gastrointestinal decontamination, observation for 4 to 6 hours, and psychiatric evaluation, if needed.
- From the hospital. Patients may be discharged when hematologic toxicity is recovering and serial methemoglobin levels are not rising.

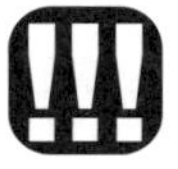

Pitfalls

DIAGNOSIS

- Arterial blood gases should be determined using a cooximeter because calculated oxygen saturations may not accurately reflect the true oxygen saturation in the presence of methemoglobin.
- Because most pulse oximeters detect only oxyhemoglobin and deoxyhemoglobin, a normal oxygen saturation by pulse oximetry does not rule out methemoglobinemia.

FOLLOW-UP

Hemolysis and methemoglobinemia may persist for several days following an acute exposure due to continued gastrointestinal absorption.

ICD-9-CM 964

Poisoning by agents affecting blood constituents.

See also: SECTION III, Methylene Blue chapter.

RECOMMENDED READING

Hall AH, Kulig KW, Rumack BH. Drug and chemical-induced methaemoglobinemia: clinical features and management. *Med Toxicol* 1986;1:253–260.

Author: Edwin K. Kuffner

Reviewer: Katherine M. Hurlbut

Dextromethorphan

Basics

DESCRIPTION

Dextromethorphan is a codeine analog and narcotic analgesic.

FORMS AND USES

- Dextromethorphan is commonly used as an antitussive in over-the-counter cough and cold preparations.
- A therapeutic dose has no analgesic, sedative, or respiratory depressant properties.

TOXIC DOSE

Ingestion of more than 10 times the therapeutic dose may cause toxicity.

PATHOPHYSIOLOGY

- In overdose, dextromethorphan has mild opioid effects.
- Dextromethorphan also inhibits reuptake of serotonin and may contribute to development of serotonin syndrome.

EPIDEMIOLOGY

- Poisoning is uncommon.
- Severe intoxication is rare.

CAUSES

- Ingestion is usually intentional.
- Child neglect or abuse should be considered if the patient is less than 1 year of age, suicide attempt if the patient is over 6 years of age.

DRUG AND DISEASE INTERACTIONS

Dextromethorphan ingested with monoamine oxidase (MAO) inhibitor or selective serotonin reuptake inhibitor may rarely induce the serotonin syndrome.

PREGNANCY AND LACTATION

Dextromethorphan has not been reported to produce teratogenic effects.

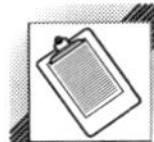

Diagnosis

DIFFERENTIAL DIAGNOSIS

Toxicologic causes of respiratory and CNS depression include sedatives, narcotics, ethanol, antidepressants, and many others.

SIGNS AND SYMPTOMS

HEENT

Blurred vision, mydriasis or miosis, and nystagmus may occur.

Cardiovascular

Tachycardia and hypertension may occur.

Gastrointestinal

Nausea, vomiting, diarrhea, or constipation have been reported.

Pulmonary

Respiratory depression may develop after a large dose.

Neurologic

- Bizarre and hyperactive behavior, hyperreflexia, hypertonia, hallucinations (auditory, tactile, and visual), psychosis, somnolence, ataxia, slurred speech, and seizures have occurred.
- Stupor and coma may develop in severe intoxication.

PROCEDURES AND LABORATORY TESTS

Essential Tests

No tests are usually needed in asymptomatic patients.

Recommended Tests

- Serum electrolytes, BUN, and creatinine are measured to assess other causes of altered mental status.
- Blood ethanol and acetaminophen levels are tested if it is suspected that the preparation is a combination product.
- Pulse oximetry or measurement of arterial blood gases is done if respiratory depression is present.
- Other studies should be ordered as indicated for altered mental status.
- ECG and serum levels of serum acetaminophen and salicylate should be measured in patients with intentional ingestion.

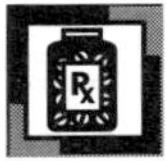

Treatment

Treatment should focus on supportive care and advanced cardiac life support.

DIRECTING PATIENT COURSE

The health-care professional should call the poison control center when:

- Hallucinations, altered mental status, or other serious effects are present.
- Toxic effects are inconsistent with dextromethorphan.
- Any toxic effects develop.
- Coingestant, drug interaction, or underlying disease presents an unusual problem.

The patient should be referred to a health-care facility when:

- Attempted suicide or homicide is possible.
- Patient or caregiver seems unreliable.
- Any toxic effects develop.
- Coingestant, drug interaction, or underlying disease presents an unusual problem.

ADMISSION CONSIDERATIONS

Patients with persistent signs or symptoms should be evaluated for further evaluation.

DECONTAMINATION

Out of Hospital

Ipecac should be administered to induce emesis within 1 hour of ingestion for the alert pediatric or adult patient if health-care evaluation will be delayed.

In Hospital

- Ipecac should be administered to induce emesis within 1 hour of ingestion for the alert patient who is too small to undergo effective gastric lavage.
- Gastric lavage should be performed in pediatric (tube size 24–32 French) or adult (tube size 36–42 French) patients presenting within 1 hour of a large ingestion or if serious effects are present.
- One dose of activated charcoal (1–2 g/kg) should be administered without a cathartic if a substantial ingestion has occurred within the previous few hours.

ANTIDOTES

Naloxone has been helpful in some cases to reverse CNS and respiratory depression, but has not been consistently beneficial, even at high doses.

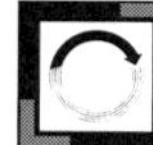

Follow-Up

PATIENT MONITORING

- With severe intoxication or coingestion of an MAO inhibitor or selective serotonin reuptake inhibitor, the airway may be compromised and requires monitoring.
- Body temperature also should be monitored.

EXPECTED COURSE AND PROGNOSIS

- Most patients will have mild symptoms.
- Symptoms resolve within 24 hours.

DISCHARGE CRITERIA/INSTRUCTIONS

Asymptomatic patients may be discharged from the emergency department or hospital after observation for 4 to 6 hours and psychiatric evaluation, if needed.

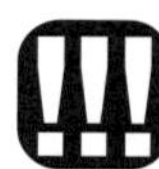

Pitfalls

DIAGNOSIS

It is important to evaluate for other causes of altered mental status.

ICD-9-CM 965.09

Expectorants and cough preparations: codeine derivatives.

See also SECTION II, Neuroleptic Malignant Syndrome and Serotonin Syndrome chapter; and SECTION III, Naloxone and Nalmephene chapter.

RECOMMENDED READING

Nierenberg DW, Semprebon M. The central nervous system serotonin syndrome. *Clin Pharm Ther* 1993;53:84–88.

Wolfe TR, Caravati EM. Massive dextromethorphan ingestion and abuse. *Am J Emerg Med* 1995;13:174–176.

Authors: Michael D. Jankoviak

Reviewer: Richard C. Dart

Diethylstilbestrol (DES)

Basics

DESCRIPTION

Diethylstilbestrol (DES; Stilphostrol) is a synthetic nonsteroidal stilbene-derivative similar to estrogen.

FORMS AND USES

- DES is available as an oral tablet (0.1, 0.25, 0.5, 1.0, and 5.0 mg), rectal suppository, or intravenous administration (250 mg/5 ml).
- Therapeutic uses include:

—Palliative treatment of advanced inoperable prostate cancer, and breast cancer in men and postmenopausal women.
—Postcoital contraception (within 72 hours of intercourse).
—Treatment of vasomotor symptoms of menopause or postpartum breast engorgement.
—Suppression of postpartum lactation.
—Transsexual hormonal feminization.

TOXIC DOSE

- Large acute overdose produces only nausea, vomiting, and diarrhea.
- Chronic ingestion of therapeutic amounts is typically associated with adverse drug events and may injure the fetus if the patient is pregnant.

PATHOPHYSIOLOGY

During chronic therapy, DES produces effects similar to endogenous estrogen.

EPIDEMIOLOGY

- Females exposed *in utero* before the 18th week of gestation may have increased incidence of oligomenorrhea, infertility, spontaneous abortion, and premature delivery.
- Males exposed *in utero* before the 18th week of gestation may have increased incidence of epididymal cysts, cryptorchidism, hypogonadism, and decreased spermatogenesis.
- Females exposed *in utero* before the 18th week of gestation and females prescribed DES have an increased incidence of vaginal clear cell adenocarcinoma and cervical adenocarcinoma.
- Causal relationships for other cancers have not been established.

RISK FACTORS

Administration of DES to pregnant women.

DRUG AND DISEASE INTERACTIONS

DES may accelerate growth of cancer in premenopausal females.

PREGNANCY AND LACTATION

FDA Pregnancy Category X. Studies in animals or humans have demonstrated fetal abnormalities or there is evidence of fetal risk based on human experience, or both, and the risk clearly outweighs any possible benefit.

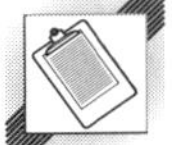

Diagnosis

SIGNS AND SYMPTOMS

Dermatologic

Skin rashes have developed.

Cardiovascular

- Incidence of myocardial ischemia is increased with chronic use.
- There is an increased incidence of thrombotic events with chronic use: cerebrovascular accidents, deep vein thrombosis, pulmonary embolism, and mesenteric and retinal thrombosis.

Gastrointestinal

Nausea, vomiting, abdominal pain, and abdominal distension are common following acute overdose.

Hepatic

Hepatitis with cholestatic jaundice may occur during chronic use.

Renal

Urethral strictures and porphyria may develop during chronic use.

Fluids and Electrolytes

Fluid retention and edema have been reported with chronic therapy.

Genitourinary

Vaginal bleeding, dysmenorrhea, and amenorrhea are common during chronic use.

Musculoskeletal

Hypercalcemia may occur, especially in immobilized patients who have osteoporosis, renal insufficiency, or bony metastases.

Hormonal

Gynecomastia, hirsutism, alopecia, and breast tenderness may develop in males with chronic use.

PROCEDURES AND LABORATORY TESTS

Essential Tests

No tests may be needed in asymptomatic patients or patients with acute single ingestion.

Recommended Tests

In asymptomatic patients on chronic therapy:

- Blood count to assess for bone marrow suppression
- Serum calcium to assess for hypocalcemia or hypercalcemia.
- ECG, chest radiograph, and other tests as appropriate to evaluate for thromboembolic or ischemic cardiac disease
- Liver enzyme tests to assess for chemical hepatitis
- Serum acetaminophen and aspirin levels in overdose setting to detect occult ingestion

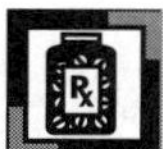

Treatment

DIRECTING PATIENT COURSE

The health-care professional should call the poison control center when:

- Severe or persistent effects develop.
- Coingestant, drug interaction, or underlying disease presents an unusual problem.

The patient should be referred to a health-care facility when:

- Toxic effects develop.
- Coingestant, drug interaction, or underlying disease presents an unusual problem.

Admission Considerations

- Inpatient management is warranted if the patient is suicidal or develops hematologic or cardiovascular complications.
- Following single accidental ingestion, children and adults can be safely observed at home.

DECONTAMINATION

Out of Hospital

Ipecac should be avoided due to low toxicity associated with a single ingestion.

In Hospital

- Ipecac should be avoided due to low toxic potential.
- Gastric lavage is rarely needed due to low toxic potential of acute ingestion. When it is indicated (e.g., coingestants), it should be performed in pediatric (tube size 24–32 French) or adult (tube size 36–42 French) patients for large ingestion presenting within 1 hour of ingestion or if serious effects are present.
- One dose of activated charcoal (1–2 g/kg) should be administered without a cathartic if a substantial ingestion has occurred within the previous few hours.

ANTIDOTES

There is no specific antidote for diethylstilbestrol poisoning.

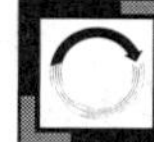

Follow-Up

PATIENT MONITORING

- Women administered DES and those exposed *in utero* need at least yearly pelvic examinations with cytologic screening.
- Monitoring appropriate for complications (e.g., pulmonary embolism) should be performed.

EXPECTED COURSE AND PROGNOSIS

- Acute overdose produces gastrointestinal effects for a few hours and then subsides.
- Prognosis is determined by complication (e.g., cardiac ischemia) for patients treated chronically with DES.

DISCHARGE CRITERIA/INSTRUCTIONS

Patients may be discharged from the emergency department or hospital when toxic effects resolve or stabilize and after psychiatric evaluation, if needed.

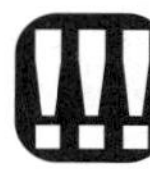

Pitfalls

DIAGNOSIS

Failure to monitor for bone marrow or gynecologic effects during chronic therapy may allow injury to develop unnoticed.

ICD-9-CM 962

Poisoning by hormones and synthetic substitutes.

RECOMMENDED READING

Ellenhorn MJ. Endocrine drugs. *Medical toxicology,* 2nd ed. Baltimore: Williams & Wilkins, 1997:716–717.

Author: Edwin K. Kuffner

Reviewer: Richard C. Dart

Diethyltoluamide (DEET)

Basics

DESCRIPTION

Products containing DEET in concentrations ranging from 5% to 100% are meant for skin application and are available without a prescription.

FORMS AND USES

DEET is an ingredient in many commercially available insect repellents, including:

- 6-12 Plus aerosol (5%) and stick (9.1%)
- Off! aerosol (15%) and towelettes (32.3%)
- Deep Woods Off! aerosol and pump spray (20%), and lotion (30%)
- Deep Woods Off! Maximum Strength liquid (100%)
- Cutter Insect Repellant spray (17.9%), stick (33%), and cream (51.75%)
- Muskol spray (40%), lotion, and liquid (100%)

TOXIC DOSE

- Ingestion of 25 to 50 ml of high concentration products or repeated skin application may cause serious toxicity.
- Dermal exposure to the recommended dose rarely produces adverse effects, although repeated and excessive application over days may produce toxicity.

PATHOPHYSIOLOGY

- The exact mechanism of DEET toxicity is unknown.
- The toxic effects of DEET primarily affect the central nervous system (CNS).
- Approximately 50% of topically applied DEET is absorbed within 6 hours. Peak plasma levels are reached in 1 hour.
- DEET and its metabolites remain in the skin and fatty tissue for 1 to 2 months after topical application, suggesting accumulation after repeated doses.

EPIDEMIOLOGY

- Although DEET is the most widely used insect repellent in the United States, reports of serious toxicity are uncommon.
- Serious toxicity or death occurs following ingestion or repeated application of excessive amounts of a high-concentration preparation.

CAUSES

- Toxicity usually results from unintentional misuse of product.
- The most common cause of toxicity is repeated excessive application of insect repellent containing DEET to young children.
- Child neglect or abuse should be considered if the patient is less than 1 year of age, suicide attempt if the patient is older than 6 years of age.

DRUG AND DISEASE INTERACTIONS

- Damaged, permeable skin may enhance absorption of DEET.
- Small children have increased skin permeability and may absorb enough DEET dermally, especially following repeated applications.
- Drugs that lower the seizure threshold may precipitate DEET-induced convulsions.
- DEET induces the cytochrome P450 system, potentially decreasing the effects of drugs metabolized by that route (e.g., phenobarbital, carbamazepine, phenytoin, rifampin, glutethimide, omeprazole, ethanol).

PREGNANCY AND LACTATION

- Experimental animal data suggest that DEET may be absorbed dermally by pregnant women, with resultant teratogenicity manifested by coarctation of the aorta.
- Pregnant women should be encouraged to use mechanical insect repellents, such as mosquito netting and protective clothing, instead of DEET or any other pesticide.

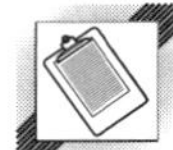

Diagnosis

DIFFERENTIAL DIAGNOSIS

- Other toxicologic causes of seizures include CNS stimulants (e.g., theophylline, amphetamine), antidysrhythmic drugs (e.g., lidocaine, disopyramide, quinine, quinidine), isoniazid (INH), tricyclic antidepressants, monoamine oxidase inhibitors, antipsychotics, and antihistamines, among many others.
- Nontoxicologic causes of seizures include electrolyte disorders (e.g., hypoglycemia, hyponatremia), hypoxia, hypothermia, hypothyroidism, or intracranial events (e.g., bleed, infection, and seizure).

SIGNS AND SYMPTOMS

The primary acute manifestations of DEET poisoning are CNS depression followed by seizures, which may be repetitive.

Vital Signs

Tachycardia, hypotension, and respiratory depression may be seen in severe overdose.

HEENT

Ocular application of DEET may result in corneal and mucosal irritation.

Dermatologic

Superficial dermatitis is the most common adverse effect of DEET use.

Cardiovascular

Sinus tachycardia with hypotension and cardiovascular collapse may occur but are rare.

Pulmonary

Respiratory failure may occur secondary to CNS depression.

Gastrointestinal

Nausea and vomiting follow ingestion or heavy dermal exposure.

Hepatic

- Acute chemical hepatitis may occur following severe toxicity.
- Idiosyncratic toxic hepatitis has been reported following repeated use.

Neurologic

- Initial CNS effects include ataxia, irritability, confusion, and disorientation, followed by CNS depression.
- In severe cases, patients may develop unresponsiveness, coma with flaccid paralysis, loss of corneal and deep tendon reflexes, seizures, and death due to respiratory failure.

PROCEDURES AND LABORATORY TESTS

Essential Tests

No tests may be needed for asymptomatic patients.

Recommended Tests

- Serum electrolytes, BUN, creatinine, and glucose to assess CNS effects.
- Arterial blood gases or pulse oximetry to assess oxygenation in symptomatic patients.
- Serum liver enzymes to assess possibility of hepatitis.
- ECG, serum acetaminophen, and aspirin in an overdose setting to detect occult ingestion.
- Head CT, lumbar puncture, bacterial cultures, and other tests as needed to determine other causes of altered mental status.

Not Recommended Tests

Serum levels of DEET are available through referral laboratories to confirm diagnosis, but their clinical utility is unclear.

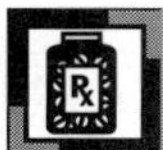

Treatment

- Initial treatment should focus on gastrointestinal and dermal decontamination, airway maintenance, and seizure control.
- Dose and time of exposure should be determined for all substances involved.

DIRECTING PATIENT COURSE

The health-care professional should call the poison control center when:

- Signs and symptoms are not consistent with DEET.
- Coingestant, drug interaction, or underlying disease presents an unusual problem.

The patient should be referred to a health-care facility when:

- Attempted suicide or homicide is possible.
- The patient or caregiver seems unreliable.
- Suspected toxic effects develop.
- Coingestant, drug interaction, or underlying disease presents an unusual problem.

Admission Considerations

Inpatient management is warranted for patients with altered mental status, respiratory depression, coma, or seizure.

DECONTAMINATION

Out of Hospital

- Ipecac-induced emesis is not recommended because seizures may develop abruptly following ingestion.
- Dermal exposures should be washed with water and soap.

In Hospital

- Dermal exposures should be washed with water and soap.
- Gastric aspiration with a nasogastric tube may be warranted for patients presenting within 1 hour of a large ingestion or if serious effects are present.
- One dose of activated charcoal (1–2 g/kg) should be administered without a cathartic if a substantial ingestion has occurred within the previous few hours.

ANTIDOTES

There is no specific antidote for DEET poisoning.

ADJUNCTIVE TREATMENT

For seizures:

- A patent airway must be ensured.
- A benzodiazepine is administered for initial control. If seizures persist or recur, another anticonvulsant such as phenobarbital may be added.

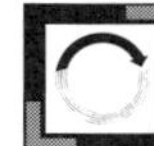

Follow-Up

PATIENT MONITORING

Cardiac and respiratory function should be monitored continuously in symptomatic patients.

EXPECTED COURSE AND PROGNOSIS

- Toxicity usually resolves within 24 hours, but patients with very severe cases may require hospitalization for more than 24 hours.
- Sequelae of repeated seizures or hypoxia are rare, but may develop.
- Subtle neuropsychiatric impairment that lasts weeks to months may develop in severe cases.

DISCHARGE CRITERIA AND INSTRUCTIONS

- From emergency department. Patients may be discharged when they are asymptomatic following decontamination, an observation period of 4 to 6 hours, and psychiatric evaluation, if needed.
- From the hospital. Patients may be discharged after toxic effects have resolved or stabilized and after psychiatric evaluation, if needed.

PATIENT EDUCATION

- Concentrated DEET preparations (more than 20%) should not be used on small children.
- To avoid accidentally overdosing of children by repeated dermal applications, parents should follow manufacturers' recommendations for products containing DEET; these provide a wide margin of safety in regard to the frequency of application and the necessity to wash DEET off children with soap and water.

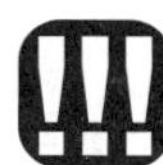

Pitfalls

DIAGNOSIS

Alternative etiologies should be considered for altered mental status and coma.

TREATMENT

The health-care provider should not fail to decontaminate the patient after dermal exposure.

ICD-9-CM 989.4

Toxic effect of other substances, chiefly nonmedicinal as to source: other pesticides, not elsewhere classified.

See also: SECTION II, Seizure chapter.

RECOMMENDED READING

Clem JR, Havemann DF, Raebel MA. Insect repellent N,N-diethyl-m-toluamide: cardiovascular toxicity in an adult. *Ann Pharmacother* 1993;27:289–293.

Snodgrass HL, Nelson DC, Weeks MH. Dermal penetration and potential for placental transfer of the insect repellent, N,N-diethyl-m-toluamide. *Am Indust Hyg Assoc J* 1982;43:747–753.

Tenenbein M. Severe toxic reactions and death following the ingestion of diethyltoluamide containing insect repellents. *JAMA* 1987;258:1509–1511.

Author: Gerald F. O'Malley

Reviewer: Katherine M. Hurlbut

Digoxin and Cardiac Glycosides

Basics

DESCRIPTION

Digoxin and digitoxin are medications used to treat heart disease.

FORMS AND USES

- Pharmaceutical preparations include deslanoside (Cedilanid-D), digoxin (Lanoxin, Lanoxicaps), digitoxin (Crystodigin, Purodigin), and powdered digitalis.
- Animal sources include several *Bufo* toad species, which contain bufogins, bufotoxin, and other toxins with cardiac glycoside activity.
- Other forms include numerous unregulated topical aphrodisiacs, including Love Stone and Rock Hard.
- Plants are discussed in SECTION IV, Plants—Cardiac Glycosides chapter.
- Digoxin and digitoxin are used to slow ventricular rate in cases of atrial fibrillation, atrial flutter, and supraventricular tachycardia.
- Digoxin and digitoxin are also used to maintain cardiac output in cases of congestive heart failure.
- Typical doses of digoxin for adults are 0.5 mg orally or 0.25 mg intravenously every 6 hours to 1 mg total dose, then 0.125 to 0.25 mg daily for maintenance.

TOXIC DOSE

Ingestion of greater than 10 mg digoxin by an adult or more than 4 mg by a child has been fatal.

PATHOPHYSIOLOGY

- Digoxin inhibits the cardiac Na^+/K^+ ATPase pump. This increases intracellular sodium, decreases calcium excretion, and produces increased intracellular calcium concentration, which augments contractility.
- Digoxin also increases vagal tone, decreasing baroreceptor sensitivity. This results in reduction of heart rate by decreasing myocardial and atrioventricular node conduction velocity and increasing atrioventricular node refractoriness.

EPIDEMIOLOGY

- Poisoning is common.
- Toxic effects following exposure are typically mild.
- Death occurs in patients with unrecognized digoxin toxicity.

CAUSES

- Poisoning usually results from suicidal ingestion.
- Child neglect or abuse should be considered in a patient under 1 year of age; suicide attempt in patients over 6 years of age.

RISK FACTORS

- Underlying cardiac disease may predispose to dysrhythmia.
- The elderly require smaller doses of digitalis and are more likely to have an underlying illness that predisposes to toxicity.

DRUG AND DISEASE INTERACTIONS

- Concurrent use of other drugs (β-receptor blocker, calcium channel blocker) can cause bradycardia or conduction delay.
- Quinidine, quinine, verapamil, diltiazem, amiodarone, erythromycin, and tetracycline may increase digitalis levels.
- Nifedipine, spironolactone, triamterene, and amiloride decrease renal clearance of digoxin.
- Warfarin can increase digoxin levels.
- Renal failure decreases digitalis elimination.
- Hepatic failure decreases digitoxin elimination.
- Hypokalemia, hypercalcemia, hypomagnesemia, increased sympathetic nervous system activity, and hypothyroidism may exacerbate digitalis toxicity.

PREGNANCY AND LACTATION

- US FDA Pregnancy Category C. The drug exerts animal teratogenic or embryocidal effects, but there are no controlled studies in women, or no studies are available in either animals or women.
- Digoxin is not contraindicated during breastfeeding.

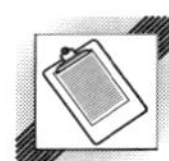

Diagnosis

DIFFERENTIAL DIAGNOSIS

- Toxic causes of nausea, hypotension, and bradycardia include cardiotoxic plants, β-receptor or calcium blockers, and type 1 antidysrhythmic agents.
- Nontoxic causes include gastroenteritis, small bowel obstruction, myocardial ischemia, hyperkalemia, or other electrolyte abnormalities.

SIGNS AND SYMPTOMS

- Early signs are nonspecific (malaise and nausea).
- As toxicity increases, interference with cardiac conduction predominates.

Vital Signs

Bradycardia, tachycardia, and hypotension may occur.

HEENT

Numerous types of visual complaints, including blurred vision, amblyopia, and colored visual halos, may occur.

Cardiovascular

Cardiac effects may include bradycardia, atrioventricular block, paroxysmal atrial tachycardia with block, intraventricular conduction delays, ventricular dysrhythmia, and congestive heart failure.

Gastrointestinal

Nausea, vomiting, anorexia, and abdominal pain are common and often precede cardiac effects.

Fluids and Electrolytes

- Hyperkalemia is common with acute overdose.
- Hypokalemia is associated with chronic toxicity or diuretic use.

Neurologic

Headache, weakness, drowsiness, hallucinations, and confusion may occur in severe cases.

PROCEDURES AND LABORATORY TESTS

Essential Tests

- Serum digoxin and digitoxin levels

—Digoxin therapeutic range is 0.5 to 2 ng/ml.
—Digitoxin therapeutic range is 18 to 22 ng/ml.
—Hypokalemia can precipitate toxicity at therapeutic levels of digoxin or digitoxin.

- ECG

—Nearly every possible dysrhythmia has been reported in cardiac glycoside toxicity.
—Prolonged PR interval and shortened QTc interval are common.
—Atrial or junctional tachydysrhythmia, sinus bradycardia, and atrioventricular block are characteristic.
—Bidirectional ventricular tachycardia, paroxysmal atrial tachycardia with 2:1 block, and junctional tachycardia are highly suggestive of digoxin toxicity.

- Serum electrolytes, calcium, magnesium, BUN, and creatinine

—Hyperkalemia in acute overdose is an indication for digoxin-specific antibodies.
—Hypokalemia disposes patients to cardiac toxicity.
—Hypercalcemia and hypomagnesemia may dispose patients to dysrhythmias.
—Renal insufficiency impairs digoxin clearance.

Recommended Tests

- Liver function tests are ordered because decreased hepatic function increases digitoxin levels.
- Serum acetaminophen and aspirin levels in an overdose setting are ordered to detect occult ingestion.

Conditions that May Alter Laboratory Results

- Treatment with digoxin immune Fab antibodies. Serum digoxin levels will be elevated because both free and bound digoxin are measured by most laboratories.
- Digoxin-like immunoreactive substance (DLIS)

—DLIS is an endogenous substance that may be detected by digoxin assays.
—It is reported in neonates and, rarely, in pregnant women or patients with renal or hepatic failure.

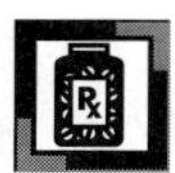

Treatment

- Treatment focuses on supportive care and administration of digoxin immune Fab, if needed.
- Dose and time of exposure should be determined for all substances involved.

DIRECTING PATIENT COURSE

The health-care provider should call the poison control center when:

- Cardiac dysrhythmia, altered mental status, or other serious effects are present.
- Toxic effects are not consistent with digitalis poisoning.
- Coingestant, drug interaction, or underlying disease presents an unusual problem.

The patient should be referred to a health-care facility when:

- Ingestion of more than 2 to 3 mg of digoxin is possible.
- Attempted suicide or homicide is possible.
- Patient or caregiver seems unreliable.
- Toxic effects develop.
- Coingestant, drug interaction, or underlying disease presents an unusual problem.

Admission Considerations

Inpatient treatment in an intensive care setting is warranted for symptomatic patients or those with new ECG abnormalities.

DECONTAMINATION

Out of Hospital

Emesis should be induced with ipecac within 1 hour of acute, single ingestion for alert pediatric or adult patients if health-care evaluation will be delayed.

In Hospital

- Emesis should be induced with ipecac within 1 hour of acute, single ingestion for pediatric patients too small to have effective gastric lavage.
- Gastric lavage should be administered in pediatric (tube size, 24–32 French) or adult patients (tube size 36–42 French) presenting within 1 hour of a large ingestion or if serious effects are present.
- One dose of activated charcoal (1–2 g/kg) should be administered without a cathartic if a substantial ingestion has occurred within the previous few hours.

ANTIDOTES

Digoxin Immune Fab Antibodies

- Indications

—Any sign of cardiovascular instability, including hypotension, symptomatic bradycardia, and other potentially unstable dysrhythmias.
—Rapid progression of toxicity, including gastrointestinal or cardiovascular symptoms.
—Serum K^+ is greater than 5.5 mEq/L.
—Digoxin immune Fab may be effective even during cardiac arrest of short duration; survival rates of up to 50% have been reported.

- Dosage and method of administration

—If the patient is critically ill in the setting of probable digoxin toxicity and the digoxin level is unknown, 10 to 20 vials should be administered empirically.
—To determine the precise amount to administer and other factors to consider, see SECTION III, Digoxin Immune Fab chapter.

ADJUNCTIVE TREATMENT

- Potassium should be replaced if patient is hypokalemic.
- Digoxin immune Fab is the preferred treatment for all dysrhythmias.
- Lidocaine and phenytoin have been used successfully for managing ventricular dysrhythmias.
- Magnesium or phenytoin may be used for supraventricular tachydysrhythmias.
- Atropine may be used for bradydysrhythmias.
- Vasopressors may be helpful during initial stabilization of the patient or until digoxin immune Fab is available

Not Recommended Therapies

- Procainamide, quinidine, disopyramide, and propranolol may worsen atrioventricular nodal block.
- Calcium is contraindicated because of the risk of cardiac tetany.

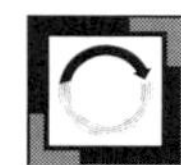

Follow-Up

PATIENT MONITORING

- Continuous cardiac and hemodynamic monitoring should be instituted and serum potassium followed closely.
- Recovery is usually complete, but often complicated by patient's underlying disease.
- Sequelae of hypotension or hypoxia may develop.

EXPECTED COURSE AND PROGNOSIS

Improvement within 30 minutes of digoxin Fab treatment is expected if complications of shock, hypoxia, or a coingestant have not occurred.

DISCHARGE CRITERIA AND INSTRUCTIONS

- From the emergency department. Asymptomatic patients with nontoxic digoxin level, normal ECG, and normal electrolytes may be discharged following gastrointestinal decontamination, 6 hours of observation, and psychiatric evaluation, if needed.
- From the hospital. Patients may be discharged following gastrointestinal decontamination, resolution of cardiac effects, and psychiatric evaluation, if needed.

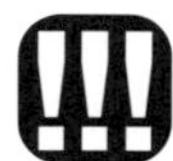

Pitfalls

DIAGNOSIS

- Symptoms of digitalis toxicity may be nonspecific, and a high index of suspicion is essential.
- Patients may exhibit digitalis toxicity at therapeutic digoxin levels.

TREATMENT

- Delay in treatment is dangerous because of acute deterioration.
- Hospital pharmacies are often inadequately stocked with digoxin immune Fab.
- Recurrence of digoxin toxicity after administration of digoxin immune Fab has occurred in patients with renal failure and in those given inadequate doses.

ICD-9-CM 972

Poisoning by agents primarily affecting the cardiovascular system.

See also: SECTION III, Digoxin Immune Fab chapter; and SECTION IV, Plants—Cardiac Glycosides chapter.

RECOMMENDED READING

Ellenhorn MJ. Digitalis. In: *Ellenhorn's medical toxicology—diagnosis and treatment of human poisoning,* 2nd ed. Baltimore: Williams & Wilkins, 1997:541–549.

POISINDEX Editorial Staff. Cardiac glycosides. In: Rumack BH, Sayre NK, Gelman CR, eds. *POISINDEX system.* Englewood, CO: Micromedex, Inc. (edition expires May 31, 1998).

Authors: Lada Kokan and Kennon Heard

Reviewer: Luke Yip

Basics

DESCRIPTION

Diphenoxylate is an oral antidiarrheal agent possessing opioid-like effects.

FORMS AND USES

- Substances include diphenoxylate, diphenoxylate hydrochloride, diphenoxylate with atropine (Lomotil), difenoxin (a metabolite of diphenoxylate) with atropine (Motofen), Diphenatrol, Lofene, Logen, Lomanate, Lonox, Lo-trol, Low-Ouel, and Nor-Mil.
- Diphenoxylate is used for treatment of diarrhea.
- A Lomotil tablet contains 2.5 mg diphenoxylate and 0.025 mg atropine.
- The adult dose is 5 mg diphenoxylate four times daily.
- Phenoxylate is not indicated for children less than 2 years of age.
- The dosage for older children is 0.3 to 0.4 mg/kg/day in four divided doses, not to exceed 6 mg daily in 2- to 5-year-olds, 8 mg in 5- to 8-year-olds, and 10 mg in 8- to 12-year-olds.

TOXIC DOSE

- As little as 15 mg has produced coma and respiratory depression in a child.
- The minimum lethal dose is unknown.

PATHOPHYSIOLOGY

- Diphenoxylate is structurally related to meperidine and produces opioid effects at high doses.
- Atropine produces anticholinergic effects that may delay absorption.
- Onset of symptoms following overdose may be delayed 6 to 8 hours or longer.
- Prolonged or cyclic effects may occur for 12 to 24 hours.

EPIDEMIOLOGY

- Poisoning is uncommon.
- Toxic effects are usually mild to moderate.
- Death is a rare event occurring in patients without adequate airway management.

CAUSES

- Poisoning usually results from accidental childhood exposure.
- Poisoning may result from substance abuse.
- The possibility of child neglect or abuse should be considered in patients under 1 year of age; suicide attempt should be considered in patients over 6 years of age.

RISK FACTORS

- In pediatric patients, there is greater susceptibility to CNS and respiratory depressant effects.
- In geriatric patients, underlying cardiac and respiratory disease may complicate management.

DRUG AND DISEASE INTERACTIONS

Diphenoxylate may have additive effects with other CNS and respiratory depressants.

PREGNANCY AND LACTATION

US FDA Pregnancy Category C. The drug exerts animal teratogenic or embryocidal effects, but there are no controlled studies in women, or no studies are available in either animals or women.

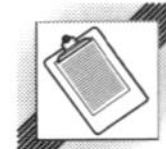

Diagnosis

DIFFERENTIAL DIAGNOSIS

- Other toxic causes of CNS depression or anticholinergic syndrome include opioids, clonidine, ethanol, sedative-hypnotics, scopolamine, diphenhydramine, cyclic antidepressants, benztropine, anticholinergic plants, and many others.
- Nontoxic causes include CNS infection or bleed, sepsis, and electrolyte abnormalities, among many others.

SIGNS AND SYMPTOMS

- Primary effects in overdose are CNS and respiratory depression.
- With large doses, anticholinergic effects may be the initial manifestation, followed by CNS depression.

Vital Signs

- Respiratory depression with bradypnea and apnea may occur.
- Transient tachycardia and mild hypertension and hyperthermia may be seen initially due to anticholinergic effect.

HEENT

Miosis is common.

Dermatologic

Flushing of the skin from anticholinergic effects may occur.

Cardiovascular

Tachycardia is a common effect.

Pulmonary

Respiratory depression with apnea may occur.

Gastrointestinal

Depressed or absent bowel sounds and constipation may develop.

Renal

Urinary retention may occur.

Neurologic/Psychiatric

- Ataxia (especially in children), drowsiness, lethargy, stupor, and coma occur; these may be delayed 6 to 8 hours or longer.
- Seizures may occur secondary to hypoxia or anticholinergic toxicity.
- Hallucinations and agitation may develop.

PROCEDURES AND LABORATORY TESTS

Essential Tests

No tests may be needed for asymptomatic patients.

Recommended Tests

- Oxygenation should be monitored by pulse oximetry in symptomatic patients to detect hypoxia.
- ECG should be performed and serum electrolytes, acetaminophen, and aspirin levels should be measured in an overdose setting to detect occult ingestion.
- Head CT, lumbar puncture, and cultures should be performed as needed to evaluate altered mental status.

Not Recommended Tests

Serum levels are not clinically useful.

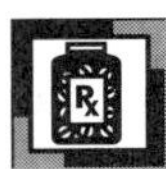

Treatment

- Treatment should focus on naloxone administration to reverse opioid effects and respiratory and cardiovascular supportive care as needed.
- Dose and time of exposure should be determined for all substances involved.

DIRECTING PATIENT COURSE

The health-care provider should call the poison control center when:

- Ingestion occurs in a child.
- Respiratory depression, seizure, or other severe effects occur.
- Toxic effects are not consistent with diphenoxylate toxicity.
- Coingestant, drug interaction, or underlying disease presents an unusual problem.

The patient should be referred to a health-care facility when:

- Ingestion occurs in a child.
- Attempted suicide or homicide is possible.
- Patient or caregiver seems unreliable.
- Any toxic effects are present.
- Coingestant, drug interaction, or underlying disease presents an unusual problem.

Admission Considerations

Inpatient treatment in an intensive care setting is warranted when:

- The patient develops hypotension, respiratory depression, seizures, or altered mental status.
- The patient is 6 years of age or younger.

DECONTAMINATION

Out of Hospital

Ipecac-induced emesis is not recommended.

In Hospital

• Gastric lavage should be performed in pediatric (tube size 24–32 French) or adult patients (tube size 36–42 French) presenting within 1 hour of a large ingestion or if serious effects are present.
• One dose of activated charcoal (1–2 g/kg) should be administered without a cathartic if a substantial ingestion has occurred within the previous few hours.

ANTIDOTES

Naloxone

• Indication. Respiratory depression from known opioid overdose.
• Contraindication. Documented naloxone allergy.
• Method of administration

—The patient should be given 2.0 mg by intravenous push and the response observed.
—If there is no response, the dose should be repeated in 2.0-mg increments up to a total dose of 10.0 mg.
—If a reversal of response occurs, the patient should be observed for 24 hours after the final dose.
—Patients with persistent or recurrent effects may be treated with a constant infusion of naloxone.

• Physostigmine

—Physostigmine is a cholinergic agonist that can be used in the treatment of a life-threatening anticholinergic syndrome.
—It is rarely required and should be considered only in patients unresponsive to supportive therapy.
—See SECTION III, Physostigmine chapter, for details of administration.

ADJUNCTIVE TREATMENT

Seizures

• Patent airway should be ensured.
• A benzodiazepine should be administered for initial control.
• If seizures persist or recur, another anticonvulsant such as phenobarbital should be added.

Hypotension

• The patient should be given 10 to 20 ml/kg 0.9% saline intravenously and placed in the Trendelenburg position.
• Further fluid therapy should be guided by central pressure monitoring to avoid volume overload.
• A vasopressor should be added if needed.

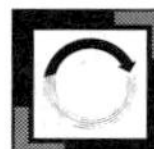

Follow-Up

PATIENT MONITORING

• Continuous respiratory and cardiovascular monitoring should be performed.
• Children 6 years of age or younger should be observed for 24 hours because toxicity may be delayed.

EXPECTED COURSE AND PROGNOSIS

• Following small doses, the onset of opioid effects is delayed, and anticholinergic effects may not develop.
• Following larger doses, anticholinergic effects predominate initially, followed by opioid effects.
• Patients generally recover completely over 24 hours unless sequelae of hypoxia intercede.

DISCHARGE CRITERIA AND INSTRUCTIONS

• From the emergency department. Asymptomatic adults may be discharged following 6 hours of observation, gastrointestinal decontamination, and psychiatric evaluation, as indicated. Patients who have a transient recovery in the emergency department may be discharged too soon.
• From the hospital. Patients may be discharged when CNS and respiratory effects have resolved for 8 to 12 hours or following 24 hours for pediatric patients undergoing observation.

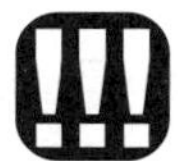

Pitfalls

DIAGNOSIS

• Early asymptomatic period does not preclude the possibility of toxic ingestion, especially in children.
• The effects of phenoxylate may be confused with those of other opioid or anticholinergic medications.
• The clinician may fail to appreciate that small doses in children are sufficient to produce significant toxicity and that the onset of symptoms may be delayed.

ICD-9-CM 973.5

Poisoning by agents primarily affecting the gastrointestinal system: antidiarrheal drugs.

See also: SECTION II, Hypotension and Seizure (Unexplained) chapters; SECTION III, Naloxone and Nalmephene, and Physostigmine chapters; SECTION IV, Anticholinergic Compounds and Narcotics chapters.

RECOMMENDED READING

Cutler EA, Barrett GA, Craven PW, et al. Delayed cardiopulmonary arrest after Lomotil ingestion. *Pediatr* 1980;65:157–158.

McCarron MA, Challoner KR, Thompson GA. Diphenoxylate-atropine (Lomotil) overdose in children: an update (report of eight cases and review of the literature). *Pediatr* 1991;87:694–700.

Moore RA, Rumack BH, Conner CS, et al. Naloxone underdosage after narcotic poisoning. *Am J Dis Child* 1980;134:156–158.

Author: Steven A. Seifert

Reviewer: Katherine M. Hurlbut

Disulfiram

Basics

DESCRIPTION

Disulfiram is an oral medication used in the treatment of alcoholism.

FORMS AND USES

- Disulfiram is used for the adjunctive treatment of alcoholism in adults.
- Disulfiram (Antabuse) is available in 250- or 500-mg tablet form, or as a suspension 25 mg/ml.
- The dose is 500 mg orally once a day for 1 to 2 weeks, then 250 mg/day.

TOXIC DOSE

- A disulfiram reaction may result when ethanol is ingested while patient is on a therapeutic dose.
- In the absence of alcohol, ingestion of several grams may produce toxicity in a child, but adults tolerate a much larger dose.

PATHOPHYSIOLOGY

- Disulfiram inhibits the hepatic enzyme acetaldehyde dehydrogenase. Accumulation of acetaldehyde during metabolism of ethanol causes the disulfiram reaction.
- Disulfiram also inhibits dopamine-β-hydroxylase, which leads to inhibition of norepinephrine synthesis and decreased reuptake of norepinephrine into adrenergic nerve terminals. This may explain the hypotension associated with disulfiram-ethanol reactions.
- The metabolites of disulfiram also have been demonstrated to inhibit acetaldehyde dehydrogenase and dopamine-β-hydroxylase.

EPIDEMIOLOGY

- Isolated disulfiram toxicity is uncommon.
- Disulfiram-ethanol reactions are common.
- Toxic effects following either isolated disulfiram ingestion or disulfiram-ethanol reactions are typically mild, with death occurring rarely.

CAUSES

- The cause of primary disulfiram poisoning is usually suicidal ingestion.
- Disulfiram-ethanol reactions may be unintentional but commonly occur in alcoholics who ingest ethanol while under treatment with disulfiram.
- The possibility of child neglect or abuse should be considered in patients less than 1 year of age; suicide attempt should be considered in patients more than 6 years of age.

DRUG AND DISEASE INTERACTIONS

Ingestion of ethanol-containing products (e.g., cologne, Listerine) may precipitate a disulfiram-ethanol reaction.

PREGNANCY AND LACTATION

US FDA Pregnancy Category C. The drug exerts animal teratogenic or embryocidal effects, but there are no controlled studies in women, or no studies are available in either animals or women.

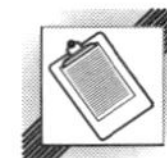

Diagnosis

DIFFERENTIAL DIAGNOSIS

A reaction resembling the ethanol-disulfiram reaction may occasionally occur following the ingestion of ethanol and another medication: antimicrobials, oral sulfonylurea agents (chlorpropamide, glipizide, others), several industrial agents (carbon disulfide, trichloroethylene, ethylene dibromide, thiuram, others), chloral hydrate, monoamine oxidase inhibitors (tranylcypromine, procarbazine), or *Coprinus* mushrooms (inky-caps).

SIGNS AND SYMPTOMS

- After acute ingestion of disulfiram alone, symptoms may require up to 12 hours to develop.
- The disulfiram-ethanol reaction usually peaks within an hour following ethanol ingestion and resolves over 2 to 4 hours.

Vital Signs

Tachycardia, hypotension, and tachypnea may follow either disulfiram overdose or the disulfiram-ethanol reaction.

HEENT

- Ketotic, garlic, or sulfur odor on breath may occur either with disulfiram overdose or during chronic therapy.
- Reversible optic neuritis may occur rarely during chronic therapy.
- Conjunctival injection is common.

Dermatologic

Flushing, erythema, skin warmth, and diaphoresis are common during the disulfiram-ethanol reaction.

Cardiovascular

- Palpitations, tachycardia, chest pain, and ECG changes of ischemia may develop during the disulfiram-ethanol reaction.
- Chronic disulfiram therapy may cause coronary atherosclerosis secondary to the carbon disulfide metabolite.

Gastrointestinal

Nausea, vomiting, and abdominal pain are common with either disulfiram overdose or the disulfiram-ethanol reaction.

Hepatic

- Chronic therapy may produce hepatic transaminase elevations that may be falsely attributed to underlying hepatic damage from alcohol.
- Idiosyncratic hepatitis is rare but has resulted in death during chronic therapy.

Hematologic

Idiosyncratic thrombocytopenia occurs rarely.

Fluids and Electrolytes

Hypokalemia may occur during the disulfiram-ethanol reaction.

Musculoskeletal

Arthritic syndromes have been reported with chronic therapy.

Neurologic

- Headache is common during the disulfiram-ethanol reaction.
- Parkinsonian syndrome, choreoathetosis, and thalamic syndrome have occurred following large ingestion.
- Peripheral neuropathy similar to Guillain-Barré syndrome has been reported after weeks to months of chronic therapy, but has also occurred following acute overdose.
- The peripheral neuropathy may progress for weeks following the discontinuation of disulfiram but eventually resolves.
- Psychosis, depression, hallucinations, encephalopathy, extrapyramidal symptoms, and seizures occur rarely either with therapeutic dosing or following overdose.
- Neurologic effects during therapeutic use or following overdose may be related to the metabolite carbon disulfide: tremor, lethargy, restlessness, headache, lightheadedness, ataxia, incoordination, dysarthria, drowsiness, confusion, memory impairment, and encephalopathy.

Reproductive

Loss of libido and sexual dysfunction may develop.

Endocrine

Elevated serum cholesterol may occur during chronic therapy.

PROCEDURES AND LABORATORY TESTS

Essential Tests

No tests are needed for minimal effects following acute overdose.

Recommended Tests

- Serum liver function tests should be performed prior to initiation of disulfiram therapy and periodically during therapy.
- Ethanol level should be measured to assess presence of ethanol and likelihood of disulfiram-ethanol reaction.

• ECG should be ordered; ischemic changes may occur with either chronic disulfiram therapy or disulfiram-ethanol reaction.
• Serum acetaminophen and aspirin levels should be measured in an overdose setting to detect occult ingestion.

Not Recommended Tests

Disulfiram, diethyldithiocarbamate, carbon disulfide, or diethylamine in plasma or urine can be measured to confirm exposure, but are not usually available.

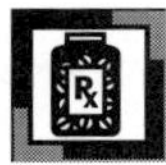

Treatment

• Treatment should focus on gastrointestinal decontamination and cardiovascular support.
• Dose and time of exposure should be determined for all substances involved.

DIRECTING PATIENT COURSE

The health-care provider should call the poison control center when:

• Hypotension, peripheral neuropathy, encephalopathy, movement disorder, hepatitis, or other serious effects are present.
• Toxic effects are not consistent with disulfiram poisoning.
• Coingestant, drug interaction, or underlying disease presents an unusual problem.

The patient should be referred to a health-care facility when:

• Attempted suicide or homicide is possible.
• Patient or caregiver seems unreliable.
• Any toxic effects develop.
• Coingestant, drug interaction, or underlying disease presents an unusual problem.

Admission Considerations

Inpatient treatment is warranted when the patient has altered mental status, persistent symptoms, cardiac ischemia, or severe hypotension.

DECONTAMINATION

Out of Hospital

• Emesis should be induced with ipecac within 1 hour of a large ingestion for alert pediatric or adult patients if health-care evaluation will be delayed.
• Ipecac should not be administered to patients who have concurrent ingestion of ethanol because of the risk of CNS depression.

In Hospital

• Gastric lavage should be performed in pediatric (tube size 24–32 French) or adult patients (tube size 36–42 French) presenting within 1 hour of a large ingestion or if serious effects are present.
• One dose of activated charcoal (1–2 g/kg) should be administered without a cathartic if a substantial ingestion has occurred within the previous few hours.

ANTIDOTES

There is no antidote for acute or chronic disulfiram toxicity.

ADJUNCTIVE TREATMENT

Persistent Vomiting

• Suggested antiemetic adult regimens include metoclopramide 0.5 to 1 mg/kg plus diphenhydramine 25 to 50 mg combined with prochlorperazine 10 mg or droperidol 2.5 mg intravenously.
• Ondansetron 8 mg intravenously infused over 15 minutes is an alternative.

Control of Agitation

• A benzodiazepine with which the provider has experience should be administered.

—Diazepam
  —Adult dose is 5 to 10 mg intravenously.
  —Pediatric dose is 0.2 to 0.5 mg/kg intravenously.
  —Doses are repeated at 10-minute intervals, titrating to effect.
—Lorazepam
  —Adult dose is 1 to 2 mg intravenously.
  —Pediatric dose is 0.05 mg/kg intravenously.
  —Doses are repeated at 10-minute intervals titrating to effect.

The airway should be monitored closely.

Hypokalemia

Potassium chloride should be administered. Adult dose is 10 to 40 mEq/h intravenously. Pediatric dose is 0.3 mEq/kg/h intravenously.

Hypotension

• The patient should be administered 10 to 20 ml/kg 0.9% saline intravenously and placed in the Trendelenburg position.
• Further fluid therapy should be guided by central pressure monitoring to avoid volume overload.
• A vasopressor should be added if needed.

Fomepizole

Anecdotal reports suggest that 4-methylpyrazole can inhibit the production of acetaldehyde, thereby decreasing acetaldehyde accumulation (see SECTION III, Fomepizole chapter, for details of administration).

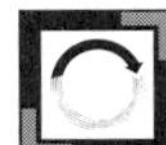

Follow-Up

PATIENT MONITORING

• Respiratory and cardiac monitoring should be performed continuously in symptomatic patients.
• Liver function tests and ECG should be performed as clinically indicated by toxic manifestations.

EXPECTED COURSE AND PROGNOSIS

• Most exposures result in only mild toxicity.
• Toxicity should occur within 12 hours of an isolated disulfiram ingestion and within 4 hours of ethanol ingestion in a patient treated with disulfiram therapeutically.
• There are typically no complications, except for idiosyncratic and potentially fatal hepatitis.

DISCHARGE CRITERIA/INSTRUCTIONS

• From the emergency department

—Following gastrointestinal decontamination, asymptomatic patients may be discharged 8 to 12 hours after an isolated disulfiram ingestion or 4 to 6 hours after a disulfiram-ethanol reaction.
—Psychiatric clearance should be obtained as appropriate.

• From the hospital. Patients may be discharged after signs of disulfiram intoxication have resolved following psychiatric clearance, if needed.

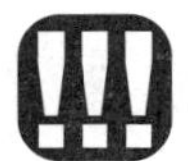

Pitfalls

DIAGNOSIS

• Patients presenting with signs or symptoms of a disulfiram-ethanol reaction may have been exposed to another drug instead of disulfiram.
• Disulfiram-ethanol reactions can occur following exposure to many drugs and chemicals containing ethanol.
• Unexpected sources of ethanol include cold and cough preparations, skin care products, mouthwash, and many intravenous medications.

FOLLOW-UP

Following termination of disulfiram therapy, the disulfiram-ethanol reaction may occur if ethanol is ingested within the subsequent 1 to 2 weeks.

ICD-9-CM 977.3

Poisoning by other and unspecified drugs and medicinal substances: alcohol deterrents.

See also: SECTION II, Hypotension chapter; and SECTION III, Fomepizol (Antizol) chapter.

RECOMMENDED READING

Mokri B. Disulfiram neuropathy. *Neurology* 1981;31:730–735.

Ryan TV, Sciara AD, Barth JT. Chronic neuropsychological impairment resulting from disulfiram overdose. *J Stud Alcohol* 1993;54:389–392.

Author: Edwin K. Kuffner

Reviewer: Luke Yip

Diuretics

Basics

DESCRIPTION

Diuretics are agents that increase urine production. Diuretics are classified according to their mechanisms of action:

- Thiazide diuretics include bendroflumethiazide (Naturetin), benzthiazide (Aquatag), chlorothiazide (Diuril), chlorthalidone (Hygroton), cyclopenthiazide, cyclothiazide, hydrochlorothiazide (HydroDiuril, Esidrix), hydroflumethiazide (Saluron), indapamide (Lozol), methyclothiazide (Enduron; Aquatensin), metolazone (Diulo; Zaroxolyn), polythiazide (Renese), quinethazone (Hydromox), and trichlormethiazide (Naqua).
- Loop diuretics include bumetanide (Bumex), ethacrynic acid (Edecrin), furosemide (Lasix), and torsemide (Demadex).
- Mercurial diuretics include mersalyl (Mersalyl-Theophylline).
- Carbonic anhydrase inhibitors include acetazolamide (Diamox), dichlorphenamide (Daranide), and methazolamide (Neptazane).
- Osmotic diuretics include glycerin (Osmoglyn, Fleet Babylax, Fleet Pain Relief Rectal Pads, Lubrin Vaginal Lubrivating Inserts), isosorbide (Ismotic), and mannitol.
- Potassium-sparing diuretics include spironolactone (Alatone, Aldactazide), amiloride hydrochloride (Midamor, Moduretic), and triamterene (Dyazide, Dyrenium).

FORMS AND USES

- Hydrochlorothiazide. For hypertension, adult dosage is 12.5 to 50 mg/day, up to 100 twice daily; pediatric dosage is 1 to 2 mg/kg/day, up to 50 mg/day.
- Acetazolamide. For diuresis, adult dosage is 250 to 375 mg (5 mg/kg) per day; pediatric dosage is 5 mg/kg/24 h; for prevention of altitude illness, adult dosage is 250 mg every 8 to 12 hours.

TOXIC DOSE

- Minimal toxicity results from acute overdose.
- Chronic ingestion of therapeutic dose can produce toxicity.

PATHOPHYSIOLOGY

- The toxic effects of diuretics arise from fluid loss and dehydration.
- Potassium-sparing diuretics may produce hyperkalemia.
- Mercurial diuretics may produce mercury toxicity, but are no longer used in many countries.

EPIDEMIOLOGY

- Acute ingestion is uncommon; overuse and misuse are common.
- Ingestion is common to lose weight or for other reasons.
- Toxic effects following acute ingestion are rare, but may occur during chronic overuse.
- Pediatric and geriatric patients are at greater risk of diuretic toxicity due to small size or underlying disease.

CAUSES

- Diuretic toxicity usually results from intentional chronic misuse or abuse.
- Child neglect or abuse should be considered if the patient is less than 1 year of age, suicide attempt if the patient is over 6 years of age.

DRUG AND DISEASE INTERACTIONS

- Underlying renal disease, gout, diabetes mellitus, and extremes of age predispose patients to diuretic toxicity.
- Concomitant use of potassium-sparing diuretic with amiloride, triamterene, or potassium may produce severe hyperkalemia.
- Concomitant use of angiotensin-converting enzyme inhibitors (e.g., captopril) or cyclosporine with amiloride can produce severe hyperkalemia.

PREGNANCY AND LACTATION

- Bendroflumethiazide, benzthiazide, bumetanide, furosemide, acetazolamide, dichlorphenamide, and methazolamide. US FDA Pregnancy Category C. The drug exerts animal teratogenic or embryocidal effects, but there are no controlled studies in women, or no studies are available in either animals or women.
- Chlorothiazide, chlorthalidone, hydrochlorothiazide, hydroflumethiazide, indapamide, methyclothiazide, metolazone, polythiazide, quinethazone, trichlormethiazide, and ethacrynic acid. US FDA Pregnancy Category D. Evidence of human fetal risk exists, but benefits in certain situations (e.g., life-threatening situations or serious diseases) may make use of the drug acceptable despite its risks.
- Furosemide, hydrochlorothiazide, and acetazolamide are excreted into breast milk, but no adverse effects in nursing infants have been reported.

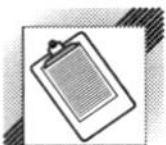

Diagnosis

DIFFERENTIAL DIAGNOSIS

- Other toxicologic agents that cause dehydration and electrolyte abnormality include lithium, salicylates, theophylline, cathartics, heavy metal ingestion, and many others
- Nontoxicologic causes of renal loss of fluid and electrolytes include diabetes insipidus, diabetes mellitus, and hypercalcemia, among others.

SIGNS AND SYMPTOMS

Vital Signs

Dehydration may cause tachycardia and hypotension.

HEENT

- Dry mucous membranes may be seen.
- Ototoxicity following a high intravenous dose of furosemide or ethacrynic acid is rare and usually reversible.

Cardiovascular

Electrolyte abnormalities may rarely become severe enough to produce ventricular dysrhythmia.

Pulmonary

Osmotic diuretics may cause pulmonary edema in patients with renal insufficiency or congestive heart failure.

Gastrointestinal

Gastrointestinal hemorrhage following a high intravenous dose of furosemide or ethacrynic acid has been reported, but is rare.

Renal

- Mannitol may cause acute renal insufficiency.
- Calcium phosphate precipitation may occur in the alkaline urine induced by acetazolamide.

Hematologic

Hemolytic anemia with hydrochlorothiazide occurs but is rare.

Fluids and Electrolytes

- Hypokalemia is common.
- A mild metabolic alkalosis (contraction alkalosis) is common with mild dehydration.
- Severe dehydration associated with compromised perfusion can result in metabolic lactic acidosis.
- Hyperkalemia may occur with potassium-sparing diuretics.
- Acetazolamide causes paradoxic metabolic acidosis with the production of an alkaline urine.

Musculoskeletal

• Severe hypokalemia can produce muscle weakness and hyporeflexia.
• Thiazides can produce hyperuricemia and exacerbate gout.

Neurologic

• Severe hyponatremia can produce altered mental status, confusion, coma, and seizures.
• Dehydration may lead to lightheadedness that can progress to syncope.

Endocrine

• Hyperglycemia can occur with glycerin and thiazides.
• Hyperlipidemia can occur with chronic thiazide therapy.

PROCEDURES AND LABORATORY TESTS

Essential Tests

Laboratory testing may not be needed in asymptomatic patients.

Recommended Tests

• Serum electrolytes, BUN, and creatinine. Hypokalemia, hyperkalemia, hyponatremia, and metabolic alkalosis or metabolic acidosis can occur.
• Serum calcium and serum magnesium. Hypocalcemia and hypomagnesemia can occur.
• Urinalysis

—The osmotic diuretics may cause elevated specific gravity, which also may occur with dehydration.
—Most potassium-sparing diuretics produce decreased specific gravity.
—Acetazolamide produces an alkaline urine.

• Complete blood count is used to detect anemia or infection.
• Arterial blood gases are measured in patients with hypoperfusion, hypoventilation, hyperventilation, or decreased serum bicarbonate.
• ECG is performed to monitor effects of electrolyte abnormalities.
• Serum acetaminophen and aspirin level are measured to detect occult ingestion.

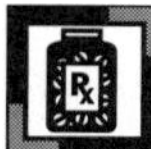

Treatment

• Treatment should focus on supportive care with maintenance of fluid and electrolyte balance.
• Dose and time of exposure should be determined for all substances involved.

DIRECTING PATIENT COURSE

The health-care professional should call a poison control center when:

• Signs and symptoms are inconsistent with diuretic poisoning.
• Coingestant, drug interaction, or underlying disease presents an unusual problem.

The patient should be referred to a health-care facility when:

• Attempted suicide or homicide is possible
• The patient or caregiver seems unreliable
• Altered mental status or other severe effects are present.
• Coingestant, drug interaction, or underlying disease presents an unusual problem.

Admission Considerations

Inpatient management is warranted for patients with dehydration or an electrolyte abnormality that requires continued intravenous therapy, or with ECG abnormalities.

DECONTAMINATION

Out of Hospital

Induction of emesis is usually not recommended because of the benign course of acute diuretic ingestion, but may be useful following a massive ingestion.

In Hospital

• Gastric lavage should be performed in pediatric (tube size 24–32 French) or adult (tube size 36–42 French) patients presenting within 1 hour of ingestion or if serious effects are present.
• One dose of activated charcoal (1–2 g/kg) should be administered without a cathartic if a substantial ingestion has occurred within the previous few hours.

ANTIDOTES

There is no specific antidote for diuretic poisoning.

ADJUNCTIVE TREATMENT

For hypotension, the patient should be treated with isotonic fluid infusion, the Trendelenburg position, and, if needed, vasopressors. Dopamine is preferred and norepinephrine is added for refractory hypotension.

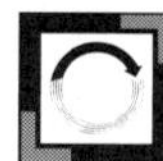

Follow-Up

PATIENT MONITORING

Vital signs, fluid balance, serum electrolytes, and ECG should be monitored in symptomatic patients.

EXPECTED COURSE AND PROGNOSIS

• After acute ingestion, patients typically develop transient polyuria lasting from 2 to 12 hours.
• Complete recovery may be expected over 24 to 48 hours, unless sequelae of electrolyte abnormality or hypotension intercedes.

DISCHARGE CRITERIA AND INSTRUCTIONS

• From emergency department. Patients may be discharged following a 4- to 6-hour observation period, if serum electrolytes and ECG are normal, and after psychiatric evaluation, if needed.
• From the hospital. Patients may be discharged when toxic effects resolve or stabilize.

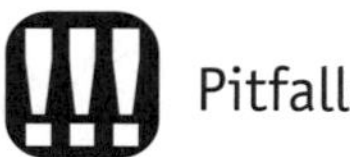

Pitfalls

TREATMENT

Most patients can be hydrated orally. In the rare instance in which fluid and electrolytes cannot be corrected by oral replacement therapy, however, intravenous replacement is warranted.

ICD-9-CM 974

Poisoning by water, mineral, and uric acid metabolism drugs.

RECOMMENDED READING

POISINDEX Editorial Staff. Diuretics. In: Rumack BH, Sayre NK, Gelman CR, eds. *POISINDEX system*. Englewood, CO: Micromedex, Inc., August 31, 1998.

Author: Edwin K. Kuffner

Reviewer: Richard C. Dart

Edrophonium

Basics

DESCRIPTION

Edrophonium chloride (Tensilon, Enlon, Reversol) is a parenteral cholinergic agonist mediator used primarily in the diagnosis of myasthenia gravis.

FORMS AND USES

- The initial dose for the differential diagnosis of myasthenia gravis is 1 to 2 mg intravenously over 15 to 30 seconds.

—If no reaction occurs after 45 seconds, the remainder of the 10-mg total dose is injected.
—In geriatric patients the maximum dose is reduced to 5 to 7 mg.

- In children over 75 pounds, the test dose is 1 mg and total dose is up to 5 mg in increments of 1 mg.
- In children under 75 pounds, the dose is 0.2 mg/kg intramuscularly.
- Adequacy of current myasthenia treatment.

—The dose is 1 to 2 mg intravenously 1 hour after ingestion of the treatment drug.
—The response is myasthenic in the undertreated patient, adequate in the controlled patient, and cholinergic in the overtreated patient.

- Differentiation of myasthenic crisis from therapeutic cholinergic excess.

—A test dose of 1 mg is administered intravenously over 15 to 30 seconds.
—If symptoms do not worsen, an additional 1 mg is given.
—If symptoms improve, no further dose is given.

- It is also used as an antagonist to nondepolarizing neuromuscular blockers.
- The bite of some neurotoxic snakes are treated with edrophonium.

PATHOPHYSIOLOGY

- Edrophonium reversibly binds acetylcholinesterase in peripheral and CNS synapses, thereby potentiating the effect of acetylcholine.
- Onset is in 30 to 60 seconds, and duration of action is 10 to 30 minutes.
- Nicotinic effects are manifested as muscle weakness and fasciculation.
- Muscarinic effects are manifested as the SLUDGE syndrome (**s**alivation, **l**acrimation, **u**rination, **d**efecation/diaphoresis, **g**astrointestinal cramping, and **e**mesis).

EPIDEMIOLOGY

Toxic effects are common but are typically mild.

CAUSES

- Poisoning may be caused by rapid injection of edrophonium or by waiting an insufficient period of time to determine the response to previous dose(s).
- Poisoning may also be caused by idiopathic hypersensitivity to anticholinesterase agents.

RISK FACTORS

- Geriatric patients are more susceptible to adverse cardiac effects.
- Dysrhythmia is more common in patients with heart disease.

DRUG AND DISEASE INTERACTIONS

- Edrophonium may cause synergistic cholinergic effects in patients already taking therapeutic anticholinesterases (neostigmine, pyridostigmine, physostigmine).
- Synergistic cholinergic effects may occur with organophosphate insecticides.
- The probability of dysrhythmia is increased with digoxin, calcium channel blockers, and β-blockers.
- Quinidine may antagonize edrophonium effects and mask diagnostic response in myasthenia gravis.
- Procainamide may antagonize effects on skeletal muscle.

PREGNANCY AND LACTATION

US FDA Pregnancy Category C. The drug exerts animal teratogenic or embryocidal effects, but there are no controlled studies in women, or no studies are available in either animals or women.

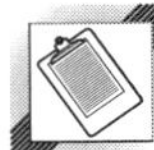

Diagnosis

DIFFERENTIAL DIAGNOSIS

Toxic causes of small pupils with signs of cholinergic excess include organophosphate or carbamate insecticides and other therapeutic cholinesterase inhibitors (neostigmine, pyridostigmine, physostigmine).

SIGNS AND SYMPTOMS

Vital Signs

Bradycardia and tachypnea may occur.

HEENT

Increased salivation and lacrimation, diplopia, and pupillary constriction may occur.

Dermatologic

Diaphoresis is common.

Cardiovascular

Bradycardia, hypotension, atrioventricular block, atrial fibrillation, atrial flutter, ventricular tachycardia, and asystole may occur.

Pulmonary

Increased pulmonary secretions, laryngospasm, bronchiolar constriction, and, in severe cases, respiratory paralysis may occur.

Gastrointestinal

Nausea, vomiting, diarrhea, abdominal cramps, and increased intestinal secretions may occur.

Renal

Urinary frequency may occur.

Musculoskeletal

Weakness and fasciculation may occur.

Neurologic

Seizures, dysarthria, dysphonia, and dysphagia may occur.

PROCEDURES AND LABORATORY TESTS

- Essential tests. ECG and continuous cardiac monitoring should be performed; bradycardia, atrioventricular block, atrial fibrillation, atrial flutter, ventricular tachycardia, and asystole may develop.
- Recommended tests. Other tests are recommended only as indicated by patient course.
- Not recommended tests. Serum levels are not clinically useful.

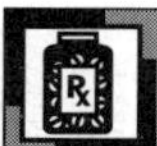

Treatment

Treatment should focus on airway management, cardiac toxicity, seizure management, and atropine administration.

DIRECTING PATIENT COURSE

The health-care provider should call the poison control center when:

- Bronchospasm, apnea, hypotension, or other severe effects are present.
- Toxic effects are not consistent with edrophonium toxicity.
- Coingestant, drug interaction, or underlying disease presents an unusual challenge.

Patients should be referred to a health-care facility when:

- Any toxic effects develop.
- Coingestant, drug interaction, or underlying disease presents an unusual challenge.

Admission Considerations

Inpatient treatment is warranted when the patient develops shock, seizure, airway compromise, or persistent dysrhythmia or has an underlying medical condition that warrants prolonged observation.

DECONTAMINATION

Decontamination is not helpful because of the intravenous route of administration.

ANTIDOTES

Atropine

- Indications. Clinically significant muscarinic symptoms: salivation, lacrimation, urination, defecation, emesis, diaphoresis, bradycardia, hypotension, and asystole.
- Contraindications. No absolute contraindications.
- Method of administration

—Adult
  —The dose is 0.5 mg up to 2 mg intravenously, then 0.5 mg every 3 to 10 minutes as needed.
—Pediatric
  —The dose is 0.01 to 0.05 mg/kg intravenously, then 0.01 to 0.05 mg/kg every 3 to 10 minutes as needed, up to 5 mg.

- Adverse effects. Anticholinergic syndrome

Pralidoxime

Indications. Severe or prolonged nicotinic symptoms (profound muscle weakness, respiratory depression, coma, seizures). For details of administration, see SECTION III, Pralidoxime chapter.

ADJUNCTIVE TREATMENT

Hypotension

- Patient should be administered 10 to 20 ml/kg 0.9% NaCl and placed in the Trendelenburg position.
- Further fluid therapy should be guided by central pressure monitoring to avoid volume overload.
- If hypotension is unresponsive, a vasopressor should be administered.

—Dopamine
  —The dose is 2 to 5 μg/kg/min, titrated to effect.
  —Infusion rates above 20 μg/kg/min should be avoided.
—Norepinephrine
  —The dose is 0.1 to 0.2 μg/kg/min, titrated to effect.
—High rates of infusion may cause tissue ischemia.

Seizures

A benzodiazepine should be administered for initial control.

- Diazepam

—Adult dose is 5 to 10 mg initially, repeated every 10 minutes if needed.
—Pediatric dose is 0.2 to 0.5 mg/kg initially, repeated every 10 minutes if needed.

- Lorazepam

—Adult dose is 2 to 4 mg by intravenous push over 2 to 5 minutes, repeated every 10 minutes if needed.
—Pediatric dose is 0.1 mg/kg by intravenous push over 2 to 5 minutes, not to exceed 4 mg/dose, repeated every 10 minutes if needed.

- The airway should be monitored closely.

Tracheostomy and Mechanical Ventilation

Required rarely for respiratory paralysis and secretions resistant to treatment.

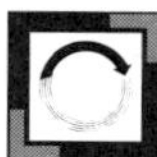

Follow-Up

PATIENT MONITORING

Cardiac and respiratory monitoring should be performed until dysrhythmias resolve and patient is stable.

EXPECTED COURSE AND PROGNOSIS

- Direct effects resolve within 10 to 30 minutes if uncomplicated unless complications of hypoxia or seizure intercede.
- Secretions and respiratory paralysis resolve over a longer period.
- Chronic renal failure may prolong duration of adverse events.

DISCHARGE CRITERIA/INSTRUCTIONS

- From the emergency department. Patient may be discharged after resolution of toxic effects, depending on the underlying medical condition and the reason for use of edrophonium.
- From the hospital. Patient may be discharged after resolution of airway compromise and as general medical condition allows.

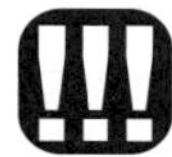

Pitfalls

DIAGNOSIS

- Myasthenia gravis may produce respiratory paralysis misinterpreted as secondary to edrophonium.
- Reversal of nondepolarizing neuromuscular blockers may wear off prematurely because of the short duration of action for edrophonium.
- Edrophonium should not be given to patients already in cholinergic excess.
- When given to reverse neuromuscular blockade, the effect of each dose should be assessed before giving additional edrophonium.

TREATMENT

Atropine may not be immediately available.

ICD-9-CM 971.0

Poisoning by drugs primarily affecting autonomic nervous system: parasympathomimetics (cholinergics).

See also: SECTION II, Hypotension and Seizure (Unexplained) chapters; and SECTION III, Pralidoxime chapter.

RECOMMENDED READING

Gilman AG, Rall TW, Nies AS, et al., eds. *Goodman and Gilman's the pharmacological basis of therapeutics,* 8th ed. New York: Pergamon, 1990.

Youngberg JA. Cardiac arrest following treatment of paroxysmal atrial tachycardia with edrophonium. *Anesthesiol* 1979;50:234–235.

Author: Steven A. Seifert

Reviewer: Richard C. Dart

Ephedrine

Basics

DESCRIPTION

- Ephedrine is an adrenergic (sympathomimetic) agent with actions similar to those of epinephrine.
- Ephedrine occurs naturally in plants of the genus *Ephedra*. Common names include Ma huang, Mexican tea, miner's tea, Mormon tea, joint fir, and squaw tea.

FORMS AND USES

- U.S. FDA approved indications include hypotension, asthma, idiopathic orthostatic hypotension, hypotension due to spinal anesthesia, nocturnal enuresis, and nasal congestion.
- Other medical uses include stress incontinence, myasthenia gravis, ejaculatory failure, obesity, diabetic neuropathy, and dysmenorrhea.
- Pharmaceutical products include generic ephedrine sulfate (0.5% oral solution, 25-mg capsules, 50 mg/ml parenteral injection), Amnesiac, Asthmalixir, Azma Aid, Bronitin, Bronkaid, Bronkolixir, Bronkotabs, Efed II, Efedron, Guiaphed, Phedral C.T., Primatene, Quelidrine, Tedral, Tedrigen, Theodrine, Theoral, and Vatronol.
- "Herbal ecstasy" is a recreational drug that contains ephedrine.
- Typical adult dosage

—Nasal congestion. 0.5% solution or 0.6% jelly every 4 hours or 25 to 50 mg orally every 6 hours.
—Urinary incontinence. 25 to 50 mg orally every 6 hours.
—Ejaculatory failure. 25 to 75 mg orally 1 hour before intercourse.

- Pediatric dosages. 0.2 to 0.3 mg/kg every 4 to 6 hours intramuscularly or intravenously, or 3 mg/kg/day in four divided doses orally or subcutaneously.

TOXIC DOSE

Just two to three times the daily dose may cause hypertension, but abusers of ephedrine may develop tolerance and therefore tolerate much larger doses without major effect.

PATHOPHYSIOLOGY

- Ephedrine is a direct α- and β-receptor agonist and an indirect adrenoreceptor agonist, releasing norepinephrine from presynaptic sympathetic neurons.
- The main effects are relaxation of bronchial smooth muscle, cardiac stimulation, constriction of arterioles, dilation of pupils, increased tone of the bladder and vesicle sphincter, and central nervous system stimulation.

EPIDEMIOLOGY

- Poisoning is uncommon.
- Toxic effects following exposure are typically mild.

CAUSES

- Poisoning is usually the result of accidental ingestion or intentional misuse.
- Child abuse should be considered if the patient is under 1 year of age.
- Attempted suicide should be considered in a patient over 6 years of age.

DRUG AND DISEASE INTERACTIONS

- Ephedrine may have a synergistic effect when interacting with other sympathomimetic agents, such as stimulants, amphetamines, and cocaine.
- Use with a monoamine oxidase (MAO) inhibitor may produce severe hypertension.

PREGNANCY AND LACTATION

- US FDA Pregnancy Category C. The drug exerts animal teratogenic or embryocidal effects, but there are no controlled studies in women, or no studies are available in animals or women.
- Ephedrine usually decreases uterine activity.
- A fetus is at risk for acceleration of heart rate if ephedrine is used intravenously to maintain blood pressure during spinal anesthesia for delivery.

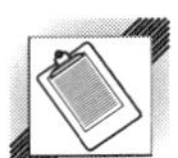

Diagnosis

DIFFERENTIAL DIAGNOSIS

- Toxic causes of hypertension and agitation include other sympathomimetic agents (e.g., cocaine, amphetamines, MAO inhibitors, phenylephrine, fenfluramine), theophylline, and others.
- Nontoxic causes include diseases with adrenergic excess, such as hyperthyroidism, manic behavior, and alcohol withdrawal.

SIGNS AND SYMPTOMS

The predominant features of acute overdose are agitation, tachycardia, and hypertension.

Vital Signs

- Hypertension (systolic and diastolic) and tachycardia are common.
- Reflex bradycardia may result from increased blood pressure.

HEENT

- Mydriasis may develop.
- Topical application constricts vessels in nasal mucosa, producing decongestion.

Dermatologic

- Mild diaphoresis may occur.
- Hypersensitivity rash has been reported.

Cardiovascular

- Positive chronotropic and inotropic effects may result in tachycardia, hypertension, increased cardiac output, and increased cardiac work.
- Ephedrine may cause anginal symptoms in patients with cardiac disease.
- Hypotension may develop in severe overdoses.
- Ephedrine may produce dysrhythmia (ventricular tachycardia, fibrillation, extrasystoles).
- Ephedrine also increases coronary, cerebral and muscle blood flow.

Gastrointestinal

- Nausea, anorexia, vomiting, and mild epigastric pain may occur.
- Intestinal necrosis occurs rarely, in severe cases.

Hepatic

Increased hepatic glycogenolysis may cause hyperglycemia.

Renal

Acute renal insufficiency may develop in serious cases.

Fluids and Electrolytes

Ephedrine may decrease plasma volume from loss of fluid to extracellular space.

Musculoskeletal

Severe poisoning may rarely cause rhabdomyolysis.

Neurologic

- Central nervous system stimulation may result in nervousness, anxiety, fear, agitation, irritability, insomnia, or seizure.
- Headache, intracranial hemorrhage, ischemic infarcts and cerebral vasculitis may occur.
- Large parenteral doses may cause confusion, delirium, hallucinations, vertigo, or dizziness.

Psychiatric

Paranoid psychosis and visual or auditory hallucinations occur in some patients, especially with chronic abuse.

PROCEDURES AND LABORATORY TESTS

Essential Tests

No tests may be needed for asymptomatic patients.

Recommended Tests

- Serum electrolytes, BUN, creatinine, creatine kinase to assess effects of dehydration, and agitation
- ECG, serum acetaminophen and aspirin levels, are used in overdose setting to detect occult ingestion
- Head CT, lumbar puncture, bacterial cultures, and other tests as needed to assess altered mental status or fever of unknown etiology
- Chest radiography in patients with hypoxia or pulmonary symptoms

Not Recommended Tests

Serum levels of ephedrine are not clinically useful.

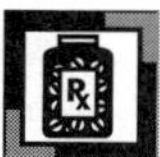

Treatment

• Treatment should focus on control of agitation, seizures, and support of hemodynamic function.
• The dose and time of exposure should be determined for all substances involved.

DIRECTING PATIENT COURSE

The health-care professional should call the poison control center when:

• Shock, dysrhythmia, altered mental status, or other serious effects are present.
• Toxic effects are not consistent with ephedrine.
• Coingestant, drug interaction, or underlying disease presents an unusual problem.

The patient should be referred to a health-care facility when:

• Attempted suicide or homicide is possible.
• The patient or caregiver seems unreliable.
• Any toxic effects are present.
• Coingestant, drug interaction, or underlying disease presents an unusual problem.

Admission Considerations

Inpatient management is appropriate for patients with refractory agitation, severe hypertension, persistent tachycardia, altered mental status, neurologic abnormality, or other end-organ dysfunction.

DECONTAMINATION

Out of Hospital

Ipecac-induced emesis is not recommended.

In Hospital

• Gastric lavage should be performed in pediatric (tube size 24–32 French) or adult (tube size 36–42 French) patients presenting within 1 hour of a large ingestion or if serious effects are present.
• One dose of activated charcoal (1–2 g/kg) should be administered without a cathartic if a substantial ingestion has occurred within the previous few hours.

Antidotes

There is no specific antidote for ephedrine toxicity.

Adjunctive Treatment

• Control of agitation or seizure

—The airway must be secured and monitored.
—A benzodiazepine familiar to the provider should be administered; for diazepam, adults should receive 5 to 10 mg intravenously, children 0.2 to 0.5 mg/kg intravenously, with doses repeated at 10-minute intervals, titrating to effect; for lorazepam, adults should receive 1 to 2 mg intravenously, children 0.05 mg/kg intravenously, repeated every 10 minutes, titrating to effect.

• Hypertension. If hypertension is not responsive to benzodiazepines or if end-organ damage develops (e.g., aortic dissection, central nervous system bleed, or myocardial infarction), a short-acting titratable agent (e.g., nitroprusside) should be administered until a desired response is seen.
• Hypotension may be treated with an isotonic fluid infusion, the Trendelenburg position, and a vasopressor such as dopamine; norepinephrine is recommended for refractory hypotension.
• Ventricular dysrhythmia

—Standard advanced cardiac life support algorithms should be used.
—Lidocaine (1 mg/kg intravenous bolus, repeated in a 0.5 mg/kg bolus if necessary and followed with 20 to 40 μg/kg/min infusion) may be used for ventricular tachycardia or frequent premature ventricular contractions.

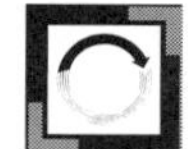

Follow-Up

PATIENT MONITORING

Respiratory and cardiac function should be monitored continuously.

EXPECTED COURSE AND PROGNOSIS

• Patients generally recover quickly unless repeated seizures, hypertension, hypoxia, or psychiatric deterioration intercede.
• Possible complications include end-organ injury from hypertension or tachydysrhythmias, as well as ischemic or hemorrhagic stroke, possibly due to drug-induced cerebral vasculitis.

DISCHARGE CRITERIA AND INSTRUCTIONS

• From the emergency department

—The patient should be discharged after effects have resolved, decontamination is complete, and mental status returns to baseline.
—Referral for substance abuse treatment should be considered.

• From the hospital

—The patient should be discharged after effects have resolved, mental status returns to baseline, and laboratory values normalize.
—Psychiatric clearance should be obtained if appropriate.

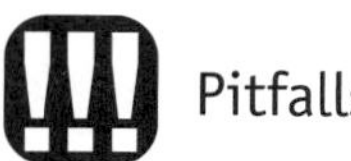

Pitfalls

DIAGNOSIS

Mental status changes, hypertension, and neurologic dysfunction should prompt evaluation for central nervous system bleed, infection, or infarct.

TREATMENT

It is important to admit patients with persistent mental status change, hypertension, or dysrhythmias.

ICD-9-CM 969.7

Poisoning by psychotropic agents: psychostimulants.

See also: SECTION II, Hypertension, Seizures, Ventricular Dysrhythmias, and Hypotension chapters; and SECTION III, Nitroprusside chapter.

RECOMMENDED READING

Bruno A, Nolte KB, Chapin J. Stroke associated with ephedrine use. *Neurology* 1993;43:1313–1316.

Sawyer DR, Conner CS, Rumack BH. Managing acute toxicity from nonprescription stimulants. *Clin Pharm* 1982;1:529–533.

Battig K. Acute and chronic cardiovascular and behavioral effects of caffeine, aspirin and ephedrine. *Int J Obesity* 1993;17:S61–S64.

Author: Melissa J. Ruyle

Reviewer: Richard C. Dart

Epinephrine

Basics

DESCRIPTION

Epinephrine is an adrenergic agonist used to treat bronchospasm, anaphylactic reactions, bradycardia, cardiac arrest, and hypotension.

FORMS AND USES

- Epinephrine for inhalation. Adrenalin, AsthmaHaler Mist, AsthmaNefrin, Bronitin Mist, Bronkaid Mist, Medihaler-Epi, Primatene Mist, MicroNefrin, Nephron, Racepinephrine, and Vaponephrin.
- Epinephrine for injection. Adrenalin, Epi-Pen, Epi-Pen Jr., and Sus-Phrine.

TOXIC DOSE

- Pharmacologically active doses are not reached with ingested dosages.
- Injection of any amount above the recommended dosage may produce toxicity.

PATHOPHYSIOLOGY

- Epinephrine stimulates α-adrenergic and β_1- and β_2-adrenergic receptors.
- There is only slight absorption via the inhaled route, and effects are generally localized to the respiratory tract.

EPIDEMIOLOGY

Poisoning is uncommon.

CAUSES

- Toxicity is usually caused by iatrogenic error or marked misuse of inhaler by patient.
- Child neglect should be considered if the patient is under 1 year of age; suicide attempt if the patient is over 6 years of age.

PREGNANCY AND LACTATION

US FDA Pregnancy Category C. The drug exerts animal teratogenic or embryocidal effects, but there are no controlled studies in women, or no studies are available in animals or women.

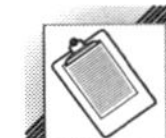

Diagnosis

DIFFERENTIAL DIAGNOSIS

Toxic causes of agitation and dysrhythmias are numerous, including stimulants, inhaled β receptor agonists, and many others.

SIGNS AND SYMPTOMS

- Rapid onset of agitation, hypertension, tachycardia, and dysrhythmias are typical.

Vital Signs

Overdosage can result in tachycardia hypertension, extreme pallor and coldness of skin.

Pulmonary

Dyspnea is common. Pulmonary arterial hypertension may result in potentially fatal pulmonary edema.

Cardiovascular

- Tachycardia may result is myocardial ischemia.
- Ventricular dysrhythmia is common after overdose.

Gastrointestinal

Vomiting is common after overdose.

Fluid and Electrolytes

Hyperglycemia is common with overdose.

Acid-Base

Lactic acidosis and reduced renal and hepatic blood flow occur due to tissue ischemia.

Neurologic

Severe hypertension may cause intracranial bleeding.
Agitation and tremulousness are common.

PROCEDURES AND LABORATORY TESTS

Essential tests

No tests may be needed for minimally symptomatic patients.

Recommended Tests

Tests should be ordered according to the manifestations that develop (e.g., ischemia, hemorrhage).

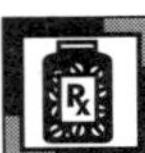

Treatment

DIRECTING PATIENT COURSE

Treatment should focus on hypertension and dysrhythmias.

The health-care professional should call the poison control center when:

- Severe or persistent effects develop.
- Coingestant, drug interaction, or underlying disease presents an unusual problem.

The patient should be referred to a health-care facility when:

- Suicide or homicide attempt is possible.
- Toxic effects develop.
- Coingestant, drug interaction, or underlying disease presents an unusual problem.

Admission Considerations

Admission is recommended for patients who develop cardiac manifestations.

DECONTAMINATION

It is not recommended because toxicity is usually caused by repeated misuse or injection of excessive dose.

ANTIDOTES

There is no specific antidote recommended for epinephrine.

ADJUNCTIVE TREATMENT

- Agitation is treated with benzodiazepines titrated to response.
- Hypertension. If end organ injury develops (aortic dissection, CNS effects, myocardial ischemia), consider administration of a short-acting agent such as nitroprusside.
- Ventricular dysrhythmia. Standard advanced cardiac life support algorithms are appropriate.
- Local tissue ischemia caused by injection of epinephrine can be treated with local infiltration of phentolamine (0.5 mg/ml concentration) around the injection site.

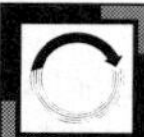

Follow-Up

PATIENT MONITORING

In cases with systemic effects, the heart rate, blood pressure, ECG, blood glucose, serum electrolytes, arterial blood gases, and serum creatinine should be monitored.

EXPECTED COURSE AND PROGNOSIS

Recovery is expected within 24 hours with supportive treatment unless sequelae of hypertension or CNS bleed intercede.

DISCHARGE CRITERIA AND INSTRUCTIONS

Patients may be discharged from the emergency room or hospital if they do not develop hypertension, tachycardia, or dysrhythmias within 6 hours of observation.

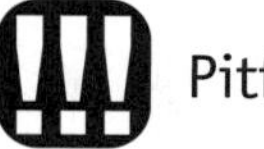

Pitfalls

DIAGNOSIS

Altered mental status should prompt investigation for CNS bleed.

TREATMENT

Use of β-receptor blocking drugs alone is not recommended as it may theoretically lead to unopposed alpha stimulation.

ICD-9-CM 971.2

Poisoning by drugs primarily affecting the autonomic nervous system: sympathomimetics (adrenergics).

See also: SECTION II, Ventricular Dysrhythmia chapter; and SECTION III, Nitroprusside chapter.

RECOMMENDED READING

Kurachek SC, Rockoff MA. Inadvertent intravenous administration of racemic epinephrine. *JAMA* 1985;253:1441–1442.

Authors: Kevin M. Lier

Reviewer: Richard C. Dart

Ergot Alkaloids

Basics

DESCRIPTION

- Ergot alkaloids are used for acute and short-term therapy for migraine or cluster headache and for treatment of uterine bleeding.
- Ergot alkaloids include ergotamine (Ergomar, Bellergal, Cafergot, Wigraine, Ergostat), ergonovine (Ergotrate), methylergonovine (Methergine), dihydroergotamine (D.H.E. 45), and methysergide (Sansert), a semisynthetic ergot alkaloid.
- Ergot alkaloids can also be found in cereal grains contaminated with the fungus *Claviceps purpurea*.

FORMS AND USES

- Migraine or cluster headache (acute and short-term therapy)

—Ergotamine is administered sublingually, 2 mg every 30 minutes. The dosage must not exceed 6 mg in 24 hours or 10 mg in 7 days.
—Dihydroergotamine is administered intravenously, 1 mg every 60 minutes. The dose must not exceed 3 mg.
—Methysergide is administered orally, 4 to 8 mg daily for prophylaxis only.

- Uterine bleeding

—Methylergonovine or ergonovine is administered intramuscularly or intravenously, 0.2 mg (1 ml), for control of uterine hemorrhage. For bleeding, 0.2 or 0.4 mg is given orally every 6 to 12 hours for 48 hours.

TOXIC DOSE

- Toxicity has occurred with 0.5 mg of parenteral ergotamine, 0.2 mg of ergonovine or methylergonovine, and less than 5 mg of sublingual or rectal ergotamine.
- A therapeutic dose can be toxic because some individuals are exquisitely sensitive.

PATHOPHYSIOLOGY

- The ergot alkaloids are direct vascular constrictors of both venous and arterial beds, decreasing blood flow to organs and tissues.
- Ergot alkaloids increase uterine contractions.

EPIDEMIOLOGY

- Poisoning is uncommon and usually associated with intermittent or chronic daily use.
- Rarely, ergot-producing fungus on grain has produced mass epidemics of ergotism (St. Anthony's Fire).
- Toxic effects after exposure are variable, with peripheral ischemic events most common and death occurring rarely.

CAUSES

- Poisoning is usually the result of accidental ingestion or drug interaction.
- Child neglect should be considered if the patient is under 1 year of age, suicide attempt if the patient is over 6 years of age.

RISK FACTORS

- Underlying hypertension, vascular disease, coronary disease, and sepsis predispose to toxicity.
- Underlying hepatic, renal, or biliary disease increases serum level of ergot alkaloids.
- In the setting of pregnancy, hypertension, preeclampsia, and toxemia are risk factors.

DRUG AND DISEASE INTERACTIONS

- Nicotine can provoke vasoconstriction, thereby increasing the potential for ischemic sequelae.
- Macrolide antibiotics (erythromycin-type) inhibit metabolism of ergot alkaloids.
- β-blockers potentiate the vasoconstrictive effects of ergot alkaloids.
- Sympathomimetics exacerbate the hypertensive effect of ergot alkaloids.
- Halothane antagonizes the effects of ergonovine and relaxes uterine smooth muscle, thereby increasing the risk of uterine bleeding.
- Use with heparin for deep venous thrombosis prophylaxis is associated with more frequent adverse effects.

PREGNANCY AND LACTATION

- Methylergonovine. US FDA Pregnancy Category C. The drug exerts animal teratogenic or embryocidal effects, but there are no controlled studies in women, or no studies are available in either animals or women.
- Ergotamine and methysergide. US FDA Pregnancy Category X. Studies have demonstrated fetal abnormalities or there is evidence of fetal risk based on human experience, or both, and the risk clearly outweighs any possible benefit.
- Fetal death has occurred following overdose.

Diagnosis

DIFFERENTIAL DIAGNOSIS

- Toxic causes of peripheral ischemia include sympathomimetic drugs (e.g., ephedrine, amphetamine, cocaine).
- Nontoxic causes include unrecognized compartment syndrome, direct vascular injury, and deep venous thrombosis.

SIGNS AND SYMPTOMS

Primary effect is tissue ischemia which may include myocardial ischemia and be associated with altered mental status.

Vital Signs

Tachycardia, bradycardia in the face of hypotension (centrally mediated), or hypertension may occur.

HEENT

Facial, lingual, or retinal artery ischemia with transient blindness may develop.

Dermatologic

Localized cyanosis and edema, pruritus, flushing, and nonspecific purpuric rash may occur.

Pulmonary

- Bronchospasm may develop acutely.
- Pleuritis, effusion, and fibrosis have developed during chronic use.

Cardiovascular

- Vasoconstriction may result in coronary, peripheral, CNS, mesenteric, or renal ischemia.
- There have been rare reports of heart valve fibrosis.
- Renal and mesenteric aneurysm formation has developed with chronic ergotism.

Gastrointestinal

- Nausea, vomiting, diarrhea, and abdominal pain are common at therapeutic doses and in overdose.
- Anorectal ulcers have occurred from one suppository.

Hepatic

Ischemic hepatitis and pancreatitis may occur.

Renal

- Hematuria may occur.
- Renal ischemia or renal failure may result from prolonged arterial spasm.
- Retroperitoneal fibrosis has developed rarely during chronic use.

Musculoskeletal

Pain and cyanosis of extremities and intermittent claudication may occur.

Neurologic

- Peripheral paresthesia, hallucinations, dysphoria, confusion, depression, and seizures may occur.
- Cerebral infarction, cranial nerve palsies, tinnitus, and vertigo have occurred.

Reproductive

- Hypertonic uterine contractions can occur.
- Spontaneous abortion may occur.
- The suppression of prolactin may inhibit lactation.

Hematologic

Neutropenia and eosinophilia can occur.

Psychological

- Dependence can develop.
- Psychosis may follow acute overdose.

PROCEDURES AND LABORATORY TESTS

Essential Tests

No tests are usually needed in asymptomatic patients.

Recommended Tests

- Serum electrolytes, BUN, creatinine to evaluate renal function
- ECG if there is evidence of cardiac ischemia
- ECG, serum acetaminophen, and aspirin levels in an overdose setting to detect occult ingestion
- Head CT, lumbar puncture, and other tests as needed to evaluate other causes of altered mental status or seizures
- Angiography to evaluate peripheral vasospasm
- Intravenous pyelogram in the setting of suspected retroperitoneal fibrosis

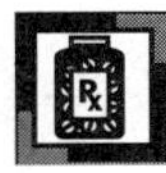

Treatment

- Treatment should focus on withdrawal of the offending agent and therapy of vasoconstriction.
- Dose and time of exposure need to be determined for all substances involved.

DIRECTING PATIENT COURSE

The health-care professional should call the poison control center when:

- Evidence of peripheral ischemia, cerebrovascular accident, myocardial infarction, or other severe effects are present.
- Toxic effects are not consistent with ergotamine poisoning.
- Coingestant, drug interaction, or underlying disease presents an unusual problem.

The patient should be referred to a health-care facility when:

- Attempted suicide or homicide is possible.
- Patient or caregiver seems unreliable.
- Any toxic effects develop.
- Coingestant, drug interaction, or underlying disease presents an unusual problem.

Admission Considerations

Inpatient management is warranted for patients with systemic effects or evidence of tissue ischemia.

DECONTAMINATION

Out of Hospital

Emesis should be induced with ipecac within 1 hour of ingestion for alert pediatric or adult patients if health-care evaluation will be delayed.

In Hospital

- Ipecac should be administered to induce emesis within 1 hour of ingestion for the alert patient who is too small to have effective gastric lavage.
- Gastric lavage should be performed in pediatric (tube size 24–32 French) or adult (tube size 36–42 French) patients presenting within 1 hour of a large ingestion or if serious effects are present.
- One dose of activated charcoal (1–2 g/kg) should be administered without a cathartic if a substantial ingestion has occurred within the previous few hours.

ANTIDOTE

There is no specific antidote for ergotamine poisoning.

ADJUNCTIVE TREATMENT

Hypertension

If end-organ damage develops (aortic dissection, CNS bleed, myocardial infarction), administer a short-acting titratable agent (see vascular spasm below).

Vascular Spasm

Multiple Modalities Have Been Used for Spasm

- Sodium nitroprusside is used most commonly.

—Adult and pediatric dose is 0.5 μg/kg/min by intravenous infusion. Infusion is increased by 0.25 to 0.5 μg/kg/min every 5 minutes, titrating dose to desired effect.
—Infusion rate over 10 μg/kg/min is rarely required and may produce cyanide toxicity.
—Nitroprusside should be tapered gradually in order to avoid rebound hypertension.

- In mild to moderate cases, captopril, nifedipine, or prazosin have been used successfully.
- Peripheral ischemia may require treatment with intraarterial phentolamine (for vasospasm) or thrombolytics (for thrombus).

Coronary Artery Spasm

- Standard techniques are used, such as sublingual or intravenous nitroglycerin.
- Heparin and aspirin are provided as indicated.
- β-blockers should be avoided to prevent unopposed α-adrenergic receptor stimulation.

Control of Agitation or Seizure

- The airway must be secured and monitored throughout.
- A benzodiazepine familiar to the provider should be administered, for example, diazepam (adult dose 5–10 mg intravenously, pediatric dose 0.2–0.5 mg/kg intravenously, repeated at 10-minute intervals, titrating to effect) or lorazepam: (adult dose 1–2 mg intravenously, pediatric dose 0.05 mg/kg, repeated every 10 minutes, titrating to effect).

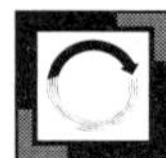

Follow-Up

PATIENT MONITORING

Cardiac, hemodynamic, and pulmonary status should be monitored continuously in symptomatic patients.

EXPECTED COURSE AND PROGNOSIS

- Possible complications include loss of extremity or other appendage, myocardial infarction, or cerebrovascular accident.
- Arterial spasm may linger for 72 hours and may end with infarction or other permanent tissue injury.

DISCHARGE CRITERIA AND INSTRUCTIONS

- From the emergency department. Asymptomatic patients with normal vital signs may be discharged after decontamination and 6 hours of observation.
- From the hospital. Patients may be discharged after vascular effects have resolved for 12 to 24 hours.

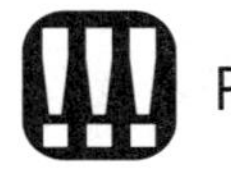

Pitfalls

TREATMENT

It is often necessary to try more than one vasodilator before vasospasm resolves.

ICD-9-CM 971

Poisoning by drugs primarily affecting the autonomic nervous system.

See also: SECTION II, Hypertension chapter; SECTION III, Nitroprusside chapter.

RECOMMENDED READING

de Groot ANJA, van Dongen PWJ, van Roosmalen J, et al. Ergotamine-induced fetal stress: review of side effects of ergot alkaloids during pregnancy. *Eur J Obstet Gynecol Reprod Biol* 1993;51:73–77.

Author: Michael Stackpool

Reviewer: Katherine M. Hurlbut

Ethchlorvynol

Basics

DESCRIPTION

Ethchlorvynol (Placidyl) is a sedative-hypnotic agent that is neither a barbiturate nor benzodiazepine.

FORMS AND USES

Available as 200-, 500-, or 750-mg capsules.

TOXIC DOSE

Acute ingestion of several grams may result in death.

PATHOPHYSIOLOGY

- Habituation occurs with chronic use.
- Withdrawal may last as long as 2 weeks following cessation of ethchlorvynol use and is similar in presentation and management to withdrawal from other sedative-hypnotic agents.

EPIDEMIOLOGY

Poisoning is uncommon.

CAUSES

- The drug is most commonly encountered as a drug of abuse.
- Child neglect should be considered if the patient is under 1 year of age; suicide attempt if the patient is over 6 years of age.

PREGNANCY AND LACTATION

- US FDA Pregnancy Category C. The drug exerts animal teratogenic or embryocidal effects, but there are no controlled studies in women, or no studies are available in either animals or women.
- Withdrawal syndrome may occur in neonates born to mother who uses ethchlorvynol.

DRUG AND DISEASE INTERACTIONS

CNS depression from ethchlorvynol is enhanced by the use of other sedative-hypnotic agents.

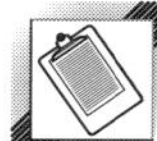

Diagnosis

DIFFERENTIAL DIAGNOSIS

Any cause of CNS and respiratory depression.

SIGNS AND SYMPTOMS

- Patients typically present with varying degrees of sedation following ethchlorvynol use.
- The patient often has a characteristic odor that is similar to a new car or shower curtain vinyl odor.
- Characteristic pink or green pills and gastric aspirate may help identify the presence of ethchlorvynol.

Vital Signs

- Hypothermia and coma may occur with severe overdose.
- Coma and respiratory depression may last several days.

HEENT

Mydriasis is common.

Dermatologic

Bullous dermal lesions also may occur.

Cardiovascular

- Tachycardia is common, but bradycardia may develop if hypertension occurs.
- Hypotension may occur with severe overdose.

Pulmonary

Respiratory depression, apnea, aspiration pneumonia, and pulmonary edema may occur with severe overdose.

Fluids and Electrolytes

Following severe overdose, patients are often dehydrated.

Musculoskeletal

Rhabdomyolysis may occur with severe overdose.

Neurologic

- CNS depression leading to coma occurs commonly following overdose.
- Delirium also may occur during recovery.

PROCEDURES AND LABORATORY TESTS

Essential Tests

No tests are usually needed in asymptomatic patients.

Recommended Tests

- Pulse oximetry or arterial blood gas to evaluate oxygenation
- Serum electrolytes, BUN, creatinine, and glucose in patients with altered mental status
- ECG, serum acetaminophen, and aspirin levels in an overdose setting to screen for occult ingestion
- Head CT, lumbar puncture, bacterial cultures, and other tests in patients with altered mental status of unknown etiology

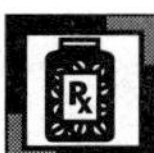

Treatment

Treatment should focus on supportive and symptomatic care.

- Oxygen should be administered and the airway closely monitored.
- The patient should be intubated if respiratory compromise occurs.
- Intravenous access must be established following severe overdose.

DIRECTING PATIENT COURSE

The health-care professional should call the poison control center when:

- Toxic effects are not consistent with ethchlorvynol toxicity.
- Severe or persistent effects develop.
- Coingestant, drug interaction, or underlying disease presents an unusual problem.

The patient should be referred to a health-care facility when:

- Suicide or homicide attempt is possible.
- Toxic effects develop.
- Coingestant, drug interaction, or underlying disease presents an unusual problem.

Admission Considerations

Admit patients who cannot care for themselves safely.

DECONTAMINATION

Out of Hospital

Emesis should not be induced.

In Hospital

One dose of activated charcoal (1–2 g/kg) should be administered without a cathartic if a substantial ingestion has occurred within the previous few hours.

ANTIDOTE

There is no specific antidote for ethchlorvynol.

ADJUNCTIVE TREATMENT

- Patients with hypotension, bradycardia, and hypothermia typically respond readily to securing the airway, administering intravenous fluids, and passive rewarming.
- Hypotension should be treated with isotonic fluid infusion and the Trendelenburg position. A vasopressor may be needed; dopamine is preferred. Norepinephrine may be added for refractory hypotension.

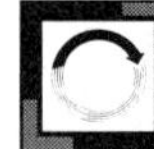

Follow-Up

PATIENT MONITORING

It is important to continuously monitor cardiovascular function and oxygen saturation.

EXPECTED COURSE AND PROGNOSIS

- Patients who have not suffered sequelae such as anoxia prior to access to medical care typically recover uneventfully.
- Withdrawal syndrome may last up to 2 weeks.

DISCHARGE CRITERIA AND INSTRUCTIONS

Patients may be discharged from the emergency department or hospital when toxic effects resolve or stabilize following decontamination, and after psychiatric evaluation, if needed.

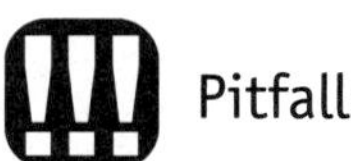

Pitfalls

DIAGNOSIS

Patient may have a flat EEG and yet fully recover.

FOLLOW-UP

Coma and respiratory compromise from ethchlorvynol poisoning may last for days following severe overdose.

ICD-9-CM 967

Poisoning by sedatives and hypnotics.

RECOMMENDED READING

Teehan BP, Maher JF, Carey JJ, et al. Acute ethchlorvynol (Placidyl) intoxication. *Ann Intern Med* 1970;72:875–882.

Author: Lada Kokan

Reviewer: Richard C. Dart

Ethylene Glycol

Basics

DESCRIPTION

Ethylene glycol is a sweet, odorless, and colorless liquid used in a wide range of consumer and commercial products.

FORMS AND USES

- Ethylene glycol (1,2-ethanediol, 1,2-dihydroxyethane, monoethylene glycol, glycol alcohol, glycol) is a common component of antifreeze used in heating and cooling systems, brake fluid, inks, and soybean foam.
- It is used as an industrial solvent in paints and plastics and is used in the manufacturing of resins, plasticizers, and synthetic fibers and waxes.

TOXIC DOSE

One or two sips or gulps can produce potentially toxic ethylene glycol levels in children and adults.

PATHOPHYSIOLOGY

- Ethylene glycol is metabolized by alcohol dehydrogenase to toxic organic acids, which produce an increased anion gap metabolic acidosis.
- The metabolite oxalic acid combines with calcium to form calcium oxalate crystals, which can be deposited in the renal tubules and cause renal damage.

EPIDEMIOLOGY

- Poisoning is uncommon.
- Death occurs in patients who do not receive medical care.

CAUSES

- Poisoning most commonly occurs after the accidental ingestion of antifreeze or attempted suicide.
- The possibility of child abuse or neglect should be considered if the patient is less than 1 year of age; suicide attempt should be considered if the patient is more than 6 years of age.

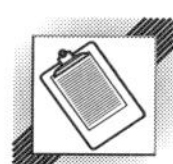

Diagnosis

DIFFERENTIAL DIAGNOSIS

- Toxic causes of an increased anion gap metabolic acidosis include methanol, salicylates, and alcoholic ketoacidosis, as well as lactic acidosis from any source.
- Nontoxic causes include diabetic ketoacidosis as well as lactic acidosis from any source.

SIGNS AND SYMPTOMS

- Inebriation may develop initially.
- Over several hours, an anion gap metabolic acidosis may develop, followed over 24 to 72 hours by progressively worsening renal injury.

Vital Signs

Tachypnea, tachycardia, and hypotension may occur in serious poisoning.

Cardiovascular

- Hypocalcemia with QT prolongation is possible in severe poisoning.
- Myocarditis occurs rarely.

Pulmonary

Pulmonary edema occurs rarely.

Gastrointestinal

- Nausea and vomiting are common.
- Pancreatitis and gastritis may occur.

Renal

Acute renal failure 24 to 72 hours after ingestion is common in patients without prompt treatment.

Fluids and Electrolytes

- Anion gap metabolic acidosis appears over several hours.
- Hypocalcemia can occur due to formation of calcium oxalate.

Musculoskeletal

Myalgia with elevated levels of creatine kinase may occur.

Neurologic

- CNS depression, ataxia, and slurred speech are common and resemble symptoms of ethanol toxicity.
- Seizures occur rarely.

PROCEDURES AND LABORATORY TESTS

Essential Tests

- Serum ethylene glycol level

—Levels should be obtained in all patients with a history of ingestion.
  —A level of over 20 mg/dl is an indication for fomepizole or ethanol infusion.
  —A level of over 50 mg/dl is an indication for hemodialysis.

- Serum electrolytes, BUN, creatinine

—As metabolism occurs, an increased anion gap metabolic acidosis will develop.
—The absence of a gap soon after ingestion does not exclude toxicity because the patient may not have metabolized enough to develop acidosis.
—Acidosis is an indication for fomepizole or ethanol infusion and hemodialysis.

- Urinalysis with microscopic examination

—The presence of calcium oxalate crystals with a history of ingestion or metabolic acidosis is strong evidence of poisoning.
—The absence of crystals does not exclude the diagnosis.
—Patients often have proteinuria and hematuria.

Recommended Tests

- Measured serum osmolality, using freezing point depression method

—Serum osmolality is not a substitute for an ethylene glycol level.
—If a delay is expected before an ethylene glycol level can be obtained, serum osmolality can be used as a screening test to rule in (but not to rule out) the possibility of ethylene glycol poisoning.
—An elevated osmolal gap suggests the presence of an unmeasured solute such as ethylene glycol.
—Osmolal gap is calculated as follows:

$$\text{Osmolal gap} = (\text{calculated serum osmolality}) - (\text{measured osmolality})$$

—The cause of a gap greater than 15 mEq/l must be determined.
—The patient should be treated with ethanol infusion until the cause is determined.
—The measured osmolality is determined by the laboratory.
—The calculated osmolality is determined as follows:

$$2 \times [\text{Na (mEq/L)}] + [\text{BUN (mg/dl)}/2.8] + [\text{glucose (mg/dl)}/18]$$

—Drugs and disorders that may alter these laboratory results include acetone, ethanol, isopropyl alcohol, mannitol, methanol, propylene glycol, renal failure, lactic acidosis, and alcoholic ketoacidosis.

- Arterial blood gases should be measured in patients with a low serum bicarbonate to assess acidosis.
- Serum ionized calcium should be followed closely after significant ingestion.
- ECG and cardiac monitoring should be performed to detect dysrhythmias and effects of hypocalcemia.
- Blood ethanol concentration

—Ethanol will delay the onset of symptoms and sequelae of ethylene glycol toxicity.
—Patients on ethanol infusions should have ethanol levels followed hourly until stable for 4 hours, then every 4 hours.

- Serum acetaminophen and aspirin levels are used in overdose setting to detect occult ingestion.

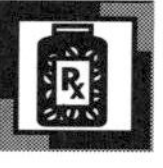

Treatment

- Focus treatment on supportive care, control of airway, and treatment with fomepizole or ethanol and hemodialysis as indicated.
- Dose and time of exposure should be determined for all substances involved.
- Consultation with a toxicologist and nephrologist should be considered early in symptomatic patients.

DIRECTING PATIENT COURSE

The health-care professional should call the poison control center when:

- Acidosis, renal failure, or other serious effects are present.
- Toxic effects are not consistent with ethylene glycol toxicity.
- Coingestant, drug interaction, or underlying disease presents an unusual problem.

The patient should be referred to a health-care facility when:

- Attempted suicide or homicide is possible.
- Patient or caregiver seems unreliable.
- Any signs of toxicity develop.
- Coingestant, drug interaction, or underlying disease presents an unusual problem.

Admission Considerations

Inpatient treatment is warranted when patient has altered mental status, acidosis, ethylene glycol levels over 20 mg/dl, or renal injury.

DECONTAMINATION

In Hospital

- Nasogastric aspiration using a nasogastric tube within the first 30 to 60 minutes following a large ingestion may be beneficial.
- If there is concern for a coingestant, then gastric lavage with a large-bore orogastric tube may be indicated.
- If the presence of a coingestant is suspected, then one dose of activated charcoal (1–2 g/kg) should be administered without a cathartic.

ANTIDOTES

Fomepizole

Fomepizole is the preferred agent for treatment.

- Indications

—History of possible ethylene glycol ingestion and evidence of toxicity (increased anion gap, metabolic acidosis, hematuria, proteinuria) or increased osmolal gap
—Serum ethylene glycol level above 20 mg/dl

- Contraindications

—History of documented allergic response to fomepizole

- Method of administration

—Loading dose for adult or pediatric patient is 15 mg/kg intravenously.
—Maintenance dose for all age groups is 10 mg/kg every 12 hours for four doses and then 15 mg/kg every 12 hours until ethylene glycol level is less than 20 mg/dl.
—Each dose is diluted in 100 ml normal saline or D5W and infused over 30 minutes.
—For further details (e.g., use during hemodialysis), see SECTION III, Fomepizole chapter.

Ethanol

10% solution in D5W.

- Indications

—Ethanol treatment is recommended if fomepizole is not available.
—Ethylene glycol level more than 20 mg/dl
—If levels are not immediately available, therapy should be instituted if there is:
  —A reliable history of significant ingestion
  —Unexplained anion gap acidosis
  —Unexplained osmolar gap

- Contraindications. Preexisting ethanol level more than 100 mg/dl obviates need for the ethanol loading dose.
- Method of administration.

—Consult SECTION III, Ethanol chapter, for details of administration.
  —Loading dose is 10 cc/kg of a 10% ethanol solution infused intravenously over 1 hour.
  —Maintenance dose is 1.0 to 2.0 ml/kg/hr of 10% ethanol solution.

ADJUNCTIVE TREATMENT

Pyridoxine and thiamine have been proposed to hasten elimination of toxic ethylene glycol metabolites. Because the safety margin is large, they may be administered at the discretion of the treating physician. Indications for use have not been established.

- Pyridoxine

—Adult dose is 50 to 100 mg administered intravenously every 6 hours until ethylene glycol level is undetectable.
—Pediatric dose is 1 to 2 mg/kg administered intravenously every 6 hours until ethylene glycol level is undetectable.

- Thiamine

—Adult dose is 100 mg administered intravenously over 5 minutes every 6 hours until ethylene glycol level is undetectable.
—Pediatric dose is 50 mg administered intravenously over 5 minutes every 6 hours until ethylene glycol level is undetectable.

- Sodium bicarbonate should not be routinely administered, but may be used as a temporizing measure for life-threatening acidosis and acidemia prior to hemodialysis.
- Hemodialysis is recommended for a serum ethylene glycol level of more than 50 mg/dl (and should be considered for levels in the 25 to 50 mg/dl range) or if signs of end-organ injury are apparent (increased anion gap acidosis, renal failure, or mental status changes).

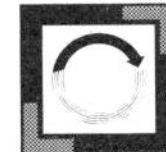

Follow-Up

PATIENT MONITORING

- Serum electrolytes and arterial blood gases should be monitored every 2 to 4 hours until acidosis begins to resolve.
- Serum ethylene glycol concentrations should be monitored until they are below 10 mg/dl.
- If hemodialysis is performed, fomepizole or ethanol administration should be continued until a postdialysis ethylene glycol concentration is known to be less than 20 mg/dl.
- When ethanol is administered, blood ethanol concentrations should be monitored every hour and the infusion rate should be adjusted to maintain a concentration of 100 to 130 mg/dl.
- Serum glucose concentrations should also be monitored every 1 to 2 hours, especially in children (ethanol may cause hypoglycemia).

EXPECTED COURSE AND PROGNOSIS

- Toxicity may take several hours to develop.
- Peak toxicity usually occurs within 24 hours.
- Patients with renal injury may suffer residual renal dysfunction.

DISCHARGE CRITERIA AND INSTRUCTIONS

- From the emergency department. Asymptomatic patients with undetectable serum ethylene glycol levels and no anion gap metabolic acidosis may be discharged after psychiatric evaluation, if needed.
- From the hospital. Patient may be discharged with serum ethylene glycol level less than 20 mg/dl, normal anion gap, and stable renal function, following psychiatric clearance, if needed.

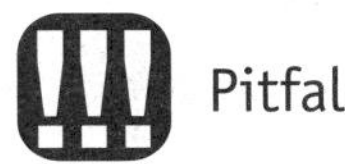

Pitfalls

DIAGNOSIS

- Ethylene glycol toxicity **cannot** be ruled out by a normal osmolal gap or absence of an anion gap metabolic acidosis.
- Patients with potentially toxic ethylene glycol levels may be asymptomatic initially.
- Serum ethylene glycol levels must be measured in all patients with a history of ingestion.

TREATMENT

- If an endotracheal intubation is performed, the increased minute ventilation (compensation for acidosis) that was present before intubation should be maintained.
- Blood ethanol levels should be monitored closely and maintained at 100 to 130 mg/dl.

ICD-9-CM 980

Toxic effect of alcohol.

See also: SECTION II, Osmolar Gap; SECTION III, Ethanol, Fomepizole (Antizol), Pyridoxine, and Thiamine chapters.

RECOMMENDED READING

Baud FJ, Galliot M, Astier A, et al. Treatment of ethylene glycol poisoning with intravenous 4-methylpyrazole. *N Engl J Med* 1988;319:97–100.

Author: Edwin K. Kuffner

Reviewer: Luke Yip

Ethylene Oxide

Basics

DESCRIPTION

Ethylene oxide is a colorless, flammable, and explosive gas with an ether-like odor.

FORMS AND USES

• It is used most commonly in cold gas sterilization of medical equipment and the manufacture of ethylene glycol, detergents, nonionic surfactants, and polyester fiber and film.
• It is also used as a fungicide for the treatment of soil and plants and a fumigant for food, drugs, paper, textiles, and furs.

TOXIC DOSE

• The acute toxic dose has not been established.
• Exposure to 800 ppm is considered immediately dangerous.

PATHOPHYSIOLOGY

• Ethylene oxide is an alkylating agent that reacts with nearly all organic molecules.
• Most common route of exposure is inhalation, although dermal absorption may occur.
• Brief exposure to concentrated vapor often causes systemic symptoms.

EPIDEMIOLOGY

Poisoning is uncommon.

CAUSES

• Ethylene toxicity usually results from an occupational exposure.
• Child neglect or abuse should be considered if the patient is less than 1 year of age, suicide attempt if the patient is over 6 years of age.

DRUG AND DISEASE INTERACTIONS

Ethylene oxide exposure would be expected to exacerbate reactive airway disorder.

PREGNANCY AND LACTATION

• Ethylene oxide is considered a human teratogen.
• In animals, exposure leads to stillbirths.

WORKPLACE STANDARDS

• OSHA. Not listed.
• ACGIH. TLV is 1 ppm, no short-term exposure limit.
• NIOSH. IDLH is 800 ppm.

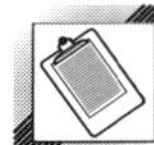

Diagnosis

DIFFERENTIAL DIAGNOSIS

Other toxicologic causes of acute respiratory complaints include chlorine or other halides, phosgene, oxides of nitrogen, or other pulmonary irritants.

SIGNS AND SYMPTOMS

Vital Signs

• Tachycardia, tachypnea, and hypoxemia are common following inhalation.
• Fever may accompany chemical pneumonitis and pulmonary edema.

HEENT

• Mucous membrane irritation (conjunctivitis, rhinorrhea, blepharospasm, drooling) is common even at low-level inhalation exposure.
• Ethylene oxide is implicated in cataract formation following chronic exposure.

Dermatologic

• Burns have been reported following acute dermal exposure.
• Frostbite injury can occur from exposure to liquid form.

Pulmonary

• Cough, chest pain, dyspnea, and bronchospasm are common following inhalation.
• Noncardiogenic pulmonary edema has been reported following inhalation exposure at high concentrations.

Gastrointestinal

• Nausea and vomiting are common following either inhalation or ingestion.
• Caustic gastrointestinal injury may follow ingestion.

Neurologic

• Headache, disorientation, lethargy, and coma have been reported following acute exposure.
• Peripheral neuropathy (axonopathy) may occur with chronic exposure.
• Cognitive deficits, including memory impairment, irritability, clumsiness, and ataxia, have been reported.

PROCEDURES AND LABORATORY TESTS

Essential Tests

Arterial blood gases or pulse oximetry are used to assess pulmonary injury due to acute exposure.

Recommended Tests

• Serum electrolytes, BUN, creatinine and other tests should be ordered as clinically indicated in symptomatic patients.
• Pulmonary function testing following symptomatic inhalation may be used.
• Chest radiograph may be helpful in acutely symptomatic patients to evaluate pulmonary effects; delayed pulmonary injury also has been reported.

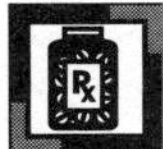

Treatment

- Treatment should focus on aggressive respiratory support.
- The dose and time of exposure should be determined for all substances involved.

DIRECTING PATIENT COURSE

The health-care professional should call the poison control center when:

- Severe or persistent effects develop.
- Coingestant, drug interaction, or underlying disease presents an unusual problem.

The patient should be referred to a health-care facility when:

- Attempted suicide or homicide is possible.
- Patient or caregiver seems unreliable.
- Toxic effects develop.
- Coingestant, drug interaction, or underlying disease presents an unusual problem.

Admission Considerations

Inpatient management is warranted for patients with respiratory distress, evidence of upper airway edema, second- or third-degree burns, pulmonary edema, hypoxia, or caustic gastrointestinal injury.

DECONTAMINATION

Out of Hospital

- Patients should be removed from source of exposure to fresh air and administered 100% oxygen.
- Exposed areas should be decontaminated by copiously irrigating with water.

In Hospital

- Gastric lavage should not be performed. However, simple aspiration with a small-bore nasogastric tube may be useful.
- One dose of activated charcoal (1–2 g/kg) should be administered without a cathartic if a substantial ingestion has occurred within the previous few hours.

ANTIDOTE

There is no specific antidote for ethylene oxide poisoning.

ADJUNCTIVE TREATMENT

- Following ingestion, the patient should be managed like a caustic ingestion. (See SECTION IV, Caustics–Basic chapter.)
- Case reports suggest that corticosteroids may be beneficial in preventing pulmonary edema, but their efficacy has not been tested in clinical trials.
- Bronchospasm should be treated with inhaled β_2-agonists such as albuterol.

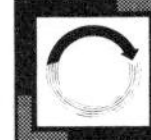

Follow-Up

PATIENT MONITORING

Respiratory and neurologic function should be monitored continuously.

EXPECTED COURSE AND PROGNOSIS

- Toxic effects occur soon after exposure and resolve over hours to days or weeks, depending on severity (e.g., a severe burn will require time to heal).
- Pulmonary edema may not appear for 24 to 72 hours.

DISCHARGE CRITERIA AND INSTRUCTIONS

- From the emergency department. Asymptomatic patients with brief exposure may be discharged after a 4- to 6-hour observation period.
- From the hospital. Patient may be discharged when toxic effects resolve or at 72 hours if observation reveals no injury.

PATIENT EDUCATION

Patients should be instructed to return if they develop persistent cough, difficulty in breathing, or chest pain.

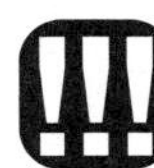

Pitfalls

DIAGNOSIS

- It may be necessary to observe patients for delayed-onset pulmonary edema.
- A normal chest radiograph shortly after exposure does not preclude the development of delayed pulmonary edema.

See also: SECTION IV, Caustics–Basic chapter.

ICD-9-CM 987.9

Toxic effect of other gases, fumes, or vapors: unspecified gas, fume, or vapor.

RECOMMENDED READING

Ellenhorn MJ. *Medical toxicology,* 2nd ed. Baltimore: Williams & Wilkins, 1997:1211–1214.

Author: Edwin K. Kuffner

Reviewer: Richard C. Dart

Felbamate

Basics

DESCRIPTION

Felbamate is an oral anticonvulsant.

FORMS AND USES

- Felbamate (Felbatol) is available as 400- and 600-mg tablets or 600 mg/5 ml suspension.
- Typical dosages are 15 to 45 mg/kg/day in divided doses two to four times/day for children, 1,200 to 3,600 mg orally in divided doses two to four times/day for adults.
- Therapeutic uses include monotherapy for partial seizures with and without secondary generalization, adjunctive therapy for seizures poorly controlled with other antiepileptic medications, and pediatric seizures associated with the Lennox-Gastaut syndrome.

TOXIC DOSE

Insufficient information is available to establish a toxic dose.

PATHOPHYSIOLOGY

- Therapeutic mechanism is unknown. Does not interact with the benzodiazepine or GABA receptor complex.
- Metabolism of felbamate will induce the cytochrome P450 system.

DRUG AND DISEASE INTERACTIONS

- Increases phenytoin, phenobarbital, and valproic acid levels.
- Decreases carbamazepine level, but increases the concentration of the active form of carbamazepine, carbamazepine epoxide.
- May increase the effects of warfarin.

PREGNANCY AND LACTATION

- US FDA Pregnancy Category C. The drug exerts animal teratogenic or embryocidal effects, but there are no controlled studies in women, or no studies are available in either animals or women.

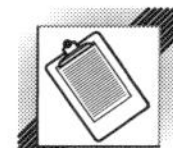

Diagnosis

DIFFERENTIAL DIAGNOSIS

Toxic causes of CNS depression include narcotics, benzodiazepines, anticonvulsants, and many others.

SIGNS AND SYMPTOMS

Central nervous system effects predominate following acute overdose or toxic accumulation during chronic therapy.

Cardiovascular

Palpitations have been reported during chronic therapy, but life-threatening dysrhythmia has not been described.

Gastrointestinal

- Nausea and vomiting are common.
- Increased hepatic transaminases have developed during chronic therapy.
- Acute liver failure has been reported but is rare.

Hematologic

- Isolated leukopenia, anemia, and thrombocytopenia have been reported.
- Aplastic anemia occurs rarely during chronic therapy.

Neurologic

- Mild CNS depression, ataxia, and nystagmus are the most common effects following acute overdose.
- Headache, agitation, blurred vision, diplopia, drowsiness, sleep disturbances, and subtle memory impairment are common during chronic therapy.
- Movement disorders including dystonia and choreoathetosis have been reported during chronic therapy.

Psychiatric

Hallucinations have been reported with chronic therapy.

PROCEDURES AND LABORATORY TESTS

Essential Tests

No tests may be needed for asymptomatic patients.

Recommended Tests

- A complete blood count and liver function tests should be checked routinely on all patients receiving chronic felbamate therapy.
- Felbamate levels are not commonly available nor are they useful for management of acute overdose. Therapeutic levels are not well established but have been reported in the range of 20 to 50 μg/ml.
- ECG, acetaminophen, and aspirin levels are used to detect occult ingestion.
- Head CT, lumbar puncture, and cultures should be performed as needed to evaluate altered mental status.

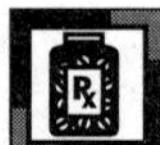

Treatment

Treatment should focus on airway control and general supportive care.

DECONTAMINATION

- Induction of emesis with ipecac or gastric lavage are rarely indicated for isolated felbamate ingestion because the effects following acute overdose are usually mild.
- Administer one dose of activated charcoal (1–2 g/kg) without a cathartic if a substantial ingestion has occurred within the previous few hours.

ANTIDOTE

There is no specific antidote for felbamate poisoning.

ADJUNCTIVE TREATMENT

- Oxygen should be administered to patients with CNS depression.
- Nausea and vomiting may be treated with typical antiemetic agents.

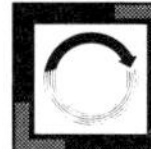

Follow-Up

EXPECTED COURSE AND PROGNOSIS

- Toxic effects following acute overdose are typically mild and peak within the first few hours.
- Complete recovery is expected unless concomitant ingestion is present.

DISCHARGE CRITERIA/INSTRUCTIONS

Patients may be discharged from the emergency department or hospital if CNS abnormalities do not develop within 4–6 hours of acute ingestion.

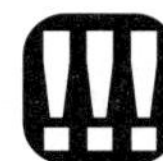

Pitfalls

DIAGNOSIS

If major toxic manifestations develop, it is likely a coingestant is present.

ICD-9-CM 966

Poisoning by anticonvulsants and antiparkinsonism drugs.

RECOMMENDED READING

Nagel TR, Schunk JE. Felbamate overdose: A case report and discussion of a new antiepileptic drug. *Pediatr Emerg Care* 1995;11:369–371.

Author: Edwin K. Kuffner

Reviewer: Richard C. Dart

Fenfluramine and Dexfenfluramine

Basics

DESCRIPTION

Fenfluramine and dexfenfluramine are oral diet agents.

FORMS AND USES

- Substances include fenfluramine (Pondimin), dexfenfluramine (Redux), and fen-phen (fenfluramine and phentermine used in combination).
- Fenfluramine and dexfenfluramine have been withdrawn from the market by the U.S. FDA.
- Phentermine remains available.
- Fenfluramine dose is 20 to 40 mg three times daily orally.
- Dexfenfluramine dose is 15 mg twice a day orally.
- Phentermine dose is 30 mg/day orally.

TOXIC DOSE

Following acute ingestion, 3 mg/kg of fenfluramine has been associated with minimal toxic effects. Death has been reported following ingestion of more than 20 mg/kg.

PATHOPHYSIOLOGY

- Fenfluramine is an amphetamine congener.
- Dexfenfluramine is the dextro isomer of fenfluramine.
- Both drugs produce less CNS excitation than do amphetamines and may cause mild CNS depression at therapeutic doses.

EPIDEMIOLOGY

- Poisoning is uncommon.
- Toxic effects following exposure are typically mild.
- Death occurs after large overdoses.

CAUSES

- The cause is usually suicidal ingestion.
- The possibility of child neglect should be considered if the patient is less than 1 year of age; suicide attempt should be considered in patients over 6 years of age.

DRUG AND DISEASE INTERACTIONS

- Serotonin syndrome may develop following use of fenfluramine with another serotonin agonist or within 2 weeks of therapy with a monoamine oxidase (MAO) inhibitor.
- Fenfluramine and dexfenfluramine may cause urine toxicology screens to be positive for amphetamines.

PREGNANCY AND LACTATION

Dexfenfluramine, fenfluramine, and phentermine. US FDA Pregnancy Category C. The drug exerts animal teratogenic or embryocidal effects, but there are no controlled studies in women, or no studies are available in either animals or women.

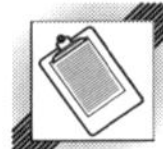

Diagnosis

DIFFERENTIAL DIAGNOSIS

- Toxic causes of agitation and seizure include amphetamine, methamphetamine, theophylline, cocaine, isoniazid, tricyclic antidepressants, and MAO inhibitors.
- Nontoxic causes include alcohol withdrawal, meningitis, intracranial hemorrhage, hyperthyroidism, and manic disorder.

SIGNS AND SYMPTOMS

- Primary toxicity is neurologic, with initial sedation followed by excitation and seizures.
- Most patients develop symptoms within 4 hours.
- Serotonin syndrome may occur rarely.

Vital Signs

Tachycardia, hypertension, and hyperthermia occur commonly.

HEENT

Mydriasis is common.

Dermatologic

Diaphoresis and facial flushing occur commonly.

Cardiovascular

- Tachycardia is common soon after ingestion.
- Ventricular ectopy and, in severe cases, cardiac arrest may occur.
- Valvular heart disease, occasionally necessitating surgical repair, has been reported in patients on dexfenfluramine.

Pulmonary

- Tachypnea can occur.
- Respiratory depression occurs as overdose amount increases.
- Pulmonary hypertension has been reported during therapeutic use.

Gastrointestinal

Nausea, vomiting, and diarrhea occur in overdose.

Musculoskeletal

- Muscle twitching often precedes other toxic effects.
- This may be followed by stiffness or opisthotonos.

Neurologic

Drowsiness followed by coma and seizures usually occurs within 4 hours of serious ingestion.

PROCEDURES AND LABORATORY TESTS

Essential Tests

No tests may be needed in asymptomatic patients.

Recommended Tests

- Serum electrolytes, BUN, creatinine, and glucose should be determined to evaluate other causes of seizures or altered mental status.
- Liver function, coagulation studies, and serum creatine kinase may be elevated in patients with hyperthermia or agitation.
- ECG, serum acetaminophen, and aspirin levels should be ordered in an overdose setting to detect occult ingestion.
- Head CT, lumbar puncture, and cultures, should be performed as needed to evaluate other causes of seizure and altered mental status.

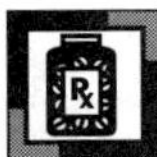

Treatment

• Treatment should focus on airway control and treatment of seizures and dysrhythmias.
• Dose and time of exposure should be determined for all substances involved.

DIRECTING PATIENT COURSE

The health-care provider should call the poison control center when:

• Seizures or other severe effects are present.
• Toxic effects are not consistent with fenfluramine poisoning.
• Coingestant, drug interaction, or underlying disease presents an unusual problem.

The patient should be referred to a health-care facility when:

• Attempted suicide or homicide is possible.
• Patient or caregiver seems unreliable.
• Any toxic effects are present.
• Coingestant, drug interaction, or underlying disease presents an unusual problem.

Admission Considerations

Inpatient treatment is warranted when patient has refractory agitation, seizure, hyperthermia, persistent tachycardia, or other end-organ injury.

DECONTAMINATION

Out of Hospital

Emesis with ipecac should not be induced because of the potential for seizures.

In Hospital

• Gastric lavage should be performed in pediatric (tube size 24–32 French) or adult (tube size 36–42 French) patients presenting within 1 hour of a large ingestion or if serious effects are present.
• One dose of activated charcoal (1–2 g/kg) should be administered without a cathartic if a substantial ingestion has occurred within the previous few hours.
• Whole-bowel irrigation with polyethylene glycol solution has been recommended in patients who have ingested sustained-release preparations; the usual dose is 1 to 2 L/h in adults until rectal effluent is clear.

ANTIDOTES

There is no specific antidote for fenfluramine or dexfenfluramine poisoning.

ADJUNCTIVE TREATMENT

Control of Agitation

• A benzodiazepine familiar to the provider should be administered.

—Diazepam
  —Adult dose is 5 to 10 mg intravenously.
  —Pediatric dose is 0.2 to 0.5 mg/kg intravenously.
  —Dose can be repeated at 10-minute intervals, titrating to effect.
—Lorazepam
  —Adult dose is 1 to 2 mg intravenously.
  —Pediatric dose is 0.05 to 0.1 mg/kg.
  —Dose can be repeated at 10-minute intervals, titrating to effect.

• The airway should be monitored closely.

Seizures

• Patent airway should be ensured.
• A benzodiazepine should be administered for initial control as for control of agitation.
• If seizures persist or recur, another anticonvulsant such as phenobarbital should be added.

Hypotension

• Hypotension should be treated with isotonic fluid infusion (10–20 ml/kg) and the Trendelenburg position.
• If needed, a vasopressor is used.

—Dopamine infusion is started at 5 μg/kg/min and titrated to desired effect. Dosages above 20 μg/kg/min are not recommended.
—If blood pressure does not respond, norepinephrine may be added.

NOT RECOMMENDED THERAPIES

Serum levels are not clinically useful.

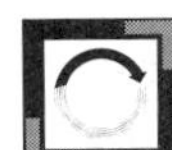

Follow-Up

PATIENT MONITORING

Continuous respiratory and hemodynamic monitoring should be provided.

EXPECTED COURSE AND PROGNOSIS

• Patients generally recover within hours of acute overdose.
• Complications are more common in patients with chronic use.
• End-organ injury from hypertension or seizures may occur.

DISCHARGE CRITERIA/INSTRUCTIONS

• From the emergency department. Asymptomatic patients who have ingested nonsustained-release formulations may be discharged after 6 hours of observation following gastrointestinal decontamination and psychiatric evaluation, if needed.
• From the hospital

—Patients may be discharged following gastrointestinal decontamination, resolution of toxicity, and psychiatric evaluation, if needed.
—Patients who have ingested a potentially toxic amount of sustained-release product should be observed for 12 to 24 hours.

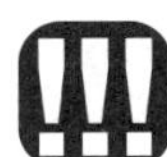

Pitfalls

TREATMENT

• Anticipatory airway management is required in patients with altered mental status.
• Seizures should be treated aggressively.

FOLLOW-UP

• Patients should be closely monitored because precipitous decompensation has been reported.
• Patients on chronic therapy should be followed for symptoms of pulmonary hypertension and valvular heart disease.

ICD-9-CM 977.0

Poisoning by other and nonspecific drugs and medicinal substances: dietetics.

See also: SECTION II, Hypotension, Neuroleptic Malignant Syndrome and Serotonin Syndrome, and Seizure (Unexplained) chapters; SECTION III, Whole-Bowel Irrigation chapter; and SECTION IV, Amphetamines chapter.

RECOMMENDED READING

Brenot F, Herve P, Petrpretz P, et al. Primary pulmonary hypertension and fenfluramine use. *Br Heart J* 1993;70:537–541.

Connolly HM, Crary JL, McGoon MD, et al. Valvular heart disease associated with fenfluramine-phentermine. *N Engl J Med* 1997;337:581–588.

Author: Kennon Heard

Reviewer: Richard C. Dart

Fire Ant

Basics

DESCRIPTION

Fire ants constitute the genus *Solenopsis*.

- Imported fire ants (*Solenopsis invicta*) are more aggressive than native fire ants, and their stings cause more serious toxic reactions.
- *S. invicta* is responsible for most envenomations of humans in the United States.

TOXIC DOSE

- One sting produces symptoms.
- Large numbers of stings may prove lethal to small children or elderly patients.

PATHOPHYSIOLOGY

Fire ants attach to the skin by biting and inject venom by inserting the stingers into the skin for 20 to 30 seconds; the ants then pivot around their heads and reinsert the stingers repeatedly, producing the characteristic circular clustering of stings.

EPIDEMIOLOGY

- Fire ants are distributed throughout the southeastern and south central United States, and stings are common in these areas.
- Fire ant nests are found in the ground or soil under mounds that vary in size according to the size of the colony and the consistency of the soil.

CAUSES

Most stings follow accidental disturbance of a fire ant nest.

RISK FACTORS

Conditions that interfere with the patient's ability to recognize an environmental danger or to remove themselves from the vicinity (age, intoxication).

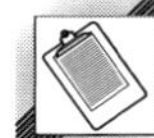

Diagnosis

DIFFERENTIAL DIAGNOSIS

The clusters of vesicles and severe pain of fire ant stings are usually diagnostic.

SIGNS AND SYMPTOMS

Envenomation causes immediate burning pain and rapid local vesicle formation; anaphylactic reactions may occur in hypersensitive patients, although rarely are these reactions fatal.

Vital Signs

- Low-grade fever may occur during the first day or two following envenomation.
- Allergic reactions can produce tachycardia, hypotension, or tachypnea.

HEENT

Angioedema is a common finding in hypersensitivity reactions.

Dermatologic

- An erythematous flare develops immediately after the sting, followed by an edematous wheal 2 to 10 mm in diameter.
- Papules appear at the site within a few hours and develop into vesicles containing clear fluid.
- The vesicles develop into umbilicated, painful, and sterile pruritic pustules surrounded by erythematous halos.
- Painful, small, red, hemorrhagic puncta may occasionally be identified at the site of attachment of the fire ant mandible.
- Bacterial superinfection is common, especially secondary to pruritus and excoriation.

Pulmonary

Allergic reactions can produce chest pain, dyspnea, and bronchospasm.

Gastrointestinal

Nausea, vomiting, and abdominal pain occur occasionally.

Hematologic

Hemolysis and coagulopathy have been reported in one neonate.

Neurologic

- Allergic reactions may produce anxiety and lightheadedness.
- Altered mental status and neuropathies are rare, but have been reported.

Immunologic

Anaphylactoid and anaphylactic reactions have been reported.

PROCEDURES AND LABORATORY TESTS

Essential Tests

No tests may be needed in mild cases.

Recommended Tests

- Complete blood count, serum electrolytes, BUN, creatinine, and other tests as clinically indicated should be performed in the rare patient with systemic manifestations.
- Wound cultures may be needed if serious bacterial superinfection develops.

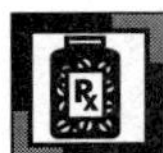

Treatment

Treatment should focus on local wound care and monitoring for rare systemic effects; supportive care with appropriate airway management is vital if angioedema develops.

DIRECTING PATIENT COURSE

The health-care professional should call the poison control center when:

- Signs and symptoms are inconsistent with fire ant envenomation.
- Coingestant, drug interaction, or underlying disease presents an unusual problem.

The patient should be referred to a health-care facility when:

- The patient or caregiver seems unreliable.
- Difficulty breathing, severe pain, or other symptoms develop.
- Coingestant, drug interaction, or underlying disease presents an unusual problem.

Admission Considerations

Inpatient management is warranted when the patient requires parenteral pain medication or treatment for anaphylaxis, infection spreading to other body areas, or other systemic effects of the sting.

DECONTAMINATION

Out of Hospital

- The patient is removed from the source of exposure and the ants are brushed off or washed off with water.
- Clothing is removed because trapped ants may continue to sting.
- Stings are washed with soap and water.

In Hospital

Any ants that were initially overlooked are removed.

ANTIDOTES

No specific antidote exists for fire ant envenomation.

ADJUNCTIVE TREATMENT

Local Vesicle

- The vesicle is treated as a local wound by washing with soap and water and covering with a bandage.
- Topical anesthetics (e.g., lidocaine 2% gel) or antihistamine (diphenhydramine; see below for allergic reaction) may be administered for pruritus and oral analgesics for pain.
- Administration of antibiotics is not recommended unless overt signs of infection appear.
- Corticosteroids provide no benefit to patients with fire ant stings.

Large Local Reactions (Coalescent Erythema and Edema Involving Much of an Extremity or More)

- Treatment is similar to that for local vesicles; oral corticosteroids (e.g., prednisone, 1.0 mg/kg for several days) and H_1-blockers (diphenhydramine, 50 mg orally, then 25–50 mg orally every 6 hours for 2–3 days) are recommended, however, and parenteral pain medication (meperidine) may be necessary.
- No credible evidence supports the use of epinephrine (except in cases of allergic reaction) or meat tenderizer to treat fire ant stings.

Allergic Reactions

- Hypersensitivity reactions are treated with diphenhydramine, steroids, and epinephrine; the combination and dose depends on the severity of reaction. Dose may be administered intravenously for the rare anaphylactic reaction.

—Diphenhydramine. Pediatric dosage 5 mg/kg/day orally divided every 4 to 6 hours; adult dosage 25 to 50 mg orally every 4 to 6 hours.
—Cimetidine. Pediatric dosage 20 to 40 mg/kg/day orally divided every 6 to 8 hours; adult dosage 300 mg orally three to four times a day.
—Methylprednisolone. Pediatric dose 1 to 2 mg/kg intravenously; adult dose 125 mg intravenously.
—Epinephrine. 0.01 ml/kg up to 0.3 to 0.5 ml of a 1:1,000 solution subcutaneously.

- Bronchospasm is treated with albuterol 0.15 mg/kg (maximum of 10 mg) in saline with humidified oxygen via nebulizer every 20 to 30 minutes.

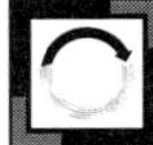

Follow-Up

PATIENT MONITORING

- Respiratory status should be monitored for deterioration.
- Secondary infection may develop.

EXPECTED COURSE AND PROGNOSIS

- Sterile pustules develop within 24 hours.
- Local reactions may continue to spread for 24 to 48 hours.
- Pustules heal within 3 to 8 days, although overlying skin sloughs from pigmented macules and fibrotic nodules may persist for weeks.
- Secondarily infected pustules can lead to cellulitis, abscess formation, and bacteremia.
- Rarely, local necrosis occurs, particularly in patients with impaired healing or circulation.

DISCHARGE CRITERIA/INSTRUCTIONS

- From the emergency department. Patients whose pain can be controlled with oral medication may be discharged after 2 to 4 hours.
- From the hospital

—Patients may be discharged when signs of infection or systemic effects have resolved.
—Patients with fire ant allergy who live in endemic areas should have injectable epinephrine available and may benefit from desensitization therapy; skin testing procedures that can help identify fire ant–sensitive individuals are available.

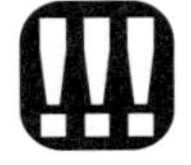

Pitfalls

DIAGNOSIS

The absence of a pustule does not rule out a fire ant sting.

ICD-9-CM 989

Toxic effect of other substances, chiefly nonmedicinal as to source.

RECOMMENDED READING

Bryson PD. Ants. In: *Comprehensive review in toxicology for emergency clinicians.* Washington, DC: Taylor & Francis, 1996:743–746.

Author: Edwin K. Kuffner

Reviewer: Richard C. Dart

Fish Stings

Basics

DESCRIPTION

• Scorpionfish (family Scorpaenidae) includes the following types:

—*Synanceja* species (stonefish) produce the most dangerous stings and are bottom dwellers of tidal pools and coral reefs in the Indian and Pacific Oceans and the Red Sea.
—*Scorpaena* species (scorpionfish, bullrout, sculpin) are bottom dwellers in shallow waters, bays, and coral reefs and along rocky coasts of tropical oceans worldwide.
—*Pterois* species (lionfish, zebrafish, butterfly cod) are free swimmers in shallow tropical oceans worldwide as well as popular specimens in home aquariums.

• Catfish species include Oriental catfish (*Plotosus lineatus*), sea catfish, coral catfish, and the freshwater catfishes of North America: brown bullhead, Carolina madtom, channel catfish, clue catfish, and white catfish.
• Weeverfish (family Trachinidae) are found partially buried in sandy or muddy bottoms in the Mediterranean basin and the eastern Atlantic Ocean.
• Spiny dogfish (*Squalus acanthias*) and surgeonfish (family Acanthuridae) also sting.
• See also SECTION IV, Stingrays chapter.

TOXIC DOSE

• One sting can cause symptoms.
• Stings of several stonefish spines can cause death, especially if medical care is unavailable.

PATHOPHYSIOLOGY

• Fish spines have surrounding integumentary sheaths.
• Each species has different spine sizes and location of venom glands.
• When the spine is forced through the skin (typically by stepping on the fish), the sheath crumples and squeezes venom into the wound along the exposed spine.
• Scorpionfish venoms are high-molecular-weight compounds that have a heat-labile component and principally affect cardiac, skeletal, and involuntary muscles.

EPIDEMIOLOGY

• The most severe and potentially life-threatening envenomation is caused by the stonefish, with the scorpionfish having moderate to severe effects and lionfish being more moderate.
• Lionfish stings are the most common due to their popularity in home aquariums.
• Death is extremely rare in humans.

CAUSES

Most cases occur during intentional handling or by accidentally stepping on the fish during swimming.

RISK FACTORS

Patients at the extremes of age may be more vulnerable to venom effects.

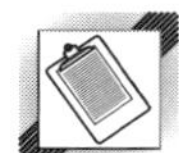

Diagnosis

DIFFERENTIAL DIAGNOSIS

• Toxic causes include painful bites or stings from sea creatures, including stingray, sea urchins, crown-of-thorns starfish, jellyfish, and sea snake or eel, as well as fire coral abrasion.
• Nontoxic causes include puncture wounds from inanimate objects.

SIGNS AND SYMPTOMS

• The severity of the envenomation depends on the species, number of stings, and amount of venom released.
• Severe pain, both local and centrally radiating, is the predominant complaint.

Vital Signs

• Hypertension and tachycardia may occur soon after the sting due to pain and agitation.
• Hypotension and dysrhythmia may soon develop, especially with stonefish.

Dermatologic

• Typically, puncture wounds or skin tears are surrounded by erythema, edema, warmth, and cyanosis.
• Vesicles may appear.
• Local necrosis and ulceration can occur.

Cardiovascular

Dysrhythmias are primarily associated with stonefish stings; bradycardia, tachycardia, and ventricular fibrillation may occur.

Pulmonary

Noncardiogenic or cardiogenic pulmonary edema may develop after a stonefish sting.

Gastrointestinal

Nausea, vomiting, and abdominal pain may occur.

Musculoskeletal

Fasciculation, spasms, and paralysis may occur with stonefish envenomation.

Neurologic

• Severe pain from stonefish stings radiating from the wound site can be so severe as to cause delirium, unconsciousness, and drowning.
• Milder pain may last several days.
• Respiratory paralysis may occur following stonefish envenomation.

PROCEDURES AND LABORATORY TESTS

Essential Tests

No tests may be needed in asymptomatic or minimally symptomatic patients, especially if the sting was not from stonefish or scorpionfish.

Recommended Tests

• ECG and cardiac monitoring is used after a stonefish sting because bradycardia, tachycardia, and ventricular fibrillation may develop.
• Complete blood count and cultures of wound and blood are ordered as clinically indicated to evaluate infection.
• Serum creatine kinase may be elevated if muscle fasciculation, spasm, or paralysis occurs.
• Soft-tissue radiographs of sting site may be useful to locate a foreign body.

Not Recommended Tests

Venom levels are not available.

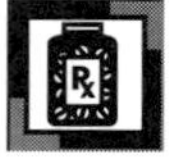

Treatment

• Treatment focuses on immersion into hot water, pain control, exploration of the wound for foreign bodies, and evaluating the need for antivenom.
• An antivenom is available for stonefish sting, but not for other fish stings.
• The time of the sting and the type of first aid measures performed should be determined.

DIRECTING PATIENT COURSE

The health-care provider should call the poison control center when:

• Shock or other severe effects are present.
• Toxic effects are not consistent with a fish sting.
• Underlying disease presents an unusual problem.

The patient should be referred to a health-care facility when:

• Severe pain or any systemic effects develop.
• Toxic effects are not consistent with a fish sting.
• Underlying disease presents an unusual problem.

Admission Considerations

Inpatient management is warranted for patients with systemic effects or pain requiring parenteral opioid therapy.

DECONTAMINATION

Out of Hospital

• The affected limb is kept lower than the heart.
• The limb is immersed in nonscalding hot water (upper limit 45°C or 113°F).

• Warm compresses are used if the wound is on the torso or face.
• Pain relief is usually prompt.
• If pain recurs after removal from water, reimmersion can offer significant relief.
• The number of punctures should be recorded and any apparent foreign bodies removed.

In Hospital

Soaking in nonscalding hot water continues for 30 to 90 minutes, with attention given to keeping the water hot, but below 45°C or 113°F.

ANTIDOTES

Stonefish antivenom (hyperimmune Fab_2 horse serum)

Indications

Any individual with symptomatic stonefish stings should receive antivenom.

Contraindications

History of allergy to this product or other horse serum products is a relative contraindication.

Method of Administration

• The antivenom is administered in an intensive care setting.
• One unit of stonefish antivenom neutralizes 0.01 mg of venom (1,000 units neutralizes 10 mg of venom).
• The dose of antivenom is based on the number of stings (5–10 mg of venom is contained in each dorsal spine of the stonefish):

—One to two punctures should be treated with 2,000 units (one ampule).
—Three to four punctures should be treated with 4,000 units (two ampules).
—Five to six punctures should be treated with 6,000 units (three ampules).

• Skin testing should be performed before antivenom infusion.
• One ampule of antivenom is diluted in 100 cc of 0.9% saline and infused intravenously over 15 to 30 minutes.
• If intravenous access is not available, undiluted antivenom is administered intramuscularly.
• If symptoms develop or persist and the identity of the stonefish is certain, the initial dose is repeated.
• Stonefish antivenom is available in the United States from the following sources and other regional centers.

—Health Services Department, Sea World, San Diego CA (619-222-6363 ext. 2201)
—Sea World, Aurora, OH (216-562-8101)
—Steinhart Aquarium, San Francisco, CA (415-221-8014)

Adverse Effects

• Acute allergic reactions, including anaphylaxis, may occur.
• Serum sickness may occur, especially if several ampules are administered.

ADJUNCTIVE TREATMENT

• Pain control is achieved with local or regional anesthesia, using 1% or 2% lidocaine without epinephrine and meperidine or morphine for severe pain.
• After soaking, the wound should be irrigated copiously with warm, sterile saline.
• The wound should be explored.

—Any previously unnoticed foreign bodies, especially spine fragments that might continue to release venom, should be removed and the wound left open to drain.
—Devitalized tissue should be debrided, but wide debridement is not typically necessary.

• If the wound is in the hand or foot or if the wound is deep, prophylactic antibiotics are recommended by some authorities.

—Freshwater wound antimicrobial therapy should be directed against *Aeromonas* species.
—Salt water wounds should be treated with therapy against *Vibrio* species.
—Although there are many organisms to consider, either ciprofloxacin 250 mg orally twice a day for 7 days or trimethoprim-sulfamethoxazole are reasonable initial regimens for either type of contamination.

• Tetanus immunization is administered, if needed.
• Not recommended therapies. Ice application, infiltration with emetine, potassium permangenate, or Congo red have not been proven effective.

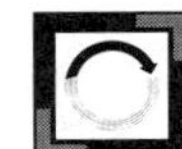

Follow-Up

PATIENT MONITORING

The patient should be monitored for pain control and neurologic effects.

EXPECTED COURSE AND PROGNOSIS

• Death in humans is rare.
• Most patients recover without complication.
• Pain control may be needed for several days.

DISCHARGE CRITERIA AND INSTRUCTIONS

• Patients may be discharged from the emergency department or hospital when systemic effects resolve and pain can be controlled with oral medication.
• An appointment for a wound recheck should be scheduled to assess for developing infection.

Pitfalls

DIAGNOSIS

It is vital to recognize the severity of a stonefish sting and to administer antivenom.

TREATMENT

• Immersion in nonscalding hot water should not be delayed.
• The clinician's own hand can be placed in the immersion water to ensure that the temperature is appropriate.

ICD-9-CM 989.5

Toxic effect of other substances, chiefly nonmedicinal as to source: venom.

See also: SECTION IV, Stingray and Jellyfish chapters.

RECOMMENDED READING

Auerbach PS. Marine envenomations. *N Engl J Med* 1991;325:486–493.

Baack BR, Kucan JO, Zook EG, et al. Hand infections secondary to catfish spines: case reports and literature review. *J Trauma* 1991;31:1432–1436.

Author: Thomas G. Burke

Reviewer: Richard C. Dart

Flunitrazepam (Rohypnol)

Basics

DESCRIPTION

Flunitrazepam (Rohypnol) is an ultra short-acting benzodiazepine.

FORMS AND USES

- US Drug Enforcement Administration (DEA) Schedule 1. Flunitrazepam is not approved for use in the United States because of its abuse potential.
- Rohypnol is widely used in Europe, Central America, and South America for induction of anesthesia and treatment of anxiety, sleep disorders, and alcohol withdrawal.
- Germany has withdrawn 2-mg tablets due to widespread abuse.
- Flunitrazepam is available in 1-mg and 2-mg scored tablets or as a solution for intravenous or intramuscular administration.
- Typical dose range is 0.5 to 2.0 mg orally.
- Current street uses include enhancing the effects of heroin, curbing the depression that follows a cocaine binge, and preying on unsuspecting people in order to rob or rape them.
- Street names include rophies, roofies, ruffies, R2, Roche, roachies, la rocha, rope, rib, and the "forget me" pill.
- It is usually taken orally, but there are reports of snorting as well.

TOXIC DOSE

- Ingestion of several milligrams can cause CNS depression in naive users; much larger doses are needed to cause toxic effects in tolerant (repeated) users.
- One pill may produce clinical effects in children.

PATHOPHYSIOLOGY

- The drug binds to CNS benzodiazepine receptors and potentiates the effect of gamma-aminobutyric acid (GABA).
- It is an ultra short-acting benzodiazepine class drug with shorter half-life and quicker onset of action after ingestion (onset 10–30 minutes, peak drug levels in 1–2 hours) than diazepam.
- Tolerance and physical dependence may occur, especially if more than 6 mg/day is taken for a month or more.

EPIDEMIOLOGY

- Poisoning is becoming more common.
- Initially smuggled into Florida and Texas from Mexico, the drug has spread into most states.
- The toxic effects are typically mild to moderate.
- Death is unusual unless the drug is coingested with other drugs, especially alcohol.

CAUSES

- The cause is usually intentional abuse.
- Children ages 8 to 10 years have been reported abusing this medication.
- Sexual assault or battery should be considered if the patient has no recollection of events, even without evidence of trauma.
- The possibility of child neglect should be considered in patients under 1 year of age; suicide attempt should be considered in patients over 6 years of age.

DRUG AND DISEASE INTERACTIONS

There is a synergistic effect with alcohol or other CNS depressants.

PREGNANCY AND LACTATION

- US FDA Pregnancy Category D. Evidence of human fetal risk exists, but benefits in certain situations (e.g., life-threatening situations or serious diseases) may make use of the drug acceptable despite its risks.
- Rohypnol appears in breast milk and may produce sedation in infants.

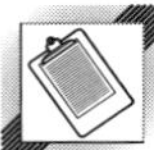

Diagnosis

DIFFERENTIAL DIAGNOSIS

- A wide variety of toxic agents produce respiratory and CNS depression, including other benzodiazepines, narcotics, ethanol, barbiturates, numerous sedative-hypnotic drugs, and tricyclic antidepressants.
- **Nontoxic causes** include hypoxia, severe electrolyte abnormality, hypoglycemia, intracranial bleed, meningitis, encephalitis, postictal state, and many others.

SIGNS AND SYMPTOMS

The predominant features are drowsiness, slurred speech, and impaired judgment and motor skills.

Vital Signs

Hypothermia, hypotension, hypertension, and bradycardia or tachycardia have been reported.

HEENT

Occasional diplopia, blurred vision, nystagmus, and miosis or mydriasis have been seen.

Cardiovascular

Collapse occurs rarely in severe overdose, usually following severe CNS depression and development of ventricular ectopy.

Pulmonary

- Respiratory depression is common.
- Aspiration may occur.

Gastrointestinal

Nausea, constipation, and decreased bowel sounds occur occasionally.

Fluids and Electrolytes

Lactic acidosis may develop if hypoxia or hypotension occurs.

Musculoskeletal

Fatigue or rhabdomyolysis may result from agitation.

Neurologic

Depression, lethargy, dysarthria, headache, ataxia, coma, amnesia, incoordination, incontinence, tremor, vertigo, rare hyperexcited states, anxiety, and hallucinations may occur.

PROCEDURES AND LABORATORY TESTS

Essential Tests

Testing may not be needed in asymptomatic patients.

Recommended Tests

- Serum electrolytes, BUN, and creatinine should be determined to assess renal injury and altered mental status.
- Pulse oximetry should be used for assessment of altered mental status.
- ECG, serum acetaminophen, aspirin, and ethanol levels may be performed in overdose setting to detect occult overdose.
- Urinalysis should be performed and serum creatine kinase determined in a comatose patient to evaluate for rhabdomyolysis.
- Chest radiographs, head CT, lumbar puncture, and cultures may be performed as needed to evaluate respiratory complications and assess other causes of CNS depression.

Not Recommended Tests

- Quantitative drug level of flunitrazepam is not recommended.
- Drugs and disorders that may cause false negative benzodiazepine screen results include Visine, hand soap, Drano, and bleach.

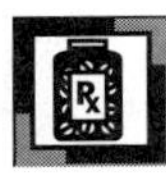

Treatment

- Treatment should focus on supportive care and early airway control.
- After decontamination, treatment is supportive.
- Dose and time of exposure should be determined for all substances involved.

DIRECTING PATIENT COURSE

The health-care provider should call the poison control center when:

- Significant CNS or respiratory depression or other severe effects are present.
- Signs and symptoms are not consistent with benzodiazepine poisoning.
- Coingestant, drug interaction, or underlying disease presents an unusual problem.

The patient should be referred to a health-care facility when:

- Attempted suicide, homicide, or sexual assault is possible.
- Patient or caregiver seems unreliable.
- Patient has symptoms.
- Coingestant, drug interaction, or underlying disease presents an unusual problem.

Admission Considerations

Inpatient treatment is warranted when patient has persistent or recurrent (after flumazenil) CNS effects or hemodynamic instability.

DECONTAMINATION

Out of Hospital

Induction of emesis is not recommended because of the potential for rapid onset of CNS depression.

In Hospital

- Induction of emesis is not recommended.
- Gastric lavage should be performed in pediatric (tube size 24–32 French) or adult (tube size 36–42 French) patients presenting within 1 hour of a large ingestion or if serious effects are present.
- One dose of activated charcoal (1–2 g/kg) should be administered without a cathartic if a substantial ingestion has occurred within the previous few hours.

ANTIDOTES

Flumazenil

- Indications. Diagnosis of benzodiazepine overdose or reversal of conscious sedation.
- Contraindications. Seizures, known flumazenil allergy, or overdose of tricyclic antidepressant drugs.
- Method of administration

—Adult dose is 0.1 to 0.2 mg by intravenous push every 1 to 2 minutes until clinical effect occurs or until 1 to 2 mg has been given.
—If resedation occurs, 1 mg may be given every 20 minutes to a maximum of 3 mg/h.
—Pediatric dose is 10 μg/kg by intravenous push, titrated to effect.

- Caution: Resedation may occur 30 to 60 minutes after administration.
- Potential adverse effects

—Agitation, vomiting, confusion, seizures, dysrhythmia, and flushing may occur.
—Flumazenil may induce withdrawal.

ADJUNCTIVE TREATMENT

Hypotension

- The patient should be given 10 to 20 ml/kg 0.9% saline intravenously and placed in the Trendelenburg position.
- Further fluid therapy should be guided by central pressure monitoring to avoid volume overload.
- If hypotension does not respond to treatment, a vasopressor is administered.

—Dopamine
  —The adult and pediatric dose is 2 to 5 μg/kg/min intravenously, titrated upward to effect.
  —Rates greater than 20 μg/kg/min are unlikely to provide further benefit.
—Norepinephrine may be added if hypotension is unresponsive.
  —The dose is 0.1 to 0.2 μg/kg/min, titrated upward to effect.
  —High rates of infusion may cause tissue ischemia.

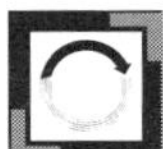

Follow-Up

PATIENT MONITORING

Patients should have continuous respiratory and cardiac monitoring.

EXPECTED COURSE AND PROGNOSIS

- Effects abate within 24 hours unless sequelae of aspiration or hypoxia develop.
- Drug effects after overdose last from 2 to 8 hours, sometimes up to 24 hours.

DISCHARGE CRITERIA AND INSTRUCTIONS

- From the emergency department

—Asymptomatic patients may be discharged after decontamination or observation for 6 hours.
—Psychiatric clearance may be indicated.

- From the hospital

—Asymptomatic patients with normal vital signs and mental status may be discharged.
—Psychiatric clearance may be indicated.

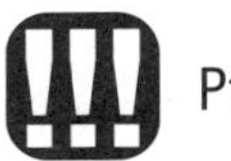

Pitfalls

DIAGNOSIS

Benzodiazepine toxicity may resemble many other conditions, including many nontoxicologic conditions.

FOLLOW-UP

Police or psychiatric counseling may be needed for suspected foul play or suicidal ideation.

ICD-9-CM 969.4

Poisoning by psychotropic agents: benzodiazepine-based tranquilizers.

See also: SECTION II, Hypotension chapter; SECTION III, Flumazenil chapter; and SECTION IV, Benzodiazepines (Including Clonazepam) and Sedative-Hypnotic Agents chapters.

RECOMMENDED READING

Flunitrazepam. DEA Publication, US Department of Justice. Taken from website: www.usdoj.gov/dea/pubs/rohypnol/rohypnol.htm on 7/2/97.

Author: Christopher Layton

Reviewer: Richard C. Dart

Basics

DESCRIPTION

- Gastroenteritis following ingestion of contaminated fried rice, milk, and cheeses is caused by *Salmonella* species, *Staphylococcus* species, *Bacillus cereus*, *Campylobacter fetus*, or *Yersinia enterocolitica*.
- Gastroenteritis following ingestion of contaminated water (or use of contaminated water to wash food items) is caused by *Escherichia coli* (both invasive and toxigenic species), *Shigella* species, *Salmonella enteritis*, *Y. enterocolitica*, *C. fetus*, or *Vibrio cholera*.

PATHOPHYSIOLOGY

Bacterial and nonbacterial pathogens produce toxicity through one of two mechanisms:

- Invasive gastroenteritis is the direct invasion of the intestinal mucosa.

—It produces local degeneration of microvilli and an intense inflammatory reaction, bloody diarrhea, vomiting, cramping, and bloating.
—It is most commonly caused by *Salmonella* species or invasive *E. coli*.

- Enterotoxin-induced gastroenteritis is caused by bacterial toxins that disrupt water and solute transport across the mucosal cell membrane.

—It results in nonbloody diarrhea, cramping, bloating, and vomiting.
—The most common pathogens include staphylococcal species, enterotoxigenic *E. coli*, *Clostridium perfringens*, *B. cereus*, and *Campylobacter jejuni*.

EPIDEMIOLOGY

- The true incidence of food poisoning is unknown because many cases are mild and unreported or misdiagnosed.
- Multiple victims presenting at the same time in roughly the same place typically result from a common exposure.

CAUSES

Food poisoning results from ingestion of contaminated vegetables, fruit, salads, fried rice, pastries, corn flour, milk, cheese, and salads, or contaminated water.

DRUG AND DISEASE INTERACTIONS

Toxic effects, especially dehydration, are more pronounced in children and the elderly, although death from shock and fluid depletion is rare even in these populations.

PREGNANCY AND LACTATION

Pregnant women are susceptible to systemic listeriosis after the ingestion of food, most commonly undercooked chicken or dairy products, contaminated with *Listeria monocytogenes*.

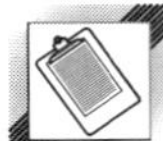

Diagnosis

Eliciting a history of ingested substances and the time of symptom onset will help elucidate pathogens.

DIFFERENTIAL DIAGNOSIS

- Other bacterial causes of acute gastroenteritis include meat, eggs, poultry, water-borne pathogens (*Giardia, Cryptosporidium*), seafood-associated poisoning, botulism, and pathogens associated with pets (*Y. enterocolitica, Plesiomonas shigelloides, Anaerobiospirillium* species).
- Nonbacterial causes of acute gastroenteritis include viruses, mushroom ingestion, plant gastrointestinal irritants, scombroid or ciguatera fish poisoning, and shellfish poisoning, among others.
- Chemical causes include pesticides, monosodium glutamate (MSG), and heavy metals.

SIGNS AND SYMPTOMS

The physical examination is nonspecific and related primarily to dehydration or local gastrointestinal effects of the toxin. Onset of symptoms and duration of illness:

- *Staphylococcus* species. Incubation period 1 to 6 hours, duration 2 to 5 days.
- *B. cereus*. Incubation period 1 to 6 hours, duration 20 to 36 hours.
- *Salmonella* species. Incubation period 8 to 40 hours, duration 2 to 5 days.
- *E. coli* (invasive). Incubation period 6 to 36 hours, duration 1 to 3 weeks.
- *E. coli* (toxigenic). Incubation period 12 to 72 hours, duration 1 to 2 weeks.
- *V. cholera*. Incubation period 9 to 72 hours, duration 3 to 4 days.
- *Shigella* species. Incubation period 12 to 50 hours, duration 4 to 7 days.
- *Y. enterocolitica*. Incubation period 3 to 7 days, duration 9 to 14 days.
- *Campylobacter* species. Incubation period 1 to 7 days, duration 1 to 7 days.

Vital Signs

- Fever suggests invasive bacterial pathogen such as *Salmonella, C. fetus*, or *E. coli*.
- Tachycardia or hypotension indicates moderate volume depletion.
- Symptoms of listeriosis include fever and pharyngitis.

Dermatologic

Dry skin with poor turgor suggests dehydration.

Gastrointestinal

- Diffuse, colicky abdominal pain, bloating, diarrhea, diffusely tender abdomen, and voluntary guarding are universal and nonspecific symptoms.
- Friable, inflamed mucosa or heme-positive rectal examination suggests an invasive bacterial agent.

Renal

Decreased urine output suggests volume depletion.

Fluids and Electrolytes

- Vomiting, diarrhea, and insensible losses may produce hypernatremia (dehydration) or hyponatremia (loss of total body sodium), hypokalemia, hypochloremia, hypomagnesemia, or hypophosphatemia.
- Metabolic alkalosis (vomiting) or acidosis (loss of bicarbonate in diarrhea) can occur.

Musculoskeletal

- Diffuse muscle cramps and myalgia are common.
- Symptoms of listeriosis include myalgia.

Neurologic

- No specific effects are expected from simple bacterial food poisoning.
- If bulbar signs or descending weakness or paralysis develop, botulism should be considered.
- Symptoms of listeriosis include severe headache.

PROCEDURES AND LABORATORY TESTS

Essential Tests

No tests may be needed in minimally symptomatic patients.

Recommended Tests

- Complete blood count may show increased polymorphonuclear cells, especially with invasive organisms.
- Microscopic stool examination may demonstrate leukocytes, bacteria, or blood, suggesting an invasive bacterial presence.
- Cultures of food, vomitus, or stool may help identify pathogen.
- Serum electrolytes, BUN, and creatinine should be obtained to assess effects of dehydration.

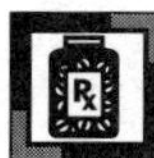

Treatment

- Treatment should focus on symptomatic relief of nausea, vomiting, and diarrhea with attention to the possible development of volume depletion and shock.
- Supportive care, including fluid resuscitation for patients with severe dehydration and shock, is vital.
- Discrimination of invasive versus noninvasive bacterial diarrhea is sufficient to direct treatment.
- If multiple cases are known, the public health department should be notified.

DIRECTING PATIENT COURSE

The health-care provider should call a poison control center when:

- Any possibility of botulism exists
- Signs and symptoms are not consistent with bacterial food poisoning.
- Dehydration, bloody diarrhea, or other severe effects are present.
- Coingestant, drug interaction, or underlying disease presents an unusual problem.

The patient should be referred to a health-care facility when:

- The patient or the caregiver seems unreliable.
- Coingestant, drug interaction, or underlying disease presents an unusual problem.

Admission Considerations

Inpatient management is warranted for:

- Patients at the extremes of age with signs of shock, and those who are unable to tolerate oral fluids despite rehydration.
- Any patient with suspected botulism should be admitted to an intensive care setting.

DECONTAMINATION

Generally, repetitive vomiting obviates the need for decontamination.

ANTIDOTES

There is no specific antidote for food poisoning.

ADJUNCTIVE TREATMENT

- In cases of suspected invasive bacterial infection, stool cultures may be falsely negative in as many as 40% of cases, and empiric therapy may be initiated:

—Ciprofloxacin, 250 mg twice a day for 5 to 7 days; or
—Trimethoprim/sulfamethoxazole, 160/800 mg tablets twice a day for 5 to 7 days

- Control of nausea and vomiting with antiemetic agents may enable the patient to retain fluids and medications orally.
- Use of antidiarrheal agents is controversial.

—Increasing gastrointestinal transit time will provide some relief but may also prolong the amount of time that bacteria and toxins are in contact with intestinal mucosa.
—Loperamide (Imodium) may be given, 2 to 4 mg initially followed by 1 to 2 mg every 4 to 6 hours; half dose is used in children over 2 years of age.

- Treatment for listeriosis is intravenous ampicillin 500 mg every 6 hours or intravenous gentamicin 5 mg/kg loading dose followed by 2 mg/kg intravenously every 8 hours, or both.

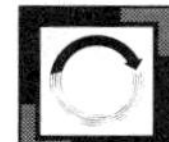

Follow-Up

PATIENT MONITORING

- Serial serum electrolytes should be monitored in patients with severe diarrhea or vomiting.
- Severe, untreated, continuing volume depletion may rarely cause shock and end-organ damage.

EXPECTED COURSE AND PROGNOSIS

Most patients are uncomfortable for several days, then will recover completely.

DISCHARGE CRITERIA AND INSTRUCTIONS

Patients with normal vital signs who are able to tolerate oral fluid administration after correction of electrolyte abnormalities and dehydration may be discharged.

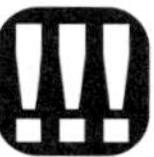

Pitfalls

DIAGNOSIS

Exhaustive attempts to identify pathogens or reservoirs definitively are unlikely to be clinically useful.

ICD-9-CM 005.0–005.9

Food poisoning (bacterial).

See also: SECTION IV, Botulism.

RECOMMENDED READING

Ellenhorn MJ. Food poisonings. In: Ellenhorn MJ, et al., eds. *Ellenhorn's medical toxicology: diagnosis and treatment of human poisoning,* 2nd ed. Baltimore: Williams & Wilkins, 1997:1036–1060.

Snydman DR. Food poisoning. In: Gorbach SL, Bartlett JG, Blacklow NR, eds. *Infectious diseases.* Philadelphia: WB Saunders, 1992:628–638.

Author: Gerald F. O'Malley

Reviewer: Richard C. Dart

Food Poisoning—Meat, Poultry, and Eggs

Basics

DESCRIPTION

Acute gastroenteritis may be caused by ingestion of contaminated meat, poultry, or egg products.

FORMS AND USES

- Some food products that are commonly implicated as carriers of gastroenteritis-causing pathogens are processed meat; undercooked, underrefrigerated, or otherwise mishandled meat; cream-filled or custard pastries; and egg salads.
- Processed beef, poultry, or other meat may be contaminated during processing. Meats, cream-filled products, and egg-containing products such as egg salad also may become toxic due to mishandling (e.g., poor refrigeration) and resultant increase in pathogen load.

PATHOPHYSIOLOGY

- Bacterial pathogens are the most common etiologic agents causing gastroenteritis associated with ingestion of meat, poultry, and eggs. Toxicity is produced through one of two different mechanisms.
- Invasive gastroenteritis results from direct invasion of the intestinal mucosa.

—It produces an intense inflammatory reaction, bloody diarrhea, vomiting, cramping, and bloating.
—It is most commonly caused by *Salmonella* species.

- Enterotoxin-induced gastroenteritis is caused by bacterial toxins that disrupt water and solute transport across the mucosal cell membrane.

—It results in voluminous, nonbloody diarrhea, cramping, bloating, and vomiting.
—The most commonly reported pathogens include *Staphylococcus* species, *Clostridium perfringens, Bacillus cereus,* and *Campylobacter jejuni.*

Mechanisms by which such pathogens reach toxic levels include the following:

- Inadequate refrigeration
- Food prepared too far in advance of consumption
- Contaminated food preparer with poor hygienic practices or dirty equipment
- Inadequate cooking, reheating, or holding temperatures
- Cross-contamination by raw materials or adjacent foods

EPIDEMIOLOGY

- The true incidence is unknown; many cases are mild and go unreported or misdiagnosed.
- Toxic effects are more pronounced in children and the elderly, although death from shock and fluid depletion is rare even in these populations.

CAUSES

Poisoning is most commonly the result of poor food handling in a home or restaurant.

RISK FACTORS

Patients at the extremes of age are particularly susceptible to dehydration.

PREGNANCY AND LACTATION

Pregnant women are susceptible to the development of systemic listeriosis after the ingestion of food contaminated with *Listeria monocytogenes* (most commonly undercooked chicken, dairy, or lettuce products). Symptoms of listeriosis include fever, severe headache, myalgias, and pharyngitis.

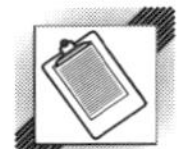

Diagnosis

DIFFERENTIAL DIAGNOSIS

- Additional food-borne bacterial causes of acute gastroenteritis include fried rice (*Shigella* species, *Yersinia enterocolitica, Campylobacter fetus*), waterborne pathogens (*Giardia lamblia*, toxigenic *Escherichia coli, Vibrio cholerae, Cryptosporidium*), shellfish (*Vibrio parahaemolyticus*), and pathogens (*Clostridium botulinum*) associated with home canning and preserves (botulism).
- Nonbacterial causes of acute gastroenteritis include viruses, some plants, seafood (scombroid or ciguatera fish poisoning, shellfish) and other compounds (pesticides, monosodium glutamate, heavy metals).

SIGNS AND SYMPTOMS

- The physical examination is generally nonspecific.
- History of substance ingested as well as temporal relationship to onset of symptoms will help elucidate pathogens.
- Onset of symptoms and duration of illness is as follows:

—*Staphylococcus* species. Incubation period 1 to 6 hours, duration 2 to 5 days.
—*C. perfringens.* Incubation period 8 to 12 hours, duration 24 hours.
—*B. cereus.* Incubation period 10 to 12 hours, duration 20 to 36 hours.
—*Salmonella* species. Incubation period 8 to 40 hours, duration 2 to 5 days
—*C. jejuni.* Incubation period 1 to 7 days, duration 1 to 7 days

Vital Signs

- Fever suggests an invasive pathogen such as *Salmonella*.
- Tachycardia indicates fever or volume depletion.
- Hypotension indicates significant (more than 10%) volume depletion and need for rehydration.

Dermatologic

Dry skin with poor turgor suggests dehydration.

Gastrointestinal

- Diffuse, colicky abdominal pain with vomiting, bloating, and diarrhea are universal.
- Signs of diffusely tender abdomen without evidence of peritonitis are universal and nonspecific.

Renal

Decrease in urine output suggests volume depletion.

Fluids and Electrolytes

Vomiting and diarrhea as well as insensible losses due to fever or tachypnea may lead to hypernatremia (dehydration) or hyponatremia (loss of total body sodium), hypokalemia, hypochloremia, hypomagnesemia, hypophosphatemia, or metabolic alkalosis (by vomiting) or acidosis (by loss of bicarbonate in diarrhea).

Musculoskeletal

Diffuse muscle cramps and myalgias are common.

Neurologic

If neurologic effects are present, botulism should be suspected (see SECTION IV, Botulism chapter).

PROCEDURES AND LABORATORY TESTS

Essential Tests

No tests may be needed in minimally symptomatic patients.

Recommended Tests

- Microscopic evaluation of stool may demonstrate leukocytes, bacteria, or blood, suggesting an invasive bacterial cause.
- Serum electrolytes, BUN, and creatinine should be assayed in markedly symptomatic cases to assess effects of fluid loss.

Not Recommended Tests

Exhaustive attempts at identification of definitive pathogens or reservoirs are unlikely to provide useful information.

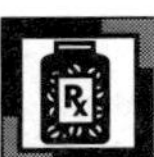

Treatment

- Treatment should focus on symptomatic relief of nausea, vomiting, and diarrhea with attention to the possible development of serious volume depletion and shock, particularly in very young and very old patients.
- Time and history of exposure should be determined for all foods ingested within the previous 48 hours.
- Discrimination of invasive versus noninvasive bacterial diarrhea with or without signs of neurologic involvement is sufficient to direct treatment.

DIRECTING PATIENT COURSE

The health-care provider should call the poison control center when:

- Concern regarding possible botulism exists.
- Toxic effects are not consistent with simple bacterial food poisoning.
- Drug interaction or underlying disease presents an unusual problem.

The patient should be referred to a health-care facility when:

- Patient or caregiver seems unreliable.
- Dehydration or other serious effects are present.
- Drug interaction or underlying disease presents an unusual problem.

Admission Considerations

Inpatient management is warranted if:

- Patients are at the extremes of age with signs of serious dehydration or shock.
- Patients are unable to tolerate oral fluids despite rehydration and control of nausea; they should receive a short inpatient course of intravenous hydration and antiemetic.

DECONTAMINATION

In general, repetitive vomiting and diarrhea eliminates the need for decontamination.

ANTIDOTES

There is no specific antidote for simple bacterial food poisoning.

ADJUNCTIVE TREATMENT

- Phenothiazines for control of nausea and vomiting

—These are not recommended for use in children.
—Prochlorperazine. Adult dose is 25 mg orally or rectally twice a day.
—Promethazine. Adult dose is 25 mg orally or rectally four times a day.

- Antibiotic therapy is generally not indicated; in cases of invasive bacterial infection, stool cultures may be falsely negative in as many as 40% of cases and empiric therapy may be initiated with one of the following.

—Ciprofloxacin, 250 mg twice a day for 5 to 7 days
—Trimethoprim/sulfamethoxazole, 160/800-mg tablets twice a day for 5 to 7 days

- Use of antidiarrheal agents is controversial; showing gastrointestinal activity will offer some relief for uncontrollable diarrhea, but will also prolong the amount of time that bacteria and toxins are in contact with intestinal mucosa.

—Diphenoxylate hydrochloride with atropine (Lomotil) may be given orally to adults, 5 mg orally two to four times a day.
—Loperamide (Imodium) dose is 2 to 4 mg orally initially, followed by 2 mg every 4 to 6 hours.

- Hypotension

—Hypotension should be treated with isotonic fluid infusion and the Trendelenburg position.
—Vasopressors may be added if needed; dopamine is preferred.
—Norepinephrine may be added for refractory hypotension.

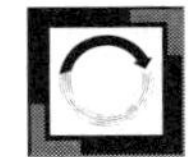

Follow-Up

PATIENT MONITORING

Serum electrolyte panel should be monitored in severe cases to assess rehydration.

EXPECTED COURSE AND PROGNOSIS

- Most patients are uncomfortable for several days, then completely recover.
- In rare cases, severe, untreated volume depletion may cause shock and end-organ damage related to dehydration.

DISCHARGE CRITERIA AND INSTRUCTIONS

Patients with normal vital signs who are able to tolerate oral fluids may be discharged.

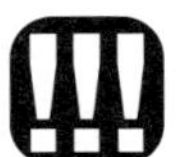

Pitfalls

DIAGNOSIS

- Failure to consider alternative possible etiologies of vomiting can lead to misdiagnosis.
- Extensive laboratory testing is generally not helpful in diagnosis or management.

TREATMENT

Overaggressive use of phenothiazines and gastrointestinal motility agents may cause dystonic reaction.

ICD-9-CM 988

Toxic effect of noxious substances eaten as food.

See also: SECTION II, Hypotension chapter; and SECTION IV, Botulism chapter.

RECOMMENDED READING

Bryan FL. Epidemiology of foodborne diseases. In: Riemann H, Bryan FL, eds. *Foodborne infections and intoxications.* New York: Academic, 1979.

POISINDEX Editorial Staff. Food poisoning. In: Ramach BH, Rider PK, Gelman CR, eds. *POISINDEX system.* Englewood, CO: Micromedex, Inc. (edition expires August 31, 1998).

Author: Gerald F. O'Malley

Reviewer: Katherine M. Hurlbut

Food Poisoning—Shellfish

Basics

DESCRIPTION

Shellfish food poisoning includes specific syndromes (paralytic, neurotoxic, and amnestic) that develop after the ingestion of shellfish.

FORMS AND USES

- Paralytic shellfish poisoning (PSP) typically begins with a brief gastrointestinal prodrome, followed by sensory disturbances and progressive paralysis.
- Neurotoxic shellfish poisoning features gastrointestinal and neurologic symptoms usually appearing simultaneously; these may include paresthesia of the face, throat, and extremities, burning sensation of the mucous membranes, abdominal pain and cramps, incoordination, seizures, and possibly coma.
- Amnestic shellfish poisoning begins with a gastrointestinal prodrome, followed by confusion, seizures, coma, and long-term memory deficits; hypotension, pulmonary edema, seizures, and coma may develop.

TOXIC DOSE

Paralytic shellfish poisoning (PSP) reportedly can cause illness with as little as 500 μg of the toxin; however, the concentration of toxin in the mollusk varies greatly.

PATHOPHYSIOLOGY

- Dinoflagellates are the major food source for bivalve mollusks such as clams and oysters; toxins produced by certain dinoflagellate species accumulate in the mollusks without injuring the mollusk.
- PSP is caused by saxitoxin and gonyautoxins, toxins that reversibly block sodium channels in nerve and muscle.
- Neurotoxic shellfish poisoning is caused by brevetoxin, a toxin that activates sodium influx into the cell.
- Amnestic shellfish poisoning is caused by domoic acid, an excitatory amino acid.

EPIDEMIOLOGY

- PSP (carried by bivalve mollusks, especially mussels, clams, oysters, scallops, or limpets) occurs on the East and West Coasts of North America, western coast of Europe, and throughout Japan; most outbreaks occur during May to August when the water temperatures are highest.
- Neurotoxic shellfish poisoning (bivalve mollusks) has occurred primarily in Florida and around the Gulf of Mexico.
- Amnestic shellfish poisoning (bivalve mollusks, and occasionally fish and crustaceans) has occurred from eating contaminated mussels from Prince Edward Island, Canada, but domoic acid has also been identified in mollusks harvested from the coastal waters of Washington and Oregon.

CAUSES

Poisoning is usually caused by inadvertent ingestion of contaminated fish.

RISK FACTORS

Children may be more sensitive to shellfish toxins.

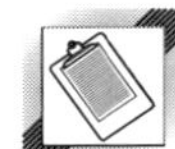

Diagnosis

DIFFERENTIAL DIAGNOSIS

- Toxic causes of gastroenteritis followed by neurologic symptoms include scombroid or puffer fish poisoning, botulism, heavy metal toxicity, diphtheria, and nicotine or hemlock poisoning, among others.
- Nontoxic causes include infectious gastroenteritis.

SIGNS AND SYMPTOMS

Vital Signs

- Paralytic. Tachycardia is common.
- Neurotoxic. Bradycardia is common.
- Amnestic. Tachycardia and hemodynamic instability may occur.

HEENT

- Paralytic. The patient may develop nystagmus, temporary blindness, loss of gag reflex, dysphagia, and difficulty speaking.
- Neurotoxic. Mydriasis, conjunctivitis, lacrimation, rhinorrhea, and sneezing may occur.
- Amnestic. The patient may exhibit miosis or mydriasis, disconjugate gaze, and ophthalmoplegia in severe cases.

Cardiovascular

- Paralytic. ECG T-wave changes may develop.
- Neurotoxic. Bradycardia may persist for up to 12 hours.
- Amnestic. Hypotension with peripheral vasodilatation or dysrhythmias may develop.

Pulmonary

- Paralytic. Respiratory failure may develop.
- Neurotoxic. Inhalation of toxin may occur when high winds aerosolize the toxin, resulting in cough, asthma attack, and respiratory irritation in nonasthmatics.
- Amnestic. Excessive pulmonary secretions and pulmonary edema are common.

Gastrointestinal

- Paralytic. Nausea, vomiting, diarrhea, and abdominal pain are common.
- Neurotoxic. Nausea, vomiting, diarrhea, cramping, abdominal pain, and rectal burning pain may occur.
- Amnestic. Nausea, vomiting, diarrhea, and hiccups are common.

Fluids and Electrolytes

All three types of shellfish poisoning may produce dehydration, as well as electrolyte abnormalities in severe cases.

Musculoskeletal

- Paralytic. Incoordination, muscle weakness, and paralysis are common.
- Neurotoxic. Myalgia, weakness, and difficulty walking may develop.

Neurologic

- Paralytic. Paresthesias ("pins and needles") and numbness of lips, tongue, throat, face, neck, and extremities may develop, as may headaches, dizziness, and sensation of lightness.
- Neurotoxic. Paresthesias of the face, lips, and extremities are common; reversal of hot/cold sensation, headache, tremor, decreased reflexes, ataxia, distorted sensorium, vertigo, seizure, and coma may develop.
- Amnestic. Confusion, agitation, seizure, coma, fasciculation, Babinski sign, neuropathy (motor and sensory), and memory loss may occur.

PROCEDURES AND LABORATORY TESTS

Essential Tests

No tests may be needed in minimally symptomatic patients.

Recommended Tests

- For all three types of shellfish poisoning

—Serum electrolytes, BUN, creatinine to assess dehydration from gastroenteritis
—Serum calcium, magnesium, phosphorus to assess other causes of symptoms.
—Serum creatine kinase to assess cardiac and muscle injury
—ECG and cardiac monitoring to monitor for ischemia and dysrhythmia

- For PSP, Electromyogram/nerve conduction velocity should be obtained to assess both motor and sensory abnormality.

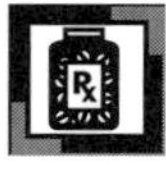

Treatment

- Treatment should focus on symptomatic and respiratory care, as well as on control of seizure and dysrhythmia.
- Patients should be intubated endotracheally if serious respiratory depression or difficulty in protecting airway develops.
- Dose and time of exposure should be determined for all substances involved.

DIRECTING PATIENT COURSE

The health-care provider should call the poison control center when:

• Shellfish poisoning is suspected.
• Toxic effects are not consistent with shellfish poisoning.
• Drug interaction or underlying disease presents an unusual problem.

The patient should be referred to a health-care facility when:

• The symptoms of shellfish poisoning or other severe effects are present.
• Patient or caregiver seems unreliable.
• Drug interaction or underlying disease presents an unusual problem.

Admission Considerations

Inpatient management in an ICU is warranted for symptomatic patients.

DECONTAMINATION

Out of Hospital

Induced emesis is not recommended.

In Hospital

• Gastric lavage should be considered in pediatric (tube size 24–32 French) or adult (tube size 36–42 French) patients presenting within 1 hour of a large ingestion or if serious effects are present.
• One dose of activated charcoal (1–2 g/kg) should be administered without a cathartic if a substantial ingestion has occurred within the previous few hours.

ANTIDOTES

There is no specific antidote for paralytic, neurotoxic, or amnestic shellfish poisoning.

ADJUNCTIVE TREATMENT

See SECTION II, Patient Presentations with Toxicologic Causes, for more detail on each of the following treatments.

Seizure

• A patent airway must be ensured.
• A benzodiazepine should be administered for initial control.
• If seizures persist or recur, another anticonvulsant such as phenobarbital may be added.

Hypotension

• Hypotension should be treated with isotonic fluid infusion and the Trendelenburg position.
• A vasopressor may be added if needed; dopamine is preferred.
• Norepinephrine may be added for refractory hypotension.

Dysrhythmias or Conduction Abnormalities

• Seizures should be controlled and acidemia corrected.
• If QRS widening or dysrhythmias persist, sodium bicarbonate (1–2 mEq/kg) may be administered in an intravenous bolus; this may be repeated as needed, but arterial pH should not exceed 7.55.
• Lidocaine may be used for ventricular tachycardia or multifocal premature ventricular contractions.

—Adult dose is 1 to 2 mg/kg in an intravenous loading dose, followed by infusion of 2 to 4 mg/min, titrated to desired effect.
—Pediatric dose is 1 mg/kg bolus followed by infusion of 20 to 50 μg/kg/min, titrated to effect.
—The initial dose may be repeated in 10 to 15 minutes at 0.5 to 1.0 mg/kg.

• Bretylium may be added for lidocaine-resistant ventricular dysrhythmia

—Dose is 5 to 10 mg/kg intravenously over 1 minute.
—If this is unsuccessful, additional doses may be administered over 1 minute and repeated as necessary to a total dose of 30 mg/kg.

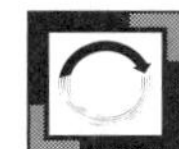

Follow-Up

PATIENT MONITORING

Cardiac and pulmonary functions should be monitored continuously in symptomatic patients.

EXPECTED COURSE AND PROGNOSIS

Paralytic

• The incubation period is usually less than 30 minutes.
• The duration of illness is hours to days; muscle weakness may last for weeks.
• In severe cases, respiratory muscle paralysis can result in respiratory failure as well as generalized muscle weakness and paralysis.

Neurotoxic

• The incubation period is usually minutes to hours.
• The illness lasts hours to days.

Amnestic

• The incubation period has ranged from 15 minutes to 38 hours.
• Long-term anterograde memory deficits and neuropathy are possible; morbidity appears to be greater in males.

DISCHARGE CRITERIA AND INSTRUCTIONS

• From the emergency department. Asymptomatic patients may be discharged after a 6-hour observation period.
• From the hospital

—PSP patients may be discharged when oral intake is adequate, and respiratory function, musculoskeletal, and neurological signs and symptoms have stabilized.
—Neurotoxic shellfish poisoning patients may be discharged when oral intake is adequate and all signs and symptoms have resolved or are improving.
—Amnestic shellfish patients may be discharged after effects of seizures, pulmonary edema, and hypotension have resolved or are improving.

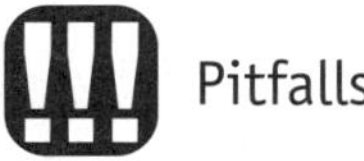

Pitfalls

DIAGNOSIS

Failure to consider that gastrointestinal and neurologic symptoms may be due to seafood poisoning is common.

TREATMENT

• Paralytic. Failure to anticipate respiratory paralysis and failure may lead to complications.
• Amnestic. Failure to anticipate pulmonary edema, dysrhythmias, and seizures may lead to unnecessary sequelae.

ICD-9-CM 988.0

Toxic effect of noxious substances eaten as food: fish and shellfish.

See also: SECTION II, Hypotension, Seizure, and Ventricular Dysrhythmias chapters.

RECOMMENDED READING

Morris PD, Campbell DS, Taylor TJ, et al. Clinical and epidemiological features of neurotoxic shellfish poisoning in North Carolina. *Am J Public Health* 1991;81:471–474.

Sakamoto Y, Lockey RF, Krzanowski JJ. Shellfish and fish poisoning related to the toxic dinoflagellates. *South Med J* 1987;80:868–872.

Teitelbaum JS, Zatorre RJ, Carpenter S, et al. Neurologic sequelae of domoic acid intoxication due to ingestion of contaminated mussels. *N Engl J Med* 1990;322:1781–1787.

Author: Luke Yip

Reviewer: Richard C. Dart

Formaldehyde

Basics

DESCRIPTION

Formaldehyde is an industrial and medical chemical used as a preservative and as an intermediary in many industrial processes.

FORMS AND USES

- Formaldehyde (methyl aldehyde, methylene oxide, formic aldehyde) is sold as an aqueous solution with concentrations varying from 37% to 56% formaldehyde by weight, with varying amounts of methanol added to retard polymerization (maximum methanol concentration is 15%).
- Medical uses of formaldehyde include antiseptics, disinfectants, tissue fixative, and embalming agents.
- Formaldehyde is used in the textile industry to attain a permanent press, wrinkle-free finish on textiles.
- Urea formaldehyde foam insulation releases formaldehyde vapor.
- Formaldehyde is a by-product of tobacco combustion.

TOXIC DOSE

- Formaldehyde solution (2%) can cause dermal or eye burns.
- Ingestion of a few gulps of 37% solution has caused death.

PATHOPHYSIOLOGY

- Formaldehyde is a direct mucosal irritant, causing rapid burning and lacrimation, as well as stimulating bronchospasm.
- Formaldehyde is rapidly metabolized to formic acid, which produces metabolic acidosis.
- The methanol contained in aqueous formaldehyde is metabolized to formic acid and contributes to the acidosis.
- Tissue necrosis with lactate production further contributes to the acidosis.

EPIDEMIOLOGY

- Ingestion of formaldehyde is rare, occupational exposure is common, and low level environmental exposure is ubiquitous.
- Toxic effects following ingestion or high-concentration dermal exposure can be severe.
- Ingestion, massive skin exposure, or inhalation of high concentrations may result in death.

CAUSES

- Ingestion of formaldehyde is usually intentional; occupational exposure is usually accidental.
- Child neglect should be considered if the patient is under 1 year of age; attempted suicide if the patient is over 6 years of age.

RISK FACTORS

Occupational formaldehyde exposures occur in the textile industry (crease-resistant finishers, fur processors, hide preservers, textile mordanters, printers, waterproofers); life sciences (anatomists, students, biologists, embalmers, histology technicians, pathologists, taxidermists); rubber and cement production (bookbinders, cosmetic formulators, electrical insulation manufacturers, glue and adhesive makers); plywood, particle board, or paper manufacturing; furniture manufacturing; and disinfectant manufacturing.

WORKPLACE STANDARDS

- OSHA: not listed.
- NIOSH REL TWA is 0.016; ceiling value is 0.1 ppm.
- ACGIH: TLV ceiling is 0.3 ppm.

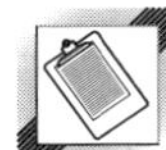

Diagnosis

DIFFERENTIAL DIAGNOSIS

- Other toxic agents that cause acute respiratory irritation include acetylene, ammonia, carbon disulfide, chloramine, chlorine, fluorine, hydrogen chloride or fluoride, and sulfur dioxide, among others.
- Other gastrointestinal irritants include strong acids or alkali.

SIGNS AND SYMPTOMS

Formaldehyde inhalation produces acute onset of respiratory irritant symptoms, and ingestion produces symptoms of acute caustic ingestion. In general, toxic effects of inhalation are less severe than those of ingestion.

Vital Signs

- Patients who have sustained significant exposure are usually anxious, as well as tachypneic and tachycardic from pain.
- In severe cases, patients present in shock with hypovolemia and hypotension.

HEENT

- Inhalation of low concentrations produces mucosal burning sensation and lacrimation.
- Inhalation of high concentrations causes mucosal burning with choking, coughing, sore throat, drooling, and difficulty in swallowing.
- Chronic inhalation causes headache, nausea and flulike symptoms.
- Ingestion may cause ulceration of the mouth, nasopharynx, esophagus, and respiratory mucosa.

Dermatologic

Acute exposure can cause dermatitis in sensitive individuals.

Pulmonary

- Respiratory effects of acute vapor inhalation are dependent on the concentration and duration of exposure.
- Prolonged high-dose exposure may cause parenchymal irritation with cough, chest pain, dyspnea, and wheezing.

Cardiovascular

Profound acidosis may cause hypotension.

Gastrointestinal

- Caustic gastrointestinal effects include hemorrhage, perforation, tissue fixation, and subsequent stricture formation.
- Severe vomiting and massive hematemesis may occur.

Renal

- Nephritis or acute tubular necrosis may develop following acute exposure.
- Chronic high-dose exposure may cause glomerulonephropathy.

Fluids and Electrolytes

Intravascular volume loss may result from massive fluid shift into injured tissues and potentially severe metabolic acidosis.

Neurologic

Limited inhalation exposure may produce headache and lightheadedness, whereas higher concentrations will have direct CNS depressant effects.

PROCEDURES AND LABORATORY TESTS

Essential Tests

- No tests may be needed for minimally symptomatic skin or inhalation exposure to formaldehyde.
- In cases of ingestion, the following should be obtained:

—Serum electrolytes, BUN, creatinine to assess fluid shifts, monitor renal function, and assess acidosis
—Complete blood count to assess blood loss
—Serum liver function tests, coagulation studies in severe cases to assess injury
—Arterial blood gas to assess acidosis and potential airway compromise

Recommended Tests

- In cases of serious skin or high-concentration formaldehyde inhalation exposure, the same tests as described as essential for ingestion should be undertaken.
- ECG, serum acetaminophen, and aspirin levels should be obtained to detect occult ingestion.
- Gastrointestinal endoscopy should be per-

formed following ingestion to evaluate for burns.
- Pulmonary peak flows should be monitored to follow progress of bronchospasm.
- Chest radiography may be useful in the hypoxic patient to evaluate pulmonary injury or possible gastric perforation.
- Gastric contrast studies should be performed to evaluate stricture formation.

Not Recommended Tests

Serum formic acid and formaldehyde levels are not clinically useful.

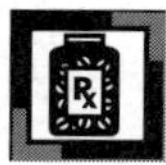

Treatment

- Following ingestion, treatment should focus on stabilization and resuscitation of patients with gastrointestinal hemorrhage and shock.
- Supportive care with appropriate airway management is vital.
- Dose and time of exposure must be determined for all substances involved.
- Vomiting and massive hematemesis may require emergent gastrectomy.

DIRECTING PATIENT COURSE

The health-care provider should call a poison control center when:

- Respiratory or gastrointestinal symptoms of formaldehyde poisoning are present.
- Signs and symptoms are not consistent with formaldehyde poisoning.
- Coingestant, drug interaction, or underlying disease presents an unusual problem.

The patient should be referred to a health-care facility when:

- Any toxic effects develop.
- Attempted suicide or homicide is possible.
- The patient or caregiver seems unreliable.
- Coingestant, drug interaction, or underlying disease presents an unusual problem.

Admission Considerations

Inpatient management is warranted in the following circumstances:

- Inhalation. Patients with hypoxia or apparent pulmonary injury, or those who remain symptomatic after a 6-hour observation period.
- Ingestion. All patients, unless they are asymptomatic after a trivial ingestion of a low-concentration formaldehyde solution.

DECONTAMINATION

Out of Hospital

- Inhalation. The patient should be removed from source of formaldehyde exposure.
- Ingestion

—Emesis should not be induced, because of its potential for caustic injury.
—Administer 4 to 6 ounces of milk or water to alert patients to reduce the corrosive effects.

- Dermal or ocular exposure. The exposed area should be irrigated with copious amounts of water.

In Hospital

- Ingestion

—Gastric lavage should be avoided because of its potential for caustic injury or perforation.
—Activated charcoal should also be avoided because it may interfere with endoscopy.

- Inhalation. Supplemental oxygen should be administered.
- Dermal or ocular exposure. The exposed area should be irrigated with copious amounts of water.

ANTIDOTES

There is no specific antidote for formaldehyde toxicity.

ADJUNCTIVE TREATMENT

- Immediate hemodialysis should be considered for severe acute ingestion to remove formaldehyde, formic acid, and methanol.
- Bronchospasm

—Albuterol 0.15 mg/kg (maximum of 10 mg) in saline with humidified oxygen via nebulizer every 20 to 30 minutes
  —If the peak respiratory flow rate is greater than 90% after the initial dose, additional doses may not be needed.
  —The patient should be continually monitored for response.
—Methylprednisolone 60 to 125 mg (1–1.5 mg/kg) given intravenously (children 1–2 mg/kg) every 6 to 8 hours; this dosage may be decreased to a single daily dose and tapered.

- Hypotension is treated with isotonic fluid infusion, the Trendelenburg position, and vasopressor if needed; dopamine is preferred, norepinephrine for refractory hypotension.

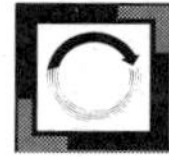

Follow-Up

PATIENT MONITORING

- Formaldehyde ingestion. Hemodynamic and respiratory function should be monitored continuously during treatment, and follow-up should include monitoring for possible stricture formation.
- Formaldehyde inhalation. Pulmonary function should be monitored continuously during treatment, and follow-up should include serial pulmonary function tests.

EXPECTED COURSE AND PROGNOSIS

- Formaldehyde ingestion is characterized by rapid onset of severe gastrointestinal effects that stabilize within hours with therapy.
- Gastrointestinal scarring, stricture, and dysfunction may occur following ingestion.
- Minor inhalational exposure resolves within hours.
- Severe inhalational exposure may lead to reactive airway disease.
- Formaldehyde hypersensitivity following toxic exposure has been reported.

DISCHARGE CRITERIA AND INSTRUCTIONS

- From the emergency department

—Formaldehyde inhalation. Asymptomatic patients with normal vital signs may be discharged 6 hours after an acute exposure.
—Formaldehyde ingestion. Asymptomatic patients who have ingested trivial amounts of low-concentration solution may be discharged following psychiatric evaluation, if needed.

- From the hospital. Patients may be discharged when toxic effects resolve or stabilize, following psychiatric evaluation, if needed.

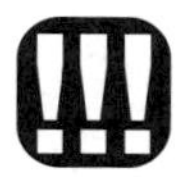

Pitfalls

FOLLOW-UP

- Hypersensitivity testing may be needed in susceptible individuals.
- The health-care provider should monitor for gastrointestinal dysfunction following ingestion.

ICD-9-CM 976

Poisoning by agents primarily affecting skin and mucous membrane, ophthalmological, otorhinolaryngological, and dental drugs.

See also: SECTION II, Caustics–Acidic and Hypotension chapters.

RECOMMENDED READING

Burge PS, Harries MG, Lam WK, et al. Occupational asthma due to formaldehyde. *Thorax* 1985;40:255–260.

Ellenhorn MJ. Antiseptics and Disinfectants. In: Ellenhorn MJ, et al., eds. *Ellenhorn's medical toxicology: diagnosis and treatment of human poisoning,* 2nd ed. Baltimore: Williams & Wilkins, 1997:1214–1217.

Gunby P. Fact or fiction about formaldehyde? *JAMA* 1980;243:1697–1703.

Author: Gerald F. O'Malley

Reviewer: Luke Yip

Freon and Fluorinated Hydrocarbons

Basics

DESCRIPTION

Fluorocarbons and fluorinated hydrocarbons are widely used as refrigerants, aerosol propellants, glass chillers, industrial solvents, and fire extinguishers.

FORMS AND USES

Compounds commonly used include bromochlorofluoromethane (BCF, Halon 1211), dibromotetrafluoroethane (Halon 2402, Fluorocarbon 114B2, CAS 124-73-2), dichlorodifluoromethane (F-12, Freon 12), trichlorofluoromethane (Fluorocarbon 11, fluorotrichloromethane, Freon 11, trichloromonofluoromethane), trichlorotrifluoroethane (Freon 13, TCTFE).

TOXIC DOSE

- Inhalation of low concentrations causes mucosal membrane irritation.
- Even brief inhalation of high concentrations can be lethal.

PATHOPHYSIOLOGY

- Most toxic exposures result from inhalation because fluorinated hydrocarbons are gases under normal conditions.
- Fluorocarbons and fluorinated hydrocarbons act as local irritants to mucous membranes and as asphyxiants causing hypoxemia.
- Following inhalation of high concentrations, alveolar membrane injury and pulmonary edema may develop.
- Hydrocarbons are thought to sensitize myocardium to endogenous catecholamines, leading to ventricular dysrhythmia.

EPIDEMIOLOGY

- Minor exposures are common.
- Toxic effects following exposure to low concentrations are typically mild.
- Death occurs following exposure to high concentrations.

CAUSES

- Poisoning is usually an occupational exposure or the result of intentional abuse.
- Low-concentration exposures are usually accidental.
- High-concentration inhalations are usually the result of intentional abuse, spills, and industrial exposures in poorly ventilated areas.
- Fluorocarbon toxicity can result from the use of fire extinguishers in closed spaces.

RISK FACTORS

The following populations are at risk for occupational exposure to fluorocarbons or fluorinated hydrocarbons: refrigerator repairers, plumbers, aerospace workers, fire fighters, and industrial workers who are exposed to fluorocarbon degreasers.

WORKPLACE STANDARDS

- Bromochlorofluoromethane. Not listed.
- Dibromoeterafluoroethane. Not listed.
- Dichlorodifluoromethane

—ACGIH TLV TWA 1000 ppm
—OSHA PEL TWA 1000 ppm
—NIOSH REL TWA 1000 ppm; IDLH 15,000 ppm.

- Trichlorofluoromethane. Not listed.
- Trichlorotrifluoroethane

—ACGIH TLV TWA 1000 ppm
—OSHA PEL TWA 1000 ppm
—NIOSH REL TWA 1000 ppm;
—STEL 1250 ppm;
—IDLH 2000 ppm.

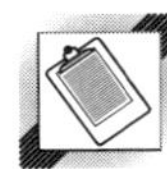

Diagnosis

DIFFERENTIAL DIAGNOSIS

- Other toxic agents that have a pulmonary irritant effect include other hydrocarbons (especially halogenated), ammonia, simple asphyxiants, carbon monoxide, hydrogen sulfide, nitrogen oxides, and pulmonary irritant gases.
- Nontoxic causes of pulmonary injury include pulmonary embolism, pneumonia, reactive airways disease, and pulmonary edema from other causes.

SIGNS AND SYMPTOMS

Pulmonary irritation is the predominant finding.

Vital Signs

Tachypnea and tachycardia are common.

HEENT

- Eye irritation and mild conjunctivitis is seen with ambient exposure.
- Corneal edema has been reported in cases involving freon application during cataract surgery.
- Nasal mucosal irritation is common.
- Frostbite of the mouth and pharynx has been reported in exposures due to intentional abuse.

Dermatologic

- Defatting, irritation, local erythema, or contact dermatitis may be seen.
- Frostbite occurs infrequently following skin exposure.
- Injection causes pain, irritation, and edema but typically little long-term tissue injury.

Pulmonary

- Respiratory irritation may cause cough, sore throat, or bronchospasm.
- Repetitive exposures increase the potential for occupational asthma.
- Pulmonary edema (which may be delayed 1 to 3 days) can occur.
- Eosinophilic pneumonia or chemical pneumonitis may develop, rarely.

Cardiovascular

Ventricular dysrhythmias and cardiac arrest may occur in high- concentration exposure.

Gastrointestinal

- Nausea or esophageal burns may result from intentional ingestion.
- Stomach necrosis has been reported following ingestion.

Hepatic

Minor transaminase elevation and jaundice may be seen following exposure to high concentrations.

Musculoskeletal

Rhabdomyolysis and compartment syndrome are rare effects of severe topical exposure.

Neurologic

- Headache, dizziness, or both are common.
- Cerebral edema has been reported following high-concentration exposure.
- Long-term occupational exposure is associated with psychomotor impairment, memory and learning deficits, and emotional lability.

PROCEDURES AND LABORATORY TESTS

Essential Tests

No tests are required following asymptomatic acute exposure.

Recommended Tests

- Patients with respiratory symptoms should undergo pulse oximetry or arterial blood gas analysis to assess oxygenation.
- ECG should be obtained in patients with tachycardia, hypotension, or chest pain.
- Carboxyhemoglobin level, methemoglobin level, and other tests (e.g., chest radiograph) as needed may be used to differentiate the cause of respiratory or cardiac effects.
- Serum electrolytes, BUN, and creatinine should be ordered as needed to assess causes of cardiac or CNS effects.
- A chest radiograph should be obtained in symptomatic patients to assess pulmonary injury or edema.

Not Recommended Tests

Serum fluorocarbon levels are not useful.

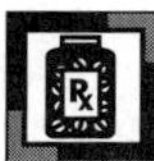

Treatment

- Treatment should focus on managing cardiopulmonary sequelae while providing supportive care and aggressive maintenance of fluid and electrolyte balance.
- Dose and time of exposure must be determined for all substances involved.

DIRECTING PATIENT COURSE

The health-care provider should call a poison control center when:

- Toxic effects develop.
- Coingestant or underlying disease presents an unusual problem.

The patient should be referred to a health-care facility when:

- Attempted suicide or homicide is possible.
- The patient or caregiver seems unreliable.
- Any toxic effects develop.
- Coingestant, drug interaction, or underlying disease presents an unusual problem.

Admission Considerations

Inpatient management is warranted for patients with a history of exposure to high concentrations of fluorocarbons, or who show evidence of cardiovascular, pulmonary, or neurologic toxicity.

DECONTAMINATION

Out of Hospital

- The patient should be removed from the area of exposure to fresh air.
- Emesis should not be induced.

In Hospital

- Following inhalation exposure, patients should receive 100% humidified oxygen, and contaminated skin and eyes should be irrigated with water.
- Gastric aspiration should be performed with a small-bore nasogastric tube for ingestion of high concentrations.
- One dose of activated charcoal (1–2 g/kg) may be administered if a substantial ingestion has occurred within the past hour or if a coingestant is involved.

ANTIDOTES

There is no specific antidote for fluorocarbon toxicity.

ADJUNCTIVE TREATMENT

- Ocular exposure should be managed with copious irrigation.
- The following considerations should be taken into account when managing dysrhythmias or conduction abnormalities:

—Seizures should be controlled and acidemia corrected.
—Ventricular dysrhythmias may be refractory to standard therapy.
—Lidocaine may be used for ventricular tachycardia or multifocal PVCs in the following dosages:
 —Adult dose, 50 to 100 mg intravenous bolus followed by infusion of 2 to 4 mg/min titrated to desired effect
 —Pediatric dose, 1 mg/kg bolus followed by infusion of 20 to 50 μg/kg/min titrated to effect
—The bolus dose may be repeated in 10 to 15 minutes.
—Bretylium 5 mg/kg may be administered intravenously over 1 minute, then 10 mg/kg may be administered over 1 minute, repeated as needed to a total of 30 mg/kg.

- Pulmonary edema should be treated with oxygen and intubation if necessary.

—Positive end-expiratory pressure or continuous positive air pressure should be added if difficulty in oxygenation develops.
—Corticosteroids have questionable benefit in the prevention of pulmonary edema.

- Bronchospasm

—Oxygen should be administered, followed by albuterol 0.15 mg/kg (maximum of 10 mg) in saline with humidified oxygen via nebulizer every 20 to 30 minutes.
—If the peak expiratory flow rate is greater than 90% after the initial dose, additional doses may not be needed.
—Response should be continually monitored.
—Methylprednisolone, 60 to 125 mg (1.0–1.5 mg/kg) may be given intravenously (children 1–2 mg/kg) every 6 to 8 hours; this may be decreased to a single daily dose and tapered.
—Initiation of prednisone, 1 to 2 mg/kg/day orally for several days, should be considered if bronchospasm persists.

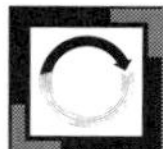

Follow-Up

PATIENT MONITORING

Cardiac and respiratory parameters should be monitored continuously.

EXPECTED COURSE AND PROGNOSIS

- Initial recovery begins within minutes once the exposure has been terminated.
- The onset of pulmonary edema may be delayed by 1 to 3 days following exposure.
- Chronic exposure can lead to impaired concentration, memory, and tremor.
- Cardiac dysrhythmias, pulmonary edema, and cerebral edema following fluorinated hydrocarbon inhalation can be fatal.

DISCHARGE CRITERIA AND INSTRUCTIONS

- From the emergency department

—Patients with normal vital signs and pulse oximetry following 6 hours of observation may be discharged.
—Patients should be instructed to return if they experience any pulmonary symptoms because even minimal respiratory symptoms are an indication for admission.

- From the hospital. Patients may be discharged after resolution of pulmonary symptoms for 24 hours.

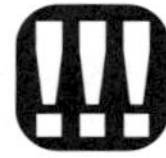

Pitfalls

DIAGNOSIS

Patients with minimal symptoms may develop pulmonary edema 12 to 24 hours after exposure.

TREATMENT

Patients with frostbite need close follow-up for wound care.

ICD-9-CM 987.4

Toxic effect of other gases, fumes, or vapors: Freon.

See also: SECTION II, Ventricular Dysrhythmias chapter.

RECOMMENDED READING

Goetting AT, Carson J, Burton BT. Freon injection injury to the hand: a report of four cases. *J Occup Med* 1992;34:775–778.

Wegener EE, Barraza KR, Das SK. Severe frostbite caused by freon gas. *South Med J* 1991;84:1143–1146.

Author: Robert Orman

Reviewer: Richard C. Dart

Gabapentin

Basics

DESCRIPTION

Gabapentin (Neurontin) is an oral anticonvulsant.

FORMS AND USES

- Gabapentin is used as adjunctive therapy in the treatment of partial complex and secondarily generalized seizure disorders.
- Typical adult dose is 300 to 600 mg orally three times daily.

TOXIC DOSE

Minimal effects have been noted with ingestions of 20 times the recommended dose.

PATHOPHYSIOLOGY

- Gabapentin is a pentamer of gamma-aminobutyric acid (GABA), an inhibitory amino acid in the CNS.
- Gabapentin primarily causes CNS depression, which resolves without sequelae unless hypoxic injury intercedes.

EPIDEMIOLOGY

Poisoning is uncommon.

CAUSES

- Toxicity typically results from therapeutic misadventure.
- Child neglect or abuse should be considered if the patient is less than 1 year of age, suicide attempt if the patient is over 6 years of age.

DRUG AND DISEASE INTERACTIONS

Toxicity of gabapentin may be increased by other CNS depressants.

PREGNANCY AND LACTATION

US FDA Pregnancy Category C. The drug exerts animal teratogenic or embryocidal effects, but there are no controlled studies in women, or no studies are available in animals or women.

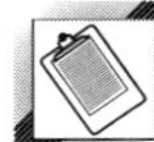

Diagnosis

DIFFERENTIAL DIAGNOSIS

Toxic causes of CNS depression include opioids, sedative-hypnotics, other anticonvulsants and many other drugs.

SIGNS AND SYMPTOMS

Vital Signs

Hypertension may develop in severe cases.

HEENT

Diplopia may develop after overdose.

Gastrointestinal

Abdominal pain and diarrhea are common.

Hematologic

Leukopenia has developed during chronic therapy.

Neurologic

- Somnolence, dizziness, ataxia, and slurred speech can occur.
- Deep coma has not been reported to date.

Genitourinary

Impotence has been reported with therapeutic doses.

PROCEDURES AND LABORATORY TESTS

Essential Tests

No tests are usually needed in asymptomatic patients.

Recommended Tests

- Blood glucose and pulse oximetry should be obtained for altered mental status.
- Complete blood count is used to monitor for leukopenia.
- Further studies should be ordered as indicated for altered mental status.
- ECG, serum acetaminophen and aspirin levels in overdose setting to detect occult ingestion.

Not Recommended Tests

Gabapentin levels are not available.

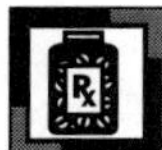

Treatment

Treatment should focus on supportive care with appropriate airway management.

DIRECTING PATIENT COURSE

The health-care professional should call the poison control center when:

- Severe or persistent effects develop.
- Coingestant, drug interaction, or underlying disease presents an unusual problem.

The patient should be referred to a health-care facility when:

- Suicide or homicide attempt is possible.
- Toxic effects develop.
- Coingestant, drug interaction, or underlying disease presents an unusual problem.

Admission Considerations

Admit patients who have persistent CNS depression following a 6-hour period.

DECONTAMINATION

Out of Hospital

Emesis should not be induced; coma or seizure may develop.

In Hospital

- Gastric lavage should be performed in pediatric (tube size 24–32 French) or adult (tube size 36–42 French) patients presenting within 1 hour of a large ingestion or if serious effects are present.
- One dose of activated charcoal (1–2 g/kg) should be administered without a cathartic if a substantial ingestion has occurred within the previous few hours.

ANTIDOTES

There is no specific antidote for gabapentin poisoning.

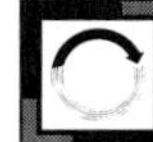

Follow-Up

PATIENT MONITORING

Cardiac and respiratory function should be monitored continuously in symptomatic patients.

EXPECTED COURSE AND PROGNOSIS

- Toxic effects typically resolve within 12 hours.
- In one case, diplopia resolved over 2 days.

DISCHARGE CRITERIA AND INSTRUCTIONS

- Patients may be discharged from the emergency department or hospital when toxic effects resolve or stabilize and after psychiatric evaluation, if needed.
- Asymptomatic patients may be discharged after decontamination and observation of 4 to 6 hours and, if needed, a psychiatric evaluation.

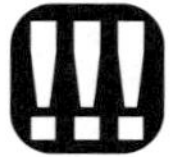

Pitfalls

DIAGNOSIS

- Coingestion of other CNS depressants would be expected to increase the toxicity of gabapentin.
- It is important to evaluate other serious causes of altered mental status.

ICD-9-CM 968

Poisoning by other central nervous system depressants and anesthetics.

RECOMMENDED READING

Fischer JH, Barr AN, Rogers SL, et al. Lack of serious toxicity following gabapentin overdose. *Neurology* 1994;44:982–983.

Garofalo E, Koto E, Feuerstein T. Experience with gabapentin overdose: five case studies. *Epilepsia* 1993;34(Suppl 2):157.

Author: Kennon Heard

Reviewer: Richard C. Dart

Gamma Hydroxybutyrate

Basics

DESCRIPTION

- Gamma hydroxybutyrate (GHB, gamma hydroxybutyric acid) is a medication that has become a popular drug of abuse.
- Precursors of GHB such as gammabutyrolactone (GBL) produce similar effects and have also become drugs of abuse.

FORMS AND USES

- Somsanit is used experimentally in the United States to treat narcolepsy; the dose for treating narcolepsy is 25 mg orally nightly, divided into two doses.
- In Europe, GHB is used as an adjunct to anesthesia and treatment of alcohol or opiate withdrawal.
- It is usually available as a white powder or clear liquid.
- Synonyms for various forms of GHB include Scoop, Somatomax PM, Sodium Oxybate, Sodium Oxybutyrate, Gamma Hydroxybutyric Sodium, Gamma-OH, 4-Hydroxy Butyrate, Gamma Hydrate, Cherry FX Bombs, Liquid X, Orange Rush, Love Potion 8.5, and Grievous Bodily Harm.

TOXIC DOSE

GHB doses over 50 mg/kg have been reported to cause coma and seizures.

PATHOPHYSIOLOGY

- GHB, an analog of gamma-aminobutyric acid, is an endogenous compound found in CNS areas that mediate sleep, temperature, memory, and emotion.
- GHB increases growth hormone release in rats, however, increased muscle mass or growth has not been demonstrated in humans.

EPIDEMIOLOGY

- GHB poisoning is increasingly common.
- GHB has been used by body builders, at "rave" parties, and as a "date rape" drug.
- Most cases that come to medical attention involve moderate toxicity, with death occurring rarely, usually before a health-care facility is reached.

CAUSES

- GHB poisoning usually results from intentional misuse.
- Due to rapid onset of CNS depression, GHB has been implicated as a date rape drug.
- Child neglect should be considered if the patient is under 1 year of age, attempted suicide if the patient is over 6 years of age.

DRUG AND DISEASE INTERACTIONS

The CNS and respiratory depression of GHB are enhanced by other depressant drugs (ethanol, opiates, benzodiazepines, barbiturates, etc.).

PREGNANCY AND LACTATION

- GHB crosses the placenta, but little data on humans are available.
- The use of GHB for obstetric anesthesia resulted in a 12% rate of poor fetal condition at birth in one study.
- Increased uterine contractions were also reported following obstetric anesthesia with GHB.

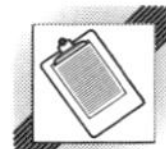

Diagnosis

DIFFERENTIAL DIAGNOSIS

- Other toxic agents that cause respiratory and CNS depression include narcotics, benzodiazepines, alcohols, barbiturates, sedative-hypnotic drugs, and tricyclic antidepressants, among others.
- Nontoxic causes of respiratory and CNS depression include hypoxia, severe electrolyte abnormality, hypoglycemia, intracranial event, meningitis, encephalitis, postictal state, and many others.

SIGNS AND SYMPTOMS

Overdose typically features CNS and respiratory depression that may be profound.

Vital Signs

- Bradypnea is typical of GHB poisoning.
- Bradycardia and hypotension occur at rest, but stimulation of the patient may provoke tachycardia and hypertension.
- Environmental hypothermia may occur due to coma.

Pulmonary

- Respiratory depression may progress to apnea rapidly.
- Aspiration pneumonia may occur.

Cardiovascular

- Chest tightness has been reported.
- Atrioventricular block has been reported.

Gastrointestinal

Nausea, vomiting, and diarrhea may occur immediately following GHB use.

Renal

Urinary urgency and incontinence have been reported.

Fluids and Electrolytes

Metabolic acidosis from seizures or agitation may occur.

Neurologic

- CNS depression with lethargy, ataxia, hypotonia and coma develop rapidly and typically resolve within several hours.
- Amnesia, dizziness, uncontrollable shaking, hallucinations, euphoria, and headaches also have been reported.
- Seizures and myoclonic movements may occur, particularly with high doses.
- Stimulation of the patient by maneuvers such as intubation often produces dramatic agitation and struggling (sometimes described as a "drowning swimmer").

PROCEDURES AND LABORATORY TESTS

Essential Tests

- All patients with altered mental status should have blood glucose determined.
- Pulse oximetry should be performed to assess oxygenation.

Recommended Tests

- Serum electrolytes, BUN, and creatinine should be obtained in patients to assess renal injury and altered mental status.
- ECG, serum acetaminophen, aspirin, and ethanol levels should be obtained in overdose settings to detect occult ingestion (note that GHB is not commonly available in toxicologic screening tests).
- Urinalysis and serum creatine kinase should be performed if the patient is comatose, to evaluate for rhabdomyolysis.
- Chest radiographs, head CT, and lumbar puncture should be performed as needed to evaluate respiratory complications and assess other causes of CNS depression particularly if CNS depression persist more than 4 hours.

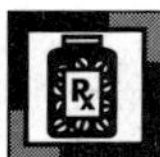

Treatment

• Therapy should focus on appropriate airway and seizure management.
• Dose and time of exposure must be determined for all substances involved.

DIRECTING PATIENT COURSE

The health-care provider should call a poison control center when:

• Life-threatening effects such as respiratory or cardiovascular collapse or seizures are present.
• Signs and symptoms are not consistent with GHB poisoning.
• Coingestant, drug interaction, or underlying disease presents an unusual problem.

The patient should be referred to a health-care facility when:

• Attempted suicide or homicide is possible.
• The patient or caregiver seems unreliable.
• Any toxic effects develop.
• Coingestant, drug interaction, or underlying disease presents an unusual problem.

Admission Considerations

Inpatient management is warranted for patients with hemodynamic instability or when symptoms do not resolve within 6 hours.

DECONTAMINATION

Out of Hospital

Emesis should not be induced because deterioration may follow rapidly.

In Hospital

• Gastric lavage should be performed in pediatric (tube size 24–32 French) or adult (tube size 36–42 French) patients who have ingested substantial amounts of GHB and present within 1 hour of ingestion or exhibit serious toxic effects.
• One dose of activated charcoal (1–2 g/kg) may be administered if a substantial ingestion has occurred within the previous few hours.

Antidote

There is no specific antidote for GHB poisoning.

ADJUNCTIVE TREATMENT

• Hypotension is treated with isotonic fluid infusion, the Trendelenburg position, and vasopressor if needed; dopamine is preferred, and norepinephrine may be administered for refractory hypotension.
• Seizures

—Patent airway must be ensured.
—A benzodiazepine should be administered for initial control.
—If seizures persist or recur, another anticonvulsant such as phenobarbital may be added.

• Coma. Flumazenil and naloxone are not recommended because they have not been demonstrated to reliably reverse GHB-induced coma.

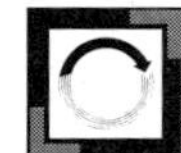

Follow-Up

PATIENT MONITORING

Patients should receive continuous respiratory and hemodynamic monitoring.

EXPECTED COURSE AND PROGNOSIS

• GHB toxicity may develop within 15 to 30 minutes and usually resolves within 6 hours.
• Patients who avoid sequelae from apnea are expected to recover fully.
• In fact, many patients recover and extubate themselves in the emergency department.
• Recovery may be prolonged up to 96 hours following severe overdose.

DISCHARGE CRITERIA AND INSTRUCTIONS

• From the emergency department. Patients who are asymptomatic after decontamination and observation for 6 hours may be discharged after psychiatric evaluation, if needed.
• From the hospital. Patients may be discharged when complications resolve or stabilize, and after psychiatric evaluation, if needed.

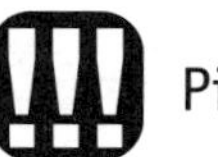

Pitfalls

DIAGNOSIS

GHB toxicity may resemble many other conditions, including many nontoxicologic causes of the same signs and symptoms.

TREATMENT

Because of agitation during intubation, rapid sequence induction may be required for successful endotracheal intubation.

FOLLOW-UP

Police evaluation or psychiatric counseling for suspected foul play (e.g., date rape) or suicidal ideation may be needed.

ICD-9-CM 968

Poisoning by other central nervous system depressants and anesthetics.

See also: SECTION II, Hypotension and Seizures chapters.

RECOMMENDED READING

Gamma hydroxybutyrate use—New York and Texas 1995–1996. *MMWR* 1997;46:281–283.

Authors: Lada Kokan and Kennon Heard

Reviewer: Richard C. Dart

Gila Monster

Basics

DESCRIPTION

- Two species of similar poisonous lizards are found on the North American continent: the Mexican beaded lizard (*Heloderma horridum*) and the Gila monster (*Heloderma suspectum*).
- Gila monsters are large (30–60 cm in length), stout, slow-moving, and nocturnal animals that feed on small mammals and the eggs of birds and other reptiles.
- Wild populations of Gila monsters are protected in the United States.

TOXIC DOSE

Brief bites rarely produce clinically important toxicity. If the Gila monster holds on, however, symptomatic envenomation is common.

PATHOPHYSIOLOGY

- Venom is as potent as rattlesnake venom, but the injection apparatus is much less effective.
- Venom is delivered to the base of specialized lower-jaw teeth and is drawn upward within dental grooves via capillary action.
- Due to the inefficient mechanism, Gila monsters hold onto the victim for a prolonged period and they are often difficult to remove.

EPIDEMIOLOGY

- Nearly all bites are the consequence of handling of a captive or confined Gila monster.
- No deaths have been reported solely from Gila monster envenomation.

CAUSES

Child neglect should be considered if the patient is less than 1 year of age.

PREGNANCY AND LACTATION

No bites in pregnant women have been reported.

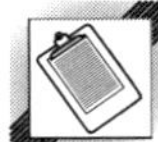

Diagnosis

SIGNS AND SYMPTOMS

Vital Signs

- After envenomation, the patient may appear diaphoretic and complain of weakness and lightheadedness.
- Hypotension and tachycardia are common.
- Hypertension soon after envenomation also has been described.

Dermatologic

- The bite usually causes multiple, small puncture wounds (2–18 in number).
- Small teeth or pieces of fractured teeth may be found in the wound.
- After envenomation, edema at the bite site may begin within 15 minutes of the bite and then progresses slowly over the next 4 to 8 hours.

Cardiovascular

ECG abnormalities, including acute myocardial infarction, have been reported in two cases.

Gastrointestinal

Nausea and vomiting may occur.

Hematologic

One case of coagulopathy has been reported.

Neurologic

- If envenomation has occurred, pain increases at the bite site, peaks in 15 to 45 minutes, and resolves over several hours.
- Pain is out of proportion to the trauma inflicted; it has been described as violent, excruciating, and burning.

Lymphatic

Tender lymphadenopathy and lymphangitis may develop.

PROCEDURES AND LABORATORY TESTS

Essential Tests

No tests are usually needed in asymptomatic or minimally symptomatic patients.

Recommended Tests

- ECG may indicate myocardial ischemia.
- Soft-tissue radiographs of the bite area may help identify teeth left in the wound.
- Wound cultures may be needed if signs of infection develop.

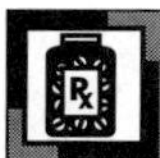

Treatment

Treatment should focus on removal of the animal and general supportive care.

DIRECTING PATIENT COURSE

The health-care professional should call the poison control center when:

- Severe or persistent effects develop.
- Coingestant, drug interaction, or underlying disease presents an unusual problem.

The patient should be referred to a health-care facility when:

- Toxic effects develop.
- Coingestant, drug interaction, or underlying disease presents an unusual problem.

Admission Considerations

Patients who develop persistent pain and swelling or systemic signs of toxicity should be admitted.

DECONTAMINATION

- The Gila monster must be removed from the victim. Several of the less dangerous methods proposed include:
- Immersion in cold water
- Placing a stick, crowbar, or pliers into the mouth to pry open the jaws
- Placing the Gila monster on a solid surface (it may release its grip if no longer suspended in mid-air)
- Applying a flame to the underside of its chin

After removal, the bite site should be cleaned and irrigated as any laceration.

ADJUNCTIVE TREATMENT

- Parenteral analgesia is usually required.
- Local wound care includes copious irrigation, gentle debridement if necessary, and exploration for foreign bodies.
- Tetanus prophylaxis should be provided if immunization status is not current.
- Hypotension usually responds to crystalloid resuscitation.
- Antibiotics are warranted if cellulitis or wound infection develops.

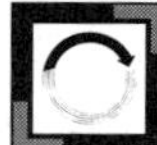

Follow-Up

PATIENT MONITORING

- Respiratory and cardiac function should be monitored continuously.
- At least 6 hours of observation is recommended in order to assess potential systemic toxicity accurately.

EXPECTED COURSE AND PROGNOSIS

Most patients can be discharged home the same day with appropriate follow-up.

DISCHARGE CRITERIA AND INSTRUCTIONS

Patients without evidence of systemic toxicity may be discharged from the emergency department or hospital after at least 6 hours of observation, when the patient returns to normal cardiovascular and neurologic status, and there is no evidence of compromised neurovascular supply of affected limb.

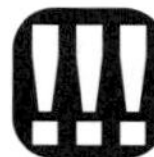

Pitfalls

DIAGNOSIS

Because teeth may not be visible on the radiograph, it is important to explore the wound adequately.

ICD-CM-9 989.5

See also: SECTION II, Hypotension chapter.

RECOMMENDED READING

Hooker KR, Caravati EM. Gila monster envenomation. *Ann Emerg Med* 1994;24:731–735.

Author: Bill Sevcik

Reviewer: Richard C. Dart

Glycopyrrolate

Basics

DESCRIPTION

Glycopyrrolate (Robinul, Robinul Forte) is an anticholinergic agent used as a premedication for anesthesia and bronchoscopy, as an adjunct in the treatment of peptic ulcer disease, and in the management of reactive airway disease.

FORMS AND USES

- The usual oral dose is 1 to 2 mg three times a day.
- The parenteral preparation may be used by nebulization in a dose of 0.4 to 0.8 mg for exacerbation of reactive airway disease.

TOXIC DOSE

Variable. Depends on individual patient and symptom complex. A therapeutic dose has been associated with central anticholinergic effects.

PATHOPHYSIOLOGY

- Glycopyrrolate is a synthetic antimuscarinic agent that has vagolytic activity. It is an effective antisalivation agent.
- Anticholinergic effects may persist for 8 to 12 hours, even in therapeutic doses.
- Although glycopyrrolate does not cross the blood-brain barrier, central anticholinergic symptoms have been described.

EPIDEMIOLOGY

Poisoning is uncommon.

CAUSES

Overdose is likely to be iatrogenic.

DRUG AND DISEASE INTERACTIONS

- Glycopyrrolate has additive effects with other anticholinergic agents.
- Cardiac dysrhythmias have been reported with the combination of glycopyrrolate and several compounds, including marijuana, ritodrine, and certain anesthetic agents.

PREGNANCY AND LACTATION

US FDA Pregnancy Category B. Animal studies indicate no fetal risk and there are no controlled human studies, or animal studies show an adverse fetal effect but well-controlled studies in women do not.

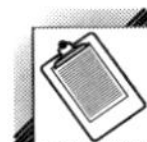

Diagnosis

DIFFERENTIAL DIAGNOSIS

Other toxic causes of anticholinergic syndrome include atropine, antihistamines, jimson weed, and many others.

SIGNS AND SYMPTOMS

Glycopyrrolate causes rapid onset of anticholinergic syndrome.

Vital Signs

Fever and tachycardia.

HEENT

Mydriasis and dry mucous membranes.

Dermatologic

Skin is warm, dry, and flushed.

Renal

Urinary retention.

Neurologic

Confusion, agitation, hallucinosis and, in severe cases, seizures and psychosis.

PROCEDURES AND LABORATORY TESTS

Essential Tests

No specific laboratory tests are necessary in minimally symptomatic patients.

Recommended Tests

- ECG monitoring, electrolytes, glucose, renal functions, complete blood count, and arterial blood gases should be obtained in symptomatic patients.
- Serum acetaminophen and aspirin levels should be determined in overdose setting to detect occult ingestion.
- Physostigmine may be used as a diagnostic agent.

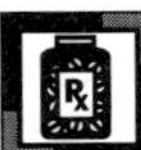

Treatment

- Treatment should focus on symptomatic and supportive care.
- The dose and time of exposure must be determined for all substances involved.
- Patients demonstrating dysrhythmias, mental status changes, or confusing symptoms and signs should be referred to a toxicologist.

DIRECTING PATIENT COURSE

The health-care professional should call the poison control center when:

- Severe or persistent effects develop.
- Coingestant, drug interaction, or underlying disease presents an unusual problem.

The patient should be referred to a health-care facility when:

- Suicide or homicide attempt is possible.
- Toxic effects develop.
- Coingestant, drug interaction, or underlying disease presents an unusual problem.

Admission Considerations

- Any patient with mental status changes requires ICU admission.
- Minimally symptomatic patients may only require decontamination and observation.
- Because symptoms may last for 12 to 24 hours, prolonged observation may be required.

DECONTAMINATION

Out of Hospital

Emesis should be induced with ipecac within 1 hour of ingestion for alert pediatric or adult patients, if medical care will be delayed.

In Hospital

- Gastric lavage should be performed in pediatric (tube size 24–32 French) or adult (tube size 36–42 French) patients presenting within 1 hour of a large ingestion or if serious effects are present.
- One dose of activated charcoal (1–2 g/kg) should be administered without a cathartic if a substantial ingestion has occurred within the previous few hours.
- Both procedures may be effective longer after ingestion than usual due to anticholinergic effects.

ANTIDOTES

There is no specific antidote to glycopyrrolate.

ADJUNCTIVE TREATMENT

- Phenothiazines should be avoided because of their anticholinergic effects and potential to cause seizures.
- Seizures are treated initially with benzodiazepines, followed by phenobarbital, if needed.
- Sinus tachycardia will often respond to benzodiazepines.
- Ventricular dysrhythmias should be treated with lidocaine.
- Hyperthermia is treated in the standard manner with external cooling measures.
- CNS agitation and hallucinosis. The patient should be sedated with benzodiazepines.
- Urinary retention may require catheterization.
- For symptomatic mydriasis, ocular pilocarpine may be used.

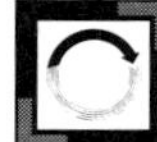

Follow-Up

PATIENT MONITORING

Symptomatic patients require cardiac monitoring, pulse oximetry, and supervision to prevent self-harm.

EXPECTED COURSE AND PROGNOSIS

Most patients recover over 24 hours with supportive care.

DISCHARGE CRITERIA AND INSTRUCTIONS

Patients may be discharged from the emergency department or hospital after central and peripheral anticholinergic effects have resolved, after decontamination has been performed, and after a psychiatric evaluation, if needed.

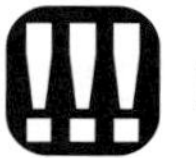

Pitfalls

TREATMENT

- Physostigmine use in the face of tricyclic antidepressant coingestion pay precipitate seizures.
- Anticholinergic agents slow gastrointestinal motility and may prolong absorption.

ICD-9-CM 971.1

Poisoning by drugs affecting the autonomic nervous system: parasympatholytics (anticholinergics and antimuscarinics) and spasmolytics.

See also: SECTION II, Anticholinergic Syndrome, Hyperthermia, Seizures, and Ventricular Dysrhythmias chapters; and SECTION III, Physostigmine chapter.

RECOMMENDED READING

Grum DF, Osborne LR. Central anticholinergic syndrome following glycopyrrolate. *Anesthesiology* 1991;74:191–193.

Author: Steven A. Seifert

Reviewer: Gerald O'Malley

Basics

DESCRIPTION

Gold compounds are anti-inflammatory medications used orally and parenterally in the treatment of rheumatoid arthritis.

FORMS AND USES

Therapeutic forms of gold include auranofin (Ridaura), gold thiopolypeptide (GTPP), gold sodium thioglucose (Solganal), gold sodium thiomalate (Myochrysine), gold thiosulfate (Sanocrysin), and gold thioglycanide.

TOXIC DOSE

For unknown reasons, there is little correlation between the cumulative dose of a gold compound and clinical toxicity.

PATHOPHYSIOLOGY

- Gold compounds inhibit the activity of enzymes in lysosomes, but the full mechanism of action is unknown.
- Toxicity results from bone marrow suppression and may form immune complexes.

EPIDEMIOLOGY

Poisoning is uncommon.

CAUSES

- Toxicity is usually an adverse drug reaction during therapeutic use.
- Child neglect or abuse should be considered if the patient is less than 1 year of age, suicide attempt if the patient is over 6 years of age.

PREGNANCY AND LACTATION

US FDA Pregnancy Category C. The drug exerts animal teratogenic or embryocidal effects, but there are no controlled studies in women, or no studies are available in animals or women.

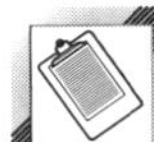

Diagnosis

DIFFERENTIAL DIAGNOSIS

Other causes of mucous membrane inflammation include colchicine and several antineoplastic drugs.

SIGNS AND SYMPTOMS

HEENT

- Stomatitis is the second most commonly observed reaction.
- Glossitis, gingivitis, keratitis, and corneal deposits have been noted.

Dermatologic

- Nonspecific dermatitis is the most common toxic effect.
- Alopecia also occurs.

Cardiovascular

- Peripheral vasodilation may produce syncope and hypotension.
- In one case, ventricular tachycardia occurred after acute ingestion.

Pulmonary

Interstitial pneumonitis and fibrosis have occurred during chronic use.

Gastrointestinal

Diarrhea, enteritis, and colitis are common effects.

Hepatic

Hepatitis and cholestasis develop rarely.

Renal

- Nephrotic proteinuria is not an uncommon effect.
- Nephritis occurs less commonly.

Hematologic

- Eosinophilia is the most common abnormality.
- Thrombocytopenia is also common and may occur months after the last dose.
- Granulocytopenia may develop.
- Aplastic anemia occurs rarely.

Neurologic

Toxicity occurs rarely and includes Guillain-Barré syndrome, encephalopathy, and stroke.

PROCEDURES AND LABORATORY TESTS

Essential Tests

Complete blood count and urinalysis should be obtained throughout therapy to evaluate hematopoietic effects of exposure.

Recommended Tests

- Creatinine and BUN should be obtained to evaluate renal injury.
- Liver function tests are used to monitor for possible hepatic and cholestatic effects.

Not Recommended Tests

Serum levels of gold are highly variable and do not correlate well with toxic reactions.

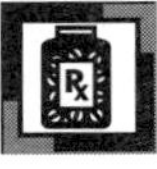

Treatment

- Treatment should focus on termination of drug exposure followed by general symptomatic care.
- Discontinuation of the drug is usually sufficient to reverse mild toxicity.

DIRECTING PATIENT COURSE

The health-care professional should call the poison control center when:

- Severe or persistent effects develop.
- Toxic effects are not consistent with gold toxicity.
- Coingestant, drug interaction, or underlying disease presents an unusual problem.

The patient should be referred to a health-care facility when:

- Suicide or homicide attempt is possible.
- Toxic effects develop.
- Coingestant, drug interaction, or underlying disease presents an unusual problem.

Admission Considerations

Patients with acute toxicity, or those with chronic toxicity causing clinically significant bone marrow depression, should be admitted.

DECONTAMINATION

Out of Hospital

Emesis should be induced with ipecac within 1 hour of ingestion for either pediatric or adult patients, if health-care evaluation will be delayed.

In Hospital

- Gastric lavage should be performed in pediatric (tube size 24–32 French) or adult (tube size 36–42 French) patients presenting within 1 hour of a large ingestion or if serious effects are present.
- Administration of activated charcoal also may be useful, especially if a coingestant may be involved.

—One dose (1–2 g/kg) should be administered without a cathartic if a substantial ingestion has occurred within the previous few hours.
—Metallic gold is poorly absorbed by charcoal, and its effectiveness is unknown.

ANTIDOTES

Chelation can be achieved with the following substances, which all require 10 to 14 days of therapy. See individual chapters for further details of chelator administration.

- Dimercaprol (British anti-Lewisite) is the most commonly used chelation agent but may produce hypertension, fever, and urticaria.
- D-penicillamine increases urinary excretion but cannot be used in penicillin-allergic or pregnant patients and may produce multiple side-effects.
- *N*-acetylcysteine also enhances excretion.

ADJUNCTIVE TREATMENT

- Hemodialysis is not effective.
- Immunosuppressive therapy using cyclophosphamide and prednisone has been used for bone marrow toxicity.

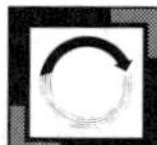

Follow-Up

PATIENT MONITORING

Serial laboratory studies should be obtained to confirm reversal of toxicity.

EXPECTED COURSE AND PROGNOSIS

- The slow absorption and elimination of gold compounds requires patients to be treated beyond their acute presentation.
- Chelation agents require 1 to 2 weeks of therapy to eliminate gold effectively.
- Immunosuppressive therapy may require weeks to reverse hematopoietic effects.

DISCHARGE CRITERIA/INSTRUCTIONS

Patients may be discharged from the emergency department or hospital when toxic effects resolve or stabilize and after psychiatric evaluation, if needed.

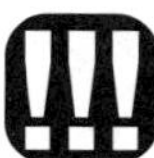

Pitfalls

TREATMENT

- Bone marrow function must be monitored closely and suppression may be refractory to therapy.
- Treatment must extend beyond the initial episode.

ICD-9-CM 961.2

Poisoning by antiinfectives: heavy metal antiinfectives.

See also: SECTION III, British Antilewisite and penicillamine chapters.

RECOMMENDED READING

Felson DT, et al. The comparative efficacy and toxicity of second-line drugs in rheumatoid arthritis; results of two metaanalyses. *Arthritis Rheum* 1990;33:1449–1461.

Schumacher HR, ed. *Primer on the rheumatic diseases,* 9th ed. Atlanta: The Arthritis Foundation, 1995.

Author: John P. Marshall

Reviewer: Richard C. Dart

Griseofulvin

Basics

DESCRIPTION

Griseofulvin is an oral antifungal medication.

FORMS AND USES

- Griseofulvin is available as Gris-PEG, Grisown, Fulvicin P/G, Grifulvin, and Grisactin.
- Uses include treatment of fungal infections (*Trichophyton, Microsporum* and *Epidermophyton* species) of the skin, hair, and nails.
- Therapeutic dosages are 500 mg to 1 g/day for adults and 10 to 20 mg/kg/day for children.

TOXIC DOSE

The toxic dose has not been established. Large doses would be expected to be tolerated well.

EPIDEMIOLOGY

Poisoning is uncommon.

CAUSES

Child neglect or abuse should be considered if the patient is less than 1 year of age, suicide attempt if the patient is over 6 years of age.

DRUG AND DISEASE INTERACTIONS

- Decreased warfarin activity
- Disulfiram-like reaction with ethanol
- Decreased estrogenic effect of birth control pills, decreasing reliability of contraception, and irregular menses

PREGNANCY AND LACTATION

U.S. FDA category C. Animal studies indicate no fetal risk and there are no controlled human studies, or animal studies show adverse fetal effect, but well-controlled studies in women do not.

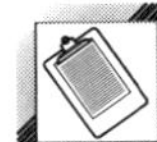

Diagnosis

SIGNS AND SYMPTOMS

Rare hypersensitivity reactions are the primary adverse effects and include photosensitivity and exacerbation of lupus erythematosus.

Dermatologic

Epidermal necrolysis, urticaria, angioneurotic edema, and other skin rashes.

Gastrointestinal

Nausea, vomiting, and diarrhea.

Hepatic

Hepatic toxicity.

Renal

Proteinuria.

Hematologic

Porphyria and leukopenia, in some reports.

Neurologic

Headache, mental fatigue, vertigo, blurred vision, and peripheral paresthesia.

PROCEDURES AND LABORATORY TESTS

Essential Tests

No tests are usually needed in asymptomatic patients.

Recommended Tests

- Complete blood count, renal function, and hepatic function tests may be useful in symptomatic patients.
- ECG, serum acetaminophen, and aspirin levels in overdose setting to detect occult ingestion.

Not Recommended Tests

Plasma levels are not available or helpful.

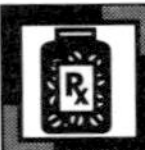

Treatment

- Treatment should focus on symptomatic and supportive care.
- Dose and time of exposure should be determined for all substances involved.

DIRECTING PATIENT COURSE

The health-care professional should call the poison control center when:

- Severe or persistent effects develop.
- Coingestant, drug interaction, or underlying disease presents an unusual problem.

The patient should be referred to a health-care facility when:

- Suicide or homicide is possible.
- Toxic effects develop.
- Coingestant, drug interaction, or underlying disease presents an unusual problem.

DECONTAMINATION

Out of Hospital

Ipecac should be administered to induce emesis within 1 hour of large ingestion for alert pediatric or adult patient if health-care evaluation will be delayed.

Admission Considerations

Patients with persistent effects should be admitted.

In Hospital

- Gastric lavage should be performed in pediatric (tube size 24–32 French) or adult (tube size 36–42 French) patients presenting within 1 hour of a large ingestion or if serious effects are present.
- One dose of activated charcoal (1–2 g/kg) should be administered without a cathartic if a substantial ingestion has occurred within the previous few hours.

ANTIDOTES

There is no specific antidote for griseofulvin poisoning.

ADJUNCTIVE THERAPY

Discontinuation of griseofulvin therapy and symptomatic care of gastrointestinal and dermal effects.

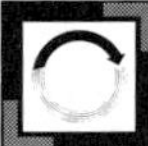

Follow-Up

PATIENT MONITORING

Complete blood count as well as renal and hepatic function tests should be monitored in symptomatic patients.

EXPECTED COURSE AND PROGNOSIS

Effects of acute ingestion resolve over several hours.

DISCHARGE CRITERIA/INSTRUCTIONS

Patients may be discharged from the emergency department or hospital after acute effects resolve, decontamination is complete, and psychiatric evaluation has been performed, if needed.

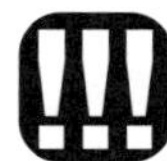

Pitfalls

DIAGNOSIS

Certain assays of vanillylmandelic acid may be falsely elevated in patients on griseofulvin.

ICD-9-CM 960.1

Poisoning by antibiotics: antifungal antibiotics.

RECOMMENDED READING

Feinstein A, Sofer E, Trau H, et al. Urticaria and fixed drug eruption in a patient treated with griseofulvin. *J Am Acad Dermatol* 1984;10:915–917.

Mion G, Verdon R, Le Gulluche Y, et al. Fatal toxic epidermal necrolysis after griseofulvin [Letter]. *Lancet* 1989;2:1331.

Author: Steven A. Seifert

Reviewer: Richard C. Dart

Guaifenesin

Basics

DESCRIPTION

Guaifenesin is an oral expectorant used in the treatment of cough.

FORMS AND USES

- Guaifenesin is available as Anti-Tuss, Breonesin, Diabetic Tussin Ex, Fenesin, Gee-Gee, Genatuss, GG-Cen, Glyate, Glycotuss, Glytuss, Guia-Cough Expectorant, Guiatuss, Halotussin, Humibid LA, Humibid Sprinkle, Hytuss, Luquibid, Malotuss, Medi-Tuss, Mytussin, Naldecon Senior EX, pneumomist, Respa-GF, Robitussin, Scot-Tussin, Silutussin, Sinumist-SR Capsulets, TouroEx, and Uni-Tussin.
- Many products contain alcohol, dextromethorphan, or opioids in addition to guaifenesin.

TOXIC DOSE

The toxic dose for guaifenesin alone is unknown, but it is very high.

PATHOPHYSIOLOGY

Guaifenesin acts by stimulating respiratory tract secretions.

PREGNANCY

US FDA Pregnancy Category C. The drug exerts animal teratogenic or embryocidal effects, but there are no controlled studies in women, or no studies are available in animals or women.

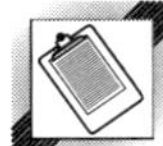

Diagnosis

DIFFERENTIAL DIAGNOSIS

Other toxic causes of CNS depression include opioids, ethanol and many other agents.

SIGNS AND SYMPTOMS

Nausea, vomiting and lethargy may be observed. In severe cases, depression and coma may develop.

LABORATORY TESTS

Essential Tests

- No tests may be needed for asymptomatic patients.
- Serum electrolytes, BUN, glucose and creatinine are ordered to assess causes of altered mental status.
- ECG, serum acetaminophen and aspirin levels should be determined to detect occult overdose.

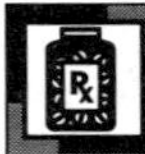

Treatment

- Treatment should focus on decontamination and supportive care of respiration.
- Dose and time of ingestion must be determined for all substances involved.

DIRECTING PATIENT COURSE

The health-care professional should call the poison control center when:

- Toxic effects are not consistent with gold toxicity.
- Coingestant, drug interaction, or underlying disease presents an unusual problem.

The patient should be referred to a health-care facility when:

- Suicide or homicide attempt is possible.
- Coingestant, drug interaction, or underlying disease presents an unusual problem.

DECONTAMINATION

Out of Hospital

Emesis need not be induced unless toxic coingestant is present.

In Hospital

- Emesis should not be induced.
- Gastric lavage would not be expected to be helfpul, because these products are typically liquids.
- One dose of activated charcoal (1–2 g/kg) should be considered if a substantial ingestion has occurred within the past hour.

ANTIDOTES

There is no specific antidote for guaifenesin poisoning.

ADJUNCTIVE TREATMENT

General supportive care is provided.

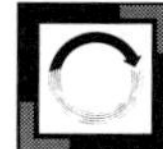

Follow-Up

PATIENT MONITORING

In severe cases, heart rate, blood pressure, ECG, serum electrolytes, arterial blood gases, and serum creatinine should be monitored.

EXPECTED COURSE AND PROGNOSIS

Symptoms rarely appear unless large amounts are ingested. Prognosis is excellent, and recovery is expected within 24 hours with supportive treatment.

DISCHARGE CRITERIA/INSTRUCTIONS

Patients may be discharged from the emergency department or hospital provided they do not develop symptoms of toxicity after 6 hours of observation and have undergone a psychiatric evaluation, if needed.

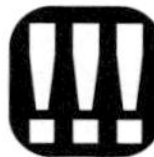

Pitfalls

Guaifenesin-containing products often also contain alcohol, dextromethorphan, or opioids.

ICD-9-CM 976

Poisoning by agents primarily affecting skin and mucous membrane: ophthalmologic, otorhinolaryngologic, and dental drugs.

Author: Kevin M. Lier

Reviewer: Richard C. Dart

Guanabenz

Basics

DESCRIPTION

Guanabenz (Wytensin) is an oral antihypertensive drug.

FORMS AND USES

The usual therapeutic dose in adults is 4 mg twice a day, increased each week by 4 to 8 mg per day to a maximum of 32 to 96 mg twice a day.

TOXIC DOSE

- Ingestion of more than 1 to 2 mg/kg may be associated with toxicity.

PATHOPHYSIOLOGY

- Similar to clonidine, guanabenz is a central α_2 agonist.
- Similar to guanethidine, guanabenz is an inhibitor of postganglionic peripheral adrenergic neurons.

EPIDEMIOLOGY

Poisoning is uncommon.

CAUSES

- Toxicity usually results from intentional ingestion.
- Child neglect or abuse should be considered if the patient is less than 1 year of age, suicide attempt if the patient is over 6 years of age.

DRUG AND DISEASE INTERACTIONS

Other hypotensive agents would be expected to exacerbate hypotensive effects.

PREGNANCY AND LACTATION

US FDA Pregnancy Category C. The drug exerts animal teratogenic or embryocidal effects, but there are no controlled studies in women, or no studies are available in animals or women.

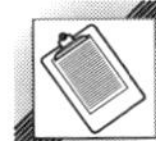

Diagnosis

DIFFERENTIAL DIAGNOSIS

Toxicologic causes of hypotension, respiratory depression, and small pupils include other α-adrenergic agonists (clonidine), all types of narcotics, imidazoline derivatives, and olanzapine, among others.

SIGNS AND SYMPTOMS

Vital Signs

- Bradycardia and hypotension may develop following acute overdose.
- Orthostatic hypotension is common.

HEENT

Miosis may occur following acute overdose.

Cardiovascular

Transient hypertension shortly after ingestion of large acute overdose has been reported, but is rare.

Pulmonary

Decreased respiratory effort and apnea following acute overdose have been reported; they usually respond to tactile stimulation.

Gastrointestinal

Nausea and vomiting are common.

Neurologic

- CNS depression progressing to coma has been reported following acute overdose.
- Sedation is common during chronic therapy.

PROCEDURES AND LABORATORY TESTS

Essential Tests

Laboratory testing may not be needed in asymptomatic patients.

Recommended Tests

- Serum electrolytes, BUN, creatinine, and complete blood count are indicated in symptomatic patients to assess other causes of hypotension and altered mental status.
- Pulse oximetry or arterial blood gases are used to assess respiratory depression.
- ECG, serum acetaminophen and aspirin levels in overdose setting to detect occult ingestion.
- Head CT and/or lumbar puncture cultures may be needed to assess altered mental status.

Not Recommended Tests

Guanabenz plasma levels are not clinically useful.

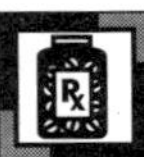

Treatment

- Treatment should focus on airway management and blood pressure support.
- The dose and time of exposure should be determined for all substances involved.

DIRECTING PATIENT COURSE

The health-care professional should call the poison control center when:

- Severe or persistent effects develop.
- Coingestant, drug interaction, or underlying disease presents an unusual problem.

The patient should be referred to a health-care facility when:

- Attempted suicide or homicide are possible.
- The patient or caregiver seems unreliable.
- Toxic effects develop.
- Coingestant, drug interaction, or underlying disease presents an unusual problem.

Admission Considerations

- Inpatient management is warranted for patients who develop bradycardia, respiratory depression, or hypotension.
- Because hypotensive effects can be delayed, admission should be considered for asymptomatic patients following large intentional ingestion for 12 to 24 hours of observation.

DECONTAMINATION

Out of Hospital

Emesis should not be induced.

In Hospital

- Gastric lavage should be performed in pediatric (tube size 24–32 French) or adult (tube size 36–42 French) patients presenting within 1 hour of a large ingestion or if serious effects are present.
- One dose of activated charcoal (1–2 g/kg) should be administered without a cathartic if a substantial ingestion has occurred within the previous few hours.

ANTIDOTES

There is no specific antidote for guanabenz poisoning.

ADJUNCTIVE TREATMENT

- Naloxone in standard doses may be effective in reducing CNS depression.
- Patients who are unable to protect their airway must be intubated.
- Hypotension should be treated with an intravenous crystalloid infusion and placement of the patient in the Trendelenburg position. A vasopressor should be added if needed.
- Bradycardia is initially treated with atropine. Symptomatic bradycardia that does not respond to atropine may require cardiac pacing.

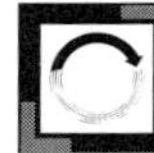

Follow-Up

PATIENT MONITORING

Cardiac and hemodynamic status should be monitored continuously.

EXPECTED COURSE AND PROGNOSIS

- Toxic effects usually develop within hours and resolve over 24 to 48 hours if effects of hypoxia intercede.
- However, hypotension may be delayed 12 to 24 hours.

DISCHARGE CRITERIA AND INSTRUCTIONS

- From the emergency department

—Asymptomatic patients may be discharged if they have no documented CNS or cardiovascular abnormality for at least 4 to 6 hours postingestion.
—Patients with large ingestion should be monitored 12 to 24 hours.

- From the hospital. Patient may be discharged when toxic effects have resolved or following 12 to 24 hour observation period.

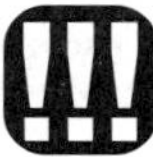

Pitfalls

DIAGNOSIS

Guanabenz toxicity may be confused with opioid effects.

ICD-9-CM 972.6

Poisoning by agents primarily affecting the cardiovascular system: antihypertensive agents.

See also: SECTION II, Bradycardia and Hypotension chapters; SECTION III, Naloxone and Nalmephene chapters.

RECOMMENDED READING

Hall AH, Smolinske SC, Kulig KW, et al. Guanabenz overdose. *Ann Intern Med* 1985;102:787–788.

Author: Edwin K. Kuffner

Reviewer: Richard C. Dart

Guanethidine

Basics

DESCRIPTION

Guanethidine and guanadrel are oral anti-hypertensive medications.

FORMS AND USES

- Guanethidine (Ismelin) is available in 10- and 25-mg tablets.

—Adult dose is 10 mg once daily initially, with 10- to 25-mg increases in daily dosing every 5 to 7 days, titrated to anti-hypertensive effect.
—Pediatric dose is 0.2 mg/kg once daily initially, with 0.2 mg/kg increases in daily dosing every 5 to 7 days, titrated to anti-hypertensive effect.
—Guanethidine is also an investigational agent for sympathetic nerve block for chronic joint pain syndromes.

- Guanadrel (Hylorel) is available in 10- and 25-mg tablets. Initial adult dosage is 10 mg/day, increased slowly to 20 to 75 mg/day.

PATHOPHYSIOLOGY

- Guanethidine is a postganglionic adrenergic neuron inhibitor that affects sympathetic neurons only.
- It acts at peripheral sympathetic nerve terminals by inhibiting norepinephrine release and depleting norepinephrine stores by blocking reuptake of norepinephrine into vesicles.
- Peripheral sympathetic blockade produces relaxation of vascular smooth muscle and decreased blood pressure.

EPIDEMIOLOGY

- Because of limited therapeutic use, poisoning is rare.
- Toxic effects following exposure are typically mild to moderate.
- Death may occur following large suicidal ingestion.

CAUSES

- The cause is usually suicidal ingestion.
- The possibility of child neglect or abuse should be considered if the patient is less than 1 year of age; suicide attempt in patients over 6 years of age.

RISK FACTORS

In geriatric patients, lower initial doses and lower and slower increases in daily dosing are recommended because of the increased risk of orthostatic hypotension.

DRUG AND DISEASE INTERACTIONS

- Guanethidine may potentiate other antihypertensive agents.
- Severe hypertension may result from the concurrent administration of sympathomimetic agents, such as epinephrine, norepinephrine, phenylephrine, phenylpropanolamine, ephedrine, or pseudoephedrine.
- Decreased antihypertensive effects may result from the concurrent administration of tricyclic antidepressants, phenothiazines, or amphetamines.

PREGNANCY AND LACTATION

- Guanadrel. US FDA Pregnancy Category B. Animal studies indicate no fetal risk and there are no controlled human studies, or animal studies show an adverse fetal effect but well-controlled studies in pregnant women do not.
- Guanethidine. US FDA Pregnancy Category C. The drug exerts animal teratogenic or embryocidal effects, but there are no controlled studies in women, or no studies are available in either animals or women.

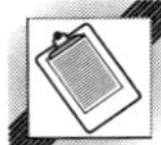

Diagnosis

DIFFERENTIAL DIAGNOSIS

- Toxic agents that predominantly cause hypotension but may initially cause transient hypertension soon after ingestion include:

—Other inhibitors of norepinephrine vesicular reuptake, including tricyclic antidepressants, reserpine, tetrabenazine, and others.
—Centrally acting α_2-receptor agonists, such as clonidine, imidazolines, α-methyldopa, guanfacine, and guanabenz
—Monamine oxidase inhibitors

- Other agents that predominantly cause hypotension include β-blockers, calcium channel blockers, and many others.

SIGNS AND SYMPTOMS

- Following initiation of therapy or within a few hours of an overdose, transient sympathomimetic effects may occur.
- However, the predominant feature of overdose is hypotension.

Vital Signs

- Hypotension and reflex tachycardia are common in overdose.
- Orthostatic hypotension may occur with therapeutic doses.

HEENT

Blurred vision is common and may be secondary to decreased intraocular pressure.

Cardiovascular

- Transient hypertension followed by hypotension is common.
- Collagen vascular disease has been reported in association with chronic therapy.

Pulmonary

Apnea has occurred following intravenous administration.

Gastrointestinal

Nausea, vomiting, and diarrhea are common.

Renal

Renal injury secondary to hypotension may occur.

Reproductive

- Male sexual dysfunction may occur.
- Sexual dysfunction usually responds to dose reduction.

Endocrine

Discontinuation of chronic therapy may cause hyperglycemia in diabetic patients.

PROCEDURES AND LABORATORY TESTS

- Essential tests. No tests may be needed in asymptomatic patients.
- Recommended tests

—Serum electrolytes, BUN, and creatinine should be measured in symptomatic patients to evaluate impaired renal function as a cause of toxicity.
—ECG, serum acetaminophen and aspirin levels in an overdose setting to detect occult ingestion.

- Not recommended tests. Serum guanethidine levels are not clinically useful.

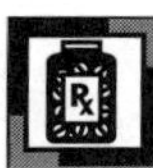

Treatment

- Treatment focuses on monitoring and maintaining blood pressure.
- Dose and time of exposure should be determined for all substances involved.

DIRECTING PATIENT COURSE

The health-care provider should call the poison control center when:

- Hypotension or other severe effects are present.
- Toxic effects are not consistent with guanethidine poisoning.
- Coingestant, drug interaction, or underlying disease presents an unusual problem.

The patient should be referred to a health-care facility when:

- Attempted suicide or homicide is possible.
- Patient or caregiver seems unreliable.
- Symptoms are present.
- Coingestant, drug interaction, or underlying disease presents an unusual problem.

Admission Considerations

Inpatient treatment:

- Is warranted when the patient has documented hypotension or symptomatic orthostatic hypotension.
- Should be considered for asymptomatic patients following large intentional ingestion so that they may be observed for 12 to 24 hours (hypotensive effects can be delayed).

DECONTAMINATION

Out of Hospital

Emesis with ipecac is not recommended.

In Hospital

- Gastric lavage should be performed in pediatric (tube size 24–32 French) or adult (tube size 36–42 French) patients for large ingestion presenting within 1 hour of ingestion or if serious effects are present.
- One dose of activated charcoal (1–2 g/kg) should be administered without a cathartic if a substantial ingestion has occurred within the previous few hours.
- Use of an intraaortic balloon pump may be considered in patients who have refractory severe hypotension.

ANTIDOTES

There is no specific antidote for guanethidine poisoning.

ADJUNCTIVE TREATMENT

Hypotension

- The patient should be given 10 to 20 ml/kg 0.9% saline intravenously and placed in the Trendelenburg position.
- Further fluid therapy should be guided by central pressure monitoring to avoid volume overload.
- If hypotension does not respond to treatment, a vasopressor is administered.

—Dopamine
  —The dose is 2 to 5 μg/kg/min, titrated to effect.
  —Rates greater than 20 μg/kg/min are unlikely to provide further benefit.
—Norepinephrine
  —The dose is 0.1 to 0.2 μg/kg/min, titrated to effect.
—High rates of infusion may cause tissue ischemia.

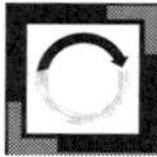

Follow-Up

PATIENT MONITORING

Continuous respiratory and hemodynamic monitoring should be performed during the observation period.

EXPECTED COURSE AND PROGNOSIS

- Hypotension resolves over 24 to 72 hours postingestion, but may persist for several days following a large overdose.
- Complications of CNS, heart, and kidneys related to hypotension may occur in severe cases.

DISCHARGE CRITERIA/INSTRUCTIONS

- From the emergency department. Asymptomatic patients without blood pressure abnormality during a 6- to 8-hour observation period may be discharged after gastrointestinal decontamination and psychiatric evaluation, if needed.
- From the hospital. Asymptomatic patients may be discharged after hypotension has resolved for at least 12 hours and psychiatric evaluation has been obtained, if needed.

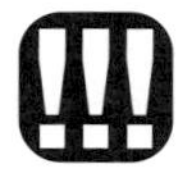

Pitfalls

DIAGNOSIS

- Initial hypertension is consistent with guanethidine toxicity and will be followed by hypotension; it should be treated only if severe or if end-organ damage has developed.
- The clinician may fail to check for orthostatic hypotension.

TREATMENT

The clinician may fail to admit patients with hypotension for 24 hours of observation.

ICD-9-CM 972.6

Poisoning by agents primarily affecting the cardiovascular system: anti-hypertensive agents.

See also: SECTION II, Hypotension chapter.

RECOMMENDED READING

Finnerty FA, Brogden RN. Guanadrel: A review of its pharmacodynamic and pharmacokinetic properties and therapeutic use in hypertension. *Drugs* 1985;30:22–31.

Author: Edwin K. Kuffner

Reviewer: Richard C. Dart

Guanfacine

Basics

DESCRIPTION

Guanfacine hydrochloride (Tenex) is used as an antihypertensive medication.

FORMS AND USES

The usual initial oral dose is 1 mg daily at bedtime, which may be increased to 2 mg if needed.

TOXIC DOSE

- Adverse reactions are more common with daily doses greater than 3 mg, but therapeutic doses up to 40 mg/day have been used.
- A 2-year-old child developed mental status depression and bradycardia after ingestion of 4 mg.

PATHOPHYSIOLOGY

- Guanfacine is an α_2-adrenoceptor agonist structurally related to clonidine, guanabenz, and methyldopa.
- It reduces blood pressure and pulse rate and may cause drowsiness.
- If guanfacine is abruptly discontinued, a rebound phenomenon may occur: anxiety, other symptoms of increased endogenous catecholamine release, and possibly an increase in blood pressure.
- Adverse reactions increase significantly with doses above 3 mg per day.

EPIDEMIOLOGY

Poisoning is uncommon.

CAUSES

Child neglect or abuse should be considered if the patient is less than 1 year of age, suicide attempt if the patient is over 6 years of age.

DRUG AND DISEASE INTERACTIONS

Guanfacine has an additive effect to other CNS depressants and antihypertensives.

PREGNANCY AND LACTATION

US FDA Pregnancy Category B. Animal studies indicate no fetal risk and there are no controlled human studies, or animal studies show an adverse fetal effect but well-controlled studies in women do not.

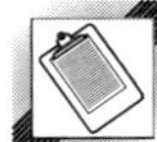

Diagnosis

DIFFERENTIAL DIAGNOSIS

Toxic causes of mental status depression include CNS depressants, clonidine, opiates, antihypertensives, and cholinergics among many others.

SIGNS AND SYMPTOMS

Drowsiness, lethargy, bradycardia, and hypotension predominate.

HEENT

Dry mouth has been reported in patients on long-term therapy.

Cardiovascular

- Bradycardia is seen within 2 hours of ingestion in most patients.
- Transient, paradoxical hypertension may develop, followed by hypotension. Hypotension may persist up to 36 hours.

Gastrointestinal

Constipation has been reported in patients on long-term therapy.

Neurologic

- Drowsiness, lethargy, and mental status depression may occur.
- Seizures have been reported in animal studies.
- Generalized weakness has been reported in patients on long-term therapy.

PROCEDURES AND LABORATORY TESTS

Essential Tests

No specific laboratory tests are usually needed in asymptomatic patients.

Recommended Tests

- ECG monitoring, serum electrolytes, glucose, renal function, complete blood count, arterial blood gases, and pregnancy test (if indicated) are recommended in significant or symptomatic overdose.
- Serum acetaminophen and salicylate level should be determined in an overdose setting to detect occult coingestion.
- CT head, lumbar puncture, cultures are used as clinically indicated to assess CNS depression.

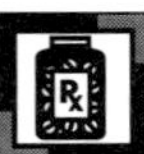

Treatment

- Symptomatic and supportive care with appropriate airway management is the mainstay of therapy.
- Dose and time of exposure need to be determined for all substances that could be involved.

DIRECTING PATIENT COURSE

The health-care professional should call the poison control center when:

- Severe or persistent effects develop.
- Coingestant, drug interaction, or underlying disease presents an unusual problem.

The patient should be referred to a health-care facility when:

- Suicide or homicide is possible.
- Toxic effects develop.
- Coingestant, drug interaction, or underlying disease presents an unusual problem.

Admission Considerations

Patients requiring treatment for hypotension, bradycardia, or altered mental status should be admitted to an ICU.

DECONTAMINATION

Out of Hospital

Induced emesis is not recommended because of risk of CNS depression.

In Hospital

- Gastric lavage should be performed in pediatric (tube size 24–32 French) or adult (tube size 36–42 French) patients presenting within 1 hour of a large ingestion or if serious effects are present.
- One dose of activated charcoal (1–2 g/kg) should be administered without a cathartic if a substantial ingestion has occurred within the previous few hours.

ANTIDOTES

There is no specific antidote for guanfacine poisoning.

ADJUNCTIVE TREATMENT

- Bradycardia. Atropine is administered: adult dose, 0.5 to 1.0 mg intravenously; pediatric dose, 0.02 mg/kg intravenously with 0.1 mg minimum and 1 mg maximum in children, 2 mg maximum in adolescents. Rarely, patients may require cardiac pacing.
- Hypotension is managed by treating bradycardia and infusion of isotonic fluid (10 to 20 ml/kg). If pressure does not respond, a vasopressor may be added.
- Hypertension is transient. It should not be treated unless clear end-organ injury develops.

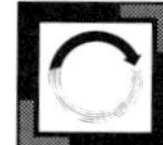

Follow-Up

PATIENT MONITORING

Cardiac rhythm and blood pressure should be monitored.

EXPECTED COURSE AND PROGNOSIS

Most patients recover over 24 to 36 hours with supportive and symptomatic care.

DISCHARGE CRITERIA/INSTRUCTIONS

- Asymptomatic patients may be discharged from the emergency department or hospital after gastrointestinal decontamination, observation for several hours, and psychiatric evaluation, if needed.
- Symptomatic patients should be observed for at least 24 hours.

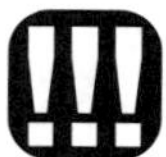

Pitfalls

DIAGNOSIS

Paradoxical transient hypertension may obscure diagnosis.

TREATMENT

Pharmacologic treatment of transient hypertension may exacerbate subsequent hypotension.

ICD-9-CM 972.6

Poisoning by agents primarily affecting the cardiovascular system: other antihypertensive agents.

See also: SECTION II, Bradycardia, Hypotension and Hypertension chapters; and SECTION III, Atropine chapter.

RECOMMENDED READING

Van Dyke MW, Bonace AL. Guanfacine overdose in a pediatric patient. *Vet Hum Toxicol* 1990;32:46–47.

Author: Steven A. Seifert

Reviewer: Kennon Heard

Heparins—Standard and Fractionated

Basics

DESCRIPTION

- Heparin medications are used to produce anticoagulation.
- Standard heparin is a family of mucopolysaccharides with molecular weights ranging from 6,000 to 20,000 daltons.
- Low-molecular-weight heparins are fractionated from heparin; molecular weights range from 4,000 to 9,000 daltons.

FORMS AND USES

- Therapeutic uses. Prophylaxis and treatment of deep venous thrombosis, hemodialysis, pulmonary embolus, myocardial ischemia, and ischemic stroke.
- Unfractionated standard heparin: anticoagulation dose

—Pediatric dose is 50 units/kg bolus followed by 25 units/kg/h to maintain partial thromboplastin time (PTT) of 1.5 to 2.5 times control.
—Adult dose is 80 to 100 units/kg bolus followed by 15 to 20 units/kg/h to maintain partial thromboplastin time of 1.5 to 2.5 times control.

- Unfractionated standard heparin: prophylaxis dose

—Typical subcutaneous adult dose is 5,000 units every 8 to 12 hours.
—Unfractionated (standard) heparin should not be administered intramuscularly.

- Low-molecular-weight heparins include ardeparin (Normiflo), dalteparin (Fragmin), enoxaparin (Lovenox), nadroparin (Fraxiparine), parnaparin, reviparin, and tinzaparin (Logiparin).

—Dalteparin dose is 2,500 to 5,000 IU subcutaneously once per day.
—Enoxaparin adult subcutaneous dose is 30 mg twice daily or 2 mg/kg/day in two divided doses.

TOXIC DOSE

- Standard heparin

—Heparin is not absorbed orally.
—Parenteral administration of more than 1,000 units/kg may produce spontaneous hemorrhage.
—There is wide interindividual variability.

- Enoxaparin

—Overdose experience is very limited.
—Similar to heparin, however, severe coagulopathy and spontaneous hemorrhage are anticipated following large parenteral overdose.

PATHOPHYSIOLOGY

- Standard heparin

—Standard heparin binds antithrombin III, causing a conformational change that accelerates the inactivation of thrombin and factors IX, X, XI, and XII.
—It inactivates thrombin to a greater extent than factor Xa, thereby causing an elevation of activated PTT (aPTT) and PTT.
—It has high affinity for vascular endothelium and von Willebrand factor, thereby inhibiting platelet aggregation.

- Low-molecular-weight heparin

—Low-molecular-weight heparin inactivates factor Xa to a greater extent than thrombin.
—It does not significantly affect either the aPTT or PTT at therapeutic doses.
—It inhibits platelet aggregation to a lesser degree than heparin.

EPIDEMIOLOGY

- Poisoning is common.
- Toxic effects following exposure are typically mild.

CAUSES

The cause is usually therapeutic error.

DRUG AND DISEASE INTERACTIONS

- Administration with other drugs that affect platelet function (aspirin, nonsteroidal anti-inflammatory drugs, dipyridamole, dextran) or thrombolytics may increase risk of hemorrhage.
- Combination of heparin and dihydroergotamine may cause vasospasm and ischemia.
- Oral anticoagulants can potentiate the anticoagulant effects of both standard heparin and low-molecular-weight heparins.

PREGNANCY AND LACTATION

- Dalteparin and enoxaparin. US FDA Pregnancy Category B. Animal studies indicate no fetal risk and there are no controlled human studies, or animal studies show an adverse fetal effect but well-controlled studies in pregnant women do not.
- Standard heparin and ardeparin. US FDA Pregnancy Category C. The drug exerts animal teratogenic or embryocidal effects, but there are no controlled studies in women, or no studies are available in either animals or women.
- Both standard heparin and low-molecular-weight heparins cross the placenta.
- Excretion in breast milk has been reported.

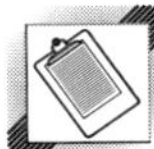

Diagnosis

DIFFERENTIAL DIAGNOSIS

- Toxic causes of coagulopathy include aspirin, coumadin, brodifacoum, snake envenomation, and severe hepatic injury from a variety of causes.
- Nontoxic causes of coagulopathy include inherited clotting factor deficiencies, sepsis, and severe head injury.

SIGNS AND SYMPTOMS

Heparin causes relatively few effects except for coagulation abnormality.

Vital Signs

Signs of hypovolemia from blood loss include tachycardia, hypotension, and tachypnea.

HEENT

Epistaxis and bleeding from the gums are common.

Dermatologic

- Ecchymosis and hematomas are common.
- Petechiae may be associated with thrombocytopenia.
- Necrosis has been reported with either standard heparin or low-molecular-weight heparin and resembles toxic epidermal necrolysis.

Fluids and Electrolytes

Hyperkalemia due to aldosterone suppression has been reported with chronic therapy with standard or low-molecular-weight heparins.

Gastrointestinal

Hematemesis, hematochezia, and melena may occur.

Genitourinary

Microscopic hematuria is common.

Hematologic

- Thrombocytopenia developing during the first weeks of use has been reported both with standard heparin and with low-molecular-weight heparin.
- Arterial thrombosis is a rare but catastrophic complication; it has been reported with both standard and low-molecular-weight heparin.

Hepatic

Transient elevations in hepatic enzymes have been reported with either type of heparin, usually during the first few days of therapy.

Musculoskeletal

Osteoporosis has been reported following chronic therapy with standard heparin.

PROCEDURES AND LABORATORY TESTS

Essential Tests

- Standard heparin

—PTT is commonly prolonged and prothrombin time (PT) may become prolonged in overdose; the therapeutic PTT is generally 1.5 to 2.5 times control value.
—Complete blood count (CBC) and platelet count should be performed to detect thrombocytopenia and assess effects of blood loss.
—Urinalysis and stool guaiac test to detect occult bleeding should be performed.

- Low-molecular-weight heparin

—The usual measures of anticoagulation effect cannot be used.
—PT, PTT, and platelet count should be determined in overdose. The precise role of these measurements in management is unclear, but marked abnormalities should be considered a sign of toxicity.
—Urinalysis and stool guaiac test to detect occult bleeding should be performed.

Recommended Tests

- Anti-IIa (thrombin) activity monitoring should be considered in high-risk patients.
- ECG, serum acetaminophen and aspirin levels are measured in an overdose setting to detect occult ingestion.
- Imaging should be performed as needed to detect complications of hemorrhage.

Not Recommended Tests

Plasma levels of either standard or low-molecular-weight heparins are not clinically useful.

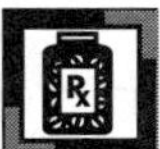

Treatment

Treatment focuses on management of the hemorrhagic complications and general supportive care.

DIRECTING PATIENT COURSE

The health-care provider should call the poison control center when:

- Signs of hemorrhage or other severe effects are present.
- Toxic effects are not consistent with heparin.
- Coingestant, drug interaction, or underlying disease presents an unusual problem.

The patient should be referred to a health-care facility when:

- Patient or caregiver seems unreliable.
- Any toxic effect is present.
- Coingestant, drug interaction, or underlying disease presents an unusual problem.

Admission Considerations

ICU admission is warranted for patients with rapid blood loss or serious complications such as intracranial hemorrhage.

DECONTAMINATION

Gastrointestinal decontamination should not be performed following ingestion of either type of heparin because neither is absorbed orally.

ANTIDOTES

- Protamine sulfate is the specific antidote for poisoning with standard heparin.
- It does not neutralize low-molecular-weight heparin as reliably but does appear to have some effect (see SECTION III, Protamine chapter, for further details).
- Indications, standard heparin

—Hemorrhage in patient treated with heparin
—Markedly elevated aPTT in patient, or presence of clinically significant hemorrhage (e.g., frank bleeding)

- Indications, low-molecular-weight heparin. Clinically significant hemorrhage.
- Contraindications. History of allergic reaction to protamine precludes use.
- Method of administration

—Standard heparin
  —Dose is 1 mg of protamine sulfate for every 100 units of heparin administered.
  —It is recommended that the rate of infusion not exceed 5 mg/minute.
—Low-molecular-weight heparin. Empiric dosing of protamine sulfate is recommended.
—Potential adverse effects. Rapid administration may produce bradycardia, dyspnea, a sensation of warmth, flushing, and severe hypotension.

ADJUNCTIVE TREATMENT

Blood component therapy may be needed to reverse anticoagulation or replace blood loss.

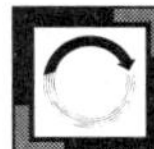

Follow-Up

PATIENT MONITORING

- Hemodynamic monitoring, serial CBC, and PTT should be performed for patients with hemorrhage.
- CBC and liver function tests should be performed for patients on chronic therapy.

EXPECTED COURSE AND PROGNOSIS

Nearly all patients do well with supportive care unless intracranial hemorrhage occurs.

DISCHARGE CRITERIA/INSTRUCTIONS

From the emergency department or hospital

- Standard heparin. Asymptomatic patients with normal to moderately elevated (in therapeutic range of 1.5 to 2.5 times control value) PTT or aPTT may be discharged at 4 hours postexposure (if not at increased risk of hemorrhage).
- Low-molecular-weight heparin. Asymptomatic patients without evidence of hemorrhage may be discharged at 4 hours postexposure.

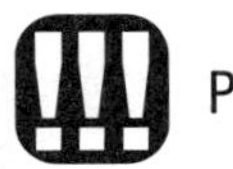

Pitfalls

TREATMENT

- Because the various low-molecular-weight heparin preparations have different binding affinities for factor Xa and antithrombin III, they may require different empiric doses of protamine for neutralization.
- Low-molecular-weight heparin has a longer duration of anticoagulation than standard heparin and may require repeated doses of protamine over time.

ICD-9-CM 964.2

Poisoning by agents primarily affecting blood constituents: anticoagulants.

See also: SECTION III, Protamine chapter.

RECOMMENDED READING

Ellenhorn MJ. Anticoagulants, antifibrinolytic agents and thrombolytic agents. In: *Ellenhorn's medical toxicology—diagnosis and treatment of human poisoning,* 2nd ed. Baltimore: Williams & Wilkins, 1997:460–463.

Author: Edwin K. Kuffner

Reviewer: Richard C. Dart

Basics

DESCRIPTION

Heroin is an addictive drug of abuse that stimulates opioid receptors.

FORMS AND USES

- Heroin, also known by the street names of black tar, china white, crank, "H," or horse, is used intravenously, intranasally, or by smoking; anal exposure may occur in an attempt to conceal the drug.
- Heroin is also mixed with cocaine or amphetamine (speedballing).
- Heroin is a U.S. Drug Enforcement Agency Schedule I substance; it has no accepted therapeutic use in the United States.
- See also SECTION II, Body Packer/Body Stuffer chapter.

TOXIC DOSE

- The toxic dose cannot be estimated because of variation in heroin potency and tolerance in the user.
- Small amounts may produce respiratory depression in naive users.
- The street drug contains variable amounts of the active drug (generally 21%–60%).

PATHOPHYSIOLOGY

- Primary effects in overdose are caused by binding to μ, κ, and σ opioid receptors, producing CNS and respiratory depression.
- Direct pulmonary toxicity results in noncardiogenic pulmonary edema.
- Some elements of toxicity may result from:

—Adulterants such as amphetamine, cocaine, dextromethorphan, quinine, scopolamine, strychnine, thiamine, or vinegar.
—Bacterial or viral contamination.
—Physical impurities.

- "Cotton fever" refers to a febrile reaction following injection of drug filtered through cotton balls.

EPIDEMIOLOGY

- Poisoning is common.
- Toxic effects following exposure are typically moderate to severe.
- Death occurs in patients with severe respiratory depression.

CAUSES

Overdose usually occurs during abuse and results from an unknown concentration of drug or from resumption of prior dose after a period of abstinence and loss of acquired tolerance.

DRUG INTERACTIONS

Heroin has an additive effect with drugs that produce CNS or respiratory depression.

PREGNANCY AND LACTATION

- US FDA Pregnancy Category B. Animal studies indicate no fetal risk, and there are no controlled human studies, or animal studies show an adverse fetal effect but well-controlled studies in pregnant women do not.
- Heroin enters breast milk and may produce addiction in the fetus or infant.

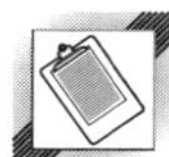

Diagnosis

DIFFERENTIAL DIAGNOSIS

- Drugs that produce CNS and respiratory depression include benzodiazepines, barbiturates, neuroleptics, alcohol, antidepressants, and other opioids, as well as many other medications.
- Other agents that produce miosis include organophosphate insecticides, carbamates, and nicotine, among others.
- Conditions that depress mental status include postictal states, hypoglycemia, cerebrovascular accident, and respiratory arrest, among others.

SIGNS AND SYMPTOMS

- Rapid onset of miosis, coma, apnea, and, possibly, pulmonary edema.
- Following ingestion, however, toxic effects may be delayed.

Vital Signs

Bradycardia, hypotension, apnea, or hyper- or hypothermia may occur.

HEENT

Pinpoint pupils occur, but they may be dilated after severe hypoxia or acidosis.

Dermatologic

Needle tracks are usually present in intravenous abusers.

Cardiovascular

Dysrhythmia from hypoxia or adulterants may occur.

Pulmonary

- Noncardiogenic pulmonary edema usually presents within 2 hours of intravenous use, but may be delayed 24 to 72 hours with smoking or ingestion.
- Talc from impurities can cause granulomatous reactions in the lung following intravenous use.

Gastrointestinal

- Decreased bowel sounds and functional bowel obstruction may develop.
- Constipation may occur in chronic users.

Renal

Rhabdomyolysis may cause acute renal failure.

Musculoskeletal

Rhabdomyolysis from localized muscle compression may occur if prolonged coma develops.

Neurologic

- CNS depression with lethargy or coma may occur.
- Seizures may occur.

PROCEDURES AND LABORATORY TESTS

Essential Tests

Pulse oximetry is used to monitor for hypoxia; persistent hypoxia after naloxone may indicate insufficient naloxone, another toxicologic agent, or pulmonary edema.

Recommended Tests

- Serum electrolytes, BUN, and creatinine are measured in symptomatic patients to assess other causes of CNS depression.
- ECG, serum acetaminophen, and aspirin levels in an overdose setting detect occult overdose.
- Head CT and lumbar puncture are used as needed to evaluate causes of altered mental status.
- Cultures of blood, urine, wounds, and sputum are ordered as clinically indicated to detect complications from intravenous drug abuse.
- Chest radiography is ordered in patients with respiratory signs or symptoms to detect pulmonary edema.
- Urine test for opioids may show positive results after ingestion of foods containing poppy seeds.

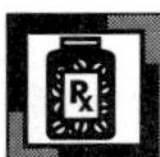

Treatment

- Treatment should focus on airway management, naloxone administration, and decontamination, if needed.
- Dose and time of exposure should be determined for all substances involved.

DIRECTING PATIENT COURSE

The health-care provider should call the poison control center when:

- Persistent apnea or hypotension, or other severe effects occur.
- Toxic effects are not consistent with heroin.
- Coingestant, drug interaction, or underlying disease presents an unusual problem.

The patient should be referred to a health-care facility when:

- Undesired effects are present.
- Attempted suicide or homicide is possible.
- Patient or caregiver seems unreliable.
- Coingestant, drug interaction, or underlying disease presents an unusual problem.

Admission Considerations

Inpatient treatment is warranted for patients who develop pulmonary edema or who have persistent respiratory, cardiac, or CNS effects despite naloxone therapy.

DECONTAMINATION

Out of Hospital

Emesis should not be induced because CNS depression may develop abruptly.

In Hospital

- Decontamination after intravenous injection or inhalation is not needed.
- Oral ingestion is classified as a "body stuffer" or "body packer."

ANTIDOTES

Naloxone

- Indications

—Naloxone is used for respiratory depression from known opioid overdose. (See SECTION III, Naloxone chapter, for information on the use of naloxone for less severe manifestations.)
—It may be prudent to observe patients who can maintain their airway and oxygenation rather than treat them, so that discharge may occur without concern for recurrent opioid toxicity.

- Contraindications. Documented naloxone allergy
- Dose and method of administration

—A dose of 2.0 mg intravenous push is administered and the response is observed.
—If no response, dose is repeated in 2.0 mg increments to a total dose of 10 mg.
—Although less desirable, naloxone may also be administered by endotracheal, intramuscular, intralingual, intraosseous, or subcutaneous injection.
—If reversal response occurs, patients should be observed for 4 hours after final dose.
—Patients with persistent or recurrent effects may be treated with constant infusion of naloxone.

Nalmefene

Nalmefene has been proposed for use when prolonged reversal of opioid effect is desired.

Dose and Method of Administration

- Starting dose of 0.5 mg intravenous push is administered; if no effect, an additional 1 mg is given.
- Higher doses of nalmefene appear to give prolonged activity; 1.5 mg of nalmefene blocks opioid activity for up to 8 hours.
- If repeat dosing is required, the patient should be admitted.

ADJUNCTIVE THERAPIES

- Pulmonary edema

—Endotracheal intubation is often needed to provide adequate ventilation and oxygenation.
—If adequate oxygenation cannot be maintained on 60% FiO_2, positive end-expiratory pressure or continuous positive airway pressure should be considered.
—Care should be taken to avoid fluid overload.

- Hypotension

—The primary treatment is correction of narcotic effects and dysrhythmia.
—In addition, 10 to 20 ml/kg 0.9% saline may be administered, the patient placed in Trendelenburg position, and, if needed, a vasopressor is administered.

- Seizures

—Seizures should be controlled with benzodiazepine, followed by phenobarbital or phenytoin, if needed.

- Complications of intraarterial injection may require heparin, vasodilators, and/or fibrinolysis; intraarterial reserpine use also has been reported.

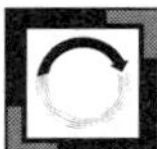

Follow-Up

PATIENT MONITORING

CNS, cardiovascular, and respiratory functions should be monitored continuously.

EXPECTED COURSE AND PROGNOSIS

- Complete recovery from hypoxia is expected if its duration is short.
- Sequelae of hypoxia may occur if apnea develops.
- Sequelae of intravenous drug abuse are common: endocarditis, abscess, human immunodeficiency virus, sepsis, hepatitis, and tetanus.

DISCHARGE CRITERIA/INSTRUCTIONS

- From the emergency department

—Patients in whom toxic effects abate may be discharged following decontamination and observation for 4 hours beyond the last dose of naloxone.
—Psychiatric evaluation and substance abuse counseling, if needed, should be obtained.

- From the hospital. Patients may be discharged after resolution of pulmonary edema and other complications such as rhabdomyolysis.

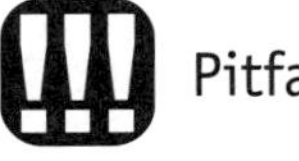

Pitfalls

DIAGNOSIS

Heroin is frequently mixed with scopolamine or other anticholinergics, which may mask opioid toxicity.

TREATMENT

- The patient must be observed beyond the expected duration of action of naloxone because respiratory depression may recur.
- The onset of pulmonary edema may be delayed for 24 to 72 hours.

ICD-9-CM 965.01

Poisoning by analgesics, antipyretics, and antirheumatics: heroin.

See also: SECTION II, Body Packers and Body Stuffers, Hypotension, and Seizure chapters; and SECTION III, Naloxone and Nalmephene, and Whole-Bowel Irrigation chapters.

RECOMMENDED READING

Duberstein JL, Kaufman DM. A clinical study of an epidemic of heroin intoxication and heroin-induced pulmonary edema. *Am J Med* 1971;51:704–714.

Harrison DW, Walls RM. "Cotton fever": a benign febrile syndrome in intravenous drug abusers. *J Emerg Med* 1990;8:135–139.

Author: Steven A. Seifert

Reviewer: Richard C. Dart

Hexachlorophene

Basics

DESCRIPTION

Hexachlorophene is used as an antibacterial soapless skin cleanser.

FORMS AND USES

- Hexachlorophene (Phisohex, Bilevon, Dermadex, Exofene, many others) is sold as a 3% or 0.75% emulsion.
- FDA regulations limit the concentration of hexachlorophene in cosmetics to less than 0.1%, and less than 0.75% in over-the-counter preparations.

TOXIC DOSE

- Ingestion of from 1 to 4 ounces of 3% solution has caused severe symptoms and death.
- The minimal lethal dose is unknown but is estimated to be 1 to 10 g.

PATHOPHYSIOLOGY

- Hexachlorophene is absorbed through the skin and may reach toxic blood levels, especially in neonates and patients with generalized dermatologic disorders.
- Systemic toxicity is primarily manifested by CNS stimulation.
- Repeated prolonged dermal exposure has resulted in toxicity and death, particularly in neonates.

EPIDEMIOLOGY

Poisoning is uncommon.

CAUSES

- Repeated, prolonged dermal exposure in patients with poor skin integrity.
- Ingestions have resulted in serious toxicity and death.

PREGNANCY AND LACTATION

US FDA Pregnancy Category C. The drug exerts animal teratogenic or embryocidal effects, but there are no controlled studies in women, or no studies are available in animals or women.

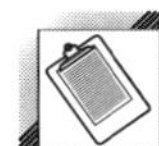

Diagnosis

DIFFERENTIAL DIAGNOSIS

- Toxic causes of pathologic CNS stimulation include sympathomimetic agents, theophylline, and epileptogenic agents, among others.
- Nontoxic causes include seizure (trauma, infection, or hemorrhage) and endocrine or electrolyte abnormalities.

SIGNS AND SYMPTOMS

Vital Signs

Low-grade fever is common.

HEENT

Optic atrophy and blindness may occur rarely following acute or chronic ingestion.

Dermatologic

- An erythematous rash followed by desquamation may occur rarely following skin application.
- Dermal reactions also may occur following oral ingestion.

Cardiovascular

Bradycardia, hypotension, and shock may occur.

Gastrointestinal

Following ingestion, severe anorexia, nausea, vomiting, abdominal cramps, and diarrhea leading to dehydration may occur.

Neurologic

- Lethargy, muscle fasciculation, weakness, irritability, coma, or seizures may occur.
- Increased intracranial pressure with cerebral edema is usually present with significant CNS symptoms.

PROCEDURES AND LABORATORY TESTS

Essential Tests

No tests are usually needed in asymptomatic patients.

Recommended Tests

- Serum electrolytes, BUN, creatinine, calcium, and magnesium should be measured in patients with seizures or altered mental status.
- Head CT, lumbar puncture, and bacterial cultures are used to evaluate altered mental status.
- ECG, serum acetaminophen and aspirin levels in overdose setting to detect occult ingestion.

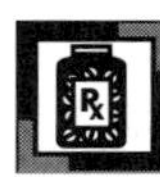

Treatment

- Supportive care with appropriate airway management is vital.
- Dose and time of exposure should be determined for all substances involved.

DIRECTING PATIENT COURSE

The health-care professional should call the poison control center when:

- Severe or persistent effects develop.
- Coingestant, drug interaction, or underlying disease presents an unusual problem.

The patient should be referred to a health-care facility when:

- Suicide or homicide are possible
- Toxic effects develop.
- Coingestant, drug interaction, or underlying disease presents an unusual problem.

Admission Considerations

Inpatient treatment is warranted for patients with an altered mental status, seizures, severe abdominal distress, hypotension or persistent vomiting and diarrhea.

DECONTAMINATION

- Skin exposure. Any residual material should be washed off with soap and water, followed by washing with olive oil or isopropanol and a second vigorous soap and water cleansing.
- Ingestion

—Gastric lavage should be performed in pediatric (tube size 24–32 French) or adult (tube size 36–42 French) patients presenting within 1 hour of a large ingestion or if serious effects are present.
—One dose of activated charcoal (1–2 g/kg) should be administered without a cathartic if a substantial ingestion has occurred within the previous few hours.

- Eye exposure. The eye is irrigated with water copiously for 15 minutes.

ANTIDOTES

There is no specific antidote for hexachlorophene poisoning.

ADJUNCTIVE TREATMENT

- Hypotension is treated with isotonic fluid infusion, the Trendelenburg position, and vasopressors if needed; dopamine is preferred, and norepinephrine is used for refractory hypotension.
- Seizures

—A patent airway must be ensured.
—A benzodiazepine should be administered for initial control. If seizures persist or recur, another anticonvulsant such as phenobarbital should be added.

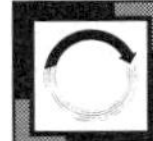

Follow-Up

PATIENT MONITORING

All patients admitted to the hospital should be placed in the ICU; management should include cardiac monitoring, pulse oximetry, and seizure precautions.

EXPECTED COURSE AND PROGNOSIS

- Most patients recover with supportive and symptomatic care.
- Severe toxicity may result in death.

DISCHARGE CRITERIA/INSTRUCTIONS

- Patients may be discharged from the emergency department if they are asymptomatic after decontamination, 6 hours of observation, and no abnormal laboratory results are found.
- Patients may be discharged from the ICU if they are asymptomatic after 24 hours or if CNS irritability, seizures, gastrointestinal symptoms, and hypotension have resolved.

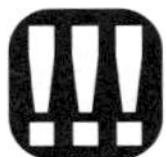

Pitfalls

DIAGNOSIS

Failure to consider hexachlorophene as an etiology for intractable seizures or CNS depression.

TREATMENT

Failure to adequately manage the airway.

ICD-9-CM 976

Poisoning by agents primarily affecting skin and mucous membrane, ophthalmological, otorhinolaryngological, and dental drugs.

See also: SECTION II, Hypotension and Seizures chapters.

RECOMMENDED READING

Goutieres F, Aicardi J. Accidental percutaneous hexachlorophene intoxication in children. *BMJ* 1977;2:663–665.

Herskowitz J, Rosman NP. Acute hexachlorophene poisoning by mouth in a neonate. *J Pediatr* 1979;94:495–496.

Author: Steven A. Seifert

Reviewer: Gerald F. O'Malley

Hydrocarbons—General

Basics

DESCRIPTION

- Hydrocarbons are a large class of organic molecules consisting of carbon, hydrogen, and oxygen.
- The types of hydrocarbons are aliphatic (straight-chain) and cyclic.
- The addition of halogens (fluoride and chlorine) and the form of conjugated aromatic ring structures are covered in following chapters.

FORMS AND USES

- Aliphatic hydrocarbons (straight-chain molecules)

—Short-chain forms include methane, ethane, propane, and butane.
—Longer chain molecules are pentane, hexane, heptane, and octane.

- Cyclic hydrocarbons

—Bitumens, creosotes, gasoline, kerosene, mineral seal oil, motor oil, naphtha, petroleum, shole oils, soots, Stoddard solvent, and other products are mixtures of various hydrocarbons, which usually do not include active functional groups such as halogens (chloride, fluoride).

- Organic hydrocarbon solvents are used for extracting, dissolving, or suspending materials, such as fats, waxes, and resins, that are not soluble in water.
- Solvents are components of paints, adhesives, glues, coatings, and degreasing/cleaning agents, and are used in the production of dyes, polymers, plastics, textiles, printing inks, agricultural products, and pharmaceuticals.

TOXIC DOSE

- Aspiration of just a few drops can cause aspiration pneumonitis.
- Conversely, ingestion requires large amounts to produce serious toxicity, unless the hydrocarbon product contains other toxins (halogens, pesticides).

PATHOPHYSIOLOGY

- Hydrocarbon solvents may be absorbed by the pulmonary, oral, or dermal route.
- Short-chain aliphatic hydrocarbons function as simple asphyxiants by displacing oxygen in the inhaled atmosphere.
- Longer chain organic solvents depress the CNS.
- Toxicity results from either local or systemic effects, but local and systemic effects may exist simultaneously.
- The most common serious effect is pulmonary aspiration.

—The risk of aspiration is largely determined by the viscosity of the hydrocarbon.
—The less viscous group of compounds [Saybolt Universal Seconds (SUS) <100], which includes gasoline, mineral seal oil, petroleum naphtha, and kerosene, are much easier to aspirate than more viscous compounds.
—More viscous, less volatile (SUS >100) compounds, such as petroleum jelly, motor oil, and mineral oil, are less likely to be aspirated, and are also poorly absorbed from the gastrointestinal tract, decreasing the likelihood of systemic toxicity.

- Ingestion of large amounts is needed to cause clinically significant systemic toxicity.

EPIDEMIOLOGY

- Hydrocarbon poisoning is common.
- Toxic effects following exposure are typically mild to moderate.
- Death is rare and usually associated with pulmonary aspiration.

CAUSES

- Hydrocarbon poisoning is usually accidental.
- Child neglect should be considered if the patient is under 1 year of age; attempted suicide if the patient is over 6 years of age.

PREGNANCY AND LACTATION

Hydrocarbon exposure possibly increases the risk of spontaneous abortion.

WORKPLACE STANDARDS

- Gasoline. ACGIH: TLV TWA is 300 ppm; STEL is 500 ppm.
- Hexane. ACGIH (n-hexane): TLV TWA is 50 ppm. NIOSH (n-hexane): REL TWA is 50 ppm; IDLH is 1100 ppm. OSHA: PEL TWA is 500 ppm.

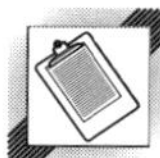

Diagnosis

DIFFERENTIAL DIAGNOSIS

Other toxic agents that cause hypoxia without other clinically apparent effects may include carbon monoxide, hydrogen sulfide, methemoglobinemia, and less common poisons.

SIGNS AND SYMPTOMS

Acute toxic exposure can produce CNS depression and cardiac dysrhythmias, and chronic exposure primarily affects the CNS and hepatic function.

HEENT

Headache, eye pain, irritation, lacrimation, or blurred vision may occur with inhalational or splash exposure.

Dermatologic

Erythema, contact dermatitis, burns, or frostbite all may occur secondary to contact with release of compressed gases such as butane or propane.

Cardiovascular

Dysrhythmias such as ventricular fibrillation occur rarely, but may develop suddenly.

Pulmonary

- Dyspnea, cough, hypoxia, and chest tightness may be seen initially after inhalation.
- Acute toxicity after respiratory exposure may include acute bronchitis, interstitial pneumonitis, aspiration pneumonia, and pulmonary edema.
- Low-viscosity compounds such as gasoline are easily aspirated, causing chemical pneumonitis or pulmonary edema.
- The first sign of aspiration may be a persistent mild cough for a few hours after exposure, followed by development of infiltrates and hypoxia.

Gastrointestinal

Nausea, vomiting, pancreatitis, diarrhea, and abdominal pain may develop.

Hepatic

Liver enzyme elevation may occur occasionally but is much more common with the chlorinated hydrocarbons.

Hematologic

Disseminated intravascular coagulation may complicate serious cases of aspiration.

Genitourinary

Acute renal failure occurs rarely.

Neurologic

- Mild CNS depression or excitation may occur after ingestion or vapor inhalation.
- See separate chapters for CNS effects that can occur secondary to additives and contaminants (i.e., aniline, heavy metals, camphor, or pesticides).

PROCEDURES AND LABORATORY TESTS

Essential Tests

No tests may be needed for minimally symptomatic patients who recover quickly.

Recommended Tests

- Symptomatic patients or patients with chronic exposure should undergo a complete blood count to assess bone marrow production.
- Serum electrolytes, BUN, and serum creatinine should be obtained to evaluate renal injury.
- Serum liver enzymes should be obtained to assess hepatic injury.
- Arterial blood gas, pulse oximetry, spirometry, or peak flow measurements should be performed for symptomatic patients to assess oxygenation and ventilation.
- A chest radiograph should be obtained if aspiration or noncardiogenic pulmonary edema is suspected.
- ECG, serum acetaminophen and aspirin levels should be obtained in suspected overdose to detect occult ingestion.

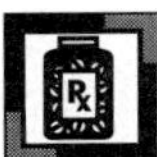

Treatment

- Therapy should focus on supportive respiratory care.
- Dose and time of exposure must be determined for all substances involved.

DIRECTING PATIENT COURSE

The health-care provider should call a poison center when:

- Signs and symptoms are not consistent with hydrocarbon exposure.
- Respiratory symptoms, altered mental status, or other serious effects are present.
- Coingestant, drug interaction, or underlying disease presents an unusual problem.

The patient should be referred to a health-care facility when:

- Attempted suicide or homicide is possible.
- The patient or caregiver seems unreliable.
- Coingestant, drug interaction, or underlying disease presents an unusual problem.

Admission Considerations

Inpatient management is warranted for symptomatic patients who develop more than nausea and vomiting.

DECONTAMINATION

Out of Hospital

- Emesis should not be induced owing to the risk of aspiration.
- Inhalation. The patient should be removed from the source of exposure.
- Skin contamination. The exposed area should be washed gently with soap and water.

In Hospital

- Gastric aspiration with a nasogastric tube should be performed in patients presenting within 1 hour of a large ingestion or if serious effects are present.
- One dose of activated charcoal (1–2 g/kg) should be administered if a substantial coingestion has occurred.
- If skin contamination occurs, the exposed area should be washed gently with soap and water.

ANTIDOTES

There is no specific antidote for hydrocarbon toxicity.

ADJUNCTIVE TREATMENT

Aspiration Pneumonia

- In mild cases with small infiltrates, administration of supplemental oxygen and observation are sufficient; antibiotics are probably not needed.
- For severe cases, endotracheal intubation and mechanical ventilation are often needed.
- Antibiotics are indicated if evidence of infection develops.
- Corticosteroids are very controversial, but probably offer no benefit.
- Extracorporeal membrane oxygenation and high frequency jet ventilation have been used successfully in pediatric patients.

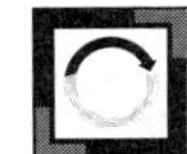

Follow-Up

PATIENT MONITORING

Cardiac and respiratory function should be monitored continuously.

EXPECTED COURSE AND PROGNOSIS

- Respiratory system toxicity may develop within hours of acute pulmonary aspiration.
- Recovery from ingestion is usually rapid unless aspiration occurs.
- The prognosis of inhalation or aspiration depends on the degree of pulmonary injury.
- Systemic poisoning is possible from pulmonary absorption.
- Permanent CNS, pulmonary, or hepatic damage is possible in severe cases, especially if complicated by hypoxia.

DISCHARGE CRITERIA/INSTRUCTIONS

Patients with normal vital signs who are asymptomatic may be discharged from the emergency department or the hospital following decontamination and 6-hour observation.

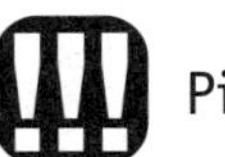

Pitfalls

DIAGNOSIS

- It is important to identify correctly the hydrocarbon-containing product involved in the exposure.
- Persistent minor cough often indicates that aspiration has occurred.

TREATMENT

Overaggressive gastrointestinal decontamination attempts may result in aspiration.

FOLLOW-UP

It is important to observe a patient with inhalation exposure for delayed symptoms.

ICD-9-CM 987.0

Toxic effect of other gases, fumes, or vapors: liquified petroleum gases.

See also: SECTION IV, Benzene, Hydrocarbons—Aromatic, Hydrocarbons—Chlorinated, Freon and Fluorinated Hydrocarbons, Toluene, and Camphor chapters.

RECOMMENDED READING

Banner W, Walson PD. Systemic toxicity following gasoline ingestion. *Am J Emerg Med* 1983;3:292–294.

Snyder R, Andrews LS. Toxic effect of solvents and vapors. In: Klaassen CD, Amdur MO, Doull J, eds. *Casarett and Doull's toxicology: the basic science of poisons,* 5th ed. New York: McGraw-Hill, 1996:737–771.

US Department of Health and Human Services. ATSDR case studies in environmental medicine: gasoline toxicity. September 1993, Monograph 31.

Author: Alvin C. Bronstein

Reviewer: Richard C. Dart

Hydrocarbons—Aniline and Xylene

Basics

DESCRIPTION

Aromatic hydrocarbons are those containing a benzene ring structure. Benzene, phenol, and toluene are discussed in separate chapters.

FORMS AND USES

• Aniline (aminobenzene) is used as a chemical intermediary to make dyes, resins, varnishes, perfumes, shoe blacks, vulcanizing rubber, inks, paint removers, herbicides, fungicides, explosives, photographic chemicals, isocyanates, and rigid polyurethanes.
• Xylene (dimethyl benzene, ortho-xylene, metaxylene, para-xylene) is used in the production of paints, varnishes, degreasers, paint thinners, pesticides, and some pharmaceutical preparations.

—Xylene is an additive to aviation fuels and is used in the synthesis of dyes.
—Xylene is used in microscopy as a solvent and clarifier.
—Xylene may be contaminated with benzene, which can cause benzene toxicity.
—Other potential contaminants include ethylbenzene, toluene, phenol, thiophene, and pyridine.

TOXIC DOSE

• Aniline is toxic in doses above approximately 0.15 mg/kg in adults.
• Xylene is lethal in oral doses of approximately 50 mg/kg in adults.

PATHOPHYSIOLOGY

• Aromatic hydrocarbon solvents cause direct cellular toxicity to the lung and gastrointestinal tract, and toxic metabolites cause injury in the CNS and in the renal, cardiac, hepatic, and hematopoietic systems.
• Sudden death following acute inhalation is believed to be related to sensitization of the myocardium to catecholamines and to hypoxia induced by simple asphyxiant effects.
• Inhalation is the most common route of exposure.
• Aniline is well absorbed through the skin, whereas xylene is less well absorbed dermally.

EPIDEMIOLOGY

• Exposure is common and underreported.
• Death is rare (generally occurring before arrival at the hospital) and is attributable to cardiac dysrhythmia or respiratory depression.

CAUSES

• Exposure occurs primarily by occupational inhalation.
• Child neglect should be considered if the patient is under 1 year of age, and attempted suicide should be considered if the patient is over 6 years of age.

RISK FACTORS

• Workers in chemical, petroleum, plastics, and agricultural industries are commonly exposed.
• The skin of infants is more permeable than the skin of older children and adults, and may allow methemoglobinemia to develop from small dermal exposures to aniline.

PREGNANCY

Both aniline and xylene are associated with an increased incidence of spontaneous abortions and preterm delivery.

WORKPLACE STANDARDS

Aniline

• ACGIH. TLV TWA is 2 ppm.
• OSHA. PEL TWA is 5 ppm.
• NIOSH. IDLH value is 100 ppm.

Xylene (Ortho-xylene, Meta-xylene, Para-xylene)

• ACGIH. PEL TWA is 100 ppm, and its PEL STEL is 150 ppm.
• OSHA. PEL TWA is 100 ppm.
• NIOSH. IDLH is 900 ppm.

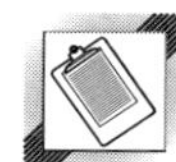

Diagnosis

DIFFERENTIAL DIAGNOSIS

• Other toxic agents that cause CNS depression include opioids, sedative-hypnotics, ethanol, gamma hydroxybutyrate, rohypnol, clonidine, tricyclic antidepressants, methanol, anticonvulsants, and ethylene glycol, among many others.
• Nontoxic causes of altered mental status include intracranial trauma or infection, hypoglycemia or other metabolic disturbances, and electrolyte abnormalities.

SIGNS AND SYMPTOMS

Primary symptoms are CNS depression, dyspnea, and mucous membrane irritation.

Vital Signs

Fever and tachycardia are common findings in aromatic hydrocarbon poisoning.

HEENT

Splash contact causes eye and mucous membrane irritation, and may cause corneal ulceration in severe cases.

Dermatologic

Prolonged skin exposure can cause dermatitis, defatting of the skin, and, rarely, burns.

Cardiovascular

Sudden cardiac death after acute inhalation is possible.

Pulmonary

• Upper airway irritation and, in severe cases, pulmonary edema or asphyxiation may occur.
• Aspiration or intravenous injection of xylene can cause pneumonitis, pulmonary edema, or respiratory failure.
• Chronic exposure may cause chronic bronchitis.

Hematologic

Aniline may cause methemoglobinemia, which may be followed by hemolysis 2 to 7 days after the exposure.

Gastrointestinal

Vomiting, abdominal cramps, and diarrhea are common following ingestion.

Hepatic

Acute chemical hepatitis with increased transaminases may occur.

Neurologic

• Headache is common.
• Initial mild euphoria is followed by CNS depression ranging from somnolence or confusion to coma.
• Tremors have been reported from aniline poisoning.

Renal

• Xylene causes proteinuria, hematuria, or renal insufficiency, and prolonged or repeated exposure may cause permanent renal injury.
• Aniline causes rapid onset of hematuria, and a large exposure may cause renal failure.

PROCEDURES AND LABORATORY TESTS

Essential Tests

No test is essential for all patients.

Recommended Tests

• Serum electrolytes, BUN, creatinine, and urinalysis should be performed to rule out other causes of CNS alteration and to detect renal injury.
• A methemoglobin level should be obtained following aniline exposure.
• Complete blood count, serum transaminase, creatine kinase, serum lactate, and arterial blood gas should be obtained to assess acidosis and liver or muscle injury.
• Arterial blood gases should be obtained to assess oxygenation in symptomatic patients.
• Serum acetaminophen, ECG, and salicylate levels should be obtained in overdose settings to evaluate occult ingestion.
• A chest radiograph should be obtained in symptomatic patients to assess pulmonary edema.

Not Recommended Tests

Levels of specific metabolites are not clinically useful for diagnosis but are used for workplace monitoring.

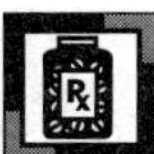

Treatment

- Treatment should focus on termination of exposure and treatment of methemoglobinemia (aniline).
- Dose and time of exposure must be determined for all substances involved.

DIRECTING PATIENT COURSE

The health-care provider should call a poison control center when:

- Severe or persistent effects develop.
- Coingestant, drug interaction, or underlying disease presents an unusual problem.

The patient should be referred to a health-care facility when:

- Suicide or homicide attempt is possible.
- Toxic effects develop.
- Coingestant, drug interaction, or underlying disease presents an unusual problem.

ADMISSION CONSIDERATIONS

Inpatient management is warranted for patients with persistent mental status depression, cardiac or pulmonary (e.g., dysrhythmia, infiltrates) toxicity, or methemoglobinemia.

DECONTAMINATION

Out of Hospital

- Inhalation. The patient should be removed from the source of exposure, and oxygen should be administered.
- Ingestion. Emesis should not be induced because of the risk of rapid onset of CNS depression.
- Dermal exposure. The exposed area should be washed gently with soap and water and rinsed thoroughly.

In Hospital

- Emesis should not be induced.
- Because these products are liquids, a small nasogastric tube may be used to aspirate stomach contents.
- Activated charcoal is not recommended.
- In cases of dermal exposure, the exposed area should be washed gently with soap and water and rinsed thoroughly

ANTIDOTES

Methylene blue is the antidote for methemoglobinemia induced by aniline.

- Indications. Methylene blue is prescribed for symptoms of hypoxia attributable to methemoglobinemia.
- Contraindications. The drug should not be prescribed for patients with known NADH methemoglobin reductase deficiency or 100% glucose-6-phosphate-dehydrogenase (G6PD) deficiency.
- Method of administration

—One dose of 1 to 2 mg/kg should be administered intravenously over 5 minutes.
—The methemoglobin level should be checked 30 minutes after the initial dose.
—If the methemoglobin level remains elevated and the patient is still symptomatic, a repeat dose of 1 to 2 mg/kg may be given.

- Adverse effects. Patients with G6PD deficiency may develop hemolysis, and paradoxical worsening of methemoglobinemia may be seen with large doses.

ADJUNCTIVE TREATMENT

- Extracorporeal membrane oxygenation. In cases of severe pulmonary aspiration with hypoxemia, treatment with bypass methods of oxygenation have been successful.
- Hypotension

—Hypotension is treated with isotonic fluid infusion, the Trendelenburg position, and vasopressors if needed; dopamine is preferred; norepinephrine is used for refractory hypotension.

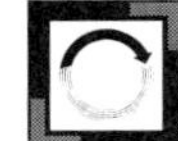

Follow-Up

PATIENT MONITORING

- Respiratory function, cardiac rhythm, methemoglobin level (in cases of aniline poisoning), and electrolytes should be monitored in symptomatic patients.
- Severe exposure may lead to sequelae of hypoxia due to methemoglobinemia (in cases of aniline poisoning) or to pulmonary edema if aspiration occurs.

EXPECTED COURSE AND PROGNOSIS

- Toxic effects develop rapidly, within minutes of inhalation.
- Methemoglobinemia may require several hours to develop.
- Complete recovery can be expected, unless sequelae of prolonged hypoxia occur.

DISCHARGE CRITERIA/INSTRUCTIONS

- From the emergency department. Asymptomatic patients with normal neurologic examination results and without cardiac effects or signs of methemoglobinemia after a 6-hour observation period may be discharged after psychiatric evaluation, if needed.
- From the hospital. Patients may be discharged after toxic effects have resolved or stabilized and psychiatric evaluation, if needed, has been completed.

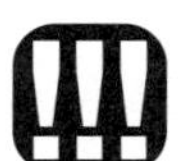

Pitfalls

DIAGNOSIS

- Alternative diagnoses for alteration and depression in mental status should be evaluated.
- It is important to check for renal injury or methemoglobinemia.

TREATMENT

Fetal monitoring should be instituted in pregnant patients acutely exposed to aromatic hydrocarbons.

ICD-9-CM 989.9

Toxic effect of other substances, chiefly nonmedicinal as to source: unspecified substance, chiefly nonmedicinal as to source.

See also: SECTION II, Hypotension, and Methemoglobinemia chapters; SECTION III, Methylene Blue chapter; SECTION IV, Benzene, Phenol, and Toluene chapters.

RECOMMENDED READING

Snyder R, Andrews LS. Toxic effect of solvents and vapors. In: Klaassen CD, Amdur MO, Doull J, eds. *Casarett and Doull's toxicology: the basic science of poisons,* 5th ed. New York: McGraw-Hill, 1996:737–771.

Author: Alvin C. Bronstein

Reviewer: Kennon Heard

Hydrocarbons—Chlorinated

Basics

DESCRIPTION

The chlorinated hydrocarbons are aliphatic or aromatic hydrocarbons, which include chlorine in their structure.

FORMS AND USES

- The chlorinated hydrocarbons include benzyl chloride; carbon tetrachloride; chlorobenzene; chloromethane; chloroform; *o*-dichlorobenzene; *p*-dichlorobenzene; 1,1-dichloroethane; 1,2-dichloroethane; dichloromethane; 1,2-dichloroethylene; ethylene dichloride; trichloroethylene; hexachloroethane; methylene chloride; 1,1,1-trichloroethane; tetrachloroethylene; 1,1,2-trichloroethane; trichloromethane; and 1,2,3-trichloropropane.
- Chlorinated hydrocarbons are used as refrigerants, solvents, dry cleaning agents, degreasers, inks, varnishes, lacquers, paints, and paint removers.
- Solvents such as trichloroethylene have been abused as inhalants.

TOXIC DOSE

- Toxic dose varies widely by compound and concentration in product.
- Ingestion of small amounts (e.g., 3 cc of carbon tetrachloride in adults) may cause massive hepatic injury and death.

PATHOPHYSIOLOGY

- Inhalation of chlorinated hydrocarbons poses a major life threat due to CNS depression and dysrhythmias.
- Trichloroethylene and trichloroethane produce direct CNS depression through their general anesthetic properties.
- Methylene chloride is metabolized in the liver to carbon monoxide.
- Many chlorinated hydrocarbons are metabolized in the liver to reactive compounds that cause liver necrosis.
- Sudden death following acute inhalation is believed to be related to sensitization of the myocardium to catecholamines and to hypoxia induced by simple asphyxiant effects.
- NIOSH considers trichloroethylene; ethylene dichloride; hexachloroethane; 1,1,2,2-tetrachloroethane; and 1,1,2-trichloroethane to be potential occupational carcinogens.

EPIDEMIOLOGY

- Chlorinated hydrocarbon exposure is widespread in occupational settings.
- Death is rare and is usually due to cardiac dysrhythmia, CNS depression, or fulminant hepatic failure.
- Both pediatric and elderly patients are more sensitive to chlorinated hydrocarbon solvent exposure effects.

CAUSES

- Exposure primarily occurs accidentally by occupational inhalation or intentionally by abusive inhalation ("sniffing" or "huffing").
- Child neglect should be considered if the patient is under 1 year of age, and attempted suicide should be considered if the patient is over 6 years of age.

RISK FACTORS

Workers at risk of chlorinated hydrocarbon exposure include painters, mechanics, dry cleaners, laboratory workers, petrochemical workers, plastic manufacturers, printers, and plumbers.

PREGNANCY AND LACTATION

Exposure to chlorinated hydrocarbons during pregnancy is probably teratogenic and increases the risk of spontaneous abortion.

WORKPLACE STANDARDS

Carbon Tetrachloride

- ACGIH. TLV TWA 5 ppm; STEL 10 ppm.
- OSHA. PEL TWA is 10 ppm; ceiling is 25 ppm.
- NIOSH. IDLH is 200 ppm.

Chlorobenzene

ACGIH. TLV TWA is 10 ppm.
OSHA. PEL TWA is 75 ppm.
NIOSH. IDLH is 1000 ppm.

Chloroform

- ACGIH. TLV TWA is 10 ppm.
- NIOSH. IDLH concentration value is 500 ppm.
- OSHA. Ceiling is 50 ppm.

Diagnosis

DIFFERENTIAL DIAGNOSIS

- Other toxic agents that cause altered mental status include opiates, sedative-hypnotics, ethanol, gamma-hydroxybutyrate, rohypnol, clonidine, tricyclic antidepressants, methanol, anticonvulsants, ethylene glycol, and other hydrocarbons, among others.
- Nontoxic causes of altered mental status include intracranial trauma or infection, hypoglycemia or other metabolic disturbances, and electrolyte abnormalities.

SIGNS AND SYMPTOMS

Vital Signs

Fever or tachycardia may occur in chlorinated hydrocarbon poisonings.

HEENT

Eye and mucous membrane irritation is common with inhalation exposure.

Dermatologic

Contact dermatitis, irritant dermatitis, or chemical burns may occur following topical exposure.

Cardiovascular

- Dilated cardiomyopathy and myocardial infarction may be seen in chronic abusers.
- Vasodilation (centrally mediated) leading to hypotension may occur.
- Cardiovascular collapse or ventricular dysrhythmias including ventricular fibrillation may develop during inhalation abuse.

Pulmonary

- Inhalation causes mucous membrane irritation, dyspnea, tachypnea, cough, and chest tightness, followed by hypoxia and pulmonary edema in severe cases.
- Ingestion may cause pulmonary effects if aspiration occurs.

Neurologic

- Initial CNS excitation includes euphoria, nervousness, tremor, insomnia, nystagmus, and headache.
- CNS excitation is followed by depression ranging from somnolence and confusion to vertigo, ataxia, seizures, and coma.
- Cognitive deficits, memory impairment, psychiatric disorders, encephalopathy, and emotional lability may develop during chronic exposure.

Gastrointestinal

Nausea, vomiting, diarrhea, and abdominal pain may occur, particularly following ingestion.

Hepatic

- Liver enzyme elevation may occur.
- Massive necrosis and hepatorenal syndrome may occur in severe cases.

PROCEDURES AND LABORATORY TESTS

Essential Tests

No test is essential for all patients.

Recommended Tests

- Serum electrolytes, BUN, creatinine, and urinalysis should be ordered to assess causes of CNS depression and renal effects.
- Complete blood count should be obtained to detect bone marrow injury.
- Serum liver transaminase levels should be assessed to detect hepatic injury.
- ECG and cardiac enzymes should be obtained in severe cases to follow cardiac injury and dysrhythmias.
- Carbon monoxide produced by methylene chloride metabolism may result in elevated carboxyhemoglobin levels.
- Serum acetaminophen and aspirin levels should be obtained in overdose settings to detect occult ingestion.

• Head CT, MRI, lumbar puncture, bacterial cultures, urine toxicology screen, and other tests should be ordered as needed to assess cognitive deficits, altered mental status, or seizures.

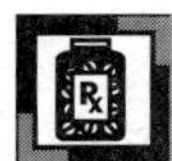

Treatment

• Therapy should focus on supportive care, particularly hemodynamic support and airway management.
• Dose and time of exposure must be determined for all substances involved.

DIRECTING PATIENT COURSE

The health-care provider should call a poison control center when:

• Altered mental status or other serious effects are present.
• Signs and symptoms are not consistent with chlorinated hydrocarbon exposure.
• Coingestant, drug interaction, or underlying disease presents an unusual problem.

The patient should be referred to a health-care facility when:

• Attempted suicide or homicide is possible.
• The patient or caregiver seems unreliable.
• Symptoms are present.
• Coingestant, drug interaction, or underlying disease presents an unusual problem.

Admission Considerations

• All patients who have ingested chlorinated hydrocarbons should be admitted because hepatic injury is likely in such cases.
• Patients with inhalation exposure should be admitted if mental status depression, seizure activity, cardiac toxicity, or serious metabolic abnormality is present.

DECONTAMINATION

Out of Hospital

• Emesis should not be induced because CNS depression may develop.
• The patient should be removed from the source of the exposure.
• Exposed areas of skin should be washed thoroughly with soap and water.

In Hospital

• Gastric aspiration with a nasogastric tube should be performed in patients presenting within 1 hour of ingestion or if serious effects are present.
• One dose of activated charcoal (1–2 g/kg) may be administered if a substantial ingestion has occurred within the previous hour.

ANTIDOTES

There is no specific antidote for chlorinated hydrocarbon toxicity.

ADJUNCTIVE TREATMENT

• There is no specific therapy for pulmonary edema (see SECTION II, Pulmonary Edema chapter, for general management).
• Cardiac dysrhythmias are managed using standard ACLS algorithms.
• Although there is concern that catecholamines may help induce ventricular dysrhythmia, it is unknown whether it is detrimental in resuscitation.
• Hepatic injury is managed by standard management of liver failure.

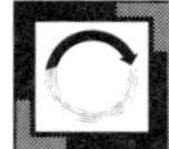

Follow-Up

PATIENT MONITORING

Respiratory function, cardiac rhythm, and CNS status should be monitored.

EXPECTED COURSE AND PROGNOSIS

Acute Inhalation

• Symptoms of respiratory irritation are followed by CNS depression in severe cases; cardiac dysrhythmia, cardiovascular collapse, or hepatic injury also may occur.
• CNS and airway symptoms peak rapidly and resolve over several hours; other effects may require days to weeks to resolve.

Chronic Inhalation

• Chronic inhalation results in cognitive and memory deficits; liver and renal injury also may occur.
• CNS symptoms may only be partially reversible; permanent liver damage or carcinoma may develop.

Acute Ingestion

• The primary result of acute ingestion is hepatic injury.
• Onset occurs quickly, followed by a prolonged course of days to weeks.

DISCHARGE CRITERIA/INSTRUCTIONS

• From the emergency department.

—Acute inhalation exposure. Patients who are asymptomatic and have normal neurologic and cardiac examination results may be discharged after a 6-hour observation period and psychiatric evaluation, if needed.
—Chronic inhalation exposure. Patients without severe liver or renal function abnormalities or altered level of consciousness may be discharged after psychiatric evaluation, if needed.

• From the hospital. Patients may be discharged after toxic effects have resolved or stabilized; psychiatric evaluation should be obtained if needed.

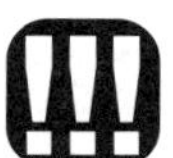

Pitfalls

DIAGNOSIS

Alternative diagnoses for CNS depression should be considered.

FOLLOW-UP

Hepatic, renal, and CNS status should be monitored following chronic or symptomatic acute exposure.

ICD-9-CM 982.3

Toxic effect of solvents other than petroleum-based: other chlorinated hydrocarbon solvents.

See also: SECTION II, Hypotension and Pulmonary Edema chapters.

RECOMMENDED READING

Snyder R, Andrews LS. Toxic effects of solvents and vapors. In: Klaassen CD, Amdur MO, Doull J, eds. *Casarett and Doull's toxicology: the basic science of poisons,* 5th ed. New York: McGraw-Hill, 1996:737–771.

US Department of Health and Human Services. ATSDR case studies in environmental medicine: carbon tetrachloride toxicity. March 1992, Monograph 18.

US Department of Health and Human Services. ATSDR case studies in environmental medicine: tetrachloroethylene toxicity. March 1990, Monograph 9.

Author: Alvin C. Bronstein

Reviewer: Richard C. Dart

Hydrofluoric Acid and Ammonium Bifluoride

Basics

DESCRIPTION

Hydrogen fluoride (HF), ammonium fluoride (NH_4F), and ammonium bifluoride (NH_4HF_2) are chemicals used in household and industrial products.

FORMS AND USES

Hydrogen Fluoride

- HF is available as a concentrated solution (for glass etching) or in more dilute household products (rust remover and automotive cleaning products).
- Concentration ranges from 6% or 8% to 90%.

Ammonium Bifluoride and Ammonium Fluoride

- Ammonium bifluoride is found in products used to clean wheels, in dairy equipment, and in beer-processing equipment.
- It is used in the manufacture of magnesium and its alloys, in the porcelain and glass industries, and in aluminum production.
- Effects of ammonium bifluoride or fluoride ingestion are similar to those of HF ingestion.

TOXIC DOSE

- Ingestion of more than 30 ml of low-concentration rust remover by an adult has been fatal.
- Dermal exposure to HF at more than 50% concentration over 1% body surface area may cause rapid deterioration and death.

PATHOPHYSIOLOGY

- Fluoride-containing compounds cause toxicity primarily by the binding and precipitation of calcium ions.
- This produces local tissue injury as well as systemic hypocalcemia.
- The direct skin injury is not as rapid and severe as caustics such as lye, unless the concentration is greater than 50%.

EPIDEMIOLOGY

- Poisoning is uncommon.
- Toxic effects following exposure are typically mild.
- Death occurs following exposure to high concentrations, large dermal exposure, or ingestion.

CAUSES

- Poisoning usually occurs by accidental skin exposure or ingestion.
- The possibility of child neglect should be considered in patients under 1 year of age; suicide attempt in patients over 6 years of age.

RISK FACTORS

Children have a larger surface area-to-volume ratio, which may increase the risk of systemic symptoms from dermal exposure.

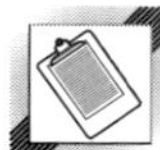

Diagnosis

DIFFERENTIAL DIAGNOSIS

Toxic causes of skin burns include acid or alkali burns and phenol.

SIGNS AND SYMPTOMS

- Skin exposure is initially asymptomatic (unless a concentrated solution is involved), followed by severe unremitting burning pain hours later.
- Following ingestion, sudden cardiac dysrhythmia and death may occur within the first few hours after ingestion.

Vital Signs

Pain may cause tachycardia and hypertension.

HEENT

- Unless a high-concentration product has been ingested, patients usually do not have clinically significant oral burns.
- Eye exposure may cause severe corneal injury.

Dermatologic

- Over time, erythema and burns may develop; time to onset is inversely related to the concentration of product.
- Exposure to HF at 6% to 8% concentration may not produce injury for several hours.
- Exposure to HF at more than 50% concentration produces injury quickly.

Cardiovascular

Ventricular dysrhythmia may develop in severe dermal exposure or following ingestion.

Pulmonary

Inhalation may cause bronchospasm, hypoxia, and pulmonary edema; upper airway burns may develop in severe exposure.

Gastrointestinal

- Ingestion of HF or ammonium bifluoride at low concentrations (<10%–20%) causes minor gastrointestinal symptoms.
- Ingestion of HF at high concentration may result in esophageal or gastric burns.

Fluids and Electrolytes

Hypocalcemia and hypomagnesemia can result from either dermal exposure or ingestion; rapidity of onset appears to be directly related to amount and concentration.

Neurologic

Tetany can develop from hypocalcemia.

PROCEDURES AND LABORATORY TESTS

Essential Tests

No tests may be needed for small dermal burns from HF at 6% to 8% concentration.

Recommended Tests

- Skin exposure. Serum electrolytes, BUN, creatinine, calcium, and magnesium levels are needed only following exposure to HF or ammonium fluoride at more than 10% concentration that involves at least 1% of body surface area, or 6% to 8% concentration that involves more than 5% body surface area.
- Ingestion

—Serum electrolytes, BUN, creatinine, calcium and magnesium levels should be measured if the patient has ingested a concentration of more than 10% or has taken more than a sip (approximately 2–5 ml) of solution at less than 10% concentration.
—Serum calcium and magnesium should be repeated hourly; decreasing or mildly decreased calcium levels should be treated immediately because the patient may deteriorate abruptly.
—ECG should be obtained at arrival and every 15 to 30 minutes for at least 2 hours for significant exposures; QT interval prolongation is a sign of cardiac toxicity.

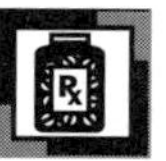

Treatment

- Treatment should focus on decontamination, close monitoring, and prompt treatment of hypocalcemia.
- Dose and time of exposure should be determined for substances involved.

DIRECTING PATIENT COURSE

The health-care provider should call the poison control center when:

- Hypocalcemia, dysrhythmia, significant burns, or other severe effects are present.
- The patient has ingested a concentration of more than 10% or has taken more than a sip (approximately 2–5 ml) of solution at less than 10% concentration.
- Toxic effects not consistent with hydrogen fluoride poisoning are present.
- Coingestant, drug interaction, or underlying disease presents unusual problems.

The patient should be referred to a health-care facility when:

- Attempted suicide or homicide is possible.
- Patient or caregiver seems unreliable.
- History of ingestion of any fluoride-containing product is obtained.
- Coingestant, drug interaction, or underlying disease presents unusual problems.

Admission Considerations

Inpatient treatment in the ICU is warranted when:

- Patient with skin exposure has hypocalcemia or burns of large surface area.
- Patient with ingestion shows any clinical effect during several hours of observation.
- Large or complicated burns (e.g., of the face or perineum) are present, which should be evaluated at a burn facility.

DECONTAMINATION

Out of Hospital

- Skin should be washed copiously with water for 20 to 30 minutes.
- Following ingestion, 30 cc of a magnesium antacid (e.g., milk of magnesia) or calcium carbonate (e.g., Tums) should be administered.

In Hospital

- Skin should be washed copiously with water for 20 to 30 minutes.
- Following ingestion, stomach contents should be aspirated if patient arrives within 30 minutes.
- Following ingestion, 30 cc of a magnesium antacid (e.g., milk of magnesia) or calcium carbonate (e.g., Tums) should be administered.

ANTIDOTES

Skin Burns

- Small burns (e.g., on a finger) can be treated with a topical paste or subcutaneous injection of calcium gluconate.
- Calcium chloride is caustic and should be used only intravenously, not topically or by infiltration.

Calcium Gluconate Paste

- Indication. Pain after any HF exposure indicates use.
- Contraindications. There are none.
- Method of administration

—Paste should be applied liberally to the affected area (for hand injury, placement of paste in latex glove allows convenient application).
—To make the paste, 3.5 g of calcium gluconate powder is mixed with 5 ounces of a water-soluble lubricant (e.g., K-Y jelly) or ten 10-grain tablets (6.5 g) of calcium carbonate (e.g., Os-Cal) are crushed in a minimum of 20 ml of water-soluble lubricant.

Calcium Gluconate 10% Solution for Injection

- Indication. Pain not responding to topical calcium indicates use.
- Method of administration

—Local infiltration of digit involved or 1 ml for each 2 cm^2 of burned area using a 30-gauge needle.
—Intravenous infusion using a Bier block technique; intraarterial infusion has been used for difficult cases; consultation with a poison center or medical toxicologist is advised.

- Adverse reactions

—Infiltration of large amounts of fluid may result in local tissue injury.
—Calcium chloride should not be used for infiltration.

Ingestion

Calcium Chloride 10% Solution

- Indications

—Indications are systemic hypocalcemia, prolonged QTc, or other evidence of hypocalcemia (e.g., paresthesias or hyperactive reflexes).
—Prophylactic use should be considered for high-risk situations (large surface area exposure, large or suicidal ingestion).

- Method of administration

—The dose is 5 to 10 cc infused intravenously over 10 minutes.
—The pediatric dose is 10 to 25 mg/kg, up to one ampule per dose.
—Dose is repeated based on narrowing of QTc interval to normal ($<$0.47 seconds in adults).

- Adverse reactions

—Calcium chloride is caustic to tissue and should not be given by local injection or topically.
—Hypotension and dysrhythmias may occur with rapid injection.

Magnesium Sulfate

- Indications

—Indication is systemic hypomagnesemia.
—Prophylactic use should be considered for high-risk situations (e.g., large surface area, large or suicidal ingestion).

- Method of administration

—The dose is 2 to 4 g infused intravenously over 10 minutes.
—Pediatric dose is 25 mg/kg, up to 2 g.
—Dose is repeated hourly as needed.

- Adverse reactions

—Rapid infusion may cause vasodilatation and hypotension.
—Hypermagnesemia may cause CNS and respiratory depression.

ADJUNCTIVE TREATMENT

Patients with digital burns may need to have fingernails removed to allow treatment of the nailbed.

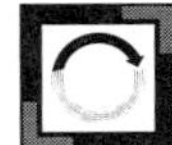

Follow-Up

PATIENT MONITORING

Patients with ingestion of any amount, high-concentration skin exposure, or large surface area skin exposure should have close cardiac monitoring because rapid cardiovascular collapse may develop.

EXPECTED COURSE AND PROGNOSIS

- Patients with low-concentration skin burns generally respond well to topical calcium, and symptoms resolve completely over several days.
- Patients with high-concentration burns usually develop immediate symptoms and may have extensive tissue injury despite rapid treatment.
- Patients with hypocalcemia may have rapid cardiovascular collapse and not respond to even high-dose calcium and magnesium.
- Local burns may require skin grafting.

DISCHARGE CRITERIA/INSTRUCTIONS

- From the emergency department. Patients with small dermal burns that improve with treatment may be discharged following 6 hours of observation and provision of follow-up for burn care.
- From the hospital. Patients may be discharged following recovery of normal cardiac function, with adequate pain control and good burn care follow-up.

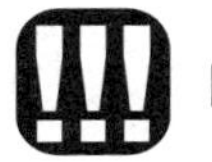

Pitfalls

DIAGNOSIS

- Ingestion may not produce the typical signs of corrosive ingestion.
- Sudden cardiac arrest may occur following ingestion of more than an ounce.

TREATMENT

- Even mildly depressed calcium or prolongation of the QTc interval may portend rapid deterioration.
- Very high doses of calcium and magnesium may be required.

ICD-9-CM 983

Toxic effect of corrosive aromatics, acids, and caustic alkalis.

See also: SECTION III, Calcium Gluconate and Chloride, and Magnesium Sulfate chapters.

RECOMMENDED READING

Caravati EM. Acute hydrofluoric acid exposure. *Am J Emerg Med* 1988;6:143–250.

Stremski ES, Grande GA, Ling LJ. Survival following hydrofluoric acid ingestion. *Ann Emerg Med* 1992;21:1396–1399.

Authors: Lada Kokan and Kennon Heard

Reviewer: Katherine M. Hurlbut

Hydrogen Peroxide

Basics

DESCRIPTION

- Hydrogen peroxide (H_2O_2) is a colorless liquid with a bitter taste. It releases oxygen bubbles on contact with tissues.
- Synonyms of hydrogen peroxide include albone, carbamide peroxide, hydrogen dioxide, hydroperite, hydroperoxide, inhibine, perhydrol, peroxan, peroxide, urea hydrogen peroxide, and urea peroxide.

FORMS AND USES

- Hydrogen peroxide 3%

—Commonly used as a topical antiseptic and household cleanser
—Used in plastic manufacturing, printing, bleaching, renovating paintings and engravings, refining oils and fats, dyes, photography, cleaning metals, and as an oxidizer and disinfectant

- Hydrogen peroxide 35%, also known as "food grade," is sold in health food stores as a remedy for a variety of medical conditions.
- Hydrogen peroxide 90% is used in rocket propulsion and the manufacture of foam rubber, and as a bleaching agent and dough conditioner.

TOXIC DOSE

- A few ounces (several gulps) of hydrogen peroxide in concentrations greater than 35% has resulted in widespread gas embolization and death in both adults and children.
- Hydrogen peroxide 3% is a local irritant; 35% can cause severe tissue injury and burns.

PATHOPHYSIOLOGY

Hydrogen peroxide releases oxygen upon contact, which may lead to perforated viscus and oxygen embolization into the tissues of the portal, gastric, and superior mesenteric venous systems when high concentrations are ingested.

EPIDEMIOLOGY

- Incidents are common with the 3% concentration, rare with 35% or greater concentration.
- Toxic effects following exposure are typically mild, with death occurring in patients exposed to concentrations of 35% or greater.

CAUSES

- Hydrogen peroxide poisonings are usually accidental ingestions in children and industrial accidents in adults.
- Child neglect should be considered if the patient is under 1 year of age; attempted suicide if the patient is over 6 years of age.

WORKPLACE STANDARDS

- OSHA. PEL TWA is 1 ppm.
- NIOSH. IDLH value is 75 ppm.
- ACGIH. TLV TWA is 1 ppm.

Diagnosis

DIFFERENTIAL DIAGNOSIS

- Other tissue irritants include hypochlorites and most household cleaners and corrosives such as strong acids, bases, ammonia, drain cleaners, flux, heavy metals, and many others.
- Other causes of abdominal pain and bleeding include gastritis, ulcer, and varices.

SIGNS AND SYMPTOMS

- Ingestion of 3% concentration typically causes mild, self-limited tissue irritation and no permanent injury.
- Ingestion of concentrations higher than 3% may cause caustic injury to the gastrointestinal tract, bleeding, and shock.

—Dermal contact may cause severe burns.
—Ocular exposure may cause ulceration or perforation.
—Inhalation exposure may cause pulmonary edema.
—Hydrogen peroxide causes gastrointestinal tumors in animals at 30% concentration.

Vital Signs

- Tachypnea and tachycardia followed by hypotension may occur in severe cases.
- Sepsis has occurred following irrigation of the colon or wounds with peroxide.

HEENT

- Hydrogen peroxide 3% causes self-limited eye irritation.
- Concentrations higher than 10% may cause corneal erosions and perforation.

Skin

- Hydrogen peroxide 3% produces bleaching and irritation.
- Concentrations higher than 10% may cause burns.

Pulmonary

Concentrations higher than 10% can cause irritation or cough leading to pulmonary edema, and may cause apnea in severe cases and in high-concentration ingestions.

Cardiovascular

Hypotension, ischemic ECG changes, and cardiac arrest have occurred after ingestion of hydrogen peroxide 35%.

Gastrointestinal

- Ingestion of hydrogen peroxide 3% causes minor irritation, bloating, nausea, and vomiting.
- Rectal administration of (or irrigation of wounds or fistulas) hydrogen peroxide 3% has caused colonic perforation.
- Ingestion of concentrations higher than 10% may cause burns, gas emboli, intestinal gangrene, hemorrhage, and perforation.

Neurologic

Ingestion of hydrogen peroxide 35% has been followed by seizures and, rarely, permanent neurologic injury, probably related to gas embolization.

PROCEDURES AND LABORATORY TESTS

Essential Tests

No tests may be needed for asymptomatic patients, especially if 3% concentration is involved.

Recommended Tests

- Arterial blood gases and ECG should be obtained in patients with suspected embolization; hypoxia or ischemic ECG changes suggest a life-threatening exposure.
- Serum electrolytes, acetaminophen, and salicylate levels should be obtained in overdose settings to assess occult ingestion.
- Abdominal radiographs should be obtained if a large amount or a high concentration was ingested, to detect perforation or gas embolization. CT or MRI should be performed if CNS effects develop.
- Endoscopy is recommended for patients who ingest concentrations of 10% or greater to detect gastrointestinal burns.

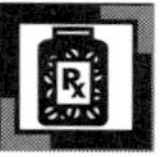

Treatment

- Initial treatment should focus on managing gastric perforation or gas embolization while continuing supportive care.
- Dose and time of exposure must be determined for all substances involved.

DIRECTING PATIENT COURSE

The health-care provider should call a poison control center when:

- Exposure involves concentration greater than 10%.
- Gastrointestinal burns or bleeding, gas embolization, pulmonary edema, shock, or other serious effects are present.
- Toxic effects are not consistent with hydrogen peroxide.
- Coingestant, drug interaction, or underlying disease presents an unusual problem.

The patient should be referred to a health-care facility when:

- Attempted suicide or homicide is possible.
- The patient or caregiver seems unreliable.
- Any toxic effects develop
- Hydrogen peroxide 10% or higher concentration has been ingested.
- Coingestant, drug interaction, or underlying disease presents an unusual problem.

Admission Considerations

Inpatient management is warranted for all patients with gastrointestinal burns, gas embolization, or hemodynamic instability.

DECONTAMINATION

Out of Hospital

- Emesis must not be induced because of the risk of burns and seizures.
- A small amount of water may be used to dilute the hydrogen peroxide.
- Exposed eyes or skin should be irrigated with copious amounts of water.
- Administer 100% oxygen after inhalation exposure.

In Hospital

- Gastric lavage is not recommended because of the risk of further gastrointestinal injury.
- Activated charcoal is not recommended unless another significant toxic coingestant is involved because the charcoal may obscure endoscopy results.
- Gastric aspiration with a small nasogastric tube may be considered if gastric distension is a potential problem, particularly after ingestion of concentrations higher than 10%.
- Exposed eyes or skin should be irrigated with copious amounts of water or 0.9% NaCl and examined for burns.
- Administer 100% oxygen after inhalation exposure.

ANTIDOTES

There is no antidote for hydrogen peroxide ingestion.

ADJUNCTIVE TREATMENT

- Hypotension is treated with isotonic fluid infusion, the Trendelenburg position, and vasopressor if needed; dopamine is preferred, and norepinephrine is used for refractory hypotension.
- Although no data specific to hydrogen peroxide are available, corticosteroids have been shown to reduce the incidence of strictures following grade 2 burns from acids and alkaline corrosives in some animal studies and a meta-analysis of human studies.
- Corticosteroids are not recommended for grade 0 or 1 burns, which have a low incidence of strictures, or for grade 3 burns, which have a high incidence of strictures regardless of therapy and bear an increased risk of perforation.
- Hyperbaric oxygen has been proposed as treatment of gas embolization, but has not been studied.
- Prophylactic antibiotics have not been shown to be of benefit; antibiotics should be reserved for patients with suspected or demonstrated perforation or infection.

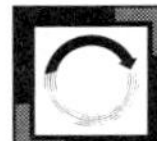

Follow-Up

PATIENT MONITORING

Pulmonary and hemodynamic function should be monitored closely if the concentration of hydrogen peroxide ingested is higher than 10%, or if pulmonary symptoms develop.

EXPECTED COURSE AND PROGNOSIS

- If the concentration of hydrogen peroxide is lower than 3%, most patients develop minimal effects that resolve over several hours.
- If the concentration is higher than 10%, acute effects develop rapidly, and gastrointestinal perforation or oxygen embolization may occur, leading to permanent neurologic injury or death.

DISCHARGE CRITERIA/INSTRUCTIONS

- From the emergency department

—If the concentration of hydrogen peroxide is lower than 3%, patients who develop no or minimal symptoms over 2 to 4 hours may be discharged after psychiatric evaluation, if needed.
—If the concentration is higher than 10%, patients without hemodynamic instability, CNS effects, clinical or radiographic evidence of emboli or perforation, and normal results or grade 1 burns on endoscopy (in cases of ingestion) may be discharged after 6 hours of observation and psychiatric evaluation, if needed.

- From the hospital. Patients may be discharged after hemodynamic condition has stabilized, CNS function is normal or improving, and enteral or parenteral feedings are tolerated (in cases of grade 2 or 3 burns or perforation).

PATIENT EDUCATION

Serious inadvertent ingestion of concentrated products has occurred because they were stored in the refrigerator and mistaken for water.

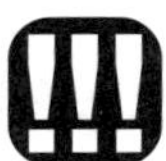

Pitfalls

DIAGNOSIS

- Oxygen embolization has occurred after use of 3% hydrogen peroxide for wound, fistula, and colonic irrigation.
- The provider should be vigilant for signs of perforated viscus, gas embolization, or both.

FOLLOW-UP

Strictures are reported to develop weeks after grade 2 or 3 esophageal burns from ingestion of other caustic products, and might develop after burns from concentrated (greater than 10%) hydrogen peroxide.

ICD-9-CM 976

Poisoning by agents primarily affecting skin and mucous membrane, ophthalmologic, otorhinolaryngological, and dental drugs.

See also: SECTION II, Hypotension chapter; and SECTION IV, Caustics—Basic chapter.

RECOMMENDED READING

Cina SJ, Downs JCU, Conradi SE. Hydrogen peroxide—a source of lethal oxygen embolism—case report and review of the literature. *Am J Forensic Med Pathol* 1994;15:44–50.

Henry MC, Wheeler J, Mofenson HC, et al. Hydrogen peroxide 3% exposures. *J Toxicol Clin Toxicol* 1996;34:323–327.

Author: Katherine M. Hurlbut

Reviewer: Richard C. Dart

Hydrogen Sulfide

Basics

DESCRIPTION

- Hydrogen sulfide (H_2S, hydrosulfuric acid) is a colorless gas with a characteristic "rotten eggs" odor.
- H_2S is heavier than air and is found naturally in caves, volcanoes, sulfur springs, natural gas, and swamps.
- Synonyms of H_2S include sewer gas, sour gas, and knock-down gas.

FORMS AND USES

- H_2S is a by-product of the decomposition of organic materials (sewage).
- Industrial sources include petroleum distillation/refining, paper production, heavy water production, leather finishing and manufacturing, and rubber vulcanizing processes.

TOXIC DOSE

H_2S is a "one-whiff" knock-down chemical; a few breaths of high concentration gas may be fatal immediately.

PATHOPHYSIOLOGY

- Toxic effects following exposure are typically severe, with coma and death occurring rapidly.
- H_2S inhibits cytochrome oxidase a_3, which results in interruption of oxidative phosphorylation and thereby of adenosine triphosphate production; this interruption forces a shift to anaerobic glycolysis, which results in rapid lactate accumulation and profound metabolic acidosis.

EPIDEMIOLOGY

- H_2S poisoning is an infrequent but important cause of sudden death in the workplace.
- Exposure results in multiple victims because rescuers attempt to retrieve the initial victim only to succumb to the gas themselves.
- Children may be at increased risk for exposure because of their tendency to explore potentially hazardous enclosed areas.

CAUSES

H_2S poisonings are usually the result of accidental occupational exposure during cleaning or servicing of septic tanks.

PREGNANCY AND LACTATION

Severe maternal poisoning with hypoxia may produce fetal hypoxia and distress.

WORKPLACE STANDARDS

- ACGIH. TLV TWA is 10 ppm; STEL is 15 ppm.
- OSHA. PEL TWA is 10 ppm; PEL STEL is 15 ppm.
- NIOSH. IDLH is 300 ppm.

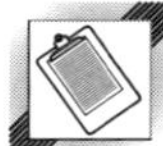

Diagnosis

DIFFERENTIAL DIAGNOSIS

- Other toxic agents that cause sudden knock-down effects include cyanide gas, very high concentrations of carbon monoxide, or asphyxiant gases.
- Nontoxic causes of sudden knock-down effects include pulmonary embolus, ventricular dysrhythmia, and catastrophic intracranial event, among others.

SIGNS AND SYMPTOMS

Most fatalities occur at the scene. If the patient rapidly recovers consciousness, recovery is usually complete if cerebral anoxic injury has not already occurred.

Vital Signs

Bradycardia or tachycardia and tachypnea may be followed quickly by respiratory arrest, hypotension, and coma.

HEENT

- Exposure results in intense mucous membrane irritation, including corneal abrasions (gas eye) and corneal ulceration.
- The characteristic odor serves as an olfactory warning for gas; the ability to smell the gas, however, is lost at higher concentrations because of paralysis of the olfactory nerve.
- Mydriasis may occur as a preterminal event.

Skin

Diaphoresis may occur.

Pulmonary

Cough and respiratory distress may be followed quickly by respiratory arrest.

Cardiovascular

Tachycardia or bradycardia may precede rapid onset of cardiovascular collapse and cardiac arrest.

Gastrointestinal

Nausea and vomiting are common.

Musculoskeletal

- Profound weakness with loss of reflexes may occur.
- Trauma secondary to a "quick knock-down" effect is common.

Neurologic

- Acute exposure. Headache and confusion may rapidly progress to seizures and coma; loss of consciousness may be transient if exposure is brief.
- Repeated exposure. Patients who experience repeated sublethal exposures are at risk for the development of cognitive function abnormalities, personality changes, and anosmia.

PROCEDURES AND LABORATORY TESTS

Essential Tests

- Arterial blood gases should be obtained to evaluate oxygenation and ventilation deficits caused by H_2S, a coingestant, aspiration pneumonia, or pulmonary edema.
- Serum electrolytes, BUN, creatinine, glucose, and lactate studies are warranted for patients with altered mental status.

Recommended Tests

- ECG, CT, lumbar puncture, blood, and cerebrospinal fluid cultures should be ordered as needed to evaluate altered mental status.
- Carboxyhemoglobin or methemoglobin level should be determined if coexposure may have occurred.
- Blood cyanide level should be considered to exclude cyanide exposure.
- A chest radiograph should be obtained for patients presenting after significant exposure or patients who remain symptomatic in the emergency department after minor exposure.

Not Recommended Tests

A sulfhemoglobin level is not useful, because acute H_2S exposure is not expected to produce sulfhemoglobin.

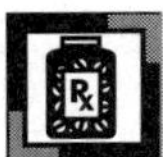

Treatment

• Treatment should focus on airway management and oxygen administration.
• The dose and time of exposure for all substances involved should be determined.

DIRECTING PATIENT COURSE

The health-care provider should call a poison control center when:

• Signs and symptoms are not consistent with H_2S poisoning.
• Drug interaction, or underlying disease presents an unusual problem.

The patient should be referred to a health-care facility when:

• Suspicion of H_2S exposure exists.
• Attempted suicide or homicide is possible.
• Respiratory arrest, altered mental status, hypotension, or other severe effects are present.
• Drug interaction or underlying disease presents an unusual problem.

Admission Considerations

Inpatient management for at least 24 hours is warranted for all patients with significant exposure to H_2S gas or persistent symptoms to observe and evaluate for delayed pulmonary edema or CNS symptoms.

DECONTAMINATION

Out of Hospital

The patient should be removed from the source of exposure, but rescuers should not attempt retrieval of the victim unless equipped with self-contained breathing apparatus.

In Hospital

H_2S toxicity does not result from dermal or ingestion exposure, so decontamination is unnecessary.

ANTIDOTES

• There is no proven antidote for H_2S poisoning.
• Cyanide antidote kit. Administration of only the sodium nitrite component of the kit in conjunction with supportive therapy within 15 to 20 minutes of exposure is supported by anecdotal reports (see SECTION III, Cyanide Antidote Package chapter). Because 85% of the sulfide is eliminated from the blood within minutes of exposure, however, this procedure is often of no benefit.

ADJUNCTIVE TREATMENT

• Hyperbaric oxygen has been described as effective in reversing CNS depression and acidosis in anecdotal reports and may be a reasonable intervention in serious cases.
• Hypotension is treated with isotonic fluid infusion, the Trendelenburg position, and vasopressor if needed; dopamine is preferred, and norepinephrine is used for refractory hypotension.
• There is no specific treatment for metabolic acidosis resulting from H_2S poisoning; the health-care provider should optimize hemodynamic parameters with intensive supportive care.

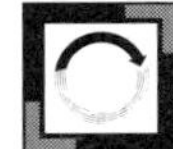

Follow-Up

PATIENT MONITORING

• Patients who have sustained significant exposure to H_2S gas should be observed for at least 24 hours with cardiac monitoring and attention primarily focused on the possible development of pulmonary edema.
• The health-care provider should be vigilant for sequelae of hypoxia.

EXPECTED COURSE AND PROGNOSIS

• Prognosis is directly related to the concentration of the exposure and, to a lesser extent, the length of time of the exposure.
• If the patient rapidly regains consciousness, recovery is usually complete, provided cerebral anoxic injury has not already occurred.
• Prolonged unconsciousness indicates a poor prognosis.

DISCHARGE CRITERIA/INSTRUCTIONS

• From the emergency department

—Patients who have not sustained a significant H_2S exposure and who remain asymptomatic after a 4- to 6-hour observation period may be discharged.
—Patients who have sustained a significant H_2S exposure or have local airway irritative effects should not be discharged.

• From the hospital. Patients may be discharged after sequelae of poisoning have resolved or remained stable for at least 24 hours.

PATIENT EDUCATION

• Patients should be aware of the risk of brain injury as a result of the cumulative effects of multiple knock-downs.
• Workers who come into contact with gases from sewage or other organic matter should avoid entering enclosed areas or areas with poor ventilation until quantitative air sampling can be performed to exclude the presence of H_2S gas or other toxic gases.
• Workers in high-risk industries need to be cognizant of the dangers of entering an enclosed area to retrieve a fallen comrade.

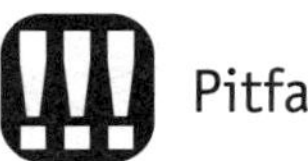

Pitfalls

DIAGNOSIS

It is important to consider exposure to another toxic gas, such as methane, ammonia, chlorine, carbon monoxide, cyanide, or sulfur dioxide, as well as alternative causes for altered level of consciousness, including metabolic, infectious, and traumatic events.

TREATMENT

It is important to treat the victim for possible comorbid conditions such as traumatic injury to the spine or myocardial ischemia secondary to hypoxia.

ICD-9-CM 987

Toxic effect of other gases, fumes, or vapors.

See also: SECTION II, Hypotension chapter; SECTION III, Cyanide Antidote Package chapter; and SECTION IV, Cyanide chapter.

RECOMMENDED READING

Hoffman HE, Guidotti TL. Natural gases. In: Greenberg MI et al., eds. *Occupational, industrial and environmental toxicology.* St. Louis: Mosby, 1997:359–366.

Smith RP, Gosselin RE. Hydrogen sulfide poisoning. *J Occup Med* 1979;21:93–97.

Author: Gerald F. O'Malley

Reviewer: Richard C. Dart

Imidazoline Decongestants

Basics

DESCRIPTION

The imidazoline derivatives are peripheral α_2 receptor agonists; local application results in vasoconstriction.

FORMS AND USES

- Imidazolines are used for nasal or ophthalmic decongestion.
- Imidazolines have been used as "knock-out drops" to induce CNS depression.

Tetrahydrozoline

- Nasal solutions of 0.10% and 0.05% (Tyzine): adult dosage is two to four drops of 0.10% into each nostril every 3 to 4 hours; pediatric (2–6 years old) dosage is two to three drops of 0.05% into each nostril every 4 to 6 hours.
- Ophthalmic solution of 0.05% (Visine Eye Drops): adult dosage is one to two drops of 0.05% into each eye two to four times daily.

Naphazoline

- Nasal solution of 0.05%
- Ophthalmic solutions of 0.012%, 0.020%, 0.025%, 0.030%, and 0.100% (Ak-Con, Albalon, Clear eyes, Comfort, Degest 2, Estivin 11, Inaphline, Muro's Opcon, Nafazair, Naphcon, Napholine, Ocu-Zoline, Opcon, VasoClear)

Oxymetazoline

- Nasal solutions of 0.025% and 0.05%
- Ophthalmic solution of 0.025% (Afrin 12 Hour, Allerest, 12 Hour Dristan Long Lasting Nasal Spray, Duration 12 Hour, Neo-Synephrine 12 Hour, Sinarest 12 Hour Nasal Spray, Vicks Sinex); adult dosage is one to two drops of 0.025% into each eye every 6 hours

Xylometazoline

Nasal solutions of 0.05% and 0.1%

TOXIC DOSE

- Death has been reported following intravenous injection of oxymetazoline.
- Mild drowsiness might occur in children following ingestion of one to two drops of tetrahydrozoline, but in one reported study no child ingesting less than 7.5 ml of 0.05% solution developed toxicity.
- Tetrahydroxoline has not been reported to cause major toxic effects in adults.

PATHOPHYSIOLOGY

- Most accidental pediatric ingestions result only in sedation, which responds to tactile stimulation.
- Systemic effects are mediated by activation of central α_2 receptors, resulting in inhibition of central sympathetic outflow in the brainstem and medulla.

EPIDEMIOLOGY

- Poisoning is common.
- Toxic effects following exposure are typically mild.
- Infants appear to be more susceptible to toxicity from topical use, and small ingestions in children have been reported to cause toxicity.

CAUSES

- Imidazoline poisonings usually result from accidental pediatric ingestion.
- Child neglect or abuse should be considered if the patient is less than 1 year of age, suicide attempt if the patient is older than 6 years of age.

DRUG AND DISEASE INTERACTIONS

- The effects of imidazolines may be enhanced by other CNS depressants.
- Hypotension may be enhanced by antihypertensive agents.
- Use of imidazolines with monoamine oxidase inhibitors may result in hypertension.
- Ocular application of imidazolines should be avoided in patients with known narrow-angle glaucoma.
- Imidazolines should be used cautiously in patients with diabetes mellitus or prostatic hypertrophy.

PREGNANCY AND LACTATION

US FDA Pregnancy Category C. The drug exerts animal teratogenic or embryocidal effects, but there are no controlled studies in women, or no studies are available in either animals or women.

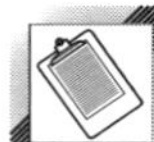

Diagnosis

DIFFERENTIAL DIAGNOSIS

- Other toxicologic agents that cause CNS and respiratory depression include other α_2 agonists (clonidine), anticonvulsants, alcohols, benzodiazepines, barbiturates, narcotics, gamma-hydroxybutyrate, and others.
- Nontoxicologic causes of CNS depression include electrolyte abnormalities, hypoxia, hypothermia, postictal states, CNS infection, or trauma.

SIGNS AND SYMPTOMS

Intentional adult and large pediatric ingestions can result in miosis, sedation, apnea, bradycardia and hypotension.

Vital Signs

- Hypotension, bradycardia, and hypoventilation are common following large exposure.
- Hypothermia has been reported following severe overdose.

HEENT

- Miosis is common.
- Rebound nasal mucosal edema is common following nasal application for more than 3 to 5 days.
- Chemical conjunctivitis and rhinitis have been reported.

Dermatologic

Pallor may reflect poor peripheral perfusion.

Cardiovascular

- Initial transient hypertension occurs but is rarely observed because it usually resolves prior to health-care evaluation.
- Hypotension and bradycardia are common following large exposures.
- Atrioventricular nodal blocks occur rarely.
- Myocardial ischemia has occurred but is rare.

Pulmonary

Hypoventilation is common and may progress to apnea.

Musculoskeletal

Hyporeflexia and hypotonia may develop in severe cases.

Neurologic

- CNS depression is common and may range from mild sedation to coma.
- Ataxia, headaches, and tremors have been reported.
- Subarachnoid hemorrhage and cerebral infarction are rare but have been reported following chronic use.

Psychiatric

Hallucinations and psychosis have been reported after acute or chronic use.

PROCEDURES AND LABORATORY TESTS

Essential Tests

No tests are usually needed in asymptomatic patients.

Recommended Tests

- ECG and cardiac monitoring should be ordered because bradycardia and atriventricular nodal blocks may occur, and cardiac ischemia may occur in hypotensive patients.
- Serum electrolytes, BUN, and creatinine should be obtained to assess renal injury, or altered mental status.
- Arterial blood gases or pulse oximetry is useful for assessment of respiratory depression or altered mental status.
- Serum acetaminophen and aspirin levels should be obtained in an overdose setting to detect occult ingestion.
- Head CT, lumbar puncture, and bacterial cultures may be ordered to assess altered mental status.

Not Recommended Tests

Tests to measure serum imidazoline levels are not clinically useful.

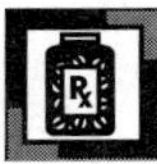

Treatment

- Treatment should focus on airway management and blood pressure support.
- The dose and time of exposure should be determined for all substances involved.

DIRECTING PATIENT COURSE

The health-care professional should call the poison control center when:

- A history of imidazoline ingestion is obtained.
- Signs and symptoms are not consistent with imidazoline toxicity.
- Coingestant, drug interaction, or underlying disease presents an unusual problem.

The patient should be referred to a health-care facility when:

- Attempted suicide or homicide is possible.
- The patient or caregiver seems unreliable.
- Any toxic effects develop.
- Coingestant, drug interaction, or underlying disease presents an unusual problem.

Admission Considerations

Inpatient management is warranted for patients with bradycardia, hypotension, or persistent CNS depression.

DECONTAMINATION

Out of Hospital

Emesis should not be induced because CNS depression may develop rapidly.

In Hospital

- Because of the small amounts of toxin involved, gastric lavage or aspiration is not recommended.
- One dose of activated charcoal (1–2 g/kg) may be administered if a substantial ingestion has occurred within the previous 30 to 60 minutes.
- Activated charcoal is also indicated for symptomatic patients following nasal or ophthalmic exposures because the solution may subsequently be swallowed.

ANTIDOTES

There is no specific antidote for imidazoline decongestant poisoning.

ADJUNCTIVE TREATMENT

- Patients with imidazoline-induced apnea often resume normal breathing patterns following tactile stimulation; some patients may require repetitive tactile stimulation.
- Naloxone is used to treat depressed mental status of unknown etiology.

—Naloxone has been reported to reverse the effects of imidazoline toxicity, but this reversal has never been demonstrated in a well-controlled clinical trial. Therefore, although administration of naloxone is safe, it is not routinely recommended in the absence of severe CNS and respiratory symptoms.
—The dose of naloxone in patients with coma and respiratory depression is 2 mg intravenously; if no clinical improvement occurs, the dose may be repeated once, but it is unlikely that more naloxone will have any effect.

- Hypotension. The patient should be treated with isotonic fluid infusion, the Trendelenburg position, and, if needed, vasopressors. Dopamine is preferred, and norepinephrine is added for refractory hypotension.
- Initial, transient hypertension usually does not require treatment; if treatment is required, however, a short-acting titratable antihypertensive agent such as intravenous nitroprusside, nitroglycerin, or esmolol should be used because hypotension may follow.

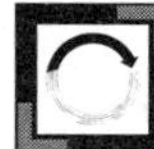

Follow-Up

PATIENT MONITORING

Cardiac and hemodynamic parameters should be monitored continuously.

EXPECTED COURSE AND PROGNOSIS

- Toxic effects typically develop within an hour, and most patients will recover uneventfully with simple supportive care.
- CNS depression, bradycardia, hypotension, and hypoventilation, however, may persist for more than 24 hours following severe overdose.
- Complications related to hypoxia and hypotension occur rarely, primarily in patients who do not reach health care promptly.

DISCHARGE CRITERIA/INSTRUCTIONS

- From the emergency department. Patients who are asymptomatic after observation for 4 to 6 hours postingestion may be discharged after psychiatric evaluation, if needed.
- From the hospital. Patients may be discharged after toxic effects have resolved and psychiatric evaluation, if needed.

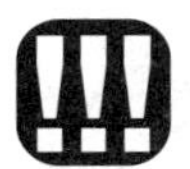

Pitfalls

DIAGNOSIS

- Imidazoline toxicity may be confused with opioid overdose.
- It is important to remember that initial, transient hypertension is consistent with imidazoline toxicity.

TREATMENT

- Aggressive management of the airway is vital.
- Treating initial and transient hypertension with a long-acting antihypertensive agent may exacerbate subsequent hypotension.

ICD-9-CM 963

Poisoning by primarily systemic agents.

See also: SECTION II, Bradycardia and Hypotension chapters.

RECOMMENDED READING

Mahieu LM, et al. Imidazoline intoxication in children. *Eur J Pediatr* 1993;152:944–946.

Author: Edwin K. Kuffner

Reviewer: Richard C. Dart

Insulin

Basics

DESCRIPTION

Insulin is an endogenous peptide that regulates blood glucose.

FORMS AND USES

- Insulin is available in many forms and preparations.
- Among the many trademarked preparations are Iletin, Lente insulin, NPH insulin, Humulin, Novalin, and Velosulin.
- Treatment of hyperglycemia. The dose varies by individual; the usual route is subcutaneous.
- Diabetic ketoacidosis. 0.1 U/kg regular insulin intravenously, then infusion of 0.1 U/kg/h.
- Hyperkalemia. Concurrent intravenous administration of 0.1 U/kg regular insulin and glucose can be used to treat hyperkalemia in normoglycemic patients.

TOXIC DOSE

- Toxic dose is relative to the patient's underlying glucose level.
- When insulin-dependent patients take their usual dose of insulin and either do not eat regularly or undergo an unusual amount of activity, they may experience hypoglycemic episodes.
- Deliberate insulin overdose can result in profound and prolonged hypoglycemia because the injected insulin can serve as a depot that results in a sustained release of insulin over several days.
- Orally administered insulin is broken down in the stomach and is nontoxic.

PATHOPHYSIOLOGY

Insulin lowers blood glucose by increasing uptake of glucose by skeletal muscle, increasing the formation of fat in adipose tissue and increasing hepatic formation of glycogen.

EPIDEMIOLOGY

- Hypoglycemia from insulin is very common, but insulin overdose is uncommon.
- Toxic effects following exposure are typically moderate.
- Death occurs rarely, usually following deliberate overdose and before medical care is reached.

CAUSES

- Insulin toxicity is usually an accidental incident.
- Child abuse should be considered if the patient is under 1 year of age; suicide if the patient is over 6 years of age.

RISK FACTORS

- Infants and children have small glycogen stores and are especially prone to develop hypoglycemia.
- Elderly patients may have decreased glycogen stores and thus are predisposed to hypoglycemia.

DRUG AND DISEASE INTERACTIONS

- Concurrent sulfonylurea ingestion increases the risk of hypoglycemia.
- Beta-blockers may mask symptoms of hypoglycemia, allowing hypoglycemia to develop unnoticed.

PREGNANCY AND LACTATION

- US FDA Pregnancy Category B. Animal studies do not indicate a risk to the fetus, and there are no controlled human studies, or animal studies do show an adverse effect on the fetus but well-controlled studies in pregnant women do not.
- Insulin does not cross the placenta; maternal hypoglycemia, however, may lead to fetal hypoglycemia and injury.

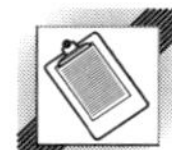

Diagnosis

DIFFERENTIAL DIAGNOSIS

- Other toxic agents that cause hypoglycemia include sulfonylurea overdose, akee fruit, ethanol, salicylate, propranolol, or any substance that causes massive hepatic necrosis.
- Nontoxic causes of hypoglycemia include insulinoma, sepsis, rapidly growing tumors, and hepatic failure from other causes.
- Hypoglycemia also may be triggered by infection, myocardial infarction, or other systemic processes.

SIGNS AND SYMPTOMS

- Insulin toxicity results in hypoglycemia, which may be delayed, prolonged, or recurrent.
- With severe hypoglycemia, anxiety, diaphoresis, tremor, tachycardia, lethargy, slurred speech, coma, and seizures may develop.
- Neurologic effects may be focal or nonfocal.

Vital Signs

Hypoglycemia initially causes tachycardia, tachypnea, and hypertension, followed by hypotension, hypothermia, and respiratory depression in severe and prolonged cases.

HEENT

Pupils may be dilated.

Dermatologic

Diaphoresis is common.

Cardiovascular

Tachycardia and hypertension occur.

Pulmonary

- Tachypnea can occur.
- Acute respiratory distress syndrome has been reported but may be related to prolonged hypoglycemia or aspiration during coma.

Gastrointestinal

Hunger, nausea, and vomiting may occur.

Fluids and Electrolytes

- Hypoglycemia is universal in significant overdose unless preexisting chronic hyperglycemia was present.
- Hypokalemia can occur due to a shift of potassium from outside to inside cells.

Musculoskeletal

- Muscle weakness may result from a lack of substrate.
- Rhabdomyolysis can occur because of prolonged immobility.

Neurologic

- Disorientation, agitation, lethargy, slurred speech, paresthesia, anxiety, headache, tremors, weakness, and ataxia may occur early, followed by coma and seizures.
- Focal neurologic signs such as paraplegia are uncommon, but may occur.
- Permanent neurologic impairment may follow prolonged hypoglycemia.

PROCEDURES AND LABORATORY TESTS

Essential Tests

Blood glucose levels should be obtained hourly, whenever the patient becomes symptomatic, and following each treatment with dextrose.

Recommended Tests

- ECG, serum acetaminophen and aspirin levels should be obtained to detect occult ingestion.
- Serum electrolytes, BUN, creatinine, liver function tests, CT, and lumbar puncture should be performed as needed to rule out other causes of altered mental status.
- Serum insulin, proinsulin, and C-peptide levels should be obtained if surreptitious use of insulin is suspected.

—C-peptide is a section of the insulin peptide that is not present in exogenous insulin but is present in secreted insulin.
—Factitious hypoglycemia can be diagnosed by documentation of a low serum C-peptide level during a hypoglycemic episode.
—Patients with a potential diagnosis of factitious hypoglycemia may require admission and serial fasting glucose levels.

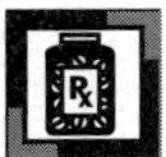

Treatment

- Management should focus on immediate dextrose administration, airway protection, serum glucose monitoring, and determination of cause for hypoglycemia.
- Dose and time of exposure should be determined for all substances involved.

DIRECTING PATIENT COURSE

The health-care provider should call a poison control center when:

- The patient or caregiver indicates that an insulin overdose has occurred.
- Coingestant, drug interaction, or underlying disease presents an unusual problem.

The patient should be referred to a health-care facility when:

- Attempted suicide or homicide is possible.
- Signs and symptoms are not consistent with hypoglycemia.
- The patient or caregiver seems unreliable.
- Altered mental status, diaphoresis, or other toxic effects are present.
- Coingestant, drug interaction, or underlying disease presents an unusual problem.

Admission Considerations

Inpatient management is warranted for patients who suffer possible parenteral overdose or who develop persistent or recurrent hypoglycemia.

DECONTAMINATION

- Oral decontamination is not necessary in cases of isolated insulin overdose.
- If coingestion of another toxic substance is possible, one dose of activated charcoal (1–2 g/kg) should be administered if a substantial ingestion has occurred within the previous few hours.
- After a massive subcutaneous insulin injection or injection of any amount of long-acting insulin, surgical excision of the site may be effective if it is performed soon after injection.

ANTIDOTES

Dextrose is the specific antidote for insulin poisoning.

Indications

Dextrose should be administered upon appearance of symptoms of hypoglycemia or glucose level below 60 mg/dl.

Method of Administration and Dosage

- Adults. 50 mL D50W by bolus intravenous infusion.
- Children. D25W 2 to 4 ml/kg (D10W 1–2 ml/kg for neonate).
- Dextrose dose should be repeated until blood glucose level is above 100 mg/dl.
- Blood glucose should be followed at least hourly to guide further therapy.
- Initiate infusion of D5W, D10W, or D20W dextrose as needed if recurrent hypoglycemia develops.
- Dextrose infusions of 20% or higher require a central venous line to avoid venous irritation.

ADJUNCTIVE TREATMENT

- Potassium replacement may be required and should be based on serum levels.
- Glucagon should not be used for insulin overdose.

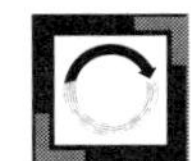

Follow-Up

PATIENT MONITORING

- Cardiac and respiratory function should be monitored continuously.
- Glucose levels should be monitored hourly, or more frequently as needed initially.

EXPECTED COURSE AND PROGNOSIS

- Full recovery is expected if prolonged hypoglycemia is avoided.
- Permanent neurologic injury may result from prolonged hypoglycemia.

DISCHARGE CRITERIA/INSTRUCTIONS

- From the emergency department. Patients who are asymptomatic may be discharged when they maintain serum glucose levels above 60 mg/dl (without dextrose treatment) during 6 to 8 hours of observation and following a psychiatric evaluation, if needed.
- From the hospital. Patients who are asymptomatic, are euglycemic without supplemental dextrose administration for 6 to 8 hours, and tolerate food may be discharged following psychiatric evaluation, if needed.

Pitfalls

DIAGNOSIS

- Early infusion of dextrose to an asymptomatic patient may maintain normal blood glucose and obscure the diagnosis of serious poisoning.
- It is important to determine whether an oral hypoglycemic is involved in addition to injected insulin.
- Multiple cases of psychiatric patients who induce hypoglycemia by injecting insulin have been reported.

TREATMENT

Patients requiring large dextrose doses should have central access established to allow infusion of D20W or greater concentrations.

FOLLOW-UP

Hypoglycemia may recur despite dextrose infusion.

ICD-9-CM 962.3

Poisoning by hormones and synthetic substitutes: insulins and antidiabetic agents.

See also: SECTION III, Dextrose chapter.

RECOMMENDED READING

Arem R, Zoghbi W. Insulin overdose in eight patients: insulin pharmacokinetics and review of the literature. *Medicine* 1985;64:323–332.

Author: Kennon Heard

Reviewer: Richard C. Dart

Interferons

Basics

DESCRIPTION

Interferons are parenteral medications that are used to treat a variety of immune system-mediated disorders.

FORMS AND USES

Substances included are human leukocyte interferon; interferon-α; interferon-β; interferon-γ; interferon-α-A3 (Alferon-N); β-1A (Aronex); β-1B (Betaseron); γ-1B (Actimmune); interferon-α-2A, recombinant (Roferon-A); interferon-α-2B.

TOXIC DOSE

Administration of more than 100 million units as a single dose or 1 million units on a daily basis may result in toxicity; there is marked interindividual variability.

PATHOPHYSIOLOGY

The mechanisms of interferon toxicity have not been described.

EPIDEMIOLOGY

Poisoning is uncommon.

CAUSES

No overdoses have been reported; all adverse events have occurred during therapeutic use.

PREGNANCY AND LACTATION

Safety in pregnancy is not known.

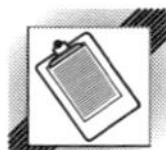

Diagnosis

- The diagnosis is based on symptoms and signs and their temporal relationship to interferon infusion.
- Adverse effects of therapeutic use include an acute flulike syndrome during infusion.

SIGNS AND SYMPTOMS

Vital signs

- Fever, chills, headache, malaise, myalgia, and tachycardia can occur.
- Dizziness and lightheadedness also may occur.
- Transient hypotension has been reported.

Dermatologic

Rash and hair loss may occur.

Pulmonary

Nasal congestion occurs.

Gastrointestinal

Diarrhea has been reported.

Hepatic

Transient elevation of liver function test results has been reported.

Renal

- Urinary urgency may occur.
- Acute renal insufficiency, hyperkalemia, and hypocalcemia have been reported.

Hematologic

Other reported effects include anemia, leukocytopenia, coagulopathy, and thrombocytopenia.

Reproductive

Impaired spermatogenesis and decreased libido have been reported.

Musculoskeletal

Arthralgias have been reported.

PROCEDURES AND LABORATORY TESTS

Essential Tests

No tests may be needed in minimally symptomatic patients.

Recommended Tests

Monitoring of cardiovascular, hepatic, renal, and hematologic organ systems (complete blood count, electrolytes, creatinine, BUN, liver function tests, ECG) are recommended in symptomatic patients.

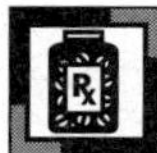

Treatment

Treatment should focus on supportive care.

DIRECTING PATIENT COURSE

The health-care professional should call the poison control center when:

- Severe or persistent effects develop.
- Coingestant, drug interaction, or underlying disease presents an unusual problem.

The patient should be referred to a health-care facility when:

- Toxic effects develop.
- Coingestant, drug interaction, or underlying disease presents an unusual problem.

Admission Considerations

Symptomatic patients should be observed or admitted until effects resolve, depending on the severity of the reaction.

DECONTAMINATION

Due to parenteral administration, no decontamination method is needed.

ANTIDOTES

There is no specific antidote for interferon toxicity.

ADJUNCTIVE TREATMENT

- Standard treatment for fever, arthralgias, and mild hypotension may be needed
- Hemodialysis does not enhance elimination.

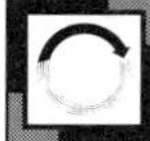

Follow-Up

PATIENT MONITORING

Symptomatic patients should have cardiac monitoring and renal evaluations until effects have resolved.

DISCHARGE CRITERIA/INSTRUCTIONS

Patients may be discharged from the emergency department or hospital when toxic effects resolve or stabilize.

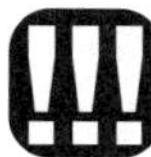

Pitfalls

DIAGNOSIS

Initial "flu-like" syndrome may be difficult to differentiate from more serious conditions such as infection, pulmonary embolus, allergic reaction, etc.

ICD-9-CM 977

Poisoning by other and unspecified drugs and medicinal substances.

RECOMMENDED READING

Wills RJ, Ennis S, Spiegel HE, et al. Interferon kinetics and adverse reactions after intravenous, intramuscular, and subcutaneous injection. *Clin Pharmacol Ther* 1984;35:722–727.

Author: Richard C. Dart

Reviewer: Katherine M. Hurlbut

Iodine and Iodide

Basics

DESCRIPTION

- Iodine-containing products are antiseptic agents (topical) or medications for treatment of thyroid conditions.
- Iodine-containing products are classified into three general categories.

—Iodine (I_2) is the most toxic and rapidly causes direct caustic injury to tissues, especially at high concentration.
—Iodides are the salt form of iodine.
—Iodophors are iodine connected to a high-molecular-weight moiety.

FORMS AND USES

- Topical preparations (solutions, ointments, foams, surgical scrubs, vaginal preparations)

—Tincture of iodine contains 2% iodine and 2% sodium iodide in 50% ethanol, 100 mg iodine/5 ml; 7% iodine and 5% potassium iodide in 83% ethanol, 350 mg iodine/5 ml.
—Iodine ointment contains 4% iodine.
—Iodophor
  —Povidone-iodine contains 0.5% to 10% iodine (Betadine, Isodine).
  —Iodine (I_2) is available in complex with polyvinylpyrrolidone (Povidone).

- Oral preparations. Inorganic iodine, potassium iodide, sodium iodide, and Lugol's solution (aqueous 5% iodine and 10% potassium iodide).
- Organic iodine is used in radiographic contrast dyes and iodinated glycerol (Organidin).
- Sclerodine is used for venous sclerosis.

TOXIC DOSE

- The lethal ingested dose of iodine for an adult may be as little as 2 to 4 g.
- A 7% topical solution of iodine is caustic, but 2% usually is not toxic unless a large volume is involved.

PATHOPHYSIOLOGY

- Iodide and iodophor compounds are usually less toxic than iodine, although large exposure can still produce acute effects.
- The primary initial effect of iodine ingestion is corrosive gastroenteritis with prostration in severe cases; pulmonary effects develop in severe cases.
- Inhalation of iodine causes acute mucous membrane irritation with pulmonary injury in severe cases.

EPIDEMIOLOGY

- Iodine or iodide poisoning of any kind is rare.
- Toxic effects of dermal exposure are typically mild, with death occurring rarely.
- Toxic effects following ingestion are usually mild; serious toxicity is possible with a high-concentration iodine product.

CAUSES

- Iodine or iodide poisoning is usually by accidental ingestion.
- Child neglect should be considered if the patient is under 1 year of age; suicide if the patient is over 6 years of age.

PREGNANCY AND LACTATION

- Iodine, iopodate, povidone-iodine, and ethiodized oil. US FDA Pregnancy Category D. Evidence of human fetal risk exists, but benefits in certain situations (e.g., life-threatening situation or serious diseases) may make use of the drug acceptable despite its risks.
- Iodinated glycerol. US FDA Pregnancy Category X. Studies have demonstrated fetal abnormalities or there is evidence of fetal risk based on human experience, or both, and the risk clearly outweighs any possible benefit.
- Hypothyroidism and congenital goiter may occur in neonates born to mothers treated with iodide.

WORKPLACE STANDARDS

- Iodine

—ACGIH. TLV TWA is 0.1 ppm ceiling.
—OSHA. PEL TWA is 0.1 ppm (1.0 mg/m^3).
—NIOSH. IDLH is 2 ppm.

- Iodoform

—ACGIH. TLV TWA is 0.6 ppm.

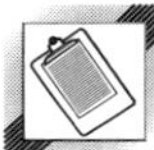

Diagnosis

DIFFERENTIAL DIAGNOSIS

Toxic causes of acute hemorrhagic gastroenteritis that mimic iodine ingestion include caustic agents, iron, arsenic, mercuric chloride, and several others.

SIGNS AND SYMPTOMS

Iodine

- Ingestion. The primary initial effect is corrosive gastroenteritis with prostration in severe cases; pulmonary effects develop in severe cases.
- Inhalation. Acute mucous membrane irritation occurs, with pulmonary injury in severe cases.

Iodide

- Chronic exposure may cause signs and symptoms of either hyper- or hypothyroidism.
- Chronic exposure by any route may produce iodism: oral soreness, sialorrhea, headache, coryza, productive cough, eosinophilia, and salivary gland enlargement. Acne-like skin eruption (iododerma) also may develop.

Iodophor

- Acute exposure may produce acute iodine poisoning as described above.
- Poisoning occurs primarily as a result of large ingestions or mucosal application (e.g., vaginal), from wound or burn exposure, or when used in neonates.

Vital Signs

Iodine ingestion may produce tachycardia, hypotension, and tachypnea.

HEENT

- Iodine ingestion

—Mucosal irritation and salivation occur.
—Oral burns may compromise airway patency.
—Discoloration of the oral mucosa is common following ingestion but cannot be used to exclude an ingestion.

- Iodine inhalation. Rhinorrhea and lacrimation commonly occur.
- Ocular exposure to iodine may result in conjunctivitis and corneal ulceration.

Dermatologic

Prolonged exposure to topical iodine or iodophor preparations can cause local dermatitis and burns.

Cardiovascular

Cardiovascular collapse may follow a large iodine ingestion.

Pulmonary

- Iodine ingestion. Pulmonary edema may occur in severe cases.
- Iodine inhalation. Pulmonary irritation with cough, dyspnea, and chest pain may develop; pulmonary edema may follow a large inhalation.

Gastrointestinal

- Iodine ingestion. Vomiting, hematemesis, and hematochezia may occur.

—Vomitus may have a brownish discoloration (which also may occur with a large iodoform ingestion).
—Mucosal burns may occur and result in gastrointestinal strictures and stenosis.

- Iodide ingestion. Mild nausea and vomiting may occur.

Hepatic

Increased liver enzymes have been reported if severe toxicity develops from iodine ingestion.

Immunologic

Allergic reactions may occur with exposure to any iodine or iodide compound.

Renal

Renal failure may develop 1 to 3 days following a large iodine ingestion.

Fluids and Electrolytes

Metabolic acidosis, decreased anion gap, increased osmolal gap, and hypernatremia may occur with iodine ingestion.

Neurologic

Iodine ingestion may cause headache and lightheadedness as well as agitation, confusion, and hallucinations.

Endocrine

- Iodine-induced thyrotoxicosis can result from high-dose iodine ingestion.
- Hypothyroidism and iodide goiter have been reported in neonates, children, and adults.

PROCEDURES AND LABORATORY TESTS

Essential Tests

- For iodine or large iodophor exposures, serum electrolyte, BUN, and creatinine levels should be obtained to assess the effects of gastroenteritis and renal insufficiency.

—Hypokalemia, hypernatremia, and metabolic acidosis may develop.
—Chloride levels are often falsely elevated due to interference in chloride assays.

- For acute iodide exposures, no tests are essential.

Recommended Tests

- For iodine or large iodophor inhalation exposure, arterial blood gases can be studied to assess pulmonary injury and severity of acidosis.
- For chronic iodide exposures, thyroid function tests to evaluate hyper- or hypothyroidism should be performed.
- For all cases, ECG and serum acetaminophen and aspirin level screens should be obtained in overdose settings to detect occult ingestion.
- Starch may turn vomitus blue, helping to confirm an ingestion.
- Patients with signs of caustic gastrointestinal injury (drooling, oral burns, persistent vomiting, abdominal tenderness), should have endoscopy performed.

Not Recommended Tests

Serum iodine concentration is not clinically useful.

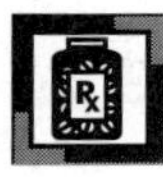

Treatment

- Therapy should focus on airway management, need for intubation, and fluid resuscitation.
- Dose and time of exposure should be determined for all substances involved.

DIRECTING PATIENT COURSE

The health-care provider should call a poison control center when:

- Signs and symptoms are not consistent with iodine poisoning.
- Coingestant, drug interaction, or underlying disease presents an unusual problem.

The patient should be referred to a health-care facility when:

- Attempted suicide or homicide is possible.
- The patient or caregiver seems unreliable.
- Any toxic effects develop.
- Coingestant, drug interaction, or underlying disease presents an unusual problem.

Admission Considerations

Inpatient management is warranted for iodine exposure patients with persistent gastrointestinal, cardiovascular, or severe fluid or electrolyte effects.

DECONTAMINATION

Out of Hospital

- Iodine or iodophor

—In cases of ingestion, emesis should not be induced; a small amount of starchy food may be administered.
—In cases of skin exposure, the affected area should be irrigated with copious amounts of water.
—In cases of inhalation, the patient should be moved to fresh air.

- In cases of chronic iodide exposure, decontamination is not needed.

In Hospital

- Ingestion

—The health-care provider should consider cautious aspiration of gastric contents with a small tube following a large ingestion.
—One dose of activated charcoal (1–2 g/kg) may be administered; activated charcoal should not be administered, however, to patients who may need endoscopy.
—If available, soluble starch should be administered (except to patients who need endoscopy).

- Skin exposure. The affected area should be irrigated with copious amounts of water.
- Inhalation. The health-care provider should administer 100% oxygen.

ANTIDOTES

There is no specific antidote for iodine toxicity.

ADJUNCTIVE TREATMENT

- Hypotension should be treated with isotonic fluid infusion, the Trendelenburg position, and vasopressors if needed; dopamine is preferred, and norepinephrine may be used for refractory hypotension.
- Hemodialysis is not recommended unless renal failure develops.

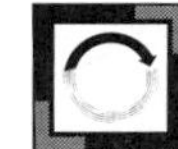

Follow-Up

PATIENT MONITORING

- In cases of iodine ingestion, fluids and electrolytes should be monitored and replaced as needed.
- In cases of inhalation, respiratory status should be monitored closely.
- Evaluation for stricture formation should be performed several weeks after ingestion of iodine or an iodophor.

EXPECTED COURSE AND PROGNOSIS

- Most patients will have self-limited nausea and vomiting.
- Ingestion of a large amount or concentrated solutions may produce serious gastroenteritis with life-threatening dehydration and hypovolemia.
- With aggressive fluid and electrolyte replacement, most patients recover, although iodine ingestion may cause mucosal burns, resulting in esophageal and gastric strictures and stenosis.

DISCHARGE CRITERIA/INSTRUCTIONS

- From the emergency department

—Following iodine or iodophor ingestion, patients who are asymptomatic and can tolerate oral fluids after 4 to 6 hours of observation may be discharged after psychiatric evaluation, if needed.
—Following inhalation, patients who are asymptomatic at 4 to 6 hours postingestion may be discharged.

- From the hospital

—Following iodine or iodophor ingestion, patients who can tolerate oral fluids may be discharged after gastrointestinal burns have resolved and follow-up endoscopy has been arranged.
—Following inhalation, patients may be discharged when pulmonary effects resolve or stabilize.

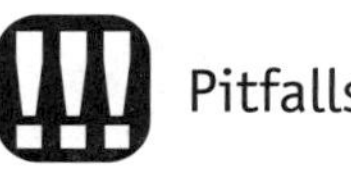

Pitfalls

DIAGNOSIS

- It is important to be alert for airway compromise or the subtle signs of a gastrointestinal caustic injury.
- Absorption of topical iodine is increased in the presence of damaged skin.

ICD-9-CM 962.8

Poisoning by hormones and synthetic substitutes: antithyroid agents.

See also: SECTION II, Hypotension chapter.

RECOMMENDED READING

Shannon MW. Bromine and iodine compounds. In: Haddad LM, Shannon MW, Winchester JF, eds. *Clinical management of poisoning and drug overdose,* 3rd ed. Philadelphia: WB Saunders, 1998:803–812.

Author: Edwin K. Kuffner

Reviewer: Luke Yip

Ipecac Syrup

Basics

DESCRIPTION

Ipecac syrup is an oral, over-the-counter medication that induces vomiting.

FORMS AND USES

- Syrup of ipecac is composed of cephaeline and emetine in a 2.5:1 to 1:1 ratio.
- Typical doses are 10 ml for patients 6 to 12 months of age, 15 ml for those 1 to 5 years of age, and 30 ml for anyone over 5 years of age.

PATHOPHYSIOLOGY

- Cephaeline stimulates the central vomiting center, and emetine activates sensory receptors in the proximal small intestine.
- Acute ingestion leads to a self-limited episode of repeated vomiting.
- A major potential adverse event of ipecac administration is esophageal tear.
- Chronic abuse is often occult and produces nutritional disease without major acute complications.
- Cardiomyopathy may develop with chronic abuse.

EPIDEMIOLOGY

- Poisoning or abuse is common.
- Abuse involves patients with behavioral disease such as bulimia, other eating disorders, and Munchausen syndrome by proxy.
- Toxic effects following acute ingestion are typically mild.
- Death is rare and occurs following chronic abuse.

CAUSES

- Child neglect should be considered if the patient is under 1 year of age; attempted suicide if the patient is over 6 years of age.
- Ipecac is a common drug used in Munchausen syndrome by proxy, in which an adult induces the appearance of illness in a child by repeated administration of ipecac.

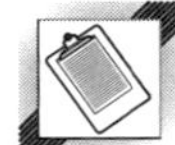

Diagnosis

DIFFERENTIAL DIAGNOSIS

Any condition that causes recurrent vomiting without major signs or symptoms involving other organ systems should be considered as a possible cause.

SIGNS AND SYMPTOMS

- Acute ingestion leads to self-limited episodes of recurrent vomiting; a major potential adverse effect is esophageal tear.
- Chronic abuse is often occult and produces nutritional disease without major acute complications.

Vital Signs

A large overdose or chronic abuse may produce tachycardia or hypotension.

Cardiovascular

- A therapeutic dose does not cause dysrhythmia.
- Chronic abuse may produce cardiomyopathy and congestive heart failure.

Gastrointestinal

- Vomiting is the primary effect of ipecac.
- Complications are rare, but may be serious: protracted vomiting, Mallory-Weiss tear, pneumomediastinum, gastric rupture, or herniation through diaphragmatic defect.
- Chronic abuse has produced hemorrhagic colitis.

Fluids and Electrolytes

Repeated vomiting may produce hypokalemia or dehydration.

Musculoskeletal

Chronic ingestion may produce hypotonia and myopathy requiring weeks to months for resolution.

Neurologic

Intracranial hemorrhage occurs rarely.

PROCEDURES AND LABORATORY TESTS

Essential Tests

- In cases of acute ingestion without excessive vomiting, no tests are needed unless the patient manifests toxicity in addition to emesis (e.g., hematemesis, chest pain, persistent tachycardia).
- In cases of chronic ingestion, serum electrolytes, BUN, and creatinine should be obtained to detect volume depletion or hypokalemia.

Recommended Tests

- Acute ingestion. Serum electrolytes, BUN, and creatinine should be performed if repeated vomiting occurs to detect volume depletion or hypokalemia.
- Serum acetaminophen and aspirin levels should be obtained in overdose settings to detect occult ingestion.
- In cases of chronic ingestion or very large acute ingestion, ECG may reveal dysrhythmia: tachycardia, T-wave flattening or inversion, prolonged PR interval, ventricular tachycardia, or ventricular fibrillation.
- Imaging studies should be ordered as needed for complications (e.g., Mallory-Weiss tear).

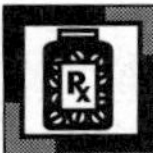

Treatment

- Treatment should focus on supportive care, correction of electrolyte abnormalities, and psychiatric evaluation.
- Dose and time of exposure should be determined for all substances that could be involved.

DIRECTING PATIENT COURSE

The health-care provider should call a poison control center when:

- Protracted vomiting, hematemesis, or other serious effects develop.
- Toxic effects are not consistent with ipecac syrup.
- Coingestant, drug interaction, or underlying disease presents an unusual problem.

The patient should be referred to a health-care facility when:

- Attempted suicide, homicide, or abuse is possible.
- The patient or caregiver seems unreliable.
- Recurrent vomiting or other serious effects are present.
- Coingestant, drug interaction, or underlying disease presents an unusual problem.

Admission Considerations

Inpatient management is warranted for patients with protracted vomiting (lasting longer than 4 hours), complications of vomiting, or chronic abuse with cardiac or electrolyte abnormalities.

DECONTAMINATION

Out of Hospital

No decontamination is needed.

In Hospital

- If inadvertent overdose has been administered, the health-care provider should attempt to aspirate syrup using a small nasogastric tube.
- A single dose of activated charcoal (1–2 g/kg) without a cathartic may be administered if a substantial ingestion has occurred within the previous few minutes.

ANTIDOTES

There is no specific antidote for syrup of ipecac.

ADJUNCTIVE TREATMENT

Hypotension

- The patient should receive 10 to 20 ml/kg 0.9% saline and be placed in the Trendelenburg position.
- Further fluid therapy should be guided by central pressure monitoring to avoid volume overload.
- A vasopressor may be given if needed. Dopamine is used initially. Norepinephrine may be added in refractory cases.

Cardiac Dysrhythmia

Advanced cardiac life support guidelines should be followed.

Electrolyte Abnormalities

Potassium, magnesium, and phosphate should be replenished as indicated by serum levels.

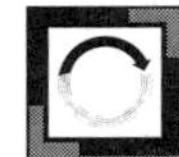

Follow-Up

EXPECTED COURSE AND PROGNOSIS

- Following acute ingestion, vomiting begins in under 30 minutes in 88% of cases; the mean number of episodes of vomiting is three (range one to eight), and duration of vomiting is 23 to 60 minutes.
- Residual cardiomyopathy may persist following chronic abuse.

DISCHARGE CRITERIA/INSTRUCTIONS

- From the emergency department

—After acute ingestion, patients may be discharged when vomiting remits and psychiatric evaluation is complete.
—After chronic ingestion, patients without significant cardiac or electrolyte disturbances may be discharged after psychiatric evaluation.

- From the hospital. Patients may be discharged when significant cardiac or electrolyte disturbances have resolved and after psychiatric evaluation.

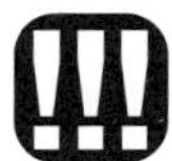

Pitfalls

DIAGNOSIS

- Many cases of chronic abuse are overlooked for months or years.
- The possibility of Munchausen syndrome by proxy should be considered for young children with repeated vomiting and dehydration that eludes diagnosis.
- Ipecac rarely causes emesis lasting longer than 2 hours; if vomiting persists, other causes should be considered.

ICD-9-CM 973.6

Poisoning by agents primarily affecting the gastrointestinal system: emetics.

See also: SECTION II, Hypotension chapter.

RECOMMENDED READING

Kunkel DB. The toxic toll of keeping thin. *Emerg Med* 1985;17:176–180.

POISINDEX Editorial Staff. Ipecac. In: Rumack BH, Hess AJ, Gelman CR, eds. POISINDEX system. Englewood, CO: Micromedex, Inc. (edition expires May 30, 1998).

Author: David Magilner

Reviewer: Richard C. Dart

Iron

Basics

DESCRIPTION

Iron is a commonly used oral medication and dietary supplement.

FORMS AND USES

- Iron (ferrous) fumarate 200 mg contains 66 mg elemental iron.
- Iron (ferrous) gluconate 325 mg contains 37 mg elemental iron.
- Iron (ferrous) sulfate 325 mg contains 65 mg elemental iron.
- A typical child's multivitamin tablet with iron contains 10 to 18 mg elemental iron; adult or prenatal multivitamins may contain up to 65 mg of iron.
- Iron dextran rarely causes iron toxicity.

TOXIC DOSE

Signs of toxicity begin to develop at doses above 20 mg/kg.

PATHOPHYSIOLOGY

- Initial toxicity is caused by direct irritation of the gastrointestinal mucosa.
- After absorption, the normal defense mechanisms are to bind iron tightly to serum proteins (e.g., transferrin, ferritin).
- In overdose, free iron exceeds defenses and produces widespread cellular injury.
- Mechanisms of cell toxicity include uncoupling of oxidative phosphorylation, free radical production, direct consumption of bicarbonate, direct depression of the myocardium, and disruption of production of coagulation proteins.

EPIDEMIOLOGY

- Poisoning is common.
- Toxic effects following exposure are typically mild to moderate.
- Death occurs as a result of large ingestions with delayed presentation.

CAUSES

- Acute overdose is usually suicidal in adults and accidental in children.
- The possibility of child neglect should be considered in patients under 1 year of age; suicide attempt in patients over 6 years of age.

WORKPLACE STANDARDS

No standards are available for iron.

PREGNANCY AND LACTATION

- US FDA Pregnancy Risk Category. Not categorized.
- Use of deferoxamine for iron poisoning improves maternal condition and thereby improves conditions for the fetus.

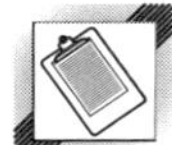

Diagnosis

DIFFERENTIAL DIAGNOSIS

- Other toxic causes of acute gastrointestinal injury include isopropyl alcohol, caustics, mushrooms, inorganic heavy metals, theophylline, and severe reactions to nonsteroidal antiinflammatory drugs and salicylates, among others.
- Other causes of anion gap metabolic acidosis are methanol, uremia, diabetic ketoacidosis, isoniazid, lactic acidosis, ethylene glycol, salicylate, toluene, and others.

SIGNS AND SYMPTOMS

- Initial symptoms are primarily vomiting, abdominal pain, diarrhea, and mild lethargy.
- In more severe cases, marked lethargy, anion gap metabolic acidosis, gastrointestinal bleeding, and shock will follow within hours.

Vital Signs

Tachycardia and tachypnea are common.

Cardiovascular

Hypotension and shock may develop in severe cases.

Pulmonary

- Hyperpnea to compensate for metabolic acidosis is common.
- Adult respiratory distress syndrome may develop in severe cases.

Gastrointestinal

- Early vomiting and diarrhea are common.
- Abdominal pain, hematemesis, and hematochezia occur early.

Hepatic

Mild to severe hepatic necrosis may occur in severe cases.

Renal

Renal failure may occur in association with shock or liver injury.

Hematologic

- Increased white blood cell count may occur early but is not a reliable marker for toxicity.
- Increased prothrombin time (PT) or international normalized ratio (INR) is common and may become severe.

Fluids and Electrolytes

- Increased anion gap acidosis may appear early in larger ingestions.
- Intravascular volume depletion is common and may become severe.

Neurologic

- Lethargy is common.
- Seizures and coma may occur in severe cases.

Endocrine

Hyperglycemia may occur early but is not a reliable marker for toxicity.

PROCEDURES AND LABORATORY TESTS

Essential Tests

- The serum iron level should be determined 4 to 6 hours after ingestion if the patient is asymptomatic or upon arrival if the patient is symptomatic.

—A level of less than 300 μg/dl is rarely symptomatic; 300 to 500 μg/dl is potentially toxic; over 500 μg/dl is usually treated with chelation.
—The normal course of serum iron levels is to peak in the first few hours and then decline as iron is taken into cells.
—A decreasing level does not assure improvement.
—Serial levels are needed when tablets are found on abdominal radiographs.
—Increasing levels should prompt further decontamination attempts.
—Iron levels become uninterpretable after deferoxamine treatment.

- Serum electrolytes, BUN, and creatinine should be measured.

—Tests should be determined at 4 to 6 hours after ingestion if the patient is asymptomatic or upon arrival if the patient is symptomatic.
—Low serum bicarbonate or anion gap metabolic acidosis indicates clinically significant poisoning.

Recommended Tests

- Complete blood count (CBC) may be obtained to assess blood loss in symptomatic cases.
- ECG, serum acetaminophen and aspirin levels are determined in an overdose setting to detect occult overdose.
- Iron tablets may be visible on abdominal radiographs.

—The radiograph is used to evaluate the effect of decontamination, but cannot rule out the continued presence of tablets.
—Chewable tablets are usually not visible.

Not Recommended Tests

- The ratio of serum iron to total iron-binding capacity is not useful.
- The deferoxamine challenge test is no longer recommended to assess toxicity.

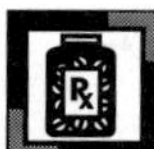

Treatment

• Treatment should focus on gastrointestinal decontamination, intensive supportive care, and administration of deferoxamine, if needed.
• Dose and time of exposure of elemental iron and possible coingestants should be determined for all substances involved.

DIRECTING PATIENT COURSE

The health-care provider should call the poison control center when:

• Gastrointestinal bleeding, acidosis, or hypotension is present, pills are seen on radiographs, or the patient worsens despite therapy.
• Signs and symptoms are not consistent with iron poisoning.
• Deferoxamine administration is needed.
• Coingestant, drug interaction, or underlying disease presents unusual challenges.

The patient should be referred to a health-care facility when:

• More than 60 mg/kg elemental iron was ingested, or the patient is symptomatic.
• Attempted suicide or homicide is possible.
• Patient or caregiver seems unreliable.
• Coingestant, drug interaction, or underlying disease presents unusual problems.

Admission Considerations

Inpatient treatment is warranted for patients with gastrointestinal bleeding, shock, or altered mental status; when gastrointestinal decontamination is unsuccessful; or if the patient is receiving deferoxamine.

DECONTAMINATION

Out of Hospital

Emesis should be induced with ipecac within 1 hour of ingestion for alert pediatric or adult patients or if more than 20 mg/kg was ingested (unless patient has already vomited).

In Hospital

• Emesis should be induced with ipecac for the pediatric patient who is too small to have effective lavage (unless the child has already vomited repeatedly).
• Gastric lavage should be performed in pediatric (tube size 24–32 French) or adult (tube size 36–42 French) patients who present after a large ingestion or if signs of toxicity are present.
• Whole-bowel irrigation is used in patients with rising iron levels or with pills evident on KUB radiographs.

—Adult dose is 1 to 2 L/h until rectal effluent is clear.
—Pediatric dose is 25 ml/kg/h until rectal effluent is clear.

• Activated charcoal binds iron poorly but may be used if coingestion is suspected; if gastrointestinal bleeding is present, the use of charcoal should be avoided to allow endoscopy.
• Bicarbonate, phosphate, and milk of magnesia should not be used.

ANTIDOTES

Deferoxamine

• Indications. Treatment should be given to any patient with toxic effects (repeated vomiting or diarrhea, increased anion gap metabolic acidosis, gastrointestinal bleeding, altered mental status, or hypotension) or serum iron levels of more than 500 μg/dl on blood drawn 4 to 6 hours after ingestion.
• Contraindications. Renal insufficiency or oliguric renal failure are relative contraindications. The deferoxamine–iron complex may be dialyzed in patients with renal failure.
• Method of administration. The initial adult or pediatric dose is 15 mg/kg/h by continuous infusion. The rate may be titrated upward to 25 to 40 mg/kg/h based on the patients course (see SECTION III, Deferoxamine chapter, for further details.)
• Potential adverse effects

—Rapid infusion may cause hypotension.
—Anaphylactoid reactions occur rarely.

ADJUNCTIVE TREATMENT

• Hypotension

—The patient should be given 10 to 20 ml/kg 0.9% saline intravenously and placed in the Trendelenburg position.
—Larger volumes will often be needed.
—Further fluid therapy should be guided by central pressure monitoring to avoid volume overload.
—If hypotension does not respond to treatment, a vasopressor is administered.
  —The dose for dopamine is 2 to 5 μg/kg/min, titrated to effect; rates greater than 20 μg/kg/min are unlikely to provide further benefit.
  —If pressure does not respond, norepinephrine (0.1–0.2 μg/kg/min) may be added and titrated to effect.
  —High rates of infusion may cause tissue ischemia.

• Blood component therapy may be needed for the treatment of bleeding.
• An exchange transfusion should be considered for critically ill young children with high serum iron levels who deteriorate despite deferoxamine therapy.

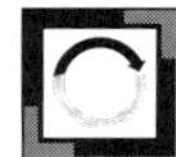

Follow-Up

PATIENT MONITORING

• Iron level, CBC, serum electrolytes, and hemodynamic monitoring should be repeated frequently over the first few hours in patients with toxic effects to assess response to therapy.
• If abdominal radiographs reveal tablets, repeat radiographs are indicated to assess decontamination.

EXPECTED COURSE AND PROGNOSIS

• Most patients develop gastrointestinal effects, are treated with deferoxamine, and recover over 12 to 48 hours.
• In severe cases, effects develop rapidly and may lead to a course lasting several days and complicated by multiple effects of shock.
• In patients without shock or coma, mortality is less than 1%.
• Shock or coma predicts mortality of 50% with supportive treatment, 10% with supportive treatment and deferoxamine.
• Scarring from local corrosive effects may result in gastrointestinal obstruction 4 to 6 weeks after severe iron poisoning.

DISCHARGE CRITERIA/INSTRUCTIONS

• From the emergency department. Asymptomatic patients with iron level less than 500 μg/ml, negative abdominal radiographs, and psychiatric evaluation may be discharged following decontamination and 4 to 6 hours of observation.
• From the hospital. Patients who receive deferoxamine may be discharged 4 hours after discontinuation of deferoxamine when they are asymptomatic, iron levels are decreasing, and serum bicarbonate level is normal.

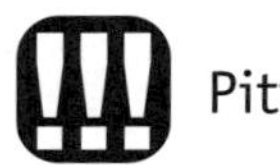

Pitfalls

DIAGNOSIS

• Iron ingestion must be evaluated based on elemental iron content.
• An iron level drawn more than 8 hours after ingestion may be misleading because iron is now intracellular and therefore unmeasured.
• Indirect tests (such as for glucose) should not be substituted for iron level tests to exclude toxicity.

ICD-9-CM 964.0

Poisoning by iron and its compounds.

See also: SECTION II, Hypotension chapter; and SECTION III, Deferoxamine and Whole-Bowel Irrigation chapters.

RECOMMENDED READING

Curry S. Iron. In: Tintanalli JE, Krome RL, Ruiz E, eds. *Emergency medicine.* New York, McGraw Hill, 1992:598–601.

Gruber JE. Iron poisoning. In: Rosen P. *Emergency medicine: concepts and clinical practice.* St. Louis: Mosby, 1992:2593–2602.

Author: Kennon Heard

Reviewer: Richard C. Dart

Isocyanates

Basics

DESCRIPTION

Isocyanates are chemicals primarily used in the manufacture of polyurethane products, including adhesives, sealants, foams, upholstery, spray paints, plastic films, and rubber.

FORMS AND USES

- Monomer forms include toluene diisocyanate (TDI), methylene diphenyl diisocyanate (MDI), hexamethylene diisocyanate (HDI), naphthalene diisocyanate (NDI), isophorone diisocyanate (IPDI), and hydrogenate dicyclohexyl methane diisocyanate (HMDI).
- Polymer forms include polymethylene polyphenylisocyanate.

TOXIC DOSE

Inhalation of TDI at 2.5 ppm concentration may cause immediate toxicity and possible death.

PATHOPHYSIOLOGY

Isocyanates are acute pulmonary irritants that may also cause:

- Acute or chronic asthma following a single exposure.
- Chronic respiratory effects secondary to low-level, extended-duration exposure.
- Occupational asthma.
- Hypersensitivity pneumonitis.

There are two types of pulmonary reaction to isocyanates:

- Primary irritation or pharmacodynamic reaction, to which all exposed persons are susceptible to some degree
- Sensitization reaction or allergic response in those persons who have become sensitized to isocyanate during earlier exposure

The monomer forms of isocyanate are much more volatile and toxic than polymers. Isocyanate is classified as an IARC 2B carcinogen (evidence of carcinogenesis in animals, but none in humans).

EPIDEMIOLOGY

- Although more than 100,000 workers are at risk of exposure in the United States, poisoning is uncommon.
- Toxic effects following exposure are typically mild to moderate, with death occurring rarely.

CAUSES

Isocyanate poisoning is usually an accidental incident in the workplace.

RISK FACTORS

Occupational exposure and prior allergy to isocyanates increase individuals' risk for toxicity.

WORKPLACE STANDARDS

CHEMICAL	ACGIH (ppm)	OSHA (ppm)	NIOSH (ppm)
TDI	0.036	0.020 (STEL)	*****
MDI	0.051	0.020 (STEL)	0.050
HDI	0.034	*****	0.035
NDI	*****	*****	0.040

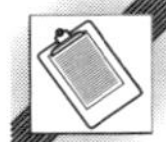

Diagnosis

DIFFERENTIAL DIAGNOSIS

- Other toxic agents that cause acute respiratory and mucous membrane irritation in an occupational setting include chlorine, trimellitic anhydride, pyrethrum, Pauli's reagent (sodium diazobenzene sulfate), copper sulfate, and many others.
- Nontoxic causes of respiratory and mucous membrane irritation include asthma and other forms of reactive airway disease.

SIGNS AND SYMPTOMS

Vital Signs

Fever, tachypnea, and tachycardia are common.

HEENT

- Irritation of the mucous membranes and rhinitis are common.
- Glaucoma and iridocyclitis have occurred following a splash to the eye.

Skin

Irritation and dermatitis (allergic and nonallergic) may be seen.

Pulmonary

- Irritation, cough, chest pain, hemoptysis, and asthma syndrome may develop.
- Asthma has been seen 4 to 6 hours after high-level exposure (over 0.5 mg/m^3).
- Bronchitis and chronic asthma may develop.
- Hypersensitivity pneumonitis may develop with chronic exposure.

Cardiovascular

Cor pulmonale has been reported after high-dose chronic exposure.

Gastrointestinal

Nausea, vomiting, and abdominal pain may develop after fume inhalation.

Neurologic

CNS depression, irritability, euphoria, loss of consciousness, and incoordination may occur.

PROCEDURES AND LABORATORY TESTS

Essential Tests

No tests may be needed in asymptomatic patients.

Recommended Tests

- No laboratory test accurately differentiates isocyanate-induced asthma from other etiologies; the diagnosis is based on the development of asthma following a subirritant exposure to isocyanates.
- Pulse oximetry, arterial blood gas, and pulmonary function tests should be performed in symptomatic patients to assess bronchospasm or pulmonary injury; findings consistent with isocyanate poisoning reveal decreases in airflow (FEV_1, FVC, FEV_1/FVC, FEF_{25-75}) similar to that observed in typical asthma.
- A chest radiograph should be obtained to rule out pneumothorax and other causes of bronchoconstriction.
- Isocyanate-specific antibodies have been found in some individuals by radioallergosorbent testing, but their clinical utility is unknown.

Provocation Testing

Specific diagnosis can be made with bronchoprovocation testing, either by pre- and post-workplace exposure with peak flow measures and symptom log, or by chamber challenge.

Challenge Technique

- The patient is tested in an environmental chamber using the suspected agent or saline and given subirritant doses in a blinded manner.
- Pulmonary functions are measured at baseline, with a control solution, and with the isocyanate in question.
- This technique is not widely available and, if undertaken, requires controls for accurate interpretation.

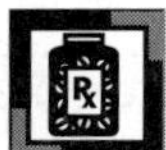

Treatment

- Treatment should focus on providing oxygen and treating bronchospasm.
- Dose and time of exposure should be determined for all substances involved.

DIRECTING PATIENT COURSE

The health-care provider should call a poison control center when:

- Signs and symptoms are not consistent with isocyanate exposure.
- Underlying disease precludes or complicates initial treatment measures.
- Bronchospasm or other serious effects are present.

The patient should be referred to a health-care professional when:

- Attempted suicide or homicide is possible.
- The patient or caregiver seems unreliable.
- Bronchospasm or other serious effects are present.
- Underlying disease presents an unusual problem.

Admissions Considerations

Inpatient management is warranted for patients with a poor or partial response of bronchospasm after 2 to 4 hours of treatment.

DECONTAMINATION

Out of Hospital

- Induced emesis is not recommended because of irritant effects.
- The patient should be moved to fresh air.
- Eyes or exposed areas should be irrigated with water.

In Hospital

- Aspiration of stomach contents should be considered in the unusual event of isocyanate ingestion.
- One dose of activated charcoal (1–2 g/kg) should be administered if a substantial ingestion has occurred within the previous few hours.

ANTIDOTES

There is no specific antidote available for isocyanate poisoning.

ADJUNCTIVE TREATMENT

Supplemental oxygen should be administered as guided by pulse oximetry.

Treatment of Bronchospasm

- Albuterol. 0.15 mg/kg (maximum of 10 mg) in saline with humidified oxygen is administered via nebulizer every 20 to 30 minutes; if the peak expiratory flow rate (PEFR) is greater than 90% after the initial dose, additional doses may not be needed.
- Methylprednisolone. 60 to 125 mg (1.0–1.5 mg/kg) is given intravenously (pediatric 1–2 mg/kg) every 6 to 8 hours; the dosage may be decreased to a single daily dose and tapered.

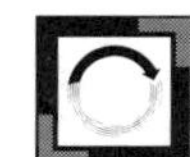

Follow-Up

PATIENT MONITORING

Pulmonary function response to therapy should be monitored continually.

EXPECTED COURSE AND PROGNOSIS

- Bronchospasm typically occurs within hours of exposure and usually responds to therapy, but cases of reactive airway disease have occurred.
- Other complications that may result from isocyanate toxicity include respiratory failure, pneumonia, pneumothorax, and other pulmonary complications that are seen in asthmatics.

DISCHARGE CRITERIA/INSTRUCTIONS

- Patients should be observed for at least 2 hours after the last dose of the bronchodilator for signs of relapse.
- Patients who have noted relief of symptoms, and whose PEFR or FEV_1 is greater than 70% of predicted values, may be discharged.

PATIENT EDUCATION

- On discharge, the health-care provider should review with the patient all medication doses, side effects, and routes and arrange for follow-up.
- Every patient should be given a PEFR meter with instructions for use.

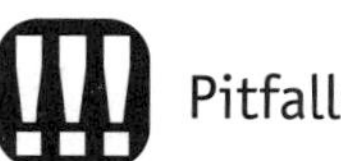

Pitfalls

DIAGNOSIS

- It is important to diagnose signs of bronchospasm.
- The health-care provider should appreciate isocyanates as asthmogenic substances.

TREATMENT

- The health-care provider must not fail to maintain an adequate airway and oxygenation.
- It is important to administer sufficient doses of bronchodilators or steroids.

FOLLOW-UP

Individuals sensitized to isocyanates should not return to work in an exposed area without full respiratory protection.

ICD-9-CM 987

Toxic effect of other gases, fumes, or vapors.

RECOMMENDED READING

Banks D, Sastre J, Butcher BT, et al. Role of inhalation challenge testing in the diagnosis of isocyanate asthma. *Chest* 1989;95:414–423.

Moller D, McKay RT, Bernstein IL, et al. Persistent airway disease caused by toluene diisocyanate. *Ann Rev Respir Dis* 1986;134:175–176.

Moller D, McKay R, Casady K, et al. Chronic asthma due to toluene diisocyanate. *Chest* 1986;90:494–499.

Author: Scott D. Phillips

Reviewer: Luke Yip

Isoniazid

Basics

DESCRIPTION

Isoniazid (INH) is an antimicrobial used mainly in the treatment of tuberculosis.

FORMS AND USES

- INH (Laniazid, Nydrazid) is available in 50-, 150-, and 300-mg capsules and as a 50 mg/5 cc syrup.
- Rifamate capsules are composed of 150 mg INH with 300 mg rifampin.
- Rafater capsules are composed of 150 mg INH with 300 mg rifampin and 300 mg pyrazinamide.
- INH is used for treatment of active tuberculosis or prophylactic therapy of positive tuberculosis skin test. Adult dose is 300 mg orally per day; a typical pediatric dose is 10 mg/kg/day up to 300 mg.

TOXIC DOSE

Seizures may follow ingestion of 30 to 40 mg/kg (2–3 g in a 70-kg adult).

PATHOPHYSIOLOGY

- INH produces pyridoxine deficiency by three mechanisms:

—Enhanced excretion of pyridoxine
—Competitive inhibition of the enzyme that converts pyridoxine to its physiologically active form (pyridoxal 5′ phosphate)
—Direct binding of pyridoxine to form inactive complex

- Pyridoxine depletion causes decreased levels of the inhibitory neurotransmitter γ-aminobutyric acid (GABA). GABA deficiency can cause seizures.
- INH also promotes lactic acidosis by blocking the conversion of lactate to pyruvate.

EPIDEMIOLOGY

- Poisoning is uncommon.
- Toxic effects following exposure range from mild to severe.
- Death may occur in untreated cases.

CAUSES

- Acute INH poisoning usually results from suicidal ingestion.
- Child neglect should be considered if the patient is under 1 year of age; attempted suicide if the patient is over 6 years of age.

DRUG AND DISEASE INTERACTIONS

- Hepatotoxicity/hepatitis risk is increased by concurrent use of carbamazepine, alcohol, phenobarbital, or rifampin.
- Concurrent disulfiram use can lead to coordination difficulties, ataxia, and psychotic episodes.

PREGNANCY AND LACTATION

- US FDA Pregnancy Category C. The drug exerts animal teratogenic or embryocidal effects, but there are no controlled studies in women, or no studies are available in either animals or women.
- INH crosses the placenta and achieves fetal blood levels similar to maternal blood levels, although INH does not appear to be a teratogen.

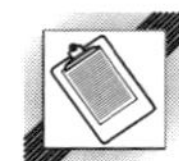

Diagnosis

DIFFERENTIAL DIAGNOSIS

- Other toxic agents that cause seizures and anion gap acidosis include hypoglycemic agents, sympathomimetic agents (e.g., cocaine, amphetamines), lidocaine, local anesthetics, methylxanthines, neuroleptic drugs, and tricyclic antidepressants, among others.
- Nontoxic causes of seizures and anion gap acidosis include hypoglycemia, hypoxia from any cause, alcohol withdrawal, meningitis, intracranial hemorrhage, and noncompliance with seizure medications.

SIGNS AND SYMPTOMS

- Initial effects of INH toxicity include nausea, vomiting, and progressive altered mental status.
- Sudden onset of seizures is common and often refractory to standard therapy.

Vital Signs

Hyperthermia and tachycardia are common with seizures.

HEENT

Optic neuritis and atrophy may be noted with chronic treatment.

Dermatologic

Rashes occur rarely.

Cardiovascular

- Hypotension may develop in patients with severe intoxication.
- Tachycardia is common.

Pulmonary

- Respiratory depression frequently accompanies seizure activity.
- Tachypnea and Kussmaul type respirations may be noted between seizure episodes.

Gastrointestinal

Nausea and vomiting are common prior to the onset of seizures.

Hepatic

- Mild hepatic injury has been reported with overdose.
- Asymptomatic elevation of liver enzyme test results may develop in 20% to 40% of patients taking INH in therapeutic doses.
- Hepatitis occurs in 0.3% to 1.3% of patients, and hepatic failure is a rare complication.

Fluids and Electrolytes

Severe anion gap acidosis is common if seizures develop.

Musculoskeletal

Rhabdomyolysis may develop following protracted seizures.

Neurologic

- Dizziness and slurred speech may be the earliest symptoms of INH poisoning, followed by seizures and coma.
- Chronic use of INH may produce peripheral neuropathy.

PROCEDURES AND LABORATORY TESTS

Essential Tests

No tests may be needed in asymptomatic patients.

Recommended Tests

- Serum electrolytes, calcium, magnesium, BUN, creatinine, and glucose should be obtained to assess renal injury and metabolic acidosis.
- Pulse oximetry should be performed for assessment of oxygenation.
- ECG, serum acetaminophen, aspirin, and ethanol levels should be obtained in overdose settings to detect occult ingestion.
- Urinalysis and serum creatine kinase should be obtained to evaluate for rhabdomyolysis.
- INH serum levels or urine strips may be available to confirm diagnosis but cannot be obtained in a clinically useful time frame.
- Chest radiographs, head CT, and lumbar puncture should be performed as needed to evaluate respiratory complications and assess other causes of seizures.

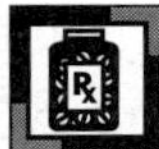

Treatment

- Treatment should focus on immediate airway management and treatment of seizures.
- Dose and time of exposure should be determined for all substances involved.

DIRECTING PATIENT COURSE

The health-care provider should call the poison control center when:

- Signs and symptoms are not consistent with INH toxicity.
- Coingestant, drug interaction, or underlying disease presents an unusual problem.

The patient should be referred to a health-care facility when:

- Attempted suicide or homicide is possible.
- The patient or caregiver seems unreliable.
- Any toxic effects develop acutely.
- Coingestant, drug interaction, or underlying disease presents an unusual problem.

Admission Considerations

Inpatient management is warranted for all patients who develop altered mental status, seizure, acidosis or other serious effects.

DECONTAMINATION

Out of Hospital

Emesis should not be induced; seizures may develop abruptly.

In Hospital

- Gastric lavage should be performed in pediatric (tube size 24–32 French) or adult (tube size 36–42 French) patients presenting within 1 hour of a large ingestion or if serious effects are present.
- One dose of activated charcoal (1–2 g/kg) should be administered if a substantial ingestion has occurred within the previous few hours.

ANTIDOTES

Pyridoxine

- Indications. Pyridoxine is used in conjunction with benzodiazepines for treatment of seizures induced by INH overdose and should be used empirically in patients with seizure of unknown etiology.
- Contraindications. Pyridoxine is contraindicated in patients with known pyridoxine hypersensitivity.
- Dose. If quantity of INH ingested is known, pyridoxine should be administered intravenously over 5 minutes on a gram-for-gram basis (e.g., 5 g pyridoxine for a 5-g INH ingestion).
- If quantity of INH ingested is not known, 5 g of pyridoxine should be administered intravenously over 5 minutes

—If seizures persist, a second dose of 5 g is administered.
—If seizures are not controlled after 10 g and the INH dose is unknown, then the diagnosis should be reconsidered.

- In pediatric patients, the initial dose of pyridoxine is reduced and should not exceed 70 mg/kg.
- Tachypnea, incoordination, ataxia, reflex abnormalities, paralysis, and convulsions may follow excessive pyridoxine administration.

ADJUNCTIVE TREATMENT

- Anion gap acidosis

—Anion gap acidosis resulting from seizures may be refractory to sodium bicarbonate but resolves with pyridoxine therapy.
—Acidosis should remit following termination of seizures with pyridoxine without further therapy.

- If seizures occur, a benzodiazepine familiar to the provider should be administered in addition to pyridoxine.

—Diazepam. Adult dose is 5–10 mg initially; pediatric dose is 0.2–0.5 mg/kg.
—Lorazepam. Adult dose is 2–4 mg intravenous push over 2–5 minutes; pediatric dose is 0.1 mg/kg intravenous push over 2–5 minutes.
—Benzodiazepine dose may be repeated every 10 minutes, if needed.
—The need for endotracheal intubation should be monitored frequently.

- Hemodialysis may be useful if pyridoxine and anticonvulsant therapy fail to correct metabolic acidosis.

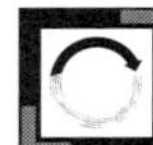

Follow-Up

PATIENT MONITORING

EEG (seizure activity), vital signs, serum electrolytes, glucose, renal and hepatic function, arterial blood gases, neurologic function, and mental status should be monitored.

EXPECTED COURSE AND PROGNOSIS

- With prompt appropriate treatment, prognosis is good and recovery is expected.
- Failure to treat seizures with pyridoxine can result in prolonged hypoxia and brain injury.

DISCHARGE CRITERIA/INSTRUCTIONS

- From the emergency department. Patients may be discharged after gastrointestinal decontamination, 4 hours of observation, and psychiatric evaluation, if necessary.
- From the hospital. Patients may be discharged when liver function tests, serum electrolytes, ECG, and neurologic status are normal and metabolic acidosis is no longer present.

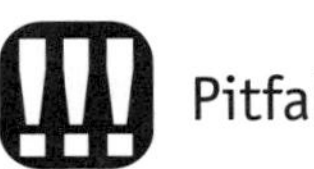

Pitfalls

TREATMENT

Pyridoxine should be administered immediately when INH-induced seizures are possible.

ICD-9-CM 961.8

Poisoning by other anti-infectives: other antimycobacterial drugs.

See also: SECTION II, Seizure chapter; and SECTION III, Pyridoxine chapter.

RECOMMENDED READING

Bryson PD. Isoniazid. In: *Comprehensive review in toxicology for emergency clinicians.* Washington, DC: Taylor & Francis, 1996:664–667.

Wason S, Lacouture PG, Lovejoy FH. Single high-dose pyridoxine treatment for isoniazid overdose. *JAMA* 1981;246:1102–1104.

Author: Kevin M. Lier

Reviewer: Katherine M. Hurlbut

Isopropyl Alcohol

Basics

DESCRIPTION

Isopropyl alcohol (isopropanol, rubbing alcohol) is a short-chain alcohol with the formula $CH_3CHOHCH_3$.

FORMS AND USES

- Not all rubbing alcohol products contain isopropanol.
- Isopropyl alcohol is used as a rubefacient, solvent, cleaning agent, disinfectant, and preservative.
- Isopropyl alcohol is a component of some window cleaners, liquid soaps, cosmetics, pharmaceuticals, and antifreezes, and is used in chemical manufacturing.

TOXIC DOSE

- Ingestion of 2 to 3 ounces of 70% isopropanol (typical rubbing alcohol or some window de-icers) may produce profound CNS depression in adults.
- Toxicity may develop after ingestion, inhalation, or dermal application.
- In children, exposure to all alcohols predispose to hypoglycemia due to suppression of gluconeogenesis.

PATHOPHYSIOLOGY

- In children, any ingestion is potentially toxic.
- Intoxication has developed both in children sponged with isopropanol and following application of isopropyl alcohol to the umbilical cord.
- Children may be more susceptible to intoxication after dermal application of isopropanol because of their increased skin permeability and greater relative body surface area.
- Isopropanol is metabolized to acetone, and is metabolized much slower than ethanol; thus, isopropanol persists in the blood much longer than ethanol.

EPIDEMIOLOGY

- Exposure is common; poisoning is uncommon.
- Toxic effects following exposure are typically moderate, with death occurring rarely after large exposures in patients without adequate airway protection.

CAUSES

- Isopropyl alcohol poisoning usually results from accidental exposure in children or intentional ingestion as an ethanol substitute by alcoholic patients.
- Child neglect should be considered if the patient is under 1 year of age; attempted suicide if the patient is over 6 years of age.

WORKPLACE STANDARDS

- ACGIH. TLV TWA is 400 ppm; STEL is 500 ppm.
- NIOSH. IDLH is 2,000 ppm.
- OSHA. PEL TWA is 400 ppm.

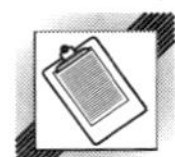

Diagnosis

DIFFERENTIAL DIAGNOSIS

- Other toxic agents that cause alcohol-like intoxication include ethanol, acetone, and sedative-hypnotic agents, among others.
- Nontoxic causes of alcohol-like intoxication include hypoxia, hypoglycemia, or CNS events (infection, thromboembolic disease, etc.).

SIGNS AND SYMPTOMS

- CNS depression, ataxia, dysarthria, and gastrointestinal irritation are the most common effects.
- Isopropanol causes inebriation, as do other alcohols; the depth of CNS depression in isopropyl alcohol intoxication, however, is considered to be more intense than that of other alcohols.

Vital Signs

- Tachycardia is common.
- Hypotension and hypothermia may develop with severe poisoning.

HEENT

Eye and upper airway irritation may develop.

Skin

Dermal irritation or 1st degree burns may develop with prolonged exposure.

Pulmonary

- Inhalation may cause respiratory irritation.
- Respiratory depression may develop with severe poisoning.
- Absorption may occur by inhalation.

Cardiovascular

- Tachycardia is common.
- Hypotension is rare but develops in severe poisoning.

Gastrointestinal

- Nausea and vomiting are common.
- Gastritis and hematemesis may develop.
- Abdominal pain may be substantial and mimic acute abdomen.

Hepatic

Mild elevation of hepatic enzymes may develop.

Renal

Renal failure occurs rarely, following rhabdomyolysis or hypotension.

Fluids and Electrolytes

- Unlike ethylene glycol or methanol toxicity, significant metabolic acidosis does not develop.
- Acetonemia and ketonuria are common.

Musculoskeletal

Rhabdomyolysis occurs rarely, and may develop with prolonged coma.

Neurologic

CNS depression, ataxia, nystagmus, dysarthria, hypotonia, hyporeflexia, and, in severe cases, coma may develop.

Endocrine

- Mild hyperglycemia has been reported in adults.
- Hypoglycemia may develop, especially in children.

PROCEDURES AND LABORATORY TESTS

Essential Tests

- Serum isopropanol level and glucose level should be obtained in symptomatic patients.
- Intoxication is generally evident at serum isopropanol levels of 50 to 100 mg/dl, and coma may develop at levels higher than 150 mg/dl.

Recommended Tests

- Serum electrolytes, BUN, and creatinine should be obtained to assess other causes of altered mental status.

—If metabolic acidosis is present, other etiologies should be considered.
—Serum creatinine may be falsely elevated in the presence of elevated serum acetone levels, if measured by colorimetric assays.

- Serum acetone level should be markedly elevated in symptomatic patients.
- Serum osmolar gap may be elevated early in the course of isopropyl alcohol toxicity.
- ECG, serum acetaminophen, and salicylate levels should be obtained in overdose setting to detect occult ingestion.

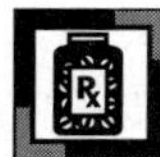

Treatment

- Supportive care, including maintenance of hydration and support of cardiovascular function, with appropriate airway management is vital.
- The dose and time of exposure should be determined for all substances involved.

DIRECTING PATIENT COURSE

The health-care provider should call a poison control center when:

- Signs and symptoms are not consistent with isopropanol poisoning.
- Coingestant, drug interaction, or underlying disease precludes or complicates initial treatment measures.
- Any toxic effects, especially coma, hypotension or other severe effects, are present.

The patient should be referred to a health-care professional when:

- Attempted suicide or homicide is possible.
- The patient or caregiver seems unreliable.
- Any toxic effects, especially coma, hypotension, or other severe effects, are present.
- Coingestant, drug interaction or underlying disease presents an unusual problem.

Admission Considerations

Inpatient management in an ICU is warranted for patients with hypotension, respiratory compromise, or CNS effects that do not clear over 4 to 8 hours of observation.

DECONTAMINATION

Out of Hospital

- Induction of emesis with ipecac should be avoided because of the risk of CNS depression.
- Exposed skin should be washed with soap and water.

In Hospital

- Aspiration of gastric contents may reduce isopropanol ingestion. Gastric lavage with a large bore tube may be needed if a coingestant is possible.
- Activated charcoal is not routinely recommended because it does not absorb isopropanol well; one dose of activated charcoal (1–2 g/kg) may be administered, however, if a coingestant is suspected.
- Exposed skin areas should be washed with soap and water.

ANTIDOTES

There is no specific antidote for isopropanol poisoning.

ADJUNCTIVE TREATMENT

- Hypotension

—The health-care provider should administer 10 to 20 ml/kg of 0.9% saline and place the patient in the Trendelenburg position.
—Further fluid therapy is guided by central pressure monitoring to avoid volume overload.
—Vasopressors should be added if needed.

- Ethanol infusion, which is used for methanol or ethylene glycol toxicity, is not indicated for isopropanol toxicity.
- Hemodialysis

—Hemodialysis increases isopropanol clearance, but is rarely necessary; it should be considered in patients with hemodynamic instability or prolonged coma.

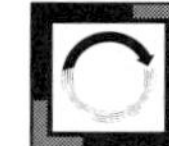

Follow-Up

PATIENT MONITORING

Glucose level and hemodynamic and respiratory parameters should be monitored in patients with mental status depression.

EXPECTED COURSE AND PROGNOSIS

- Aspiration occurs relatively commonly.
- Inadequate airway management may result in hypoxic injury.
- Most patients recover within 4 to 24 hours with supportive care, unless sequelae of hypoxia or hypotension supervene.

DISCHARGE CRITERIA/INSTRUCTIONS

- From the emergency department

—Patients who have returned to baseline mental status after 4 to 8 hours of observation and continued normoglycemia may be discharged after decontamination.
—Psychiatric or substance abuse referral should be considered.

- From the hospital

—Patients may be discharged when toxic effects have resolved or stabilized.
—Psychiatric or substance abuse referral should be considered.

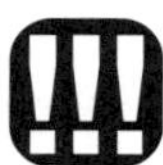

Pitfalls

DIAGNOSIS

- Isopropyl alcohol intoxication may be difficult to diagnose because of its similarity to ethanol intoxication.
- If metabolic acidosis occurs, another cause such as hypotension (lactic acidosis) or methanol or ethylene glycol toxicity should be considered.
- Severe gastritis and substantial hematemesis may develop.

ICD-9-CM 980.2

Toxic effect of alcohol: isopropyl alcohol.

See also: SECTION II, Hypotension chapter; SECTION III, Ethylene Glycol and Methanol chapters.

RECOMMENDED READING

Goldfrank LR, Flomenbaum NE, Howland MA. Methanol, ethylene glycol, and isopropanol. In: Goldfrank LR, Flomenbaum NE, Lewin NA, et al., eds. *Goldfrank's toxicologic emergencies,* 6th ed. Norwalk, CT: Appleton & Lange, 1998.

Pappas AA, Ackerman BH, Olsen KM, et al. Isopropanol ingestion: a report of six episodes with isopropanol and acetone serum concentration time data. *J Toxicol Clin Toxicol* 1991;29:11–21.

Author: Katherine M. Hurlbut

Reviewer: Richard C. Dart

Jellyfish

Basics

DESCRIPTION

- Members of the phylum Cnidaria include the Indo-Pacific box jellyfish (*Chironex fleckeri*), Portuguese man-of-war (*Physalia physalis*), moon jellyfish, Irukandji (*Carukia barnesii*), thimble jellyfish, sea wasp, sea nettle, fire coral, and sea anemones.
- *Sea lice* refers to sea bather's dermatitis caused by thimble jellyfish.
- The box jellyfish is found in the South Pacific waters near Australia and in the Indian Ocean.
- The Portuguese man-of-war is found in temperate waters worldwide.

TOXIC DOSE

- Box jellyfish. A few feet of tentacles can produce severe skin lesions, scarring, and death.
- Portuguese man-of-war. Death is rare, but has been reported following a large surface area exposure.

PATHOPHYSIOLOGY

- Jellyfish consist of two cellular layers with a jellylike substance between the layers.
- The stinging organelles (nematocysts) are located on the outer surfaces of the tentacles or near the mouth.
- Nematocysts are triggered by contact with the victim's body surface and inject a pointed thread tube, which penetrates the dermis and injects venom.
- The tentacle nematocysts can still discharge after the death of a jellyfish.

EPIDEMIOLOGY

- Poisoning is common; tens of thousands of bathers are stung on beaches around the world each year.
- The toxic effects following exposure are typically mild to moderate with the Portuguese man-of-war, and severe with the box jellyfish.
- Death is common following serious box jellyfish envenomation.

CAUSES

- Poisoning is usually an accidental incident while swimming.
- Most cases occur in the warmer summer months.

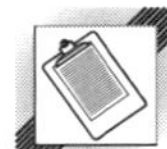

Diagnosis

DIFFERENTIAL DIAGNOSIS

Jellyfish envenomations are usually obvious due to the typical setting of ocean bathing and immediate onset of pain and skin lesions.

SIGNS AND SYMPTOMS

- Box jellyfish stings produce intense local pain and erythema that may be quickly followed by cardiovascular collapse in severe cases.
- Portuguese man-of-war produces primarily local effects of stinging pain followed by erythema and papular urticaria that gradually worsens over the next 24 hours; linear purple-red marks or "tentacle prints" can persist for months.
- Anaphylaxis may occur with any type of jellyfish sting.
- The Irukandji syndrome classically follows the sting of the irukandji jellyfish (*Carukia barnesii*).

—The Irukandji causes unremarkable initial pain and inflammation, sometimes associated with nausea and vomiting, but can then progress, after 30 to 45 minutes, to severe hypertension; chest, back, and abdominal pain; and, rarely, pulmonary edema.
—The syndrome sometimes occurs (in less severe form) in association with other species of jellyfish.

Vital Signs

Tachycardia is common and hypotension may develop in severe cases.

Dermatologic

- Box jellyfish. Skin blistering and necrosis is common, and a pathognomonic "frosted" and cross-hatched pattern may occur.
- Portuguese man-of-war

—Skin erythema occurs, and blistering may develop in severe cases.
—Generalized piloerection has been noted as a possible diagnostic clue.
—Pruritic lesions distant from the initial exposure site often occur.

- Thimble jellyfish

—The tiny larval form of this jellyfish causes "seabather's eruption" when it lodges between oceangoers and their swimwear, causing an intensely pruritic, vesicular, or maculopapular eruption of the skin.
—This usually begins within 24 hours, lasts 3 to 5 days, and resolves spontaneously.

Cardiovascular

Cardiovascular collapse may occur following box jellyfish stings, and it occurs rarely following stings from Portuguese man-of-war.

Pulmonary

- Box jellyfish. Wheezing or pulmonary edema may develop in severe stings.
- Portuguese man-of-war. Difficulty in breathing and chest wall pain have been reported with severe stings.

Gastrointestinal

- Nausea is common.
- Severe cramping and abdominal pain have occurred following jellyfish ingestion.

Musculoskeletal

- Muscular cramping in extremities and other large muscle groups is common and may become severe.
- Muscle necrosis and compartment syndromes have been reported in extremities following severe stings.

Neurologic

- Agitation and confusion may occur due to severe pain and hypoxia.
- Generalized weakness or vertigo may occur.

PROCEDURES AND LABORATORY TESTS

Essential Tests

No tests may be needed in patients without systemic effects.

Recommended Tests

- ECG and continuous cardiac monitoring are used in patients with systemic effects. Various dysrhythmias may develop with severe stings.
- Serum electrolytes, BUN, creatinine, and creatine kinase are studied in patients with systemic effects to detect electrolyte abnormalities and muscle injury.
- Specialized tests (e.g., compartment pressure monitoring) may be needed depending on clinical circumstances.

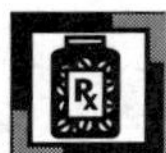

Treatment

Treatment should focus on decontamination, airway management, and supportive care.

DIRECTING PATIENT COURSE

The health-care provider should call the poison control center when:

- Systemic effects are present.
- Toxic effects are not consistent with jellyfish envenomation.
- Drug interaction or underlying disease presents an unusual problem.

The patient should be referred to a health-care facility when:

- Box jellyfish is involved.
- Patient or caregiver seems unreliable.
- Systemic effects are present.
- Drug interaction or underlying disease presents an unusual problem.

Admission Considerations

Inpatient management is warranted for patients with systemic effects or serious local effects (e.g., large surface area, infection) that cannot be managed as outpatients.

DECONTAMINATION

- The affected area should not be rubbed because this may cause the embedded nematocysts to discharge more venom.
- The affected area should be soaked thoroughly with sea water (fresh water may cause further discharge) followed immediately by liberal application of 5% acetic acid (household vinegar) to inactivate the nematocyst stinging apparatus.
- Tentacles should then be removed carefully with a gloved hand; alternatively, the area can be shaved with a razor.

ANTIDOTES

Box Jellyfish Antivenom

- Indications. Any envenomation by box jellyfish indicates use. There is no antivenom for other species of jellyfish.
- Contraindications. There are no absolute contraindications.
- Method of administration

—One ampule is administered intravenously immediately, or three ampules are administered intramuscularly.
—Antivenom treatment should be repeated one to two times at intervals of 2 to 4 hours for worsening effects.

- Adverse effects. Anaphylaxis occurs rarely.

ADJUNCTIVE TREATMENT

- Pain. A parenteral narcotic is administered for severe pain; morphine sulfate 2 to 5 mg is administered intravenously every 15 to 60 minutes as needed for adults; 0.05 to 0.1 mg/kg up to 5 mg every 15 to 60 minutes is administered as needed for children.
- Hypotension is treated with isotonic fluid infusion, the Trendelenburg position, and a vasopressor if needed; dopamine is preferred, and norepinephrine may be administered for refractory hypotension (see SECTION II, Hypotension chapter, for further details).
- Dysrhythmias or conduction abnormalities are treated using standard procedures (see SECTION II, Ventricular Dysrhythmia chapter, for further details).
- Skin eruption. Topical steroids, such as 1% hydrocortisone or 0.1% triamcinolone cream, and topical anesthetics are useful for symptomatic relief.

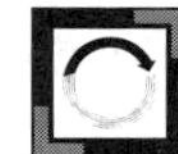

Follow-Up

PATIENT MONITORING

Continuous respiratory and hemodynamic monitoring should be performed when systemic effects develop.

EXPECTED COURSE AND PROGNOSIS

- Following box jellyfish envenomation, toxic effects peak rapidly and death may occur within minutes to hours. Permanent scarring from skin injury is common.
- Portuguese-man-of-war envenomation is less severe; most patients improve over 24 hours. Permanent scarring from local injury may occur.

DISCHARGE CRITERIA/INSTRUCTIONS

- From the emergency department. Patients may be discharged after 4 to 6 hours of observation if only minimal effects develop or mild systemic effects resolve completely.
- From the hospital. Patients may be discharged after cardiovascular effects resolve and local wounds are improving.

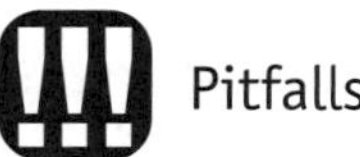

Pitfalls

TREATMENT

Rubbing the affected area or washing with fresh water may stimulate more nematocysts to fire.

ICD-9-CM 989.5

Toxic effect of other substances, chiefly nonmedicinal as to source: venom.

See also: SECTION II, Hypotension and Ventricular Dysrhythmias chapters.

RECOMMENDED READING

Auerbach PS. Marine envenomation. In: Auerback PS, ed. *Wilderness medicine,* 3rd ed. St. Louis: Mosby, 1989:953–964.

Burnett JW, Calton GJ. Jellyfish envenomation syndromes updated. *Ann Emerg Med* 1987;16: 1000–1005.

Fenner PJ, Williamson JA. Worldwide deaths and severe envenomation from jellyfish stings. *Med J Aust* 1996;165:658–661.

Tomchik RS, Russell MT, Szmant AM, et al. Clinical perspectives on seabather's eruption, also known as "sea lice." *JAMA* 1993;269:1669–1672.

Author: Robert E. Vander Leest

Reviewer: Richard C. Dart

Lamotrigine

Basics

DESCRIPTION

Lamotrigine (Lamictal) is used in the treatment of partial and generalized seizure disorders.

FORMS AND USES

- The maintenance dose is 100 to 250 mg orally twice daily.
- The dose must be adjusted when used with other antiseizure medications.

TOXIC DOSE

- Lethal dose is unknown.
- Ingestion of 4 g has caused coma followed by recovery.

PATHOPHYSIOLOGY

Lamotrigine blocks presynaptic voltage-dependent Na^+ channels, inhibiting the release of the excitatory neurotransmitter glutamate.

EPIDEMIOLOGY

- Poisoning is uncommon.
- Death is unlikely unless coingestant is present.

CAUSES

Toxicity is usually caused by therapeutic misuse or drug interaction.

DRUG AND DISEASE INTERACTIONS

- Phenytoin, carbamazepine, and phenobarbital increase the metabolism of lamotrigine.
- Valproate inhibits lamotrigine metabolism.

PREGNANCY AND LACTATION

US FDA Pregnancy Category C. The drug exerts animal teratogenic or embryocidal effects, but there are no controlled studies in women, or no studies are available in animals or women.

Diagnosis

DIFFERENTIAL DIAGNOSIS

Lamotrigine may cause QRS prolongation and may resemble toxicity of other sodium channel-blocking drugs, such as tricyclic antidepressants, phenothiazines, or carbamazepine.

SIGNS AND SYMPTOMS

HEENT

Headache, blurred vision, and diplopia may occur.

Dermatologic

- Rash may occur in 3% of patients.
- Stevens-Johnson syndrome and angioedema develop rarely.

Cardiovascular

QRS prolongation has been reported in overdose.

Gastrointestinal

Nausea and vomiting are common.

Hepatic

Increased liver enzymes may develop during therapy.

Hematologic

Leukopenia and disseminated intravascular coagulation have been reported.

Fluids and Electrolytes

Hypokalemia has been reported in an overdose setting.

Musculoskeletal

Rhabdomyolysis in the absence of seizures has been reported.

Neurologic

- Dizziness and ataxia may occur.
- Nystagmus (vertical and horizontal), hyperreflexia or hyporeflexia, hypertonicity, tremor, somnolence, and coma have all been reported with therapeutic use of lamotrigine, as well as in overdose.

PROCEDURES AND LABORATORY TESTS

Essential Tests

No tests may be needed in asymptomatic patients.

Recommended Tests

- Serum electrolytes, BUN, creatinine are measured to assess other causes of altered mental status.
- Creatine kinase in symptomatic patients to detect myopathy
- Serum liver enzymes in symptomatic patients to detect hepatitis
- Complete blood count and coagulation studies in symptomatic patients to detect leukopenia or coagulation abnormality
- ECG, serum acetaminophen and aspirin levels, and urine toxicology screen in overdose setting to detect occult ingestion

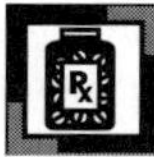

Treatment

- Treatment should focus on airway protection and control of seizures, as well as detection and correction of cardiac dysrhythmias and metabolic abnormalities.
- Dose and time of exposure should be determined for all substances involved.

DIRECTING PATIENT COURSE

The health-care professional should call the poison control center when:

- Severe or persistent effects develop.
- Coingestant, drug interaction, or underlying disease presents an unusual problem.

The patient should be referred to a health-care facility when:

- Suicide or homicide are possible.
- Toxic effects develop.
- Coingestant, drug interaction, or underlying disease presents an unusual problem.

Admission Considerations

Inpatient management is warranted for patients with significant neurologic symptoms, including seizures and coma, leukopenia, rhabdomyolysis, or metabolic abnormalities.

DECONTAMINATION

Out of Hospital

Emesis should be induced with ipecac within 1 hour of ingestion for either pediatric or adult patients, if health-care evaluation will be delayed.

In Hospital

- Emesis should be induced with ipecac within 1 hour of ingestion for pediatric patients who are too small to have effective gastric lavage.
- Gastric lavage should be administered to pediatric (tube size 24-32 French) or adult (tube size 36-42 French) patients presenting within 1 hour of a large ingestion or if serious effects are present.
- One dose of activated charcoal (1-2 g/kg) should be administered without a cathartic if a substantial ingestion has occurred within the previous few hours.

ANTIDOTES

There is no specific antidote for lamotrigine poisoning.

ADJUNCTIVE TREATMENT

- Seizures and hypotension should be treated in the standard manner.
- Dysrhythmias or conduction abnormalities

—Sodium bicarbonate has been reported as effective for the treatment of lamotrigine-associated cardiac conduction prolongation.
—Seizures should be controlled and acidemia corrected.
—If QRS widening or dysrhythmias persist, an intravenous bolus of sodium bicarbonate (1 to 2 mEq/kg) should be administered, repeated as needed but not to exceed arterial pH of 7.55.
—Lidocaine is used for ventricular tachycardia or multifocal premature ventricular contractions; adult dose, 50 to 100 mg intravenous bolus followed by infusion of 2 to 4 mg/min, titrated to desired effect; pediatric dose, 1 mg/kg bolus followed by infusion of 20 to 50 μg/kg/min, titrated to effect; bolus dose may be repeated in 10 to 15 minutes.
—Bretylium is administered at 5 mg/kg over 1 minute; if unsuccessful, it is administered 10 mg/kg over 1 minute, repeated as necessary to total dose of 30 mg/kg.

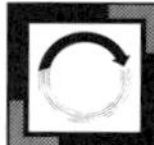

Follow-Up

PATIENT MONITORING

Cardiac and respiratory function should be monitored continuously.

EXPECTED COURSE AND PROGNOSIS

- Toxic effects typically occur within first few hours.
- Complete recovery is expected unless sequelae of hypoxia or hypotension intercede.

DISCHARGE CRITERIA/INSTRUCTIONS

Patients may be discharged from the emergency department or hospital when toxic effects resolve or stabilize and after psychiatric evaluation, if needed.

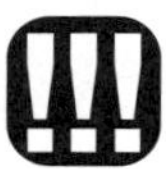

Pitfalls

DIAGNOSIS

CNS depression is easily confused with many other causes.

ICD-9-CM 966

Poisoning by anticonvulsants and antiparkinsonism drugs.

See also: SECTION II, Hypotension and Seizures chapters; SECTION III, Sodium Bicarbonate.

RECOMMENDED READING

Brodie MJ. Lamotrigine. *Lancet* 1992;339:1397–1400.

Buckley NA, Whyte IM, Dawson AH. Self-poisoning with lamotrigine. *Lancet* 1993;342:1552–1553.

Author: Edward W. Cetaruk

Reviewer: Richard C. Dart

Lead Poisoning—Adult

Basics

DESCRIPTION

Lead is a heavy metal used in a wide variety of consumer products and occupational settings.

FORMS AND USES

- Substances discussed in this chapter include lead and other lead compounds, such as galena (PbS), lead acetate, lead arsenate, lead azide, lead carbonate, lead chloride, lead chromate, lead molybdate, lead nitrate, lead monoxide, lead oxide, lead suboxide, lead peroxide, lead oxychloride, lead silicate, lead sulfate, lead sulfide, lead stearate, tetraethyl lead, and tetramethyl lead.
- Lead is used in many different industries: lead smelting, battery manufacturing, welding, construction and demolition, printing, firing ranges, radiator repair, soldering, zinc smelting, and frit manufacturing.
- Approximately half of all lead produced goes into lead storage batteries.
- Lead is used in paints and coatings, particularly white lead (lead carbonate) and red lead (lead oxide).
- Less common uses are lead azide in explosives and organo-lead compounds as anti-knock additives.
- Leaded gasoline remains available in some countries.

TOXIC DOSE

Blood lead levels of above 40 μg/dl may be associated with symptoms.

PATHOPHYSIOLOGY

- Fumes and fine lead particulates are absorbed readily through the lungs.
- Adults absorb a smaller portion of lead from the gastrointestinal tract (20%–30%) than do children (50%).
- Organo-lead compounds (e.g., tetraethyl lead) may be absorbed through intact skin.
- Once absorbed, lead is distributed throughout soft tissues; however, bone is the principal storage area.
- Lead also crosses the blood–brain barrier and concentrates in unmyelinated areas.
- Lead inhibits two enzyme systems in hematopoiesis—δ-aminolevulinic acid dehydratase and ferrochelatase—resulting in anemia.

EPIDEMIOLOGY

- Lead poisoning is common.
- Toxic effects following exposure are typically mild to moderate.
- Death occurs in repeated high-dose exposures, resulting in CNS toxicity.
- Carcinogenesis. Lead is currently an IARC-2B carcinogen (possibly carcinogenic).

CAUSES

- Exposures typically involve occupational inhalation.
- A common example would be the use of a cutting torch in burning lead-containing paint.

PREGNANCY AND LACTATION

- Chronic lead poisoning in the female working population has been associated with decreased fertility, spontaneous abortions, stillbirths, and increased infant mortality.
- Infants born to lead-poisoned mothers may suffer delayed neurologic development.

WORKPLACE STANDARDS

- Air sample

—OSHA. Not listed.
—ACGIH. TLV TWA. 0.05 mg/m^3.
—NIOSH. IDLH 100 mg/m^3.

- Water sample. EPA: MCL is 0.015 mg (15 μg) Pb/m^3.
- Blood lead level (BLL)

—OSHA. BLL of 60 μg/dl requires removal from work until level falls below 40 μg/dl on two consecutive levels.

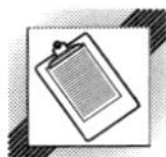

Diagnosis

DIFFERENTIAL DIAGNOSIS

Other toxic causes of CNS injury, renal injury, and peripheral neuropathy: include heavy metals, mercury (arsenic, thallium, hexane), methybutylhetone, and acrylamide.

SIGNS AND SYMPTOMS

- Lead poisoning is usually a chronic condition that primarily affects erythrocyte production, as well as the kidneys and nervous system.
- Inhalational abuse of organic lead compounds like gasoline may cause CNS toxicity (irritability, tremor, ataxia, nystagmus, delusions, seizures, or coma).

HEENT

Lead lines are distinguished by blue-black stippling that develops along the gum margins after chronic exposure, usually most evident along the lower incisors.

Cardiovascular

Hypertension may occur with chronic exposure.

Gastrointestinal

- Anorexia, dyspepsia, and constipation are common.
- Lead colic refers to rare, severe, and paroxysmal abdominal pain.

Renal

A Fanconi-like syndrome (proteinuria, amino aciduria, and phosphaturia) may occur, ultimately leading to chronic interstitial nephritis and renal failure.

Hematologic

- Hemoglobin levels may remain normal despite moderate lead poisoning.
- In severe lead poisoning, a normocytic, normochromic anemia develops.

Neurologic

- CNS symptoms include headache, difficulty in concentrating, altered mental status, and, rarely, seizure.
- Motor neuropathy may develop, affecting upper extremities more than lower extremities.
- In addition, lead poisoning may lead to nerve entrapment such as carpal tunnel or tarsal tunnel syndrome.

Reproductive

Lead poisoning may produce decreased sperm count or an increased number of abnormal sperm.

PROCEDURES AND LABORATORY TESTS

Essential Tests

- Complete blood count is drawn to assess the presence of anemia.
- Serum electrolytes, BUN, and creatinine are used to assess renal injury.
- Blood lead level

—A normal level is less than 10 μg/dl.
—Employees with a blood lead level greater than or equal to 60 μg/dl should be removed from exposure until their blood lead is less than 40 μg/dl.
—Other state or federal regulations may apply to the management of increased lead level in the occupational setting.

- Urinalysis with microscopic examination is used to assess renal effects.

Recommended Tests

- Urinary β_2-microglobulin or *n*-acetylglucosaminidase may be increased.
- An abdominal radiograph may detect ingested lead objects.
- Electromyogram and nerve conduction velocity may be used to assess peripheral neuropathy.
- A head CT or MR, lumbar puncture, and cultures should be considered to assess other causes of altered mental status.

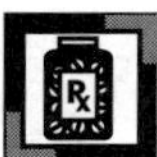

Treatment

- Treatment should focus on terminating exposure and administering a lead-chelating drug, if appropriate.
- The dose and time of exposure must be determined for all substances involved.

DIRECTING PATIENT COURSE

The health-care provider should call the poison control center when:

- Seizure, altered mental status, or other serious effects develop.
- Toxic effects are not consistent with lead poisoning.
- Drug interaction or underlying disease presents an unusual problem.

The patient should be referred to a health-care facility when:

- Patient or caregiver seems unreliable.
- Any toxic effects are present.
- Drug interaction or underlying disease presents an unusual problem.

Admission Considerations

Inpatient management is warranted for patients with CNS toxicity or those who require parenteral chelation.

DECONTAMINATION

Out of Hospital

The affected skin areas are washed.

In Hospital

- Gastrointestinal decontamination is not recommended unless lead is visible on abdominal radiographs.
- If lead is seen on the radiographs, whole-bowel irrigation should be considered.

—The usual adult dose is 1 to 2 L per hour until rectal effluent is clear.
—Abdominal films are followed to assess the clearing of lead.

ANTIDOTES

British Anti-Lewisite (BAL, Dimercaprol)

- Indications. Parenteral treatment of severe poisoning with evidence of encephalopathy or inability to tolerate oral medication.
- Contraindications

—Allergy to BAL or peanuts, as well as hepatic dysfunction, precludes use.
—BAL may cause hemolysis in glucose-6-phosphate dehydrogenase–deficient patients.

- Method of administration

—The dose of BAL is 3 to 5 mg/kg intramuscularly every 4 to 6 hours, and then tapered over 1 to 2 days to intervals of every 6 to 12 hours until an oral antidote can be tolerated.
—It is discontinued after 5 days or sooner if severe adverse effects develop.

- Adverse effects include headache, hypertension, tachycardia, fever, nausea, vomiting, and pain at the injection site.

EDTA (Calcium Disodium EDTA)

- Indications. Severe lead toxicity with lead encephalopathy indicates use.
- Contraindications. Documented allergy or renal failure precludes use.
- Method of administration

—BAL therapy should be initiated first.
—EDTA is then administered, 1,500 mg/m^2/day as a continuous infusion over 24 hours.

- Adverse effects. Dose-related acute tubular necrosis may occur rarely; the recommended dose should not be exceeded.

Succimer (Chemet)

- Indications

—Lead poisoning without encephalopathy.
—Succimer also has been used in conjunction with a parenteral chelator in some encephalopathy patients under the guidance of a medical toxicologist.

- Contraindications. Documented allergy to succimer precludes use.
- Method of administration

—First it must be ensured that the lead exposure has ended and that there is no lead visible on the abdominal radiograph prior to treatment.
—A dose of 10 mg/kg (or 350 mg/m^2) orally three times a day for 5 days is followed by 10 mg/kg twice a day for 14 days.
—The blood lead level is repeated several days after completion of therapy and every 2 to 4 weeks thereafter until the level stabilizes.
  —If the blood lead level rebounds to more than or equal to 45 μg/dl, the clinician should investigate whether a repeat exposure has occurred.
  —If a repeat exposure has occurred, the patient should be moved to a lead-free environment and the course of chelation repeated.
  —If it has not, the course of chelation should be repeated.
  —If the level rebounds to 20 to 45 μg/dl, the treatment recommendations are uncertain.
—Adverse effects. Nausea, vomiting, and a sulfur odor of body fluids occurs commonly; mild transient elevation of transaminase levels or rash occur rarely.

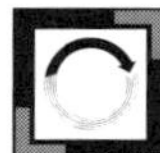

Follow-Up

PATIENT MONITORING

Blood lead levels need to be reassessed 2 weeks after chelation and periodically thereafter to detect rebound or reexposure.

EXPECTED COURSE AND PROGNOSIS

- Most patients recover over days to weeks to apparent baseline function.
- If encephalopathy develops, sequelae include those of increased intracranial pressure.

DISCHARGE CRITERIA/INSTRUCTIONS

- From the emergency department. Patients without CNS effects may be discharged after gastrointestinal decontamination and if the abdominal radiograph reveals no lead opacities.
- From the hospital. Patients may be discharged after encephalopathy has improved and gastrointestinal decontamination has been completed.

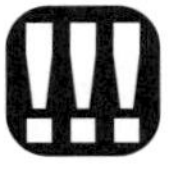

Pitfalls

DIAGNOSIS

The most common pitfall is failure to consider lead as a possibility of anemia, altered mental status, or peripheral motor neuropathy.

TREATMENT

Repeat courses are often needed because levels usually rebound even after chelation.

ICD-9-CM 984

Toxic effect of lead and its compounds.

See also: SECTION III, British Anti-Lewisite, EDTA, Penicillamine, Succimer, and Whole-Bowel Irrigation chapters; SECTION IV, Lead Poisoning—Pediatric.

RECOMMENDED READING

Cooper WC, Wong O, Kheifets L. Mortality among employees of lead battery plants and lead-producing plants, 1947-1980. *Scand J Work Environ Health* 1985;11:331–345.

Cullen MR, Robins JM, Eskenazi B. Adult inorganic lead intoxication: presentation of 31 new cases and a review of recent advances in the literature. *Medicine* 1983;62:221–247.

Landrigan P. Current issues in the epidemiology and toxicology of occupational exposure to lead. *Environ Health Perspect* 1990;89:61–66.

Author: Scott D. Phillips

Reviewer: Katherine M. Hurlbut

Lead Poisoning—Pediatric

Basics

DESCRIPTION

Lead is a poisonous heavy metal.

FORMS AND USES

Sources of lead exposure:

- Paint. The most common source of lead exposure in children is dust and peeling paint from pre-World War II homes or homes painted before 1980.
- Parental occupation. A parent's clothing may be contaminated during smelting, battery manufacturing or recycling, painting, construction, mining, soldering, art work or restoration, welding, capacitor manufacturing, plumbing, radiator repair, metal refining, or bridge repair.
- Hobbies. Art, jewelry making, stained glass, painting, home renovation, target shooting, and ceramic work may all involve lead.
- Food. Lead can be found in ceramic dishes made outside the United States (especially from Mexico), lead crystal, water (lead pipes), wine, or canned foods sealed with lead solder.
- Folk remedies may contain lead.

—Mexican. Azarcon, greta, abayalde, rueda, coral, alarcon, Maria Luisa.
—Southeast Asian. Pay-loo-ah.
—India. Maha yogran guggulu, ayurvedic herbal medications.
—China. Hau ge fen.
—Traditional remedies from Korea, Pakistan, and the Middle East have also been implicated.

- Foreign bodies. Bullets (ingested or retained near joints), curtain weights, fishing sinkers, and contaminated soil may all lead to lead poisoning.

TOXIC DOSE

Blood lead levels (BLL) are used instead of ingested amount.

- BLL greater than 10 μg/dl causes delayed cognitive development.
- BLL greater than 45 μg/dl may also cause gastrointestinal effects.
- BLL greater than 100 μg/dl may be life-threatening.

PATHOPHYSIOLOGY

- Lead combines with sulfhydryl groups (R-SH) and thereby inhibits the function of many enzymes.
- CNS development is altered by lead through undescribed mechanisms.
- Anemia is caused by interference with heme-biosynthesis.
- Iron deficiency increases the absorption of lead from the gastrointestinal tract.

EPIDEMIOLOGY

- Poisoning is common in poor children in cities with old deteriorated housing, but is generally uncommon in the western United States.
- Toxic effects following acute exposure are typically mild.
- Death occurs in young children with severe chronic exposure.

CAUSES

- Poisoning is usually caused by accidental chronic exposure.
- An unusual source of exposure (food, traditional remedy, water) should be considered, particularly if the patient is less than 1 year of age.

RISK FACTORS

- Children younger than 3 years of age are at greatest risk of lead poisoning because of hand-to-mouth behavior, increased bioavailability of lead, and an immature blood–brain barrier.
- Iron-deficient children are at risk because of increased pica behavior and increased gastrointestinal absorption of lead.

PREGNANCY AND LACTATION

An elevated cord blood lead level is associated with delayed neurologic development in the infant.

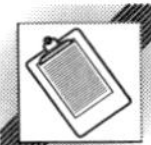

Diagnosis

DIFFERENTIAL DIAGNOSIS

- Toxic causes of encephalopathy appearing like lead encephalopathy include theophylline or salicylate toxicity.
- Nontoxic causes include encephalitis, meningitis, fulminant hepatic failure, or CNS mass or bleed.

SIGNS AND SYMPTOMS

- Patients are usually asymptomatic.
- Abdominal pain, headache, anemia, and fatigue may develop with a BLL of 45 to 60 μg/dl.
- CNS depression, seizures, and encephalopathy are rare and usually are associated with a BLL of more than 100 μg/dl.

HEENT

- Mild hearing loss may occur.
- Blue-black lines ("lead lines") may develop on the gums but are rare in children under 5 years of age.

Gastrointestinal

- Abdominal pain and constipation may develop with chronic intoxication.
- Nausea, vomiting, and diarrhea may develop with acute poisoning from lead salts.

Renal

Nephropathy, interstitial nephritis, decreased glomerular filtration rate, and proximal tubular dysfunction may develop with chronic poisoning.

Hematologic

- Anemia may develop from chronic exposure if the BLL is more than 40 μg/dl.
- Basophilic stippling may develop in patients with chronic exposure.

Musculoskeletal

- Muscle and joint pain may develop with chronic poisoning.
- Lead lines (radiodense areas in the metaphyses of growing bones) may develop with chronic lead poisoning.

Neurologic

- Subclinical cognitive dysfunction, decreased IQ, and difficulties with attention are reported in children with chronic poisoning and BLL higher than 10 μg/dl; irritability, headache, and fatigue also may develop.
- Encephalopathy, coma, and seizures occur rarely and typically with a BLL above 100 μg/dl.
- Peripheral neuropathy is unusual in children.

Endocrine

Chronic poisoning is associated with decreased levels of growth hormone and 1,25 dihydroxy vitamin D in children.

PROCEDURES AND LABORATORY TESTS

Essential Tests

- Blood lead level

—BLL of 10 to 14 μg/dl. The family should be educated to avoid future lead exposure, and the BLL reassessed after 3 months.
—BLL of 15 to 19 μg/dl. The family should be educated to avoid future lead exposure, and the BLL reassessed after 2 months.
—BLL of 20 to 44 μg/dl. A complete assessment of the child and the home environment should be performed. The family should be educated to avoid lead exposure, and the BLL reassessed within 1 month (if BLL is 20 to 29 μg/dl) or within 1 week (if BLL is 29 to 44 μg/dl).
—BLL of 45 to 69 μg/dl. A complete assessment of the child should be performed and chelation treatment initiated. If the home is the likely source, the patient should be moved to other housing immediately.
—BLL of more than 69 μg/dl. The patient should be hospitalized and chelation treatment started. Environmental assessment should be performed immediately and the source remediated before the child can return.

- Environmental assessment

—Although the mechanism varies geographically, it is critical to perform assessment of the child's environmental source of lead.
—The county or state health department should be contacted for further information.

- Complete blood count. Hypochromic microcytic anemia may indicate the need for iron supplementation.
- Serum iron, ferritin, and total iron-binding capacity are measured to determine iron deficiency (which will increase lead absorption).

Recommended Tests

- Abdominal or kidney-ureter-bladder (KUB) radiography should be performed to evaluate for radiopaque foreign bodies in any child who has a suspected recent ingestion, whose BLL has recently increased, in whom oral chelation is considered, or whose BLL is greater than 45 μg/dl.
- A radiograph of long bones (tibia or radius) may reveal lead lines: linear areas of increased density that develop at the metaphyses of growing bones in chronically lead-poisoned children.

—Lead lines have no prognostic value.
—Generally they are not present in children with BLLs of less than 30 to 40 μg/dl.

- X-ray fluorescence is a procedure being developed to measure lead in bone noninvasively; it is not widely available.

Not Recommended Tests

Free erythrocyte protoporphyrin and zinc protoporphyrin are not sensitive nor specific tools for screening.

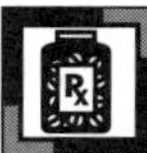

Treatment

- Treatment focuses on determining the source of exposure; eliminating lead exposure; initiating chelation in appropriate patients; and educating parents on sources of lead exposure, hygiene measures to limit exposures, and dietary measures to reduce lead exposure.
- In cases of lead encephalopathy, supportive care with appropriate airway management is vital.
- Temporary relocation of the patient is an important component of therapy when the home environment may be the source of exposure.

DIRECTING PATIENT COURSE

- Consultation with a physician experienced in the management of pediatric lead poisoning is strongly encouraged.

The health-care provider should call the poison control center when:

- Seizure, encephalopathy, or other severe effects are present.
- Toxic effects are not consistent with lead poisoning.
- Coingestant, drug interaction, or underlying disease presents an unusual problem.

The patient should be referred to a health-care facility when:

- Environmental exposure to lead cannot be stopped.
- BLL is higher than 45 μg/dl.
- Seizure, encephalopathy, or other severe effects are present.
- Oral chelation is necessary, and the patient is not in a lead-free environment.

Lead Poisoning—Pediatric

Admission Considerations

Inpatient management is warranted for:

- Patients who have seizure, encephalopathy, or other severe effects.
- Patients who require parenteral chelation.
- Patients who require oral chelation but are not in a lead-free environment.

DECONTAMINATION

- Whole-bowel irrigation is recommended before initiating chelation for patients who have evidence of radiopaque matter on KUB radiographs.
- A polyethylene glycol solution is administered orally at a rate of 10 to 20 ml/kg/h until the rectal effluent is clear and radiopacities have resolved.

ANTIDOTES

Succimer (Chemet)

- Indications

—Succimer is the preferred treatment in children with BLLs higher than 45 μg/dl and less than 100 μg/dl without evidence of encephalopathy.
—It is also used for treatment of children with BLLs of 25 to 45 μg/dl in many centers, but the precise application for this use varies.
—In severe poisoning, succimer is used orally after initial stabilization with a parenteral chelator.

- Contraindications. Documented allergy to succimer precludes use.
- Method of administration

—The clinician should ensure that lead exposure has ended and that there are no radiopacities on KUB radiographs prior to initiation.
—The dose is 10 mg/kg (or 350 mg/m^2) administered orally three times a day for 5 days followed by 10 mg/kg twice a day for 14 days. (The capsules contain microspheres that may be mixed into food or drink for consumption by small children.)
—BLL is reassessed several days after completion of therapy and every 2 to 4 weeks thereafter until level stabilizes.
  —If BLL rebounds to 45 μg/dl or higher, the clinician should investigate whether repeat exposure has occurred.
  —If repeat exposure may have occurred, the patient is moved to lead-free housing and the course of chelation is repeated.
  —If repeat exposure has not occurred, the course of chelation is repeated.
  —If BLL rebounds to 20 to 45 μg/dl, treatment recommendations are uncertain; many centers would perform at least one more course of chelation.

- Adverse effects: Nausea, vomiting, sulfur odor to body fluids, mild transient elevation of transaminase levels, and rash.

EDTA (Calcium Disodium EDTA)

- Indications

—Lead toxicity without CNS toxicity
—Treatment of patients whose BLL is less than 100 μg/dl and who cannot tolerate oral medication
—Severe lead toxicity or lead encephalopathy
  —EDTA should be used in conjunction with BAL (see SECTION III, British Anti-Lewisite chapter).
  —Severe lead poisoning is defined as (1) lead level higher than 100 μg/dl in a child, (2) evidence of CNS toxicity (seizure, altered mental status, encephalopathy), or (3) severe gastrointestinal effects precluding oral administration (severe abdominal pain and dehydration from recurrent vomiting).

- Contraindications. Documented allergy or renal failure.
- Method of administration

—Lead poisoning without CNS toxicity
  —A continuous infusion of 1,000 mg/m^2/day is administered over 24 hours or divided every 8 to 12 hours.
  —Dosage should not exceed 50 mg/kg/day.
  —EDTA is continued for 5 days, then is interrupted for 2 days to reassess the need for further chelation.
  —BLL is reassessed several days after completion of therapy and every 2 to 4 weeks thereafter until level stabilizes.
  —If BLL increases substantially, the clinician should investigate whether repeat exposure could have occurred in the interim.
  —If repeat exposure has not occurred, the course of chelation is repeated; however, succimer is the preferred drug if the patient can take medication orally.
  —If repeat exposure has occurred, the patient should be moved to lead-free housing and chelation repeated.
—With CNS effects
  —First, BAL therapy is initiated (see SECTION III, British Anti-Lewisite chapter).
  —A continuous infusion of EDTA, 1,500 mg/m^2/day, is administered over 24 hours.
  —A total dose of 75 mg/kg/day should not be exceeded.

- Adverse effects

—Redistribution of lead to the brain. BAL is administered prior to EDTA, and EDTA is administered by continuous infusion if BLL is higher than 100 μg/dl or if there is evidence of encephalopathy.
—Dose-related acute tubular necrosis. The recommended dose should not be exceeded.

British Anti-Lewisite (BAL, Dimercaprol)

- Indications. Parenteral treatment of severe poisoning with BLL higher than 100 μg/dl or evidence of encephalopathy.
- Contraindications

—Allergy to BAL or peanuts or hepatic dysfunction precludes use.
—BAL may cause hemolysis in glucose-6-phosphate dehydrogenase-deficient patients.

• Method of administration

—A dose of 2.5 to 5 mg/kg is administered intramuscularly every 4 to 6 hours or 75 mg/m^2 intramuscularly every 4 hours.
—The dose is tapered over 1 to 2 days to intervals of every 6 to 12 hours until an oral antidote can be tolerated.
—It is discontinued after 5 days; sooner if severe adverse effects develop.

• Adverse effects. Headache, hypertension, tachycardia, fever, nausea, vomiting, pain at injection site.

D-Penicillamine

• Indications

—It is a less effective, more toxic, and less expensive alternative to succimer.
—It is used in some areas for treatment of children with BLL less than 100 μg/dl and without evidence of encephalopathy.
—It is used after initial stabilization with parenteral chelator in patients with severe poisoning in some centers.

• Contraindications. Allergy, encephalopathy, or BLL higher than 100 μg/dl precludes use.
• Method of administration. A dose of 20 to 30 mg/kg/day is administered orally, divided four times a day up to 250 to 500 mg/dose.
• Adverse effects. Rash, fever, leukopenia, thrombocytopenia, eosinophilia, or hemolytic anemia may occur.

ADJUNCTIVE TREATMENT

• Encephalopathy is treated, as in other causes, with osmotic diuretics, corticosteroids, and control of fluid balance.
• Seizures are treated in the standard manner, beginning with benzodiazepine administration (see SECTION II, Seizure chapter).

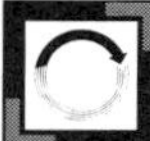

Follow-Up

PATIENT MONITORING

• BLL is repeated several days to 2 weeks after chelation and periodically thereafter to detect rebound or reexposure.
• Follow serial BLL in children with BLL higher than 10 μg/dl as indicated in Essential Tests section.

EXPECTED COURSE AND PROGNOSIS

• Children with mild to moderate poisoning (levels less than 60 or 70 μg/dl) have nonspecific symptoms but may sustain permanent, subtle intellectual impairment.
• Children with severe poisoning (BLL higher than 70 μg/dl, seizures, encephalopathy) are often left with neurologic impairment.
• Without aggressive chelation, children with encephalopathy may die.
• Developmental delay, hyperactivity, and learning disabilities are possible complications.

DISCHARGE CRITERIA AND INSTRUCTIONS

Patients may be discharged from the hospital to continue oral chelation when BLL is lower than 50 μg/dl, evidence of encephalopathy has resolved or stabilized, and a lead-free environment has been arranged.

PATIENT EDUCATION

• Homes with chipping, peeling leaded paint require remediation.
• Caregivers who work in the lead industry or who have hobbies that involve lead should shower and change clothes before returning home.
• Caregivers should avoid vacuuming hard floors and surfaces (because it stirs up lead dust) and to wash hard surfaces with phosphate-based detergents.
• Caregivers need to control pica behavior and make sure the children wash hands frequently especially before eating and avoid taking toys or other equipment outdoors.

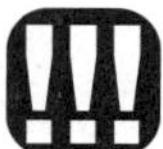

Pitfalls

DIAGNOSIS

• A low threshold for evaluation of potential lead poisoning is important because children with BLL less than 60 μg/dl may suffer CNS injury but typically have few symptoms.
• Blood obtained by capillary stick may be contaminated with lead on skin; venipuncture is preferred.
• Screening children at risk is the most effective way to detect lead poisoning.

TREATMENT

BLL usually rebounds even after chelation; repeat courses are often needed.

FOLLOW-UP

• Ensuring a lead-free environment is often difficult and must be pursued vigorously.
• Levels may rebound even after repeated courses of chelation over months because most of the body burden of lead is stored in bone.

ICD-9-CM 984

Toxic effect of lead and its compounds.

See also: SECTION II, Seizure chapter. SECTION III, British Anti-Lewisite, EDTA, d-penicillamine, Succimer, and Whole-Bowel Irrigation chapters.

RECOMMENDED READING

Bellinger DC, Leviton A, Waternaux C, et al. Longitudinal analysis of prenatal and postnatal lead exposure and early cognitive development. *N Engl J Med* 1987;316:1037–1043.

Bellinger DC, Stiles KM, Needleman HL. Low-level lead exposure, intelligence and academic achievement: a long-term follow-up study. *Pediatr* 1992;90:855–861.

Centers for Disease Control. *Screening young children for lead poisoning: guidance for state and local public health officials.* Atlanta, GA: Centers for Disease Control, February 1997.

Author: Katherine M. Hurlbut

Reviewer: Richard C. Dart

Levamisole

Basics

DESCRIPTION

Levamisole is an antihelmintic and cancer chemotherapeutic agent.

FORMS AND USES

- Levamisole (Ergamisol, Ketrax) is indicated for use with 5-fluorouracil in the treatment of adenocarcinoma of the colon.
- It has been used in combination with other chemotherapeutics for a variety of cancers.
- Typical antihelmintic dose is 2 to 3 mg/kg.

TOXIC DOSE

There are reports of fatalities in children at a dose of 15 mg/kg and in adults at 32 mg/kg.

PATHOPHYSIOLOGY

- Levamisole has complex immune-modulating effects.

—It restores macrophages and T-lymphocytes to normal immune function.
—It also may stimulate the formation of antibodies and potentiate chemotaxis and phagocytosis.

- It has both nicotinic and muscarinic cholinergic activity and may inhibit alkaline phosphatase.

EPIDEMIOLOGY

Poisoning is uncommon.

CAUSES

Most cases of toxicity arise from therapeutic use.

PREGNANCY AND LACTATION

US FDA Pregnancy Category C. The drug exerts animal teratogenic or embryocidal effects, but there are no controlled studies in women, or no studies are available in either animals or women.

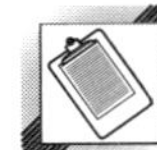

Diagnosis

DIFFERENTIAL DIAGNOSIS

Other causes of increased nicotinic receptor stimulation, including tobacco, organophosphates, or carbamate insecticides, and certain mushrooms.

SIGNS AND SYMPTOMS

After acute ingestion, the patient may develop nicotine-like syndrome with vomiting, diarrhea, and fasciculation ranging to pulmonary edema, seizure, and coma.

HEENT

Increased salivation may occur.

Dermatologic

Rashes (dermatitis, alopecia, urticaria, skin discoloration) may be present.

Gastrointestinal

Abdominal pain, cramping, nausea, vomiting, anorexia, and taste perversion may occur.

Neurologic

Headache, nervousness, irritability, insomnia, and smell perversion may occur.

Hematologic

Granulocytopenia occurs in about 20% of patients (when used as a chemotherapeutic agent), and agranulocytosis, anemia, and thrombocytopenia also have been observed.

PROCEDURES AND LABORATORY TESTS

Essential Tests

Complete blood count, liver function, and kidney function should be monitored.

Recommended Tests

ECG, serum acetaminophen and aspirin levels in overdose setting to detect occult ingestion.

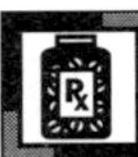

Treatment

- Supportive care with appropriate airway management is vital.
- Dose and time of exposure must be determined for all substances involved.

DIRECTING PATIENT COURSE

The health-care professional should call the poison control center when:

- Severe or persistent effects develop.
- Coingestant, drug interaction, or underlying disease presents an unusual problem.

The patient should be referred to a health-care facility when:

- Attempted suicide or homicide is possible.
- Toxic effects develop.
- Coingestant, drug interaction, or underlying disease presents an unusual problem.

Admission Considerations

Patients usually should be admitted if granulocytopenia develops or persistent nicotinic effects are present.

DECONTAMINATION

Out of Hospital

Emesis should be induced with ipecac for alert pediatric or adult patient if health-care evaluation will be delayed.

In Hospital

- Gastric lavage should be performed in pediatric (tube size 24–32 French) or adult (tube size 36–42 French) patients presenting within 1 hour of a large ingestion or if serious effects are present.
- One dose of activated charcoal (1–2 g/kg) should be administered without a cathartic if a substantial ingestion has occurred within the previous few hours.

ADJUNCTIVE TREATMENT

- Seizures are treated in the standard manner with airway management, benzodiazepine administration, and other antiseizure medications as needed.
- Atropine (0.02 mg/kg) intravenously may be used to control nicotinic cholinergic effects.

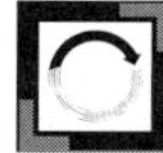

Follow-Up

PATIENT MONITORING

- Patients should be closely monitored until vital signs are normal and the patient is asymptomatic.
- Follow-up visits should be arranged for possible delayed hematologic effects.

EXPECTED COURSE AND PROGNOSIS

- Symptom onset is usually rapid following acute ingestion.
- Most cases resolve spontaneously.
- Granulocytopenia may require antibiotics or cytokine therapy.

DISCHARGE CRITERIA/INSTRUCTIONS

Patients may be discharged from the emergency department or hospital when toxic effects resolve or stabilize and after psychiatric evaluation, if needed.

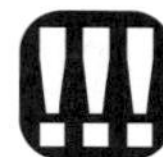

Pitfalls

DIAGNOSIS

- Due to infrequent occurrence, levamisole toxicity may be misdiagnosed even in the presence of nicotinic signs.
- Patient should be monitored for low white blood cell counts after acute episode has resolved.

ICD-9-CM 963.1

Poisoning by primarily systemic agents: antineoplastic and immunosuppressive drugs.

971.0

Poisoning by drugs primarily affecting the autonomic nervous system: parasympathomimetics (cholinergics).

See also: SECTION III, Atropine chapter; SECTION IV, Nicotine chapter.

RECOMMENDED READING

Parkinson DR, Cano PO, Jerry LM, et al. Complications of cancer immunotherapy with levamisole. *Lancet* 1977;1:1129–1132.

Author: Scott D. Phillips

Reviewer: Katherine M. Hurlbut

Levodopa

Basics

DESCRIPTION

Levodopa and carbidopa are used to treat Parkinson's disease.

FORMS AND USES

- Levodopa is available as a single agent or in combination with carbidopa (Bendopa, Dopar, Larodopa, Sinemet).
- The usual therapeutic dose of levodopa is 500 to 1,000 mg/day given in two to three divided doses, with dosage increases titrated to effect up to a maximum of 8 g per day.

TOXIC DOSE

- The lethal dose in humans is unknown.
- Ingestion of more than 10 to 20 g is often associated with mild to moderate toxicity.

PATHOPHYSIOLOGY

- Levodopa is converted to dopamine by the pyridoxine-dependent enzyme L-amino acid decarboxylase.
- Carbidopa decreases the side effects of levodopa by decreasing the conversion of levodopa to dopamine outside of the CNS.

EPIDEMIOLOGY

Poisoning is uncommon, but adverse effects during chronic therapy are common.

CAUSES

Child neglect or abuse should be considered if the patient is less than 1 year of age, suicide attempt if the patient is over 6 years of age.

DRUG AND DISEASE INTERACTIONS

- Levodopa may exacerbate the effects of other drugs that cause hypotension.
- Levodopa may be associated with serotonin syndrome, particularly when combined with another agent that increases the relative amount of serotonergic activity.

PREGNANCY AND LACTATION

US FDA Pregnancy Category C. The drug exerts animal teratogenic or embryocidal effects, but there are no controlled studies in women, or no studies are available in animals or women.

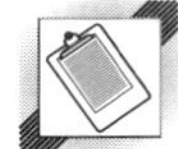

Diagnosis

DIFFERENTIAL DIAGNOSIS

Other toxicologic causes of adrenergic excess (agitation, hypertension, altered mental status) include tricyclic antidepressants, all types of stimulants, neuroleptic malignant syndrome, and serotonin syndrome, among others.

SIGNS AND SYMPTOMS

Vital Signs

- Tachycardia and hypertension are common following acute overdose.
- Orthostatic hypotension is common during chronic therapy.
- Malignant hyperthermia has occurred rarely following discontinuation of chronic therapy.

Cardiovascular

Transient hypertension may be followed by hypotension after acute overdose.

Gastrointestinal

Anorexia, nausea, and vomiting are common after either acute overdose or initiation of chronic therapy.

Neurologic

- Confusion, agitation, insomnia, and restlessness have been reported following acute overdose and during chronic therapy.
- Involuntary movement disorders, especially choreoathetosis, are common following acute overdose and during chronic therapy.
- Dystonia has been reported with chronic therapy.

Psychiatric

Depression, paranoia, hallucinations, anxiety, and mania are common during chronic therapy.

PROCEDURES AND LABORATORY TESTS

Essential Tests

ECG and hemodynamic monitoring should be performed on symptomatic patients.

Recommended Tests

- Serum electrolytes, BUN, and creatinine are used to assess other causes of altered mental status.
- Serum acetaminophen and aspirin levels should be checked in the overdose setting to detect occult ingestion.
- Head CT, blood and CSF cultures, and lumbar puncture should be considered in severe cases to evaluate other causes of altered mental status.

Not Recommended Tests

Levodopa plasma levels are not clinically useful.

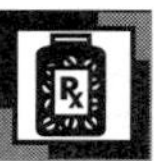

Treatment

- Treatment should focus on supportive care with appropriate airway management and treatment of hyper- or hypotension.
- Dose and time of exposure should be determined for all substances involved.

DIRECTING PATIENT COURSE

The health-care professional should call the poison control center when:

- Severe or persistent effects develop.
- Signs and symptoms are not consistent with levodopa poisoning.
- Coingestant, drug interaction, or underlying disease presents an unusual problem.

The patient should be referred to a health-care facility when:

- Attempted suicide or homicide is possible.
- Toxic effects develop.
- The patient or caregiver seems unreliable.
- Coingestant, drug interaction, or underlying disease presents an unusual problem.

Admission Considerations

Inpatient management is warranted for patients who have persistent CNS alterations or cardiovascular instability.

DECONTAMINATION

Out of Hospital

Ipecac-induced emesis is not recommended owing to the potential for CNS depression and cardiovascular instability.

In Hospital

- Ipecac-induced emesis is not recommended.
- Gastric lavage should be performed in pediatric (tube size 24–32 French) or adult (tube size 36–42 French) patients presenting within 1 hour of a large ingestion or if serious effects are present.
- One dose of activated charcoal (1–2 g/kg) should be administered without a cathartic if a substantial ingestion has occurred within the previous few hours.

ANTIDOTES

There is no specific antidote for levodopa poisoning.

ADJUNCTIVE TREATMENT

- Pyridoxine has been used to reverse choreoathetosis and dyskinesia.

—This may occur by increasing the peripheral conversion of levodopa to dopamine, thereby making less levodopa available to the CNS.
—Adult dose of pyridoxine is 5 g intravenously over 5 minutes. An additional 5 g may be given if no response is noted within 1 hour.

- Hypertension does not usually require treatment. If end-organ damage develops, a short-acting titratable anti-hypertensive agent such as nitroglycerin, nitroprusside, or esmolol should be used, due to the likelihood of subsequent hypotension.
- Hypotension is treated with 10–20 cc/kg normal saline, Trendelenburg position and, if needed, vasopressors. Dopamine is used initially and norepinephrine is added for refractory hypotension.

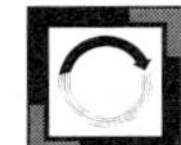

Follow-Up

PATIENT MONITORING

Cardiac and respiratory monitoring should be performed continuously.

EXPECTED COURSE AND PROGNOSIS

Toxic effects typically peak within hours of an acute single ingestion unless sequelae of hypotension intercede.

DISCHARGE CRITERIA/INSTRUCTIONS

- From the emergency department. Asymptomatic patients may be discharged with no documented CNS or cardiovascular abnormality for at least 4 to 6 hours postingestion and after psychiatric evaluation if needed.
- From the hospital. Patient may be discharged after CNS or cardiovascular abnormality has resolved for at least 12 hours.

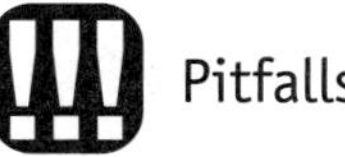

Pitfalls

DIAGNOSIS

- Due to psychological dependence, patients may increase their daily dosages until toxic effects are experienced.
- Peripheral neuropathy may develop with large doses and chronic therapy.

TREATMENT

Hypertension may be quickly followed by hypotension. Hypertension should be treated with short-acting agents.

FOLLOW-UP

This drug should not be administered concurrently or within 2 weeks of administration of a monamine oxidase inhibitor.

ICD-9-CM 966.4

Poisoning by anti-parkinsonism drugs.

See also: SECTION II, Hypertension, Hypotension chapters; SECTION III, Pyridoxine chapter.

RECOMMENDED READING

Mills KC. Serotonin syndrome: a clinical update. *Med Toxicol* 1997;13:763–783.

Author: Edwin K. Kuffner

Reviewer: Richard C. Dart

Levorphanol

Basics

DESCRIPTION

Levorphanol (Levo-Dromoran) is a synthetic opiate analgesic, the levo-isomer of dextromethorphan.

FORMS AND USES

Levorphanol is available as a tablet and for subcutaneous injection.

TOXIC DOSE

Respiratory depression can occur at therapeutic doses (2 mg).

PATHOPHYSIOLOGY

- Levorphanol is an opiate receptor agonist with a duration of action similar to that of morphine.
- It may accumulate during repeated administration, leading to toxicity.

EPIDEMIOLOGY

Poisoning is uncommon.

CAUSES

Child neglect or abuse should be considered if the patient is less than 1 year of age, suicide attempt if the patient is over 6 years of age.

PREGNANCY AND LACTATION

- U.S. FDA Category B. Animal studies do indicate a fetal risk and there are no controlled human studies, or animal studies to show an adverse fetal effect, but well-controlled studies in pregnant women do not.
- FDA classification becomes D if used at term.
- Neonatal withdrawal may occur 12–72 hours after delivery.

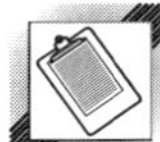

Diagnosis

DIFFERENTIAL DIAGNOSIS

- Other toxic causes of CNS depression include: Alcohol, other narcotics, clonidine, benzodiazepines, barbiturates, tricyclic antidepressants
- Nontoxic causes of CNS depression: Hypoxia, severe electrolyte abnormalities, hypoglycemia, intracranial bleed, meningitis, encephalitis, postictal state.

SIGNS AND SYMPTOMS

Vital Signs

Bradycardia, hypotension, and bradypnea may occur.

HEENT

Miosis usually occurs with overdose.

Dermatologic

Skin may be cool.

Cardiovascular

Bradycardia, hypotension, and vasodilation may occur.

Pulmonary

- Dose-related respiratory depression is common and may be prolonged in overdose.
- Pulmonary edema can occur with overdose.

Gastrointestinal

- Nausea and vomiting can occur but reportedly less than with morphine.
- Constipation may occur in therapeutic doses.

Neurologic

- Somnolence progressing to coma occurs with overdose.
- There may be less CNS depression than with a morphine overdose.

PROCEDURES AND LABORATORY TESTS

Essential Tests

No tests may be needed in asymptomatic patients.

Recommended Tests

- All patients with altered mental status should have blood glucose level determined.
- Serum electrolytes, BUN, creatinine to assess cause of altered mental status.
- Pulse oximetry or arterial blood gases should be obtained to evaluate oxygenation.
- Head CT, lumbar puncture, urine toxicology, and other studies should be performed as needed to evaluate other causes of altered mental status.

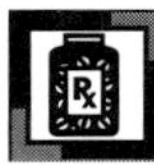

Treatment

- Treatment should focus on control of airway and administration of naloxone.
- Dose and time of exposure need to be determined for all substances involved.

DIRECTING PATIENT COURSE

The health-care professional should call the poison control center when:

- Severe or persistent effects develop.
- Coingestant, drug interaction, or underlying disease presents an unusual problem.

The patient should be referred to a health-care facility when:

- Suicide or homicide attempt is possible.
- Toxic effects develop.
- Coingestant, drug interaction, or underlying disease presents an unusual problem.

Admission Considerations

Patients should be admitted if they have persistently altered mental status or require a second dose of opiate antagonist during their 6-hour observation period.

DECONTAMINATION

Out of Hospital

Emesis should not be induced.

In Hospital

- Gastric lavage (after appropriate airway management) should be performed in pediatric (tube size 24–32 French) or adult (tube size 36–42 French) patients presenting within 1 hour of a large ingestion or if serious effects are present.
- One dose of activated charcoal (1–2 g/kg) should be administered without a cathartic if a substantial ingestion has occurred within the previous few hours.

ANTIDOTES

Naloxone is a specific antidote for levorphanol poisoning.

- An adult or child should be administered 2 mg intravenously for respiratory depression.
- The dose may be repeated up to 10 mg, but most patients will respond to 2 mg.
- Naloxone may precipitate withdrawal in dependent patients.

ADJUNCTIVE TREATMENT

Patients should be placed on a cardiac monitor, receive oxygen, and have intravenous access established.

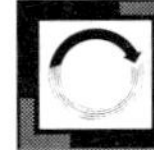

Follow-Up

PATIENT MONITORING

Cardiac and respiratory function should be monitored continuously.

EXPECTED COURSE AND PROGNOSIS

Complete recovery is expected unless sequelae of hypoxia develop before medical treatment can be provided.

DISCHARGE CRITERIA/INSTRUCTIONS

An asymptomatic patient may be discharged from the emergency deparment or hospital after adequate decontamination and 4 hours of observation after the administration of naloxone.

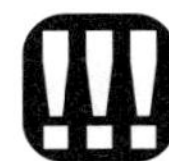

Pitfalls

TREATMENT

Naloxone effect may dissipate over 30–60 minutes, allowing CNS and respiratory depression to recur.

ICD-9-CM 965

Poisoning by analgesics, antipyretics, and antirheumatics.

970.1

Poisoning by central nervous system stimulants: opiate antagonists.

See also: SECTION III, Naloxone and Nalmephene chapter.

RECOMMENDED READING

Ellenhorn MJ. The opiates. *Medical toxicology.* Baltimore: Williams & Wilkins, 1997:405–412.

Author: Kennon Heard

Reviewer: Richard C. Dart

Lipid-Lowering Agents

Basics

DESCRIPTION

Lipid-lowering agents are oral drugs used to treat hyperlipidemia, hyperlipoproteinemia, and hypercholesterolemia.

FORMS AND USES

There are four types:

- Bile acid-binding resins

—Colestipol dosage is 5 to 30 g orally per day (single or divided dose).
—Cholestyramine dosage is 4 g of resin orally three or four times a day (doses larger than 24 g/day of resin are associated with increased incidence of adverse reactions).

- Fibric acid derivatives

—Clofibrate dosage is 2 g orally per day (divided into two to four doses).
—Gemfibrozil dosage is 600 mg orally twice a day to 1,500 mg per day (in divided doses).

- Hydroxymethylglutaryl (HMG)-coenzyme A (CoA) reductase inhibitors

—Atorvastatin dosage is 10 to 80 mg orally per day; fluvastatin dosage is 20 to 80 mg orally per day (doses of more than 60 mg are divided into two doses).
—Lovastatin dosage is 20 to 80 mg orally per day (doses of more than 60 mg are divided into two doses).
—Pravastatin dosage is 10 to 40 mg orally per day
—Simvastatin dosage is 10 to 40 mg orally per day.

- Niacin dosage is 1.5 to 9.0 g orally per day, in divided doses (although doses larger than 6 g daily are generally not recommended).

TOXIC DOSE

- A 7-year-old child recovered without sequelae after ingesting 9 g of gemfibrozil.
- Although a few accidental lovastatin overdose cases have been reported, all patients fully recovered; doses up to 200 mg of lovastatin have been administered to healthy adults without clinically significant toxicity.

PATHOPHYSIOLOGY

- Bile acid-binding resins (colestipol, cholestyramine) increase sterol excretion and low-density lipoprotein (LDL) removal, thereby decreasing LDL with a slight increase in high-density lipoproteins (HDL).
- Fibric acid derivatives (gemfibrozil, clofibrate) increase lipoprotein lipase activity and very low-density lipoprotein (VLDL) catabolism, decrease VLDL synthesis, and increase HDL.
- HMG-CoA reductase inhibitors (atorvastatin, fluvastatin, lovastatin, pravastatin, and simvastatin) inhibit HMG-CoA reductase, the rate-determining enzyme in cholesterol synthesis, thereby increasing LDL receptor activity, significantly decreasing LDL, slightly decreasing triglycerides, and slightly increasing HDL.
- Nicotinic acid (niacin) decreases hepatic lipase and VLDL synthesis, decreases adipocyte lipolysis and APO B, significantly decreases LDL and triglycerides, and significantly increases HDL.
- Because of the relatively nontoxic nature of the lipid-lowering agents in acute overdose, little is known of their toxic mechanism.

EPIDEMIOLOGY

- Poisoning is uncommon.
- Toxic effects following exposure are typically mild.
- Death is unlikely unless a coingestant is present.

CAUSES

- Lipid-lowering agent poisoning is usually by accidental ingestion.
- Child neglect should be considered if the patient is under 1 year of age; attempted suicide if the patient is over 6 years of age.

DRUG AND DISEASE INTERACTIONS

- Colestipol or cholestyramine may interfere with the absorption of other drugs.
- Clofibrate or gemfibrozil:

—May cause pancreatitis, rhabdomyolysis, and renal failure when used concurrently with HMG-CoA reductase inhibitors (e.g., lovastatin).
—May potentiate the anticoagulant effects of warfarin or dicoumerol.
—May increase the diuretic effects of furosemide and the hypoglycemic effects of sulfonylureas.

- HMG-CoA reductase inhibitors

—Myopathy and renal failure have occurred when HMG-CoA reductase inhibitors were used concurrently with immunosuppressants (e.g., cyclosporine), erythromycin, or itraconazole.
—Concurrent use with clofibrate or gemfibrozil may cause myositis, rhabdomyolysis, renal failure (rare), and pancreatitis.
—Coadministration with niacin has also been reported to cause myopathy and rhabdomyolysis.

- Niacin may potentiate the effects of ganglionic blocking drugs (e.g., guanethidine, reserpine); coadministration with HMG-CoA reductase inhibitors may cause myopathy and rhabdomyolysis.

PREGNANCY AND LACTATION

- Cholestyramine, gemfibrozil, clofibrate, and niacin. US FDA Pregnancy Category C. The drug exerts animal teratogenic or embryocidal effects, but there are no controlled studies in women, or no studies are available in either animals or women.
- HMG-CoA reductase inhibitors. US FDA Pregnancy Category X. Studies in animals or humans have demonstrated fetal abnormalities or there is evidence of fetal risk based on human experience, or both, and the risk clearly outweighs any possible benefit.

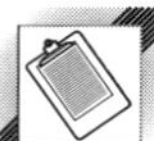

Diagnosis

SIGNS AND SYMPTOMS

Adverse Reactions to Therapeutic Dosages

- Colestipol and cholestyramine may cause constipation, abdominal pain, flatulence, nausea, vomiting, hyperchloremic acidosis, increased urinary excretion of calcium, and elevated liver function test results (LFTs).
- Clofibrate and gemfibrozil may cause gastrointestinal disturbance, abdominal pain, acute appendicitis in some instances, elevated LFTs, cholelithiasis, headache, dizziness, and blood dyscrasia.
- HMG-CoA reductase inhibitors may cause diarrhea, elevated LFTs, cholestatic jaundice, hepatitis, peripheral neuropathy, hyperkalemia, myopathy, acute renal failure, rhabdomyolysis (rarely), lens opacities, and insomnia.
- Niacin may cause gastrointestinal disturbances, flushing (especially in the face and neck), pruritus, hypotension, dizziness, tachycardia, hyperuricemia, elevated LFTs, hepatotoxicity, glucose intolerance, and exacerbation of peptic ulcer disease.
- Sustained-release niacin preparations are associated with a significantly higher incidence of hepatotoxicity than the immediate-release crystalline preparations.

Adverse Reactions to Toxic Dosages

- For colestipol and cholestyramine, the primary concern is gastrointestinal obstruction; high doses have been associated with steatorrhea, interference with fat-soluble vitamin absorption, and hypoprothrombinemia.
- Effects following overdose of gemfibrozil include incoordination, depression, flaccid prostration, dyspnea, and slight hepatocellular enlargement (in animal models).
- Megadoses of niacin are associated with atrial fibrillation, other cardiac dysrhythmias, and acanthosis nigricans.

PROCEDURES AND LABORATORY TESTS

Essential Tests

No tests may be needed in asymptomatic patients.

Recommended Tests

- Serum electrolytes, BUN, and creatinine should be obtained for symptomatic patients.
- Serum LFTs and prothrombin time should be obtained for symptomatic patients.
- ECG, serum acetaminophen and aspirin levels should be obtained in overdose setting to detect occult ingestion.

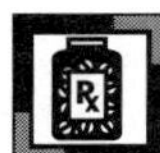

Treatment

- Supportive care is the mainstay of therapy.
- The dose and time of exposure should be determined for all substances involved.

DIRECTING PATIENT COURSE

The health-care provider should call a poison control center when:

- Severe effects are present.
- Toxic effects are not consistent with lipid-lowering agents.
- Coingestant, drug interaction, or underlying disease presents an unusual problem.

The patient should be referred to a health-care facility when:

- Attempted suicide or homicide is possible.
- The patient or caregiver seems unreliable.
- Acute toxic effects develop.
- Coingestant, drug interaction, or underlying disease presents an unusual problem.

Admission Considerations

Inpatient management is warranted for patients who develop complications of mechanical gastrointestinal tract obstruction or exhibit persistent toxic effects of coingestants.

DECONTAMINATION

Out of Hospital

Decontamination is not recommended unless a coingestant is present.

In Hospital

- Gastric lavage should be initiated in pediatric patients (tube size 24–32 French) or adult (tube size 36–42 French) patients in cases of large ingestion presenting within 1 hour of ingestion or if serious effects are present.
- One dose of activated charcoal (1–2 g/kg) may be administered without a cathartic if a substantial ingestion has occurred within the previous few hours.

ANTIDOTE

There are no antidotes for poisoning with lipid-lowering agents.

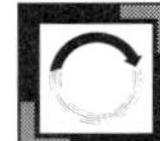

Follow-Up

PATIENT MONITORING

In patients with symptoms, serum creatinine, BUN, creatine kinase, LFTs, and urine analysis should be monitored as indicated by clinical condition.

EXPECTED COURSE AND PROGNOSIS

Acute toxic effects typically develop quickly and resolve within hours.

DISCHARGE CRITERIA/INSTRUCTIONS

Patients may be discharged from the emergency department or hospital when their symptoms resolve and following psychiatric evaluation, if needed.

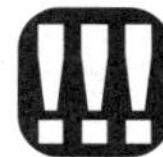

Pitfalls

DIAGNOSIS

If major toxicity develops acutely, a coingestant should be suspected.

ICD-9-CM 963

Poisoning by primarily systemic agents.

RECOMMENDED READING

Division of Drugs and Toxicology, American Medical Association. *AMA drug evaluations.* Chicago: AMA, 1995.

Facts Comparisons Staff. *Drug facts and comparisons,* 51st ed. St. Louis: Facts & Co., 1997.

Jacobson TA, Amorosa LF. Combination therapy with fluvastatin niacin in hypercholesterolemia: a preliminary report on safety. *Am J Cardiol* 1994;73:25D–29D.

McEvoy GK, ed. *AHFS drug information.* New York: Facts on File, 1995.

Mitchel YB. The long-term tolerability profile of lovastatin and simvastatin. *Atherosclerosis* 1992;97:S33–S39.

Author: Jana Vander Leest

Reviewer: Kennon Heard

Lithium

Basics

DESCRIPTION

Lithium is an oral medication used in the treatment of a variety of psychiatric disorders.

FORMS AND USES

Substances include lithium carbonate (Eskalith, Lithotabs, Lithonate, Eskalith, Lithobid) and lithium citrate.

Therapeutic Uses and Dosage

- Lithium is used for treatment of bipolar affective disorder.
- It is less often used for schizoaffective disorder, attention deficit disorder, aggressive disorders, alcoholism, cluster headaches, anorexia nervosa, and induction of leukocytosis.
- It is generally not used in children under 12 years of age.
- Typical adult dose is 900 to 1,200 mg/day orally.

TOXIC DOSE

- Due to variable absorption, the ingested dose is not a reliable indicator of toxicity. A serum lithium level above 2.0 mEq/L is often associated with toxic effects.
- Toxicity is based on clinical manifestations.

PATHOPHYSIOLOGY

- The mechanism of toxicity is poorly understood.
- Lithium may alter cell membrane conductivity, decrease neurotransmitter levels, and inhibit adenylate cyclase activity.
- Lithium is filtered and reabsorbed in the proximal tubule, much like sodium.
- Chronic intoxication during therapeutic dosing may occur if renal resorption of sodium is increased (e.g., by dehydration or drug interactions).

EPIDEMIOLOGY

- Poisoning is common.
- Toxic effects following acute overdose are typically mild to moderate.
- Death is rare.

CAUSES

- Acute intoxication is usually intentional.
- Chronic intoxication is usually due to intercurrent illness.
- The possibility of child neglect should be considered in patients under 1 year of age; suicide attempt in patients over 6 years of age.

RISK FACTORS

Elderly patients or those with dehydration, renal insufficiency, hyponatremia, low sodium diet, metabolic stress, or infection are at risk for chronic intoxication.

DRUG AND DISEASE INTERACTIONS

- Concurrent neuroleptic use may increase risk of toxic effects or neuroleptic malignant syndrome.
- Calcium channel blockers increase the risk of lithium neurotoxicity.
- Drugs that decrease lithium excretion include diuretics (especially thiazides and spironolactone), nonsteroidal antiinflammatory drugs, angiotensin-converting enzyme inhibitors, and metronidazole.

PREGNANCY AND LACTATION

- US FDA Pregnancy Category D. Positive evidence of human fetal risk exists, but benefits in certain situations (e.g., life-threatening situations or serious diseases) may make use of the drug acceptable despite its risks.
- Maternal use is associated with cardiac abnormalities in the infant.
- Infants born to mothers with lithium toxicity may have increased lithium levels and clinical toxicity.

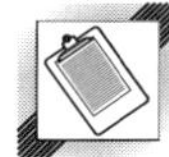

Diagnosis

DIFFERENTIAL DIAGNOSIS

- Toxic causes of altered mental status, tremors, and movement disorders include sympathomimetic drugs, and withdrawal from ethanol, sedative-hypnotic agents.
- Nontoxic causes include thyrotoxicosis and catecholamine excess.

SIGNS AND SYMPTOMS

- Acute overdose generally causes nausea and vomiting.
- CNS effects (tremor, hyperreflexia, altered mental status) may develop over hours or days if a large ingestion has occurred.
- In chronic overdose, CNS effects predominate: confusion, hyperreflexia, cogwheeling, tremor, nystagmus, seizures, and coma.
- Hypotension and dysrhythmias occur in exceptional cases.

Vital Signs

Hypotension occurs in severe cases.

HEENT

Nystagmus and extraocular muscle abnormalities may develop.

Cardiovascular

ECG changes (primarily T-wave flattening or inversion) and dysrhythmias (conduction delays, sinus node dysfunction) occur in more severe cases.

Pulmonary

Respiratory failure and adult respiratory distress syndrome occur with severe intoxication.

Gastrointestinal

Nausea, vomiting, and diarrhea are common.

Renal

Diabetes insipidus may develop.

Fluids and Electrolytes

- Dehydration is a common precipitant of chronic intoxication.
- Hypernatremia may develop with diabetes insipidus.
- Decreased anion gap is common.

Neurologic

- Lethargy, confusion, tremor, ataxia, slurred speech, hyperreflexia, clonus, choreoathetosis, dystonia, cogwheel rigidity, and fasciculations may develop.
- Coma and seizures may occur with severe toxicity.
- Sensory-motor peripheral neuropathy and neuroleptic malignant syndrome occur rarely.
- Permanent neurologic effects may include ataxia, cerebellar atrophy, basal ganglia degeneration, parkinsonism, and altered mental status.

Endocrine

- Therapeutic use is associated with hypothyroidism.
- Diabetes insipidus may develop with acute or chronic intoxication.

Hematologic

Leukocytosis is common.

PROCEDURES AND LABORATORY TESTS

Essential Tests

- Serum electrolytes, BUN, and creatinine should be determined; dehydration or renal insufficiency suggests etiology of chronic intoxication.
- Serum lithium levels should be determined every 2 to 4 hours until levels decline and symptoms improve. The normal range is typically 0.6 to 1.2 mEq/L.

—Patients with chronic or acute-on-chronic (supratherapeutic ingestion while on therapy with lithium) intoxication may have neurologic effects at levels only slightly above or within the therapeutic range.
—Patients with high levels following acute overdose may be initially asymptomatic only to become toxic over the next 12 to 24 hours.
—Peak levels may be delayed more than 8 hours with sustained-release products.

Recommended Tests

- Serum creatine kinase should be determined in patients with seizure or persistent fasciculation to assess muscle injury.
- ECG, serum acetaminophen and aspirin levels are measured in overdose setting to detect occult ingestion.
- CT, lumbar puncture, cultures, and other tests may be performed as needed to rule out other causes of altered mental status.
- Tablets may be visible on plain abdominal radiographs or abdominal radiographs, but the absence of radiopacity does not rule out lithium ingestion.

Drugs and Disorders that May Alter Laboratory Results

Green-top Vacutainer tubes contain lithium heparin, resulting in spuriously elevated lithium levels.

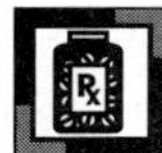

Treatment

- Treatment should focus on decontamination, hydration, and initiating hemodialysis if appropriate.
- Dose and time of exposure should be determined for substances involved.

DIRECTING PATIENT COURSE

The health-care provider should call the poison control center when:

- Altered mental status, seizure, or other severe effects are present.
- Hemodialysis is being considered.
- Toxic effects are not consistent with lithium poisoning.
- Coingestant, drug interaction, or underlying disease presents unusual problems.

The patient should be referred to a health-care facility when:

- Attempted suicide or homicide is possible.
- Patient or caregiver seems unreliable.
- Any toxic effects are present.
- Coingestant, drug interaction, or underlying disease presents unusual problems.

Admission Considerations

Inpatient treatment is warranted when the patient has signs of toxicity (other than mild gastrointestinal upset), the serum lithium level is rising, or a sustained-release preparation was ingested.

DECONTAMINATION

Out of Hospital

Emesis should be induced with ipecac within 1 hour of single ingestion for alert pediatric or adult patients if health care evaluation will be delayed.

In Hospital

- Emesis should be induced with ipecac within 1 hour of ingestion for the pediatric patient who is too small to have effective gastric lavage due to orogastric tube size constraints.
- Gastric lavage should be performed in pediatric (tube size 24–32 French) or adult (tube size 36–42 French) patients presenting within 1 hour of a large ingestion or if serious effects are present.
- Activated charcoal does not bind lithium efficiently, but is used if a coingestant is possible.
- Whole-bowel irrigation should be considered for large ingestion or ingestion of a sustained-release preparation (see SECTION III, Whole-Bowel Irrigation chapter, for details).

ANTIDOTES

There is no specific antidote for lithium intoxication.

ADJUNCTIVE TREATMENT

Hydration

- Lithium renal elimination is increased by hydration.
- A bolus of 10 to 20 ml/kg 0.9% saline should be administered intravenously, followed by infusion at twice the maintenance rate.
- The dose is adjusted as needed to maintain urine output of 2 to 3 ml/kg/h.
- Serum electrolytes should be monitored, potassium administered as needed, and volume overload avoided.

Hemodialysis

- Hemodialysis increases lithium clearance.
- It is most effective following a single ingestion, when it can prevent further distribution of lithium into the CNS.
- Hemodialysis for chronic intoxication is controversial, but is recommended for life-threatening toxicity, rising levels despite decontamination, renal insufficiency, pulmonary edema or neurologic effects, and levels that do not fall with aggressive hydration.
- Hemodialysis should be continued until the serum lithium level is less than 0.5 mEq/L.
- Lithium levels rebound after hemodialysis due to redistribution of the agent from peripheral sites.
- Hemodialysis should be repeated if severe symptoms persist (and level is elevated).
- Peritoneal dialysis and hemofiltration increase clearance but are much slower than hemodialysis; they may be useful if hemodialysis is not available.

Diuretics

- Furosemide increases lithium elimination slightly, but is not routinely recommended.
- It also may be used in patients who are volume overloaded due to hydration therapy.
- The dose is 10 to 40 mg intravenously for patients not under chronic treatment with furosemide.

Seizures

Seizures are treated in the standard manner, starting with benzodiazepine administration (see SECTION II, Seizures chapter, for further details).

Sodium Polystyrene Sulfonate

- Sodium polystyrene sulfonate increases lithium clearance in animal models and human volunteers, but has not been shown to affect outcome after overdose.
- Its use is not routinely recommended.

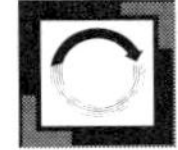

Follow-Up

PATIENT MONITORING

- ECG, hemodynamics, and electrolytes should be monitored serially in symptomatic patients.
- Serial lithium levels are used to help guide therapy.

EXPECTED COURSE AND PROGNOSIS

- Patients with acute ingestion generally recover over 1 to 2 days.
- Patients with chronic intoxication require days to months to recover, and permanent neurologic sequelae may develop (ataxia, cerebellar atrophy, basal ganglia degeneration, parkinsonism, and altered mental status).

DISCHARGE CRITERIA/INSTRUCTIONS

- From the emergency department. Asymptomatic patients who have ingested an immediate-release product may be discharged following gastrointestinal decontamination, 6 hours of observation, documentation of falling lithium level, and psychiatric evaluation, if needed.
- From the hospital. Patients may be discharged when serum lithium levels are falling, neurologic and renal effects are improving, and psychiatric clearance has been obtained, if needed.

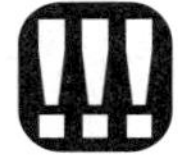

Pitfalls

DIAGNOSIS

- A serum level at the upper end of the therapeutic range may produce chronic intoxication.
- Peak levels may be delayed more than 8 hours after ingestion of a sustained-release preparation.

TREATMENT

- Lithium therapy should not be resumed until all neurologic effects have resolved, even if serum levels are below the limits of detection.
- Substitution of another agent should be considered, particularly in the elderly or those with repeated chronic intoxication.

FOLLOW-UP

- Neurologic effects may require weeks or months to resolve.
- Some patients sustain permanent cerebellar or basal ganglia injury.

ICD-9-CM 969

Poisoning by psychotropic agents.

See also: SECTION II, Seizures chapter; and SECTION III, Whole-Bowel Irrigation chapter.

RECOMMENDED READING

Henry GC, Osborn H, Weisman R. Lithium. In: *Goldfrank's toxicologic emergencies,* 6th ed. Norwalk, CT: Appleton & Lange, 1998.

Author: Edwin K. Kuffner

Reviewer: Katherine M. Hurlbut

Local Anesthetics

Basics

DESCRIPTION

Local anesthetics are used for minor surgical procedures, regional anesthesia, spinal anesthesia, and treatment of cardiac dysrhythmias.

FORMS AND USES

- Local anesthetics are available in a wide variety of formulations, including chloroprocaine (Nesacaine), procaine (Anuject, Novacaine), proparacaine, propoxycaine (Rovocaine), tetracaine (Pontocaine, Niphaoid, Ak-taine, Kainaii, Occucaine, Opthaine, Opthetic, Fluorocaine, Ocufluorocaine), bupivacaine (Marcaine, Sensorcaine), etidocaine (Duranest), lidocaine (Xylocaine), mepivacaine (Carbocaine), prilocaine (Citanest), pramoxine (Tronolane, Fleet Relief, Proctofoam, Prax, Tronothane, Itch-X, Pramagel), and dyclonine (Dyclone, Tanaco, Sucrets).
- Dosage varies with each specific agent.
- Agents used for infiltrative anesthesia may be mixed with epinephrine to prolong action and provide local hemostasis.
- Agents used only as topical agents include benzocaine (Unguentine, Foille, Aerocaine, Aerotherm, Americaine, Burntame, Dermoplast, Lanacaine, Solarcaine, Benzocol, Ivarest, Rhulicream, Bicozeze, Chiggarex, Anacaine, Chiggertox, Campophenique), butanilicaine, carticaine, and dibucaine (Nupercainal).

TOXIC DOSE

Lidocaine

- Ingestion of more than 5 mg/kg (e.g., 3.0 ml of 2% solution in a 15-kg child) may result in seizure.
- Skin infiltration greater than approximately 4.0 mg/kg should be avoided (amount may be increased to 7.0 mg/kg if epinephrine-containing solution is used).

PATHOPHYSIOLOGY

- Local anesthetic agents interrupt electrical impulse transmission by blocking sodium channels in nerves.
- Systemic absorption of local anesthetics may lead to suppression of inhibitory centers in the brain, resulting in agitation, anxiety, and seizures.
- Blockade of the cardiac sodium channels may cause progressive heart block and asystole; however, cardiac effects only occur when levels are above those that produce neurologic effects (although bupivacaine reportedly produces cardiovascular collapse without warning signs of CNS toxicity).
- Methemoglobinemia has been reported frequently as a side effect of benzocaine use and occasionally with prilocaine, tetracaine, or lidocaine.
- Systemic effects of coadministered epinephrine may cause agitation or anxiety and mimic toxicity.
- Allergic reactions may occur, but most are due to paraben added to multidose vials as a preservative; when true allergic reaction occurs, agents in another class (e.g., amide instead of ester) may be used.

EPIDEMIOLOGY

- Poisoning from local anesthetics is uncommon and often iatrogenic.
- Toxic effects are usually mild to moderate and self-limited.
- Neonates and infants are at increased risk for methemoglobinemia.

CAUSES

- Most poisonings result from inadvertent injection of a therapeutic dose into a blood vessel, repeated use of therapeutic dose, or unintentional administration of a toxic dose.
- Child neglect or abuse should be considered if the patient is less than 1 year of age, suicide attempt if the patient is over 6 years of age.

RISK FACTORS

Advanced age and liver disease increase the likelihood of toxicity.

DRUG AND DISEASE INTERACTIONS

- Use of lidocaine with other class Ib antidysrhythmic agents (phenytoin, tocainide) may produce additive cardiac depression.
- Lidocaine and β-blockers produce additive cardiac effects.

PREGNANCY AND LACTATION

- Lidocaine. US FDA Pregnancy Category B. Animal studies indicate no fetal risk, and there are no controlled human studies, or animal studies show an adverse fetal effect, but well-controlled studies in pregnant women do not.
- Bupivacaine. US FDA Pregnancy Category C. The drug exerts animal teratogenic or embryocidal effects, but there are no controlled studies in women, or no studies are available in either animals or women.
- Toxicity may develop in mother or fetus following paracervical or pudendal block.

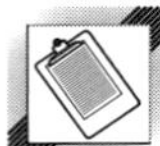

Diagnosis

DIFFERENTIAL DIAGNOSIS

- Other toxicologic agents that cause agitation and seizure include sympathomimetic drugs (cocaine, ephedrine, etc.), type 1 antiarrhythmics, theophylline, and a variety of stimulants, among others.
- Nontoxicologic causes of agitation and seizure include allergic reactions, hypoxia from any cause, and withdrawal from alcohol or sedative-hypnotics.

SIGNS AND SYMPTOMS

- Severe overdose may involve abrupt onset of CNS depression and seizure, sometimes accompanied by dysrhythmia and hypotension.
- Methemoglobinemia has been reported frequently with high doses of benzocaine and occasionally with tetracaine and lidocaine.

Vital Signs

Tachycardia and hypertension are initial signs of toxicity but may be quickly followed by bradycardia and hypotension in severe overdose.

HEENT

- Vision loss has been reported after intranasal local anesthesia.
- Tinnitus may occur with toxic doses.

Cardiovascular

- Mild intoxication may cause tachycardia and hypertension.
- Overdose may cause bradycardia, ventricular dysrhythmia, and hypotension.

Pulmonary

Respiratory depression occurs with severe overdose.

Gastrointestinal

Nausea and vomiting are common.

Hematologic

Methemoglobinemia may occur.

Fluids and Electrolytes

Hyponatremia has been reported after ingestion.

Neurologic

- Agitation, anxiety, seizures, and, ultimately, coma may develop.
- Parasthesias may occur.
- Abrupt onset of numbness and seizures occur in severe overdose.

PROCEDURES AND LABORATORY TESTS

Essential Tests

ECG and cardiac monitoring are performed to detect dysrhythmia.

Recommended Tests

- Serum electrolytes, BUN, and creatinine should be obtained to assess the cause of cardiac dysrhythmia.
- Methemoglobin level should be obtained in symptomatic patients with cyanosis; serial levels may be needed if methemoglobinemia is present.

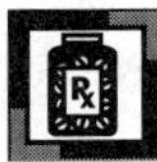

Treatment

- Treatment should focus on airway management, blood pressure support, treatment of seizures, and dysrhythmias.
- Dose and time of exposure should be determined for all substances involved.

DIRECTING PATIENT COURSE

The health-care professional should call the poison control center when:

- Hypotension or other severe effects occur.
- Signs and symptoms are not consistent with local anesthetic poisoning.
- Coingestant, drug interaction, or underlying disease presents an unusual problem.

The patient should be referred to a health-care facility when:

- Attempted suicide or homicide is possible.
- The patient or caregiver seems unreliable.
- Any toxic effects develop.
- Coingestant, drug interaction, or underlying disease presents an unusual problem.

Admission Considerations

Inpatient management is warranted for patients who develop altered mental status, seizure, or dysrhythmia.

DECONTAMINATION

Out of Hospital

Ipecac-induced emesis is not recommended because of the potential for seizures.

In Hospital

- Decontamination is not needed for parenteral exposure.
- Gastric aspiration with a nasogastric tube should be performed in patients with large ingestion presenting within 1 hour of ingestion or if serious effects are present.
- One dose of activated charcoal (1–2 g/kg) should be administered without a cathartic if a substantial ingestion has occurred within the previous few hours.

ANTIDOTES

There is no specific antidote for local anesthetic poisoning.

ADJUNCTIVE TREATMENT

- Cardiopulmonary bypass has been used successfully to treat massive lidocaine exposure with refractory dysrhythmia, allowing hepatic metabolism of lidocaine despite hypotension.
- Symptomatic methemoglobinemia is treated with methylene blue (see SECTION III, Methylene Blue chapter).
- Dialysis has been used to increase clearance of lidocaine.

Seizure

- A patent airway must be ensured.
- A benzodiazepine is administered for initial control. If seizures persist or recur, another anticonvulsant such as phenobarbital may be added.

Dysrhythmias or Conduction Abnormalities

- Seizures must be controlled and acidemia corrected.
- Treatment for stable patients begins with drug therapy; unstable patients receive defibrillation followed by pharmacologic therapy.
- Sodium bicarbonate should be administered in a 1 to 2 mEq/kg intravenous bolus and repeated as needed to maintain a narrow QRS interval.

—Arterial pH should not exceed 7.55.
—Simultaneous hyperventilation and bicarbonate therapy must be undertaken cautiously because it may cause severe alkalemia.
—Seizure control should continue during sodium bicarbonate therapy.

- Cardiac bypass may be used to maintain perfusion and allow continued lidocaine metabolism in patients with refractory dysrhythmia or hypotension.
- Bretylium should be avoided because its alpha-blocking effects may worsen hypotension.
- Other class I antiarrhythmic agents should be avoided because they may worsen dysrhythmias.

Hypotension

- Primary treatment for hypotension in local anesthetic poisoning is correction of dysrhythmia.
- In addition, 10 to 20 ml/kg 0.9% saline may be administered followed by a vasopressor, if needed. Dopamine is preferred, and norepinephrine may be added for refractory hypotension.

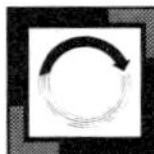

Follow-Up

PATIENT MONITORING

Cardiac and respiratory monitoring should be performed continuously.

EXPECTED COURSE AND PROGNOSIS

- Toxic effects develop rapidly within minutes of iatrogenic parenteral overdose.
- Recovery generally occurs within minutes to hours, except in massive overdose, unless sequelae of hypoxia and hypotension intercede.

DISCHARGE CRITERIA/INSTRUCTIONS

- From emergency department. Asymptomatic patients without CNS or cardiac affects for 4 to 6 hours may be discharged after gastrointestinal decontamination and psychiatric evaluation, if needed.
- From the hospital. Patients may be discharged after mental status and cardiac conduction return to normal, and gastrointestinal decontamination and psychiatric evaluation, if needed.

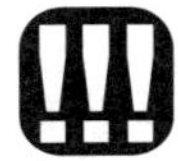

Pitfalls

DIAGNOSIS

- Cardiac toxicity may develop suddenly with bupivacaine, whereas it is heralded by neurotoxicity with lidocaine.
- It is important to consider local anesthetic toxicity in patients who develop neurologic symptoms during minor procedures.

TREATMENT

It is important to manage the airway adequately to avoid hypoxia and aspiration.

FOLLOW-UP

To avoid toxic exposure, maximal recommended doses of local anesthetics should be determined prior to administration.

ICD-9-CM 968.3

Intravenous anesthetics.

See also: SECTION II, Hypotension, Methemoglobinemia, and Seizure chapters; and SECTION IV, Benzocaine chapter.

RECOMMENDED READING

Cardiotoxicity of local anesthetic drugs. *Lancet* 1986;2:1192–1194.

Noble J, Kennedy J, Latimer RD, et al. Massive lignocaine overdose during cardiopulmonary bypass. *Br J Anaesth* 1984;56:1439–1441.

Norris RL. Local anesthetics. *Emerg Med Clin North Am* 1992;10:707–717.

Author: Kennon Heard

Reviewer: Luke Yip

Loperamide

Basics

DESCRIPTION

Loperamide (Imodium, Imodium A-D) is an oral antidiarrheal drug chemically related to haloperidol.

PATHOPHYSIOLOGY

- Loperamide directly inhibits peristalsis and intestinal secretion.
- Children may be more susceptible than adults.

EPIDEMIOLOGY

Poisoning is uncommon.

CAUSES

- In children, poisoning usually results from unintentional ingestion.
- Child neglect should be considered if the patient is under 1 year of age; suicide attempt if over 6 years of age.

PREGNANCY

US FDA Pregnancy Category B. Animal studies indicate no fetal risk and there are no controlled human studies, or animal studies show an adverse fetal effect, but well-controlled studies in women do not.

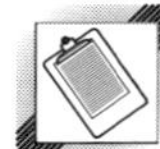

Diagnosis

DIFFERENTIAL DIAGNOSIS

Toxicologic causes of miosis and respiratory depression include numerous types of opioids as well as olanzapine.

SIGNS AND SYMPTOMS

HEENT

Miosis and rarely, dystonic reactions.

Respiratory

- Large overdose may lead to bradycardia, respiratory depression, and apnea.
- Pulmonary edema may develop.
- Onset may be delayed for several hours.

Gastrointestinal

- Decreased motility is common.
- Paralytic ileus and necrotizing enterocolitis have been reported.

Metabolic

Hyperglycemia may occur.

Neurologic

Drowsiness and coma may occur after a large overdose.

PROCEDURES AND LABORATORY TESTS

Essential Tests

No tests may be needed in asymptomatic patients.

Recommended Tests

- Arterial blood gases in symptomatic patients to detect hypoxia and hypoventilation.
- Serum electrolytes, glucose, BUN, creatinine to assess other causes of CNS depression.
- ECG, serum acetaminophen and aspirin levels in overdose setting to detect occult ingestion.

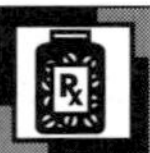

Treatment

- Treatment should focus on control of airway and administration of naloxone.
- Dose and time of exposure should be determined for all substances involved.

DIRECTING PATIENT COURSE

The health-care provider should call a poison control center when:

- Signs and symptoms are not consistent with loperamide poisoning.
- Coingestant, drug interaction, or underlying disease presents an unusual problem.

The patient should be referred to a health-care facility when:

- Attempted suicide or homicide is possible.
- Any toxic effects develop.
- Coingestant, drug interaction, or underlying disease presents an unusual problem.

Admission Considerations

Significant overdose, manifested by apnea with acidosis or pulmonary edema, should be managed in an ICU setting.

DECONTAMINATION

- Emesis should be avoided after large ingestions because of the possibility of rapid obtundation and aspiration.
- Gastric lavage and activated charcoal plus cathartic are indicated up to 4 to 6 hours after ingestion because of slowed gastrointestinal motility.
- Airway protection, including intubation, may be necessary during lavage if respiratory depression does not respond to naloxone.

ANTIDOTES

Naloxone

- Indication. Respiratory depression from known opioid overdose.
- Contraindication. Documented naloxone allergy.
- Method of administration

—The initial dose is 2.0 mg by intravenous push.
—If there is no response, the dose should be repeated in 2.0 mg increments to a total of 10 mg.
—Patients with recurrent effects may be treated with a naloxone infusion.

ADJUNCTIVE TREATMENT

- Noncardiogenic pulmonary edema is treated with naloxone, oxygen (increased fraction inspired oxygen FiO_2, and positive end-expiratory pressure or continuous positive airway pressure, as necessary) and respiratory support.
- Administration of intravenous fluids should be minimized.

DYSTONIC REACTIONS

These should be treated for 2 to 3 days postreaction with diphenhydramine or benztropine (adult, 1 to 2 mg twice a day).

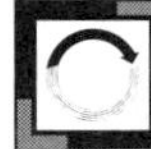

Follow-Up

PATIENT MONITORING

Respiratory and cardiac function should be monitored continuously.

DISCHARGE CRITERIA/INSTRUCTIONS

- From the emergency department. Asymptomatic patient may be discharged after 4 to 6 hour observation period, decontamination and psychiatric evaluation, if needed.
- From the hospital. Patient may be discharged when respiratory and CNS effects have resolved (with patient off naloxone therapy).

EXPECTED COURSE AND PROGNOSIS

Peak effects usually develop within hours and resolve within 24 hours.

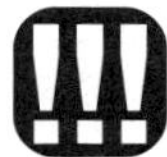

Pitfalls

TREATMENT

Antidiarrheal effect may not be reversed by naloxone.

ICD-9-CM 973.5

Poisoning by agents primarily affecting the gastrointestinal system: antidiarrheal drugs.

See also: SECTION III, Naloxone and Nalmephene chapter.

RECOMMENDED READING

Gilman AG, Rall TW, Nies AS, et al., eds. *Goodman and Gilman's the pharmacological basis of therapeutics,* 8th ed. New York: Pergamon, 1990.

Author: Steven A. Seifert

Reviewer: Richard C. Dart

LSD and Other Psychedelic Compounds

Basics

DESCRIPTION

- Lysergic acid diethylamide (LSD) is colorless, odorless, and tasteless.
- Other hallucinogens with similar structure and toxic effects are kava-kava, mate, mescaline, morning glory, nutmeg, periwinkle, peyote, psilocin, psilocybin, and yohimbine.

FORMS AND USES

The psychedelic dose for LSD is 100 to 750 μg, for mescaline is 5 mg/kg, and for nutmeg about 5 to 10 g (1 tablespoon).

TOXIC DOSE

The lethal dose is unknown, but death has occurred rarely from hallucinogen overdose.

PATHOPHYSIOLOGY

- The psychedelic effect of hallucinogens is thought to be caused by agonistic actions at presynaptic serotonin receptors in the midbrain.
- One hypothesis suggests that they prevent the inhibitory effects of serotonin, allowing increased neuronal activity and causing distortions of perception and thought.

EPIDEMIOLOGY

- Poisoning is common, and use of hallucinogens has increased in recent years.
- Death from hallucinogen abuse is rare and usually due to trauma or complications of hyperthermia, hypertension, or rhabdomyolysis.

CAUSES

- Poisoning usually results from intentional abuse.
- Child neglect or abuse should be considered in children under 1 year of age.

DRUG AND DISEASE INTERACTIONS

- A combination of lithium, fluoxetine, and LSD or a combination of fluoxetine and LSD has resulted in seizures.
- Hallucinogens are usually serotonergic compounds and may precipitate serotonin syndrome, especially if the patient is under treatment with another serotonergic compound such as a selective serotonin reuptake inhibitor (SSRI).

PREGNANCY AND LACTATION

- LSD and nutmeg. US FDA Pregnancy Category C. The drug exerts animal teratogenic or embryocidal effects, but there are no controlled studies in women, or no studies are available in either animals or women.
- Prolonged seizures can compromise the fetus via hypoxia and trauma.
- Mescaline has produced teratogenic effects in animals.

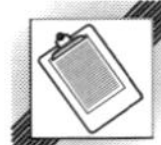

Diagnosis

DIFFERENTIAL DIAGNOSIS

- Toxic causes of hallucinations include amphetamines, anticholinergics, high-dose corticosteroid, phencyclidine, peyote, psilocybin, mescaline, and several others.
- Nontoxic causes include CNS trauma, meningitis, AIDS-related illness, hypoglycemia, electrolyte imbalance, heat-related illness, hypoxia, alcohol withdrawal, or sedative-hypnotic withdrawal.

SIGNS AND SYMPTOMS

- Diagnosis is clinical, based primarily on a medical history and the exclusion of other causes in the hallucinating patient.
- Soon after ingestion, diaphoresis, mydriasis, dizziness, twitching, flushing, hyperreflexia, and hypertension develop.
- Psychosis can occur within 15 to 20 minutes; auditory and visual hallucinations can occur after 30 minutes; behavioral changes, emotional lability, euphoria or dysphoria, paranoia, and depersonalization can occur after several hours.

Vital Signs

Hypertension, hypotension, hyperthermia, tachycardia, and tachypnea may develop with any of these agents.

HEENT

- Mydriasis and blurred vision are common with all agents.
- Repeated visual illusions are common.

Dermatologic

Diaphoresis is common, and piloerection may occur.

Cardiovascular

Hypertension and tachycardia may occur.

Pulmonary

Bronchospasm develops rarely.

Gastrointestinal

Vomiting, diarrhea, salivation, and anorexia may develop.

Renal

Renal failure may develop rarely, due to rhabdomyolysis.

Fluids and Electrolytes

Metabolic acidosis may develop rarely, secondary to seizures.

Musculoskeletal

Rhabdomyolysis may develop rarely, secondary to seizures.

Neurologic

- Restlessness, incoordination, tremors, and ataxia may develop.
- Behavioral changes characterized by mild apprehension to panic and depersonalization may develop 2 to 12 hours after ingestion.
- Seizures, coma, and weakness are rare, but have been reported.

Reproductive

LSD causes uterine contractions.

PROCEDURES AND LABORATORY TESTS

Essential Tests

No tests are usually needed in asymptomatic or minimally symptomatic patients.

Recommended Tests

- Serum electrolytes, BUN, and creatinine levels are used to assess other causes of altered mental status, seizures, or cardiac effects.
- Urinalysis. Rhabdomyolysis or hypotension may produce renal injury.
- Arterial blood gases. Metabolic acidosis may develop with prolonged seizures.
- A urine drug screen is used in patients with hallucinations of unknown cause to determine other ingestant or causes of seizures and cardiac effects.
- Head CT, lumbar puncture, blood, and CSF cultures are ordered as needed to evaluate infection or cranial bleed as a cause of altered mental status.

Not Recommended Tests

Serum levels of hallucinogens are not clinically useful.

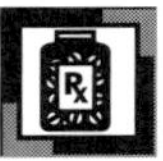

Treatment

- Treatment focuses on managing the airway and controlling activity associated with hallucinations, psychosis, or panic reaction.
- The dose and time of exposure must be determined for all substances involved.

DIRECTING PATIENT COURSE

The health-care provider should call the poison control center when:

- Seizures, coma, hyperthermia, hypotension, acidemia, or other severe effects are present.
- Toxic effects are not consistent with hallucinogen poisoning.
- Coingestant, drug interaction, or underlying disease presents an unusual problem.

The patient should be referred to a health-care facility when:

- Attempted suicide or homicide is possible.
- Patient or caregiver seems unreliable.
- Undesired effects develop.
- Coingestant, drug interaction, or underlying disease presents an unusual challenge.

Admission Considerations

Inpatient management is warranted for patients with persistent alteration in mental status or end-organ complications such as rhabdomyolysis or renal failure.

DECONTAMINATION

- Gastrointestinal decontamination is not usually recommended because a very small amount of LSD is needed to produce hallucination and it is rapidly absorbed.
- If another hallucinogen was ingested or coingestants are possible, one dose of activated charcoal (1–2 g/kg) without cathartic should be administered.

ANTIDOTES

There is no specific antidote available for hallucinogens.

ADJUNCTIVE TREATMENT

Hallucinogen-induced Agitation or Psychosis

- The patient is placed in a dimly lit room, offered counseling and companionship, and "talked down."
- A benzodiazepine familiar to the provider should be administered.

—Diazepam. Adult dose is 5 to 10 mg intravenously; pediatric dose is 0.2 to 0.5 mg/kg intravenously; doses are repeated at 10-minute intervals and titrated to effect.
—Lorazepam is an alternative. Adult dose is 1 to 2 mg intravenously; pediatric dose is 0.05 mg/kg; doses are repeated at 10-minute intervals and titrated to effect.
—The airway is monitored closely.
—A neuroleptic agent such as droperidol should be used only in refractory cases because neuroleptics may induce seizure by lowering seizure threshold.

Seizure

A patent airway is ensured and a benzodiazepine is administered for initial control in the same method described above for agitation. If seizures persist, phenytoin or phenobarbital may be added.

Hyperthermia

- Clothing should be removed, and intravenous infusion of isotonic crystalloid started; agitation must be controlled.
- Fluid losses may be severe and should be replenished until a urine output of 1 to 2 ml/kg/h is reached; the fluid infusion needs to be monitored carefully to avoid overload.
- Cooling fans and wet sheets are effective, especially in a dry climate.
- Application of ice may be more effective in humid climates.
- The core temperature should be monitored frequently, and cooling should be discontinued when body temperature decreases to 39°C.

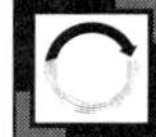

Follow-Up

EXPECTED COURSE AND PROGNOSIS

- Effects usually peak within several hours and then abate over 24 hours or more.
- Patients with repeated seizures or hyperthermia are more likely to die or sustain permanent neurologic injury.
- Possible complications include renal failure and CNS injury due to prolonged seizures.
- Flashbacks are generally uncommon, but they may occur in chronic, frequent LSD abusers.

DISCHARGE CRITERIA/INSTRUCTIONS

- From the emergency department

—Asymptomatic patients may be discharged after 6 hours of observation.
—The patient must be cautioned that the continued use of drugs may precipitate flashbacks and should be avoided.
—The patient should be referred for substance abuse treatment.

- From the hospital

—Patients may be discharged to a responsible friend or family member, after complications have resolved and vital signs have returned to normal.
—The patient should be referred for substance abuse treatment.

PATIENT EDUCATION

Patients should be cautioned that drug use may precipitate flashbacks and should be avoided.

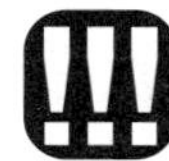

Pitfalls

DIAGNOSIS

- Before attributing hallucinations to LSD, other causes must be excluded.
- Standard urine drug screening may not detect LSD.

TREATMENT

- Large amounts of benzodiazepines may be needed to control agitation.
- Prompt seizure control is mandatory; general anesthesia or neuromuscular paralysis and EEG monitoring may be required.

ICD-9-CM 969.6

Poisoning by psychotropic agents: psychodysleptics (hallucinogens).

See also: SECTION II, Hyperthermia and Seizures chapters.

RECOMMENDED READING

Aaron CK, Ferm RP. Lysergic acid diethylamide and other psychedelics. In: Goldfrank LR, Flomenbaum NE, Lewin NA, et al., eds. *Goldfrank's toxicologic emergencies,* 6th ed. Norwalk, CT: Appleton & Lange, 1998.

Lewin NA, Howland MA, Goldfrank LR. Herbal preparations. In: Goldfrank LR, Flomenbaum NE, Lewin NA, et al.; eds. *Goldfrank's toxicologic emergencies,* 6th ed. Norwalk, CT: Appleton & Lange, 1998.

Author: Robin Millin

Reviewer: Luke Yip

Manganese

Basics

DESCRIPTION

Manganese is an essential element used in a variety of occupational settings.

FORMS AND USES

- Manganese is used in foundry work and electroplating, as well as in the manufacture of batteries, permanganate, fertilizers, ceramics, and matches.
- Methylcyclopentadienyl manganese tricarbonyl (MMT) was used as a gasoline anti-knock agent, but this use has been curtailed because of MMT's interference with catalytic converters in exhaust.
- Potassium permanganate is a strongly corrosive oxidant.

TOXIC DOSE

- Acute ingestion of inorganic manganese salts does not produce toxicity.
- Chronic inhalation leads to toxic effects, but with variable individual susceptibility.

PATHOPHYSIOLOGY

Neurologic toxicity of manganese is related to CNS dopamine depletion and formation of toxic compounds (dopamine quinone, hydrogen peroxide).

EPIDEMIOLOGY

- Poisoning is rare.
- Toxic effects are mild after acute ingestion.

CAUSES

Toxicity most often results from chronic occupational exposure to dust.

WORKPLACE STANDARDS

- ACGIH. TLV TWA 0.2 mg/m^3.
- OSHA. PEL TWA is 5 mg/m^3; evidence suggests, however, that chronic exposure at this level may result in pulmonary and neurologic symptoms.
- NIOSH. REL TWA is 1 mg/m^3 of manganese; STEL is 3 mg/m^3; IDLH is 500 mg/m^3.

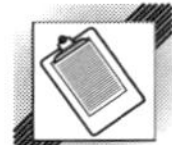

Diagnosis

SIGNS AND SYMPTOMS

- Potassium permanganate ingestion often causes hemorrhagic gastritis, abdominal pain, and vomiting.
- Metal fume fever is a flulike syndrome that may occur 4 to 8 hours following inhalation of fumes from welding or melting manganese-containing compounds (see SECTION II, Metal Fume Fever).

Manganese Dioxide Dust

- Acute exposure may cause dermatitis, conjunctivitis, and sinusitis.
- Pneumonitis and bronchitis may occur after inhalation with dyspnea and cough.
- Abdominal pain, hepatic dysfunction, and pancreatitis also may occur with ingestion or dialysate contamination.
- Pulmonary symptoms resemble asthma or chronic obstructive pulmonary disease, and changes on lung ventilation tests may develop.

Manganese Madness

A syndrome that follows chronic high-level exposure to manganese dioxide. It includes

- emotional lability and psychosis with bizarre or compulsive behavior
- visual hallucinations and confusion
- lumbosacral pain
- urinary urgency and incontinence
- dysarthria, nystagmus
- increased sweating, salivation
- changes in gait

A Parkinson's-like Neurologic Disease

May occur following chronic exposure. It involves the insidious development of apathy, fatigue, changes in sleep, decreased libido, headache, paresthesia, muscle cramps, and leg weakness.

PROCEDURES AND LABORATORY TESTS

Essential Tests

No tests are usually needed after acute exposure.

Recommended Tests

- MRI sometimes reveals lesions in the globus pallidum and striatum following chronic exposure.
- Pulmonary function testing should be performed in patients with respiratory symptoms.
- Chest radiographs are used to assess other causes of pulmonary symptoms.
- For potassium permanganate ingestion, tests should be ordered as for caustic base ingestion.
- Following chronic, high-level exposure with personality changes, complete evaluation for altered mental status should be performed.

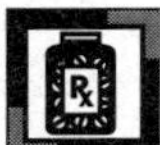

Treatment

- Treatment is largely supportive, with emphasis on removal of the patient from exposure.
- Further care depends on the severity of exposure and development of systemic effects.

DIRECTING PATIENT COURSE

The health-care professional should call the poison control center when:

- Severe or persistent effects develop.
- Underlying disease presents an unusual problem.

The patient should be referred to a health-care facility when:

- Toxic effects develop.
- Underlying disease presents an unusual problem.

Admission Considerations

- Inpatient therapy may be needed if patients cannot care for themselves.
- Following potassium permanganate ingestion, any symptomatic patient should be admitted.

DECONTAMINATION

- Immediate irrigation is recommended following ocular or dermal exposure.
- Following inhalation, the patient should be moved to fresh air, and oxygen should be administered.
- Ingestion may be diluted with a small amount (4 oz) of milk or water.
- Gastric lavage and activated charcoal are not recommended because of caustic properties.

ANTIDOTES

There is no antidote for manganese poisoning.

ADJUNCTIVE TREATMENT

- Therapy with chelating agents has been proposed, but there is little evidence to support their use.
- Amelioration of symptoms from chronic exposure has been reported with the use of intravenous p-aminosalicylic acid; spontaneous improvement without treatment, however, is typical.
- L-dopa and trihexyphenidyl may relieve symptoms such as tremor and bradykinesia.

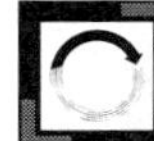

Follow-Up

EXPECTED COURSE AND PROGNOSIS

- The symptoms of manganese dioxide dust exposure usually resolve, but severe exposures may be fatal.
- Psychosis associated with manganese madness typically resolves following removal from exposure.
- Symptoms of metal fume fever typically resolve spontaneously within 1 to 2 days.

DISCHARGE CRITERIA/INSTRUCTIONS

- Patients with acute exposures can usually be discharged after appropriate decontamination.
- Patients with chronic exposure can be discharged with appropriate follow-up arranged, providing they can care for themselves.

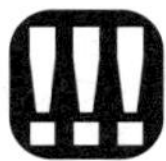

Pitfalls

TREATMENT

Potassium permanganate is treated as a caustic ingestion rather than manganese ingestion.

ICD-9-CM 985.2

Toxic effect of other metals: manganese and its compounds.

See also: SECTION III, Metal Fume Fever chapter; and SECTION IV, Caustics-Basic.

RECOMMENDED READING

Brown DSO, Wills CE, Yousefi V, et al. Neurotoxic effects of chronic exposure to manganese dust. *Neuropsychol Behav Neurol* 1991;4:238–250.

Author: Lada Kokan

Reviewer: Richard C. Dart

Maprotiline

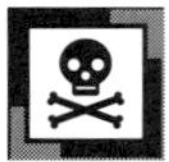

Basics

DESCRIPTION

Maprotiline is a pharmaceutical preparation, known as Ludiomil.

FORMS AND USES

For depression, adults are treated with 75 mg/day initially, increasing to 150 to 225 mg/day over several weeks; children should take 10 mg/day initially, increasing to 75 mg/day over several weeks.

PATHOPHYSIOLOGY

- Maprotiline is similar to tricyclic antidepressants in that it increases the synaptic concentration of serotonin and norepinephrine by decreasing their presynaptic reuptake.
- Maprotiline also causes a peripheral α-receptor blockade and has direct membrane stabilization effects.

EPIDEMIOLOGY

- Poisoning is uncommon.
- Toxic effects following exposure are typically mild to moderate.
- Death occurs rarely, primarily after massive ingestion.

CAUSES

- Poisoning is usually a suicidal gesture or a therapeutic misadventure.
- Child neglect should be considered if the patient is under 1 year of age; attempted suicide should be considered if the patient is over 6 years of age.

RISK FACTORS

Drug interactions include the following:

- The combination of maprotiline with a monoamine oxidase inhibitor may produce effects similar to serotonin syndrome.
- Addition of cimetidine can increase the maprotiline level.
- Maprotiline will potentiate the effects of sympathomimetic drugs and warfarin.

PREGNANCY AND LACTATION

- US FDA Pregnancy Category B. Animal studies do not indicate fetal risk, and there are no controlled human studies, or animal studies show an adverse fetal effect, but well-controlled studies in pregnant women have failed to demonstrate a fetal risk.
- Maprotiline is excreted in breast milk, but adverse effects have not been reported.

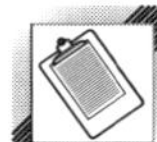

Diagnosis

DIFFERENTIAL DIAGNOSIS

Any compound that depresses mental status may initially appear to be maprotiline, especially if seizures occur.

SIGNS AND SYMPTOMS

Maprotiline toxicity is characterized by depression of mental status, seizures, and potential for abnormal cardiac conduction.

Vital Signs

- Tachycardia is common.
- Mild hypertension may occur, followed by hypotension if serious cardiac effects develop.
- Hypothermia occurs rarely.
- Hyperthermia may occur.

HEENT

- Blurred vision and tinnitus may occur.
- Maprotiline may cause dental erosions and increased intraocular pressure.

Dermatologic

Sweating may be present.

Cardiovascular

- Palpitations and hypertension may occur initially.
- QTc prolongation, QRS widening, and atrioventricular block may occur rarely.
- Hypotension may accompany serious cardiac effects.

Gastrointestinal

Nausea and vomiting, dry mouth, decreased bowel sounds, and constipation sometimes occur.

Renal

Urinary retention may occur.

Fluids and Electrolytes

Syndrome of inappropriate antidiuretic hormone secretion may develop.

Musculoskeletal

Tremor, myoclonus, and rhabdomyolysis may occur if prolonged seizures develop.

Neurologic

Headache, hallucinations, and agitation may progress to confusion and mental status depression.

PROCEDURES AND LABORATORY TESTS

Essential Tests

- Serum electrolytes, BUN, and creatinine levels to evaluate altered mental status or ECG abnormalities.
- ECG to detect prolonged conduction (QRS, QTc) and atrioventricular block.

Recommended Tests

- Pulse oximetry to evaluate altered mental status.
- Complete blood count to evaluate bone marrow suppression.
- Serum acetaminophen and aspirin levels in overdose setting to detect occult overdose.

Not Recommended Tests

Serum drug levels are not clinically helpful.

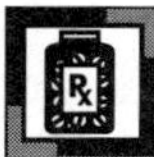

Treatment

- Treatment should focus on cardiac monitoring and treatment of seizures, hypotension, or dysrhythmia.
- The dose and time of exposure should be determined for all substances involved.

DIRECTING PATIENT COURSE

The health-care professional should call a poison center when:

- Cardiac, central nervous system, or other clinically significant effects are present.
- Signs and symptoms are not consistent with maprotiline toxicity.
- Coingestant, drug interaction, or underlying disease presents an unusual problem.

Patients should be referred to a health-care professional when:

- Attempted suicide or homicide is possible.
- The patient or caregiver seems unreliable.
- Symptoms of toxicity are present.
- Coingestant, drug interaction, or underlying disease presents an unusual problem.

Admission Considerations

Inpatient management is warranted when patients have major effects, such as altered mental status, seizure, or cardiac conduction abnormality.

DECONTAMINATION

Out of Hospital

Induction of emesis is not recommended due to the potential for rapid mental status depression.

In Hospital

- Gastric lavage should be performed in pediatric (tube size 24–32 French) or adult (tube size 36–42 French) patients presenting within 1 hour of a large ingestion or if serious effects are present.
- A single dose of activated charcoal (1–2 g/kg) should be administered without a cathartic if a substantial ingestion has occurred within the previous few hours.

ANTIDOTES

There are no specific antidotes for maprotiline poisoning.

ADJUNCTIVE THERAPIES

Hemodialysis and hemoperfusion are not useful.

Dysrhythmia or Conduction Abnormality

- First, seizures should be controlled; if QRS widening or dysrhythmia persists, sodium bicarbonate should be administered (1 to 2 mEq/kg intravenous bolus) and repeated as needed to narrow the QRS and suppress dysrhythmia. Arterial pH should not exceed 7.55.
- Lidocaine is used for ventricular tachycardia or multifocal premature ventricular contractions.

—Adult dose is 50 to 100 mg intravenous bolus followed by an infusion of 2 to 4 mg/min titrated to desired effect.
—Pediatric dose is 1 mg/kg bolus followed by an infusion of 20 to 50 μg/kg/min titrated to effect.
—One-half of the bolus dose may be repeated in 15 minutes, if needed.

- Bretylium. Five mg/kg can be administered over 1 minute; if unsuccessful, 10 mg/kg can be given over 1 minute and repeated as necessary to a total dose of 30 mg/kg.

Seizure

Concurrent with airway management, benzodiazepine should be administered for initial control.

- Diazepam. Adult dose is 5 to 10 mg initially; pediatric dose is 0.2 to 0.5 mg/kg.
- Lorazepam. Adult dose is 2 to 4 mg intravenous push over 2 to 5 minutes; pediatric dose is 0.1 mg/kg intravenous push over 2 to 5 minutes, not to exceed 4 mg/dose.
- Benzodiazepine dose for adults or children can be repeated every 10 minutes if needed.
- The need for intubation should be monitored closely.
- If seizures persist or recur, another anticonvulsant, such as phenobarbital or phenytoin, can be added.

Hypotension

- Patient should be given 10 to 20 ml/kg 0.9% saline and placed in the Trendelenburg position.
- Further fluid therapy should be guided by central venous pressure monitoring or right heart catheterization to avoid volume overload.
- If hypotension is unresponsive to fluid bolus, a vasopressor may be administered.
- Dopamine. Infusion should begin at 2 to 5 μg/kg/min and be titrated upward to desired effect; rates above 20 μg/kg/min are unlikely to provide further benefit.
- Norepinephrine

—Infusion should be administered at 0.1 to 0.2 μg/kg/min and be titrated to desired effect.
—A high rate of infusion of the vasopressor may cause tissue ischemia.

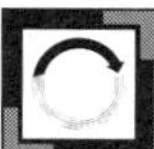

Follow-Up

Asymptomatic patients should receive continuous cardiac monitoring for at least 6 hours. If adverse effects develop, cardiac monitoring should continue until health effects have resolved.

EXPECTED COURSE AND PROGNOSIS

- Most patients demonstrate toxic effects within the first few hours.
- Effects peak within 24 hours and resolve within 24 to 48 hours unless sequelae of seizures or hypotension intercede.

DISCHARGE CRITERIA/INSTRUCTIONS

- From the emergency department. Patients may be discharged after decontamination, resolution of symptoms, normal ECG at 6 hours post-ingestion, and psychiatric assessment.
- From the hospital

—Patients with cardiac or substantial central nervous system effects should be monitored for 24 hours after toxic effects resolve.
—Patients may be discharged after decontamination has been performed, symptoms have resolved, ECG is normal, and psychiatric assessment has been performed.

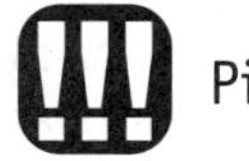

Pitfalls

FOLLOW-UP

Because maprotiline has anticholinergic effects, delayed drug absorption and onset of cardiac effects is possible.

ICD-9-CM 969.0

Poisoning by antidepressants.

See also: SECTION II, Hypotension, Seizures, and Serotonin Syndrome chapters; and SECTION III, Sodium Bicarbonate chapter.

RECOMMENDED READING

Bergman RN, Watson WA. Cardiac toxicity associated with acute maprotiline self-poisoning. *Am J Emerg Med* 1983;2:144–146.

Knudsen K, Heath A. Effects of self poisoning with maprotiline. *BMJ* 1984;288:601–603.

Author: Richard C. Dart

Reviewer: Katherine M. Hurlbut

Marijuana

Basics

DESCRIPTION

Marijuana is the popular name for the dried flowering leaves of *Cannabis sativa, C. indica,* and *C. ruderalis,* the active ingredient of which is Δ9-tetrahydrocannabinol (THC).

FORMS AND USES

- Other names for illicit marijuana are pot, weed, grass, ganja, hashish, bhang, charas, dagga, kif, reefer, mary jane, honey oil, fimble, and gallow grass; marijuana is sometimes named according to its place of origin and color (e.g., Panama red or Acapulco gold).
- Sensemilla marijuana refers to the flowering tops of the female plant, which contain the greatest resin content.
- Hashish has a high content of THC and is obtained by extracting marijuana with a nonpolar solvent.
- Marijuana products may be added to food (e.g., cookies or brownies) or dissolved for intravenous use.
- Pharmaceutical preparations include dronabinol (Marinol) and nabilone (Cesamet).
- Marijuana cigarettes and synthetic cannabinoids may be used as antiemetics for chemotherapy-induced nausea.
- Other proposed indications for using THC include pain, seizures, asthma, glaucoma, and ulcerative colitis.
- Typical adult doses are dronabinol, 2.5 mg orally twice a day, and nabilone, 1 to 2 mg orally twice a day.

TOXIC DOSE

- Acute oral toxicity is extremely low.
- The estimated human toxic dose following ingestion is 30 mg/kg of marijuana; 15 mg/m^2 of THC has produced central nervous system toxicity in cancer patients.

PATHOPHYSIOLOGY

- Marijuana has at least 60 cannabinoid molecules, including the most active compound, THC.
- The concentration of THC in marijuana cigarettes varies from 1% to 8%; hashish may contain 5% to 10% and hash oil up to 50%.
- After smoking marijuana, approximately 20% to 50% of the THC is absorbed, the onset of effects is 6 to 12 minutes, and symptoms may last up to 3 hours.
- After ingestion, only 5% to 20% of THC is bioavailable due to first-pass liver metabolism. The onset of symptoms is 30 to 60 minutes and persists for 4 to 6 hours.
- Comparing marijuana and tobacco smokers, marijuana use was associated with a fivefold increase in carboxyhemoglobin levels and a threefold increase in inhaled tar.
- Carcinogenesis. Marijuana is implicated in increasing risk for mouth, head, neck, and bronchial cancer.

EPIDEMIOLOGY

- Poisoning is common.
- Toxic effects following exposure are typically mild.
- Death is rare and is usually attributable to trauma arising from impaired judgment.

CAUSES

- Use is nearly always intentional.
- Child neglect or abuse should be considered in pediatric intoxication.
- Significant toxicity can be seen with pediatric ingestion or intravenous injection of marijuana extracts.

DRUG INTERACTIONS

- Marijuana may act synergistically with other central nervous system depressants.
- Marijuana may potentiate cocaine-induced tachycardia and a subjective high.

PREGNANCY

- Dronabinol and nabilone. US FDA Pregnancy Category B. Animal studies indicate no fetal risk and there are no controlled human studies, or animal studies show an adverse fetal effect but well-controlled studies in pregnant women do not.
- Marijuana. US FDA Pregnancy Category C. The drug exerts animal teratogenic or embryocidal effects, but there are no controlled studies in women, or no studies are available in either animals or women.
- Incidence of preterm labor and low birth weight in babies is increased by marijuana abuse.

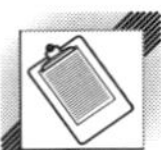

Diagnosis

DIFFERENTIAL DIAGNOSIS

- Toxic causes of altered mental status include anticholinergic toxicity, sedative-hypnotic toxicity, toluene, and ethanol, among others.
- Nontoxic causes include hypoxia and hypoglycemia or electrolyte disorders.

SIGNS AND SYMPTOMS

- Oral or inhalational abuse produces primarily desirable CNS effects (a "high").
- Intravenous infusion of dissolved marijuana extract can cause severe multiorgan toxicity, including gastroenteritis, hepatitis, acute renal failure, anemia, thrombocytopenia, and leukocytosis.

Vital Signs

Hypothermia or hyperthermia, tachycardia or bradycardia, hypotension or hypertension, and bradypnea have been observed.

HEENT

Conjunctival injection, decreased intraocular pressure, mydriasis, nystagmus, photophobia, uvula edema, and dry mouth can occur.

Pulmonary

Bradypnea, irritation, coughing, and bronchodilation may occur.

Cardiovascular

Hypertension or hypotension, tachycardia or bradycardia, and a sensation of tightness in the chest may occur.

Gastrointestinal

Increased appetite, reduced gut motility, and constipation may occur.

Renal

Urinary retention may occur.

Musculoskeletal

Skeletal muscle jerking and weakness may occur.

Neurologic

- Antimotivational syndrome may occur in chronic users.
- Seizures may occur in patients with a history of seizure disorder.
- Mild intoxication involves euphoria, somnolence, heightened awareness, relaxation, altered time perception, and increased appetite also may occur.
- Moderate intoxication involves short-term memory loss, poor concentration and attention, inability to perform multi-step tasks, mood alterations including laughing episodes and de-

pression, altered thought patterns, and disorientation may occur.
- Extreme intoxication involves decreased strength and coordination, lethargy, ataxia, slurred speech, anxiety and fears of death, muscle jerking, respiratory depression, and coma have been observed.

Reproductive

Decreased sperm generation and motility, increased abnormal sperm, and decreased ovulation may occur.

Endocrine

Gynecomastia, as well as decreased levels of testosterone, luteinizing hormone, growth hormone, and follicle-stimulating hormone may be observed.

PROCEDURES AND LABORATORY TESTS

Essential Tests

No tests are needed in minimally symptomatic patients.

Recommended Tests

- Serum electrolytes, BUN, creatinine, and glucose may be needed to evaluate other causes of seizures or altered mental status.
- Liver function, coagulation studies, and serum creatine kinase may be elevated in patients with hyperthermia or agitation.
- ECG, serum acetaminophen, and aspirin levels should be obtained in an overdose setting to detect occult ingestion.
- Head CT, lumbar puncture, and toxicology studies should be ordered as needed to evaluate other causes of seizure and altered mental status.
- Urine drug screens for marijuana may remain positive for several weeks after clinical effects have resolved.

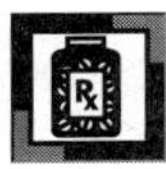

Treatment

- Treatment should focus on airway management and supportive care.
- For paranoia or panic attacks, the patient should be placed in a quiet room and treated with reassurance in a nonthreatening manner.
- The dose and time of exposure should be determined for all substances involved.

DIRECTING PATIENT COURSE

Health-care professionals should call a poison control center when:

- Severe effects are present.
- The toxic effects are not consistent with marijuana toxicity.
- Coingestant, drug interaction, or underlying disease presents an unusual problem.

Patients should be referred to a health-care professional when:

- Attempted suicide or homicide is possible.
- Patients or caregivers seem unreliable.
- Severe effects are present.
- The toxic effects are not consistent with marijuana poisoning.
- Coingestant, drug interaction, or underlying disease presents an unusual problem.

Admission Considerations

Inpatient management is warranted for persistently abnormal vital signs, altered mental status, or other clinically significant organ toxicity.

DECONTAMINATION

Out of Hospital

Emesis should be induced with ipecac within 1 hour of ingestion for alert pediatric or adult patients if health-care evaluation will be delayed.

In Hospital

- Emesis should be induced with ipecac within 1 hour of ingestion for alert pediatric patients who are too small to have effective gastric lavage due to orogastric tube size constraints.
- Gastric lavage (adult tube size 36–42 French) is recommended if the patient presents within 1 hour of a large ingestion or if serious effects are present.
- A dose of activated charcoal (1–2 g/kg) should be administered if the patient has ingested a substantial amount within the previous few hours.

ANTIDOTES

There are no specific antidotes for marijuana poisoning.

ADJUNCTIVE TREATMENT

To control agitation, the health-care provider should administer a benzodiazepine with which he has experience.

- For diazepam, the adult dose is 5 to 10 mg intravenously; the pediatric dose is 0.2 to 0.5 mg/kg intravenously, and doses are repeated at 10-minute intervals, titrating to effect.
- For lorazepam, the adult dose is 1 to 2 mg intravenously; the pediatric dose is 0.05 to 0.1 mg/kg intravenously. Doses are repeated at 10-minute intervals, titrating to effect.
- The patient's airway should be closely monitored.

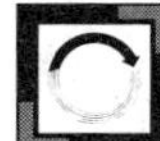

Follow-Up

PATIENT MONITORING

If severe manifestations or complications develop, electrolytes, renal function, and other tests indicated by the patient's clinical condition should be monitored.

EXPECTED COURSE AND PROGNOSIS

- Effects peak rapidly and persist for several hours, followed by complete recovery unless complications develop.
- Inhalation has been associated with pneumothorax and pneumomediastinum.

DISCHARGE CRITERIA/INSTRUCTIONS

From the emergency department or hospital, discharge is warranted for alert patients with normal vital signs, good ambulation, and a reliable caregiver, following psychiatric evaluation, if needed.

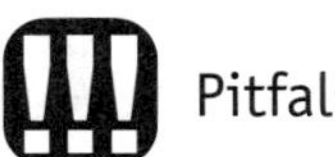

Pitfalls

DIAGNOSIS

It is important to recognize other serious or treatable causes of altered mental status.

FOLLOW-UP

Patients should be referred for substance abuse treatment.

ICD-9-CM 969.6

Poisoning by psychotropic agents: psychodysleptics (hallucinogens).

RECOMMENDED READING

Bryson PD. Marijuana. In: *Comprehensive review in toxicology for emergency clinicians.* Washington, DC: Taylor & Francis, 1996:531–534.

Author: Dan Stillman

Reviewer: Richard C. Dart

Mefenamic Acid

Basics

DESCRIPTION

Mefenamic acid (Ponstel) is an antipyretic and antiinflammatory agent.

FORMS AND USES

Adult dose is 500 mg initially, followed by 250 mg every 6 hours up to 1.5 g/day. It is not recommended for children under 14 years of age.

TOXIC DOSE

Seizures have been associated with ingestion of at least 2.5 to 5.0 grams.

PATHOPHYSIOLOGY

- Mefenamic acid inhibits prostaglandin synthesis as do other nonsteroidal antiinflammatory drugs.
- The cause of seizures is unknown.

EPIDEMIOLOGY

Poisoning is uncommon.

CAUSES

- Poisoning usually involves suicidal ingestion.
- Child abuse or neglect should be considered if the patient is less than 1 year of age, suicide attempt if over 6 years of age.

PREGNANCY AND LACTATION

US FDA Pregnancy Category C. The drug exerts animal teratogenic or embryocidal effects, but there are no controlled studies in women, or no studies are available in either animals or humans.

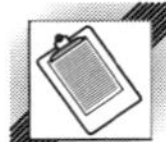

Diagnosis

DIFFERENTIAL DIAGNOSIS

Toxicologic causes of seizure include tricyclic antidepressants, camphor, theophylline, withdrawal from alcohol or sedative-hypnotic, and others.

SIGNS AND SYMPTOMS

Seizures are common and unique to mefenamic acid among the nonsteroidal antiinflammatory drugs (NSAIDS).

Gastrointestinal

- Nausea, vomiting, and diarrhea have been reported after overdose.
- Abdominal pain, gastritis, and ulcers are associated with therapeutic use.

Renal

- Renal failure occurs rarely after overdose.
- Renal papillary necrosis, interstitial nephritis, fibrosis, and renal insufficiency are associated with long-term therapeutic use.

Acid-Base

Metabolic acidosis may develop with seizures.

Neurologic

Seizures are common with substantial overdose and are usually preceded by muscle twitching; dyskinesia, CNS depression, and agitation are less common.

Hematologic

Hemolytic anemia, agranulocytosis, pancytopenia, and thrombocytopenic purpura are rare adverse effects at therapeutic dose.

PROCEDURES AND LABORATORY TESTS

Essential Tests

No tests may be needed.

Recommended Tests

- ECG, serum acetaminophen and aspirin levels, and serum electrolytes should be monitored in an overdose setting to detect occult ingestions.
- Serum electrolytes, BUN, creatinine, glucose in patients with seizure or altered mental status.
- Head CT, lumbar punctures, cultures as needed to assess other causes of seizure or altered mental status.

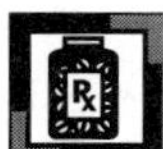

Treatment

- Treatment should focus on supportive care with appropriate airway management.
- Dose and time of exposure should be determined for all substances involved.

DIRECTING PATIENT COURSE

The health-care professional should call the poison control center when:

- Toxic effects are not consistent with mefenamic acid poisoning.
- Coingestant, drug interaction, or underlying disease presents an unusual problem.

The patient should be referred to a health-care facility when:

- Attempted suicide or homicide is possible.
- Seizure or other toxic effects develop.
- Coingestant, drug interaction, or underlying disease presents an unusual problem.

Admission Considerations

Inpatient management is warranted in patients with seizure or acid-base disorder.

DECONTAMINATION

Out of Hospital

Emesis should not be induced.

In Hospital

- Gastric lavage should be performed in pediatric (tube size 24–32 French) or adult (36–42 French) patients presenting within 1 hour of a large ingestion or if serious effects are present.
- One dose of activated charcoal (1–2 g/kg) should be administered without a cathartic if a substantial ingestion has occurred within the previous few hours.

ANTIDOTES

A specific antidote is not available for mefenamic acid poisoning.

ADJUNCTIVE TREATMENT

Seizure

- Adequate airway and oxygenation are essential.
- Initial treatment is a benzodiazepine familiar to the provider.

—Diazepam. Adult dosage is 5 to 10 mg intravenous push, repeated every 10 minutes, as needed; pediatric dosage is 0.2 to 0.5 mg/kg every 10 minutes, as needed.
—Lorazepam. Adult dosage is 2 to 4 mg intravenous push, repeated every 10 minutes, as needed; pediatric dosage is 0.1 mg/kg repeated every 10 minutes, as needed.
—Airway must be monitored closely.

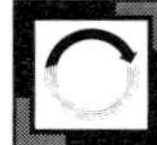

Follow-Up

PATIENT MONITORING

Patients with seizures or altered mental status should be admitted to a monitored setting.

EXPECTED COURSE AND PROGNOSIS

Patients usually recover within 24 hours with supportive care.

DISCHARGE CRITERIA/INSTRUCTIONS

- From emergency department. Patients who do not develop seizures or altered mental status within 6 hours of observation after gastrointestinal decontamination and psychiatric evaluation, if needed, may be discharged.
- From hospital. Patients may be discharged when seizures have ceased and mental status has returned to baseline, and after psychiatric evaluation, if needed.

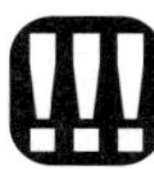

Pitfalls

DIAGNOSIS

Other NSAIDS do not cause seizures, and the diagnosis may be difficult to make if the specific agent is not known.

ICD-9-CM 965

Poisoning by analgesics, antipyretics, and antirheumatics.

See also: SECTION II, Seizures chapter; and SECTION IV, Nonsteroidal Antiinflammatory Drugs chapter.

Author: Katherine M. Hurlbut

Reviewer: Richard C. Dart

Mercury—Elemental

Basics

DESCRIPTION

Elemental mercury (Hg) exists as a silver-colored liquid. Inorganic and organic mercury are covered in following chapters.

FORMS AND USES

- Other names for elemental mercury include colloidal mercury, hydrargyrum, liquid silver, metallic mercury, and quicksilver.
- It is used in dental amalgams, thermometers, calibration of instruments, ceramics, electrical apparatus, fluorescent light bulbs, and silver and gold extraction, among others.

TOXIC DOSE

- Death has occurred after inhalation of fumes, usually in a closed space.
- The lethal concentration is unknown.

PATHOPHYSIOLOGY

- Elemental mercury is volatile at room temperature and easily inhaled, with 80% of the inhaled dose absorbed.
- Toxicity is caused by binding to enzyme and protein sulfhydryl groups.
- Toxicity to the respiratory system is the major acute life threat; a spectrum ranging from pneumonitis to necrotizing bronchiolitis to pulmonary edema occurs, depending on severity of exposure.
- Elemental mercury is very poorly absorbed by ingestion or across intact skin; however, inflammatory bowel disease or gastrointestinal obstruction may allow clinically significant absorption to occur.

EPIDEMIOLOGY

- Poisoning is common.
- Toxic effects following exposure are typically mild to moderate.
- Death is rare.

CAUSES

- Toxicity is usually the result of an accidental incident.
- Child abuse or neglect must be considered if the patient is less than 1 year of age; suicide attempt if the child is over 6 years of age.

RISK FACTORS

- Pediatric patients are considered more sensitive to elemental mercury exposure.
- Geriatric patients are considered more sensitive to elemental mercury exposure due to possible reduced functioning of renal, pulmonary, and CNS systems.

PREGNANCY AND LACTATION

Mercury is a probable teratogen that easily passes placental and blood-brain barriers.

WORKPLACE STANDARDS

- ACGIH. TLV TWA is 0.025 mg/m^3.
- OSHA. Not listed.
- NIOSH. REL TWA is 0.05 mg/m^3; IDLH is 10 mg/m^3.
- NIOSH. REL is 0.05 mg/m^3; IDLH 10 mg/m^3.

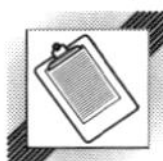

Diagnosis

A thorough history of exposure generally reveals the source of toxicity.

DIFFERENTIAL DIAGNOSIS

Toxic causes of acute pulmonary injury and altered mental status include smoke inhalation and other respiratory irritants (e.g., chlorine, nitrogen dioxide).

SIGNS AND SYMPTOMS

- Acute inhalation is most common and may produce pulmonary edema within hours of exposure.
- Chronic respiratory exposure primarily produces CNS effects.
- Intravenous, intramuscular, or subcutaneous injection allows prolonged absorption and may lead to chronic poisoning.

HEENT

Headache, metallic taste, visual disturbances, weakness, and chills may occur after acute exposure.

Dermatologic

- Stomatitis and contact dermatitis may develop following acute exposure or during chronic exposure.
- Acrodynia (pink disease) is a rare effect of chronic exposure featuring pink discoloration and desquamation of fingers, nose, and toes; irritability; sweating; and miliary-type diffuse rash.

Pulmonary

Dyspnea, cough and chest tightness may be seen acutely after inhalation, followed by bronchitis, pneumonitis, necrotizing bronchiolitis, and pulmonary edema in more serious cases.

Gastrointestinal

Gingivitis, stomatitis, nausea, vomiting, abdominal pain, and diarrhea may develop with chronic exposure.

Hepatic

Liver enzyme abnormalities may occur.

Genitourinary

- Proteinuria and nephrotic syndrome have been reported.
- Acute tubular necrosis and renal failure may occur.

Neurologic

Acute inhalation may cause tremor, confusion, and excitability.

- Early symptoms may be nonspecific: malaise, blurred vision, or hearing loss.
- Irreversible brain damage may result after massive exposure.
- Chronic exposure may produce personality changes, weakness, tremor, headache, short-term memory loss, decreased appetite, insomnia, emotional instability, paresthesia, and sensory and motor nerve conduction delays.
- Chronic intoxication from inhalation may produce erethism, the classic triad of gingivostomatitis, tremor, and neuropsychiatric effects (excitability, agitation, and withdrawal).

PROCEDURES AND LABORATORY TESTS

Essential Tests

No tests may be needed in asymptomatic patients or following ingestion.

Recommended Tests

- Whole blood mercury may be useful in confirming acute exposure if level is elevated; normal level is below 1.5 μg/dl.
- Urinary mercury, 24-hour collection, is used for chronic exposure.

—Recent ingestion of seafood may temporarily increase urinary mercury level. This form of mercury is not toxic.
—There is no clinical effect from urine mercury levels below 20 μg/L.
—Decreased verbal skills and decreased nerve conduction may be evident at mercury levels from 20 to 100 μg/L.
—Irritability, depression, memory loss, tremor, CNS dysfunction, and kidney damage occur at mercury levels ranging from 100 to 500 μg/L.
—Kidney damage, swollen gums, and marked tremor and CNS dysfunction occur at mercury levels from 500 to 1,000 μg/L.

- Serum electrolytes, BUN, and creatinine should be assayed to evaluate renal injury.
- Elemental mercury is radio-opaque and is often apparent on radiographs.

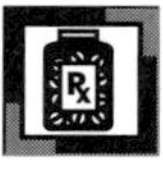

Treatment

- Treatment should focus on supportive respiratory care after inhalation exposure and on initiating early chelation.
- Dose and time of exposure should be determined for all substances involved.

DIRECTING PATIENT COURSE

The health-care provider should call the poison control center when:

- Respiratory symptoms, altered mental status, or other severe effects are present.
- Toxic effects are not consistent with elemental mercury poisoning.
- Coingestant, drug interaction, or underlying disease presents an unusual problem.

The patient should be referred to a health-care facility when:

- Attempted suicide or homicide is possible.
- Patient or caregiver seems unreliable.
- Toxic effects develop.
- Coingestant, drug interaction, or underlying disease presents an unusual problem.

Admission Considerations

Inpatient management is warranted if the patient exhibits any symptoms after mercury inhalation or injection.

DECONTAMINATION

Out of Hospital

- Emesis should not be induced due to low toxicity of ingestion.
- Patient must be removed from source of mercury fumes.
- Clean-up of large elemental mercury spills should not be attempted except by the local fire department; elemental mercury should not be vacuumed because of mercury aerosol production.

In Hospital

Emesis, gastric lavage, and activated charcoal are not needed, unless coingestant is suspected.

ANTIDOTES

Specific chelators are available for mercury poisoning (see individual chelator chapters in SECTION III for further details).

Succimer

Succimer is the preferred chelating agent.

- Indications. Succimer should be considered for symptomatic acute mercury exposure or increased urinary excretion of mercury.
- Contraindications. Known hypersensitivity to succimer contraindicates its use.
- Method of administration

—Adult dose is 10 mg/kg (350 mg/m^2 for a child) orally three times a day for 5 days, followed by 10 mg/kg twice a day for 14 days; a repeat course may be given if the need is indicated by continuing symptoms and elevated urinary mercury levels.

Penicillamine

- Indications. Penicillamine also may be considered for symptomatic acute mercury exposure or increased urinary excretion of mercury.
- Contraindications. Known hypersensitivity to penicillin or penicillamine contraindicates its use.
- Method of administration

—Adult dose is 15 to 40 mg/kg/day, up to a maximum of 250 to 500 mg orally four times a day, before meals.
—Pediatric dose is 20 to 30 mg/kg per day, given orally once or twice daily before meals, for 5 to 10 days.
—Urinary excretion of mercury should be monitored; if urine mercury falls rapidly, body burden is probably small.
—After 10 days, baseline urine mercury should be repeated; if it is still elevated, another course of chelation may be required.

- Adverse effects. Nephrotic syndrome, hypersensitivity reactions, transient blood dyscrasia, aplastic anemia, agranulocytosis, and various autoimmune responses are possible.

British Anti-Lewisite

In the rare case in which oral treatment is not possible, parenteral therapy with British anti-Lewisite should be considered.

ADJUNCTIVE TREATMENT

Pulmonary edema occurs rarely and is managed as noncardiogenic pulmonary edema (see SECTION II, Pulmonary Edema chapter).

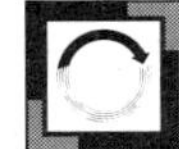

Follow-Up

PATIENT MONITORING

- Clinical symptoms should be monitored closely.
- Serial urine mercury levels are used to guide therapy.

EXPECTED COURSE AND PROGNOSIS

- Ingestion. Unless a preexisting gastrointestinal obstruction or perforation is present, ingestion causes no effects.
- Inhalation

—High-concentration exposure rapidly produces pulmonary symptoms; prognosis depends on the degree of pulmonary injury.
—Permanent CNS, pulmonary, or renal system damage may occur in severe cases.
—Less severe exposure may produce systemic mercury poisoning, which will take weeks or months to resolve.

- Chronic exposure is possible; symptoms of CNS, respiratory tract, and renal damage may be reversible if exposure is stopped before severe damage develops.

DISCHARGE CRITERIA/INSTRUCTIONS

From emergency department or hospital. After inhalation exposure, patient may be discharged when asymptomatic and when major organ involvement has been assessed and does not require hospitalization.

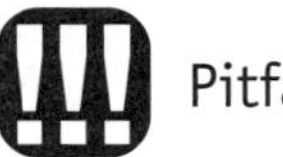

Pitfalls

DIAGNOSIS

A single elevated mercury level does not prove toxicity in an asymptomatic patient.

FOLLOW-UP

In patients with inflammatory bowel disease, fistula formation may absorb elemental mercury if mercury remains in the gastrointestinal tract due to obstruction.

ICD-9-CM 985.0

Toxic effect of other metals: mercury and its compounds.

See also: SECTION II, Pulmonary Edema chapter; SECTION III, British Anti-Lewisite, Penicillamine, Succimer; and SECTION IV, Mercury—Inorganic chapters.

RECOMMENDED READING

Goyer RA. Toxic effect of metals. In: Klaassen CD, Amdur MO, Doull J, eds. *Casarett and Doull's toxicology: the basic science of poisons,* 5th ed. New York: McGraw-Hill, 1996:712.

US Department of Health and Human Services. ATSDR case studies in environmental medicine: mercury toxicity, monograph 17, March 1992.

Author: Alvin C. Bronstein

Reviewer: Luke Yip

Mercury—Inorganic

Basics

DESCRIPTION

The inorganic mercury salts are typically solid compounds used in industrial processes.

FORMS AND USES

- Inorganic mercury compounds are of two types.
- Mercuric compounds include mercuric chloride, acetate, arsenate, bromide, chloride, cyanide, iodide, nitrate, oxide, oxycyanide, potassium cyanide, potassium iodide, and mercuric sulfide.
- Mercurous compounds include mercurous acetate bromide, chloride (calomel), iodide, nitrate, oxide, sulfate, and ammoniated mercury.

TOXIC DOSE

The potentially lethal dose of mercuric chloride is 10 to 50 mg/kg orally; mercuric salts are more toxic than mercurous salts.

PATHOPHYSIOLOGY

- Mercury acts by binding to enzyme and protein sulfhydryl groups, producing cell dysfunction and death.
- Inorganic mercury salts have corrosive gastrointestinal effects.

EPIDEMIOLOGY

- Poisoning is uncommon.
- Toxic effects following exposure are typically mild to moderate.
- Death is rare, usually due to large suicidal ingestion.
- Carcinogenesis. Inorganic mercury is characterized as IARC group 3: inadequate human evidence.

CAUSES

- Toxic exposure is usually an accidental incident.
- Child abuse or neglect must be considered if the patient is under 1 year of age; suicide attempt if the child is over 6 years of age.

RISK FACTORS

Pediatric and geriatric patients are considered more sensitive to inorganic mercury exposure.

PREGNANCY AND LACTATION

- Inorganic mercury is a probable teratogen that easily passes placental and blood-brain barriers.
- Mercuric chloride has been associated with spontaneous abortions in humans.

WORKPLACE STANDARDS

- OSHA. TLV TWA: none given. PEL (ceiling) is 0.1 mg/m^3 or 12 ppm.
- ACGIH. TLV TWA is 0.025 mg/m^3.
- NIOSH. IDLH is 10 mg/m^3.

Diagnosis

DIFFERENTIAL DIAGNOSIS

- Toxic causes of acute corrosive gastroenteritis include ingestion of acids or alkaline corrosives or another metal salt, such as arsenic or thallium.
- Other causes include any food poisoning or infectious gastroenteritis.

SIGNS AND SYMPTOMS

- Ingestion may cause severe corrosive damage to the gastrointestinal tract, which may be complicated by hemorrhage and shock; acute renal failure may develop within 24 hours.
- Inhalation causes acute respiratory distress.
- Chronic low-level inhalational exposure can produce tremor and neuropsychological changes.

HEENT

- Acute ingestion can cause oral burns.
- Chronic exposure may cause headache, metallic taste, gum swelling, salivation, visual disturbances, decreased visual acuity, and mercurialentis (discoloration of the lens and cornea, usually without visual impairment).

Dermatologic

- Chronic exposure may cause stomatitis and contact dermatitis.
- Acrodynia (pink disease) occurs rarely, primarily in children; leg cramps; painful and peeling skin; and pinkish color of fingers, hands, nose, and feet.

Cardiovascular

Ingestion may cause shock secondary to gastrointestinal hemorrhage.

Pulmonary

Inhalation may quickly produce dyspnea, cough, and chest tightness with edema of the trachea, bronchi, lungs, as well as pulmonary edema or adult respiratory distress syndrome in severe cases.

Gastrointestinal

- Ingestion may cause potentially massive gastrointestinal hemorrhage.
- Gingivitis, stomatitis, dysphagia, hematemesis, nausea, vomiting, abdominal pain, gastrointestinal mucosa necrosis, and diarrhea with melena can occur.

Genitourinary

- Acute exposure may cause proteinuria (albuminuria) and nephrotic syndrome.
- Hematuria, glycosuria, casts, oliguria, and aminoaciduria leading to renal failure may occur; onset is often within 24 hours of ingestion, but may be delayed.
- Chronic exposure may cause membranous glomerulonephropathy with nephrotic syndrome.

Fluids and Electrolytes

Recurrent vomiting or renal failure may cause electrolyte abnormality.

Hematologic

- Acute exposure may cause blood loss secondary to a gastrointestinal hemorrhage.
- Acute severe exposure may be complicated by disseminated intravascular coagulation.

Neurologic

- Acute inhalation exposure may cause tremor, irritability, loss of coordination, confusion, anxiety, and insomnia.
- Hyperreflexia, CNS excitation, and personality changes can occur.
- Irreversible brain damage may result.
- Acute exposure has been reported to cause a syndrome resembling amyotrophic lateral sclerosis; these symptoms may be associated with decreased mental function.
- Chronic exposure may cause personality changes, weakness, tremors, headache, short-term memory loss, decreased appetite, shyness, insomnia, emotional instability, paresthesia, and peripheral neuropathy.

PROCEDURES AND LABORATORY TESTS

Essential Tests

- Whole-blood mercury may be useful in confirming acute exposure if the level is elevated; normal level is below 5 μg/dl.
- Urinary mercury, 24-hour collection, is used for acute or chronic exposure

—In chronic exposure, no clinical effect is expected with urine mercury levels below 20 μg/L, the normal level.

—Decreased verbal skills, tremor, and decreased nerve conduction may be evident at mercury levels from 20 to 100 μg/L.

—Irritability, depression, memory loss, tremor, CNS dysfunction, and kidney damage occur at mercury levels ranging from 100 to 500 μg/L.

—Kidney inflammation, gingivitis, and marked tremor and CNS dysfunction occur at mercury levels from 500 to 1000 μg/L.

—In acute exposure, urinary levels are performed serially to assess mercury excretion; they do not correlate well with clinical effects.

Recommended Tests

- Complete blood count (CBC), serum electrolytes, BUN, and creatinine should be assayed to detect anemia or renal injury.
- Abdominal radiographs may help assess adequacy of gastrointestinal decontamination because mercury is radiopaque.
- Electromyography/NCV in symptomatic patients may demonstrate decreased motor and sensory conduction.

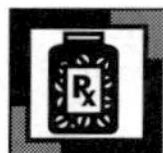

Treatment

• Following acute exposure, treatment should focus on hemodynamic support and chelation.
• Dose and time of exposure should be determined for all substances involved.

DIRECTING PATIENT COURSE

The health-care provider should call the poison control center when:

• Toxic effects develop.
• Coingestant, drug interaction, or underlying disease presents an unusual problem.

The patient should be referred to a health-care facility when:

• History of inorganic mercury ingestion is obtained.
• Coingestant, drug interaction, or underlying disease presents an unusual problem.

Admission Considerations

Inpatient management is usually warranted if the patient exhibits any symptoms.

DECONTAMINATION

Out of Hospital

• Emesis should not be induced.
• Patient should be removed from source of inhalation exposure.

In Hospital

• Gastric lavage is generally not useful unless the patient presents before vomiting develops.
• One dose of activated charcoal (1–2 g/kg) should be administered without a cathartic if a substantial recent ingestion has occurred and recurrent vomiting has not developed.

ANTIDOTES

Succimer

Succimer is the preferred oral chelating agent.

Indications

Symptomatic acute mercury exposure or increased urinary excretion of mercury.

Contraindications

Known hypersensitivity to succimer.

Method of Administration

Adult dose is 10 mg/kg (350 mg/m^2 for a child) orally three times a day for 5 days, followed by 10 mg/kg twice a day for 14 days; a repeat course may be given if need is indicated by continuing symptoms and elevated mercury levels.

Penicillamine

Indications

A second line oral agent for symptomatic acute mercury exposure or documented increased urinary excretion of mercury.

Contraindications

Known hypersensitivity to penicillin or penicillamine.

Method of Administration

• Adult dose is 15 to 40 mg/kg per day, up to a maximum of 500 mg four times a day, orally before meals, for 5 to 10 days.
• Pediatric dose is 20 to 30 mg/kg per day, up to 250 to 500 mg/day, given orally once or twice daily before meals, for 5 to 10 days.
• Blood and urine mercury levels should be monitored to determine whether additional courses of chelation are required.

Adverse Effects

Nephrotic syndrome, hypersensitivity reactions, blood dyscrasia, aplastic anemia, agranulocytosis, and various autoimmune responses are possible.

British Anti-Lewisite (BAL)

Indications

In acute mercury exposures when oral treatment is not possible (e.g., in the case of emesis or gastrointestinal burns), BAL should be considered.

Contraindications

Hypersensitivity to BAL or peanuts, glucose-6-phosphate dehydrogenase deficiency, or hepatic insufficiency contraindicate its use.

Method of Administration

Dose is 2.5 to 5 mg/kg intramuscularly every 4 hours tapering to every 6 to 12 hours over several days, until an oral chelator can be tolerated.

Adverse Effects

Headache, hypertension, pain at injection site, allergic reaction, and fever are possible.

ADJUNCTIVE TREATMENT

Hemodialysis may be needed as supportive therapy of renal failure.

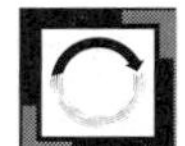

Follow-Up

PATIENT MONITORING

• Continuous cardiac and respiratory monitoring should be performed in symptomatic patients following acute exposure.
• In patients with chronic or symptomatic acute exposure, blood and urine mercury levels should be monitored, along with CBC and tests of renal function such as electrolytes, BUN, and creatinine.

EXPECTED COURSE AND PROGNOSIS

• Toxic effects after acute exposure usually improve and may return to baseline.
• Chronic exposure is more likely to produce slow gradual improvement over months and may not improve to baseline.
• Permanent CNS or renal damage is possible in severe cases.

DISCHARGE CRITERIA/INSTRUCTIONS

• From the emergency department. Asymptomatic and reliable patients with acute ingestion may be discharged after 4 to 6 hours of observation and psychiatric evaluation (if needed).
• From the hospital. Patient may be discharged when CNS, pulmonary, and renal injury are stable or improving and management as an outpatient is possible.

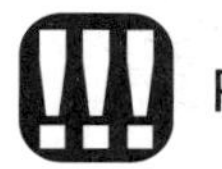

Pitfalls

DIAGNOSIS

Clinical symptoms must be correlated with history and mercury levels; presence of mercury in blood or urine sample does not necessarily indicate mercury poisoning.

TREATMENT

Side effects from chelation therapy are common; consultation with medical toxicologist is recommended.

ICD-9-CM 985.0

Toxic effect of other metals: mercury and its compounds.

See also: SECTION II, Pulmonary Edema chapter; SECTION III, British Anti-Lewisite, Penicillamine, and Succimer chapters; and SECTION IV, Caustic—Basic and Mercury—Elemental chapters.

RECOMMENDED READING

Clarkson TW, Hursh JB, Sager PR, Syversen TLM. Mercury. In: *Biological monitoring of toxic metals.* New York: Plenum, 1988:199–246.

Goyer RA. Toxic effect of metals. In: Klaassen CD, Amdur MO, Doull J, eds. *Casarett and Doull's toxicology: the basic science of poisons,* 5th ed. New York: McGraw-Hill, 1996:712.

US Department of Health and Human Services. ATSDR Case Studies in Environmental Medicine: mercury toxicity, monograph 17, March 1992.

Author: Alvin C. Bronstein

Reviewer: Katherine M. Hurlbut

Mercury—Organic

Basics

DESCRIPTION

- Substances include short-chain alkyl (methyl, ethyl, dimethyl, n-propyl, etc.), long-chain alkyl, aryl (e.g., phenyl), and alkoxyalkyl mercury compounds.
- Aryl, long-chain alkyl, and alkoxyalkyl mercury compounds produce a clinical picture similar to that of inorganic mercury salts and are discussed in the Mercury—Inorganic chapter.

FORMS AND USES

- Sources of exposure include fungicides, herbicides, germicides, and timber preservatives.
- Occupations associated with exposure include chemists, researchers, embalmers, paper workers, and seed and wood handlers.
- Other uses include preservatives in eye drops, tetanus toxoid, ointments, and vaccines; mercurochrome and thimerosal are topical antiseptics that contain organic mercury.
- Consumption of fish from contaminated sources is a common source of chronic, low-level exposure.

TOXIC DOSE

- Acute ingestion of 10 to 60 mg/kg of methyl mercury may be lethal.
- Sip ingestions of mercurochrome and thimerosal are nontoxic; a large ingestion can produce neuropathy and renal injury.

PATHOPHYSIOLOGY

- Mercury binds to protein sulfhydryl groups, interfering with cellular processes and producing cellular damage and death.
- Clinical experience with organic mercury has been primarily based on mass exposure to methyl mercury; available information is mainly based on anecdotal reports.
- Methyl mercury is well absorbed following inhalation, ingestion, or dermal exposure and has an average half-life of 70 days.
- The primary target organs of methyl mercury are the brain and kidney.
- Carcinogenesis. Methyl mercury is possibly carcinogenic to humans and is rated IARC group 2B.

EPIDEMIOLOGY

Poisoning is uncommon, but chronic toxic effects may be severe.

CAUSES

- Poisoning usually is the result of an occupational incident.
- Child neglect should be considered if patients are under 1 year of age; attempted suicide if patients are over 6 years of age.

RISK FACTORS

Pediatric and geriatric patients are considered more sensitive than others to organic mercury exposure.

PREGNANCY AND LACTATION

- Methyl mercury crosses the placenta and is excreted in breast milk.
- Perinatal exposure to methyl mercury has caused mental retardation and cerebral palsy type syndrome.

WORKPLACE STANDARDS

Among the alkyl compounds, including methyl mercury:

- OSHA. PEL TWA not listed; ceiling is 0.1 mg/m^3.
- NIOSH. REL TWA is 0.05 mg/m^3; IDLH is 10 mg/m^3.
- ACGIH. TLV TWA is 0.01 mg/m^3.

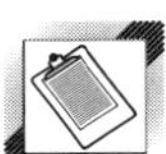

Diagnosis

DIFFERENTIAL DIAGNOSIS

- Toxic causes of CNS and renal injury primarily include other heavy metal poisonings (arsenic, gold, lead, copper) as well as toluene and other solvents.
- Nontoxic causes include sepsis and collagen vascular disease.

SIGNS AND SYMPTOMS

- Symptoms of methyl mercury poisoning are often delayed for weeks to months; early symptoms are usually nonspecific; progression of toxicity produces a triad of dysarthria, ataxia, and constricted visual fields.
- For chronic long chain or aryl ingestion see SECTION IV, Mercury—Inorganic.

HEENT

Chronic exposure may cause loss of taste and smell, constricted visual fields, and hearing impairment.

Dermatologic

Acute or chronic exposure may cause irritation and dermatitis.

Gastrointestinal

Following acute ingestion, dysphagia, nausea, vomiting, diarrhea, and abdominal pain may occur.

Hepatic

Chronic exposure may cause abnormal liver function tests.

Genitourinary

Renal injury and insufficiency may develop.

Neurologic

- Short-chain alkyl mercury compounds primarily affect the CNS.
- Typically, repeated exposure is needed to produce CNS toxicity.
- Over time, the patient may develop paresthesia, ataxia, dysphagia, speech problems, blurred vision and hearing loss, impaired taste and smell, mental status changes, learning deficits, neurasthenia, intention tremor, hyperreflexia, spasticity, coma, and death.

PROCEDURES AND LABORATORY TESTS

Essential Tests

- Whole-blood mercury titers may be useful if drawn within a day of exposure. Normal methyl mercury level is less than 2.0 μg/dl; more than 5 to 10 μg/dl have been associated with symptoms.
- 24-hour urine mercury collection is the usual method for assessment of aryl, long-chain, and alkoxyalkyl mercury compounds, which are primarily excreted in the urine.
  - —The normal level is 10 μg/L in adults.
  - —Quantitative 24-hour urinary mercury excretion should be less than 50 μg/24 h.
- Complete blood count, serum electrolytes, glucose, BUN, creatinine, head CT, and lumbar puncture to assess other causes of altered mental status should be undertaken.

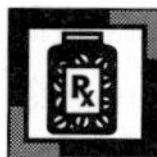

Treatment

- Treatment should focus on supportive care.
- Primary treatment is to eradicate the source of exposure and prevent continued intoxication; others may be poisoned as well.
- The dose and time of exposure should be determined for all substances involved.

DIRECTING PATIENT COURSE

The health-care professional should call the poison control center when:

- The history of the exposure is obtained.
- Toxic effects are not consistent with organic mercury.
- Coingestant, drug interaction, or underlying disease presents an unusual problem.

The patient should be referred to a health-care facility when:

- Attempted suicide or homicide is possible.
- Patients or caregivers seem unreliable.
- Symptoms are present.
- Coingestant, drug interaction, or underlying disease presents an unusual problem.

Admission Considerations

Inpatient admission is recommended for acutely symptomatic individuals; however, most cases are evaluated in an office setting.

DECONTAMINATION

Out of Hospital

- For inhalation, patients should be removed from the source.
- For acute ingestion, emesis should be induced with ipecac within 1 hour of ingestion for alert pediatric or adult patients, if health-care evaluation will be delayed.

In Hospital

- For inhalation, symptomatic treatment is recommended.
- For ingestion, gastric aspiration with a nasogastric tube is indicated for substantial ingestion presenting within 1 hour of ingestion.
- One dose of activated charcoal (1–2 g/kg) should be administered if the patient has ingested a substantial amount within the previous few hours.

ANTIDOTES

Consultation with a physician experienced in the use of heavy metal chelators is recommended before initiating therapy.

- Chelation therapy has been used to aid in elimination of mercury. Even though the clinical efficacy of chelators in the prevention or treatment of neuropsychiatric toxicity resulting from methylmercury poisoning has not been well evaluated, therapy is recommended.
- Succimer is used.

—Indication. Symptomatic patient with elevated whole blood mercury level or documented elevated 24-hour urine mercury excretion.
—Contraindications. Known hypersensitivity to succimer.
—Method of administration. 10 mg/kg orally three times daily for 5 days followed by 10 mg/kg twice daily for 14 days; repeating the course may be indicated if symptoms continue and elevated whole-blood mercury levels or elevated urine mercury levels persist or recur.

- Dimercaptopropane sulfonic acid also increases excretion, but is not yet approved for human use in the United States.

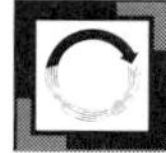

Follow-Up

PATIENT MONITORING

- The patient should be monitored for development of clinical symptoms, and blood and urine mercury levels should be followed for several weeks.
- Neuropsychiatric testing may be indicated.

EXPECTED COURSE AND PROGNOSIS

Persistent CNS impairment following a large acute or chronic exposure is possible.

DISCHARGE CRITERIA/INSTRUCTIONS

Patients should be discharged from the emergency department or hospital following decontamination and psychiatric evaluation, if needed.

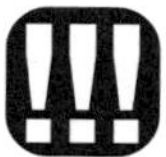

Pitfalls

DIAGNOSIS

- An elevated mercury level alone does not prove mercury poisoning.
- Clinical symptoms should be correlated with history, blood, and urine levels.
- For organic mercury exposures, it is important to distinguish between short- and long-chain and aryl mercury compounds.

ICD-9-CM 985.0

Toxic effect of other metals: mercury and its compounds.

See also: SECTION III, Succimer chapter; and SECTION IV, Mercury—Inorganic chapter.

RECOMMENDED READING

Clarkson TW, Hursh JB, Sager PR, Syversen TLM. Mercury. In: *Biological monitoring of toxic metals.* New York: Plenum, 1988:199–246.

Goyer RA. Toxic effect of metals. In: Klaassen CD, Amdur MO, Doull J, eds. *Casarett and Doull's toxicology: the basic science of poisons,* 5th ed. New York: McGraw-Hill, 1996:712.

US Department of Health and Human Services. ATSDR Case Studies in Environmental Medicine: mercury toxicity, monograph 17, March 1992.

Author: Alvin C. Bronstein

Reviewer: Luke Yip

Metformin and Biguanide Hypoglycemic Agents

Basics

DESCRIPTION

Metformin and biguanide hypoglycemic agents are used to treat non–insulin-dependent diabetes mellitus and to reduce insulin requirements in patients with insulin-dependent diabetes.

FORMS AND USES

- Substances include metformin (Glucophage) and phenformin.
- Metformin is available in 500- and 850-mg tablets; adult dosage is 500 mg twice daily, up to 2,500 mg/day divided three times a day.

TOXIC DOSE

The toxic dose is unknown; metformin is thought to be less likely than sulfonylurea agents to produce hypoglycemia in nondiabetic patients who ingest a single pill.

PATHOPHYSIOLOGY

- The mechanism of the action is unclear; biguanides may increase glucose reuptake by cells, decrease gluconeogenesis, and increase glucose turnover.
- Lactic acidosis may be secondary to impaired adenosine triphosphate production due to actions on mitochondrial membranes.

EPIDEMIOLOGY

- Poisoning is uncommon, but increasing in incidence.
- Toxic effects are typically mild.
- Death occurs rarely, primarily in patients with underlying renal or hepatic disease who develop lactic acidosis.

CAUSES

- Acute overdose is usually caused by intentional ingestion.
- Child neglect should be considered in patients under 1 year of age; suicide attempt in patients over 6 years of age.

DRUG AND DISEASE INTERACTIONS

- Patients with underlying hepatic or renal dysfunction are at risk for metformin-induced lactic acidosis.
- Enhanced hypoglycemic effects occur with other oral hypoglycemics or insulin.

PREGNANCY AND LACTATION

US FDA Pregnancy Category B. Animal studies indicate no fetal risk, and there are no controlled human studies, or animal studies show an adverse fetal effect but well-controlled studies in pregnant women do not.

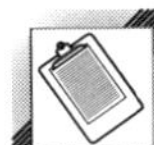

Diagnosis

DIFFERENTIAL DIAGNOSIS

- Toxic causes of metabolic acidosis include isoniazid, iron, methanol, ethylene glycol, and salicylates, among others.
- Nontoxic causes include diabetic ketoacidosis, sepsis, renal failure, seizure, and renal tubular acidosis.

SIGNS AND SYMPTOMS

- Severe lactic acidosis may develop after either an overdose or chronic excessive dosing of any biguanide.
- Metabolic acidosis or hypoglycemia suggest a serious overdose and a need for immediate therapy.

Vital Signs

- Hypothermia may develop in patients with coma and acidosis.
- Tachycardia may develop from volume depletion.

Cardiovascular

- Hypotension, bradycardia, and dysrhythmia may appear in patients with severe acidosis.
- Myocardial infarction may be either the precipitating factor or the result of severe acidosis during chronic therapy.

Pulmonary

- Kussmaul respirations may occur with lactic acidosis.
- Pulmonary edema may occur after severe overdose.

Gastrointestinal

- Nausea, vomiting, and abdominal pain develop as side effects with an acute overdose or with lactic acidosis.
- Gastrointestinal bleeding is a rare effect.

Renal

Acute renal failure may develop in patients with acidosis and hypotension.

Fluids and Electrolytes

- Lactic acidosis may develop after an acute overdose or chronic excessive dosing of any biguanide hypoglycemic agent.
- Lactic acidosis from chronic therapeutic use of metformin has been reported in patients with underlying renal or hepatic insufficiency.

Neurologic

- CNS depression, coma, and abnormal reflexes are seen in patients with hypoglycemia or severe acidosis.
- Seizures rarely occur.

Endocrine

Hypoglycemia may develop after an overdose or with acidosis.

PROCEDURES AND LABORATORY TESTS

Essential Tests

Serum electrolytes, glucose, BUN, creatinine, and arterial blood gas may be monitored to assess the presence and severity of acidosis.

Recommended Tests

- Liver function tests are recommended for patients with acidosis; patients with hepatic insufficiency are susceptible to metformin-induced acidosis.
- Serum iron, methanol, ethylene glycol, salicylate, and lactate levels may be needed to evaluate other causes of acidosis.
- Blood cultures, a lumbar puncture, and a head CT may be needed to rule out other causes of altered mental status.
- An ECG may be useful for patients with acidosis; severe acidosis may precipitate myocardial infarction.
- Serum acetaminophen and aspirin levels in overdose setting to detect occult ingestion.

Not Recommended Tests

Serum levels of biguanides are not readily available or useful.

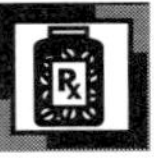

Treatment

- Treatment should focus on managing the airway, supporting cardiovascular function, correcting hypoglycemia, and reversing acidosis as clinically indicated.
- The dose and time of exposure should be determined for all substances involved.

DIRECTING PATIENT COURSE

The health-care professional should call the poison control center when:

- Metabolic acidosis, hypotension, dysrhythmia, or other severe effects are present.
- Toxic effects are not consistent with metformin toxicity.
- Coingestant, drug interaction, or underlying disease presents an unusual problem.

The patient should be referred to a health-care facility when:

- Attempted suicide or homicide is possible.
- Patients or caregivers seem unreliable.
- Toxic effects develop.
- Coingestant, drug interaction, or underlying disease presents an unusual problem.

Admission Considerations

Inpatient treatment is warranted when the patient has altered mental status, hypoglycemia, acidosis, hypotension, or dysrhythmia.

DECONTAMINATION

Out of Hospital

Emesis should be induced with ipecac within 1 hour of ingestion for alert pediatric or adult patients if health-care evaluation will be delayed.

In Hospital

- Gastric lavage should be performed in pediatric (tube size 24–32 French) or adult (tube size 36–42 French) patients presenting within 1 hour of a large ingestion or if serious effects are present.
- A dose of activated charcoal (1–2 g/kg) should be administered if a substantial ingestion has occurred within the previous few hours.

ANTIDOTES

There are no specific antidotes available for metformin poisoning.

ADJUNCTIVE TREATMENT

- Hemodialysis using a sodium bicarbonate buffer has been used for biguanide-induced metabolic acidosis.
- Dextrose is indicated for symptoms of hypoglycemia or a serum glucose less than 60 mg/dl.

—Adults should receive 50 ml of D50W by bolus intravenous infusion.
—Children should receive 2 to 4 ml/kg D25W (1–2 ml/kg D10W for neonates).
—The dextrose dose should be repeated until the blood glucose is more than 100 mg/dl.
—The patient's blood glucose level should be followed hourly to guide further therapy.
—An infusion of 5%, 10%, or 20% dextrose should be initiated as needed if recurrent hypoglycemia develops.
—Dextrose infusions of D20W or more require a central venous line to reduce venous injury.

- Insulin and dextrose infusion is indicated for severe biguanide-induced lactic acidosis; retrospective data suggest that the survival rate is better with insulin and dextrose infusion than with bicarbonate or hemodialysis; however, no well-controlled studies have been published.

—Dose for adults. Insulin should be administered 2 to 5 U/h, dextrose 1 to 3 g/h intravenously; titration is indicated to maintain euglycemia and improve acidosis.
—Adverse effects include hypoglycemia and hyperglycemia.

- Sodium bicarbonate may be indicated for severe metabolic acidosis (pH less than 7.1).

—Dose. 1 to 2 mEq/kg intravenous push is a reasonable starting dose in adults or children, repeated as needed to correct pH; arterial blood gases and electrolytes should be monitored frequently.
—Adverse effects include hypernatremia, volume overload, hyperosmolality, and alkalosis.

- Hypotension should be treated with isotonic fluid infusion (10–20 mg/kg), Trendelenburg positioning, and a vasopressor if needed (preferably dopamine). Norepinephrine may be added for refractory hypotension.

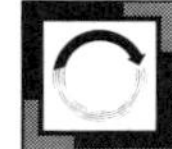

Follow-Up

PATIENT MONITORING

Any patient with acidosis, hypotension, altered mental status, hypoglycemia, or dysrhythmias should be monitored in an intensive care setting.

EXPECTED COURSE AND PROGNOSIS

- Hypoglycemia or mild acidosis usually resolves over 1 to 2 days.
- Sequelae of severe prolonged acidosis or hypoglycemia may develop.
- Severe acidosis is often associated with underlying illness (myocardial infarction, sepsis, renal failure), and mortality has approached 50% in some series.

DISCHARGE CRITERIA/INSTRUCTIONS

- From the emergency department. Discharge is recommended for asymptomatic patients who do not develop hypoglycemia, acidosis, hypotension, dysrhythmias, mental status changes during 6 hours of observation, decontamination, and psychiatric evaluation if needed.
- From the hospital. Patients may be discharged after resolution of hypoglycemia and metabolic acidosis, dysrhythmia, and hypotension, and after stabilization of any precipitating factors (e.g., sepsis, myocardial infarction, and renal failure).

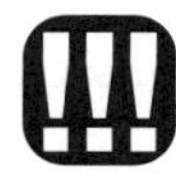

Pitfalls

DIAGNOSIS

Acidosis may develop without a change in the dose in patients with underlying disease states.

ICD-9-CM 962.3

Poisoning by hormones and synthetic substitutes: Insulins and antidiabetic agents.

See also: SECTION II, Hypotension chapter; SECTION III, Dextrose chapter.

RECOMMENDED READING

Luft D, Schmulling RM, Eggstein M. Lactic acidosis in biguanide-treated diabetics. *Diabetologia* 1978;14:75–87.

Misbin RI. Phenformin-associated lactic acidosis: pathogenesis and treatment. *Ann Intern Med* 1977;87:591–595.

Wilholm PE, Myrhed M. Metformin-associated lactic acidosis in Sweden 1977–1991. *Eur J Clin Pharmacol* 1993;44:589–591.

Author: Katherine M. Hurlbut

Reviewer: Richard C. Dart

Methamphetamine

Basics

DESCRIPTION

- Methamphetamine is a class II controlled substance and a common drug of abuse.
- Slang terms include meth, speed, crank, ice, crystal, and crystal meth.

FORMS AND USES

Methamphetamine is available by prescription as 5-mg tablets (Desoxyn), 10-mg tablets (Methampex), and 5-, 10-, or 15-mg long-acting tablets (Desoxyn Gradumet).

- FDA-approved indications are attention deficit disorder with hyperactivity and exogenous obesity.
- The typical dosage for adults is 2.5 to 5.0 mg/day.
- Illicit methamphetamine is smoked, ingested, or injected. Ice is a clear crystalline form of illicit methamphetamine that may be smoked. Compounds sold illicitly often contain other minor sympathomimetics instead of methamphetamine.

TOXIC DOSE

For the naive user, 1 mg/kg may cause serious toxicity. Much higher doses may be tolerated by chronic users.

PATHOPHYSIOLOGY

- Methamphetamine is a potent, synthetic sympathomimetic structurally related to norepinephrine.
- Peripherally, methamphetamine stimulates the release of norepinephrine from adrenergic neurons and the adrenal cortex, as well as directly stimulating α- and β-adrenergic receptors.
- Centrally, methamphetamine is a potent stimulator of the cerebral cortex, medullary respiratory center, and reticular activating system.
- Methamphetamine is more potent than amphetamine in its central effects and less potent in its peripheral effects.

EPIDEMIOLOGY

- Poisoning is common, with large regional variation in the incidence of abuse.
- Toxic effects following exposure are typically mild.
- Death occurs in patients who take escalating doses.

CAUSES

- Overdose is usually the result of recreational abuse.
- The possibility of child abuse should be considered in patients under 1 year of age; suicide attempt in patients over 6 years of age.

RISK FACTORS

- In geriatric patients, preexisting liver or kidney dysfunction increases toxic potential.
- A history of cardiovascular disease, cerebrovascular disease, seizure disorder, or psychosis predisposes to toxicity.

DRUG AND DISEASE INTERACTIONS

- All stimulants have an additive effects when used together.
- Use with monoamine oxidase inhibitors may cause hypertensive crisis.

PREGNANCY AND LACTATION

- US FDA Pregnancy Category C. The drug exerts animal teratogenic or embryocidal effects, but there are no controlled studies in women, or no studies are available in either animals or women.
- Birth defects reportedly associated with methamphetamine use during pregnancy include cardiac malformations, cleft palate, exencephaly, microcephaly, and mental retardation.
- Neonatal withdrawal symptoms have been reported.
- Infants exposed to methamphetamine have been reported to have low birth weight and to be prone to prematurity.

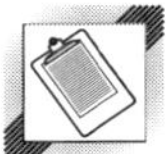

Diagnosis

DIFFERENTIAL DIAGNOSIS

- Toxic causes of agitation and seizure include amphetamine, theophylline, cocaine, isoniazid, tricyclic antidepressants, and monoamine oxidase inhibitors, among others.
- Nontoxic causes include alcohol withdrawal, meningitis, intracranial hemorrhage, hyperthyroidism, manic behavior, psychotic episode, seizure disorder, and cardiovascular crisis.
- Metabolic disorders and infectious processes also must be excluded.

SIGNS AND SYMPTOMS

- Toxicity is manifested by initial hypertension, hyperpyrexia, agitation, and hyperactivity.
- Fasciculation, seizures, and coma may develop.
- Toxic effects are persistent because of the drug's long half-life.
- Methamphetamine may cause serotonin syndrome (see SECTION II, Neuromalignant Syndrome and Serotonin Syndrome chapter).

Vital Signs

Hypertension, hyperthermia, and tachycardia are common.

Dermatologic

Skin is usually pale and diaphoretic.

Cardiovascular

A variety of dysrhythmias, myocardial ischemia or infarction, and aortic dissection have been reported.

Pulmonary

- Use of "Ice" has been associated with acute onset of pulmonary edema.
- Pulmonary hypertension may develop.

Genitourinary

- Increased sphincter tone may cause dysuria or acute urinary retention.
- Renal failure can occur secondary to dehydration or rhabdomyolysis.

Gastrointestinal

Anorexia, vomiting, diarrhea, and gastrointestinal hemorrhage have been reported.

Musculoskeletal

Rhabdomyolysis may occur.

Neurologic

- Symptoms range from restlessness, hyperactivity, talkativeness, insomnia, and headache to seizures and coma.
- Stroke and cerebral vasculitis have been reported.

Psychiatric

- Delusions, paranoia, and aggressive behavior are most common.
- Paranoid psychosis is the classic manifestation of chronic abuse.
- Visual, tactile, or auditory hallucinations may occur.
- Patients may also present with dyskinesia (bruxism, tics) and compulsive, repetitive, or stereotypical behavior.

PROCEDURES AND LABORATORY TESTS

Essential Tests

Laboratory testing may not be needed in asymptomatic patients.

Recommended Tests

- Serum electrolytes, glucose, BUN, and creatinine should be measured to assess the presence of metabolic acidosis or renal injury.
- ECG may reveal sinus tachycardia; other dysrhythmia suggests severe intoxication; ischemia may occur.
- Liver function, coagulation studies, and serum creatine kinase may be abnormal in patients with hyperthermia or agitation.
- Serum acetaminophen and aspirin levels and urine toxicology screen should be performed in overdose setting to detect occult ingestion.
- Head CT, lumbar puncture, and cultures should be performed in patients with altered mental status, headache, seizures, or fever.
- Chest radiograph should be obtained in patients with hypoxia or pulmonary symptoms.

Not Recommended Tests

Serum levels are not available or useful.

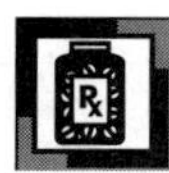

Treatment

- After decontamination, treatment is supportive and symptomatic, focusing on airway control and prompt treatment of hyperthermia, seizures, and dysrhythmias.
- Dose and time of exposure should be determined for all substances involved.

DIRECTING PATIENT COURSE

The health-care provider should call the poison control center when:

- Altered mental status, seizure, cardiac dysrhythmia, or other severe effects are present.
- Toxic effects are not consistent with the reported poisoning.
- Coingestant, drug interaction, or underlying disease presents unusual problems.

The patient should be referred to a health-care facility when:

- Attempted suicide or homicide is possible.
- Patient or caregiver seems unreliable.
- Signs of toxicity develop.
- Coingestant, drug interaction, or underlying disease presents unusual problems.

Admission Considerations

Inpatient treatment in an intensive care setting is warranted when a patient develops persistent acidosis or CNS or cardiac toxicity.

DECONTAMINATION

Out of Hospital

Emesis with ipecac should not be induced due to the potential for seizures.

In Hospital

- Gastric lavage should be administered in pediatric (tube size 24–32 French) or adult (tube size 36–42 French) patients presenting within 1 hour of a substantial ingestion or if serious effects are present.
- One dose of activated charcoal (1–2 g/kg) should be administered without a cathartic if a substantial ingestion has occurred within the previous few hours.

ANTIDOTES

There is no specific antidote available for methamphetamine poisoning.

ADJUNCTIVE TREATMENT

Agitation

A benzodiazepine familiar to the provider should be administered to control agitation.

- Diazepam

—The adult dose is 5 to 10 mg administered intravenously.
—The pediatric dose is 0.2 to 0.5 mg/kg administered intravenously.
—Doses are repeated at 10-minute intervals, titrated to effect.

- Lorazepam

—The adult dose is 1 to 2 mg administered intravenously.
—The pediatric dose is 0.05 mg/kg administered intravenously.
—Doses are repeated at 10-minute intervals, titrating to effect.

- The airway should be monitored closely.

Seizure

- Patent airway should be ensured.
- A benzodiazepine should be administered for initial control.
- If seizures persist or recur, another anticonvulsant, such as phenobarbital, should be added.

Hypertension

If hypertension is not responsive to treatment of agitation with benzodiazepines or if end-organ damage develops (aortic dissection, CNS bleed, myocardial infarction), a short-acting titratable agent, such as nitroprusside, should be administered.

Hypotension

- Hypotension should be treated with isotonic fluid infusion, Trendelenburg positioning, and a vasopressor if needed.
- Dopamine is preferred; norepinephrine is added for refractory hypotension.

Ventricular Dysrhythmia

Standard treatment should be initiated (see SECTION II, Ventricular Dysrhythmia chapter).

Rhabdomyolysis

- Adequate hydration and urine output (1–2 ml/kg/h) should be ensured.
- Urinary alkalinization has not proven beneficial.

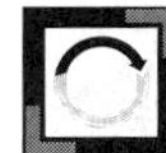

Follow-Up

PATIENT MONITORING

Respiratory and cardiac function should be monitored continuously for at least 24 hours, or as long as dysrhythmia is present.

EXPECTED COURSE AND PROGNOSIS

- Many cases of methamphetamine toxicity can be managed conservatively.
- Admitted patients can be usually be discharged within 48 hours.
- Complete recovery usually occurs over 1 to 2 days unless complications of rhabdomyolysis, seizures, or hyperthermia develop.

DISCHARGE CRITERIA/INSTRUCTIONS

- From the emergency department. Asymptomatic or minimally symptomatic patients may be discharged after 6 hours of observation, following gastrointestinal decontamination and psychiatric evaluation, if needed.
- From the hospital

—Patients may be discharged after monitoring for at least 24 hours, when a normal mental status and ECG have been achieved.
—Patients should be referred for substance abuse treatment.

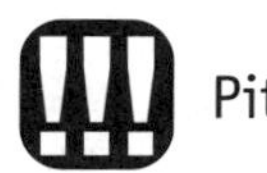

Pitfalls

DIAGNOSIS

- Methamphetamine abuse should be considered in any patient presenting with psychosis, violence, seizures, or cardiovascular abnormalities.
- Intravenous drug abusers should always be examined for infectious complications of abuse.

TREATMENT

Many methamphetamine users are polydrug abusers.

FOLLOW-UP

After abrupt cessation of methamphetamine use, withdrawal symptoms peak in 2 to 3 days (headaches, lethargy, dyspnea, and severe depression).

ICD-9-CM 971.2

Poisoning by drugs primarily affecting the autonomic nervous system: Sympathomimetics (adrenergics).

See also: SECTION II, Hypertension, Hypotension, Seizure (Unexplained), Neuroleptic Malignant Syndrome and Serotonin Syndrome, and Ventricular Dysrhythmias chapters; and SECTION III, Nitroprusside chapter.

RECOMMENDED READING

Beebe DK, Walley E. Smokable methamphetamine ("ice"): an old drug in a different form. *Am Fam Phys* 1995;51:449–453.

Derlet RW, Heischober B. Methamphetamine: stimulant of the 90's? *West J Med* 1990;153:625–628.

Author: David Nyman

Reviewer: Richard C. Dart

Methanol

Basics

DESCRIPTION

- Methanol (methyl alcohol, wood alcohol) is present in windshield wiper fluid, Sterno, industrial solvents, and other products.
- The most common source is windshield wiper fluid, which may contain 95% methanol.
- Methanol is commonly added to ethanol for denaturation and may contaminate bootleg liquor (moonshine).

TOXIC DOSE

Ingestion of just 0.15 ml/kg of 100% methanol may cause toxicity (1.5 ml in a 10-kg child, 10 ml in a 65-kg adult).

PATHOPHYSIOLOGY

- Methanol is metabolized by the enzyme alcohol dehydrogenase to formaldehyde, which is then metabolized to formic acid.
- Retinal toxicity is caused by formic acid accumulation.
- Ethanol is a preferred substrate for alcohol dehydrogenase and will delay formation of formaldehyde and formic acid.
- Folic acid or tetrahydrofolate (Leucovorin) enhances the elimination of formic acid.

EPIDEMIOLOGY

- Poisoning is common.
- Toxic effects are typically severe, if untreated.
- Death may occur in untreated patients.

CAUSES

- Pediatric cases are usually accidental.
- Adult cases usually involve suicidal ingestion or ingestion of methanol as an alcohol substitute.
- The possibility of child abuse should be considered if the patient is under 1 year of age; suicide attempt if the patient is over 6 years of age.
- Inhalation or dermal absorption can produce toxicity under some conditions.

PREGNANCY AND LACTATION

Methanol is a proven teratogen in animals.

WORKPLACE STANDARDS

- ACGIH. TLV TWA is 200 ppm; STEL is 250 ppm.
- OSHA. PEL (ceiling limit) is 200 ppm; PEL TWA is 250 ppm, no ceiling limit.
- NIOSH. IDLH is 6000 ppm.

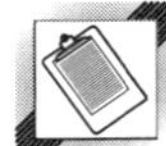

Diagnosis

DIFFERENTIAL DIAGNOSIS

- Toxic causes of increased anion gap metabolic acidosis include iron, isoniazid, lactic acidosis, ethylene glycol, salicylic acid, and toluene.
- Nontoxic causes of metabolic acidosis are uremia, diabetic ketoacidosis, and alcoholic ketoacidosis.
- Other causes of visual disturbances include ethambutol or quinine poisoning.

SIGNS AND SYMPTOMS

- After ingestion, mild inebriation may be apparent early, followed by worsening metabolic acidosis in untreated patients.
- Development of metabolic acidosis is usually delayed for 8 to 12 hours postingestion.
- Onset may be further delayed by concurrent ethanol intoxication.

Vital Signs

- Hyperpnea usually develops to compensate for metabolic acidosis.
- Hypotension may develop late in severe cases.

HEENT

- Blurred, double, or hazy vision begins several hours after ingestion.
- Constricted visual fields, dilated pupils, hyperemic optic disk and retinal edema, and transient or permanent blindness may develop.

Gastrointestinal

Nausea, vomiting, and abdominal pain may develop.

Renal

Hematuria and acute renal insufficiency have been reported.

Fluids and Electrolytes

Hypokalemia, hypomagnesemia, and elevated anion gap metabolic acidosis are common and may become severe.

Neurologic

- The earliest sign is inebriation, which progresses to ataxia, seizures, and coma in severe cases.
- Parkinsonism may develop as a sequela of severe intoxication.

PROCEDURES AND LABORATORY TESTS

Essential Tests

- Serum electrolytes, BUN, creatinine, and glucose should be measured.
- Elevated anion gap acidosis supports the diagnosis.
- Hypoglycemia may occur during ethanol therapy.
- Arterial blood gases should be measured to assess metabolic acidosis.
- Serum methanol level greater than 50 mg/dl indicates need for hemodialysis; 25 to 50 mg/dl is controversial, and dialysis usually is advised.

Recommended Tests

- Serum ethanol level may be needed to assess intoxication; concurrent ethanol ingestion may delay onset of methanol toxicity for 24 hours or more.
- Serum osmolarity may be measured (by freezing point depression method), if serum methanol level is not readily available.

—An elevated osmolarity gap is consistent with methanol poisoning.
—A normal osmolarity gap cannot exclude methanol poisoning.

- ECG, serum acetaminophen, and aspirin levels may be ordered in an overdose setting to detect occult ingestion.
- Head CT, lumbar puncture, and cultures may be performed as indicated in patients with altered mental status, headache, seizure, or fever.

Not Recommended Tests

Serum osmolarity measurement is not recommended if serum methanol level is available within several hours.

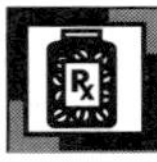

Treatment

- Treatment should focus on correction of acid-base abnormality and fomepizole or ethanol administration, followed by hemodialysis in serious cases.
- The dose and time of exposure should be determined for all substances.
- Consultation with a toxicologist and nephrologist should be considered early in symptomatic patients.

DIRECTING PATIENT COURSE

The health-care provider should call the poison control center when:

- Acidosis, visual changes, or other serious effects are present.
- Toxic effects are not consistent with methanol.
- Coingestant, drug interaction, or underlying disease presents an unusual challenge.

The patient should be referred to a health-care facility when:

- Methanol ingestion may have occurred or when any toxic effects are present.
- Attempted suicide or homicide is possible.
- Patient or caregiver seems unreliable.
- Coingestant, drug interaction, or underlying disease presents an unusual challenge.

Admission Considerations

Inpatient treatment is warranted when the patient has methanol levels greater than 20 mg/dl or evidence of organ injury produced by methanol (e.g., elevated anion gap acidosis, visual or mental status changes).

DECONTAMINATION

Out of Hospital

Emesis with ipecac should be considered within 1 hour of ingestion for an alert pediatric or adult patient if health-care evaluation will be delayed.

In Hospital

- Gastric aspiration with nasogastric tube should be considered in pediatric or adult patients presenting within 1 hour of ingestion or if serious effects are present.
- Large-bore tube should be used for gastric aspiration and lavage if coingestion is possible.
- One dose of activated charcoal (1–2 g/kg) should be administered without a cathartic if coingestion is possible.

ANTIDOTES

Fomepizole (Antizol)

Fomepizole is the preferred agent for treatment.

Indications

History of possible methanol ingestion and clinical evidence of toxicity (e.g., increased anion gas metabolic acidosis, visual complaints) or increased osmolal gap, and serum methanol level greater than 20 mg/dl indicate the need for fomepizole administration.

Contraindications

Patients with a history of documented allergic reaction to fomepizole should receive a different type of therapy.

Method of Administration

- Loading dose for adult or pediatric patient is 15 mg/kg intravenously.
- Maintenance dose for all age groups is 10 mg/kg every 12 hours for four doses, then 15 mg every 12 hours thereafter until the methanol level is less than 20 mg/dl.
- Each dose is diluted in 100 ml normal saline or D5W and infused over 30 minutes.
- For further details (e.g., dosing during hemodialysis), see SECTION III, Fomepizole chapter.

Ethanol

Ethanol is administered as a 10% solution in D5W.

Indications

Ethanol infusion may be used if fomepizole is not available; indications are the same as for use of fomepizole.

Contraindications

Preexisting ethanol level greater than 125 mg/dl obviates the need for the ethanol loading dose.

Method of Administration

See SECTION III, Ethanol chapter, for details of administration.

- Loading dose is 10 cc/kg of a 10% ethanol solution infused intravenously over 1 hour.
- Maintenance dose is 1.0 to 2.0 ml/kg/h of 10% ethanol solution infused intravenously.
- Target blood ethanol level is 100–125 mg/dl.
- Oral treatment may be used when intravenous formulation is not available.

ADJUNCTIVE TREATMENT

- Folate or tetrahydrofolate (Leucovorin) has been recommended to hasten elimination of formic acid.
- Leucovorin 1 to 2 mg/kg may be administered intravenously every 4 to 6 hours until methanol becomes undetectable.
- Hemodialysis is recommended for serum methanol levels greater than 50 mg/dl (and should be considered for patients with levels in the 25 to 50 mg/dl range) or if signs of end-organ injury are apparent (elevated anion gap acidosis, visual or mental status changes).

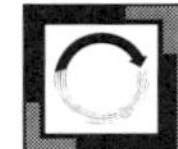

Follow-Up

PATIENT MONITORING

- Hourly evaluation of acid-base status and glucose and methanol levels is performed initially to determine whether condition is deteriorating despite therapy.
- Hourly serum ethanol levels are measured to guide ethanol infusion.

EXPECTED COURSE AND PROGNOSIS

- Full recovery is expected if appropriate management is initiated before severe effects develop.
- Permanent visual deficits may develop.
- Renal failure subsequent to myoglobinuria may develop.
- Parkinsonism occurs rarely, associated with basal ganglia infarcts.
- Polyneuropathy occurs rarely.

DISCHARGE CRITERIA/INSTRUCTIONS

- From the emergency department. Asymptomatic patients may be discharged when the following conditions are met:

—Normal electrolytes, BUN, and creatinine
—Serum ethanol and methanol levels of zero
—Eight hours of observation
—Completed psychiatric evaluation, if needed

- From hospital

—An asymptomatic patient with normal or stable laboratory values may be discharged following psychiatric evaluation, if needed.
—Serum methanol and ethanol levels must be zero before discharge.

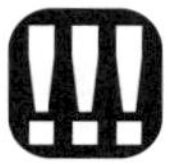

Pitfalls

DIAGNOSIS

- An anion gap metabolic acidosis may not be apparent within the first 8 to 12 hours of acute poisoning.
- An elevated osmolarity gap is consistent with methanol poisoning, but a normal osmolarity gap cannot exclude methanol poisoning.
- In late presentations of methanol poisoning, the osmolarity gap may be "normal" while the anion gap is elevated.

TREATMENT

- Serum glucose should be monitored during ethanol infusion to detect hypoglycemia.
- If endotracheal intubation is performed, the increased minute ventilation (compensation for acidosis) that was present before intubation should be maintained.

ICD-9-CM 980.1

Toxic effect of methyl alcohol.

See also: SECTION II, Anion Gap Metabolic Acidosis (Unexplained) chapter; and SECTION III, Ethanol, Folic Acid/Leucovorin, and Fomepizol (4-Methylpyrazole) chapters.

RECOMMENDED READING

Jacobsen D, McMartin KE. Methanol and ethylene glycol poisonings: mechanism of toxicity, clinical course, diagnosis and treatment. *Med Toxicol* 1986;1:309–334.

Author: Luke Yip

Reviewer: Katherine M. Hurlbut

Methenamine

Basics

DESCRIPTION

Methenamine hippurate and methenamine mandelate are antimicrobial agents for the treatment of urinary tract infections.

FORMS AND USES

- Adult, 1 g twice a day orally with ascorbic acid
- Pediatric, for children over 6 years, 40 mg/kg/day twice a day of methenamine hippurate or 0.05 to 0.1 g/kg/day three times a day of methenamine mandelate

TOXIC DOSE

The toxic dose is unknown, but is expected to be large.

PATHOPHYSIOLOGY

- Methenamine is inactive until excreted in the urine, where it is converted at a pH of less than 5.5 to ammonia and formaldehyde, which exert its antibacterial effect.
- Patients with moderate to severe renal insufficiency do not concentrate enough of the drug for it to be clinically effective.

EPIDEMIOLOGY

Poisoning is uncommon.

CAUSES

Child neglect or abuse should be considered if the patient is less than 1 year of age, suicide attempt if the patient is over 6 years of age.

DRUG AND DISEASE INTERACTIONS

Use of drugs or food that alkalinize the urine inhibit the conversion of methenamine.

PREGNANCY AND LACTATION

US FDA Pregnancy Category C. The drug exerts animal teratogenic or embryocidal effects, but there are no controlled studies in women, or no studies are available in animals or women.

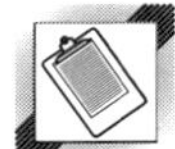

Diagnosis

DIFFERENTIAL DIAGNOSIS

- Toxic causes of gastroenteritis include:

—Bacterial food poisoning
—Early lithium toxicity
—Arsenic, selenium, mercury, or other heavy-metal poisoning

- Nontoxic causes include

—Bacterial, viral, or parasitic gastroenteritis
—Inflammatory bowel disease

SIGNS AND SYMPTOMS

Toxicity is manifested primarily as nausea, vomiting, diarrhea, abdominal cramps, abdominal discomfort, and stomatitis.

Pulmonary

Lipoid pneumonia is seen in dysphagic patients taking the oil-based suspension.

Gastrointestinal

Acute ingestion causes nausea, vomiting, diarrhea, and so forth.

Renal

- Dysuria may occur with therapeutic use.
- Hematuria has been reported following accidental overdose.

PROCEDURES AND LABORATORY TESTS

Essential Tests

No specific laboratory tests are needed in asymptomatic patients.

Recommended Tests

- Serum electrolytes, BUN, creatinine in symptomatic patients to assess fluid and electrolyte status and potential renal injury.
- ECG, serum acetaminophen, and aspirin level screen in overdose setting should be used to detect occult ingestion.

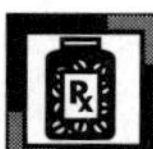

Treatment

- Treatment should focus on supportive care of acute gastrointestinal fluid losses.
- Dose and time of exposure should be determined for all substances involved.

DIRECTING PATIENT COURSE

The health-care professional should call the poison control center when:

- Severe or persistent effects develop.
- Coingestant, drug interaction, or underlying disease presents an unusual problem.

The patient should be referred to a health-care facility when:

- Suicide or homicide attempt is possible.
- Toxic effects develop.
- Coingestant, drug interaction, or underlying disease presents an unusual problem.

Admission Considerations

Inpatient management is warranted if the patient has persistent severe gastrointestinal effects.

DECONTAMINATION

Out of Hospital

Ipecac-induced emesis is not recommended.

In Hospital

- Following ingestion, one dose of activated charcoal (1–2 g/kg) should be administered without a cathartic if a substantial ingestion has occurred within the previous few hours.
- Gastric lavage is not indicated for isolated ingestions.

ANTIDOTES

There is no specific antidote for methenamine poisoning.

ADJUNCTIVE TREATMENT

Symptomatic care may include intravenous fluids and antiemetics.

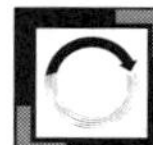

Follow-Up

PATIENT MONITORING

Urinalysis with urine pH should be followed during therapeutic use.

EXPECTED COURSE AND PROGNOSIS

Prompt recovery is expected with supportive and symptomatic care.

DISCHARGE CRITERIA/INSTRUCTIONS

Patients may be discharged from the emergency department or hospital when toxic effects resolve or stabilize and after psychiatric evaluation, if needed.

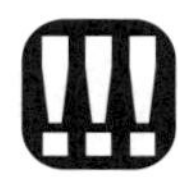

Pitfalls

DIAGNOSIS

Rare therapeutic use of methenamine may lead to misdiagnosis.

ICD-9-CM 961

Poisoning by other anti-infectives.

RECOMMENDED READING

Timmerman RJ, Schroer JA. Lipoid pneumonia caused by methenamine mandelate suspension. *JAMA* 1973;225:1524.

Author: Steven A. Seifert

Reviewer: Richard C. Dart

Methocarbamol

Basics

DESCRIPTION

Methocarbamol (Robaxin, Robaxisal) is a centrally acting skeletal muscle relaxant.

FORMS AND USES

- Methocarbamol is used in the treatment of painful musculoskeletal conditions (strains, sprains, muscle spasm) as well as for tetanus and black widow spider envenomation.
- Oral adult dosage is 4 to 8 grams a day in divided doses
- Parenteral adult dosage is 10 ml (1000 mg) administered at different intramuscular sites every 8 hours, or 10 to 30 ml intravenously every 6 hours, to a maximum rate of 3 ml/min.
- Pediatric use is recommended only for tetanus; intravenous rate of infusion at 15 mg/kg every 6 hours

TOXIC DOSE

There is no established toxic dose. Minor effects may develop just above the therapeutic dose.

PATHOPHYSIOLOGY

- The mechanism of action of methocarbamol is unknown.
- Methocarbamol does not act directly on skeletal muscles or peripheral nerves.

EPIDEMIOLOGY

Poisoning is uncommon.

CAUSES

- Toxicity is usually caused by intentional ingestion.
- Child neglect or abuse should be considered if the patient is less than 1 year of age, suicide attempt if the patient is over 6 years of age.

DRUG AND DISEASE INTERACTIONS

- The intravenous formulation contains polyethylene glycol 300 in the vehicle and is thus contraindicated in patients with renal pathology.
- CNS depressant medications have an additive effect with methocarbamol.

PREGNANCY AND LACTATION

US FDA Pregnancy Category C. The drug exerts animal teratogenic or embryocidal effects, but there are no controlled studies in women, or no studies are available in either animals or women.

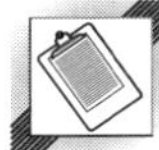

Diagnosis

DIFFERENTIAL DIAGNOSIS

Toxic causes of CNS depression include barbiturates, benzodiazepines, baclofen, GHB, opiates, and many others.

SIGNS AND SYMPTOMS

The primary symptom is CNS depression.

Vital Signs

Respiratory depression may develop with large dosage.

HEENT

Nystagmus and blurred vision may occur.

Cardiovascular

Tachycardia and hypotension may occur.

Neurologic

CNS depression, leading in rare cases to coma, may occur.

PROCEDURES AND LABORATORY TESTS

Essential Tests

No tests may be needed in asymptomatic patients.

Recommended Tests

- Arterial blood gas or pulse oximetry should be assessed in symptomatic patients.
- ECG, serum acetaminophen, and aspirin levels should be monitored in an overdose setting to detect occult ingestion.
- Salicylate level should be checked if the patient ingested Robaxisal.
- Serum electrolytes, glucose, BUN, creatinine to assess other potential causes of CNS depression.
- Head CT, lumbar puncture, cultures to CNS depression.
- Serum and plasma levels are not useful.

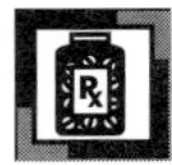

Treatment

- Treatment should focus on supportive care with appropriate airway management.
- Dose and time of exposure for all substances involved should be determined.

DIRECTING PATIENT COURSE

The health-care professional should call the poison control center when:

- Severe or persistent effects develop.
- Coingestant, drug interaction, or underlying disease presents an unusual problem.

The patient should be referred to a health-care facility when:

- Suicide or homicide attempt is possible.
- Toxic effects develop.
- Coingestant, drug interaction, or underlying disease presents an unusual problem.

Admission Considerations

Admit any patient that demonstrates altered mental status, nystagmus, or abnormal vital signs.

DECONTAMINATION

Out of Hospital

Emesis should not be induced.

In Hospital

• Gastric lavage should be performed in pediatric (tube size 24–32 French) or adult (tube size 36–42 French) patients presenting within 1 hour of a large ingestion or if serious effects are present.
• One dose of activated charcoal (1–2 g/kg) should be administered without a cathartic if a substantial ingestion has occurred within the previous few hours.

ANTIDOTES

There is no specific antidote for methocarbamol poisoning.

ADJUNCTIVE TREATMENT

• Hemodialysis, hemoperfusion, or plasmapheresis are not necessary and are unlikely to be effective.
• Hypotension

—The patient should be placed in Trendelenburg position and 10–20 ml/kg of normal saline infused.
—A vasopressor is used, if needed; dopamine is preferred and norepinephrine may be added for refractory hypotension.

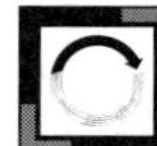

Follow-Up

PATIENT MONITORING

Respiratory and cardiac monitoring should be performed continuously in symptomatic patients.

EXPECTED COURSE AND PROGNOSIS

Patients that receive adequate supportive care and airway maintenance are expected to recover.

DISCHARGE CRITERIA/INSTRUCTIONS

Patients may be discharged from the emergency department or hospital after a 6-hour observation period and following decontamination and psychiatric evaluation, if needed.

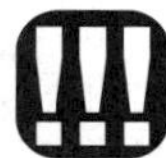

Pitfalls

TREATMENT

• Robaxisal contains salicylate (325 mg per tablet); significant salicylate toxicity may occur.
• Patients with musculoskeletal pain may be taking more than one pain and muscle-relaxant medication.

ICD-9-CM 968.0

Poisoning by other central nervous system depressants and anesthetics: central nervous system muscle-tone depressants.

See also: SECTION II, Hypotension chapter; and SECTION IV, Salicylates chapter.

RECOMMENDED READING

De Lee JC, Rockwood CA. Skeletal muscle spasm and a review of muscle relaxants. *Curr Ther Res* 1980;27:64–74.

Kemal M, Imami R, Poklis A. A fatal methocarbamol intoxication. *J Forensic Sci* 1982;217–222.

Author: Steven A. Seifert

Reviewer: Gerald F. O'Malley

Methoxamine

Basics

DESCRIPTION

- Methoxamine hydrochloride (Vasoxyl) is a sympathomimetic agent used to reverse hypotension during spinal and general anesthesia.
- It was used in the past to terminate supraventricular tachycardia not responsive to other modes of therapy.

FORMS AND USES

- Methoxamine is available only in parenteral form.
- The usual therapeutic dose for intraoperative hypotension is 3 to 5 mg slow intravenous push.

PATHOPHYSIOLOGY

- Methoxamine is a sympathomimetic amine with potent α-adrenergic receptor agonist effect.
- Onset of action is 1 to 2 minutes following intravenous administration; duration of action is 60 to 90 minutes.
- The mechanism of pressor effect is peripheral vasoconstriction without inotropic or chronotropic effects; reflex bradycardia is common.
- Toxic effects may occur at therapeutic doses secondary to underlying medical conditions.

RISK FACTORS

Drug interactions. Effects are additive with other sympathomimetic drugs (monoamine oxidase inhibitors, tricyclic antidepressants, vasopressin, other sympathomimetics or ergot alkaloids) or conditions (hyperthyroidism).

PREGNANCY AND LACTATION

- US FDA Pregnancy Category D. Positive evidence of fetal risk exists, but benefits in certain situations (e.g., life-threatening situations or serious disease) may make use of this drug acceptable despite its risks.
- Methoxamine may cause uterine hypertonus.
- Methoxamine may cause fetal bradycardia.

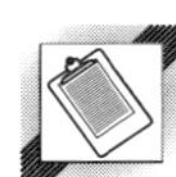

Diagnosis

SIGNS AND SYMPTOMS

Vital Signs

Rapid and prolonged increase in blood pressure, often associated with reflex bradycardia may occur

Cardiac

- Hypertension and bradycardia may occur.
- Myocardial infarction may occur in patients with coronary artery disease.
- Methoxamine may exacerbate preexisting bradycardia, heart block, or peripheral vasoconstriction.

Gastrointestinal

Nausea and vomiting may occur.

Neurologic

Headaches and tingling of extremities may occur.

PROCEDURES AND LABORATORY TESTS

Essential Tests

No tests may be needed in asymptomatic patient.

Recommended Tests

- Electrolytes, ECG, and cardiac monitoring is advised in symptomatic patients.
- Plasma cortisol and adrenocorticotropic hormone levels may be increased.

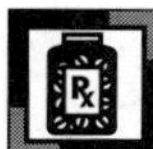

Treatment

Treatment should focus on termination of methoxamine infusion.

DIRECTING PATIENT COURSE

The health-care provider should call the poison control center when:

- Hypertension becomes uncontrolled.
- Drug interaction or underlying disease presents an unusual problem.

Admission Considerations

Inpatient management is warranted if injury from hypertension develops or if hypertension cannot be controlled.

ANTIDOTES

There is no specific antidote for methoxamine poisoning.

ADJUNCTIVE TREATMENT

- Severe or prolonged hypertension can be treated using an agent such as nitroprusside.
- Symptomatic bradycardia can be treated with atropine (but is often not needed if patient is hypertensive).

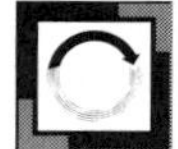

Follow-Up

PATIENT MONITORING

Electrocardiogram and blood pressure should be monitored continuously.

EXPECTED COURSE AND PROGNOSIS

Recovery is likely, with control of excessive hypertension, and in the absence of complications of cardiac ischemia or intracranial pathology.

DISCHARGE CRITERIA/INSTRUCTIONS

The patient may be discharged after adverse effects have resolved.

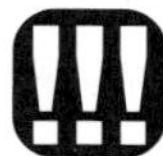

Pitfalls

TREATMENT

Methoxamine contains potassium metabisulfite, which may cause allergic and anaphylactic sulfite reactions in sensitive individuals.

ICD-9-CM 971.2

Poisoning by drugs primarily affecting the autonomic nervous system: sympathomimetics.

See also: SECTION II, Bradycardia and Hypertension chapters; and SECTION III, Atropine and Nitroprusside chapters.

RECOMMENDED READING

King BD, Dripps RD. The use of methoxamine for maintenance of the circulation during spinal anesthesia. *Surg Gynecol Obstet* 1950;90:659–665.

Smith NT, Whitcher C. Acute hemodynamic effects of methoxamine in man. *Anesthesiology* 1967;28:735–748.

Author: Steven A. Seifert

Reviewer: Richard C. Dart

Methyl Bromide

Basics

DESCRIPTION

Methyl bromide (bromomethane) is a colorless and odorless gas used as a fumigant.

FORMS AND USES

- Methyl bromide is used primarily as an insecticide fumigant of agricultural and residential dwellings.
- It is also used in ionization chambers, for degreasing wool, and for extracting oil from flowers, seeds, and nuts.

TOXIC DOSE

- Acute injury has resulted from inhalation of under 500 ppm for many hours.
- Death has occurred following brief exposure to 60,000 ppm.

PATHOPHYSIOLOGY

- Because it lacks odor and does not cause immediate irritation of mucous membranes, methyl bromide poisoning may not be noticed initially.
- The precise mechanism of toxicity is unknown.
- The primary target organ is the CNS.

EPIDEMIOLOGY

- Poisoning is rare.
- Toxic effects are typically moderate.
- Death occurs in severe exposure, generally from work-related accidents.
- Carcinogenesis. Animal data indicate that methyl bromide is a possible carcinogen.

PREGNANCY AND LACTATION

Severe fetotoxicity develops in animals.

WORKPLACE STANDARDS

- ACGIH. TLV TWA is 1 ppm; no STEL.
- OSHA. PEL TWA is 5 ppm.
- NIOSH. IDLH is 2,000 ppm.

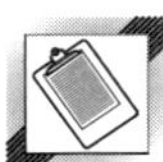

Diagnosis

DIFFERENTIAL DIAGNOSIS

- Toxic causes of mental status depression and seizures are numerous, including organochlorine insecticides, heavy metals, carbon monoxide, carbon disulfide, hydrogen sulfide, and isoniazid, among others.
- Nontoxic causes include seizure disorder, head trauma, intracranial bleed, tumor or infection, severe electrolyte disturbance, or any cause of hypoxia.

SIGNS AND SYMPTOMS

- Lethal exposure may occur at concentrations that do not cause an initial irritation.
- Initial symptoms following serious exposure begin with nausea and headache and progress to tremors, myoclonus, and seizures; symptom onset may be delayed 1 to 36 hours post-exposure.
- Chronic exposure may produce symptoms of acute exposure plus visual and hearing complaints, incoordination, and ataxia, as well as loss of libido and personality changes.

HEENT

Conjunctivitis and throat irritation may develop after inhalation.

Dermatologic

Dermal erythema and bullae may develop after exposure, and corneal injury may occur.

Cardiovascular

Dysrhythmias leading to ventricular fibrillation may develop in severe cases.

Pulmonary

- Respiratory irritation is common after inhalation.
- Pulmonary edema may develop after severe exposure and may be delayed.

Gastrointestinal

Nausea and vomiting are common.

Hepatic

Elevations in liver enzymes may develop.

Musculoskeletal

Rhabdomyolysis may develop with prolonged myoclonus or seizures.

Renal

Acute tubular necrosis may develop in severe poisoning.

Neurologic

- CNS excitation, myoclonus, and repeated seizures develop with severe intoxication.
- CNS depression and coma also may occur.
- Peripheral neuropathy occurs rarely.
- Sequelae include depression, ataxia, sensory neuropathy, and myoclonus.

PROCEDURES AND LABORATORY TESTS

Essential Tests

No tests may be needed for asymptomatic patients with minor exposure.

Recommended Tests

- Serum electrolytes, BUN, creatinine

—Elevated serum chloride and depressed anion gap suggest bromide intoxication because bromide is measured as chloride in many assays.
—Acidosis suggests serious toxicity with seizures, prolonged myoclonus, or agitation.

- Serum liver enzymes. Mild elevation in liver enzymes suggests exposure.
- Measurement of arterial blood gases or pulse oximetry is recommended in patients with respiratory complaints.
- Serum creatine kinase may be elevated in patients with prolonged myoclonus or seizures.
- Serum bromide level is used to confirm diagnosis.
- Head CT, lumbar puncture, complete blood count, blood cultures, and urine toxicology screen are recommended as needed to rule out other etiologies of seizures and altered mental status.
- Chest radiograph is recommended in patients with respiratory complaints.

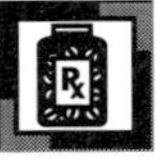

Treatment

- Treatment should focus on control of airway and seizures.
- Dose and time of exposure should be determined for all substances involved.

DIRECTING PATIENT COURSE

The health-care provider should call the poison control center when:

- Myoclonus, seizures, CNS depression, or other severe effects are present.
- Signs and symptoms are not consistent with methyl bromide poisoning.
- Coingestant, drug interaction, or underlying disease presents an unusual problem.

The patient should be referred to a health-care facility when:

- Attempted suicide or homicide is possible.
- Patient or caregiver seems unreliable.
- Toxic effects are present.
- Coingestant, drug interaction, or underlying disease presents an unusual problem.

Admission Considerations

Inpatient treatment is warranted when the patient has CNS effects or respiratory effects (e.g., persistent cough, infiltrates).

DECONTAMINATION

Out of Hospital

- The patient should be removed from the contaminated environment.
- Oxygen should be administered.
- Contaminated clothing should be removed and the skin washed.
- Exposed eyes or skin should be irrigated with copious amounts of water.

In Hospital

- Oxygen should be administered.
- Contaminated clothing should be removed and the skin washed.
- Exposed eyes or skin should be irrigated with copious amounts of water.

ANTIDOTES

There is no specific antidote for methyl bromide toxicity.

ADJUNCTIVE TREATMENT

Seizure

- Adequate airway and oxygenation should be ensured.
- A benzodiazepine should be administered for initial control.

—Diazepam
 —The adult dose is 5 to 10 mg intravenously, repeated every 10 minutes if needed.
 —The pediatric dose is 0.2 to 0.5 mg/kg intravenously, repeated every 10 minutes if needed.
 —The need for intubation should be monitored closely.

—Lorazepam
 —The adult dose is 2 to 4 mg by intravenous push over 2 to 5 minutes, repeated every 10 minutes if needed.
 —The pediatric dose is 0.1 mg/kg by intravenous push over 2 to 5 minutes, not to exceed 4 mg/dose, repeated every 10 minutes if needed.
 —The need for intubation should be monitored closely.

- If seizures persist or recur, another anticonvulsant such as phenobarbital or phenytoin should be added.
- In severe cases refractory to treatment, endotracheal intubation and neuromuscular paralysis may be needed.

Diuresis

- Anecdotal reports and animal studies suggest that diuretics increase urinary bromide excretion over the administration of intravenous chloride alone.
- Furosemide 10 mg intravenously every 6 to 12 hours has been recommended.
- No study has shown any effect on clinical outcome, and dehydration is a potential complication if fluid status is not carefully monitored.
- Hemodialysis has been used to rapidly reduce serum bromide levels after methyl bromide exposure.

Hypotension

- Hypotension should be treated with isotonic fluid infusion, Trendelenburg positioning, and a vasopressor if needed.
- Dopamine is preferred.
- Norepinephrine may be used for refractory hypotension.

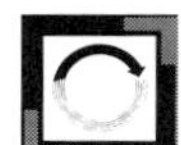

Follow-Up

PATIENT MONITORING

Continuous cardiac and respiratory monitoring should be undertaken in symptomatic patients.

EXPECTED COURSE AND PROGNOSIS

- Patients with mild to moderate intoxication generally recover promptly with supportive care.
- Those with prolonged seizures and myoclonus may develop permanent neurologic impairment.

DISCHARGE CRITERIA/INSTRUCTIONS

- From the emergency department. Because of the potential for delayed deterioration, most patients with known exposure should be admitted to the hospital.
- From the hospital. The patient may be discharged when CNS depression, myoclonus, and seizures have resolved and oxygenation is normal.

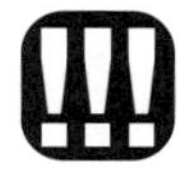

Pitfalls

DIAGNOSIS

- Methyl bromide should be considered when diagnosing seizure in a patient without a history of seizure disorder.
- Lethal poisoning can occur at air concentrations that do not produce immediate pulmonary irritation.
- Initial chest radiograph may be negative in the face of hypoxia.

ICD-9-CM 989

Toxic effect of other substances, chiefly nonmedicinal as to source.

See also: SECTION II, Hypotension and Seizures chapters.

RECOMMENDED READING

Henzstein J, Cullen MR. Methyl bromide intoxication in 4 field-workers during removal of soil fumigation sheets. *Am J Ind Med* 1990;17:321–326.

Hezemans-Boer M, Toonstra J, Meulenbelt J, et al. Skin lesions due to exposure to methyl bromide. *Arch Dermatol* 1988;124:917–921.

Hustinx WNM, van der Laar RTH, van Huffelen AC, et al. Systemic effects of inhalational methyl bromide poisoning: a study of nine cases occupationally exposed due to inadvertent spread during fumigation. *Br J Ind Med* 1993;50:155–159.

Author: Katherine M. Hurlbut

Reviewer: Luke Yip

Methyldopa

Basics

DESCRIPTION

Methyldopa is an antihypertensive agent.

FORMS AND USES

- Methyldopa is available as a tablet, suspension, intravenous solution, or in combination with a diuretic.
- It is available as methyldopa, alpha methyldopa, Aldomet, Aldoril, and Aldoclor.

TOXIC DOSE

- The lethal dose is unknown.
- Adult ingestion of several grams typically causes toxicity.

PATHOPHYSIOLOGY

- Mechanism of action is poorly understood but is believed to have central α_2 receptor agonist activity similar to clonidine.
- Methyldopa also reduces adrenergic activity by inhibiting dopa-decarboxylase.
- Peak effects are usually seen within 4 to 6 hours.

EPIDEMIOLOGY

Poisoning is uncommon.

CAUSES

- Poisoning is typically caused by inadvertent ingestion.
- Child neglect or abuse should be considered if the patient is less than 1 year of age, suicide attempt if the patient is over 6 years of age.

DRUG AND DISEASE INTERACTIONS

- Preexisting liver disease prediposes to hepatic injury during chronic use.
- Concurrent ingestion with other agents that cause hypotension increases the likelihood of hypotension.

PREGNANCY AND LACTATION

- US FDA Pregnancy Category C. The drug exerts animal teratogenic or embryocidal effects, but there are no controlled studies in women, or no studies are available in animals or women.
- Excretion in breast milk has been reported.

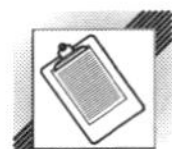

Diagnosis

DIFFERENTIAL DIAGNOSIS

- Other toxicologic causes of hypotension and CNS depression are numerous.
- Other than obtaining a history, there is no other method for differentiation from other causes.

SIGNS AND SYMPTOMS

Vital Signs

- Bradycardia, hypotension, and hypertension may occur with acute overdose.
- Orthostatic hypotension may occur following acute overdose or during chronic therapy.
- Fever has been reported during chronic therapy.
- Paradoxical hypertension is rare and may be more common following intravenous administration.

HEENT

Dry mouth is common.

Gastrointestinal

Nausea and vomiting are common.

Hepatic

- Hepatitis develops rarely.
- Mild elevations in liver function tests are common during the first 6 months of therapy.

Hematologic

Depression of red blood cell, white blood cell, and platelet production may occur during chronic therapy.

Immunologic

Positive results of lupus erythematosus cell, rheumatoid factor, and antinuclear antibody tests may occur on chronic therapy.

Neurologic

CNS depression progressing to coma may occur following acute overdose. Generalized weakness has been reported following acute overdose and during chronic therapy.

Psychiatric

Depression and decreased mental acuity may occur.

PROCEDURES AND LABORATORY TESTS

Essential Tests

ECG and hemodynamic monitoring should be undertaken for all patients with acute overdose and for symptomatic patients on chronic therapy.

Recommended Tests

- Serum electrolytes, BUN, and creatinine are used to assess other causes of altered mental status.
- Positive direct Coombs test develops in 10% of patients during chronic therapy.
- Serum acetaminophen and aspirin levels should be checked in the overdose setting to detect occult ingestion.
- Head CT, blood and CSF cultures, and lumbar puncture should be considered to evaluate other causes of coma.

Not Recommended Tests

Serum methyldopa levels are not useful in treatment of acute overdose.

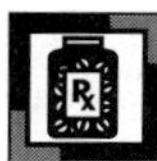

Treatment

- Treatment should focus on airway management and hemodynamic support.
- The dose and time of exposure should be determined for all substances involved.

DIRECTING PATIENT COURSE

The health-care professional should call the poison control center when:

- Severe or persistent effects develop.
- Toxic effects are not consistent with methyldopa poisoning.
- Coingestant, drug interaction, or underlying disease presents an unusual problem.

The patient should be referred to a health-care facility when:

- Attempted suicide or homicide is possible.
- The patient or caregiver seems unreliable.
- Toxic effects develop.
- Coingestant, drug interaction, or underlying disease presents an unusual problem.

Admission Considerations

- Inpatient management is warranted if the patient has documented bradycardia or hypotension, or persistent and symptomatic orthostatic hypotension.
- Following large intentional ingestion, an asymptomatic patient should be considered for admission for 12 to 24 hours of observation because hypotensive effects can be delayed.

DECONTAMINATION

Out of Hospital

Induction of emesis with ipecac is not recommended.

In Hospital

- Gastric lavage should be performed in pediatric (tube size 24–32 French) or adult (tube size 36–42 French) patients presenting within 1 hour of a large ingestion or if serious effects are present.
- One dose of activated charcoal (1–2 g/kg) should be administered without a cathartic if a substantial ingestion has occurred within the previous few hours.

ANTIDOTES

There is no specific antidote for methyldopa poisoning.

ADJUNCTIVE TREATMENT

- Hypotension. The patient should be treated with isotonic fluid infusion, Trendelenburg positioning, and, if needed, vasopressors. Dopamine is preferred and norepinephrine is added for refractory hypotension.
- Bradycardia should initially be treated with atropine administration, followed by cardiac pacing in severe cases, if needed.

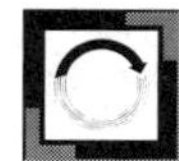

Follow-Up

PATIENT MONITORING

- Cardiac and respiratory monitoring should be performed continuously in symptomatic patients or following large ingestions.
- Complete blood count and platelet level should be monitored in patients on chronic therapy.

EXPECTED COURSE AND PROGNOSIS

Toxicity usually develops within hours after acute ingestion, but has been delayed 12 hours or more in some reports.

DISCHARGE CRITERIA/INSTRUCTIONS

- From the emergency department. Asymptomatic patients without CNS or cardiovascular abnormality for at least 4 to 6 hours post-ingestion can be discharged following decontamination and psychiatric evaluation, if needed.
- From the hospital. Patients may be discharged when mental status and vital signs return to normal, and decontamination and psychiatric evaluation are complete, if needed.

PATIENT EDUCATION

Patients should be warned of the orthostatic hypotensive effects accompanying use of methyldopa.

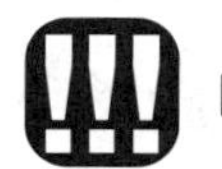

Pitfalls

TREATMENT

Failure to monitor liver function tests on patients receiving chronic therapy can result in missed diagnosis.

ICD-9-CM 972

Poisoning by agents affecting the cardiovascular system.

See also: SECTION II, Hypotension and Bradycardia chapters.

RECOMMENDED READING

Poisindex editorial staff. Methyldopa. In: Rumack DBH, Toll LL, Gelman CR, eds. Poisindex System. Englewood, CO: Micromedex Inc. (edition expires August 31, 1997).

Author: Edwin K. Kuffner

Reviewer: Richard C. Dart

Methylphenidate (Ritalin)

Basics

DESCRIPTION

• Methylphenidate (Ritalin, Ritalin S) is an amphetamine derivative used in the treatment of patients with attention deficit disorder (ADD) and narcolepsy.
• The phrase "T's and blues" refers to a combination of crushed pentazocine (Talwin) tablets and methyphenidate that is typically used illicitly by intravenous injection.

FORMS AND USES

• A typical dose for children with ADD is 5 mg orally twice a day initially, with a possible increase to maximum of 30 mg/day total.
• Adults with narcolepsy are treated with 30 to 40 mg orally per day.

TOXIC DOSE

Ingestion of 1 to 2 mg/kg may result in hyperactivity and mydriasis in children.

PATHOPHYSIOLOGY

Methylphenidate overdose produces a hyperadrenergic state similar to that induced by amphetamines.

EPIDEMIOLOGY

• Poisoning is uncommon.
• Toxic effects following exposure are typically mild to moderate.
• Death has occurred following intravenous abuse.

CAUSES

• Methylphenidate toxicity usually results from illicit use or therapeutic misadventures.
• Methylphenidate is commonly abused by adolescents without ADD for the sympathomimetic effects.
• Child abuse should be considered if the patient is under 1 year of age; attempted suicide if the patient is over 6 years of age.

DRUG AND DISEASE INTERACTIONS

• Use with monoamine oxidase (MAO) inhibitors may result in serotonin syndrome.
• Additive stimulant effects with other amphetamines are expected.

PREGNANCY AND LACTATION

• US FDA Pregnancy Category C. The drug exerts animal teratogenic or embryocidal effects, but there are no controlled studies in women, or no studies are available in either animals or women.
• Intrauterine growth retardation and withdrawal symptoms may occur in infants chronically exposed to amphetamines *in utero*.

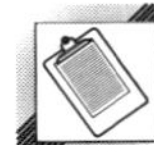

Diagnosis

DIFFERENTIAL DIAGNOSIS

• Toxic causes of agitation and seizure include amphetamine, methamphetamine, theophylline, cocaine, isoniazid, tricyclic antidepressants, MAO inhibitors, and phencyclidine (PCP).
• Nontoxic causes include alcohol withdrawal, meningitis, intracranial hemorrhage, hyperthyroidism, hypoxia from any cause, and manic behavior.

SIGNS AND SYMPTOMS

Acute intoxication is characterized by agitation, tachycardia, hypertension, and mydriasis.

Vital Signs

Tachycardia, hypertension, and hyperthermia occur with moderate to severe overdose.

HEENT

• Mydriasis and a dry mouth are common.
• Talc retinopathy may occur in methylphenidate abusers who crush tablets for intravenous use.

Dermatologic

Diaphoresis is common early in the course of moderate to severe overdose.

Pulmonary

• Precocious emphysema has rarely been reported in intravenous users of crushed tablets.
• Noncardiogenic pulmonary edema may occur.

Cardiovascular

• Tachycardia and hypertension are common.
• Ventricular dysrhythmias are rare but may occur with intravenous use.
• Cardiomyopathy may occur with chronic abuse.

Gastrointestinal

Nausea, vomiting, anorexia, and abdominal pain may occur.

Hepatic

Hepatitis occurs rarely.

Renal

Acute renal failure may result from dehydration, seizures, rhabdomyolysis, or hypotension.

Fluids and Electrolytes

Dehydration, hypokalemia, and lactic acidosis may occur.

Musculoskeletal

Agitation may lead to rhabdomyolysis.

Neurologic

• Agitation, hyperactivity, insomnia, euphoria, dizziness, and paranoid ideation can occur.
• Social withdrawal that resolves following discontinuation has been reported in children.
• Delirium, hallucinations, psychosis, and stereotypic behavior may occur.
• Psychosis may develop and persist beyond discontinuation.
• Tremors and seizures may occur with severe intoxication.

PROCEDURES AND LABORATORY TESTS

Essential Tests

No tests may be needed in asymptomatic patients.

Recommended Tests

• Serum electrolytes, BUN, creatinine, and glucose are recommended to evaluate other causes of seizure and altered mental status.
• Liver function, coagulation studies, and serum creatine kinase may be elevated in patients with hyperthermia or agitation.
• ECG, serum acetaminophen and aspirin levels are advised in an overdose setting to detect occult ingestion.
• Head CT, lumbar puncture, pulse oximetry, and toxicology studies may be needed to evaluate other causes of seizure and altered mental status.
• Chest radiographs may show infiltrates and signs of pulmonary hypertension in intravenous users of crushed tablets; precocious emphysema also has been reported.
• An abdominal radiograph may reveal radiopaque sustained-release preparations; however, their absence on a radiograph cannot exclude ingestion.

Not Recommended Tests

Serum methylphenidate levels are not clinically useful.

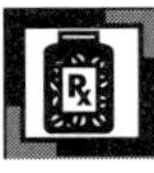

Treatment

• Treatment should focus on control of agitation, hyperthermia, seizures, and dysrhythmias, and on supporting hemodynamic function.
• The dose and time of exposure should be determined for all substances involved.

DIRECTING PATIENT COURSE

The health-care provider should call a poison control center when:

• Seizure, shock, hyperthermia, or other severe effects develop.
• Toxic effects are not consistent with methylphenidate poisoning.

• Coingestant, drug interaction, or underlying disease presents an unusual problem.

The patient should be referred to a health-care facility when:

• Attempted suicide or homicide is possible.
• Patients or caregivers seem unreliable.
• Coingestant, drug interaction, or underlying disease presents an unusual problem.

Admission Considerations

Inpatient treatment is warranted when patients present with refractory agitation, seizure, hyperthermia, persistent tachycardia, or other end-organ injury.

DECONTAMINATION

Out of Hospital

Induction of emesis is not recommended due to seizure potential.

In Hospital

• Gastric lavage should be performed in pediatric (tube size 24–32 French) or adult (tube size 36–42 French) patients presenting within 1 hour of a large ingestion or if serious effects are present.
• One dose of activated charcoal (1–2 g/kg) should be administered if the patient has ingested a substantial amount within the previous few hours.
• Whole-bowel irrigation with polyethylene glycol has been recommended in patients who have ingested sustained-release preparations.

ANTIDOTES

There are no specific antidotes for methylphenidate poisoning.

ADJUNCTIVE TREATMENT

Agitation

• While closely monitoring the patient's airway, a benzodiazepine should be administered.
• For diazepam, the adult dose is 5 to 10 mg intravenously, and the pediatric dose is 0.2 to 0.5 mg/kg intravenously, with doses repeated at 10-minute intervals, titrating to effect.
• For lorazepam, the adult dose is 1 to 2 mg intravenously; the pediatric dose is 0.05 mg/kg, with doses repeated at 10-minute intervals, titrating to effect.

Seizures

• After the patient's airway has been assured, a benzodiazepine should be administered in the same dose as described above for initial control of agitation.
• If seizures persist or recur, another anticonvulsant should be added, such as phenobarbital.

Hypertension

If hypertension persists after treatment of agitation with benzodiazepine or end-organ damage develops (e.g., aortic dissection, central nervous system bleed, myocardial infarction), a short-acting titratable agent such as nitroprusside should be administered.

Hypotension

• Hypotension should be treated with isotonic fluid infusion, Trendelenburg positioning, and a vasopressor if needed (preferably dopamine).
• Norepinephrine is recommended for refractory hypotension.

Ventricular Dysrhythmia

See SECTION II, Ventricular Dysrhythmias chapter.

Rhabdomyolysis

Adequate hydration and urine output (1–2 ml/kg/h) should be ensured. Urinary alkalinization may be beneficial, but definitive data are not available.

Not Recommended Therapies

β-blocker therapy for tachycardias or hypertension may result in unopposed α-adrenergic receptor stimulation and worsening of hypertension.

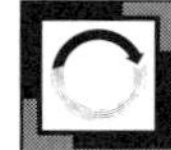

Follow-Up

PATIENT MONITORING

ECG, respiratory and hemodynamic function, and core temperature should be monitored.

EXPECTED COURSE AND PROGNOSIS

• Toxic effects occur soon after ingestion.
• Recovery is usually complete with no sequelae.
• Complications are more common in patients with massive or chronic intravenous abuse.
• Pulmonary granulomatosis may occur following chronic intravenous use of crushed tablets.
• End-organ injury may occur from hypertension or seizures.
• Acute renal failure can result from severe rhabdomyolysis or hypotension.

DISCHARGE CRITERIA/INSTRUCTIONS

• From the emergency department

—Asymptomatic patients who have ingested non–sustained-release formulations may be discharged after observation for 6 hours, gastrointestinal decontamination, and psychiatric evaluation, if needed.
—Symptomatic patients should be discharged after resolution of effects and referral for psychiatric evaluation, if needed.

• From the hospital

—Patients should be discharged after resolution of symptoms, normalization of laboratory values, and psychiatric evaluation, if needed.
—Patients should be referred for substance abuse treatment, if needed.

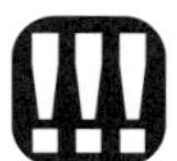

Pitfalls

DIAGNOSIS

• It is important to evaluate other causes of mental status change, such as hypoglycemia; hypoxia; CNS bleed, infection, or infarct; and infection.
• Methylphenidate may be detected as amphetamine by some urine toxicology screens.

TREATMENT

Intravenous abusers are at risk for the complications of intravenous drug use.

ICD-9-CM 969.7

Poisoning by psychotropic agents: psychostimulants.

See also: SECTION II, Hypotension, Seizures, and Ventricular Dysrhythmias chapters; and SECTION III, Nitroprusside and Whole-Bowel Irrigation chapters.

RECOMMENDED READING

Sherman CB, Hudson LD, Pierson DJ. Severe precocious emphysema in intravenous methylphenidate (Ritalin) abusers. *Chest* 1987;92:1085–1087.

Stecyk O, Loludice TA, Demeter S, et al. Multiple organ failure resulting from intravenous abuse of methylphenidate hydrochloride. *Ann Emerg Med* 1985;14:597–599.

Authors: Lada Kokan and Steven A. Seifert

Reviewer: Luke Yip

Metoclopramide

Basics

DESCRIPTION

Metoclopramide (Reglan, Maxolon) is an oral and intravenous medication used in the treatment of gastroesophageal reflux disease and diabetic gastroparesis, and as an antiemetic.

FORMS AND USES

- Diabetic gastroparesis. Adult dosage is 10 mg orally 30 minutes before meals and at bedtime.
- Antiemetic. Adult or child, 0.5 to 2 mg/kg/dose.
- Gastroesophageal reflux disease. Adult dosage is 10 to 20 mg orally every 4 to 6 hours. Pediatric dosage is 0.1 mg/kg/day orally in three divided doses.

TOXIC DOSE

- Dystonic reactions may occur at therapeutic doses.
- Ingestion of several times the daily dose may produce toxicity.

PATHOPHYSIOLOGY

Metoclopramide causes central and peripheral dopaminergic receptor blockade, directly affecting the chemoreceptor trigger zone and preventing vomiting; increases esophageal peristalsis; increases gastric emptying; and accelerates intestinal transit.

EPIDEMIOLOGY

- Poisoning is rare.
- CNS adverse effects such as drowsiness and fatigue may occur in 10% of patients taking therapeutic doses.
- Dystonic reactions occur in less than 1% of patients taking therapeutic doses.

CAUSES

- Poisoning is usually intentional in adults.
- Child neglect or abuse should be considered if the patient is less than 1 year of age, suicide attempt if the patient is over 6 years of age.

RISK FACTORS

- Renal insufficiency allows drug accumulation.
- Dystonic reactions are more common in children and young adults.
- Tardive dyskinesia and parkinsonism are more common in the elderly.

DRUG AND DISEASE INTERACTIONS

- Patients with a history of seizures should avoid taking metoclopramide because frequency and severity of seizures may be increased.
- Metoclopramide should not be given to patients taking other drugs that may cause extrapyramidal reactions.
- Patients with pheochromocytoma should not take metoclopramide because it may cause a hypertensive crisis secondary to catecholamine release.

PREGNANCY AND LACTATION

- US FDA Pregnancy Category B. Studies indicate no fetal risk, and there are no controlled human studies, or animal studies show an adverse fetal effect but well-controlled studies in pregnant women do not.
- Excretion in breast milk has been reported.

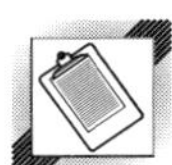

Diagnosis

DIFFERENTIAL DIAGNOSIS

- Other toxicants that cause CNS depressions are anticholinergics, barbiturates, benzodiazepines, ethanol, phenothiazines, sedative-hypnotics, tricyclic antidepressants, opiates, clonidine, and carbon monoxide.
- Other agents that cause methemoglobinemia are benzocaine, dapsone, sulfonamides, amyl nitrite, chloroquine, and nitroglycerine.
- Other drugs associated with extrapyramidal symptoms, including haloperidol, butyrophenones, and phenothiazines, should be ruled out.

SIGNS AND SYMPTOMS

Vital Signs

Hypotension occurs rarely, following rapid intravenous administration.

HEENT

- Acute dystonic reactions (trismus, torticollis, facial spasm, opisthotonos, oculogyric crisis) may occur after therapeutic dosing, overdose, or chronic therapy. This reaction is more common in children and young adults.
- Tardive dyskinesia also has been reported following chronic therapy with large daily doses.

Cardiovascular

Although structurally related to procainamide, few cardiac effects have been reported (heart block and dysrhythmias).

Endocrine

Hyperaldosteronism, hyperprolactinemia, and galactorrhea have been reported with chronic therapy.

Hematologic

Methemoglobinemia occurs rarely in infants after overdose.

Neurologic

- Mild CNS depression is common following overdose.
- Extrapyramidal symptoms (agitation, dystonic reactions, and parkinsonian-like signs) are rare (<1%) but well reported following therapeutic dosing, chronic therapy, and overdose.
- Neuroleptic malignant syndrome and seizure have been reported but are extremely rare.

PROCEDURES AND LABORATORY TESTS

Essential Tests

No laboratory tests are recommended in asymptomatic patients or in dystonic reactions that resolve with treatment.

Recommended Tests

- Metoclopramide serum levels are not clinically useful.
- Serum electrolytes, BUN, creatinine, and ECG are assessed in patients with altered mental status.
- ECG, serum acetaminophen, and aspirin levels are measured in the overdose setting to detect occult ingestion.

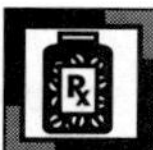

Treatment

OVERVIEW

- Treatment should focus on supportive care with appropriate airway management.
- The dose and time of exposure should be determined for all substances involved.

DIRECTING PATIENT COURSE

The health-care professional should consult the poison control center when:

- Severe or persistent effects develop.
- The signs and symptoms are not consistent with metoclopramide.
- Coingestion, drug interaction, or underlying disease presents an unusual problem.

The patient should be referred to a health-care facility when:

- Attempted suicide or homicide is possible.
- Patient or caregiver seems unreliable.
- Any symptoms are present.
- Coingestion, drug interaction, or underlying disease presents an unusual problem.

Admission Considerations

All patients who have persistent CNS depression, hypotension, or cardiac dysrythmias should be admitted.

DECONTAMINATION

Out of Hospital

Ipecac is not recommended because most ingestions are not problematic.

In Hospital

- Gastric lavage should be performed in pediatric (tube size 24–32 French) or adult (tube size 36–42 French) patients presenting within 1 hour of a large ingestion or if serious effects are present.
- One dose of activated charcoal (1–2 g/kg) should be administered orally without a cathartic if a substantial ingestion has occurred within the previous few hours.

ANTIDOTES

There is no specific antidote for metoclopramide poisoning.

ADJUNCTIVE THERAPIES

- Acute dystonic reactions should be treated with diphenhydramine: children 0.5 to 1 mg/kg/dose intravenously (maximum 5 mg/kg/day), adults 1 mg/kg/dose intravenously (maximum 50 mg/dose) to symptom resolution.
- Tardive dyskinesia and parkinsonian symptoms are treated by decreasing the dose or withdrawing treatment.

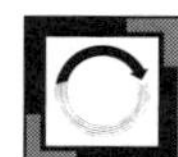

Follow-Up

EXPECTED COURSE AND PROGNOSIS

- Most patients manifest few effects and suffer no permanent effects.
- Dystonic reactions usually respond rapidly to treatment.

DISCHARGE CRITERIA/INSTRUCTIONS

- From the emergency department. Patients who are asymptomatic for 6 hours following overdose and who have undergone gastrointestinal decontamination may be discharged following psychiatric evaluation as appropriate.
- From the hospital. Patients may be discharged from the hospital after mental status, neurologic, and vital signs have returned to normal, and psychiatric evaluation is complete.

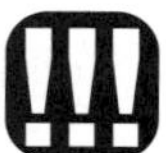

Pitfalls

TREATMENT

The use of metoclopramide should be avoided when increased gastrointestinal motility could be harmful (e.g., gastrointestinal hemorrhage, bowel perforation, or mechanical obstruction).

ICD-9-CM 973.4

Poisoning by digestants.

RECOMMENDED READING

Reglan (metoclopramide), product information. A.H. Robins Company, 1999.

POISINDEX Editorial Staff. Metoclopramide. In: Rumack BH, Sayre NK, Gelman CR, eds. *POISINDEX system*. Volume 101. Englewood, CO: MICROMEDEX, Inc., 1999.

Authors: Heath Jolliff and Edwin K. Kuffner

Reviewer: Richard C. Dart

Minoxidil

Basics

DESCRIPTION

Minoxidil is a medication used orally for control of hypertension and topically to stimulate hair growth.

FORMS AND USES

- Hypertension. 5 mg orally daily increased to a maximum of 100 mg daily.
- Hair regrowth. 1 ml of 2% solution to dry scalp twice a day.
- Pharmaceutical preparations include minoxidil in 2.5-mg tablets, Loniten in 10-mg tablets, and Rogaine in a 2% solution.

TOXIC DOSE

Experience with overdose is limited. However, the topical solution contains a large amount (2 g/100 ml) of drug, and significant toxicity has been reported.

PATHOPHYSIOLOGY

- Minoxidil is a prodrug that is metabolized by the liver to its active form, causes direct vasodilation, and affects arterioles more than veins.
- Arteriolar vasodilation can result in orthostatic hypotension at therapeutic doses and profound hypotension in overdose.

EPIDEMIOLOGY

- Poisoning is rare.
- Toxic effects are typically mild.
- Death occurs rarely, even in large overdose.
- No reports of death following acute ingestion of minoxidil alone could be found.

CAUSES

- Poisoning occurs usually through accidental ingestion.
- Child neglect should be considered if the patient is less than 1 year of age, suicide attempt if the patient is over 6 years of age.

DRUG AND DISEASE INTERACTIONS

Coingestion of other antihypertensive agents could exacerbate hypotension.

PREGNANCY

US FDA Pregnancy Category C. The drug exerts animal teratogenic or embryocidal effects, but there are no controlled studies in women, or no studies are available in either animals or women.

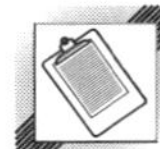

Diagnosis

DIFFERENTIAL DIAGNOSIS

- Toxicologic causes of hypotension include β-receptor or calcium channel blockers, class 1a antidysrythmics, tricyclic antidepressant drugs, monoamine oxidase inhibitors, clonidine, imidazolines, α-methyldopa, nitrates, and α_1-receptor blocking agents.
- Nontoxic causes include sepsis, adrenal insufficiency, hypovolemia, and autonomic dysfunction from diabetes or alcohol.

SIGNS AND SYMPTOMS

Vital Signs

Peripheral vasodilatation causes hypotension and reflex tachycardia.

Dermatologic

- Diaphoresis follows acute ingestion.
- Contact dermatitis from minoxidil-containing topical products occurs rarely.
- Hypertrichosis is common during chronic use.

Cardiovascular

- Tachycardia, hypotension, and palpitations may occur.
- Pericardial effusions have been reported with chronic use.

Gastrointestinal

Nausea and vomiting occur with overdose.

Fluids and Electrolytes

Sodium retention has been reported with chronic use.

Neurologic

After a large overdose, lethargy, disorientation, dizziness, slurred speech, and coma may occur.

Reproductive

Breast tenderness and gynecomastia have been reported with chronic use.

PROCEDURES AND LABORATORY TESTS

Essential Tests

No test may be needed for asymptomatic patients.

Recommended Tests

- Serum electrolytes, BUN, creatinine, glucose to evaluate other causes of hypotension
- ECG, serum acetaminophen and aspirin levels in overdose setting to detect occult ingestion
- Adrenocorticotropic hormone stimulation test in patients with suspected adrenal in sufficiency

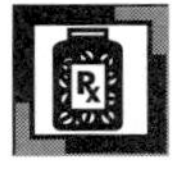

Treatment

- Treatment should focus on hemodynamic monitoring and maintaining blood pressure.
- Dose and time of exposure should be determined for all substances involved.

DIRECTING PATIENT COURSE

The health-care provider should call the poison control center when:

- Hypotension, altered mental status, or other serious effects are present.
- Toxic effects are not consistent with minoxidil poisoning.
- Coingestant, drug interaction, or underlying disease presents an unusual problem.

The patient should be referred to a health-care professional when:

- Attempted suicide or homicide is possible.
- Patient or caregiver seems unreliable.
- Toxic effects develop.
- Coingestant, drug interaction, or underlying disease presents an unusual problem.

Admission Considerations

Inpatient treatment is warranted for patients with hypotension or other clinically significant effects.

DECONTAMINATION

Out of Hospital

Emesis should be induced with ipecac within 1 hour of ingestion for alert pediatric or adult patients if health-care evaluation will be delayed.

In Hospital

- Emesis should be induced with ipecac within 1 hour of ingestion for the patient who is too small to undergo effective gastric lavage.
- Gastric lavage should be performed in pediatric (tube size 24–32 French) or adult (tube size 36–42 French) patients presenting within 1 hour of a large ingestion or if serious effects are present.
- One dose of activated charcoal (1–2 g/kg) is administered if a substantial ingestion has occurred within the previous few hours.

ANTIDOTES

There is no specific antidote for minoxidil poisoning.

ADJUNCTIVE THERAPIES

Hypotension

- Treatment includes infusion and isotonic fluid infusion (10–20 ml/kg) and placement in the Trendelenburg position.
- If needed, a vasopressor is used; dopamine is preferred, and norepinephrine is used for refractory hypotension.

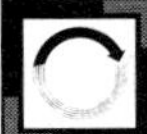

Follow-Up

PATIENT MONITORING

All patients should undergo hemodynamic and cardiac monitoring.

EXPECTED COURSE AND PROGNOSIS

- Hemodynamic effects may last 1 to 2 days following ingestion.
- Possible complications related to prolonged hypotension may occur, although this is rare.

DISCHARGE CRITERIA/INSTRUCTIONS

- From the emergency department. Asymptomatic patients (with orthostatic hypotension) following decontamination, observation for 6 to 10 hours, and, if needed, a psychiatric evaluation.
- From the hospital. The patient may be discharged when: signs of toxicity have resolved, blood pressure has been normal for 12 hours, and the psychiatric evaluation, if needed, is complete.

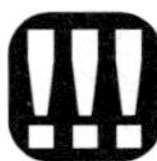

Pitfalls

TREATMENT

Tachycardia is a compensatory mechanism due to vasodilatation. Therefore, control of heart rate may be detrimental.

FOLLOW-UP

For geriatric patients, lower initial doses and slower increases in daily dose are recommended due to the increased risk of orthostatic hypotension.

ICD-9-CM 972.6

Poisoning by agents primarily affecting the cardiovascular system: other antihypertensive agents.

976.4

See also: SECTION II, Hypotension chapter.

RECOMMENDED READING

MacMillan AR, Warshawski FG, Steinberg RA. Minoxidil overdose. *Chest* 1993;103:1290–1291.

McCormick MA, Forman MH, Manoguerra AS. Severe toxicity from ingestion of a topical minoxidil preparation. *Am J Emerg Med* 1989;7:419–421.

Author: Lada Kokan

Reviewers: Gerald F. O'Malley and Kennon Heard

Misoprostol

Basics

DESCRIPTION

Misoprostol (Cytotec) is a synthetic prostaglandin E_1 analog that inhibits gastric acid secretion and stimulates gastric mucus secretion.

FORMS AND USES

Therapeutic uses of misoprostol include the following:

- Gastric and duodenal ulcers. Adult dose is 200 μg orally four times a day or 400 μg twice a day.
- Prevention of nonsteroidal antiinflammatory drug (NSAID)-induced ulcers. Adult dose is 100 to 200 μg orally four times a day.
- Hemorrhagic gastritis
- Induction of labor. Oral or intravaginal (50 to 800 μg) administration results in cervical ripening and myometrial contraction.
- Abortifacient. Misoprostol does not reliably produce complete abortion.

TOXIC DOSE

Ingestion of a few milligrams has produced toxicity.

PATHOPHYSIOLOGY

- Misoprostol is an analog of prostaglandin E_1, an endogenous cellular messenger.
- Its primary effects are smooth muscle contraction and decreased gastric acid secretion.

EPIDEMIOLOGY

Poisoning is uncommon.

CAUSES

- Exposure is usually intentional; occasionally to induce abortion.
- Child neglect or abuse should be considered if the patient is less than 1 year of age, suicide attempt if the patient is over 6 years of age.

PREGNANCY AND LACTATION

- US FDA Pregnancy Category X. Studies in animals or humans have demonstrated fetal abnormalities or there is evidence of fetal risk based on human experience, or both, and the risk clearly outweighs any possible benefit.
- It is unknown if misoprostol is excreted in breast milk; use is not recommended for nursing mothers.
- Misoprostol is an abortifacient and is contraindicated in pregnancy.
- Prostaglandins of the E and F series can induce uterine contractions.
- Case reports suggest that misoprostol may be teratogenic in humans.
- Fetal death has been reported following acute maternal overdose.

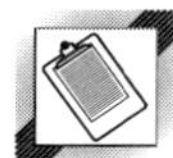

Diagnosis

DIFFERENTIAL DIAGNOSIS

Toxic causes of gastrointestinal distress include organophosphate/carbamate insecticides, heavy metals, nonsteroidal antiinflammatory drugs, and others.

SIGNS AND SYMPTOMS

Vital Signs

Fever, tachycardia, hypertension, and tachypnea have been reported following acute overdose but are mild and rare.

Gastrointestinal

Nausea, vomiting, diarrhea, flatulence, dyspepsia, abdominal cramping, and constipation may occur.

Musculoskeletal

Rhabdomyolysis has been reported in acute overdose.

Neurologic

- Headache, fatigue, and lightheadedness occur during chronic therapy.
- Delirium has been reported but is rare.

Gynecologic

Menorrhagia, uterine contractions, and dysmenorrhea may develop.

PROCEDURES AND LABORATORY TESTS

Essential Tests

No tests may be needed in asymptomatic patients.

Recommended Tests

- Blood chemistry and serum creatine kinase are indicated in symptomatic patients.
- ECG, serum acetaminophen and aspirin levels are indicated in overdose situations to detect occult ingestion.

Not Recommended Tests

Misoprostol levels are not clinically useful in overdose.

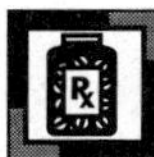

Treatment

• Treatment should focus on symptomatic treatment of gastrointestinal effects.
• The dose and time of exposure should be determined for all substances involved.

DIRECTING PATIENT COURSE

The health-care professional should call the poison control center when:

• Severe or persistent effects develop.
• Coingestant, drug interaction, or underlying disease presents an unusual problem.

The patient should be referred to a health-care facility when:

• Suicide or homicide attempt is possible.
• Toxic effects develop.
• Coingestant, drug interaction, or underlying disease presents an unusual problem.

Admission Considerations

Admission is rarely needed, except for pregnant patients and those with severe volume depletion.

DECONTAMINATION

• Induction of emesis or gastric lavage are rarely needed for isolated misoprostol ingestion due to the limited toxicity.
• One dose of activated charcoal (1–2 g/kg) should be administered without a cathartic if a substantial ingestion has occurred within the previous few hours.

ANTIDOTES

There is no specific antidote for misoprostol poisoning.

ADJUNCTIVE TREATMENT

Administration of intravenous isotonic fluids may be needed in volume-depleted patients.

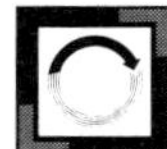

Follow-Up

PATIENT MONITORING

All pregnant patients should be observed for 6 to 8 hours following ingestion and absence of fetal distress documented.

EXPECTED COURSE AND PROGNOSIS

Most adverse effects resolve rapidly upon discontinuation of misoprostol therapy.

DISCHARGE CRITERIA/INSTRUCTIONS

• Asymptomatic patients may be discharged from emergency department or hospital after observation for 4 to 8 hours.
• Symptomatic patients may be discharged from the emergency department or hospital when toxic effects resolve or stabilize and after psychiatric evaluation, if needed.

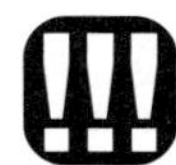

Pitfalls

TREATMENT

Women of childbearing potential should have a negative pregnancy test result and should be placed on oral contraceptives prior to initiating therapy with misoprostol.

ICD-9-CM 973.4

Poisoning by agents primarily affecting the gastrointestinal system: digestants.

RECOMMENDED READING

Bond GR, Van Zee A. Intentional misoprostol overdose in pregnancy. *Vet Hum Toxicol* 1990;32:352.

Author: Edwin K. Kuffner

Reviewer: Richard C. Dart

Molindone

Basics

DESCRIPTION

Molindone is an oral antipsychotic medication.

FORMS AND USES

- Substances include molindone (Moban).
- Treatment of psychotic disorders. Usual starting dosage is 50 to 75 mg/day, divided into three or four doses a day, and titrated to a maximum of 225 mg/day.

TOXIC DOSE

- Acutely toxic dose of molindone is unknown due to insufficient evidence.
- The therapeutic dose can approach 500 mg/day in some patients.

PATHOPHYSIOLOGY

Molindone blocks postsynaptic dopamine receptors but has little affinity for cholinergic, noradrenergic, and histaminic receptors.

DRUG AND DISEASE INTERACTIONS

Recent or concomitant use of neuroleptic or other dopamine antagonists may predispose to neuroleptic malignant syndrome (NMS) at therapeutic dose.

PREGNANCY AND LACTATION

US FDA Pregnancy Category C. The drug exerts animal teratogenic or embryocidal effects, but there are no controlled studies in women, or no studies are available in animals or women.

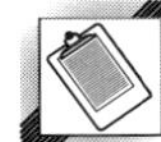

Diagnosis

DIFFERENTIAL DIAGNOSIS

Toxic causes of extrapyramidal effects include phenothiazine or butyrophenone medications.

SIGNS AND SYMPTOMS

NMS is possible, particularly in patients exposed to other dopamine antagonists. Fever and autonomic instability can occur with NMS.

Vital Signs

Mild hypotension, tachycardia, and extrapyramidal effects can occur.

Cardiovascular

Tachycardia, hypotension, nonspecific T-wave changes may occur.

Hepatic

Elevated levels on liver function tests are possible with therapeutic use.

Musculoskeletal

Rhabdomyolysis can occur with NMS.

Neurologic

- Rigidity, dystonia, tremor, and other extrapyramidal effects can occur with therapeutic use.
- Altered mental status and coma can occur with NMS.

Endocrine

Hypothyroidism and galactorrhea may result with therapeutic use.

PROCEDURES AND LABORATORY TESTS

Essential Tests

No tests may be needed for asymptomatic patients.

Recommended Tests

- Serum electrolytes, BUN, creatinine should be ordered in patients with altered mental status.
- Head CT, lumbar puncture, cultures may be needed to assess CNS depression.
- ECG, acetaminophen and salicylate levels should be obtained in overdose setting to detect occult ingestion.

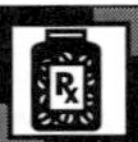

Treatment

- Focus therapy on supportive care and airway management.
- Dose and time of exposure should be determined for all substances involved.

DIRECTING PATIENT COURSE

The health-care professional should call the poison control center when:

- Toxic effects are not consistent with molindone toxicity.
- Coingestant, drug interaction, or underlying disease presents an unusual problem.

The patient should be referred to a health-care facility when:

- Attempted suicide or homicide is possible.
- Coingestant, drug interaction, or underlying disease presents an unusual problem.

Admission Considerations

Inpatient management is warranted if patient develops altered mental status, hypotension, or evidence of NMS.

DECONTAMINATION

Out of Hospital

Emesis should be induced within 1 hour of ingestion for alert pediatric or adult patients if health-care evaluation will be delayed.

In Hospital

- Gastric lavage should be used for patients presenting within 1 hour of a substantial ingestion or if serious effects are present.
- One dose of activated charcoal (1–2 g/kg) should be administered if a substantial ingestion has occurred within the previous few hours.

ANTIDOTES

There is no specific antidote for molindone poisoning.

ADJUNCTIVE THERAPIES

- Hypotension should be treated with isotonic fluid infusion, Trendelenburg positioning, and vasopressors if needed.
- NMS should be treated by lowering of temperature, vasopressor administration, and fluid resuscitation.
- Dystonic reactions are treated with diphenhydramine or benztropine.

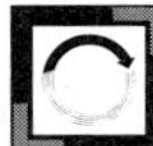

Follow-Up

PATIENT MONITORING

Symptomatic patients should have continuous cardiac and respiratory monitoring.

EXPECTED COURSE AND PROGNOSIS

Most patients recover within 12 to 24 hours with supportive care if NMS does not develop.

DISCHARGE CRITERIA/INSTRUCTIONS

- From the emergency department. Asymptomatic patients may be discharged after 6 hours of observation following appropriate decontamination and psychiatric evaluation, if needed.
- From the hospital. The patient may be discharged when hemodynamically stable, mental status is baseline, and evidence of NMS has resolved.

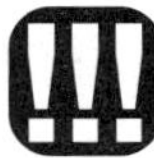

Pitfalls

DIAGNOSIS

Toxic symptoms are similar to overdose with phenothiazine or butyrophenone.

ICD-9-CM 969

Poisoning by psychotropic agents.

See also: SECTION II, Hypotension, and Neuroleptic Malignant Syndrome and Serotonin Syndrome chapters.

RECOMMENDED READING

Gradon JD. Neuroleptic malignant syndrome possibly caused by molindone hydrochloride. *DICP* 1991;25:1071–1072.

Author: Katherine M. Hurlbut

Reviewer: Richard C. Dart

Monoamine Oxidase Inhibitors

Basics

DESCRIPTION

Monoamine oxidase inhibitors are oral antihypertensive and antidepressant agents.

FORMS AND USES

- Pharmaceutical preparations include selegiline (Deprenyl), clorgyline, nialimide, isocarboxazid (Marplan), pargyline (Eutonyl), phenelzine (Nardil), moclobemide, tranylcypromine (Parnate), furazolidone (Furoxone), and procarbazine (Matulane).
- Selegiline (Deprenyl), isocarboxazid, pargyline, phenelzine, and tranylcypromine are approved for use in treating anxiety, phobias, bulimia, treatment-resistant or atypical depression, migraines, obsessive-compulsive disorders, narcolepsy, and Parkinson's disease.
- Approved indications for furazolidone include bacterial or protozoal diarrhea and enteritis caused by the majority of gastrointestinal pathogens.
- Tranylcypromine. Adult dosage, 10 to 30 mg/day orally.
- Phenelzine. Adult dosage, 15 to 90 mg/day orally.
- Moclobemide. Adult dosage, 300 to 450 mg, given in two to three divided doses orally.
- Furazolidone. Adult dosage, one tablet four times per day or 2 tablespoons four times per day; children 5 years of age or older, 25 to 50 mg four times per day; children 1 to 4 years of age, 1 to 1½ tablespoons four times per day orally.

TOXIC DOSE

Ingestion of 2 to 3 mg/kg of any MAO inhibitor may produce serious toxicity.

PATHOPHYSIOLOGY

- Inhibition of the enzyme monoamine oxidase results in the increase of norepinephrine, dopamine, and serotonin in the synapse, producing an antidepressant effect.
- In overdose, overstimulation of the postsynaptic receptors results in toxicity.

EPIDEMIOLOGY

- Toxicity from MAO inhibitors is uncommon.
- Toxic effects are typically mild to moderate.
- Death occurs infrequently, related to a large overdose or an adverse drug interaction.

CAUSES

- Overdose is usually the result of intentional ingestion.
- Child neglect should be considered if the patient is under 1 year of age; attempted suicide should be considered in patients over 6 years of age.

RISK FACTORS

Drug Interactions

MAO inhibitors may interact with many drugs or foods to produce life-threatening hypertension, neuroleptic malignant syndrome (NMS), or serotonin syndrome (SS).

- All sympathomimetic agents
- Opioids
- Tricyclic antidepressants
- Lithium
- Selective serotonin reuptake inhibitors (SSRIs)
- Levodopa, methyldopa, and tryptophan
- Guanethidine
- Theophylline, caffeine
- Various foods, including chocolate, aged cheese, chianti, vermouth, pickled fish, and concentrated yeast extracts

Pregnancy and Lactation

- US FDA Pregnancy Category C. The drug exerts animal teratogenic or embryocidal effects, but there are no controlled studies in women, or no studies are available in either animals or women.
- Abruptio placentae may occur if severe hypertension develops.

DIAGNOSIS

Differential Diagnosis

- Toxic causes of hypertension include stimulants (amphetamine, cocaine, etc.), and theophylline, among others.
- Primary causes of hypertension associated with hyperthermia and altered mental status are NMS (phenothiazines, many other drugs), SS, SSRIs, stimulants, hallucinogens, and many other drugs.
- Nontoxic causes include hypertensive crisis, noncompliance with antihypertensive medications, and alcohol or sedative-hypnotic withdrawal, among others.

SIGNS AND SYMPTOMS

The primary effects associated with overdose are hyperadrenergic and include agitation and hypertension; severe cases may involve multiple organ failure.

Vital Signs

- Hypertension is followed by hypotension in serious cases.
- Hyperthermia should raise concern for NMS or SS.

HEENT

Headaches, dilated pupils, blurry vision or tinnitus may occur.

Pulmonary

Tachypnea and pulmonary edema may develop in severe cases.

Cardiovascular

Hypertension may cause myocardial ischemia and dysrhythmias.

Gastrointestinal

Nausea, diarrhea, abdominal pain, and constipation may occur.

Hepatic

Hepatitis occurs rarely.

Renal

Renal failure and syndrome of inappropriate antidiuretic hormone secretion have been reported.

Musculoskeletal

- Weakness, muscle spasm, and myoclonic jerks have been reported.
- If stiffness or rhabdomyolysis develop, diagnosis of NMS or SS should be considered.

Neurologic

- Tinnitus, numbness, paresthesia, akinesia, restlessness or insomnia occur.
- Weakness and drowsiness may progress to agitation, confusion, seizures, and coma.
- Headache and focal neurologic deficits may indicate intracranial hemorrhage.

Urologic

Urinary retention, retarded ejaculation, and impotence may occur.

Hematologic

Anemia, leukopenia, thrombocytopenia, and agranulocytosis have been reported.

PROCEDURES AND LABORATORY TESTS

Essential Tests

No tests may be needed in asymptomatic patients.

Recommended Tests

- Serum electrolytes, BUN, creatinine, and urinalysis are recommended to assess acidosis, renal injury, and electrolyte abnormalities.
- Serum creatine kinase and liver enzyme tests may be done to assess rhabdomyolysis and chest pain.
- An ECG should be performed if symptoms of myocardial ischemia occur.
- Arterial blood gases may show respiratory alkalosis, respiratory acidosis, or metabolic acidosis.
- A complete blood count often reveals leukocytosis.
- Serum acetaminophen and aspirin levels in overdose setting to detect occult ingestion.
- Head CT, lumbar puncture, and bacterial cultures should be ordered as needed to evaluate patients with altered mental status of unknown etiology.

Not Recommended Tests

Drug levels are not clinically useful.

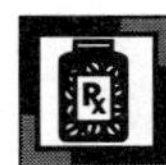

Treatment

- Treatment should focus on intensive supportive care of hypertension, airway, and temperature.
- Dose and time of exposure should be determined for all substances involved.

DIRECTING PATIENT COURSE

Health-care professionals should call a poison control center when:

- Evidence of hypertension with end-organ damage, hypotension, hyperthermia, or rigidity develops.
- Toxic effects are not consistent with the MAO inhibitor.
- A coingestant, drug interaction, or underlying disease presents an unusual problem.

Patients should be referred to a health-care professional when:

- Attempted suicide or homicide is possible.
- Patients or caregivers seem unreliable.
- Any toxic effects develop.
- A coingestant, drug interaction, or underlying disease presents an unusual problem.

Admission Considerations

Patients with a suspected MAO inhibitor overdose should be admitted to a monitored unit for at least 24 hours, even if asymptomatic.

DECONTAMINATION

Out of Hospital

Emesis should not be induced because abrupt deterioration may occur.

In Hospital

- Gastric lavage should be performed in pediatric (tube size 24–32 French) or adult (tube size 36–42 French) patients presenting within 1 hour of a large ingestion or if serious effects are present.
- One dose of activated charcoal (1–2 g/kg) should be administered if the patient has ingested a substantial amount within the previous few hours.

ANTIDOTES

There are no specific antidotes for MAO inhibitors.

ADJUNCTIVE TREATMENT

Hypertension

If hypertension does not respond to initial therapy or end-organ damage develops (e.g., aortic dissection, central nervous system bleed, myocardial infarction), a short-acting titratable agent such as nitroprusside should be administered.

Hypotension

- The patient should be placed in Trendelenburg position and 10 to 20 ml/kg of 0.9% saline should be infused.
- Further fluid therapy should be guided by central pressure monitoring to avoid volume overload.
- A vasopressor should be cautiously added if needed.

Tachydysrhythmia

- Only tachydysrhythmias involving hypotension or myocardial ischemia should be treated.
- The recommended dose of esmolol for adults is an intravenous bolus of 500 μg/kg infused over 1 minute followed by an infusion of 50 μg/kg/min for 4 minutes.
- After reassessment, the loading dose may be repeated if needed, accompanied by an increase in infusion rate to 100 μg/kg/min for 4 minutes.
- This titration process should be repeated as needed until a rate is reached that controls the heart rate or toxicity (hypotension) develops.
- Unopposed α-receptor stimulation is a theoretical concern during β-blockade; if the heart rate or blood pressure increases dangerously during infusion, α-receptor stimulation may be the cause and the infusion should be stopped.

Seizures

- After the patient's airway is assured, a benzodiazepine should be administered for initial control.
- If seizures persist or recur, another anticonvulsant should be added, such as phenobarbital.

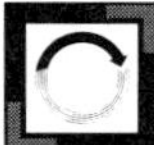

Follow-Up

PATIENT MONITORING

Vital signs, neurologic effects, liver and renal function, creatine kinase, acid-base, and fluid and electrolyte balance should be closely monitored in serious cases.

EXPECTED COURSE AND PROGNOSIS

- Toxic effects usually peak within several hours, but may be delayed 12 to 24 hours.
- If severe effects develop, they often require a few days to resolve or stabilize.
- End-organ complications of hypertension or hyperthermia may be permanent.

DISCHARGE CRITERIA/INSTRUCTIONS

- From the emergency department. If MAO inhibitor overdose is likely or symptoms have developed, the patient should not be discharged.
- From the hospital. Patients should be discharged following the resolution or stabilization of toxic effects and after psychiatric evaluation, if needed.

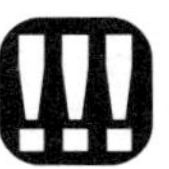

Pitfalls

DIAGNOSIS

- Toxic effects may be delayed 12 hours or more.
- Newer "selective" MAO inhibitors, such as selegiline, lose their receptor specificity in overdose.
- It is important to rule out other causes of altered mental status.

TREATMENT

Hyperthermia must be treated rapidly and aggressively.

ICD-9-CM 969.0

Poisoning by psychotropic agents: antidepressants.

See also: SECTION II, Hypertension, Hyperthermia, Hypotension, Neuroleptic Malignant Syndrome and Serotonin Syndrome, and Seizures chapters; and SECTION III, Nitroprusside chapter.

RECOMMENDED READING

Bryson P. Monoamine oxidase inhibitors. In: *Comprehensive review in toxicology for emergency clinicians,* 3rd ed. Washington, DC: Taylor & Francis, 1996:209–215.

Author: Wyatt J. Hall

Reviewer: Katherine M. Hurlbut

Mothballs

Basics

DESCRIPTION

The active ingredient in mothballs, flakes, and crystals is paradichlorobenzene or naphthalene.

FORMS AND USES

Mothballs are used to repel moths, but also other insects and small animals.

TOXIC DOSE

One naphthalene mothball can produce hemolysis in glucose-6-phosphate dehydrogenase (G-6-PD)-deficient children.

PATHOPHYSIOLOGY

Paradichlorobenzene

- Accidental acute ingestion is inconsequential.
- Although methemoglobinemia and red cell hemolysis have been reported, they have not been convincingly demonstrated.
- Hepatotoxicity following chronic exposure has been reported.

Naphthalene

- This polycyclic aromatic hydrocarbon is readily absorbed and can cause toxicity from oral, inhalational, or dermal exposure.
- Gastrointestinal distress may occur shortly after ingestion.
- Toxicity consists of hemolysis and methemoglobinemia 1 to 5 days after ingestion.
- Toxicity is usually delayed for several days as naphthalene is metabolized to α-naphthol, a potent hemolytic agent.

EPIDEMIOLOGY

Poisoning is uncommon.

CAUSES

- In a child, exposure usually results from accidental ingestion.
- Child neglect or abuse should be considered if the patient is less than 1 year of age, suicide attempt if the patient is over 6 years of age.

DRUG AND DISEASE INTERACTIONS

- Less than one naphthalene mothball in a patient with G-6-PD deficiency can cause significant toxicity.
- Neonatal inability to conjugate naphthalene metabolites may lead to hemolysis in the presence of normal G-6-PD levels.

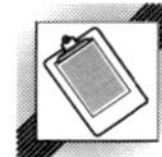

Diagnosis

DIFFERENTIAL DIAGNOSIS

Toxicologic causes of methemoglobinemia and hemolysis include nitrites, benzocaine, other topical anesthetics, dapsone, many others.

SIGNS AND SYMPTOMS

- Acute

—Most patients develop no toxicity from a single mothball.
—Large ingestion may result in fever, nausea, vomiting, abdominal pain, and diarrhea 24 to 48 hours later.
—Nausea and vomiting may occur in chronic exposure.
—Lethargy and seizures may develop in severe cases.
—Signs of hemolysis may include pallor, weakness, hemoglobinuria, jaundice, and cyanosis.

- Chronic

—Nausea, vomiting, aplastic anemia, hepatic necrosis, and jaundice may occur.

PROCEDURES AND LABORATORY TESTS

Essential Tests

No tests may be needed in asymptomatic patients with acute single ingestion.

Recommended Tests

Rapid determination of mothball components can be accomplished using the following tests. Further evaluation may not be needed if the mothball is composed of paradichlorobenzene.

- Paradichlorobenzene

—Clear white, wet, oily crystalline balls
—Densely radiopaque
—Will sink in saturated salt solution [3 tablespoons of table salt in 4 ounces (120 cc) of tepid water, stirred vigorously until the salt will not dissolve any further]

- Naphthalene

—White, dry crystalline balls
—Faintly radiopaque
—Will float in saturated salt solution

Renal function tests, methemoglobin level, and G-6-PD level are recommended after naphthalene ingestion.

Hemolysis Screening

- Initial screening for hemolysis with a complete blood count and peripheral smear should be performed after naphthalene ingestion.
- Peripheral smear may show fragmented red blood cells, anisocytosis, Heinz bodies, and poikilocytosis.

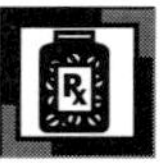

Treatment

Treatment should focus on detection and supportive care of hemolysis following naphthalene ingestion.

DIRECTING PATIENT COURSE

The health-care professional should call the poison control center when:

- Severe or persistent effects develop.
- Coingestant, drug interaction, or underlying disease presents an unusual problem.

The patient should be referred to a health-care facility when:

- Toxic effects develop.
- Coingestant, drug interaction, or underlying disease presents an unusual problem.

Admission Considerations

Persistently symptomatic patients or patients with hemolysis or methemoglobinemia should be admitted for evaluation.

DECONTAMINATION

Paradichlorobenzene

- Because of its limited toxicity, gastric lavage and activated charcoal is recommended only when large quantities are ingested.
- One dose of activated charcoal (1–2 g/kg) should be administered without a cathartic if a substantial ingestion has occurred within the previous few hours.

Naphthalene

- Patients without G-6-PD deficiency tolerate small quantities well; large ingestions may require gastric decontamination and follow-up.
- Because mothballs exceed the size of orogastric tubes, ipecac should be used, unless CNS depression has developed.
- Activated charcoal (see dose and procedure above) should be used to reduce absorption.
- Cutaneous exposure is managed by removing contaminated clothing and washing exposed skin.

ANTIDOTES

There is no specific antidote for either paradichlorobenzene or naphthalene.

ADJUNCTIVE TREATMENT

Blood transfusion may be needed in rare cases.

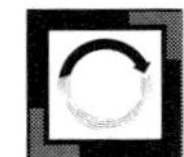

Follow-Up

EXPECTED COURSE AND PROGNOSIS

- Most patients develop no toxicity from a single mothball.
- In acute exposures, larger ingestions may produce fever, nausea, vomiting, abdominal pain, and diarrhea 24 to 48 hours later.
- Hemolysis may be delayed for days or not occur at all.

DISCHARGE CRITERIA/INSTRUCTIONS

Asymptomatic patients who can be followed closely may be discharged from the emergency department or hospital.

PATIENT EDUCATION

Instruct patient or parent about the delayed manifestations of hemolysis (anemia, hemoglobinemia, jaundice, weakness) and to return if symptoms develop.

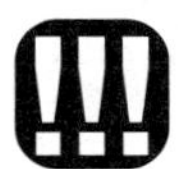

Pitfalls

DIAGNOSIS

Mothball exposure is often missed initially.

ICD-9-CM 989.8

Other substances, chiefly nonmedicinal as to source.

RECOMMENDED READING

Goldfrank LR, Bania TC. Camphor and mothballs. In: Goldfrank LR, Flomenbaum NE, Lewin NA, et al., eds. *Goldfrank's toxicologic emergencies*, 6th ed. Norwalk, CT: Appleton & Lange, 1998.

Author: Luke Yip

Reviewer: Richard C. Dart

Multivitamins

Basics

DESCRIPTION

Multivitamins are over-the-counter oral medications that provide small amounts of several vitamins in one pill.

FORMS AND USES

- Multivitamins containing iron are covered in SECTION IV, Iron.
- Although there are hundreds of formulations, the primary vitamins included here are vitamins A, C, D, E, folic acid, thiamine (B_1), riboflavin (B_2), cyanocobalamin (B_{12}), biotin, niacin, pantothenic acid, and pyridoxine (B_6).

TOXIC DOSE

- A single ingestion must be very large to cause toxicity.
- Chronic ingestion of large amounts may produce adverse effects.
- Due to the number of pills needed to ingest toxic amounts, local gastrointestinal irritant effects are the only common effect.

EPIDEMIOLOGY

Poisoning is common; toxic effects are very rare.

CAUSES

- In a child, acute poisoning is usually an unintentional overdose.
- Child neglect or abuse should be considered if the patient is less than 1 year of age, suicide attempt if the patient is over 6 years of age.

PREGNANCY AND LACTATION

U.S. FDA Pregnancy Category C. For any vitamin taken in doses that exceed the recommended daily allowance.

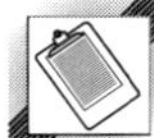

Diagnosis

DIFFERENTIAL DIAGNOSIS

The diagnosis is largely dependent on the history of vitamin supplement use or abuse.

SIGNS AND SYMPTOMS

HEENT

Scleral icterus may be seen with overdose of niacin (adults) or vitamin K (neonates).

Dermatologic

Perspiration may take on a yellow color with excess riboflavin (vitamin B_2).

Gastrointestinal

Nausea and diarrhea may occur with large ingestions.

Hepatic

Nicotinic acid has been linked with dose-dependent centrilobular hepatic cholestasis and parenchymal necrosis.

Renal

- Acute or chronic overdose of vitamin C may cause nephropathy or even frank renal failure.
- Excessive amounts of B vitamins will intensify the yellow color of urine.

Neurologic

A well-described syndrome of peripheral neurotoxicity with prolonged ingestion of large doses of pyridoxine has been seen.

PROCEDURES AND LABORATORY TESTS

Essential Tests

No tests may be needed in asymptomatic patients.

Recommended Tests

- Serum liver enzymes, coagulation parameters, and bilirubin may be helpful when niacin toxicity is considered.
- Urinalysis and renal function testing are useful for evaluation of possible vitamin C intoxication.
- An anion gap may be present on the electrolyte analysis due to the presence of the oxalic acid metabolite.
- The laboratory is not helpful in identifying or quantifying the ingested substance.

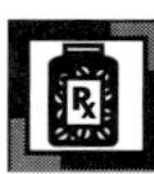

Treatment

- The primary therapy is to discontinue treatment.
- The dose and duration of exposure for all substances involved should be determined.

DIRECTING PATIENT COURSE

The health-care professional should call the poison control center when:

- Severe or persistent effects develop.
- Coingestant, drug interaction, or underlying disease presents an unusual problem.

The patient should be referred to a health-care facility when:

- Attempted suicide or homicide is possible.
- Toxic effects develop.
- Coingestant, drug interaction, or underlying disease presents an unusual problem.

Admission Considerations

- Admission is rarely needed.
- Patients with chronic ingestion leading to hepatic or renal injury may need hospitalization for evaluation.

DECONTAMINATION

Out of Hospital

Decontamination is not needed.

In Hospital

- Gastric lavage should be performed in pediatric (tube size 24–32 French) or adult (tube size 36–42 French) patients for massive ingestion presenting within 1 hour of ingestion or if serious effects are present.
- One dose of activated charcoal (1–2 g/kg) should be administered without a cathartic if a substantial ingestion has occurred within the previous few hours.

ANTIDOTES

There is no specific antidote for multivitamin poisoning.

ADJUNCTIVE TREATMENT

Supportive care of hepatic, renal, or neurologic injury may be needed.

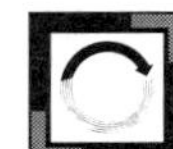

Follow-Up

EXPECTED COURSE AND PROGNOSIS

- Most patients can be expected to make a full recovery with cessation of the vitamin supplement and with supportive care.
- Patients that develop ascorbic acid–induced crystalluria or nephropathy can be expected to recover with supportive care (including hemodialysis) if necessary.

DISCHARGE CRITERIA/INSTRUCTIONS

Asymptomatic patients may be discharged from the emergency department or hospital following evaluation of coingestants and psychiatric evaluation, if needed.

PATIENT EDUCATION

The patient should be instructed to discontinue taking the formulations involved.

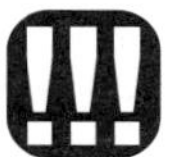

Pitfalls

DIAGNOSIS

Vitamins and "alternative" medications are often not considered a medicine by the patient. The history should actively solicit this information.

ICD-9-CM 988

Toxic effect of noxious substances eaten as food.

See also: SECTION III, Pyridoxine, Thiamine, and Vitamin K chapters; and SECTION IV, Niacin/Nicotinic acid/Nicotinamide and Vitamin A chapters.

RECOMMENDED READING

Rader JI, Calvert RJ, Hathcock JW. Hepatic toxicity of unmodified and time-release preparations of niacin. *Am J Med* 1992;92:77–81.

Author: Gerald F. O'Malley

Reviewer: Richard C. Dart

Mushrooms

Basics

DESCRIPTION

- Mushroom toxicity is classified clinically based on the time of symptom onset.
- Lethal intoxication is associated with mushrooms producing initial symptoms more than 6 hours after ingestion.
- Caution must be exercised, however, because it is possible to develop symptoms before 6 hours and still have a lethal ingestion if more than one type of mushroom was ingested.

Mushroom/Toxin Groups that Typically Produce Symptoms Within 3 Hours of Ingestion

- The disulfiram-like group (certain species of *Coprinus, Clitocybe, Boletus* mushrooms) may produce a disulfiram reaction if alcohol is later ingested; this is most commonly associated with ingestion of *Coprinus atramentarius* ("inky cap").
- The muscarine group (among which are some species of *Boletus, Clitocybe, Inocybe*) produces muscarinic receptor stimulation: salivation, lacrimation, urination, defecation, and bronchorrhea.
- The ibotenic acid and muscimol group (some species of *Amanita, Tricholoma, Panaeolus*) causes alcohol-like intoxicated delirium accompanied by jerking movements.
- The hallucinogen group (species of the genera *Conocybe, Gymnopilus, Panaeolus, Pluteus, Psilocybe,* and *Stropharia*) causes hallucination; the chief toxins are psilocybin and psilocin.

—*Psilocybe* genus contains more than 100 species of small, brown, slender-stalked mushrooms, commonly found growing in piles of dung and fertilized grasses in moist areas all over the United States; they are especially common in the South.
—A classic feature of *Psilocybe* species (and of many other toxic mushrooms) is the development of blue-green color where it is injured or handled.

- The gastrointestinal irritant group causes repeated vomiting and diarrhea.

—This group is a catch-all for mushrooms that produce gastroenteritis but do not produce systemic signs or symptoms (besides dehydration), usually resulting in a benign clinical course; toxins are varied and mostly unknown.
—One of the most common species is *Chlorophyllum molybdites;* its juvenile form is often mistaken for the edible "shaggy mane," from which it may be distinguished by faint green gills and a green spore print.

Symptoms Noted More than 6 Hours After Ingestion

- The cyclopeptide group of toxins (present in a number of *Amanita, Galerina, Lepiota,* and *Conocybe* species) produce severe hepatic injury with a high fatality rate.

—Included in this group is the "death cap" (*Amanita phalloides*) and the "destroying angel" (*A. virosa,* which superficially resembles common cultivated mushrooms), whose chief toxin is amatoxin.
—Not all mushrooms of the *Amanita* genus contain amatoxin.

- The monomethylhydrazine group (*Gyromitra* species) can produce seizures and occasionally death.

—Not all species of *Gyromitra* have been found to contain the toxin gyromitrin.
—Monomethylhydrazine has been found in *Gyromitra esculenta,* the "false morel," a mushroom that is occasionally foraged in the Pacific Northwest of the United States.

Symptoms Developing More than 24 Hours After Ingestion

The orelline- and orellanine-containing group (*Cortinarius* species) causes renal injury.

TOXIC DOSE

- One death cap (*Amanita phalloides*) can cause death.
- At least 15 to 20 *Galerina* mushrooms are needed to produce death.
- Ingestion of just a few gastrointestinal-irritant mushrooms can produce marked gastroenteritis.

PATHOPHYSIOLOGY

Cyclopeptide Group

- α-Amanitin is primarily responsible for the toxicity seen with the phalloides syndrome.
- α-Amanitin binds to nuclear RNA polymerase II of eukaryotic cells and inhibits mRNA synthesis, resulting in cell death.
- The liver and the kidney are the primary targets of α-amanitin due to high rates of protein synthesis.

Monomethylhydrazine Group

- Gyromitrin (monomethylhydrazine) causes toxicity similar to isoniazid overdose.
- Both agents deplete pyridoxine (vitamin B_6) in the brain, inhibiting production of γ-aminobutyric acid (GABA) and thereby allowing seizures to occur.

Disulfiram-like Group

Like disulfiram, coprine may inhibit the metabolism of ethanol at the acetaldehyde dehydrogenase step, resulting in an Antabuse-like reaction.

Muscarine Group

- The toxic component is muscarine, which stimulates muscarinic receptors, thereby producing cholinergic syndrome.
- Because of its quaternary configuration, muscarine cannot cross into the CNS; therefore, it causes peripheral cholinergic effects.

Ibotenic Acid and Muscimol Group

- These compounds apparently compete with the normal transmitter, GABA, and cause psychotropic symptoms.
- The peripheral effects, relatively slight, are usually more anticholinergic than cholinergic.

Hallucinogen Group

It is believed that the clinical effects are caused by the indoles such as psilocybin and psilocin, which are chemically related to serotonin.

Gastrointestinal Irritant Group

This group contains many toxins, mostly unidentified.

Orelline- and Orellanine-containing Group

- These heat-stable toxins are chemically related to diquat.
- Poisoning results in tubulo-interstitial nephritis and fibrosis.

EPIDEMIOLOGY

- Poisoning is common.
- The cyclopeptide-containing mushrooms, chiefly *Amanita* species, are responsible for over 90% of all deaths from mushroom poisoning.

CAUSES

Poisoning usually results from intentional ingestion as food.

Drug and Disease Interactions

An Antabuse-like reaction can be produced by drinking alcohol within a week or two of eating coprine-type mushrooms.

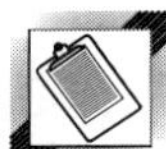

Diagnosis

DIFFERENTIAL DIAGNOSIS

- Diagnosis is based on a history of ingestion combined with clinical presentation and identification of the mushroom (if possible).
- Most poison centers can guide the identification of the mushroom.

SIGNS AND SYMPTOMS

Symptoms Developing Within 3 Hours of Ingestion

Disulfiram-like Group

- Ingestion produces disulfiram reaction: flushing of the face and trunk, palpitations, dyspnea, chest pain, diaphoresis, and hypotension (secondary to vasodilation).
- The reaction may occur after the ingestion of ethanol as long as 1 week after consumption of *Coprinus atramentarius*.

Muscarine Group

- Ingestion produces cholinergic syndrome: vomiting, miosis, salivation, lacrimation, bronchorrhea, bronchospasm, bradycardia, diarrhea, and urinary retention.
- Seizure may occur in severe cases.

Ibotenic Acid and Muscimol Group

- Ingestion produces alcohol-like intoxication, ataxia, clonus, spontaneous jerking movements, and delirium.
- Seizure and coma may develop in severe cases.

Hallucinogen Group

- In addition to a psychedelic experience, tachycardia, mydriasis, and paresthesia commonly develop; seizure occurs rarely.
- The initial episode lasts 4 to 6 hours; flashbacks may occur.
- In children, fever (102°F to 106°F) may develop with intermittent tonic-clonic seizures.

Gastrointestinal Irritant Group

- Onset of symptoms is usually within 30 minutes to 3 hours of ingestion.
- Response is variable; the same species may cause symptoms in one person at one time and not at another time.

Symptoms Noted More than 6 Hours after Ingestion

Cyclopeptide Group

Amanita poisoning develops in four stages:

- The first phase is a latent period of 6 to 12 hours and is of diagnostic value.

—Most other poisonous but less harmful mushrooms cause symptoms within 3 hours of ingestion.
—Caution. In mixed mushroom ingestion, symptoms may develop within 3 hours but still contain the deadly *Amanita*.

- The second, or gastrointestinal, phase begins in 6 to 12 hours and is characterized by nausea, vomiting, abdominal pain, and cholera-like diarrhea with concurrent dehydration; hypoglycemia may develop.
- The third phase is another period of latency.

—Although the patient feels better when the gastrointestinal phase is over, liver injury becomes evident by the rise in ALT, AST, LDH (serum glutamic-oxaloacetic transaminase, serum glutamic-pyruvic transaminase, and lactic dehydrogenase), and abnormal coagulation studies.
—A rapid fall of coagulation factors usually indicates poor prognosis.

- The fourth, or hepatic, phase follows.

—During this period, fulminant hepatic failure and possibly acute renal failure become clinically apparent.
—The patient may progress to hepatic encephalopathy, coma, and death.

Monomethylhydrazine Group

- Symptoms are usually mild and include vomiting, diarrhea, dizziness, fatigue, and muscle cramps.
- Delirium, coma, and seizures may develop in severe cases.
- Methemoglobinemia and hemolysis may be life threatening.
- Pancreatitis may develop.

Symptoms Developing More than 24 Hours after Ingestion

The orelline and orellanine group produces late-onset nausea, vomiting, oliguria, and renal failure.

PROCEDURES AND LABORATORY TESTS

Essential Tests

Symptoms Developing Within 3 Hours of Ingestion

- No tests are essential.
- Tests to evaluate fluid and electrolyte status should be considered if severe gastroenteritis develops.

Symptoms Developing More than 6 Hours after Ingestion

• If a mycologist is available, stomach contents should be saved for spore identification.
• Serum electrolytes, BUN, creatinine, glucose, and liver function tests should be performed.

—Amatoxin-containing mushrooms may produce fulminant hepatic failure.
—Elevated serum ALT, AST, LDH, and serum bilirubin are the first and best indicators of liver damage.
—Glucose, fibrinogen, and international normalized ratio (INR) or prothrombin levels are the best indicators of liver failure.

Symptoms Developing More than 24 Hours after Ingestion

Serum electrolytes, BUN, and creatinine should be assayed to detect onset of kidney injury.

Recommended Tests

Symptoms Developing Within 3 Hours of Ingestion

If mushrooms from the gastrointestinal-irritant group are suspected, serum electrolytes, BUN, and creatinine should be followed only if gastrointestinal effects are severe.

Symptoms Developing More than 6 Hours after Ingestion

If *Gyromitra* species is suspected, methemoglobin levels should be monitored.

Symptoms Developing More than 24 Hours after Ingestion

• Urinalysis reveals concentrated urine with hematuria, protein, and red blood cell casts early, followed by dilute urine with protein and a few casts later in the course.
• Other tests may be available for complicated cases, but should be guided by a mycologist experienced in poisonous mushroom identification.

Not Recommended Tests

Although some mushroom toxins can be measured in blood or urine, none are available for clinical use.

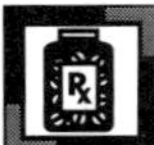

Treatment

• Treatment should focus on decontamination, identification of the mushroom if possible, and intensive supportive care.
• Dose and time of exposure should be determined for all substances involved.

DIRECTING PATIENT COURSE

The health-care provider should call the poison control center when:

• There is any opportunity to identify the mushroom involved; many certified regional poison centers have a mycologist available for difficult cases.
• Toxic effects are present.
• Coingestant, drug interaction, or underlying disease presents an unusual problem.

The patient should be referred to a health-care facility when:

• Attempted suicide or homicide is possible.
• Patient or caregiver seems unreliable.
• Toxic effects are present.
• Coingestant, drug interaction, or underlying disease presents an unusual problem.

Admission Considerations

Inpatient management is warranted if patient exhibits persistent gastrointestinal effect or if symptoms begin after 6 hours.

DECONTAMINATION

Out of Hospital

Although rarely needed, emesis should be considered within 1 hour of ingestion for alert pediatric or adult patients if health-care evaluation will be delayed.

In Hospital

• Gastric lavage should be performed in pediatric (tube size 24–32 French) or adult (tube size 36–42 French) patients presenting within 1 hour of a large ingestion or if serious effects are present.
• One dose of activated charcoal (1–2 g/kg) should be administered without a cathartic if a substantial ingestion has occurred within the previous few hours.
• Amatoxins have been reported to undergo enterohepatic recirculation, and in that case, activated charcoal may be useful for at least 24 hours postingestion.

ANTIDOTES

• There are no proven antidotes for any type of mushroom poisoning.
• Experimental treatments for severe cyclopeptide poisoning include penicillin G, silibinin, thioctic acid, steroids, and hyperbaric oxygen; consultation with a poison center and physician experienced in the care of severe *Amanita* poisoning is recommended.

ADJUNCTIVE TREATMENT

Symptoms Developing Within 3 Hours of Ingestion

Hallucinogen Group

• Treatment should consist of intensive supportive care.
• Patients who present to the emergency department usually need reassurance only; sedation with benzodiazepines may be necessary.
• See SECTION IV, LSD chapter, for more details on management.

Hypotension (Caused by Any Group)

• Patient should rapidly receive 10 to 20 ml/kg 0.9% saline intravenously and be placed in the Trendelenburg position.
• Further fluid therapy should be guided by central monitoring or right heart catheter to avoid volume overload.
• If hypotension is unresponsive, a vasopressor should be administered.

—Dopamine initial dosage for adults or children is 2 to 5 μg/kg/min, titrated to effect; administration at rates above 20 μg/kg/min is unlikely to provide further benefit.
—If hypotension is unresponsive, norepinephrine should be infused at 0.1 to 0.2 μg/kg/min and titrated to effect.

• High rates of infusion may cause tissue ischemia.

Symptoms Developing More than 6 Hours after Ingestion

Cyclopeptide Group

• Patients with severe effects will need intensive critical care support of liver and kidney function.

• Orthotopic liver transplantation has been performed successfully in some cases of severe phalloides syndrome.

—Exact criteria have not been tested.
—However, consultation with a liver transplantation center is recommended when any of the following signs of poor prognosis are present:
  —pH less than 7.3 after fluid resuscitation
  —Grade III or IV encephalopathy
  —Creatinine above 3.4 mg/dl
  —Prothrombin time above 35 to 40 seconds, or rapidly rising

Monomethylhydrazine Group

• Methylene blue should be used to treat symptomatic methemoglobinemia (see SECTION III, Methylene Blue chapter).
• Blood transfusion may be needed for hemolysis.
• Intravenous pyridoxine (5 g) and benzodiazepine should be administered for monomethylhydrazine-induced seizures; pyridoxine dose may be repeated once for recurrent seizures (see SECTION III, Pyridoxine chapter).

Symptoms Developing More than 24 Hours after Ingestion

The orelline/orellanine group may require prolonged monitoring and support of renal function. Preliminary evidence suggests that early hemodialysis or hemoperfusion may reduce kidney injury.

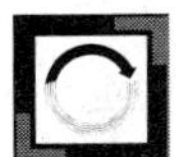

Follow-Up

PATIENT MONITORING

Symptoms Developing Within 3 Hours of Ingestion

Electrolytes should be monitored as indicated by clinical course.

Symptoms Developing More than 6 Hours after Ingestion

If signs of liver injury develop, serial electrolytes, and renal and hepatic function tests and continuous cardiac monitoring should be performed.

Symptoms Developing More than 24 Hours after Ingestion

If signs of kidney injury develop, serial electrolytes and renal function tests should be monitored.

EXPECTED COURSE AND PROGNOSIS

Symptoms Developing Within 3 Hours of Ingestion

• Gastrointestinal effects typically peak and abate within a few hours.
• Psychedelic mushroom effects peak and abate within hours, but flashbacks may rarely occur weeks to months later.
• Renal insufficiency induced by volume depletion develops rarely if adequate hydration is provided.

Symptoms Developing More than 6 Hours after Ingestion

• *Amanita* species ingestion outcome depends on severity of hepatic injury; recovery takes weeks to months and may involve liver transplantation.
• Amatoxin may produce fulminant hepatic and renal failure and death.
• Gyromitrin may produce repeated seizures and hepatorenal failure.

Symptoms Developing More than 24 Hours after Ingestion

Renal failure peaks within several days and slowly improves over weeks, but renal insufficiency may persist.

DISCHARGE CRITERIA/INSTRUCTIONS

Symptoms Developing Within 3 Hours of Ingestion

Patient may be discharged when gastrointestinal or psychedelic effects resolve, and volume depletion is corrected and patient can tolerate fluids.

Symptoms Developing More than 6 Hours after Ingestion

• Patient should not normally be discharged from emergency department.
• Patient may be discharged from hospital when liver and kidney function are stable or clearly improving.

Symptoms Developing More than 24 Hours after Ingestion

Patient may be discharged when kidney function is stable or returning to normal.

PATIENT EDUCATION

Patients should be cautioned to not eat wild mushrooms; even experienced foragers have died from misidentification.

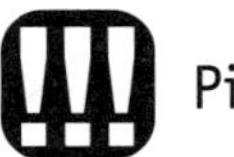

Pitfalls

DIAGNOSIS

• If more than one type of mushroom was eaten, symptoms emerging in less than 3 hours does not assure that cyclopeptide mushrooms were not ingested.
• "Mushroom poisoning" may actually be an allergic reaction or food poisoning.
• "Mushroom poisoning" may actually be a reaction secondary to pesticides sprayed on the mushroom or to edible mushrooms being laced with drugs (e.g., phencyclidine).
• Not all persons ingesting the same species of mushroom will become ill.
• All patients who experience initial symptoms more than 6 hours after ingestion should be presumed to have eaten *Amanita phalloides* or *A. virosa*.

TREATMENT

High doses of pyridoxine are known to cause peripheral neuropathy, and excessive use should be avoided.

FOLLOW-UP

Patients who appear to have recovered from their gastrointestinal symptoms when those symptoms developed more than 6 hours postingestion should not be discharged without follow-up.

ICD-9-CM 988.1

Toxic effect of noxious substances eaten as food: mushrooms.

See also: SECTION II, Hypotension and Seizures chapters; SECTION III, Methylene Blue and Pyridoxine chapters; and SECTION IV, Disulfiram and LSD chapters.

RECOMMENDED READING

Goldfrank LR. Mushrooms: toxic and hallucinogenic. In: Goldfrank LR, Flomenbaum NE, Lewin NA, et al., eds. *Goldfrank's toxicologic emergencies*, 6th ed. Norwalk, CT: Appleton & Lange, 1998.

Author: Luke Yip

Reviewer: Richard C. Dart

Narcotics

Basics

DESCRIPTION

- Pharmaceutical preparations for oral administration include morphine (MS-Contin, Roxanol), hydromorphone (Dilaudid), levorphanol (Levo-Dromoran), methadone (Dolophine), meperidine (Demerol), fentanyl (Sublimaze), codeine, hydrocodone (Vicodin, Hycodan), dihydrocodeine (Synalgos-DC), paregoric, oxycodone (Percocet, Percodan), propoxyphene (Darvon), and oxymorphone (Numorphan). Numerous other products are available and many are combination products containing acetaminophen or aspirin, and occasionally caffeine.
- Heroin is covered in a separate chapter.

FORMS AND USES

- Narcotics are used for the oral treatment of pain.

—Morphine is administered at 2.5 to 20 mg orally every 2 to 6 hours as required.
—Hydromorphone is administered at 2 to 4 mg orally every 4 to 6 hours as required.
—Meperidine is administered at 50 to 100 mg orally every 3 to 4 hours as required.

- Narcotics are also present in selected cough preparations.

TOXIC DOSE

- Codeine. The lethal dose for adults is 7 to 14 mg/kg.
- Hydrocodone. The lethal dose for adults is 100 mg.
- A tolerant individual may require much larger doses for toxicity.
- Children may have unusual sensitivity to opioids and may develop toxicity near the therapeutic dose.

PATHOPHYSIOLOGY

- The primary effects in overdose are mediated by μ, κ, and σ opioid receptors.
- μ-receptor stimulation produces agonist-type supraspinal analgesia, respiratory depression, euphoria, and decreased gastrointestinal motility.
- κ-receptor stimulation produces agonist-antagonist type spinal analgesia, sedation, and miosis.
- σ-receptor activation produces antagonist activity such as dysphoria and psychotomimetic effects (e.g., hallucinations).
- Opioids lose receptor specificity when given at high doses.
- The onset of effects may occur immediately after intravenous injection or inhalation, minutes to hours after ingestion.
- Direct pulmonary injury may produce noncardiogenic pulmonary edema.

EPIDEMIOLOGY

- Poisoning is common.
- Toxic effects following exposure are typically moderate, with death occurring from respiratory depression.

CAUSES

- Use is typically intentional in adults, accidental in children.
- Child neglect or abuse should be considered if the patient is less than 1 year of age, suicide attempt if the patient is over 6 years of age.

RISK FACTORS

Persistent pain (e.g., severe toothache or headache) may lead to overuse.

DRUG AND DISEASE INTERACTIONS

- Narcotics potentiate CNS depression of sedative-hypnotic drugs and other respiratory depressants.
- Meperidine and monoamine oxidase inhibitors may cause serotonin syndrome.
- Methadone serum levels are decreased by chronic use of carbamazepine, phenytoin, and rifampin, resulting in withdrawal.

PREGNANCY AND LACTATION

- US FDA Pregnancy Category. Pregnancy risk is category B for nearly all narcotics; however, the risk factor is category D for prolonged use or in high doses at term.
- Category D. Despite positive evidence that human fetal risk exists, benefits in certain situations (e.g., life-threatening situations or serious diseases) may make use of the drug acceptable despite its risks.
- Newborns of addicted women often suffer symptoms of withdrawal.

Diagnosis

DIFFERENTIAL DIAGNOSIS

- Other toxicologic causes of miosis include cholinergic agonist drugs such as pilocarpine or the organophosphate insecticides, but these also may cause salivation, lacrimation, urination, defecation, and bronchorrhea.
- Other toxicologic causes of CNS and respiratory depression are numerous; of note, olanzapine appears to produce miosis and altered mental status.
- Other causes. Pontine hemorrhage (which occurs rarely) may cause sudden loss of consciousness, pinpoint pupils, and cardiovascular instability.

SIGNS AND SYMPTOMS

Rapid onset of miosis, respiratory depression, and decreased mental status suggest opioid overdose.

Vital Signs

Hypothermia or hyperthermia and hypotension may develop.

HEENT

The pupils are normally pinpoint but may be dilated when acidosis or hypoxia is severe.

Cardiovascular

- Hypotension, bradycardia, pulmonary hypertension, cardiac dysrhythmia, and cyanosis can occur with all opioids.
- Norpropoxyphene, the metabolite of propoxyphene, may cause heart block, conduction delays, and ventricular dysrhythmia.
- Pentazocine overdose can cause ventricular dysrhythmia.

Pulmonary

- Respiratory depression, noncardiogenic pulmonary edema, respiratory arrest, hypoxia, bronchoconstriction, acute asthma, and pneumonitis may occur.
- Butorphanol overdose is associated with pulmonary hypertension induced by naloxone administration.

Gastrointestinal

Constipation, decreased intestinal motility, and ileus occur commonly.

Renal

Urinary retention, myoglobinuria, proteinuria, glomerulonephritis, acute tubular necrosis, and nephropathy may occur during chronic abuse.

Musculoskeletal

Rhabdomyolysis may cause acute renal failure.

Neurologic

- Lethargy and coma are common and responsive to naloxone.
- Normeperidine, a metabolite of meperidine, can cause tremors and seizures.
- Seizures can occur with propoxyphene or high doses of fentanyl.

PROCEDURES AND LABORATORY TESTS

Essential Tests

No tests may be needed for asymptomatic patients.

Recommended Tests

- Serum electrolytes, BUN, and creatinine are recommended to assess the causes of altered mental status, seizure, or cardiac effects.
- Serum creatine kinase may be elevated due to repeated seizures or rhabdomyolysis.
- An ECG and continuous cardiac monitoring for symptomatic patients are advised to detect the effects of cardiotoxic medication such as propoxyphene.

- Urinalysis is used to assess injury from rhabdomyolysis or hypotension.
- Serum acetaminophen and aspirin levels should be checked in an overdose setting to detect occult ingestion.
- Head CT, blood and CSF cultures, and lumbar puncture should be performed as needed to rule out other causes of coma or seizures.
- Chest radiography is used to evaluate persistent hypoxia.

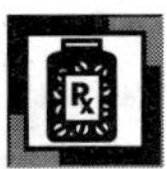

Treatment

- Treatment should focus on airway management, naloxone administration, and hemodynamic support.
- The dose and time of exposure should be determined for all substances involved.

DIRECTING PATIENT COURSE

The health-care professional should call the poison control center when:

- Seizures, dysrhythmia, hypotension, acidemia, or other severe effects are present.
- Toxic effects are not consistent with narcotic poisoning.
- Coingestant, drug interaction, or underlying disease presents an unusual problem.

The patient should be referred to a health-care facility when:

- Attempted suicide or homicide is possible.
- The patient or caregiver seems unreliable.
- Any toxic effects develop.
- Coingestant, drug interaction, or underlying disease presents an unusual problem.

Admission Considerations

Inpatient admission to an intensive care setting is warranted for patients with persistent altered mental status, persistent hypoxia, seizures, hypotension, or dysrhythmia.

DECONTAMINATION

Out of Hospital

Emesis should not be induced because coma or seizure may develop abruptly.

In Hospital

- Gastric lavage should be performed in pediatric (tube size 24–32 French) or adult (tube size 36–42 French) patients presenting within 1 hour of a large ingestion or if serious effects are present.
- One dose of activated charcoal (1–2 g/kg) should be administered without a cathartic if a substantial ingestion has occurred within the previous few hours.

ANTIDOTES

- Naloxone should be administered for respiratory depression from known opioid overdose.

—The dose is 2.0 mg intravenous push; if the patient does not respond, the dose can be repeated in 2.0-mg increments to a total dose of 10 mg.
—Although these methods are less desirable, naloxone also may be administered by endotracheal, intramuscular, intralingual, intraosseous, or subcutaneous injection.
—If a reversal response occurs, patients should be observed for 4 hours after the final dose to avoid resedation.
—Patients with persistent or recurrent effects may be treated with a constant infusion of naloxone.

- Nalmefene may be substituted for naloxone if prolonged antagonist effect is desired. The starting dose is 0.5 mg by intravenous push; if no effect is seen, an additional 1 mg may be given.

—Higher doses of nalmefene appear to give prolonged activity; 1.5 mg of nalmefene blocks opioid activity up to 8 hours.
—If repeated dosing is required, the patient should be admitted to an ICU setting.

ADJUNCTIVE TREATMENT

Pulmonary Edema

- Adequate ventilation and oxygenation should be maintained.
- Positive end-expiratory pressure (PEEP) or continuous positive airway pressure (CPAP) should be considered if adequate oxygenation cannot be maintained on 60% FiO_2.
- Care should be taken to avoid fluid overload.

Hypotension

- The primary treatment is correction of narcotic effects and dysrhythmia.
- Also, 10 to 20 ml/kg 0.9% saline should be administered, and the patient should be placed in the Trendelenburg position and given a vasopressor, if needed.

Seizures

- A patent airway must be ensured.
- A benzodiazepine is administered for initial control. If seizures persist or recur, another anticonvulsant such as phenobarbital may be added.

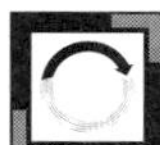

Follow-Up

PATIENT MONITORING

- Respiratory and cardiac function should be monitored continuously.
- Possible complications include renal failure and CNS injury secondary to prolonged seizure, and myocardial or CNS injury from hypoxia.

EXPECTED COURSE AND PROGNOSIS

The prognosis is determined by the hypoxic injury that occurred before treatment or the muscle injury from lying on an extremity for a prolonged period.

DISCHARGE CRITERIA/INSTRUCTIONS

- From the emergency department. For most narcotics, asymptomatic patients may be discharged following decontamination, a 6-hour observation period, and psychiatric evaluation, if needed.
- From the hospital. Patients may be discharged after mental status, ECG, and vital signs return to normal, and decontamination and psychiatric evaluation are completed, if needed.

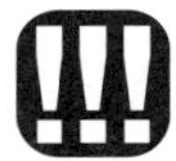

Pitfalls

DIAGNOSIS

- Pinpoint pupils may be obscured by hypoxia or agents that produce mydriasis, such as scopolamine.
- Many tablets containing narcotics also contain acetaminophen or aspirin.

FOLLOW-UP

Discharge of the patient immediately after naloxone treatment may allow the recurrence of respiratory depression outside of the emergency department.

ICD-9-CM 965.0

Poisoning by analgesics, antipyretics, and antirheumatics: opiates and related narcotics.

See also: SECTION II, Body Packer/Body Stuffer, Hypotension, Pulmonary Edema, and Seizures chapters; SECTION III, Naloxone chapter; and SECTION IV, Heroin, Acetaminophen, and Salicylates chapters.

RECOMMENDED READING

Goldfrank LR, Weisman RS. Opioids. In: Goldfrank LR, Flomenbaum NE, Lewin NA, et al., eds. *Goldfrank's toxicologic emergencies,* 6th ed. Norwalk, CT: Appleton & Lange, 1998.

Author: Robin Millin

Reviewer: Richard C. Dart

Niacin and Nicotinamide

Basics

DESCRIPTION

Niacin and nicotinamide are used in the treatment of hyperlipidemia.

FORMS AND USES

- Substances include niacin (nicotinic acid, Niacor, Nicotinex, Slo-Niacin) and nicotinamide (niacinamide).
- Nicotinamide is a metabolite of nicotinic acid that lacks the adverse effect of flushing.
- Either compound is used in the treatment and prevention of nicotinic acid deficiency; up to 500 mg daily in divided doses.
- Nicotinic acid is used as an adjunct in therapy of hyperlipidemia; up to 600 mg daily by mouth in divided doses; doses of up to 6 g daily have been used.
- Nicotinamide has been used as treatment for ingestion of pyriminil (PNU, Vacor), alloxan, or streptozotocin; the dose is 500 mg intravenously, immediately followed by 100 to 200 mg intravenously every 4 hours for up to 48 hours.
- Nicotinamide is used as a topical treatment of inflammatory acne vulgaris.
- Nicotinamide is used for newly diagnosed insulin-dependent diabetes mellitus; it also may delay the onset of disease in prediabetic children.

TOXIC DOSE

- Acute overdose of any magnitude may cause flushing.
- During chronic therapeutic use, hepatitis has occurred with doses as low as 3 to 4 g/day.

PATHOPHYSIOLOGY

- Nicotinic acid and nicotinamide are water-soluble vitamin B substances that are converted to nicotinamide adenine dinucleotide (NAD) and nicotinamide adenine dinucleotide phosphate (NADP).
- These coenzymes are involved in electron transfer reactions in the respiratory chain.
- Nicotinic acid may produce dramatic vasodilation due to release of histamine.

EPIDEMIOLOGY

Poisoning is uncommon, but the adverse effect of flushing is common.

CAUSES

Child neglect or abuse should be considered if the patient is less than 1 year of age, suicide attempt if the patient is over 6 years of age.

DRUG AND DISEASE INTERACTIONS

Nicotinic acid therapy, when given in conjunction with lovastatin or some other inhibitors of HMG CoA reductase (lipid lowering agents), has been reported to be associated with rhabdomyolysis.

PREGNANCY AND LACTATION

- US FDA Pregnancy Category A. Controlled studies in women fail to demonstrate a risk to the fetus in the first trimester, and the possibility of fetal harm appears remote.
- When used in doses above the recommended daily allowance, it is US FDA Pregnancy Category C. The drug exerts animal teratogenic or embryocidal effects, but there are no controlled studies in women, or no studies are available in animals or women.

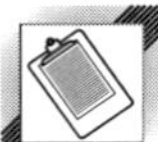

Diagnosis

DIFFERENTIAL DIAGNOSIS

The primary acute effect is sudden flushing. Other drugs that cause the effect are vancomycin or acute allergic reaction to any medication.

SIGNS AND SYMPTOMS

When given by mouth or by injection in therapeutic doses, nicotinic acid may cause transient symptoms of flushing, a sensation of heat, faintness, and pounding in the head.

HEENT

Amblyopia may occur.

Dermatologic

Dryness of the skin, pruritus, and hyperpigmentation may result.

Gastrointestinal

Abdominal cramps, diarrhea, nausea and vomiting, anorexia, and activation of peptic ulcer may occur.

Hepatic

- Chemical hepatitis occurs uncommonly.
- It is more likely to develop in patients given large increases in dosage over short periods of time or treated with sustained-release formulations.

Musculoskeletal

Myopathy also has been reported with nicotinic acid.

Endocrine

Decrease in glucose tolerance, hyperglycemia, and hyperuricemia may occur.

PROCEDURES AND LABORATORY TESTS

Essential Tests

No tests are usually needed after acute overdose ingestion.

Recommended Tests

- Liver function tests are used to detect hepatitis during therapy.
- Serum creatine kinase is measured in symptomatic patients to detect rhabdomyolysis.
- ECG, serum acetaminophen and aspirin levels in overdose setting to detect occult ingestion.

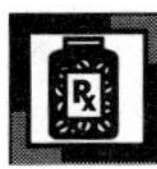

Treatment

- Focus therapy on symptomatic and supportive care.
- Dose and time of exposure should be determined for all substances involved.

DIRECTING PATIENT COURSE

The health-care professional should call the poison control center when:

- Severe or persistent effects develop.
- Coingestant, drug interaction, or underlying disease presents an unusual problem.

The patient should be referred to a health-care facility when:

- Suicide or homicide attempt is possible.
- Toxic effects develop.
- Coingestant, drug interaction, or underlying disease presents an unusual problem.

Admission Considerations

Extended observation or hospital admission is rarely needed.

DECONTAMINATION

Gastrointestinal decontamination is not usually needed unless coingestant is possible.

ANTIDOTES

There is no specific antidote available for nicotinic acid or nicotinamide poisoning.

ADJUNCTIVE TREATMENT

- The primary treatment is to discontinue the therapeutic use of nicotinic acid.
- To decrease symptoms of flushing, the clinician may substitute nicotinamide for nicotinic acid.

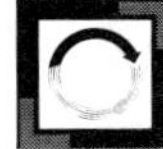

Follow-Up

EXPECTED COURSE AND PROGNOSIS

Flushing usually lasts 2 to 3 hours.

DISCHARGE CRITERIA/INSTRUCTIONS

Following acute ingestion, the patient may be discharged from the emergency department or hospital when flushing has resolved.

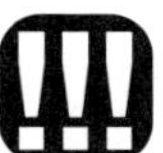

Pitfalls

FOLLOW-UP

- Nicotinic acid should be given cautiously to patients with gout, impaired liver function, or a history of peptic ulceration.
- Requirements of insulin or oral hypoglycemic agents may change when nicotinic acid is given.
- Nicotinic acid should not be substituted for niacinamide because the vasodilatory effects of nicotinic acid may exacerbate the problems of blood pressure control; nicotinic acid may be less effective and also may worsen glucose tolerance.

ICD-9-CM 972.2

Poisoning by agents primarily affecting the cardiovascular system: antilipemic and antiarteriosclerotic drugs.

RECOMMENDED READING

Rader JI, Calvert RJ, Hathcock JW. Hepatic toxicity of unmodified and time-release preparations of niacin. *Am J Med* 1992;92:77–81.

Author: Luke Yip

Reviewer: Edwin K. Kuffner

Nickel

Basics

DESCRIPTION

Nickel is an ubiquitous metal element found in a wide variety of compounds.

FORMS AND USES

- Nickel is used most commonly as a finishing agent for jewelry and as a corrosive protectant for other metal objects.
- Workers in the electroplating industry, jewelers, and those in contact with metal alloys, ceramic glazes, batteries, cement, and green glass are at risk for exposure.

PATHOPHYSIOLOGY

- Contact dermatitis secondary to nickel hypersensitivity from jewelry and watches is the most common adverse effect.
- Exposures of clinical significance involve pulmonary complications of inhalation of nickel alloys in welders, leading to asthma, fibrosis, and pulmonary edema (rare).

TOXIC DOSE

- Dermal hypersensitivity may be caused by very small amounts of nickel in metallic finish.
- Inhalation of concentration greater than 10 mg/m^3 may cause acute severe injury.

EPIDEMIOLOGY

Poisoning is uncommon.

CAUSES

Occupational exposure or exposure to jewelry containing nickel are the usual settings leading to toxicity.

PREGNANCY AND LACTATION

Nickel crosses placenta and into breast milk.

WORKPLACE STANDARDS

- ACGIH. TLV TWA is 1.5 mg/m^3 (as elemental Ni).
- OSHA. PEL TWA is 1.0 mg/m^3.
- NIOSH. IDLH 10 is 10 mg/m^3.

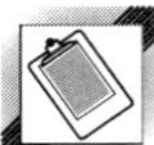

Diagnosis

DIFFERENTIAL DIAGNOSIS

Any cause of dermal hypersensitivity reaction should be ruled out.

SIGNS AND SYMPTOMS

- Almost all nickel toxicities of clinical consequence involve either allergic response to dermal exposure or pulmonary inflammation caused by chronic exposure. Severity of signs and symptoms increases as duration of exposure increases.
- Parenteral exposure (prosthetic implants) may lead to allergic reactions, osteomyelitis, tumors, and contaminated dialysate.

HEENT

Metallic taste following acute inhalation may occur.

Dermatologic

Eczematous dermatitis with irritation, generally benign and self-limited, may occur. This is typically limited to the area of contact with a nickel-containing object (jewelry).

Pulmonary

- Acute exposure. Cough, dyspnea, chest pain, pneumonitis with hyaline membrane formation, pulmonary edema and hemorrhage, and hypoxia may occur.
- Chronic exposure. Cancer of the respiratory tract, pulmonary eosinophilia (Loeffler's syndrome), and asthma may occur.

Gastrointestinal

- Ingestion often causes nausea, vomiting, abdominal pain, and hemorrhagic gastritis.
- Acute inhalation also may cause nausea and abdominal pain.

Neurologic

Acute inhalation may cause headache and vertigo.

PROCEDURES AND LABORATORY TESTS

Essential Tests

No tests may be needed in asymptomatic patients.

Recommended Tests

- Severity of poisoning may be estimated using the nickel concentration in urine collected over 8 hours:

—Mild (<10 μg/dl). Delayed symptoms will either not develop or will be mild.
—Moderate (>10 but <50 μg/dl). Delayed symptoms frequently develop, and these patients should be under careful observation for at least 1 week.
—Severe (>50 μg/dl). These patients are likely to become seriously ill and will require intensive supportive care.

- Arterial blood gases in symptomatic patients.
- Chest radiographs in symptomatic patients may show interstitial pneumonitis following inhalation.
- Pulmonary function testing may be consistent with interstitial infiltrative lung disease.
- Following ingestion, ECG, serum acetaminophen and aspirin levels should be determined if event was possible suicide attempt.

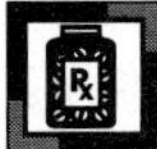

Treatment

- Treatment should focus on supportive care with appropriate airway management; endotracheal intubation may be needed to protect the airway in severe cases.
- Dose and time of exposure should be determined for all substances involved.

DIRECTING PATIENT COURSE

The health-care provider should call the poison control center when:

- Signs and symptoms are not consistent with nickel poisoning.
- Coingestant, drug interaction, or underlying disease presents an unusual challenge.

The patient should be referred to a health-care facility when:

- Attempted suicide or homicide is possible.
- Patient or caregiver seems unreliable.
- Any toxic effects develop.
- Coingestant, drug interaction, or underlying disease presents an unusual challenge.

Admission Considerations

Inpatient management is warranted if:

- Systemic signs or symptoms develop.
- Persistent vomiting develops.
- Significant inhalation exposure occurred.

DECONTAMINATION

Out of Hospital

Immediate irrigation with copious amounts of water is recommended following dermal or ocular exposure to nickel salts.

In Hospital

For ingestions, decontamination is not usually needed because spontaneous vomiting often occurs.

ANTIDOTES

Disulfiram

- Indication is urinary nickel concentration of 10 to 50 μg/dl on 8-hour collection.
- Initial dose is 1 g orally followed by 300 mg every 8 hours.
- If urinary concentration is greater than 50 μg/dl, the initial dose is 12.5 mg/kg.
- Oral disulfiram has been used successfully to treat hypersensitivity dermatitis in nickel-allergic patients after ingestion of coins or other object with high nickel content; patients should avoid alcohol while taking disulfiram.

ADJUNCTIVE TREATMENT

Intravenous hydration with crystalloid solution enhances renal nickel excretion; urine output should be maintained at 1 cc/kg/h.

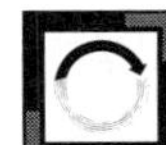

Follow-Up

PATIENT MONITORING

- Cardiac, pulmonary, renal, and hepatic functions should be monitored.
- Patient should be observed for 24 to 48 hours for onset of pneumonitis or pulmonary edema.

EXPECTED COURSE AND PROGNOSIS

- Dermatitis resolves without sequelae.
- Patients with serious nickel inhalation exposure recover unless the pulmonary damage is severe, in which case chronic respiratory insufficiency and restrictive lung disease may develop.

DISCHARGE CRITERIA/INSTRUCTIONS

Patients may be discharged from the emergency department or hospital when toxic effects resolve or stabilize and after psychiatric evaluation, if needed.

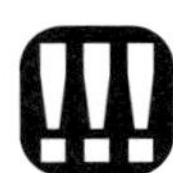

Pitfalls

DIAGNOSIS

- Initial symptoms may be mild and vague and may resolve quickly; however, the respiratory inflammatory process commonly recurs 12 to 36 hours later.
- Asymptomatic patients with seemingly insignificant exposures to vapors of inorganic nickel salts therefore require in-hospital observation for 24 to 48 hours.

ICD-9-CM 985.8

Toxic effect of other metals: other specified metals (nickel compounds).

Author: Lada Kokan

Reviewer: Gerald F. O'Malley

Nickel Carbonyl

Basics

DESCRIPTION

• Nickel carbonyl is a colorless, highly flammable liquid, volatile at room temperature, which produces a musty odor described as "sooty" or "like a damp cellar."
• It is highly explosive, and vapors in air can explode at 20°C.

FORMS AND USES

Nickel carbonyl [$Ni(CO)_4$] is used as a catalyst in the petroleum, plastic, and rubber industries.

TOXIC DOSE

Inhalation of air containing just a few parts per million of carbon disulfide can be lethal.

PATHOPHYSIOLOGY

• Nickel carbonyl and its vapor are decomposed by heat into carbon monoxide and nickel.
• Most exposures involve inhalation of the vapor leading to pulmonary parenchymal damage; secondary injury occurs in the liver and brain as well.
• Inhaled nickel carbonyl vapor is rapidly absorbed from the lungs and enters erythrocytes where it undergoes conversion to nickel (Ni^{+2}) and carbon monoxide.
• Death is usually the result of diffuse interstitial pneumonitis and cerebral edema.
• Chronic exposure has been implicated in nasal and lung cancers as well as pulmonary eosinophilia (Loeffler's syndrome) and asthma.

EPIDEMIOLOGY

Poisoning is uncommon but frequently causes severe toxicity or death.

CAUSES

Exposure is nearly always an accidental occupational inhalation.

PREGNANCY AND LACTATION

• Female workers in nickel carbonyl industry showed no reproductive or birth effects.
• Large exposure in animals has produced teratogenic effects.

WORKPLACE STANDARDS

• OSHA. PEL TWA is 0.001 ppm.
• ACGIH. TLV TWA is 0.05 ppm.
• NIOSH. REL TWA is 0.001 ppm; IDLH is 2 ppm.

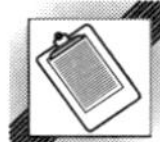

Diagnosis

DIFFERENTIAL DIAGNOSIS

Toxicologic causes of acute respiratory irritation include chlorine and other halogens, phosgene, carbon disulfide, hydrogen sulfide, smoke, and others.

SIGNS AND SYMPTOMS

The toxic presentation of nickel carbonyl poisoning occurs in two symptomatic phases.

• Initial symptoms

—Frontal headache, nausea, vomiting, and giddiness
—Hacking nonproductive cough and chest soreness
—Diaphoresis, dyspnea, and weakness
—Initial symptoms resolve quickly when the exposure is terminated.

• Symptoms of the second phase usually begin from 10 hours to 8 days later and include:

—Paroxysmal coughing, retrosternal pain, and tachypnea
—Cyanosis and lethargy
—Delirium, seizure, and hyperpyrexia

PROCEDURES AND LABORATORY TESTS

Essential Tests

Severity of poisoning should be estimated for all exposed individuals after determining an initial 8-hour urine nickel concentration:

• Mild (<10 $\mu g/dl$). Delayed symptoms will either not develop or will be mild.
• Moderate (>10 but <50 $\mu g/dl$). Delayed symptoms are likely; patient should be under careful observation for at least 1 week.
• Severe (>50 $\mu g/dl$). These patients are likely to be seriously ill and will require intensive supportive care.

Recommended Tests

• Serum electrolytes, glucose, BUN, creatinine are used to assess other causes.
• If the patient develops altered mental status, carbon monoxide poisoning (carboxyhemoglobin level) also should be considered.
• Arterial blood gases are used to assess severity of pulmonary injury.
• Chest radiographs may show interstitial pneumonitis.
• Pulmonary function testing will be consistent with interstitial infiltrative lung disease.

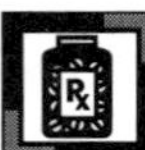

Treatment

• Treatment should focus on intensive supportive care.
• Appropriate respiratory system and airway management is vital.

DIRECTING PATIENT COURSE

The health-care professional should call the poison control center when:

• Exposure to nickel carbonyl has occurred.
• Underlying disease presents an unusual problem.

The patient should be referred to a health-care facility when:

• Exposure to nickel carbonyl has occurred.
• Underlying disease presents an unusual problem.

Admission Considerations

• Inpatient management is warranted in the case of any exposure to nickel carbonyl.
• All exposed individuals should be admitted to the ICU and given intensive supportive care.

DECONTAMINATION

• The patient should be moved to a fresh air environment.
• The patient should be given 100% humidified supplemental oxygen with assisted ventilation as required.

ANTIDOTES

There is no specific antidote for nickel carbonyl poisoning.

ADJUNCTIVE TREATMENT

Corticosteroids may be useful in reducing tissue reaction.

- Sodium diethyldithiocarbamate (Dithiocarb, Immuthiol)

—Mild or doubtful exposure. Dithiocarb 250 mg and sodium bicarbonate 250 mg with water every 30 minutes for eight doses orally, with re-evaluation.

—Moderate to severe exposure. Dithiocarb 50 mg/kg (total dosage for the first 24 hours) orally; for example, 4 g for an 80-kg patient.

—Suggested dosage schedule is 2 g (ten 200-mg capsules) at time 0, 1 g (five 200-mg capsules) at 4 hours, 600 mg (three 200-mg capsules) at 8 hours, and 400 mg (two 200-mg capsules) at 16 hours

—On subsequent days: 400 mg every 8 hours orally until patient is asymptomatic and the urine nickel concentration is in the normal range (<5.0 μg/dl)

—If patient's condition is critical, Dithiocarb should be administered intravenously.

—Solution prepared by adding 10 cc of a sterile solution of phosphate buffer (500 mg NaH_2PO_4 per 100 cc) to 1 g of sterile powdered Dithiocarb.

—Dose: 25 to 100 mg/kg during the first 24 hours with additional doses given based on patient's clinical status

- If Dithiocarb is not available, disulfiram (Antabuse) may be substituted, although it is less effective; dose is half that of Dithiocarb.

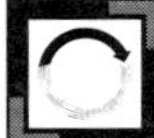

Follow-Up

PATIENT MONITORING

Continuous respiratory and cardiac monitoring should be performed in all exposed patients.

EXPECTED COURSE AND PROGNOSIS

- In patients who survive the acute poisoning, there is usually a protracted convalescence due to pulmonary insufficiency.
- Sequelae include pulmonary fibrosis.

DISCHARGE CRITERIA/INSTRUCTIONS

The patient may be discharged from hospital when asymptomatic for 24 hours or when toxic effects have stabilized.

PATIENT EDUCATION

Patients should abstain from all alcohol-containing beverages for at least 1 week after disulfiram therapy because they may produce disulfiram reaction.

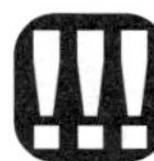

Pitfalls

DIAGNOSIS

- Many cases of accidental nickel carbonyl vapor poisoning are not recognized until days later, delaying therapy.
- Failure to admit an asymptomatic patient to the ICU may allow respiratory deterioration in an unmonitored setting.

ICD-9-CM 985.8

Toxic effect of other metals: other specified metals (nickel compounds).

See also: SECTION IV, Carbon Monoxide and Disulfiram chapters.

RECOMMENDED READING

Sunderman FW Jr. A review of the metabolism and toxicology of nickel. *Ann Clin Lab Sci* 1977;7:377–398.

Sunderman FW Sr. Chelation therapy in nickel poisoning. *Ann Clin Lab Sci* 1981;11:1–7.

Sunderman FW, Kincaid JF. Nickel poisoning II. Studies on patients suffering from acute exposure to vapors of nickel carbonyl. *JAMA* 1954;10:889–894.

Authors: Luke Yip

Reviewer: Gerald F. O'Malley

Nicotine

Basics

DESCRIPTION

Nicotine is derived from alkaloid plants of *Nicotiana* species such as wild tobacco, tree tobacco, and desert tobacco.

FORMS AND USES

- Nicotine is found in cigarettes, cigars, snuff, and chewing tobacco.
- Nicotine is used in insecticides, in veterinary applications as an ectoparasiticide, and in the leather tanning process.
- Nicotine gum (Nicorette) is used for smoking cessation and comes in 2- and 4-mg doses.
- Nicotine transdermal systems (Nicoderm, Nicotrol, Habitrol, Prostep) come in doses of 5 to 22 mg, used at intervals of 16 to 24 hours.
- Nicotine nasal spray (Nicotrol) comes as a 0.5- to 1.0-mg per metered dose spray at intervals of 30 minutes to 1 hour.
- Nicotine inhaler (Nicotrol) contains 10 mg per cartridge.

PATHOPHYSIOLOGY

- Initial stimulation of nicotinic receptors in the sympathetic and parasympathetic ganglia and neuromuscular junctions produces mild to moderate toxicity and is manifested by the classic symptoms of cholinergic excess.
- In severe toxicity, the initial stimulatory effect is followed by depolarization blockade of autonomic ganglion and neuromuscular transmission, which leads to muscle fasciculations and skeletal muscle paralysis.

TOXIC DOSE

- In a child, ingestion of one cigarette, three to five cigarette butts, a pinch of snuff, or any amount of gum, spray, or transdermal system may be toxic.
- In an adult, a lethal oral dose is estimated as more than 40 mg.

EPIDEMIOLOGY

- Poisoning is common.
- Toxic effects are typically mild to moderate.
- Severe toxicity is rare, with death occurring only after large ingestion, usually in a child who deteriorates before medical care is provided.
- Patients at the extremes of age are more susceptible to the effects of nicotine.

CAUSES

- Poisoning is usually accidental in children under 6 years of age.
- Child neglect or abuse should be considered if the patient is under 1 year of age; attempted suicide should be considered in patients over 6 years of age.

PREGNANCY

- US FDA Pregnancy Category D. Evidence of human fetal risk exists, but benefits in certain situations (e.g., life-threatening situations or serious diseases) may make use of the drug acceptable despite its risks.
- Nicotine may be a human teratogen.

WORKPLACE STANDARDS

- ACGIH. TLV TWA is 0.5 mg/m^3
- OSHA. PEL TWA is 0.5 mg/m^3.
- NIOSH. IDLH value is 5 mg/m^3.

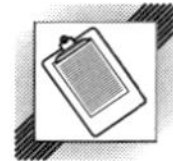

Diagnosis

DIFFERENTIAL DIAGNOSIS

- Toxic causes of cholinergic excess include organophosphate or carbamate insecticides, carbachol, methacholine, bethanechol, pilocarpine, and certain mushrooms.
- Nontoxic causes include myasthenia gravis and Eaton-Lambert syndrome.

SIGNS AND SYMPTOMS

Severe exposure may cause vomiting, confusion, agitation, and restlessness, followed by lethargy, seizures, and coma.

Vital Signs

- Tachycardia is common even with mild toxicity.
- Hypertension may be present early but progresses to hypotension in serious cases.
- Hyperthermia may develop in severe toxicity.

HEENT

- Increased salivation and lacrimation are common.
- Initial miosis followed by mydriasis may occur.
- A burning sensation in mouth and throat may occur.

Dermatologic

Diaphoresis is common.

Pulmonary

Initial tachypnea is followed by respiratory depression.

Cardiovascular

- Sinus tachycardia is common.
- Initial tachycardia and hypertension followed by hypotension and bradycardia may occur.
- Cardiac dysrhythmia may occur in severe cases.

Gastrointestinal

- Nausea and vomiting are common.
- Abdominal pain and diarrhea also may occur.

Renal

Urinary incontinence occurs, especially in severe cases.

Neurologic

Headache, dizziness, and restlessness is followed by lethargy, seizure, and coma.

PROCEDURES AND LABORATORY TESTS

Essential Tests

- Serum electrolytes, glucose, BUN, creatinine, calcium, magnesium, and phosphate to detect other causes of dysrhythmia, weakness or kidney injury
- ECG and continuous monitoring to assess potential causes of hypotension and bradycardia.

Recommended Tests

- Cotinine levels in urine, plasma, and saliva correlate with passive exposure.
- Urine cotinine levels can be used to follow occupational exposure in tobacco pickers.

Not Recommended Tests

Nicotine levels are not clinically useful.

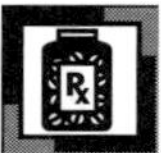

Treatment

- Treatment should focus on decontamination, control of vomiting, support of hemodynamic function, and control of agitation.
- Dose and time of exposure should be determined for all substances involved.

DIRECTING PATIENT COURSE

The health-care professional should call a poison control center when:

- Seizure, hypotension, or serious dysrhythmia develops.
- Toxic effects are not consistent with nicotine poisoning.
- Coingestant, drug interaction, or underlying disease presents an unusual problem.

The patient should be referred to a health-care facility when:

- Attempted suicide or homicide is possible.
- Patient or caregiver seems unreliable.
- Any toxic effects develop.
- Coingestant, drug interaction, or underlying disease presents an unusual problem.

Admission Considerations

Inpatient treatment is warranted when the patient develops serious effects such as cardiac dysrhythmia, seizure, hypotension, persistent vomiting, or agitation.

DECONTAMINATION

Out of Hospital

Emesis is not recommended; seizures may develop quickly.

In Hospital

- Gastric lavage should be administered in pediatric (tube size 24–32 French) or adult (tube size 36–42 French) patients presenting within 1 hour of ingestion or if serious effects are present.
- Gastric lavage is not indicated following spontaneous vomiting.
- One dose of activated charcoal (1–2 g/kg) should be administered if a substantial ingestion has occurred within the previous few hours.
- Following a large ingestion or in patients who have serious signs or symptoms, one to two extra doses of activated charcoal (0.5–1.0 gm/kg) are indicated at 2- to 4-hour intervals.

ANTIDOTES

There is no specific antidote for nicotine poisoning.

ADJUNCTIVE TREATMENT

Seizures

- Airway should be monitored.
- A benzodiazepine familiar to the provider should be administered.

—If diazepam is administered, the adult dose is 5 to 10 mg intravenously, pediatric dose 0.2 to 0.5 mg/kg intravenously, with the dose repeated at 10-minute intervals, titrating to effect.

—If lorazepam is administered, the adult dose is 1 to 2 mg intravenously, pediatric dose 0.05 mg/kg intravenously, with the dose repeated at 10-minute intervals, titrating to effect.
—If benzodiazepines do not control seizures or they recur, phenytoin or phenobarbital should be administered.

Cholinergic Excess

Atropine may be used for control of signs of cholinergic excess.

- The adult dose is 0.5 to 1.0 mg intravenously or intratracheally, repeated every 5 minutes up to a maximum of 0.04 mg/kg.
- Pediatric dose is 0.02 mg/kg intravenously, intratracheally, or intraosseously, repeated every 5 minutes up to a maximum dose of 1 mg in children and 2 mg in adolescents.

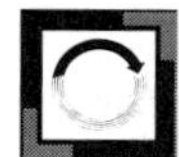

Follow-Up

PATIENT MONITORING

Symptomatic patients require continuous cardiac and respiratory monitoring until signs and symptoms of toxicity resolve.

EXPECTED COURSE AND PROGNOSIS

- Signs and symptoms typically occur within 30 to 90 minutes.
- Mild exposures peak within a few hours, but severe poisoning may produce toxicity for 18 to 24 hours.
- Most patients recover without sequelae with supportive care alone.
- Deaths are usually due to respiratory failure and may occur as early as 1 hour postingestion.

DISCHARGE CRITERIA/INSTRUCTIONS

- From the emergency department

—Patients who are asymptomatic after gastrointestinal decontamination and 4 to 6 hours of observation or after effects have resolved may be discharged.
—A psychiatric evaluation should be provided if needed.

- From the hospital. Patients should be discharged after the effects have resolved and after psychiatric evaluation, if needed.

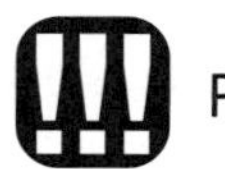

Pitfalls

DIAGNOSIS

Nicotine withdrawal symptoms may occur following chronic exposure, but would not be expected following an acute overdose.

ICD-9-CM 989

Toxic effect of other substances, chiefly nonmedicinal as to source.

See also: SECTION II, Seizures chapter; and SECTION III, Activated Charcoal chapter.

RECOMMENDED READING

Lavoie FW, Harris TM. Fatal nicotine ingestion. *J Emerg Med* 1991;9:133–136.

Woolf A, Burkhart K, Caraccio T, et al. Self-poisoning among adults using multiple transdermal nicotine patches. *Clin Toxicol* 1996;34:691–698.

Author: Benjamin Camp

Reviewer: Richard C. Dart

Nitrates and Nitrites

Basics

DESCRIPTION

- Nitrates and nitrites are used as medications to produce vasodilation or to induce methemoglobinemia.
- Nitrates and nitrites are also used as fertilizers, explosives, food preservatives, and deodorizers.

FORMS AND USES

- Amyl nitrite and sodium nitrite are components of a cyanide kit.
- Organic nitrates are used in explosives and fertilizers.
- Amyl nitrite, butyl nitrite, ethyl nitrite, and isopropyl nitrite are sold as room deodorizers under various trade names (e.g., Poppers, Locker Room).
- Pharmaceutical uses include organic nitrates (nitroglycerin and the isosorbide nitrates, including isosorbide dinitrate and isosorbide mononitrate); inorganic nitrites (sodium nitrite and amyl nitrite); and inorganic nitrates (bismuth subnitrate, sodium nitrate, and ammonium nitrate).
- Sodium and potassium nitrates and nitrites are used as food preservatives.
- High levels of nitrates may occur in well water.
- Nitroglycerin (Tridil, Nitro-Bid, Nitrol, Nitrostat, Deponit, Minitran, Nitro-Dur, Nitrodisc, Transiderm-Nitro) is given in a dose of 0.3 to 0.4 mg sublingually; as a 2.5-mg oral starting dose two to three times a day; or in the form of 0.5 to 2 inches of 2% ointment transdermally.
- Isosorbide dinitrate (Isordil, Sorbitrate) is given in a dose of 10 to 40 mg four times a day, 2.5 to 10 mg sublingually, or 40 to 80 mg two or three times a day.
- Isosorbide mononitrate (ISMO, Monoket, Imdur) is given in doses of 20 mg, 7 hours apart, 30 to 240 mg/day.

TOXIC DOSE

- Nitroglycerin. The estimated adult lethal dose is 200 to 1,200 mg.
- Amyl nitrite. Adult ingestion of 10 cc has produced serious levels of methemoglobin.
- Sodium nitrite. The estimated lethal dose in adults is 1 g.

PATHOPHYSIOLOGY

- Nitrates cause venous smooth muscle relaxation at low doses and arterial relaxation at higher doses, which may produce hypotension.
- Nitrates are converted to nitrites *in vivo*.
- Nitrites may convert hemoglobin to methemoglobin, reducing oxygen-carrying capacity and delivery.
- Nitrates and nitrites may produce toxicity after ingestion, skin absorption, or inhalation.

EPIDEMIOLOGY

- Toxicity is uncommon.
- Symptoms are usually mild.
- Death occurs rarely, usually following intentional abuse or overdose.

CAUSES

- Most cases involve unintentional ingestion.
- Hypotension may result from therapeutic doses or overdose.
- Methemoglobinemia can result from prolonged therapeutic uses or from intentional abuse.

RISK FACTORS

- Infants under the age of 4 months have greater susceptibility due to immature NADH methemoglobin reductase activity.
- Infants are more susceptible to toxicity from otherwise nontoxic doses of nitrates and nitrites in foods because of easier conversion of fetal hemoglobin to methemoglobin.
- There is an increased rate of stomach cancer in occupational nitrate fertilizer exposures.

DRUG AND DISEASE INTERACTIONS

- Profound hypotension when combined with other drugs that cause hypotension
- Enhanced toxicity of other methemoglobin-producing agents.

PREGNANCY AND LACTATION

- Isosorbide dinitrate, mononitrate, and nitroglycerin. US FDA Pregnancy Category C. The drug exerts animal teratogenic or embryocidal effects, but there are no controlled studies in women, or no studies are available in either animals or women.
- Nitrates are excreted in breast milk and may cause methemoglobinemia in infants.

WORKPLACE STANDARDS

Nitroglycerin

- ACGIH. TLV TWA is 0.05 ppm.
- NIOSH. REL is 0.1 mg/m^3 STEL; IDLH 75 mg/m^3.
- OSHA. Ceiling is 0.2 ppm.

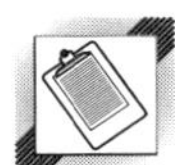

Diagnosis

DIFFERENTIAL DIAGNOSIS

- Toxic causes of methemoglobinemia include dapsone, benzocaine, chloroquine, sulfonamide, aniline dyes, naphthalene, and phenazopyridine.
- Nontoxic causes of methemoglobinemia include primarily deficiency of NADH methemoglobin reductase.

SIGNS AND SYMPTOMS

Primary effects are orthostatic hypotension and methemoglobinemia.

Vital Signs

Hypotension and tachycardia are most common toxic effects.

HEENT

Nitrate salts may be irritating to the eyes and to mucous membranes.

Dermatologic

- Visible venodilation may develop where nitrates contact the skin.
- Peripheral or central cyanosis that does not improve with oxygen administration is characteristic of methemoglobinemia.

Cardiovascular

Hypotension, dysrhythmia, syncope, and myocardial infarction may occur in severe cases.

Pulmonary

Dyspnea and tachypnea may occur if methemoglobinemia develops.

Gastrointestinal

- Nausea and vomiting are early signs after ingestion.
- Diarrhea and abdominal pain may develop.

Hematologic

- Methemoglobinemia is common.
- Hemolysis may occur.

Fluids and Electrolytes

Potassium may be elevated following exposure to potassium nitrate.

Neurologic

- Headache is common.
- Depressed mental status and coma may occur.
- Seizures may occur from hypotension or hypoxia.

PROCEDURES AND LABORATORY TESTS

Essential Tests

- Methemoglobin level

—The normal methemoglobin level is less than 3%.
—If methemoglobin level is not immediately available, a drop of the patient's blood is placed on a white sheet and compared with that of a normal control; blood with methemoglobinemia has a characteristic chocolate brown color.

Recommended Tests

- Arterial blood gases in symptomatic patients should be performed with a cooximeter because most pulse oximeters are inaccurate in the presence of methemoglobin.

- Serum electrolytes, glucose, BUN, and creatinine levels are measured to assess elevated anion gap acidosis.
- Serum glucose-6-phosphate dehydrogenase (G-6-PD) level is used to determine etiology in patients with methemoglobinemia.
- ECG and creatine kinase are used in symptomatic patients to assess cardiac effects of methemoglobinemia.
- CT, lumbar puncture, and urine toxicology screen are used to assess other causes of CNS depression.
- Unusual samples (well water, etc.) may require testing for nitrates and nitrites to determine source of exposure.

Not Recommended Tests

Blood levels of nitrates and nitrites are not useful.

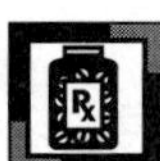

Treatment

- Treatment should focus on hypotension and methemoglobinemia.
- Supportive care, appropriate airway management, and administration of 100% oxygen are vital.
- Dose and time of exposure need to be determined for all substances involved.

DIRECTING PATIENT COURSE

The health-care provider should call the poison control center when:

- Cyanosis, acidosis, respiratory distress, or other severe effects are present.
- Toxic effects are not consistent with nitrite poisoning.
- Coingestant, drug interaction, or underlying disease presents an unusual problem.

The patient should be referred to a health-care facility when:

- Attempted suicide or homicide is possible.
- Patient or caregiver seems unreliable.
- Toxic effects develop.
- Coingestant, drug interaction or underlying disease presents an unusual problem.

Admission Considerations

Inpatient management is warranted for patients who develop symptoms greater than mucous membrane irritation.

DECONTAMINATION

Out of Hospital

- Ingestion

—Dilution should be considered to reduce mucous membrane irritation.
—Emesis should be avoided because of the risk of altered mental status from hypotension and hypoxia.

- Inhalation

—The patient should be removed from the source and administered oxygen.

- Dermal exposure

—The exposed area should be washed thoroughly.

In Hospital

- Ingestion

—Gastric lavage should be performed in pediatric (tube size 24–32 French) or adult (tube size 36–42 French) patients presenting within 1 hour of a large ingestion or if serious effects are present.
—One dose of activated charcoal (1–2 g/kg) should be administered without a cathartic if a substantial ingestion has occurred within the previous few hours.

- Dermal exposure

—The exposed area should be washed thoroughly.

ANTIDOTES

Methylene blue is the recommended antidote for methemoglobinemia.

- Indications. The decision to treat is based primarily on the patient's clinical condition. Any evidence of CNS or cardiac hypoxia (anxiety, confusion, hypotension, chest pain, etc.) indicates need for treatment.
- Contraindications are known NADH methemoglobin reductase deficiency or G-6-PD deficiency.
- Method of administration. A dose of 1 to 2 mg/kg should be infused intravenously over 5 minutes. Clinical improvement should occur shortly after administration. The methemoglobin level should be repeated 30 minutes later. If the level remains elevated and the patient is still symptomatic, a repeat dose of 0.5 to 1.0 mg/kg may be administered intravenously.
- Monitoring. Serial methemoglobin levels should be checked. Patients should be monitored until methemoglobin is declining for 6 hours to be certain that it does not recur.
- Potential adverse effects. Hemolysis may occur in patients with G-6-PD deficiency.

ADJUNCTIVE TREATMENT

- Hypotension

—Isotonic fluid infusion is used and the patient placed in the Trendelenburg position.
—A vasopressor is used if needed; dopamine is preferred, and norepinephrine may be added for refractory hypotension.

- Exchange transfusion has been used successfully when life-threatening methemoglobinemia is refractory to methylene blue therapy, patient has severe G-6-PD deficiency, or neonates are being treated.
- Hyperbaric oxygen therapy may be useful while preparing for exchange transfusion.

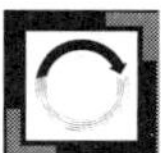

Follow-Up

PATIENT MONITORING

Cardiac and hemodynamic parameters should be monitored continuously.

EXPECTED COURSE AND PROGNOSIS

- Methemoglobinemia usually develops gradually over several hours or days.
- Hypotension may develop quickly but is usually brief and easily managed by conservative measures.
- Patients recover quickly if treatment is initiated before hypoxic injury occurs.
- Patients with hypoxic injury or G-6-PD deficiency may have prolonged course.

DISCHARGE CRITERIA/INSTRUCTIONS

- Asymptomatic patients with a normal or decreasing methemoglobin level may be discharged from the emergency department or hospital after decontamination, stable vital signs after 6 hours of observation, and completion of psychiatric evaluation, if needed.
- Patient should be instructed to return if fatigue, dyspnea, lightheadedness, shortness of breath, or cyanosis develops.

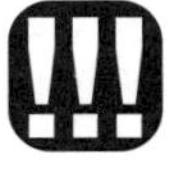

Pitfalls

DIAGNOSIS

- The arterial pO_2 reflects the partial pressure of oxygen dissolved in the blood and may be normal despite significant methemoglobinemia.
- A normal oxygen saturation by pulse oximetry does not rule out methemoglobinemia.

TREATMENT

Methemoglobinemia may recur or may be refractory to treatment, especially in the face of continued gastrointestinal or dermal absorption of the toxicant. Consultation with a toxicologist should be considered.

ICD-9-CM 972.4

Poisoning by agents primarily affecting the cardiovascular system: coronary vasodilators.

See also: SECTION II, Methemoglobinemia and Hypotension chapters; and SECTION III, Methylene Blue chapter.

RECOMMENDED READING

POISINDEX Editorial Staff. Nitrates. In: Rumack BH, Sayre NK, Gelman CR, eds. *POISINDEX system.* Englewood, CO: MICROMEDEX, Inc. (ddition expires May 31, 1998).

Author: Steven A. Seifert

Reviewer: Luke Yip

Nitrogen Oxides

Basics

DESCRIPTION

- Nitrogen oxides are components of air pollution and may be present in some occupational settings.
- Nitrogen dioxide is a reddish-brown gas, heavier than air.
- Nitric oxide is colorless and is the major nitrogen oxide in smog.
- See also SECTION IV, Nitrous Oxide chapter.

FORMS AND USES

Nitrogen oxides include nitric oxide (NO), nitrogen dioxide (NO_2), dinitrogen trioxide (N_2O_3), nitrogen pentoxide (N_2O_5), nitrogen peroxide, dinitrogen trioxide, dinitrogen tetroxide, dinitrogen pentoxide, and nitrous anhydride. Occupational exposures include:

- Fire fighting, arc welding, and work at missile sites
- Manufacturing of explosives, jet fuels, dyes, lacquers, and celluloid
- Ice rink resurfacing
- Grain silos, which release nitrogen dioxide within the first few weeks after filling
- Farm workers are at risk for silo-fillers' disease

Environmental sources include decaying organic matter, volcanic emissions, atmospheric lightning, fires, and burning of fossil fuels.

PATHOPHYSIOLOGY

- Nitrogen dioxide reacts with water within the airway and on the respiratory mucosa to form nitrous and nitric acids.
- Localized caustic mucosal injury and inflammation develop.
- Because the gas is of intermediate water solubility, inhalation causes both upper airway and lower airway injury.

EPIDEMIOLOGY

- Poisoning is uncommon.
- Most significant nitrogen dioxide exposures involve inhalation.
- Toxic effects following exposure are typically mild to moderate, with death following prolonged high-concentration inhalation exposure.
- Most serious toxicity is occupationally related.

DRUG AND DISEASE INTERACTIONS

- Children may be more severely affected because they have higher minute ventilation and because they absorb more by being closer to the ground (nitrogen dioxide is heavier than air).
- Geriatric patients with underlying pulmonary dysfunction may be at increased risk for toxicity.

CAUSES

Poisoning is usually an accidental occupational incident.

WORKPLACE STANDARDS

Nitrogen Dioxide

- ACGIH. TLV TWA is 3 ppm; STEL is 5ppm.
- NIOSH. REL TWA is 1 ppm; IDLH level is 20 ppm.

Nitric Oxide

- ACGIH. TLV TWA is 25 ppm.
- OSHA. PEL TWA is 25 ppm.
- NIOSH. IDLH level is 100 ppm.

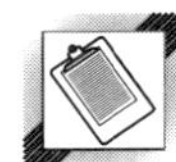

Diagnosis

DIFFERENTIAL DIAGNOSIS

Toxic causes of airway irritation include acrolein, ammonia, chlorine, formaldehyde, mercury vapor, metal fume fever, methyl bromide, natural gas, nickel carbonyl, phosgene, smoke inhalation, sulfur dioxide, zinc chloride fumes and others.

SIGNS AND SYMPTOMS

Acute Phase

- Symptoms of mucous membrane irritation as well as upper and lower airway irritation appear.
- Mild cases resolve over a few hours, but severe cases may progress to pulmonary edema (delayed 3 to 30 hours).

Delayed Phase

Noncardiogenic pulmonary edema, bronchitis, and interstitial lung disease occur days to weeks following an acute exposure.

Vital Signs

- Tachycardia and tachypnea are common following inhalation.
- Hypotension can be caused by either nitrate-induced vasodilatation or hypovolemia.

HEENT

- Conjunctivitis, rhinorrhea, blepharospasm, and sore throat may occur, but are more common following high-concentration exposure.
- Acute upper airway obstruction has occurred following inhalation exposures at high concentrations.
- Corneal burns may follow high-level exposures but are rare.

Pulmonary

- Cough, chest pain or tightness, dyspnea, and bronchospasm are common following either low- or high-concentration exposures.
- Wheezing, hemoptysis, rhonchi, and rales have all been reported.
- Noncardiogenic pulmonary edema has been reported following high-concentration prolonged exposure and may be delayed for hours to days.
- Bacterial superinfection and pneumonia may develop.
- Interstitial lung disease, pulmonary fibrosis, bronchiolitis obliterans, and reactive airway disease have occurred after either severe acute or chronic exposures.

Cardiovascular

- Tachycardia is common.
- Hypotension can be caused by either nitrate-induced vasodilatation or hypovolemia.
- Myocardial ischemia may occur.

Gastrointestinal

Nausea and vomiting are common.

Neurologic

- Headaches and lightheadedness are common following low-level exposure.
- Anxiety and agitation often reflect hypoxia.
- Syncope and loss of consciousness have been reported following high-level exposures but are rare.

Hematologic

Methemoglobinemia occurs rarely.

PROCEDURES AND LABORATORY TESTS

Essential Tests

No tests may be required following minimal exposure.

Recommended Tests

- Arterial blood gases to evaluate acid-base status and pulmonary gas exchange in patients with pulmonary symptoms
- Serum electrolytes, lactate, BUN, creatinine in serious cases
- Methemoglobin levels in patients who present with cyanosis that does not correct following the delivery of 100% oxygen
- ECG for all symptomatic patients at risk for myocardial ischemia
- Chest radiography if symptoms develop or oxygenation is abnormal (a normal radiograph obtained shortly after exposure does not preclude the development of delayed pulmonary effects)
- Serial performance of pulmonary function testing to assess course of injury
- Pulmonary scans including xenon lung scans to aid in determining the extent of injury following severe exposure

Not Recommended Tests

Levels are not clinically useful.

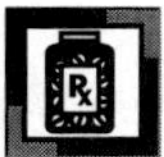

Treatment

- Treatment should focus on management of airway and on assuring oxygenation.
- The need for intubation should be evaluated.
- Wheezing should be treated symptomatically.
- Severe cases may develop life-threatening airway obstruction.

DIRECTING PATIENT COURSE

The health-care provider should call the poison control center when:

- Severe bronchospasm, upper airway obstruction, pulmonary edema, or other severe effects are present.
- Toxic effects are not consistent with nitrogen oxide poisoning.
- Coingestant, drug interaction, or underlying disease presents unusual problem.

The patient should be referred to a health-care professional when:

- Attempted suicide or homicide is possible.
- Patient or caregiver seems unreliable.
- History of significant exposure is obtained.
- Coingestant, drug interaction, or underlying disease presents unusual problems.

Admission Considerations

- Following most low-level inhalation exposures, asymptomatic patients rarely need to be evaluated in a health-care facility.
- Inpatient management is warranted for patients with persistent respiratory symptoms, upper airway edema, burns, pulmonary edema, or hypoxia.

DECONTAMINATION

Eye exposure. The eye should be irrigated with water for 15 minutes and evaluated for corneal burns.

Out of Hospital

The patient should be moved to fresh air and oxygen administered.

In Hospital

Oxygen should be administered to symptomatic patients.

ANTIDOTES

There is no specific antidote for exposure to oxides of nitrogen.

ADJUNCTIVE THERAPIES

Bronchospasm

- Oxygen is administered, followed by albuterol 0.15 mg/kg (maximum of 10 mg) in saline with humidified oxygen via nebulizer every 20 to 30 minutes. If the peak expiratory flow rate is greater than 90% of predicted after initial dose, additional doses may not be needed. Response should be continually monitored.
- Methylprednisolone is administered intravenously every 6 to 8 hours; adult dose is 60 to 125 mg (1.0–1.5 mg/kg); pediatric dose is 1 to 2 mg/kg; this may be decreased to a single daily dose and tapered.
- Initiation of prednisone, 2 mg/kg orally for several days, should be considered.
- Prophylactic antibiotic therapy is not recommended because it does not reduce morbidity or mortality.

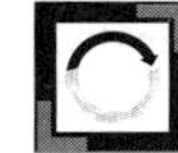

Follow-Up

PATIENT MONITORING

Pulmonary and cardiac parameters should be monitored closely until the patient recovers.

EXPECTED COURSE AND PROGNOSIS

- Delayed pulmonary edema may develop within hours of a severe prolonged inhalation exposure.
- Patients suffering high-level inhalation exposure may have a protracted hospital course.
- Resolution of chest radiographic abnormalities usually occurs within 2 months. Persistent infiltrates are sometimes present and may be consistent with bronchiolitis fibrosa obliterans or focal interstitial fibrosis.

DISCHARGE CRITERIA/INSTRUCTIONS

- From the emergency department. Asymptomatic patients may be discharged following complete resolution of cough, dyspnea, and tachypnea during a 6-hour observation period.
- From the hospital. Patient may be discharged following resolution or stabilization of toxic effects.

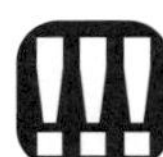

Pitfalls

DIAGNOSIS

- Patients may develop life-threatening respiratory complications following a latent period of hours to days.
- Despite a normal chest radiograph result shortly after a high-level exposure, the patient may develop delayed pulmonary edema or radiographic abnormalities.

FOLLOW-UP

- Patients discharged following an acute exposure should be instructed to follow up with their primary care physician for a recheck within 24 hours.
- Patients should be told to return immediately for health-care evaluation if they develop difficulty breathing, shortness of breath, persistent cough, or chest pain.
- Patients should be followed closely for a few weeks following significant exposures.
- Pulmonary function testing is recommended in patients with persistent respiratory complaints.

ICD-9-CM 987.2

Toxic effect of other gases, fumes, or vapors: nitrogen oxides.

See also: SECTION IV, Nitrous Oxide chapter.

RECOMMENDED READING

Kuffner EK. Athletes in Greenberg, MI. In: Hamilton RJ, Phillips SD, eds. *Occupational, industrial and environmental toxicology.* St. Louis: CV Mosby 1997:19–28.

Langley RL, Meggs WJ. Farmers and farm personnel in Greenberg, MI. In: Hamilton RJ, Phillips SD, eds. *Occupational, industrial and environmental toxicology.* St. Louis: CV Mosby, 1997:105–111.

Authors: Edwin K. Kuffner and Gerald F. O'Malley

Reviewer: Luke Yip

Nitrous Oxide

Basics

DESCRIPTION

Nitrous oxide (dinitrogen monoxide or N_2O) can be found in dental offices and operating suites where it is used extensively for its anesthetic properties after being mixed with oxygen (usually 50:50) and titrated to effect.

FORMS AND USES

- It is commonly encountered in prepackaged whipped cream containers and in metallic "chargers" or "whippets" for making whipped cream.
- It is also used as a drug of abuse.

—Inhalation produces euphoria.
—It is sold in balloons or other containers at rock concerts, etc.

- Nitrous oxide is used in metallurgy, to freeze foods, and in rocket fuel formulations.
- Synonyms include laughing gas and "nitrous."

TOXIC DOSE

- Acute toxicity is primarily related to hypoxia and thus may develop abruptly.
- Chronic toxicity may be produced by daily abuse for several weeks.

PATHOPHYSIOLOGY

- The majority of acute toxicity cases are due to the asphyxiant action of nitrous oxide (replacing oxygen in the inhaled gas), resulting in hypoxia.
- Long-term exposure may produce vitamin B_{12} deficiency states.

—In animal studies, nitrous oxide inactivates vitamin B_{12}.
—This impairs synthesis of DNA and myelin by interfering with methionine synthetase and folate metabolism.
—Subacute combined degeneration may develop.

- Nitrous oxide is a partial opioid agonist at the μ, κ, and σ opioid receptors.
- Daily occupational exposure has been associated with increased risk of cervical cancer in one study.

EPIDEMIOLOGY

- Toxicity most commonly occurs in health-care settings, where 25 million patients and 200,000 workers are exposed to the gas annually.
- Intentional abuse is also common.
- Toxicity is usually mild, and death occurs rarely.

CAUSES

Toxicity is usually due to long-term exposure, either in the workplace or from abuse.

PREGNANCY AND LACTATION

- Acute, severe hypoxia to the mother may result in fetal hypoxia and distress.
- Long-term exposure may increase the risk of abortion or teratogenesis.

WORKPLACE STANDARDS

- OSHA. PEL has not been defined for nitrous oxide.
- ACGIH. TLV TWA is 50 ppm.
- NIOSH. REL TWA is 25 ppm.

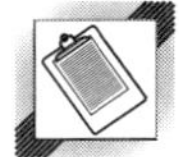

Diagnosis

DIFFERENTIAL DIAGNOSIS

- Toxic causes of acute hypoxia and CNS depression include other simple asphyxiants (methane, CO_2, inert gases), carbon monoxide, hydrocarbons, hydrogen sulfide, opiates, barbiturates, alcohol, and benzodiazepines.
- Nontoxic causes include pulmonary embolus, pneumonia, and hypoglycemia.

SIGNS AND SYMPTOMS

- Acute symptoms are those of inebriation and euphoria followed by symptoms of hypoxia with increasing exposure.
- Chronic symptoms are of sensory and motor neuropathy.

Vital Signs

Tachypnea and tachycardia are common initially, followed by bradycardia, respiratory depression, and hypotension.

HEENT

- Freezing injuries to the lips and mouth may occur if the gas is inhaled directly from a cylinder.
- Air spaces will tend to expand with nitrous administration, resulting in damage to the middle ear, obstucted sinuses, etc.

Dermatologic

Diaphoresis and cyanosis may occur with hypoxia.

Pulmonary

- Air hunger, tachypnea, and hyperpnea occur early; as hypoxia worsens, respiratory depression will develop.
- Inhaling the gas directly from whipped cream containers has caused interstitial emphysema and pneumomediastinum.

Cardiovascular

Hypotension has been reported.

Neurologic

- Acute delirium and euphoria are followed by lethargy and coma as hypoxia develops.
- Long-term abuse (>2 months) may result in subacute combined degeneration of the spinal cord, resulting in numbness, paresthesia, and ataxia.
- Further exposure may result in abnormal gait, weakness, impotence, and incontinence.
- Onset may begin months after a period of intense exposure.
- Chronic abusers also may develop depression, memory disturbances, and confusion.

Reproductive

- Long-term exposure (e.g., dental office workers) has been correlated with higher rates of infertility (in men and women), spontaneous abortions, and congenital abnormalities.
- Deranged spermatogenesis has been noted.

Hematologic

- Prolonged exposure may produce megaloblastic anemia, leukopenia, and thrombocytopenia, similar to the findings in pernicious anemia.
- Methemoglobinemia has resulted from contaminants in nitrous oxide canisters.

PROCEDURES AND LABORATORY TESTS

Essential Tests

No tests may be needed for asymptomatic patients.

Recommended Tests

Acute Exposure

- Arterial blood gases or pulse oximetry in symptomatic patients to evaluate hypoxia
- Methemoglobin level if the patient is cyanotic
- Serum electrolytes, BUN, creatinine, and glucose to assess altered mental status
- Head CT, lumbar puncture, bacterial cultures, and toxicology studies as needed to evaluate other causes of altered mental status that does not improve promptly

Chronic Abuse

- Complete blood count (CBC) and vitamin B_{12} level in symptomatic patients, especially with history of chronic use
- Nerve conduction studies (e.g., sensory and visual evoked potentials) in symptomatic patients with chronic exposure

Not Recommended Tests

Nitrous oxide levels can be performed on plasma or urine but are not clinically useful.

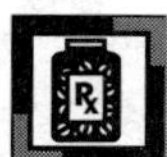

Treatment

- Oxygen therapy should be initiated while continuing supportive care and appropriate airway management.
- The dose and time of exposure should be determined for all substances involved.

DIRECTING PATIENT COURSE

The health-care provider should call the poison control center when:

- Patient does not improve with oxygen therapy or other serious effects are present (acute exposure).
- Toxic effects are not consistent with nitrous oxide.
- Coingestant, drug interaction, or underlying disease presents an unusual problem.

Patient should be referred to a health-care facility when:

- Patient or caregiver seems unreliable.
- Toxic effects develop.
- Coingestant, drug interaction, or underlying disease presents an unusual problem.

Admission Considerations

Inpatient management is warranted for patients with persistent symptoms, hypoxia, severe anemia, or disabling neuropathy.

DECONTAMINATION

The patient should be removed from exposure immediately, and oxygen therapy should be initiated.

ANTIDOTES

- There is no specific antidote for nitrous oxide poisoning.
- Methylene blue should be considered for methemoglobinemia greater than 30% (see SECTION II, Methemoglobinemia chapter)

ADJUNCTIVE THERAPIES

Administration of cyanocobalamin (vitamin B_{12}) is recommended by some authors for chronic toxicity.

Hypotension

- Patient is placed in the Trendelenburg position and administered 10 to 20 ml/kg 0.9% saline.
- Further fluid therapy is guided by central pressure monitoring to avoid volume overload.
- A vasopressor is added, if needed.

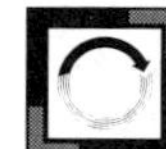

Follow-Up

PATIENT MONITORING

Acute Exposure

Cardiac and respiratory function should be continuously monitored in symptomatic patients.

Chronic Exposure

- Serial CBCs should follow resolution of anemia.
- Neurology follow-up should be obtained for all patients with neuropathic findings.

PATIENT EDUCATION

- Nitrous oxide should be used in well-ventilated areas, and a nitrous scrubber should be considered for work settings where nitrous oxide is used.
- Patients who present with nitrous abuse should be referred to a substance abuse treatment center.

EXPECTED COURSE AND PROGNOSIS

- Acute effects develop rapidly and resolve over minutes to hours unless sequelae of hypoxia intercede.
- Chronic nitrous oxide poisoning should improve if exposure to the gas is strictly avoided.
- The neuropathic symptoms may not reverse completely.

DISCHARGE CRITERIA/INSTRUCTIONS

- From the emergency department

—Asymptomatic patients may be discharged following a brief observation period.
—Patients should be referred for substance abuse counseling, if appropriate.

- From hospital

—Patient may be discharged when toxic effects resolve or stabilize.
—Patients should be referred for substance abuse counseling, if appropriate.

Pitfalls

DIAGNOSIS

- It is important to recognize other toxicities, including other asphyxiants, nitrous cylinder contaminants such as N_2 or NO_2, or drugs of abuse.
- It is vital to note potential methemoglobinemia.

ICD-9-CM 968.2

Poisoning by other central nervous system depressants and anesthetics: other gaseous anesthetics.

See also: SECTION II, Hypotension chapter; and SECTION III, Methylene Blue chapter.

RECOMMENDED READING

Brodsky JB, Cohen EN. Adverse effects of nitrous oxide. *Med Toxicol* 1986;1:362–374.

Author: John P. Marshall

Reviewer: Kennon Heard

Nonsteroidal Antiinflammatory Drugs

Basics

DESCRIPTION

Nonsteroidal antiinflammatory agents or drugs (NSAIDs) are used in a wide range of conditions involving the treatment of musculoskeletal pain and inflammation, fever, arthritis, and headache.

FORMS AND USES

- Pharmaceutical preparations include carprofen (Rimadyl), fenbufen, fenobufen (Nalfon), fenoprofen (Nalfon), flurbiprofen (Ansaid), ibuprofen (Advil, IBU, Motrin), indoprofen, ketoprofen (Orudis, Oruvail), naproxen (Aleve, Anaprox, Naprelan, Naprosyn), oxaprozin (Daypro), piroxicam (Feldene), pirprofen, tiaprofenic acid, aceclofenac, bromfenac, diclofenac (Cataflam, Voltaren, Voltaren XR), diflunisal (Dolobid), etodolac (Lodine), indomethacin (Indocin), ketorolac (Toradol), nabumetone (Relafen), sulindac (Clinoril), tolmetin (Tolectin), flufenamic, meclofenamate, isoxicam, meloxicam, piroxicam, sudoxicam, azapropazone, fenprazone, oxphyenbutazone, and phenylbutazone (Butazolidin, Tendearil).
- Mefenamic acid is covered separately in this section.

TOXIC DOSE

- Pediatric doses of ibuprofen of 200 to 400 mg/kg is associated with mild toxicity; greater than 400 mg/kg may cause severe effects.
- Phenylbutazone can result in serious toxicity in adults who have ingested more than 4 g.

PATHOPHYSIOLOGY

- NSAIDs have local irritant effects to the gastrointestinal system.
- NSAIDs inhibit prostaglandin synthesis, which weakens the gastrointestinal mucosal barriers and contributes to gastrointestinal discomfort and bleeding.
- NSAIDs inhibit thromboxane A_2 production, and this prolongs bleeding time.
- Inhibition of prostaglandins I_2 and E_2 inhibit natruresis and vasodilation of renal arteries, causing sodium retention and occasionally renal insufficiency.

EPIDEMIOLOGY

- Poisoning is common.
- Toxic effects following exposure are typically mild, with death occurring in rare cases secondary to gastrointestinal bleeding.

CAUSES

- Poisoning is usually accidental in children, intentional in adults.
- Child neglect or abuse should be considered if the patient is less than 1 year of age; suicide attempt in patients over 6 years of age.

DRUG AND DISEASE INTERACTIONS

- Alcoholics and patients with underlying ulcer disease are predisposed to gastrointestinal bleeding.
- Advanced age or preexisting renal disease predispose to kidney toxicity.
- Use with anticoagulants increases the risk of bleeding.

PREGNANCY

Flurbiprofen, Fenoprofen, Ibuprofen, Ketoprofen, Diclofenac, Indomethacin, Sulindac, Meclofenamate, and Piroxicam

US FDA Pregnancy Category B. Animal studies do not indicate a fetal risk and there are no controlled human studies, or animal studies do show an adverse fetal effect but well-controlled studies in pregnant women do not.

Carprofen, Ketorolac, Etodolac, Nabumetone, Tolmetin, and Phenylbutazone

US FDA Pregnancy Category C. The drug exerts animal teratogenic or embryocidal effects, but there are no controlled studies in women, or no studies are available in either animals or women.

Most NSAIDs if Used Near Time of Delivery

US FDA Pregnancy Category D. Positive evidence of human fetal risk exists, but benefits in certain situations (e.g., life-threatening situations or serious diseases) may make use of the drug acceptable despite its risks.

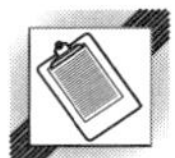

Diagnosis

DIFFERENTIAL DIAGNOSIS

- Toxic causes of acute gastrointestinal irritation or bleeding include ethanol, isopropanol, acetone, salicylate, and ingestion of irritant or caustic substances, among others.
- Nontoxic causes include upper gastrointestinal bleeding, gastritis, and ulcer disease.

SIGNS AND SYMPTOMS

- A large ingestion typically produces only nausea, vomiting, and abdominal pain.
- Massive ingestion may cause CNS depression, apnea, metabolic acidosis, seizures, acute renal failure, hypotension, and coma.

VITAL SIGNS

- Hypotension and respiratory depression are rare effects of massive overdose.
- Tachycardia, bradycardia, and mild hypothermia may occur.

HEENT

Tinnitus, nystagmus, blurred vision, diplopia, and transient hearing loss have been reported.

Pulmonary

- Respiratory depression, apnea, and adult respiratory distress syndrome are rare effects associated with large ingestion.
- Therapeutic doses may worsen bronchospasm in asthmatics.

Cardiovascular

- Hypotension is a rare effect associated with large overdose.
- Cardiogenic shock and asystole have been reported with phenylbutazone and derivatives.

Gastrointestinal

- Nausea, vomiting, and abdominal pain are common.
- Gastritis and gastrointestinal bleeding may develop after overdose or with therapeutic use.

Hepatic

- Hepatotoxicity develops rarely after ibuprofen overdose and has occasionally developed during therapeutic use of other NSAIDs.
- Delayed (>24 hours) hepatotoxicity may follow phenylbutazone overdose.

Renal

- Acute renal failure is rare after acute ingestion.
- Renal insufficiency may occur during chronic use.
- Delayed renal insufficiency may develop after phenylbutazone overdose.
- Sodium retention may develop rarely.

Fluids and Electrolytes

- Metabolic acidosis occurs rarely, following massive overdose.
- Hypokalemia, hypophosphatemia, hyponatremia, and hyperkalemia have occurred rarely after ibuprofen overdose.

Neurologic

- Mild CNS depression is common with large acute ingestion.
- Coma and seizures may develop after massive overdose.

Hematologic

- Thrombocytopenia, agranulocytosis, aplastic anemia, and pancytopenia have been reported with therapeutic use.
- Rarely, pancytopenia, and coagulopathy have occurred following acute overdose.

PROCEDURES AND LABORATORY TESTS

Essential Tests

No tests may be necessary in asymptomatic patients.

Recommended Tests

- Serum electrolytes, BUN, creatinine, calcium, magnesium, and urinalysis are measured in patients with symptoms of sodium retention, renal failure, or seizure.
- CBC, international normalized ratio (INR), and prothrombin time (PT) are used in patients with gastrointestinal or other bleeding.
- Serum liver enzymes are measured in patients with severe symptoms or after phenylbutazone overdose.
- ECG, serum acetaminophen and salicylate levels after deliberate ingestion are used to rule out occult ingestion.

Not Recommended Tests

Serum levels of NSAIDs are not clinically useful.

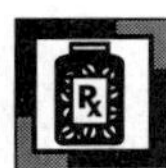

Treatment

- Treatment should focus on decontamination and general supportive care.
- Appropriate airway management in severe cases is vital.
- Dose and time of exposure should be determined for all substances involved.

DIRECTING PATIENT COURSE

The health-care provider should call the poison control center when:

- CNS depression, renal failure, or other serious effects develop.
- Toxic effects are not consistent with NSAID poisoning.
- Coingestant, drug interaction, or underlying disease presents an unusual problem.

The patient should be referred to a health-care professional when:

- Attempted suicide or homicide is possible.
- Patient or caregiver seems unreliable.
- Toxic effects are present.
- Coingestant, drug interaction, or underlying disease presents an unusual problem.

Admission Considerations

Inpatient treatment is warranted for patients with seizure, persistent CNS depression, hypotension, metabolic acidosis, or renal insufficiency.

DECONTAMINATION

Out of Hospital

Emesis should be induced with ipecac within 1 hour of ingestion for alert pediatric or adult patients if health-care evaluation will be delayed.

In Hospital

- Gastric lavage (adult tube size 36–42 French) should be used in patients presenting within 1 hour of a large ingestion or if serious effects are present.
- One dose of activated charcoal (1–2 g/kg) should be administered if a substantial ingestion has occurred within the previous few hours.

ANTIDOTES

There is no specific antidote for NSAID poisoning.

ADJUNCTIVE TREATMENT

Hypotension

- Isotonic fluid infusion is used and the patient is placed in the Trendelenburg position.
- If needed, a vasopressor is given; dopamine is preferred, and norepinephrine may be added for refractory hypotension.

Seizures

- The patency of the airway must be ensured.
- A benzodiazepine is administered for initial control; if seizures persist or recur, another anticonvulsant such as phenobarbital may be added.

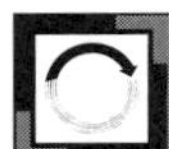

Follow-Up

PATIENT MONITORING

Respiratory function, CNS depression, and acid-base status should be monitored in symptomatic patients.

EXPECTED COURSE AND PROGNOSIS

- Peak effects usually occur within hours.
- Most patients recover within 24 hours with supportive care.
- Possible complications are gastrointestinal bleeding and renal insufficiency.

DISCHARGE CRITERIA/INSTRUCTIONS

- From the emergency department. Asymptomatic patients without evidence of metabolic acidosis may be discharged after decontamination, observation for 4 hours, and psychiatric evaluation, as appropriate.
- From hospital. Patients may be discharged when mental status has returned to normal, renal function has stabilized, and gastrointestinal bleeding has resolved.

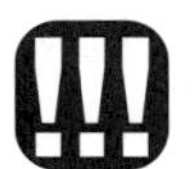

Pitfalls

DIAGNOSIS

Because patients often misidentify analgesics, the health-care provider needs to rule out acetaminophen and salicylate as coingestants.

FOLLOW-UP

Because delayed renal and hepatic toxicity may develop after phenylbutazone overdose, patients should be followed for several days.

ICD-9-CM 965.69

Other antirheumatics.

See also: SECTION II, Hypotension and Seizure chapters; and SECTION IV, Mefenamic Acid.

RECOMMENDED READING

Hall AH, Smolinske SC, Kulig KW, et al. Ibuprofen overdose: a prospective study. *West J Med* 1988;148:653–656.

Howland MA, Weisman RS. Nonsteroidal antiinflammatory agents. In: Goldfrank LS, Flomenbaum NE, Lewin NA, et al., eds. *Goldfrank's toxicologic emergencies,* 6th ed. Norwalk CT: Appleton & Lange, 1998.

Authors: Karen Brigid-Ita Holowinski and Katherine M. Hurlbut

Reviewer: Richard C. Dart

Omeprazole and Lansoprazole

Basics

DESCRIPTION

Omeprazole (Prilosec) and lansoprazole (Prevacid) are used to decrease gastric secretion.

FORMS AND USES

- Omeprazole and lansoprazole are potent proton-pump inhibitors and thus inhibit gastric acid secretion.
- The usual oral dosage is 20 to 60 mg/day of omeprazole and 15 to 30 mg/day of lansoprazole.

TOXIC DOSE

- The therapeutic index is large.
- Limited overdose experience with omeprazole has shown mild clinical effects.
- Overdose experience with lansoprazole is limited, but doses up to 1,300 times the human therapeutic dose did not produce adverse effects in animal studies.

PATHOPHYSIOLOGY

- Following an overdose of 320 mg of omeprazole, plasma levels peaked at 6 hours, and an elimination half-life of 52 minutes was measured.
- Blood gastrin levels increase, and hyperplastic gastropathy is seen with chronic therapeutic dosing.
- Omeprazole is metabolized in the liver, and its metabolites are excreted in the urine and bile.

EPIDEMIOLOGY

Poisoning is rare. Toxic effects are typically mild.

CAUSES

Child neglect or abuse should be considered if the patient is less than 1 year of age, suicide attempt if the patient is over 6 years of age.

RISK FACTORS

Omeprazole inhibits some P450 enzymes and may impair the clearance of other drugs metabolized by these enzymes, including diazepam, phenytoin, and warfarin.

PREGNANCY AND LACTATION

US FDA Pregnancy Category C. The drug exerts animal teratogenic or embryocidal effects, but there are no controlled studies in women, or no studies are available in animals or women.

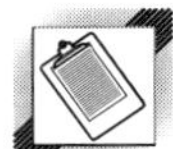

Diagnosis

SIGNS AND SYMPTOMS

Acute overdose produces mild tachycardia, mild CNS effects, and gastrointestinal effects.

Dermatologic

Rashes and an autoimmune syndrome consisting of arthritis and Raynaud's phenomena have been reported during chronic therapy.

Cardiovascular

Tachycardia and flushing may occur following acute overdose.

Gastrointestinal

Nausea, vomiting, and abdominal pain may follow acute ingestion.

Hepatic

Mild elevations of liver function tests have been reported during chronic therapy.

Neurologic

Somnolence, confusion, headache, and blurred vision may develop following acute overdose.

PROCEDURES AND LABORATORY TESTS

Essential Tests

No tests may be needed for asymptomatic or minimally symptomatic patients.

Recommended Tests

- Serum electrolytes, BUN, and creatinine are useful in patients with persistent gastrointestinal effects.
- Serum alanine transaminase, aspartate transaminase, and bilirubin are used to assess liver effects in symptomatic patients on chronic therapy.
- ECG, serum acetaminophen, and salicylate levels may be obtained in an overdose setting to detect occult ingestion.

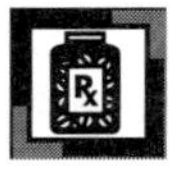

Treatment

- Supportive care is the mainstay of therapy.
- The dose and time of exposure for all substances involved should be determined.

DIRECTING PATIENT COURSE

The health-care professional should call the poison control center when:

- Severe or persistent effects develop.
- Coingestant, drug interaction, or underlying disease presents an unusual problem.

The patient should be referred to a health-care facility when:

- Suicide or homicide attempt is possible.
- Toxic effects develop.
- Coingestant, drug interaction, or underlying disease presents an unusual problem.

Admission Considerations

Patients with persistent gastrointestinal or neurologic effects should be admitted.

DECONTAMINATION

Out of Hospital

Emesis should not be induced due to low toxic potential.

In Hospital

- Gastric lavage should be performed in pediatric (tube size 24–32 French) or adult (tube size 36–42 French) patients presenting within 1 hour of a massive ingestion or if serious effects are present.
- One dose of activated charcoal (1–2 g/kg) should be administered without a cathartic if a substantial ingestion has occurred within the previous few hours.

ANTIDOTES

There is no specific antidote for omeprazole poisoning.

ADJUNCTIVE TREATMENT

- CNS symptoms of somnolence and confusion usually do not require specific therapy.
- Hypotension

—Patient should be treated with 10 to 20 mg/kg 0.9% saline intravenously. Further volume resuscitation should be guided by central pressure monitoring to avoid volume overload.
—If pressure is unresponsive, dopamine may be used. Adult dose is 2 to 5 μg/kg/min, up to 20 μg/kg/min titrated to blood pressure.
—If pressure remains unresponsive, norepinephrine (0.1–0.2 μg/kg/min) may be added and titrated to effect.

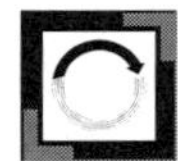

Follow-Up

PATIENT MONITORING

Respiratory and cardiac monitoring may be useful in the rare patient that develops significant toxicity.

EXPECTED COURSE AND PROGNOSIS

Recovery within 24 hours is expected.

DISCHARGE CRITERIA/INSTRUCTIONS

- From emergency department. Patient may be discharged if symptoms resolve over 4 to 6 hours following gastrointestinal decontamination and psychiatric evaluation, if needed.
- From hospital. Patient may be discharged when toxic effects resolve and following psychiatric evaluation, if needed.

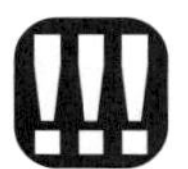

Pitfalls

DIAGNOSIS

A coingestant or drug interaction should be suspected in patients who develop toxic effects.

ICD-9-CM 973

Poisoning by agents primarily affecting the gastrointestinal system.

See also: SECTION II, Hypotension chapter.

RECOMMENDED READING

Ferner RE, Allison TR. Omeprazole overdose. *Hum Exp Toxicol* 1993;12:541–542.

Gallerani M, Lanza M, Calo G. Omeprazole overdose: a case report. *Clin Drug Invest* 1996;11:117–119.

Author: Steven A. Seifert

Reviewer: Richard C. Dart

Oral Hypoglycemic Agents

Basics

DESCRIPTION

- Oral hypoglycemic agents are used primarily in the treatment of type II diabetes mellitus.
- Substances include acetohexamide (Dymelor), carbutamide, chlorpropamide (Diabinese), gliclazide (Diamicron), glimepiride (Amaryl), glipizide (Glucotrol, Glucotrol XL), glybenclamide, glyburide (Micronase, DiaBeta, Glynase), glymidine, metahexamide, tolazamide (Tolinase, Tolamide), and tolbutamide (Orinase, Oramide).
- Metformin is discussed in a separate chapter.

FORMS AND USES

- Chlorpropamide. 100 mg orally every day up to 750 mg/day.
- Glipizide. 5 mg orally every day up to 40 mg/day.
- Glyburide. 2.5 mg orally every day up to 20 mg/day.
- Tolbutamide. 250 mg orally every day up to 3,000 mg divided twice a day.

TOXIC DOSE

One pill may cause hypoglycemia in a nondiabetic child or adult.

PATHOPHYSIOLOGY

- Sulfonylurea agents cause hypoglycemia by stimulating pancreatic insulin release and suppressing glucagon release.

EPIDEMIOLOGY

- Poisoning is common.
- Toxic effects are typically mild following accidental exposure, but may be severe after large, deliberate ingestion.
- Death is rare, occurring in untreated cases with severe hypoglycemia.
- Infants and children have smaller glycogen stores than adults and are prone to developing hypoglycemia.

CAUSES

- Poisoning is usually an accidental incident in a child.
- Therapeutic misadventures are common in adults.
- Child neglect should be considered if patient is less than 1 year of age, suicide attempt if patient is over 6 years of age.

RISK FACTORS

Conditions that decrease sulfonylurea elimination (hepatic and renal insufficiency) or that decrease glycogen stores (starvation, alcohol abuse, hepatic disease) predispose individuals to hypoglycemia.

DRUG AND DISEASE INTERACTIONS

- Hypoglycemia may be potentiated by cimetidine, ethanol, insulin, salicylates, phenylbutazone, sulfonamides, β-blockers, enalapril, chloramphenicol, gemfibrozil, ranitidine, clofibrate, and warfarin.
- A disulfiram-like reaction may occur upon ingestion of alcohol.

PREGNANCY AND LACTATION

Glimepride

US FDA Pregnancy Category C. The drug exerts animal teratogenic or embryocidal effects, but there are no controlled studies in women, or no studies are available in either animals or women.

Acetohexamide, Chlorpropamide, Glyburide, Tolazamide, and Tolbutamide

- US FDA Pregnancy Category D. Evidence of human fetal risk exists, but benefits in certain situations (e.g., life-threatening situations or serious diseases) may make use of the drug acceptable despite its risks.
- Neonatal hypoglycemia may occur in a child born to a sulfonylurea-treated mother.

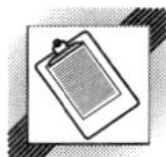

Diagnosis

DIFFERENTIAL DIAGNOSIS

- Diseases or toxicants that present with hypoglycemia (without hepatic injury) include overdose with insulin or akee fruit, and intoxication with any type of alcohol, especially in children.
- Many medications cause hypoglycemia under certain conditions.

SIGNS AND SYMPTOMS

- Hypoglycemia may be delayed, prolonged, or recurrent.
- With severe hypoglycemia, anxiety, diaphoresis, tremors, tachycardia, lethargy, slurred speech, coma, and seizures may develop.

Vital Signs

Hypoglycemia initially causes tachycardia, tachypnea, and hypertension, followed by hypotension, hypothermia, and respiratory depression with severe prolonged hypoglycemia.

Dermatologic

Hypoglycemia commonly causes diaphoresis.

Pulmonary

Tachypnea and dyspnea occur initially; respiratory depression may occur during prolonged hypoglycemia.

Gastrointestinal

Hunger, nausea, and vomiting may occur as a result of hypoglycemia.

Hepatic

Cholestatic hepatitis has been reported with therapeutic use of acetohexamide or glyburide.

Fluids and Electrolytes

Hyponatremia and inappropriate secretion of antidiuretic hormone (SIADH) have been reported with chlorpropamide and tolbutamide use.

Neurologic

- Lethargy, slurred speech, paresthesia, anxiety, headache, tremors, weakness, and ataxia may occur early, followed by disorientation, agitation, coma, and seizures.
- Focal neurologic signs such as paraplegia are uncommon but may occur.
- Permanent neurologic impairment may follow prolonged hypoglycemia.

Endocrine

Recurrent, severe hypoglycemia that lasts for days may develop after large overdose.

PROCEDURES AND LABORATORY TESTS

Essential Tests

Serum or finger-stick glucose determination should be performed immediately and then hourly.

Recommended Tests

- ECG, serum acetaminophen and aspirin levels in overdose setting to detect occult overdose.
- Serum electrolytes, renal and hepatic function tests, lumbar puncture, and urine toxicology screen as needed to rule out other causes of altered mental status
- Serum insulin, proinsulin, C peptide levels, and urinary sulfonylurea level if surreptitious use of insulin is suspected
- Head CT as needed to rule out other causes of altered mental status.

Not Recommended Tests

Serum levels of sulfonylureas are not clinically useful in overdose.

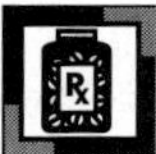

Treatment

- Immediate administration of glucose and appropriate airway management are critical.
- Dose and time of exposure should be determined for all substances involved.

DIRECTING PATIENT COURSE

The health-care provider should call the poison control center when:

- Hypoglycemia or other severe effects are present.
- Toxic effects are not consistent with oral hypoglycemic poisoning.
- Coingestant, drug interaction, or underlying disease presents an unusual problem.

The patient should be referred to a health-care facility when:

- Attempted suicide or homicide is possible.
- Patient or caregiver seems unreliable.
- A child or nondiabetic patient has ingested sulfonylurea or any individual has received a sulfonylurea overdose.
- Toxic effects are not consistent with oral hypoglycemic poisoning.
- Coingestant, drug interaction, or underlying disease presents an unusual problem.

Admission Considerations

Inpatient management for serial glucose determinations is warranted for nondiabetic patients who ingest one pill or more.

DECONTAMINATION

Out of Hospital

- Emesis should not be induced.
- The patient should ingest a glucose-containing food or drink (soda or juice with added sugar) immediately if any symptoms of hypoglycemia develop.

In Hospital

- Gastric lavage should be performed in pediatric (tube size 24–32 French) or adult (tube size 36–42 French) patients presenting within 1 hour of a large ingestion or if serious effects are present.
- One dose of activated charcoal (1–2 g/kg) should be administered without a cathartic if a substantial ingestion has occurred within the previous few hours.

ANTIDOTES

Dextrose is a specific antidote.

- Indications are symptoms of hypoglycemia following oral hypoglycemic overdose or glucose less than 60 mg/dl; routine administration of dextrose to a patient with a normal glucose level is not recommended.
- Method of administration

—Adult. 50 ml of D50W (25 grams) by bolus intravenous infusion.
—Child. 1 to 2 ml/kg of D25W.
—Neonate. 1 to 2 ml/kg of D10W.
—Dextrose dose is repeated until blood glucose is greater than 100 mg/dl.
—Blood glucose is followed hourly to guide further therapy.
—Continuous infusion of 5%, 10%, or 20% dextrose is initiated as needed if recurrent hypoglycemia develops.
—Infusion of D20W requires a central venous line to avoid venous injury.

ADJUNCTIVE TREATMENT

Octreotide Acetate

- Indications. Hypoglycemia resistant to glucose administration following sulfonylurea overdose
- Contraindications. Octreotide allergy.
- Method of administration. Continuous infusion of 30 ng/kg/min for approximately 12 to 18 hours, longer if needed due to recurrent hypoglycemia.
- For adults, a dose of 100 μg subcutaneously every 8 hours has been recommended.
- Potential adverse effects. Steatorrhea.

Diazoxide

- Indications. Hypoglycemia resistant to glucose administration following sulfonylurea overdose.
- Contraindications. Diazoxide allergy.
- Method of administration. Adult dose is 300 mg intravenously over 60 minutes, repeated as necessary.
- Potential adverse effects: Hypotension.

Not Recommended Treatment

- Glucagon is not recommended.
- Multiple-dose activated charcoal has been recommended for glipizide, but has not been shown to affect outcome and is not routinely recommended.
- Although the half-life of chlorpropamide is reduced by urinary alkalinization, this has not been shown to affect outcome and is not routinely recommended.

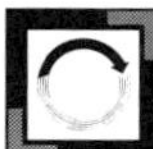

Follow-Up

EXPECTED COURSE AND PROGNOSIS

- After significant ingestion, hypoglycemia usually develops within 12 to 16 hours, may last for days and may recur when glucose is weaned.
- Full recovery is expected if prolonged hypoglycemia does not occur.
- Permanent neurologic injury may result from prolonged hypoglycemia.

DISCHARGE CRITERIA/INSTRUCTIONS

- From the emergency department. Asymptomatic patients may be discharged after gastrointestinal decontamination and psychiatric evaluation, when appropriate, and when their serial blood glucose levels are greater than 60 mg/dl without dextrose treatment during an observation period of 12 to 16 hours.
- From the hospital. Asymptomatic patients may be discharged when they are tolerating food and are euglycemic without supplemental dextrose administration for at least 6 hours following psychiatric evaluation, if needed.

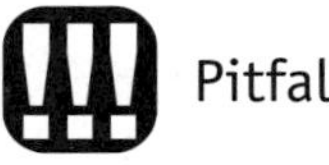

Pitfalls

DIAGNOSIS

Early infusion of D5W in an asymptomatic patient with a history of ingestion of oral hypoglycemia agents may maintain normal blood glucose and delay diagnosis of serious ingestion.

TREATMENT

Hypoglycemia may recur despite dextrose infusion.

ICD-9-CM 977

Poisoning by other and unspecified drugs and medicinal substances.

See also: SECTION III, Dextrose chapter; and SECTION IV, Insulin and Metformin chapters.

RECOMMENDED READING

Palatnick W, Meatherall RC, Tenenbein M. Clinical spectrum of sulfonylurea overdose and experience with diazoxide therapy. *Arch Intern Med* 1991;151:1859–1862.

McLaughlin SA, Crandall CS, McKinney PE. Octreotide: An antidote for sulfonylurea-induced hypoglycemia *Ann Emerg Med.* In Press.

Author: Lada Kokan

Reviewer: Katherine M. Hurlbut

Organochlorine Pesticides (Lindane)

Basics

DESCRIPTION

The organochlorine pesticides are chlorinated hydrocarbons usually in a petroleum distillate solvent base.

FORMS AND USES

- The organochlorines are composed of several subgroups.

—Dichlorodiphenylethanes. DDT (dichlorodiphenyltrichloroethane), DDD, DDE, dicofol, dienochlor, and methoxychlor.
—Hexachlorocyclohexanes. Hexachlorocyclohexane and lindane.
—Cyclodienes. Aldrin, dieldrin, chlordane, endrin, endosulfan, ethylan, heptachlor, and toxaphene.
—Others. Chlordecone, mirex, orthodichlorobenzene, hexachlorobenzene, strobane, kelthane, perthane, chloropyrolate, and chlorobenzilate.

- Once the most common insecticides, they are largely banned in the United States.
- Lindane is still used for treatment of scabies.

TOXIC DOSE

- Any ingestion of 100% lindane is likely to produce toxicity.
- A lindane ingestion of less than 1 teaspoon in a child or less than 1 tablespoon in an adult is considered nontoxic.
- Toxicity may follow ingestion, skin application, or inhalation.

PATHOPHYSIOLOGY

- Organochlorines interfere with the transmission of nerve impulses by altering neuronal ion flux.
- Exposure may result in either impairment of function (respiratory depression) or enhanced activity (seizures).
- Some evidence suggests that lindane may antagonize γ-aminobutyric acid (GABA)-mediated inhibition in the CNS.
- Carcinogenesis. None of the organochlorines are known human carcinogens.

EPIDEMIOLOGY

- Poisoning is uncommon.
- Toxic effects are typically mild to moderate, but may be severe with large exposure.
- Death occurs with massive exposure.

CAUSES

- Exposure is usually accidental or inadvertent misuse of product; intentional ingestion usually involves larger quantities.
- Child abuse/neglect must be considered if the patient is less than 1 year of age; suicide attempt if the patient is over 6 years of age.

DRUG AND DISEASE INTERACTIONS

Stimulants or other drugs that induce seizure may increase the risk of seizure from organochlorine compounds.

PREGNANCY AND LACTATION

- Lindane. US FDA Pregnancy Category B. Animal studies indicate no fetal risk and there are no controlled human studies, or animal studies show an adverse fetal effect but well-controlled studies in pregnant women do not.
- Organochlorines cross into breast milk; acute toxic effects have not been reported.

WORKPLACE STANDARDS

Aldrin and Dieldrin

- ACGIH. TLV TWA is 0.25 mg/m^3.
- OSHA. PEL TWA is 0.25 mg/m^3.
- Carcinogen status. IARC 3; EPA B2.

Chlordane and Heptachlor

- ACGIH. TLV TWA is 0.5 mg/m^3.
- OSHA. PEL TWA is 0.5 mg/m^3.
- Carcinogen status. IARC 2B; EPA B2.

DDT

- ACGIH. TLV TWA is 1 mg/m^3.
- OSHA. PEL TWA is 1 mg/m^3.
- Carcinogen status. IARC 2B; EPA B2.

Endosulfan

- ACGIH. TLV TWA is 0.1 mg/m^3,
- Carcinogen status. TLV is A4.

Endrin

- ACGIH. TLV TWA is 0.1 mg/m^3.
- OSHA. PEL TWA is 0.1 mg/m^3.
- Carcinogen status. IARC 3; EPA D.

Lindane

- ACGIH. TLV TWA is 0.5 mg/m^3.
- OSHA. PEL TWA is 0.5 mg/m^3.
- Carcinogen status. IARC 2B; TLV A3.

Methoxychlor

- ACGIH. TLV TWA is 10 mg/m^3.
- OSHA. PEL TWA is 15 mg/m^3.
- Carcinogen status. IARC 3; EPA D.

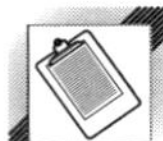

Diagnosis

DIFFERENTIAL DIAGNOSIS

- Toxic causes of agitation and seizures include sympathomimetic drugs, theophylline, lithium, monoamine oxidase inhibitors, isoniazid, and alcohol or sedative withdrawal, among others.
- Nontoxic causes include noncompliance with seizure medications, and CNS infection or injury.

SIGNS AND SYMPTOMS

CNS excitation and seizures are the principal concerns.

Vital Signs

Hypertension, tachycardia, and bradypnea may occur.

Dermatologic

Dermatitis may be present at areas of prolonged contact.

Cardiovascular

Hydrocarbons may predispose to dysrhythmia.

Pulmonary

Aspiration pneumonitis may develop from a petroleum distillate component following ingestion.

Gastrointestinal

- Nausea and vomiting are common.
- The petroleum distillates may cause diarrhea.

Hepatic

No human hepatotoxicity has been demonstrated.

Renal

Renal failure from rhabdomyolysis may follow prolonged seizure activity.

Hematologic

Porphyria cutanea tarda (hexachlorobenzene) and megaloblastic anemia (chlordane) are rare effects.

Neurologic

- Seizures are common with large ingestions or prolonged skin contact of some compounds (aldrin, chlordane, dieldrin, endrin, heptachlor, lindane, strobane, toxaphene, and DDT).
- CNS depression predominates in others (kelthane, perthane, methoxychlor, hexachlorobenzene).
- CNS irritation, agitation, amnesia, and opsoclonus (chlordecone) have been reported.

PROCEDURES AND LABORATORY TESTS

Essential Tests

No tests may be needed in asymptomatic patients or following minor inhalational exposure.

Recommended Tests

- Serum electrolytes, BUN, creatinine, glucose, calcium, and magnesium are measured if repeated vomiting or seizure develops.
- Complete blood count (CBC) in severe or chronic exposure is used to detect blood dyscrasia.
- CT, lumbar puncture, cultures, pulse oximetry, and other tests are used as needed to assess altered mental status.
- ECG, serum acetaminophen and aspirin levels are used in an overdose setting to assess occult ingestion.
- Specific levels are available as send-out test only and may be used for confirmation of exposure (e.g., lindane level).

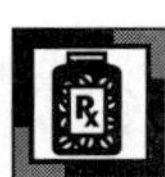

Treatment

- Treatment should focus on airway support and control of seizures.
- Dose and time of exposure should be determined for all substances that could be involved.

DIRECTING PATIENT COURSE

The health-care provider should call the poison control center when:

- Seizure, altered mental status, or other serious effects are present.
- Toxic effects are not consistent with organochlorine poisoning.
- Coingestant, drug interaction, or underlying disease presents an unusual challenge.

The patient should be referred to a health-care facility when:

- Attempted suicide or homicide is possible.
- Patient or caregiver seems unreliable.
- Any toxic effects develop.
- Coingestant, drug interaction, or underlying disease presents unusual problems.

Admission Considerations

Inpatient management is warranted if patient experiences seizures or other major toxicity.

DECONTAMINATION

Out of Hospital

Skin

The affected area should be washed with soap and water thoroughly, and patient's clothing should be discarded in a hazardous materials bag.

Ingestion

Emesis should not be induced due to the risk of seizures.

Inhalation

Patient should be moved to fresh air.

In Hospital

Skin

The affected area should be washed with soap and water repeatedly, and the patient's clothing should be discarded in a hazardous materials bag.

Ingestion

- Gastric lavage should be performed in pediatric (tube size 24–32 French) or adult (tube size 36–42 French) patients presenting within 1 hour of a large ingestion or if serious effects are present.
- One dose of activated charcoal (1–2 g/kg) should be administered without a cathartic if a substantial ingestion has occurred within the previous few hours.

ANTIDOTES

There is no specific antidote for organochlorine poisoning.

ADJUNCTIVE TREATMENT

Seizure management includes the following measures:

- Adequate airway and oxygenation are crucial.
- Benzodiazepine should be administered for initial control.

—Diazepam. Adult dosage is 5 to 10 mg intravenous push over 2 to 5 minutes initially, repeated every 10 minutes as needed; pediatric dosage is 0.2 to 0.5 mg/kg every 10 minutes as needed; airway must be monitored closely.
—Lorazepam. Adult dosage is 2 to 4 mg intravenous push over 2 to 5 minutes, repeated every 10 minutes as needed; pediatric dosage is 0.1 mg/kg intravenous push over 2 to 5 minutes, not to exceed 4 mg/dose, repeated every 10 minutes as needed; airway must be monitored closely.
—If seizures persist or recur, another anticonvulsant such as phenobarbital or phenytoin may be added.
—Other options for repeated seizures include general anesthesia and neuromuscular blockade with EEG monitoring.

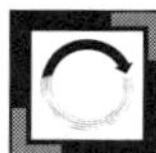

Follow-Up

PATIENT MONITORING

- Respiratory and hemodynamic status should be monitored continuously until acute effects resolve.
- CBC should be monitored in patients with chronic exposure.

EXPECTED COURSE AND PROGNOSIS

- Following ingestion, most patients become acutely ill and improve with supportive care over the next 24 to 48 hours.
- Severe cases may require several days to recover.
- Sequelae of repeated seizure activity (rhabdomyolysis, acidosis, long-term CNS injury) may develop rarely.

DISCHARGE CRITERIA/INSTRUCTIONS

- From the emergency department. Asymptomatic patients can be discharged following decontamination, observation for 6 hours, and psychiatric evaluation, if needed.
- From the hospital. Patients can be discharged following resolution of toxic effects and psychiatric evaluation, if needed.

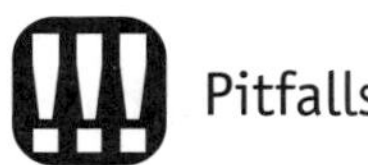

Pitfalls

DIAGNOSIS

Failure to consider organochlorine pesticides in the differential diagnosis of seizures can lead to misdiagnosis.

TREATMENT

- Failure to adequately control airway and seizures is a common pitfall.
- Multiple drug therapy may be required for adequate seizure control.

ICD-9-CM 989

Toxic effect of other substances, chiefly nonmedicinal as to source.

See also: SECTION II, Seizures chapter.

RECOMMENDED READING

Peters HH, Gocmen A, Cripps DJ, et al. Epidemiology of hexachlorobenzene-induced porphyria in Turkey: clinical and laboratory follow-up after 25 years. *Arch Neurol* 1982;39:744–749.

Rowley DL, Rab MA, Hardjotanojo W, et al. Convulsions caused by endrin poisoning in Pakistan. *Pediatrics* 1987;79:928–934.

Samuels AJ, Milby TH. Human exposure to lindane: clinical hematological and biochemical effects. *J Occup Med* 1971;13:147–151.

Author: Scott D. Phillips

Reviewer: Luke Yip

Organophosphate Insecticides

Basics

DESCRIPTION

The organophosphate insecticides include chemicals of organophosphorus structure used as pesticides in both domestic and industrial settings.

FORMS AND USES

The organophosphates are found in agricultural and large-scale landscape maintenance settings; some low-toxicity forms are found as components in home gardening products. They are also used in many industrial processes. They are classified by their relative toxicity:

- Low-toxicity (LD_{50} >1,000 mg/kg) products include bromophos (Nexagan), etrimfos (Ekamet), iodofenphos (Nuvanol N), malathion (Cythion), phoxim (Baythion), propylthiopyrophosphate (Aspon), temephos (Abate, Abathion), and tetrachlorvinphos (Gardona, Rabon).
- Moderate-toxicity (LD_{50} 50–1,000 mg/kg) products include acephate (Orthene), bensulide (Betasan), chlorpyrophos (Lorsban, Dursban), crotoxyphos (Ciodrin), cythioate (Proban), DEF (De-Green, E-Z-off D), demeton-*S*-methyl (Metasystox), diazinon (Spectracide, Basudin), dichlorovos (DDVP, Vapona), dimethoate (Cygon), dioxathion (Delnav), edifenphos (EDDP), ethion (Nialate), ethoprop (Mocap), fenitrothion (Accothion), fenthion (Baytex, Entex), formothion (Anthio), IPB (Kitazin), leptophos (Phosvel), merphos (Folex), methyl trithion, naled (Dibrom), phencapton, phosalone (Zofos), phosmet (Imidan, Prolate), pirimiphos-ethyl (Fernex), profenophos (Curacron, Ploycron, Selecron), propetamphos (Safrotin), pyrazophos (Afugan, Curamil), quinalphos (Bayrusil), sulprofos (Bolstar), thiometon (Ekatin), triazophos (Hostathion), tribufon (Butonate), and trichlorofon (Tugon, Dylox, Dipterex).
- Highly toxic (LD_{50} <50 mg/kg) organophosphate products include bomyl (Swat), carbophenothion (Trithion), chlormephos (Dotan), chlorthiophos (Celathion), chlorfenvinfos (Birlane), coumaphos (Co-ral), cyanofenphos (Surecide), dementon (Systox), dialifor (Torak), dicrotophos (Bidrin), disulfoton (Disyston), EPN, famphur (Warbex, Bo-ana), fenamiphos (Nemacur), fenophosphon (Agritox), isofenphos (Amaze, Oftanol), diisopropyl fluorophosphate, mephosfolan (Cytrolane), methamidophos (Monitor), methidathion (Supracide), mevinphos (Phosdrin), monocrotophos (Azodrin), ethylparathion, phorate (Thimet), phosfolan (Cyolane), phosphamidon (Dimecron), prothoate (Fac), sulfotep (Bladafum), terbufos (Counter), and tetraethyl pyophosphate (TEPP, Bladan, Tetron).

TOXIC DOSE

Toxicity varies by potency. Several swallows are needed to produce toxicity from low-potency compounds, whereas only a few milliliters may be needed for high-toxicity compounds.

PATHOPHYSIOLOGY

- Organophosphate insecticides reversibly bind to the enzyme acetylcholinesterase, inhibiting its activity and resulting in excessive stimulation of the acetylcholine receptor.
- The binding then "matures" and the inhibition becomes irreversible over a period of hours.
- Toxicity may manifest as nicotinic effects (muscle weakness, fasciculation, hypertension, tachycardia) or muscarinic effects (diaphoresis, vomiting, diarrhea).

EPIDEMIOLOGY

- Poisoning is common.
- Toxic effects are typically mild to moderate.
- Death is rare and usually occurs before health care is provided.

CAUSES

- Toxic ingestion or dermal exposure is usually accidental.
- Child abuse or neglect must be considered if the patient is less than 1 year of age; suicide attempt if the child is older than 6 years.

RISK FACTORS

Patients with congenital low levels of acetylcholinesterase are at increased risk of toxicity from any given exposure.

DRUG AND DISEASE INTERACTIONS

- Organophosphates prolong the activity of neurologic blocking agents.
- Gentamicin and other antibiotics may prolong organophosphate toxicity.

PREGNANCY AND LACTATION

Numerous animal studies indicate teratogenic effects of various organophosphate compounds. However, some have no effect; therefore, each agent should be addressed individually.

WORKPLACE STANDARDS

Malathion

ACGIH. TLV TWA is 10 mg/m^3.

Parathion

- ACGIH. TLV TWA is 0.1 mg/m^3.
- OSHA. PEL TWA is 0.1 mg/m^3.

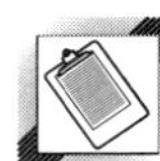

Diagnosis

DIFFERENTIAL DIAGNOSIS

- Other toxic causes of acute onset of acetylcholine effects include carbamates, nicotine, carbachol, methacholine, arecoline, bethanechol, pilocarpine, and some mushrooms, among others.
- Nontoxic causes include myasthenia gravis and Eaton-Lambert syndrome, among others.

SIGNS AND SYMPTOMS

Muscarinic effects are manifested by the DUMBELS syndrome (*d*iaphoresis and diarrhea; *u*rination; *m*iosis; *b*radycardia, bronchospasm, and bronchorrhea; *e*mesis and excess of *l*acrimation; and *s*alivation and seizures) and usually occur soon after exposure.

Vital Signs

Bradycardia, hypotension, and hypothermia may occur.

HEENT

Miosis, blurred vision, rhinorrhea, salivation, and lacrimation are common.

Dermatologic

Profuse diaphoresis is common.

Cardiovascular

- Hypotension and bradycardia may occur.
- Cardiac depression and cardiovascular collapse may occur.
- Atrial fibrillation, atrioventricular blocks, and asystole may occur.

Pulmonary

Bronchospasm and bronchorrhea are common, leading to pulmonary edema in severe cases.

Gastrointestinal

Nausea, vomiting, abdominal pain, and diarrhea are common; fecal incontinence may occur.

Renal

Urinary incontinence occurs, especially in severe cases.

Musculoskeletal

Fasciculation, weakness, paralysis, and respiratory failure may occur.

Neurologic

Confusion, seizures, and coma may occur.

PROCEDURES AND LABORATORY TESTS

Essential Tests

Red blood cell cholinesterase level correlates roughly with effects; first sample should be drawn before treatment (plasma cholinesterase can be used if red blood cell cholinesterase is unavailable).

- Latent Poisoning. No clinical manifestations are present; cholinesterase levels are 50% to 90% of baseline.
- Mild Poisoning. Patient is ambulatory, and may experience nausea, vomiting, fatigue, headache, dizziness, sweating and salivation, tightness in chest, and abdominal cramps or diarrhea; cholinesterase activity is 20% to 50% of baseline.
- Moderate Poisoning. Patient cannot walk and experiences generalized weakness, difficulty

speaking, fasciculation, and miosis; cholinesterase activity is 10% to 20% of baseline.
• Severe Poisoning. Patient is unconscious, with miosis, fasciculation, flaccid paralysis, increased secretions, moist rales, and cyanosis; cholinesterase activity is less than 10% of baseline.

Recommended Tests

• Serum electrolytes, glucose, BUN, calcium, magnesium, phosphate, and creatinine should be assayed to detect other causes of dysrhythmia, weakness, or kidney injury.
• ECG and continuous cardiac monitoring should be performed to assess potential causes of hypotension and bradycardia.
• Serum acetaminophen and aspirin levels should be measured in an overdose setting to detect occult ingestion.
• Arterial blood gases should be measured if acidosis or hypoxia develop.
• Comprehensive urine drug screen should be done if source of intoxication is unknown (abused drugs may contain contaminants).
• CT, lumbar puncture, cultures, and other tests as indicated should be performed in patients with altered mental status of unknown etiology.
• Negative inspiratory force should be followed to assess ventilatory capacity.
• Chest radiographs can assist evaluation of pulmonary edema.
• Patients with delayed polyneuropathy may demonstrate denervation on electromyography.

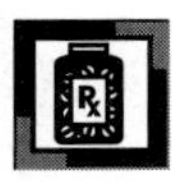

Treatment

• Treatment should focus on decontamination, airway management, and administration of atropine and pralidoxime.
• Dose and time of exposure should be determined for all substances involved.

DIRECTING PATIENT COURSE

The health-care provider should call the poison control center when:

• Breathing difficulty, hypotension, or other severe effects are present.
• Toxic effects are not consistent with organophosphate poisoning.
• Coingestant, drug interaction, or underlying disease presents an unusual problem.

The patient should be referred to a health-care facility when:

• Attempted suicide or homicide is possible.
• Patient or caregiver seems unreliable.
• Any toxic effects develop.
• Coingestant, drug interaction, or underlying disease presents an unusual problem.

Admission Considerations

Inpatient management is warranted if the patient develops toxic effects that require treatment.

DECONTAMINATION

Out of Hospital

• Emesis should not be induced.
• Providers must wear protection to prevent contamination.
• Patient's clothing should be removed and skin washed with soap and water.

In Hospital

• Patient's clothing should be removed and skin washed with soap and water; providers should wear protection to prevent contamination.
• Gastric aspiration should be performed with a nasogastric tube in the case of recent ingestion or a symptomatic patient.
• One dose of activated charcoal (1–2 g/kg) should be administered without a cathartic if a symptomatic ingestion has occurred.

ANTIDOTES

Atropine

• Indications. Control of bronchorrhea and other secretions.
• Contraindication. Preexisting atropinization (dry airway, mydriatic pupils, etc.).
• Method of administration

—Adult initial dose is 2 to 4 mg intravenously; dose (or double the dose) may be repeated every 5 to 10 minutes as needed until pulmonary secretions are controlled.
—Pediatric initial dose is 0.05 mg/kg intravenously; dose (or double the dose) may be repeated every 5 to 10 minutes as needed until pulmonary secretions are controlled.
—In severe cases, massive amounts of atropine may be needed over 12 to 24 hours.

• Adverse effects. Anticholinergic symptoms possible with excessive atropine.

Pralidoxime (2-PAM)

• Indications. Patients with nicotinic effects (weakness, fasciculations) or CNS effects should be treated.
• Method of administration

—Adult dose is 1 to 2 g intravenously over 15 to 30 minutes or as a continuous intravenous infusion at 500 mg/h.
—Pediatric dose is 25 mg/kg (up to 1 g) intravenously over 15 to 30 minutes, followed by 25 to 50 mg/kg (up to 500 mg) per hour.

ADJUNCTIVE TREATMENT

Hypotension

• Atropine should be used if hypotension is due to bradycardia.
• The patient should receive 10 to 20 ml/kg 0.9% saline intravenously and be placed in the Trendelenburg position.
• Further fluid therapy should be guided by central pressure monitoring.
• A vasopressor may be added if needed.

Seizure

• A patent airway must be assured.
• A benzodiazepine should be administered for initial control.
• If seizures persist or recur, another anticonvulsant such as phenobarbital may be added.

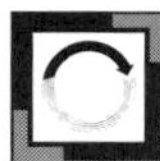

Follow-Up

PATIENT MONITORING

• Continuous cardiac and respiratory monitoring should be performed.
• Following occupational exposure, patient should not be allowed to work with organophosphate or carbamate insecticides until serum cholinesterase levels have returned to 75% of known baseline.
• If baseline levels are not available, patient should not return to work until two serum cholinesterase levels drawn 1 week apart show an increase of less than 5% (plateau level).

EXPECTED COURSE AND PROGNOSIS

• Toxicity develops rapidly and peaks within hours, but may persist for a day or more if patient does not receive antidotal treatment.
• Patients who receive early decontamination and adequate treatment usually recover without sequelae.

DISCHARGE CRITERIA/INSTRUCTIONS

• From the emergency department. Asymptomatic patients may be discharged after decontamination, a 6-hour observation period, and psychiatric evaluation, if needed.
• From the hospital. Patients who have not required atropine for 24 hours may be discharged.

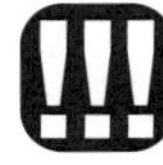

Pitfalls

TREATMENT

Failure to adequately protect health-care providers may result in secondary exposures.

ICD-9-CM 989.3

Toxic effect of other substances, chiefly nonmedicinal as to source: organophosphate and carbamate.

See also: SECTION II, Hypotension, Pulmonary Edema, and Seizures chapters; SECTION III, Atropine and Pralidoxime chapters.

RECOMMENDED READING

Aaron CK, Howland MA. Insecticides: organophosphates and carbamates. In: Goldfrank LR, Flomenbaum NE, Lewin NA, et al., eds. *Goldfrank's toxicologic emergencies,* 6th ed. Norwalk, CT: Appleton & Lange, 1998.

Willems JL, De Bisschop HC, Verstraete AG, et al. Cholinesterase reactivation in organophosphorus poisoned patients depends on the plasma concentrations of the oxime pralidoxime methylsulphate and of the organophosphate. *Arch Toxicol* 1993;67:79–84.

Author: Luke Yip

Reviewer: Richard C. Dart

Ozone

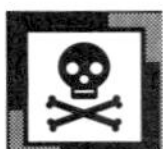

Basics

DESCRIPTION

Ozone (O_3) is a colorless gas with a sharp, pungent odor sometimes described as "electrical."

FORMS AND USES

- At low temperature, ozone is a dark blue liquid.
- Ozone is used as an oxidizing agent in organic chemical production, public water purification, and sewage treatment; for mold and bacteria control on food in cold storage rooms; as a bleaching agent in textile, paper pulp, wax, starch, and sugar production; and in mineral oil refining.

TOXIC DOSE

- The odor threshold for ozone is 0.05 ppm.
- Concentrations greater than 0.1 ppm cause irritation of the upper respiratory tract.
- At 1 ppm, exposures exceeding 30 minutes may cause headache, malaise, or tachycardia.

PATHOPHYSIOLOGY

- Ozone alters pulmonary response to infection, causes thickening of pulmonary arteries, and may enhance pulmonary allergic reactions.
- Ozone exposure may result in noncardiac pulmonary edema.
- Prolonged or cumulative exposure to low concentrations of ozone may cause a more serious clinical problem than short-term exposure to high concentrations.

EPIDEMIOLOGY

Low-level exposure is common (air pollution); high-concentration exposure is rare.

CAUSES

- Children and the elderly are considered more sensitive to ozone exposure than adults.
- Occupational exposure may occur during inert gas-shielded arc welding.

WORKPLACE STANDARDS

- ACGIH. TLV TWA is 0.05 ppm (heavy work) to 0.10 ppm (light work).
- OSHA. PEL TWA is 0.1 ppm.
- NIOSH. REL (ceiling) is 0.1 ppm (0.2 mg/m^3); IDLH level is 5 ppm.

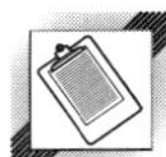

Diagnosis

DIFFERENTIAL DIAGNOSIS

Toxicologic causes of mucous membrane irritation and pulmonary injury include chlorine, nitrogen oxides, phosgene, ethylene oxide, and others.

SIGNS AND SYMPTOMS

HEENT

Headache, chemical conjunctivitis, and an acrid taste and smell may be reported.

Dermatologic

Dermatitis or burns may occur with liquid product (cryogenic) exposure; rapidly expanding gases may cause frostbite.

Pulmonary

- Dyspnea, tachypnea, cough, choking and chest tightness, substernal chest pain, wheezing, and decreased exercise tolerance may be seen.
- Pulmonary edema is possible.
- Ozone exposure potentiates asthma symptoms in asthmatic patients.

Gastrointestinal

Nausea and vomiting may occur.

Hepatic

Liver enzyme abnormalities are possible.

Hematologic

Increased red blood cell fragility may be seen.

Neurologic

Malaise, dizziness, decreased concentration, or insomnia may occur.

PROCEDURES AND LABORATORY TESTS

Essential Tests

No tests may be needed in asymptomatic patients.

Recommended Tests

- Complete blood count, serum electrolytes and renal function tests, and pulse oximetry should be ordered for symptomatic patients.
- Chest radiography and pulmonary function tests should be performed for patients with pulmonary symptoms.
- Peak flow testing is helpful in assessing pulmonary damage and in following response to therapy.
- Ozone exposure decreases inspiratory capacity, FVC (forced vital capacity), FEV_1 (forced expiratory volume in 1 second), peak flow, and tidal volume.

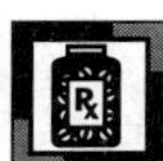

Treatment

- Treatment should focus on supportive care with appropriate airway management.
- Oxygen should be administered to symptomatic patients.
- The dose and time of exposure should be determined for all substances involved.

DIRECTING PATIENT COURSE

The health-care professional should call the poison control center when:

- Severe or persistent effects develop.
- Underlying disease presents an unusual problem.

The patient should be referred to a health-care facility when:

- Toxic effects develop.
- Underlying disease presents an unusual problem.

Admission Considerations

Inpatient management is warranted for all patients with continuing respiratory symptoms after exposure.

DECONTAMINATION

Out of Hospital

The patient should be removed from the source of the exposure.

In Hospital

High-flow oxygen should be administered.

ANTIDOTES

There is no specific antidote for ozone toxicity.

ADJUNCTIVE TREATMENT

- Bronchospasm is treated with inhaled β_2 adrenergic agents such as albuterol, 0.15 mg/kg (maximum 10 mg) in saline via nebulizer every 20 to 30 minutes, as needed.
- Pulmonary edema is treated as noncardiogenic type (see SECTION II, Pulmonary Edema chapter).

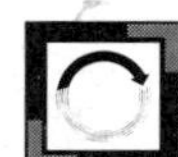

Follow-Up

PATIENT MONITORING

- Respiratory and cardiac function should be monitored continuously in symptomatic patients.
- Serial peak flow or other pulmonary tests are used to follow response to therapy.

EXPECTED COURSE AND PROGNOSIS

- Acute exposure should be self-limiting with no sequelae unless very high concentration is involved.
- Chronic inhalation may produce symptoms of CNS and renal impairment, or emphysema.

DISCHARGE CRITERIA/INSTRUCTIONS

- From emergency department. Asymptomatic patients may be discharged after 6 hours of observation.
- From hospital. Patients with significant exposure may be discharged if pulmonary effects do not develop within 24 hours.

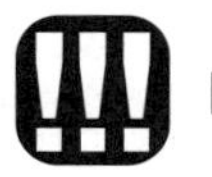

Pitfalls

DIAGNOSIS

Acute high concentration exposure may not cause pulmonary edema immediately.

ICD-9-CM 987.3

Toxic effect of other gases, fumes, or vapors: ozone.

See also: SECTION II, Pulmonary Edema chapter.

RECOMMENDED READING

Beckett WS. Ozone, air pollution and respiratory health. *Yale J Biol Med* 1991;64:167–175.

Costa DL, Amdur MO. Air pollution. In: Klaassen CD, Amdur MO, Doull J, eds. *Casarett and Doull's toxicology: the basic science of poisons,* 5th ed. New York: McGraw-Hill, 1996:857–882.

Author: Alvin C. Bronstein

Reviewer: Richard C. Dart

Paraquat and Diquat

Basics

DESCRIPTION

Paraquat and diquat are herbicides used in commercial applications.

FORMS AND USES

- Paraquat is used as a desiccant, a contact herbicide, defoliant, and plant growth regulator.
- It is a restricted herbicide in the United States and therefore not widely available.
- Paraquat-based substances include Gramoxone (S, D, W), Gramonol, Gramixel, Gramuron, Actor, Dextrone, Dexuron, Esgram, Goldquat, Herbaxon, Herboxone, Para-col, Pathelion, Pillarquat, Pillarxone, Preglone, Priglone, Sweep, Terraklene, Total, Totacol, Toxer, Toxer Total, Viologen, and Weedol.
- Diquat is a structurally similar herbicide that produces similar toxicity, except for lung injury.

TOXIC DOSE

- Death occurs in most patients who ingest 20 to 40 mg/kg of paraquat; this may be just one swallow of more concentrated forms.
- Diquat is slightly less toxic, but 25 ml of concentrated solution is estimated as a lethal dose.

PATHOPHYSIOLOGY

- Paraquat is rapidly absorbed after gastrointestinal or dermal exposure.
- Pulmonary absorption is small because aerosol droplets are too large to reach the alveolus.
- After absorption, paraquat is actively taken up by type 1 and type 2 pulmonary epithelial cells, the principal target organ for toxicity.
- Paraquat is enzymatically reduced to an unstable free radical that is then reoxidized to produce a superoxide radical, causing direct free radical cell injury to the lung.

EPIDEMIOLOGY

- Poisoning is uncommon.
- Toxic effects are typically severe, with death occurring in most patients who ingest a gulp or more.

CAUSES

- Toxic ingestion is usually intentional.
- Dermal exposure is typically occupational.
- Child abuse must be considered if the patient is less than 1 year of age; suicide attempt if the patient is over 6 years of age.

PREGNANCY AND LACTATION

- Paraquat is concentrated in the fetus.
- The value of emergent cesarean section is unproven; no fetus has ever survived.

WORKPLACE STANDARDS

Paraquat

- OSHA. PEL TWA is 0.5 mg/m^3.
- NIOSH. Not listed.
- ACGIH. TLV TWA is 0.5 mg/m^3 for total particulate.

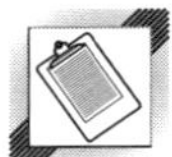

Diagnosis

DIFFERENTIAL DIAGNOSIS

- Caustic injury to mucosa and oropharyngeal membranes may be mistaken for diphtheria or ingestion of caustic agents.
- The rapid progression of multiorgan failure following serious paraquat ingestion may resemble several clinical conditions, such as sepsis, cardiogenic shock, or severe salicylate toxicity.
- Pulmonary fibrosis and restrictive lung disease may resemble silicosis, asbestosis, and sarcoidosis; however, the rapid progression of severe pulmonary fibrosis is highly characteristic of paraquat ingestion.

SIGNS AND SYMPTOMS

- Paraquat. The initial effects are caustic burns to the gastrointestinal tract or skin, depending on exposure; after a day or two, pulmonary complaints and rapidly progressive pulmonary injury develop in serious cases.
- Diquat. Symptoms begin with gastrointestinal effects similar to paraquat, but diquat does not produce pulmonary injury.

Vital Signs

- Tachycardia and hypotension may occur due to gastrointestinal toxicity.
- Tachypnea develops in patients who develop pulmonary injury.

HEENT

- Splash injuries may result in severe conjunctival and corneal lesions or uveitis from paraquat or diquat.
- Oropharyngeal burns may result from ingesting paraquat or diquat.

Dermatologic

Concentrated paraquat or diquat solutions may cause dermal burns that enhance absorption.

Cardiovascular

- Cardiovascular collapse may occur rapidly following large ingestions of paraquat or diquat.
- Myocarditis may occur with large ingestions of paraquat.

Pulmonary

- Death due to pulmonary fibrosis is common with paraquat.
- Progression of pulmonary fibrosis is refractory to treatment.

Gastrointestinal

Both diquat and paraquat produce marked gastrointestinal effects: nausea, vomiting, abdominal pain and diarrhea, followed by perforation and hemorrhage within a few days in some severe cases.

Hepatic

- Moderate centrilobular hepatocellular necrosis may occur within a few days with paraquat.
- Intrahepatic cholestasis is common.
- Diquat produces minor injury.

Renal

- Renal tubular injury evolves over a few days for both paraquat and diquat.
- Renal failure may resolve if the patient survives.

Fluids and Electrolytes

Fluid losses may be severe due to gastrointestinal burns or hemorrhage.

Musculoskeletal

Muscular necrosis has occurred after ingestion.

Neurologic

- Cerebral edema, lethargy, and coma occur in severe cases with either paraquat or diquat.
- Pontine purpura and brainstem infarct have occurred with diquat.

Endocrine

Adrenal necrosis may occur with massive ingestion.

PROCEDURES AND LABORATORY TESTS

Emergency information and analysis for paraquat:

- United States: Zeneca Inc. Agricultural Products, Wilmington, DE 19897; Telephone 1-800-327-8633 (24-hour emergency line)
- Canada: ICI Chipman, Stoney Creek, Ontario L8G 3G1; Telephone 1-800-561-3636 (24-hour emergency line)
- United Kingdom: Zeneca Agrochemicals, Femhurst, Haslemere, Surrey GU27 3JE, England; Telephone (0622) 814777 (24-hour emergency line)
- Australia: ICI Crop Care, Melbourne, Victoria 3001; Telephone 008-033-111 (24-hour emergency line)

Essential Tests

- Serum electrolytes, glucose, BUN, creatinine, and urinalysis to assess renal injury and guide replacement therapy in patients with fluid losses; paraquat may cause hypokalemia, which indicates a poor prognosis.
- Aspartate aminotransferase, alanine aminotransferase, lactic dehydrogenase, bilirubin, prothrombin time/international normalized ratio, and partial thromboplastin time are used to monitor for the development of hepatic injury.

Recommended Tests

- Serum creatine kinase assesses muscle injury.
- Serum amylase assesses pancreatic injury.
- Arterial blood gases are used to monitor the progression and treatment of pulmonary injury.
- Paraquat levels in urine and serum are possibly helpful in predicting severity of poisoning, but they are not typically available (see emergency numbers above).
- Quantitative tests are predictive of prognosis; plasma levels greater than 2 mg/L at 4 hours and greater than 0.1 mg/L at 24 hours usually indicate a fatal outcome.
- Chest radiograph may be normal initially, but bilateral massive infiltrates develop in severe cases.
- Pulmonary function tests. Impairment of diffusion and decrease in pulmonary compliance as fibrosis develops.
- Endoscopy. The presence of gastric or esophageal ulcers indicate a poor prognosis; endoscopy is also used to identify ulcerations at risk of perforation.

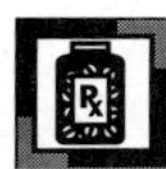

Treatment

- Initial treatment for diquat or paraquat exposure should focus on decontamination and supportive care.
- Supportive care with appropriate airway management is vital.
- Name, amount, concentration, and time of exposure should be determined for all substances involved.

DIRECTING PATIENT COURSE

The health-care professional should call the poison control center when history of paraquat or diquat exposure is obtained.

The patient should be referred to a health-care facility when:

- History of paraquat or diquat exposure is obtained.
- Patient or caregiver seems unreliable.
- Toxic effects develop.

Admission Considerations

Inpatient management is warranted for all patients who have ingested paraquat or diquat or have signs that suggest potential paraquat toxicity.

DECONTAMINATION

Out of Hospital

- Emesis should not be induced due to caustic effects.
- If delay in reaching medical care is expected, the patient should be instructed to eat 1 to 2 handfuls of dirt, food, or activated charcoal immediately in order to decrease gastrointestinal absorption as much as possible.
- Exposed skin should be irrigated with soap and water; scrubbing may enhance absorption and is not recommended.

In Hospital

- Gastric lavage is not recommended due to caustic hazard.
- Cautious aspiration with nasogastric tube for patient presenting soon after ingestion of paraquat or diquat may be reasonable due to extreme potential toxicity.
- Activated charcoal (1–2 g/kg) should be administered without a cathartic if an ingestion has occurred within the previous few hours; a second dose can be given after 4 hours.
- Both fuller's earth (1–2 g/kg of a 15% aqueous suspension) and bentonite (1–2 g/kg of a 7% aqueous slurry) have been advocated to absorb paraquat after ingestion; these are often not available and have no clear advantage over activated charcoal.
- Exposed skin should be irrigated with soap and water; scrubbing should be avoided.

ANTIDOTES

There is no specific antidote for paraquat or diquat poisoning.

ADJUNCTIVE TREATMENT

Hemodialysis is used for renal failure, but is not effective for paraquat pulmonary toxicity. The following therapies are not recommended for either paraquat or diquat toxicity:

- Hemoperfusion is not effective.
- Lung transplantation has been attempted; there have been no long-term survivors due to paraquat injury to the transplanted lung.
- Urinary alkalinization has no proven benefit.
- Whole-bowel irrigation has no proven benefit.
- None of the following therapies have yet been found effective: cyclophosphamide, D-propranolol, vitamin E, deferoxamine, selenium, superoxide dismutase, ascorbic acid (vitamin C), *N*-acetylcysteine, fibrinolytic agents, colchicine, radiotherapy, and dexamethasone.

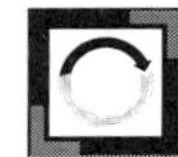

Follow-Up

PATIENT MONITORING

- Continuous cardiac and pulmonary monitoring should be performed on all patients.
- Patients should be monitored for the development of pulmonary fibrosis even after other systemic effects have resolved.

EXPECTED COURSE AND PROGNOSIS

- Large (>40 mg/kg) paraquat ingestion (more than 15 ml of 20% liquid concentrate in adult) typically causes death from multiorgan failure within a few days.
- Ingestion of 20 to 40 mg/kg (e.g., more than one sachet of 2.5% Weedol or less than 15 ml of 20% concentrate in adult). Initial gastrointestinal toxicity is followed by systemic toxicity, which may include reversible renal failure or hepatic failure, followed by death from pulmonary failure within 3 to 20 days.
- Ingestion of less than 20 mg/kg (e.g., less than one sachet of 2.5% Weedol). Patient is asymptomatic or develops some gastrointestinal effects; transient impairment of lung function may occur, but patient recovers.
- Fatal pulmonary fibrosis may occur even in patients who recover from initial toxic effects.
- Esophageal perforation and possibly mediastinitis may occur following ingestion.

DISCHARGE CRITERIA/INSTRUCTIONS

- From the emergency department. Patients with paraquat or diquat exposure should not be discharged.
- From the hospital. Asymptomatic patients may be discharged if toxic effects do not develop within a few days of exposure.

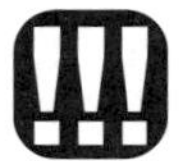

Pitfalls

DIAGNOSIS

Smoking of paraquat-treated marijuana has not been documented to cause significant toxicity; pyrolysis inactivates the paraquat.

TREATMENT

Administration of activated charcoal should not be delayed while waiting for endoscopy to be performed.

FOLLOW-UP

Patients may recover from early gastrointestinal, renal, and other effects only to develop fatal pulmonary fibrosis later.

ICD-9-CM 989

Toxic effect of other substances, chiefly nonmedicinal as to source.

RECOMMENDED READING

Ellenhorn MJ. Paraquat. *Ellenhorn's medical toxicology,* 2nd ed. Baltimore: Williams & Wilkins, 1997:1631–1637.

POISINDEX Editorial Staff. Paraquat. In: Rumack BH, Sayre NK, Gelman CR, eds. *POISINDEX system.* Englewood, CO: Micromedex Inc. (edition expires May 31, 1998).

Authors: Lada Kokan and Gerald F. O'Malley

Reviewer: Richard C. Dart

Pennyroyal

Basics

DESCRIPTION

Pennyroyal (pulegium) is an essential oil contained in the plants *Hedeoma pulegioides* (American pennyroyal) and *Mentha pulegium* (European pennyroyal) as well as some herbal products such as Broncodin tea.

FORMS AND USES

- Common names for pennyroyal plants include squawmint/squawbalm, mosquito plant, mock pennyroyal, and tickweed.
- Active constituents

—American pennyroyal contains up to 2% of the volatile oil.
—European pennyroyal contains up to 1% of the volatile oil.

- "Folk" uses of pennyroyal include control of menstruation and as an abortifacient, as well as a flea-killing bath (Latin for flea is *pulegioides*), stimulant, carminative, and diaphoretic.

TOXIC DOSE

- Toxicity may develop at a dose of 5 cc.
- Death has occurred after a single 15-cc ingestion of the essential oil.
- However, ingestion of plant parts usually produces no or minimal toxicity.

PATHOPHYSIOLOGY

- Pennyroyal oil contains pulegone, a toxic volatile oil.
- Pulegone is metabolized to a compound that is toxic to the liver and lung.

EPIDEMIOLOGY

- Poisoning is rare.
- Toxic effects following ingestion of essential oil are typically severe.
- Death occurs in a high proportion of victims.

CAUSES

- Cause is usually unintentional misuse of the product.
- Often the pulegone content is unknown to the user.
- Child neglect should be considered if the patient is less than 1 year of age; suicide attempt in patients over 6 years of age.

PREGNANCY AND LACTATION

Pennyroyal is used as an abortifacient; however, the dose needed to induce abortion is close to the lethal dose.

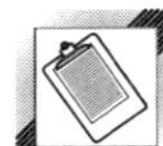

Diagnosis

- The history is the most crucial aspect of making the diagnosis.
- The patient should be questioned extensively about the use of herbal products.

DIFFERENTIAL DIAGNOSIS

Toxic causes of liver injury include acetaminophen, *Amanita* mushroom, carbamazepine, valproic acid, phenytoin, salicylate, isoniazid, carbon tetrachloride, halothane, disulfiram, procainamide, pyrrolizidine alkaloids, and methotrexate.

SIGNS AND SYMPTOMS

- Initial gastrointestinal symptoms are followed by abdominal pain and altered mental status early after exposure.
- Liver and pulmonary injury develop within hours and may result in death.

Vital Signs

Vital signs are variable but are consistent with hypotension and metabolic acidosis.

HEENT

The patient may have minty odor on the breath.

Cardiovascular

Shock develops in severe cases.

Pulmonary

Bronchiolar epithelial destruction and acute pulmonary necrosis may occur.

Gastrointestinal

Protracted emesis, abdominal pain, gastrointestinal bleeding, and hepatotoxicity with fulminant hepatic failure may occur.

Renal

- Hematuria is common.
- Acute renal failure is common in severe cases.

Hepatic

Hepatic enzyme elevation, fulminant hepatic failure, and disseminated intravascular coagulation develop in severe cases.

Fluids and Electrolytes

Severe metabolic acidosis develops in serious cases.

Neurologic

Initial dizziness, hallucinations, and seizures may occur; cerebral edema may occur in severe cases.

Reproductive

Vaginal bleeding and uterine contraction leading to abortion may develop.

PROCEDURES AND LABORATORY TESTS

Essential Tests

No tests may be needed for asymptomatic patients who ingested plant parts or if a long period has elapsed since ingestion without apparent effect.

Recommended Tests

- Serum electrolytes, glucose, BUN, and creatinine should be determined and urinalysis performed in symptomatic patients to assess for metabolic acidosis and acute renal failure.
- Serum liver function tests should be performed in symptomatic patients to assess hepatic injury.
- Platelet count, international normalized ratio (INR) or prothrombin time (PT), partial thromboplastin time (PTT), fibrinogen, and fibrin split products should be determined to assess for coagulation defect in symptomatic patients.
- Complete blood count should be performed to assess blood loss.
- ECG, serum acetaminophen and aspirin levels determined in overdose setting to detect occult ingestion.

Not Recommended Tests

Pulegone levels are not available.

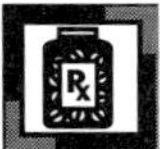

Treatment

- Treatment should focus on supportive care of renal insufficiency, hepatic injury, and coagulopathy.
- Dose and time of exposure should be determined for all substances involved.

DIRECTING PATIENT COURSE

The health-care provider should call the poison control center when:

- Altered mental status, liver injury, renal failure, or other severe effects are present.
- Toxic effects are not consistent with pennyroyal poisoning.
- Coingestant, drug interaction, or underlying disease presents an unusual problem.

The patient should be referred to a health-care facility when:

- History of pennyroyal ingestion is obtained.
- Attempted suicide or homicide is possible.
- Patient or caregiver seems unreliable.
- Coingestant, drug interaction, or underlying disease presents an unusual problem.

Admission Considerations

Inpatient treatment is warranted for symptomatic patients.

DECONTAMINATION

Out of Hospital

Emesis should be induced with ipecac within 1 hour of ingestion for alert pediatric or adult patients if health-care evaluation will be delayed and vomiting has not already occurred.

In Hospital

- Aspiration of gastric contents using a nasogastric tube should be performed in patients presenting within 1 hour of ingestion or if serious effects are present.
- One dose of activated charcoal (1-2 g/kg) should be administered without a cathartic if a substantial ingestion has occurred within the previous few hours.

ANTIDOTES

There is no specific antidote for pennyroyal toxicity.

ADJUNCTIVE TREATMENT

Patients with Coagulopathy and Active Bleeding

- Fresh-frozen plasma should be administered.

—Pediatric dose is 10 to 15 ml/kg intravenously.
—Adult dose is 2 to 4 units intravenously.
—Based on serial INR and PT determinations, further fresh-frozen plasma should be administered as needed to return values toward normal.
—Packed red blood cells should be administered as indicated for bleeding and anemia.

N-Acetylcysteine (NAC)

- Because pulegone depletes hepatic glutathione, it has been proposed that early NAC administration be used to prevent pennyroyal hepatic injury.
- This may be reasonable because the risk of NAC treatment is low; however, the dosing regimen is unknown.

Hypotension

- The patient should be given 10 to 20 ml/kg 0.9% saline intravenously and placed in the Trendelenburg position.
- Further fluid therapy should be guided by central pressure monitoring to avoid volume overload.
- If hypotension does not respond to treatment, a vasopressor is administered.

—The dose for dopamine is 2 to 5 μg/kg/min, titrated upward to effect; rates greater than 20 μg/kg/min are unlikely to provide further benefit.
—The dose for norepinephrine is 0.1 to 0.2 μg/kg/min, titrated to effect.
—High rates of infusion may cause tissue ischemia.

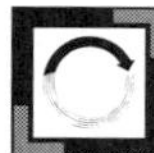

Follow-Up

PATIENT MONITORING

Indices of coagulation function and liver and renal injury should be followed.

EXPECTED COURSE AND PROGNOSIS

- Patients ingesting leaves or plant parts usually recover.
- Ingestion of oil often leads to a severe course lasting days or weeks.
- Sequelae of hypoxia or hypotension may occur in severe cases, if the patient survives.

DISCHARGE CRITERIA/INSTRUCTIONS

- From the emergency department. Asymptomatic patients who have ingested plant parts may be discharged after gastrointestinal decontamination, observation for 4 to 6 hours, and psychiatric evaluation, if needed.
- From the hospital. Patient may be discharged after liver and renal injury resolve or stabilize.

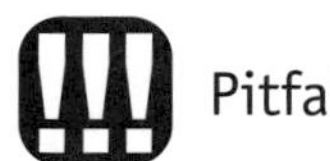

Pitfalls

DIAGNOSIS

Careful history of alternative medication use is needed to detect pennyroyal ingestion.

ICD-9-CM 988

Toxic effect of noxious substances eaten as food.

See also: SECTION II, Hypotension chapter.

RECOMMENDED READING

Bakerink JA, Gospe SM, Dimand RJ, et al. Multiple organ failure after ingestion of pennyroyal oil from herbal tea in two infants. *Pediatr* 1996;98:944–947.

Anderson IB, Mullen WH, Meeker JE, et al. Pennyroyal toxicity: measurement of toxic metabolite levels in two cases and review of the literature. *Ann Intern Med* 1996;124:726–734.

Author: Kathleen Graham

Reviewer: Richard C. Dart

Pentoxifylline

Basics

DESCRIPTION

Pentoxifylline (Trental) is a xanthine derivative used in the treatment of peripheral vascular and cerebrovascular disease.

FORMS AND USES

- Pentoxifylline is a sustained-release formulation.
- A typical adult dosage is 400 mg three times a day.

TOXIC DOSE

Toxicity has occurred at three or four times the daily dose.

PATHOPHYSIOLOGY

- Pentoxifylline increases erythrocyte flexibility and thereby reduces blood viscosity, which results in increased perfusion of the microvascular beds.
- Pentoxifylline also impairs platelet function.

EPIDEMIOLOGY

Poisoning is uncommon.

CAUSES

- Toxicity is usually an adverse drug event rather than acute ingestion.
- Child neglect or abuse should be considered if the patient is less than 1 year of age, suicide attempt if the patient is over 6 years of age.

PREGNANCY AND LACTATION

US FDA Pregnancy Category C. The drug exerts animal teratogenic or embryocidal effects, but there are no controlled studies in women, or no studies are available in animals or women.

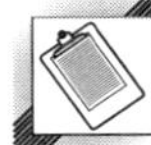

Diagnosis

DIFFERENTIAL DIAGNOSIS

Toxic causes of agitation, seizures, and CNS depression include a variety of stimulants, theophylline, and β-receptor agonists, among others.

SIGNS AND SYMPTOMS

Vital Signs

Hypotension and bradycardia have been reported.

Dermatologic

Flushing has been reported as a side effect of therapy and in overdose.

Cardiovascular

- Varying degrees of heart block have been reported after overdose.
- Angina and chest pain have been reported as side effects of therapy.

Gastrointestinal

Abdominal pain and vomiting may occur.

Hematologic

Aplastic anemia has been reported as a rare side effect of therapy.

Fluids and Electrolytes

Hypokalemia has been reported.

Neurologic

Seizures, decreased level of consciousness, and agitation have been reported in overdose.

PROCEDURES AND LABORATORY TESTS

Essential Tests

No tests may be needed in asymptomatic patients.

Recommended Tests

- Serum electrolytes, glucose, BUN, and creatinine should be obtained to evaluate for hypokalemia and causes of seizure.
- Complete blood count should be obtained to evaluate for bone marrow suppression.
- Serum magnesium and calcium to assess cause of seizure.
- ECG should be obtained to detect atrioventricular block or ischemia.
- Head CT, lumbar puncture, and cultures should be obtained as indicated for altered mental status.
- Serum acetaminophen, aspirin in overdose setting to detect occult ingestion.

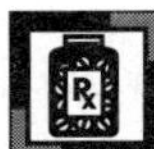

Treatment

- Treatment should focus on control of seizures, maintenance of airway, and general supportive care.
- Dose and time of exposure should be determined for all substances involved.

DIRECTING PATIENT COURSE

The health-care professional should call the poison control center when:

- Severe or persistent effects develop.
- Coingestant, drug interaction, or underlying disease presents an unusual problem.

The patient should be referred to a health-care facility when:

- Suicide or homicide attempt is possible.
- Toxic effects develop.
- Coingestant, drug interaction, or underlying disease presents an unusual problem.

Admission Considerations

Inpatient management is warranted for symptomatic patients.

DECONTAMINATION

Out of Hospital

Emesis should not be induced.

In Hospital

- Gastric lavage (after appropriate airway management) should be performed in pediatric (tube size 24–32 French) or adult (tube size 36–42 French) patients presenting within 1 hour of a large ingestion or if serious effects are present.
- One dose of activated charcoal (1–2 g/kg) should be administered without a cathartic if a substantial ingestion has occurred within the previous few hours.
- Because the standard pentoxifylline formulation is sustained release, whole-bowel irrigation may be useful in symptomatic patients.

ANTIDOTES

There is no specific antidote for pentoxifylline toxicity.

ADJUNCTIVE TREATMENT

- Hypotension and seizures should be treated using standard measures.
- Temporary pacing may be indicated for symptomatic heart block.

Hypotension

The patient should be treated with isotonic fluid infusion, Trendelenburg positioning, and, if needed, vasopressors. Dopamine is preferred, and norepinephrine is added for refractory hypotension.

Seizures

- A patent airway must be ensured.
- A benzodiazepine is administered for initial control. If seizures persist or recur, another anticonvulsant may be added.

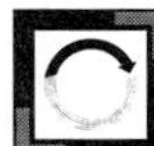

Follow-Up

PATIENT MONITORING

Respiratory and cardiac monitoring should be monitored continuously.

EXPECTED COURSE AND PROGNOSIS

Toxic effects of pentoxifylline poisoning may take 12 to 24 hours to resolve.

DISCHARGE CRITERIA/INSTRUCTIONS

Patients who are asymptomatic after decontamination, 6 hours of observation, and psychiatric evaluation may be discharged from the emergency department or hospital.

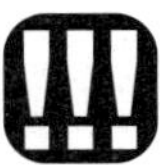

Pitfalls

DIAGNOSIS

Pentoxifylline is often overlooked as a cause of agitation.

ICD-9-CM 964

Poisoning by agents primarily affecting blood constituents.

See also: SECTION II, Hypotension and Seizures chapters.

RECOMMENDED READING

McEvoy GK, ed. Pentoxifylline. In: *AHFS drug information 94*. Bethesda, MD: American Society of Hospital Pharmacists, 1994:928–931.

Sznajder IJ, Bentur Y, Taitelman U. First and second degree atrioventricular block in pentoxifylline overdose. *BMJ* 1984;288:26.

Author: Kennon Heard

Reviewer: Richard C. Dart

Phencyclidine

Basics

DESCRIPTION

Phencyclidine is a drug of abuse that produces hallucinations.

FORMS AND USES

- Phencyclidine is commonly known as PCP.
- Slang terms include angel dust, hog, mist, peace pill, kayo jay, KJ, crystal joint, elephant tranquilizer, super grass, super weed, rocket fuel, scuffle, sheets, space basing (phencyclidine plus crack cocaine), DOA, T, cyclone, snorts, soma, goon, horse franks, and dust.
- PCP is often used to enhance the effects of other drugs (e.g., "dipping" a marijuana joint).

TOXIC DOSE

- A dose of 5 mg will usually produce euphoria.
- A dose of 150 to 200 mg has been associated with death.

PATHOPHYSIOLOGY

- Phencyclidine is a dissociative anesthetic.
- It stimulates α-adrenergic receptors, causing sympathomimetic effects.
- It also has hallucinogenic effects and is believed to potentiate the effects of serotonin.

EPIDEMIOLOGY

- Poisoning from recreational abuse is common.
- Incidence of abuse is highly regional.
- Toxic effects are typically mild to moderate.
- Death is rare and usually caused by trauma incurred due to impaired judgment.

CAUSES

- Cause is usually intentional ingestion or inhalation.
- The possibility of child neglect or abuse should be considered if the patient is less than 1 year of age; suicide attempt in patients over 6 years of age.

RISK FACTORS

Elderly patients may be less tolerant of the cardiovascular effects.

DRUG AND DISEASE INTERACTIONS

Sympathomimetic effects may be enhanced by other sympathomimetic drugs such as cocaine or amphetamines.

PREGNANCY AND LACTATION

- US FDA Pregnancy Category X. Studies demonstrate fetal abnormalities or there is evidence of fetal risk based on human experience, or both, and the risk outweighs any possible benefit.
- Phencyclidine crosses the placenta and may produce toxicity in the fetus.

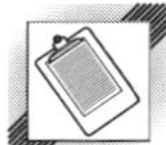

Diagnosis

DIFFERENTIAL DIAGNOSIS

- Toxic causes of hallucinations include amphetamines, anticholinergic agents, high-dose corticosteroids, LSD, peyote, psilocybin, and mescaline, among others.
- Nontoxic causes include CNS trauma, meningitis, AIDS-related illness, hypoglycemia, electrolyte imbalance, heat-related illness, hypoxia, and alcohol or sedative-hypnotic withdrawal.

SIGNS AND SYMPTOMS

- Common effects include nystagmus, hypertension, tachycardia, agitation, hallucinations, and violent behavior.
- Associated conditions are complications of drug abuse (hepatitis, abscess, HIV, endocarditis, etc.).

Vital Signs

- Hyperthermia or hypothermia may develop depending on degree of physical activity and ambient temperature.
- Tachycardia and hypertension are common.

HEENT

- Nystagmus is common and may be horizontal, vertical, or rotatory.
- Mydriasis occurs with severe intoxication.
- Miosis is more common in children.

Cardiovascular

Hypertension and mild tachycardia are common.

Pulmonary

Apnea and respiratory failure may occur after severe overdose.

Renal

Acute renal failure may develop rarely due to rhabdomyolysis.

Musculoskeletal

Rhabdomyolysis may occur due to prolonged agitation or hyperthermia.

Neurologic

- Common findings include impaired judgment, agitation, violent behavior, delusions or hallucinations, psychosis, and paranoid or self-destructive behavior.
- Coma occurs infrequently.
- Seizures, dystonia, and dyskinesia occur rarely.

Endocrine

Mild hypoglycemia is common.

PROCEDURES AND LABORATORY TESTS

Essential Tests

No tests may be needed in asymptomatic patients with a history of possible ingestion.

Recommended Tests

- Serum electrolytes, glucose, BUN, and creatine levels should be determined in symptomatic patients.

—Mild hypoglycemia is common.
—Rhabdomyolysis and renal failure imply prolonged agitation and severe intoxication.

- ECG and cardiac monitoring may reveal tachycardia; other dysrhythmias suggest severe intoxication.
- Serum creatine kinase may be determined to detect rhabdomyolysis.
- Liver function and coagulation studies are performed in symptomatic patients to assess the severity of toxicity.
- Urine drug screening may be performed in patients with hallucinations of unknown cause to determine toxic effects and the presence of other ingestants.
- Urinalysis may be performed to determine renal injury produced by rhabdomyolysis or hypotension.
- Other tests (complete blood count, blood culture, head CT, lumbar puncture) should be performed as needed to rule out other causes of mental status change.

Not Recommended Tests

Serum phencyclidine levels are not available or helpful.

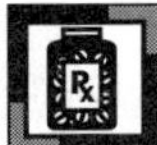

Treatment

- Treatment focuses on supporting blood pressure, managing airway, and controlling agitation.
- Dose and time of exposure should be determined for all substances involved.

DIRECTING PATIENT COURSE

The health-care provider should call the poison control center when:

- Seizure, coma, dysrhythmia, severe hypertension or hyperthermia, or other serious effects are present.
- Toxic effects are not consistent with phencyclidine poisoning.
- Coingestant, drug interaction, or underlying disease presents an unusual problem.

The patient should be referred to a health-care facility when:

- Attempted suicide or homicide is possible.
- Patient or caregiver seems unreliable.
- Toxic effects develop.
- Coingestant, drug interaction, or underlying disease presents an unusual problem.

Admission Considerations

Inpatient treatment is warranted when there is persistent alteration in mental status or when end-organ complications, such as rhabdomyolysis or renal failure, develop.

DECONTAMINATION

- Gastrointestinal decontamination is not usually recommended because of the small amount of phencyclidine needed to produce hallucinations and its rapid absorption.
- Lavage or activated charcoal may be appropriate if other drugs were ingested.

ANTIDOTES

There is no specific antidote for phencyclidine poisoning.

ADJUNCTIVE TREATMENT

Agitation or Psychosis

For control of agitation or psychosis, a number of strategies may be used:

- Naloxone and D50W should be administered if appropriate.
- The patient should be placed in a dimly lit room and offered counseling and companionship, to be "talked down."
- A benzodiazepine familiar to the provider should be administered.
- The airway should be monitored closely.

Diazepam

- Adult dose is 5 to 10 mg intravenously.
- Pediatric dose is 0.2 to 0.5 mg/kg intravenously.
- Doses are repeated at 5- to 10-minute intervals, titrating to effect.

Lorazepam

- Adult dose is 1 to 2 mg intravenously.
- Pediatric dose is 0.05 mg/kg intravenously.
- Doses are repeated at 5- to 10-minute intervals, titrating to effect.

Neuroleptics

- Neuroleptics such as droperidol should be used only in refractory cases
- Neuroleptics may induce seizure by lowering seizure threshold.

Mild Hypertension

Primary treatment is control of agitation.

Severe Hypertension

- For persistent severe hypertension or if end-organ damage is present, intravenous infusion of nitroprusside 1 μg/kg/min should be started and titrated up to 10 μg/kg/min as needed to control blood pressure.
- If infusion is required for more than 24 hours, the patient should be monitored for cyanide intoxication.

Hyperthermia

- Clothing should be removed and intravenous infusion of isotonic crystalloid begun.
- Agitation should be controlled.
- Fluid losses may be severe and should be replenished until a urine output of 1 to 2 ml/kg/h is reached.
- Fluid infusion should be monitored carefully to avoid overload.
- Cooling fans and wet sheets are effective, especially in dry climates.
- Other forms of central cooling (ice application, iced lavage fluids) are also recommended.
- Core temperature should be monitored frequently and cooling discontinued when body temperature decreases to 39°C.

Seizures

- Patent airway should be assured.
- A benzodiazepine should be administered for initial control as described for agitation, above.
- If seizures persist or recur, another anticonvulsant such as phenobarbital or phenytoin should be added.

Rhabdomyolysis

- Adequate hydration and urine output (1–2 ml/kg/h) should be ensured.
- Urinary alkalinization has not proven beneficial.

Not Recommended Therapies

Urinary acidification increases urinary excretion of phencyclidine by ion trapping, but carries a serious risk of inducing acidemia and worsening acute tubular necrosis in patients with rhabdomyolysis.

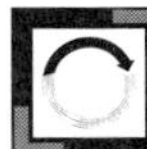

Follow-Up

EXPECTED COURSE AND PROGNOSIS

- Effects usually peak within several hours and then abate over 24 hours or more.
- Patients with repeated seizures are more likely to die or sustain permanent neurologic injury.
- Possible complications include renal failure, CNS injury due to prolonged seizures, and complications of trauma due to impaired judgment.

DISCHARGE CRITERIA/INSTRUCTIONS

- The patient may be discharged from the emergency department or hospital when tachycardia, hypertension, and hyperthermia have resolved and mental status has returned to baseline, provided there is no evidence of trauma or end-organ injury.
- The patient should be referred for substance abuse treatment.

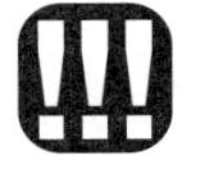

Pitfalls

DIAGNOSIS

Before attributing hallucinations to phencyclidine, other causes must be excluded.

TREATMENT

- Large amounts of benzodiazepines may be needed to control agitation.
- Severe hyperthermia may be life threatening and requires aggressive cooling and control of agitation.
- Patients may be extremely violent and a danger to themselves and others.

ICD-9-CM 968

Poisoning by other central nervous system depressants and anesthetics.

See also: SECTION II, Hyperthermia and Seizures chapters; and SECTION III, Nitroprusside chapter.

RECOMMENDED READING

McCarron MM, Schulze BW, Thompson GA, et al. Acute phencyclidine intoxication: clinical pattern, complications and treatment. *Ann Emerg Med* 1981;10:290–297.

Author: Katherine M. Hurlbut

Reviewer: Richard C. Dart

Phenol

Basics

DESCRIPTION

Phenol is a disinfectant that exists as a weak acid (carbolic acid).

FORMS AND USES

- Substances included are phenol, dinitrophenol, benzenol, carbolic acid, hydroquinone, and hydroxyquinone.
- Phenol is used as a disinfectant, dental analgesic, local anesthetic, preservative for parenteral medications, household cleaner, antiseptic, chemical face-peeling agent, and over-the-counter topical medication (skin and throat sprays, lozenges, Chloraseptic, and Sting Eze).
- It is also used in the manufacture of dyes and resins, as a chemical reagent, and in germicidal paints and slimicides.

TOXIC DOSE

In adults, a dose of 1 to 5 g has been associated with death; this would require ingesting more than 100 ml of Chloraseptic (1.4% solution).

PATHOPHYSIOLOGY

- Phenol concentrations greater than 5% denature proteins, causing mucosal and dermal burns.
- Some phenols (dinitrophenol, hydroxyquinone) are oxidizing agents, causing methemoglobinemia.
- CNS stimulation may be secondary to increased acetylcholine release.

EPIDEMIOLOGY

- Poisoning is rare.
- Toxic effects are typically mild.
- Death occurs in large exposures, primarily after ingestion.

CAUSES

- Exposure is usually accidental.
- Child neglect or abuse should be considered if the patient is less than 1 year of age; suicide attempt if the patient is over 6 years of age.

RISK FACTORS

Underlying cardiac disease may predispose to dysrhythmia.

WORKPLACE STANDARDS

- ACGIH. TLV TWA is 5 ppm.
- NIOSH. REL TWA is 5 ppm; ceiling is 15.6 ppm; IDLH level is 250 ppm.
- OSHA. PEL TWA is 5 ppm (19 mg/m^3).

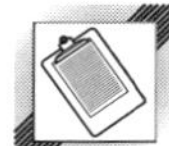

Diagnosis

DIFFERENTIAL DIAGNOSIS

- Other causes of toxic caustic ingestion include alkaline or acid solutions and numerous other agents that cause mucosal irritation.
- Other toxic causes of seizure, CNS depression, and dysrhythmia include tricyclic antidepressants (TCAs), various antidysrhythmic agents, antihistamine, cocaine, β-receptor or calcium channel blocker, camphor, and many others.
- Other causes of seizures and mental status depression include CNS bleed, mass, infection, and noncompliance with seizure medications.

SIGNS AND SYMPTOMS

- In ingestion exposures, a concentration greater than 5% may cause caustic gastrointestinal burns and upper airway edema.
- Large oral, dermal, parenteral, or inhalation exposure may cause mental status depression, seizures, coma, hypotension, and tachycardia.

Vital Signs

Hypotension and tachycardia may occur with severe intoxication.

HEENT

- Eye exposure may result in irritation, corneal injury, and burns.
- Rebound pharyngitis may develop after 7 days of using phenol lozenges.

Dermatologic

Irritation or burns may develop.

Pulmonary

- Upper airway edema and stridor may develop after ingestion.
- Respiratory failure may develop in severe cases from either inhalation or ingestion.

Cardiovascular

- Hypotension and tachycardia may develop.
- Atrial fibrillation, premature ventricular contractions, bigeminy, and ventricular tachycardia have occurred following large ingestions or dermal exposure.

Gastrointestinal

- Nausea, vomiting, and diarrhea are common after ingestion of high-concentration solution and suggest the possibility of mucosal burns.
- Esophageal burns may develop after ingestion of concentrations greater than 5%; the burns are initially white and painless and then slough after several days.

Hepatic

Liver function test elevation and jaundice may develop.

Renal

Acute renal failure is a rare complication of severe toxicity.

Fluids and Electrolytes

Metabolic acidosis may develop with hypotension or seizures.

Neurologic

CNS depression, coma, and seizures may develop after significant exposure.

Hematologic

Methemoglobinemia may develop after exposure to dinitrophenol or hydroquinone.

PROCEDURES AND LABORATORY TESTS

Essential Tests

No tests may be needed following dilute topical exposure.

Recommended Tests

- Serum electrolytes, BUN, and creatinine are measured in symptomatic patients; metabolic acidosis or renal insufficiency suggests severe poisoning.
- ECG and cardiac monitoring should be undertaken in patients with ingestion of concentrations over 5% or significant dermal, inhalation, or parenteral exposure.
- Methemoglobin level should be obtained to detect methemoglobinemia after dinitrophenol or hydroquinone exposure.
- Serum acetaminophen and aspirin levels should be obtained in an overdose setting to detect occult ingestion.
- Phenol and metabolites are detectable in urine but not useful in acute management; they may be useful to confirm exposure or for occupational monitoring.
- Endoscopy after ingestion of solutions with phenol concentrations above 5% is used to assess severity of burns, or in patients with pain, drooling, stridor, or persistent vomiting.

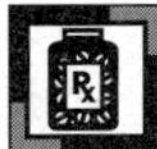

Treatment

- Treatment should focus on evaluating burns, controlling seizures and dysrhythmias, and managing the airway, if necessary.
- Dose and time of exposure should be determined for all substances involved.

DIRECTING PATIENT COURSE

The health-care professional should call the poison control center when:

- Burns, dysrhythmia, CNS toxicity, or other severe effects are present.
- Toxic effects are not consistent with phenol poisoning.
- Coingestant, drug interaction, or underlying disease presents an unusual problem.

The patient should be referred to a health-care facility when:

- Attempted suicide or homicide is possible.
- Patient or caregiver seems unreliable.
- Any toxic effects develop.
- Coingestant, drug interaction, or underlying disease presents an unusual problem.

Admission Considerations

Inpatient management is warranted if:

- Patient exhibits dysrhythmia, seizure, altered mental status, or documented grade 2 or 3 gastrointestinal burns.
- Patient has experienced significant ingestion and cannot undergo endoscopy in the emergency department.

DECONTAMINATION

Out of Hospital

- Emesis should not be induced with ipecac because of the potential for CNS depression and seizures.
- Ingestion should be diluted with 4 to 8 ounces of milk or water.
- Exposed skin or eyes should be irrigated copiously with water.

In Hospital

- Careful gastric aspiration with a small, flexible tube may be considered in patients presenting within 1 hour of a large ingestion or if serious effects are present. The risk of causing further injury to burned mucosa must be weighed against the potential benefit of reducing systemic absorption.
- One dose of activated charcoal (1–2 g/kg) without a cathartic should be considered if a substantial ingestion has occurred within the previous few hours. However, it should be avoided if endoscopy is planned.
- Exposed skin should be irrigated copiously with water, followed by soap and water; burns should be covered with a sterile dressing.
- Exposed eyes should be irrigated copiously with water or 0.9% saline.

—Patient should undergo slit-lamp examination.
—Patients with corneal burns or other ocular injury should be referred to an ophthalmologist immediately.

ANTIDOTES

There is no specific antidote for phenol poisoning.

ADJUNCTIVE THERAPIES

Seizure

- Adequate airway and oxygenation are crucial.
- Benzodiazepine should be administered for initial control.

—Diazepam. Adult dosage is 5 to 10 mg intravenous push initially, repeated every 10 minutes as needed. Pediatric dosage is 0.2 to 0.5 mg/kg every 10 minutes as needed; airway must be monitored closely
—Lorazepam. Adult dosage is 2 to 4 mg intravenous push over 2 to 5 minutes, repeated every 10 minutes as needed. Pediatric dosage is 0.1 mg/kg intravenous push over 2 to 5 minutes, not to exceed 4 mg/dose, repeated every 10 minutes as needed; airway must be monitored closely.

- If seizures persist or recur, another anticonvulsant such as phenobarbital or phenytoin can be added.
- Other options for repeated seizures include general anesthesia and neuromuscular blockade and artificial ventilation with EEG monitoring.

Hypotension

- The patient should be placed in the Trendelenburg position and administered 10 to 20 ml/kg 0.9% saline intravenously.
- Further fluid therapy should be guided with central pressure monitoring to avoid volume overload.
- If hypotension is unresponsive, a vasopressor can be administered.

—Dopamine: 2 to 5 μg/kg/min, titrated to desired effect; rates above 20 μg/kg/min are unlikely to provide further benefit.
—If hypotension is unresponsive, norepinephrine infusion of 0.1 to 0.2 μg/kg/min titrated to desired effect may be added.
—Tissue ischemia is possible with a high rate of infusion.

Cardiac Dysrhythmias

These should be treated in accordance with the guidelines specified in the chapter on Ventricular Dysrhythmias.

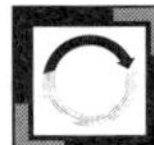

Follow-Up

Patient Monitoring

Hemodynamic and pulmonary function should be monitored continuously.

EXPECTED COURSE AND PROGNOSIS

- Acute gastrointestinal caustic injury occurs soon after ingestion.
- Recovery may take weeks; strictures may develop in patients with second- or third-degree gastrointestinal burns.
- Prolonged hypotension or hypoxia may rarely produce hypoxic brain or myocardial injury.

DISCHARGE CRITERIA/INSTRUCTIONS

- From the emergency department

—Ingestion. Following decontamination and a 6-hour observation period, patients without dysrhythmia, hypotension, or CNS effects who either have documented grade 0 or 1 burns, or have no stridor or vomiting, can be discharged.
—Inhalation. Asymptomatic patients with normal peak flow can be discharged after a 6-hour observation period.

- From the hospital. Patient may be discharged after dysrhythmias and hypotension have resolved for 24 hours, mental status has returned to baseline, and soft foods can be tolerated; follow-up for management of gastrointestinal injury should be arranged.

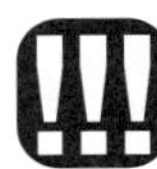

Pitfalls

FOLLOW-UP

Patients with second- or third-degree gastrointestinal burns should be evaluated for possible stricture development.

ICD-9-CM 968

Poisoning by other central nervous system depressants and anesthetics.

See also: SECTION II, Hypotension, Methemoglobinemia, Seizures, and Ventricular Dysrhythmia chapters; and SECTION IV, Caustics—Basic chapter.

RECOMMENDED READING

Spiller HA, Quadranikushnar DA, Cleveland P. A 5-year evaluation of acute exposures to phenol disinfectant (26 percent). *J Toxicol Clin Toxicol* 1993;31:307–313.

Author: Katherine M. Hurlbut

Reviewer: Luke Yip

Phenolphthalein

Basics

DESCRIPTION

Phenolphthalein is a stimulant laxative that increases peristalsis and mucous secretions in the gastrointestinal tract.

FORMS AND USES

- Phenolphthalein (Evac-U-Genr, Feen-A-Mint, Modane, Phenolax, Prulet) is used as a laxative for patients with anorectal conditions and constipation, as a postpartum laxative, and as a laxative to prepare the bowel for surgical procedures.
- The usual adult dose is 30 to 200 mg, and the usual pediatric dose is 15 to 60 mg, with yellow phenolphthalein two to three times more effective than white phenolphthalein.
- Therapeutic effect is usually seen in 6 to 8 hours.
- Phenolphthalein was withdrawn from the market in the United States in 1997; some products have been reformulated to omit phenolphthalein as an ingredient.

TOXIC DOSE

The level of toxicity ranges from 400 mg to 130 g.

PATHOPHYSIOLOGY

- Up to 15% of a dose is absorbed, conjugated, and excreted in the urine.
- Chronic laxative abuse, especially in patients with anorexia nervosa, may lead to osteomalacia, hypoproteinemia, fluid and electrolyte disorders such as hypokalemia and metabolic alkalosis, chronic diarrhea, and dependence on laxatives to induce bowel movements.

EPIDEMIOLOGY

Poisoning is uncommon.

CAUSES

Child neglect or abuse should be considered if the patient is less than 1 year of age; suicide attempt if the patient is greater than 6 years of age.

DRUG AND DISEASE INTERACTIONS

Phenolphthalein may decrease the absorption and bioavailability of anticoagulants such as anisindione, dicumarol, phenprocoumon, and warfarin because of decreased transit time in the gastrointestinal tract.

PREGNANCY AND LACTATION

US FDA Pregnancy Category C. The drug exerts animal teratogenic or embryocidal effects, but there are no controlled studies in women, or no studies are available in animals or women.

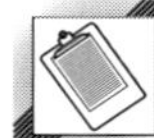

Diagnosis

DIFFERENTIAL DIAGNOSIS

Other toxic agents that cause abdominal cramps, nausea, tenesmus, and excessive bowel activity include other laxatives and numerous other substances that can cause diarrhea:

- Bisacodyl
- Calomel
- Prune concentrate
- Mineral oil
- Glycerin
- Methylcellulose
- Senna

SIGNS AND SYMPTOMS

HEENT

Brown tongue discoloration has been reported.

Dermatologic

Rashes and eruptions (including Stevens-Johnson syndrome) occur rarely.

Gastrointestinal

Primary effects are exaggeration of therapeutic effect: abdominal cramps, nausea, tenesmus, and excessive bowel activity with diarrhea.

Renal

- Nephrotic syndrome may occur during therapeutic dosing.
- Alkaline urine may develop red discoloration.
- Ammonium urate calculi and osteomalacia have been reported in phenolphthalein abusers.

PROCEDURES AND LABORATORY TESTS

Essential Tests

No tests may be needed in asymptomatic or minimally symptomatic patients.

Recommended Tests

- Stool analysis can identify the presence of phenolphthalein in cases of suspected laxative abuse.
- Serum electrolytes, BUN, and creatinine levels should be obtained in patients with prolonged effects or chronic abuse.
- ECG and serum acetaminophen and aspirin levels should be obtained in overdose setting to detect occult ingestion.

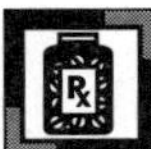

Treatment

- Symptomatic and supportive care is the mainstay of therapy.
- The dose and time of exposure for all substances involved should be determined.

DIRECTING PATIENT COURSE

The health-care professional should call the poison control center when:

- Severe or persistent effects develop.
- Coingestant, drug interaction, or underlying disease presents an unusual problem.

The patient should be referred to a health-care facility when:

- Suicide or homicide attempt is possible.
- Toxic effects develop.
- Coingestant, drug interaction, or underlying disease presents an unusual problem.

Admission Considerations

- Patients who are dehydrated or exhibit symptoms of electrolyte abnormalities, such as hypokalemia, hypocalcemia, or acidosis, should be admitted.
- Patients who demonstrate hypersensitivity eruptions also should be admitted.

DECONTAMINATION

Out of Hospital

Induction of emesis is not recommended.

In Hospital

One dose of activated charcoal (1–2 g/kg) should be administered without a cathartic if a substantial ingestion has occurred within the previous few hours.

ANTIDOTES

There is no specific antidote for phenolphthalein poisoning.

ADJUNCTIVE TREATMENT

Serious volume depletion and electrolyte abnormalities should be corrected.

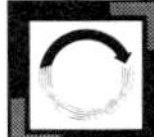

Follow-Up

PATIENT MONITORING

Dehydrated patients require repeated electrolyte monitoring.

EXPECTED COURSE AND PROGNOSIS

Complete recovery is likely with acute overdose, although at least one fatality secondary to fulminant hepatic failure and disseminated intravascular coagulation has been reported.

DISCHARGE CRITERIA/INSTRUCTIONS

Patients may be discharged from the emergency department or hospital when symptoms and fluid and electrolyte disorders have resolved, and vital signs are stable.

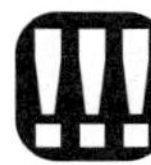

Pitfalls

DIAGNOSIS

Chronic abuse may lead to occult severe electrolyte abnormality.

ICD-9-CM 973.1

Poisoning by agents primarily affecting the gastrointestinal system: irritant cathartics.

RECOMMENDED READING

Sidhu PS, Wilkinson ML, Sladen GE, et al. Fatal phenolphthalein poisoning with fulminant hepatic failure and disseminated intravascular coagulation. *Hum Toxicol* 1989;8:381–384.

Author: Steven A. Seifert

Reviewer: Gerald F. O'Malley

Phenothiazines

Basics

DESCRIPTION

Phenothiazines are neuroleptic medications used to treat a wide range of disorders; thioridazine (Mellaril) is covered in a separate chapter.

FORMS AND USES

- Substances include chlorpromazine (Thorazine), fluphenazine (Prolixin), mesoridazine (Serentil), perphenazine (Trilafon), prochlorperazine (Compazine), promethazine (Phenergan), and trifluoperazine (Stelazine).
- Phenothiazines are used as antiemetic agents, pain medications, antipsychotic agents, and anxiolytic agents; they are also used in the treatment of allergic reactions and hiccups.

TOXIC DOSE

Toxicity varies widely by agent, but ingestion of several grams has been associated with death.

PATHOPHYSIOLOGY

- Phenothiazines competitively inhibit several types of receptors, including α_1- and α_2-adrenergic, cholinergic, dopaminergic, histaminic and serotonergic receptors.
- In overdose, the primary effects involve CNS dysfunction and cardiac conduction abnormalities combined with anticholinergic effects and peripheral α-adrenoceptor blockade.

EPIDEMIOLOGY

- Poisoning is common.
- Toxic effects following exposure are typically mild to moderate.
- Death is rare, occurring in patients with delayed treatment or coingestion.

CAUSES

- Poisoning is usually attributable to a suicidal ingestion.
- Child abuse or neglect should be considered if the patient is less than 1 year of age; suicide attempt in patients over 6 years of age.

RISK FACTORS

- Children are more susceptible to the extrapyramidal side effects of prochlorperazine.
- In geriatric patients liver disease may result in drug accumulation from therapeutic doses.

PREGNANCY AND LACTATION

For all phenothiazines available in the United States: US FDA Pregnancy Category C. Studies show animal teratogenic or embryocidal effects, but there are no controlled studies in women, or no studies are available in either animals or women.

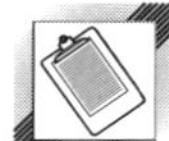

Diagnosis

DIFFERENTIAL DIAGNOSIS

- Toxic agents that produce CNS depression, especially those that also impair cardiac conduction, include type Ia antidysrhythmics, tricyclic antidepressant agents, chloroquine, antihistamines, and other agents.
- Other causes include primary CNS event (e.g., bleed, ischemia) or severe electrolyte abnormality (e.g., hypocalcemia).

SIGNS AND SYMPTOMS

- CNS depression is common.
- Seizures and cardiac dysrhythmias may develop in large overdose.

Vital Signs

- Tachycardia is common.
- In serious cases, hypertension may occur early, followed by hypotension.

HEENT

Mydriasis is common, but may be absent.

Cardiovascular

- Tachycardia, prolonged QTc, widened QRS, atrioventricular block, torsade de pointes, ventricular tachycardia or fibrillation, and sudden death may occur.
- Mesoridazine is more likely to produce cardiac effects.

Gastrointestinal

Constipation and ileus are common.

Hepatic

Cholestatic jaundice or mixed cholestatic and hepatocellular jaundice may occur after overdose or with therapeutic use.

Renal

- Urinary retention may occur.
- Priapism may occur rarely.

Hematologic

Agranulocytosis and anemia may occur with therapeutic use or after overdose.

Musculoskeletal

Rhabdomyolysis may occur in severe poisoning.

Neurologic

Agitation, CNS depression, coma, seizures, extrapyramidal symptoms, tardive dyskinesia (from acute overdose or chronic use), or neuroleptic malignant syndrome (NMS) may occur.

PROCEDURES AND LABORATORY TESTS

Essential Tests

ECG and cardiac monitoring:

- ECG effects are similar to type 1a antidysrhythmics such as quinidine (QRS or QT prolongation, ventricular dysrhythmia).
- Sinus tachycardia is common and indicates sufficient drug absorption to produce anticholinergic effects.

Recommended Tests

- Arterial blood gases should be ordered in patients with QRS widening, dysrhythmia, seizures, or mental status depression and those receiving bicarbonate therapy (pH should not exceed 7.55).
- Serum aspartate aminotransferase, alanine aminotransferase, and bilirubin are used to assess development of hepatitis or cholestatic jaundice.
- Serum creatine kinase is measured in patients with seizures or coma to assess rhabdomyolysis.
- Urinalysis may reveal pink, red, purple, orange, or rust-colored urine following overdose.
- Serum acetaminophen and aspirin levels are used in an overdose setting to detect occult overdose.
- Head CT, lumbar puncture, and bacterial cultures are ordered as needed to evaluate other causes of coma or seizures.
- Phenothiazine tablets may be radiopaque on abdominal radiography; however, the absence of visible pills does not rule out ingestion.

Not Recommended Tests

- Quantitative serum levels are not generally available or helpful.
- Phenothiazines may cross-react with tricyclic antidepressants in EMIT assay.

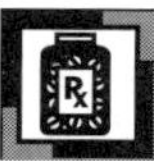

Treatment

- Treatment should focus on appropriate airway management and treatment of seizure, hypotension, and cardiac dysrhythmia.
- The dose and time of exposure must be determined for all substances involved.

DIRECTING PATIENT COURSE

The health-care provider should call the poison control center when:

- Coma, cardiovascular toxicity, or other severe effects are present.
- Toxic effects are not consistent with phenothiazine toxicity.
- Coingestant, drug interaction, or underlying disease presents an unusual challenge.

The patient should be referred to a health-care facility when:

- Attempted suicide or homicide is possible.
- Patient or caregiver seems unreliable.
- Toxic effects are apparent.
- Coingestant, drug interaction, or underlying disease presents an unusual challenge.

Admission Considerations

- Inpatient management in an intensive care setting is warranted for patients who develop seizure, CNS depression, or cardiac effects.
- Observation for 24 hours is probably warranted for patients who have ingested extended-release products.

DECONTAMINATION

Out of Hospital

Emesis should not be induced; coma or seizures may develop abruptly.

In Hospital

- Gastric lavage should be performed in pediatric (tube size 24–32 French) or adult (tube size 36–42 French) patients presenting within 1 hour of a large ingestion or if serious effects are present.
- Lavage may be reasonable even though it is performed 4 to 6 hours after ingestion, due to the medication-induced slowing of the gastrointestinal tract.
- One dose of activated charcoal (1–2 g/kg) is administered without a cathartic if a substantial ingestion has occurred within the previous few hours.

ADJUNCTIVE TREATMENT

Seizure

A benzodiazepine is administered for initial control.

- Diazepam. Adult dose is 5 to 10 mg initially, repeated every 10 minutes or longer if needed; pediatric dose is 0.2 to 0.5 mg/kg, repeated every 10 minutes or longer if needed; the airway should be monitored closely.
- Lorazepam. Adult dosage is 2 to 4 mg intravenous push over 2 to 5 minutes, repeated every 10 minutes or longer if needed. Pediatric dosage is 0.1 mg/kg intravenous push over 2 to 5 minutes, not to exceed 4 mg/dose and repeated every 10 minutes or longer if needed; the airway should be monitored closely.
- If seizures persist or recur, another anticonvulsant such as phenobarbital or phenytoin is added.

Hypotension

- The patient should receive 10 to 20 ml/kg 0.9% saline intravenously and be placed in the Trendelenburg position.
- Further fluid therapy should be guided by central pressure monitoring to avoid volume overload.
- If the hypotension is unresponsive, a vasopressor is administered.

—The dose of dopamine is 2 to 5 μg/kg/min intravenously, titrated to desired effect; rates above 20 μg/kg/min are unlikely to provide further benefit.
—If hypotension is unresponsive, norepinephrine is added, 0.1 to 0.2 μg/kg/min, and titrated to desired effect.
—A high rate of infusion may cause tissue ischemia.

Dysrhythmia or Conduction Abnormality

- Seizures must be controlled and acidemia corrected.
- If QRS widening is present, sodium bicarbonate (1–2 mEq/kg) is administered as an intravenous bolus and repeated as needed to narrow the QRS interval; arterial pH should not exceed 7.55.
- Lidocaine is used for ventricular tachycardia or multifocal premature ventricular complexes.

—Adult dosage is 50 to 100 mg as an intravenous bolus, followed by an infusion of 2 to 4 mg/min, titrated to desired effect.
—Pediatric dosage is 1 mg/kg bolus, followed by an infusion of 20 to 50 μg/kg/min, titrated to effect.
—The bolus dose may be repeated in 10 to 15 minutes.

- Cardiac pacing may be required for atrioventricular block.
- Overdrive pacing may be required for torsade de pointes.

Dystonic Reaction

- Diphenhydramine is administered, 1 mg/kg/dose intravenously over 1 to 2 minutes.
- Maintenance for 1 to 2 days of diphenhydramine or benztropine for continuing symptoms is suggested.

Not Recommended Therapies

Forced diuresis, hemodialysis, and hemoperfusion are not recommended.

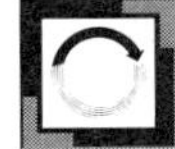

Follow-Up

PATIENT MONITORING

- Continuous respiratory and cardiac monitoring and serial ECGs should be performed.
- Fluid and electrolytes, liver and renal function, and clinical indicators of toxicity should be followed.

EXPECTED COURSE AND PROGNOSIS

- Most patients who overdose on phenothiazines recover within 24 to 48 hours.
- Death may result in severe cases involving dysrhythmia, seizures, hypotension, or hyperthermia.

DISCHARGE CRITERIA/INSTRUCTIONS

- From the emergency department. Patients may be discharged if they did not develop seizure or QRS widening, hypotension, or dysrhythmia (other than mild transient sinus tachycardia) during 6 hours of observation, and after they have received gastrointestinal decontamination and, if appropriate, a psychiatric evaluation.
- From the hospital. Patients may be discharged from the hospital after all clinical effects have resolved (hypotension, QRS widening, CNS depression, dysrhythmia) and after the ECG has been normal for 24 hours.

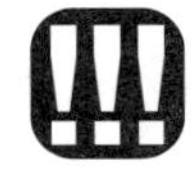

Pitfalls

DIAGNOSIS

Extended-release products may require admission and extended observation.

TREATMENT

Incomplete decontamination may result in prolonged symptoms or delayed deterioration.

FOLLOW-UP

Inadequate observation time may result in missing late complications of extrapyramidal symptoms or NMS.

ICD-9-CM 969.1

Poisoning by psychotropic agents: phenothiazine-based tranquilizers.

See also: SECTION II, Hypotension, Seizures, Neuroleptic Malignant Syndrome and Serotonin Syndrome, and Ventricular Dysrhythmia chapters.

RECOMMENDED READING

Ellenhorn MJ. Neuroleptic drugs. In: *Medical toxicology: diagnosis and treatment of human poisoning.* Baltimore: Williams & Wilkins, 1997:662–669.

Malhotra AK, Litman RE, Pickar D. Adverse effects of antipsychotic drugs. *Drug Safety* 1993;9:429–436.

Author: Steven A. Seifert

Reviewer: Richard C. Dart

Phenoxybenzamine

Basics

DESCRIPTION

Phenoxybenzamine (Dibenzyline) is an irreversible α-adrenergic receptor antagonist.

FORMS AND USES

Phenoxybenzamine is used to control episodes of hypotension and tachycardia caused by pheochromocytoma; it comes in 10-mg capsules.

TOXIC DOSE

- Toxic dose is not well established.
- Maximum dose is 40 mg, three times a day, although this is governed by the clinical signs.

PATHOPHYSIOLOGY

- Phenoxybenzamine relaxes vascular smooth muscle by antagonism of α-adrenergic receptors.
- Blood pressure decreases and reflex tachycardia typically follows smooth-muscle relaxation.
- Recovery from phenoxybenzamine exposure takes days because new α-adrenergic receptors must be generated.

EPIDEMIOLOGY

Poisoning is uncommon.

CAUSES

Child neglect or abuse should be considered if the patient is less than 1 year of age, suicide attempt if the patient is over 6 years of age.

DRUG AND DISEASE INTERACTIONS

Because phenoxybenzamine only antagonizes α-adrenergic receptors, drugs that stimulate both α and β receptors may result in an exaggerated β-agonist response.

PREGNANCY AND LACTATION

US FDA Pregnancy Category C. The drug exerts animal teratogenic or embryocidal effects, but there are no controlled studies in women, or no studies are available in animals or women.

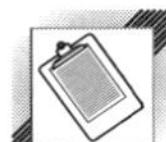

Diagnosis

DIFFERENTIAL DIAGNOSIS

Toxic causes of hypotension and tachycardia include:

- Tricyclic antidepressants
- Theophylline
- Opiates

Nontoxic causes of hypotension and tachycardia include:

- Sepsis
- Hypovolemia
- Acute myocardial infarction

SIGNS AND SYMPTOMS

Vital Signs

Orthostatic hypotension, tachycardia, miosis, and dizziness may occur.

HEENT

Flushing is common and miosis may occur.

Cardiovascular

Hypotension, dysrhythmia, cardiac ischemia, and seizures may occur following severe poisoning.

Gastrointestinal

Vomiting, diarrhea, and abdominal pain may occur.

CNS

Sedation, dizziness, and seizures may occur following severe poisoning.

PROCEDURES AND LABORATORY TESTS

Essential Tests

No tests may be needed for asymptomatic patients.

Recommended Tests

- ECG, complete blood count, electrolytes, BUN, creatinine, and pulse oximetry to assess cause of hypotension
- Serum acetaminophen and salicylate in symptomatic patients to detect occult ingestion

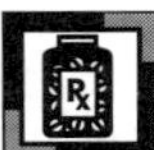

Treatment

- Treatment should focus on symptomatic and supportive care with continuous respiratory and cardiac monitoring.
- Patients with potential respiratory compromise should be intubated.

DIRECTING PATIENT COURSE

The health-care professional should call the poison control center when:

- Severe or persistent effects develop.
- Coingestant, drug interaction, or underlying disease presents an unusual problem.

The patient should be referred to a health-care facility when:

- Suicide or homicide attempt is possible.
- Toxic effects develop.
- Coingestant, drug interaction, or underlying disease presents an unusual problem.

Admission Considerations

Any symptomatic patient requires ICU admission.

DECONTAMINATION

Out of Hospital

Emesis is not recommended.

In Hospital

- Gastric lavage should be performed in pediatric (tube size 24–32 French) or adult (tube size 36–42 French) patients presenting within 1 hour of a large ingestion or if serious effects are present.
- One dose of activated charcoal (1–2 g/kg) should be administered without a cathartic if a substantial ingestion has occurred within the previous few hours.

ANTIDOTES

There is no specific antidote for phenoxybenzamine.

ADJUNCTIVE TREATMENT

Hypotension

- First-line treatment of hypotension is with intravenous isotonic crystalloid fluids.
- An α-adrenergic receptor agonist such as phenylephrine may be added, given as a 50-μg intravenous bolus, followed by intravenous infusion for severe hypotension: 20 mg in 250 ml D5W (80 μg/ml) at 40 to 180 μg/min (35–160 ml/h); 2 to 5 μg/kg/min in children.
- Pressors such as dopamine and epinephrine may be ineffective because of irreversible blockade of α-adrenergic receptors, and unopposed β_2-adrenergic activity following epinephrine use for phentolamine overdose could result in vasodilation and worsening of hypotension.
- Seizures should be treated with benzodiazepines; phenobarbital is recommended as a second-line agent.

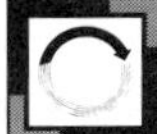

Follow-Up

PATIENT MONITORING

Respiratory and cardiac function should be monitored continuously.

EXPECTED COURSE AND PROGNOSIS

- Aggressive supportive care for a prolonged period of time (several days) may be necessary in major overdose.
- Poisoning with phenoxybenzamine can be life threatening even with supportive care.

DISCHARGE CRITERIA/INSTRUCTIONS

Patients may be discharged from the emergency department or hospital after decontamination, 6 hours of observation, and psychiatric evaluation, if needed.

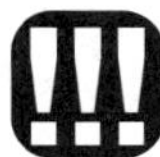

Pitfalls

TREATMENT

The α-receptor effects of epinephrine could be antagonized by phenoxybenzamine, resulting in unopposed β_2 receptor–mediated vasodilation and hypotension.

ICD-9-CM 975.1

Poisoning by agents primarily acting on the smooth and skeletal muscles and respiratory system: smooth muscle relaxants.

See also: SECTION II, Hypotension, Seizures chapters.

Author: Lada Kokan

Reviewer: Gerald F. O'Malley

Phentolamine

Basics

DESCRIPTION

Phentolamine mesylate (Regitine) is a parenteral α-adrenergic antagonist. It causes vasodilation by direct relaxation of smooth muscle.

FORMS AND USES

Catecholamine Extravasation

- Phentolamine is administered subcutaneously in doses of 5 to 10 mg diluted in 10 ml normal saline in adults; a maximum of 2 mg phentolamine in children is recommended.
- A 30-gauge needle is used to inject phentolamine locally to reverse pallor, numbness, and other symptoms of catecholamine-induced vasoconstriction.
- Care must be taken to avoid injection of excess fluid in volume-limited spaces such as fingers.

Treatment of Hypertension

- Phentolamine in 5 mg increments every 10 minutes intravenously, 0.1 to 0.2 mg/kg in children, has been used for treatment of hypertension secondary to pheochromocytoma.
- The amount used is titrated to the target blood pressure.
- Agents such as nitroprusside can be titrated much more easily and with tighter control of blood pressure, however, and are usually recommended as first-line agents following toxin-induced hypertension.

TOXIC DOSE

- A toxic dose has not been established and is dependent on the patient and clinical circumstance.
- When used subcutaneously, the dose should not exceed 10 mg.
- Intravenous infusions should not exceed 2 mg/min.

PATHOPHYSIOLOGY

- Phentolamine relaxes smooth muscle by competitive antagonism of α_1- and α_2-adrenergic receptor sites.
- It also induces the release of histamine from most cells.

EPIDEMIOLOGY

Poisoning is rare.

CAUSES

- Poisoning is most likely to be iatrogenic.
- Child abuse or neglect should be considered in patients less than 1 year of age; suicide attempt in patients over 6 years of age.

DRUG AND DISEASE INTERACTIONS

The hypotensive effect is additive to that of other hypotensive agents.

PREGNANCY AND LACTATION

US FDA Pregnancy Category C. The drug exerts animal teratogenic or embryocidal effects, but there are no controlled studies in women, or no studies are available in animals or women.

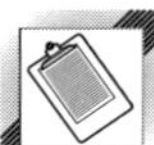

Diagnosis

DIFFERENTIAL DIAGNOSIS

Toxicologic causes of hypotension are numerous, including all cardiac drugs, all adrenergic blocking agents, and many others.

SIGNS AND SYMPTOMS

Vital Signs

Tachycardia and orthostatic hypotension are common.

HEENT

Mydriasis is a common finding.

Cardiovascular

Hypotension, dysrhythmia, and cardiac ischemia may occur with serious poisoning.

Neurologic

Dizziness, agitation, and seizures may occur.

PROCEDURES AND LABORATORY TESTS

Essential Tests

No tests may be needed in asymptomatic or minimally symptomatic patients.

Recommended Tests

- Electrolytes, glucose, BUN, and creatinine to assess effects of hypotension.
- Complete blood count to assess causes of hypotension.
- ECG to assess cardiac causes.
- Serum acetaminophen and aspirin to detect occult ingestion.

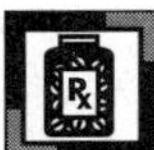

Treatment

- Treatment should focus on symptomatic and supportive care.
- Patients with a potential for respiratory compromise should be intubated.

DIRECTING PATIENT COURSE

- Patients who receive phentolamine are likely to be inpatients.
- All patients receiving phentolamine require ICU admission.

DECONTAMINATION

Patients who become symptomatic when receiving phentolamine should have the infusion stopped immediately.

ANTIDOTE

There are no antidotes specific to phentolamine.

ADJUNCTIVE TREATMENT

- First-line treatment of hypotension is with intravenous isotonic crystalloid fluids, followed by pressors if adequate response is not achieved.

—An α-adrenergic receptor agonist such as phenylephrine is preferred, given as a 50-μg intravenous bolus, followed by intravenous infusion for severe hypotension: 20 mg in 250 ml D5W (80 μg/ml) at 40 to 180 μg/min (35 to 160 ml/h); 2 to 5 μg/kg/min in children.
—Pressors such as dopamine and epinephrine may be ineffective because of blockade of α-adrenergic receptors, and unopposed β_2-adrenergic activity following epinephrine use for phentolamine overdose could result in vasodilation and worsening of hypotension.

- Symptomatic tachycardia can be treated with esmolol as a 500-μg/kg intravenous bolus, followed by an infusion of 50 to 200 μg/kg/min (5 g in 500 ml = 10 mg/ml).
- Seizures should be treated with benzodiazepines; phenobarbital is recommended as a second-line agent.

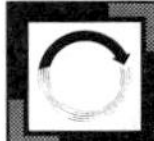

Follow-Up

PATIENT MONITORING

- All patients receiving phentolamine require ICU admission with continuous cardiac monitoring and pulse oximetry.
- Neurovascular status should be checked every hour to any area affected by catecholamine extravasation.

EXPECTED COURSE AND PROGNOSIS

- Dependent on underlying pathology
- Reversal of phentolamine-induced hypotension is rapidly accomplished by stopping the infusion and providing supportive care.
- Skin necrosis after catecholamine extravasation is generally preventable if phentolamine is injected within 12 hours.

DISCHARGE CRITERIA/INSTRUCTIONS

Patients that receive phentolamine are unlikely to be discharged until their other problems are addressed.

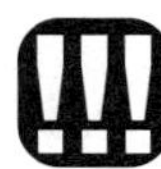

Pitfalls

TREATMENT

Infusion of α-adrenergic agonists in treatment of phentolamine toxicity should be performed in intensive care setting with close monitoring.

ICD-9-CM 975.1

Poisoning by agents primarily acting on the smooth and skeletal muscles and respiratory system: smooth muscle relaxants.

See also: SECTION II, Extravasation of Drugs, Hypotension, Seizure, and Tachycardia chapters; and SECTION IV, α_1-Adrenergic Antagonists.

RECOMMENDED READING

Siny BK, Sadove AM. Acute management of dopamine infiltration injury with regitine. *Plast Reconstr Surg* 1987;80:610–612.

Author: Lada Kokan

Reviewer: Gerald F. O'Malley

Phenylpropanolamine

Basics

DESCRIPTION

Phenylpropanolamine (PPA) is a common over-the-counter decongestant.

FORMS AND USES

PPA is used as a decongestant and appetite suppressant. Pharmaceutical preparations that contain PPA include:

- Numerous decongestants including St. Joseph Cold Tablets for Children, Allerest Maximum Strength 12-hour Caplets, Contac Maximum Strength 12-hour Caplets, Ornade Spansules, Contac 12-hour Capsules, Teldrin 12-hour Allergy Relief Capsules, Vicks DayQuil Allergy Relief 12-hour Tablets, Tavist-D Tablets, Vicks DayQuil Allergy Relief 4-hour Tablets, Demazin Syrup, Temazine Cold Syrup, Dimetapp Elixir, Triaminic Syrup, Dimetapp Cold & Allergy, Triaminic Oral Infant Drops, Naldelate Pediatric Syrup, Naldecon Pediatric Syrup, Nalgest Pediatric Syrup, Naldecon Pediatric Drops, Alka Seltzer Plus Cold Tablets, Coricidin Maximum Strength Sinus Headache Tablets, Congestant D Tablets, Drixoral Cough & Sore Throat Liquid Caps, Alka-Seltzer Plus Cold & Cough Tablets, Alka-Seltzer Plus Night Time Cold Tablets, Maximum Strength Comtrex Liqui-Gels (Capsules), Comtrex Max Strength Multi-Symptom Cold & Flu Relief Liqui-Gels, Triaminic-DM Syrup, and numerous generic forms.
- Appetite suppressants including Dexatrim, Control, and Acutrim.
- Therapeutic dosages for nasal decongestion: adult, 20 to 25 mg every 4 hours up to 150 mg/day; pediatric (6–12 years), 10 to 12.5 mg every 4 hours up to 75 mg/day
- Therapeutic dosages for appetite suppression: adult, 25 mg three times a day up to 75 mg/day; pediatric (2–6 years), 6.25 mg every 4 hours up to 37.5 mg/day

TOXIC DOSE

- Twice the maximum daily dose is tolerated well by children or adults.
- Death in adults has been reported at ingestions exceeding 500 mg.

PATHOPHYSIOLOGY

- PPA is a sympathomimetic agent that is an indirect α-receptor agonist, but may also have some direct stimulatory properties.
- The CNS, cardiovascular, and gastrointestinal systems are the target organs.

EPIDEMIOLOGY

- Poisoning is common.
- Toxic effects following exposure are typically mild to moderate.
- Death is associated with massive overdose or concurrent abuse of other drugs.

CAUSES

- Toxic ingestion is usually accidental, and by a child.
- Adolescents may purchase PPA to achieve an amphetamine-like "high."
- Child abuse or neglect must be considered if the patient is less than 1 year of age; suicide attempt if the patient is over 6 years of age.

DRUG AND DISEASE INTERACTIONS

- Persons with hypertension, atherosclerotic peripheral vascular disease, or diabetes mellitus should avoid this drug unless prescribed by their physician.
- Concurrent use with an monoamine oxidase (MAO) inhibitor may cause severe hypertension.
- Concurrent use of caffeine may enhance absorption or inhibit elimination, thereby increasing adverse effects.
- Concurrent use of bromocriptine may cause possible exacerbation of side effects.
- Indomethacin may enhance the vasoconstrictive effects of PPA.

PREGNANCY AND LACTATION

- US FDA Pregnancy Category C. The drug exerts animal teratogenic or embryocidal effects, but there are no controlled studies in women, or no studies are available in either animals or women.
- Women who are pregnant should use this drug with caution.

Diagnosis

DIFFERENTIAL DIAGNOSIS

- Toxic causes of tachycardia, hypertension, agitation, and seizures include other sympathomimetic agents (cocaine, amphetamines, MAO inhibitors, phenylephrine, fenfluramine, others), caffeine, theophylline, and others.
- Nontoxic causes include diseases with adrenergic excess: hyperthyroidism, manic behavior, alcohol or sedative-hypnotic withdrawal, and many others.

SIGNS AND SYMPTOMS

- Patients are typically anxious and nauseated, and have headache.
- Dry mouth, psychosis, and seizures are possible.
- Patient presentation with hypertension and reflex bradycardia is possible.

Vital Signs

Tachycardia and hypertension are common. Reflex bradycardia may occur instead of tachycardia.

HEENT

Blurred vision and mydriasis may occur.

Cardiovascular

- Tachycardia, bradycardia, and hypertension may occur.
- Myocardial ischemia is possible due to hypertensive crisis.

Pulmonary

Tachypnea and dry mouth may occur.

Gastrointestinal

Anorexia, vomiting, and nausea may occur.

Renal

Acute renal failure and rhabdomyolysis may occur in severe cases.

Musculoskeletal

Rhabdomyolysis can occur with seizures or severe agitation.

Neurologic

- Anxiety, restlessness, irritability, psychosis, seizures, and altered mental status may occur.
- Intracranial hemorrhage has occurred with hypertensive crisis.

PROCEDURES AND LABORATORY TESTS

Essential Tests

No tests may be needed in minimally symptomatic patients.

Recommended Tests

- ECG and cardiac enzymes in patients with possible myocardial ischemia
- Serum creatine kinase to assess muscle injury
- Serum electrolytes, BUN, and creatinine to assess acid-base balance and renal function
- Urinalysis to assess renal injury
- ECG, serum acetaminophen and aspirin levels in overdose setting to detect occult ingestion
- Head CT, lumbar puncture, bacterial cultures, other tests as needed to assess altered mental status or fever of unknown etiology

Not Recommended Tests

Serum levels of PPA are not clinically useful.

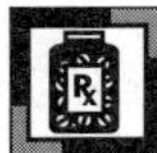

Treatment

- Treatment should focus on control of airway, agitation, seizures, and support of hemodynamic function.
- Dose and time of exposure should be determined for all substances involved.

DIRECTING PATIENT COURSE

The health-care provider should call the poison control center when:

- Seizure, dysrhythmia, or other severe effects are present.
- Toxic effects are not consistent with PPA.
- Coingestant, drug interaction, or underlying disease presents an unusual problem.

The patient should be referred to a health-care facility when:

- Attempted suicide or homicide is possible.
- Patient or caregiver seems unreliable.
- Toxic effects develop.
- Coingestant, drug interaction, or underlying disease presents an unusual problem.

Admission Considerations

Inpatient management is warranted if the patient exhibits severe or persistent cardiac or CNS toxicity.

DECONTAMINATION

Out of Hospital

Emesis should be induced with ipecac within 1 hour of ingestion in asymptomatic children who have ingested 6 to 10 mg/kg if health-care evaluation will be delayed.

In Hospital

- Gastric lavage should be performed in pediatric (tube size 24–32 French) or adult (tube size 36–42 French) patients presenting within 1 hour of a large ingestion or if serious effects are present.
- One dose of activated charcoal (1–2 g/kg) should be administered without a cathartic if a substantial ingestion has occurred within the previous few hours.

ANTIDOTES

There is no specific antidote for PPA poisoning.

ADJUNCTIVE TREATMENT

Agitation or Seizure

- Airway must be secured.
- A benzodiazepine familiar to the provider should be administered.

—Diazepam. Adult dose 5 to 10 mg intravenously; pediatric dose 0.2 to 0.5 mg/kg intravenously; doses repeated at 10-minute intervals, titrating to effect

—Lorazepam. Adult dose 2 to 4 mg intravenously; pediatric dose 0.05 to 0.1 mg/kg; doses repeated every 10 minutes, titrating to effect.

- Airway must be monitored closely.

Hypertension

If hypertension is not responsive to benzodiazepines, or end-organ damage develops (aortic dissection, CNS bleed, myocardial infarction), a short-acting titratable agent (e.g., nitroprusside) should be administered until desired response is seen.

Hypotension

- Hypotension should be treated with isotonic fluid infusion, Trendelenburg positioning, and vasopressor if needed; dopamine is preferred.
- Norepinephrine can be used for refractory hypotension.

Ventricular Dysrhythmia

- The standard Advanced Cardiac Life Support algorithms should be followed.
- Lidocaine (1 mg/kg intravenous bolus; repeat 0.5 mg/kg bolus if necessary and follow with 20 to 40 μg/kg/min infusion) may be used for ventricular tachycardia or frequent premature ventricular contractions.

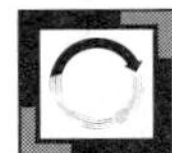

Follow-Up

PATIENT MONITORING

Cardiac and respiratory function should be monitored continuously until toxic effects resolve.

EXPECTED COURSE AND PROGNOSIS

Following acute ingestion, toxicity develops soon, peaks within hours, and patient recovers within 24 hours unless complications of hypertension, seizures, or intracranial bleeding develop.

DISCHARGE CRITERIA/INSTRUCTIONS

- From the emergency department

—Asymptomatic patients with normal blood pressure may be discharged following gastrointestinal decontamination, a 4- to 6-hour observation period, and psychiatric evaluation, if needed.
—A longer observation period should be considered for ingestions involving sustained-release products.

- From the hospital. Patients may be discharged following gastrointestinal decontamination, resolution of complications, and psychiatric evaluation, if needed.

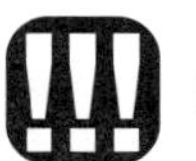

Pitfalls

DIAGNOSIS

- Combinations with other oral decongestants or antihistamines are common in overdoses.
- Due to the popularity of diet aids, there is great potential for abuse and these should be suspected.

ICD-9-CM 971.2

Poisoning by drugs primarily affecting the autonomic nervous system: sympathomimetics (adrenergics).

See also: SECTION II, Hypertension, Hypotension, Seizures, and Ventricular Dysrhythmias chapters; and SECTION III, Nitroprusside chapter.

RECOMMENDED READING

Dietz A. Amphetamine-like reactions to phenylpropanolamine. *JAMA* 1981;245:601–602.

Goldfrank LR, Lewin NA, Weisman RS. Dieting agents and regimens. In: Goldfrank LR, et al., eds. *Goldfrank's toxicologic emergencies,* 6th ed. Norwalk, CT: Appleton & Lange, 1998.

Author: Kathleen M. Wruk

Reviewer: Richard C. Dart

Phenytoin

Basics

DESCRIPTION

Phenytoin is a commonly used anticonvulsant medication.

FORMS AND USES

- Pharmaceutical preparations include phenytoin (Dilantin) and fosphenytoin (Cerebyx).
- These drugs have antiseizure and antidysrhythmic properties.
- They are also used for chronic pain and several other conditions.
- Typical dosages for adults and children are as follows:

—Phenytoin. 15 to 20 mg/kg loading, not to exceed 50 mg/min intravenous infusion rate; 3 to 5 mg/kg/day maintenance (dosage may vary).
—Fosphenytoin. 15 to 20 phenytoin equivalents intravenously or intramuscularly, not to exceed 150 mg/min intravenous (dosing based on phenytoin delivered).

TOXIC DOSE

- Acute ingestion above 20 mg/kg may cause ataxia; death is rare regardless of dose.
- Cardiac toxicity may develop if intravenous rate of administration exceeds 35 to 50 mg/min.

PATHOPHYSIOLOGY

- Phenytoin stabilizes neuronal membranes by decreasing resting membrane sodium flux and by decreasing sodium flow during action potentials; impaired cerebellar function is the initial manifestation, followed at higher levels by cortical function.
- The diluent for intravenous phenytoin contains propylene glycol.

—Rapid injection of propylene glycol may cause cardiac dysrhythmias and hypotension.
—Cardiac effects are extremely rare with oral administration.

- Fosphenytoin is a water-soluble prodrug of phenytoin. It is rapidly metabolized to phenytoin in the blood. It does not contain propylene glycol and causes fewer cardiovascular effects than phenytoin during intravenous administration.

EPIDEMIOLOGY

- Phenytoin toxicity is common.
- Toxic effects following exposure are typically mild.
- Death is rare and usually involves a coingestant.

CAUSES

- Toxicity usually involves unintentional drug accumulation during therapy.
- Child abuse must be considered if the patient is less than 1 year of age; suicide attempt if the patient is over 6 years of age.

RISK FACTORS

- Changes in dose and addition or cessation of medications that alter phenytoin metabolism can lead to toxicity.
- Dosing may require adjustment in the elderly because albumin levels may be decreased.

DRUG AND DISEASE INTERACTIONS

- Phenytoin levels are increased by dioumerol, disulfiram, cimetidine, isoniazid, and some sulfonamides.
- Phenytoin levels are decreased by concurrent use of carbamazepine.
- Interactions between phenobarbital and ethanol and phenytoin are variable.

PREGNANCY AND LACTATION

- US FDA Pregnancy Category D. Evidence of human fetal risk exists, but benefits in certain situations (e.g., life-threatening situations or serious diseases) may make use of the drug acceptable despite its risks.
- Phenytoin is generally contraindicated in pregnancy.

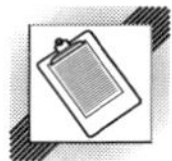

Diagnosis

DIFFERENTIAL DIAGNOSIS

- Toxic causes of nystagmus and ataxia are ethanol, phenobarbital, sedative-hypnotics, and many others.
- Nontoxic causes include cerebellar disease, middle ear disease, hypoglycemia, and electrolyte disorder.

SIGNS AND SYMPTOMS

- Ataxia and lethargy are the predominant manifestations after acute ingestion.
- Cardiovascular complications have been reported only with intravenous administration.

Vital Signs

Hypotension is common with rapid intravenous infusion.

Dermatologic

Adverse drug reactions can include erythema multiforme; rarely, Stevens-Johnson may develop, with therapeutic dosing.

Cardiovascular

Myocardial depression occurs with rapid intravenous infusion but has not been reported with oral ingestion.

Neurologic

- Cerebellar impairment results in ataxia, dysarthria, and nystagmus; this may occur with therapeutic blood levels.
- Cortical depression occurs at very high serum levels and may lead to coma.
- Toxic levels are reported to increase seizures, but data are inconclusive.

PROCEDURES AND LABORATORY TESTS

Essential Tests

- Phenytoin level

—This is typically measured on total serum level; therapeutic levels are 10 to 20 mg/L (1 to 2 mg/dl, 10 to 20 μg/ml).
—Free (not protein-bound) phenytoin levels may be obtained at reference laboratories.

- Levels of other antiseizure medications should be obtained.

Recommended Tests

- Serum albumin. In hypoalbuminemic patients the phenytoin level is corrected using the following formula: Corrected value = (concentration measured $\times$ 4.4) $\div$ (albumin level).
- Serum electrolytes, glucose, BUN, creatinine, calcium, and magnesium should be determined in patients with altered mental status.
- ECG, serum acetaminophen and aspirin levels should be screened in an overdose setting to detect occult ingestion.
- Head CT, lumbar puncture, and cultures should be performed in patents with altered mental status.

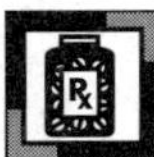

Treatment

- Treatment should focus on prevention of absorption, maintenance of airway, and prevention of falls due to ataxia.
- Dose and time of exposure should be determined for all substances involved.

DIRECTING PATIENT COURSE

The health-care professional should call the poison control center when:

- Coma or hypotension occur.
- Toxic effects are not consistent with phenytoin poisoning.
- Coingestant, drug interaction, or underlying disease presents an unusual problem.

The patient should be referred to a health-care facility when:

- Attempted suicide or homicide is possible.
- Patient or caregiver seems unreliable.
- Ataxia or other toxic effects develop.
- Toxic effects are not consistent with phenytoin poisoning.
- Coingestant, drug interaction, or underlying disease presents an unusual problem.

Admission Considerations

Inpatient management is warranted if the patient is unable to ambulate safely or perform activities of daily life.

DECONTAMINATION

Out of Hospital

Emesis should be induced with ipecac within 1 hour of ingestion for alert pediatric or adult patient if health-care evaluation will be delayed.

In Hospital

- Ipecac-induced emesis within 1 hour of ingestion is appropriate for the pediatric patient who is too small to have effective gastric lavage.
- Gastric lavage should be performed in pediatric (tube size 24–32 French) or adult (tube size 36–42 French) patients presenting within 1 hour of a large ingestion or if serious effects are present.
- One dose of activated charcoal (1–2 g/kg) should be administered without a cathartic if a substantial ingestion has occurred within the previous few hours.
- Multiple-dose charcoal decreases serum phenytoin levels more rapidly, but has not been shown to shorten clinical course.

ANTIDOTES

There is no specific antidote for phenytoin toxicity.

ADJUNCTIVE THERAPIES

- Ataxia. Bed rest with precautions for falling are needed until ataxia resolves.
- Apnea and ventricular dysrhythmias have occurred during rapid intravenous infusion.

—Immediate advanced cardiac life support (ACLS) usually produces rapid improvement.
—Infusion should be discontinued immediately; intubation may be needed.
—Normal saline should be infused for hypotension.
—Dysrhythmias should be treated according to ACLS protocols.

- Patients who become hypotensive or have dysrhythmias during intravenous infusion should have the infusion stopped immediately; endotracheal intubation and fluid resuscitation may be needed.

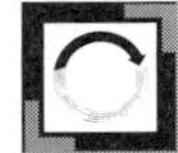

Follow-Up

PATIENT MONITORING

- Phenytoin levels should be monitored; level should be decreasing before patient is discharged.
- Continuous respiratory and cardiac monitoring should be performed in patients receiving phenytoin intravenously.

EXPECTED COURSE AND PROGNOSIS

Ataxia may last several days, but usually sufficient recovery often occurs within 24 hours.

DISCHARGE CRITERIA/INSTRUCTIONS

Patients who can ambulate safely and have decreasing serum levels can be discharged following psychiatric evaluation, if needed.

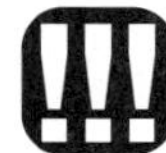

Pitfalls

DIAGNOSIS

- Patients with focal neurologic findings or CNS effects other than ataxia should be evaluated for CNS lesions.
- Hypoalbuminemic patients may be toxic at therapeutic levels of phenytoin due to reduced protein binding (e.g., high fraction of free drug).

TREATMENT

- Infusion rate greater than 50 mg/min may produce dysrhythmia or apnea.
- Failure to monitor intravenous infusion closely has resulted in death on rare occasions.

FOLLOW-UP

Patients who become toxic due to drug interactions should have the offending agent stopped.

ICD-9-CM 966.1

Poisoning by anticonvulsants and anti-Parkinsonism drugs: hydantoin derivatives.

RECOMMENDED READING

Parke-Davis. Product information: Fosphenytoin. 1996.

Wyte CD, Berk WA. Severe oral phenytoin overdose does not cause cardiovascular morbidity. *Ann Emerg Med* 1991;20:508–512.

Author: Kennon Heard

Reviewer: Richard C. Dart

Phosphine

Basics

DESCRIPTION

Phosphine is a toxic, colorless, flammable gas that has the odor of decaying fish.

FORMS AND USES

- Phosphine is used for pest control, including eradication of prairie dogs and mice, as well as for control of insects in stored grains.
- Substances include aluminum phosphide, calcium phosphide, phosphine (PH_3), Phostoxin, and zinc phosphide.

TOXIC DOSE

- Aluminum phosphide: ingestion of less than 500 mg has caused death in adults.
- Zinc phosphide: adult death has been reported with the ingestion of 4 g.

PATHOPHYSIOLOGY

- The exact mechanism of toxicity is not completely understood.
- Following ingestion of a phosphide-containing compound, phosphine gas is released during reaction with water and hydrochloric acid in the stomach.
- Phosphine is believed to be a metabolic poison that affects cytochrome C oxidase, blocking the electron transport chain and inhibiting cellular respiration. The result is inability to generate adenosine triphosphate.

EPIDEMIOLOGY

- Poisoning is not common in North America; however, countries such as India have reported epidemic suicidal ingestion of aluminum phosphide.
- Toxic effects range from mild to life threatening.
- In cases of intentional ingestion, the mortality rate is high.

CAUSES

- Toxic ingestion is usually intentional.
- Child abuse or neglect must be considered if the patient is less than 1 year of age; suicide attempt if the patient is over 6 years of age.
- Accidental exposures may occur due to grain fumigation or rodent control; due to rapid dissipation of the gas, significant exposure is unlikely except in enclosed areas.

WORKPLACE STANDARDS

- ACGIH. TLV TWA is 0.3 ppm; STEL is 1 ppm.
- OSHA. PEL TWA is 0.3 ppm.
- NIOSH. IDLH value is 50 ppm.

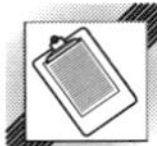

Diagnosis

DIFFERENTIAL DIAGNOSIS

- Toxic causes of acute airway irritation include inhalation of other irritants such as chlorine or other halogen gas, chloramine, ammonia, isocyanates, and others.
- Nontoxic causes include viral upper respiratory infection, cardiogenic pulmonary edema, pneumonia, or adult respiratory distress syndrome (ARDS) of various etiologies.

SIGNS AND SYMPTOMS

- Phosphine can affect nearly all organs.
- The primary target organs following ingestion are gastrointestinal and cardiovascular.
- After inhalation, the primary systems affected are pulmonary, cardiovascular, and CNS.

Vital Signs

- Tachycardia and hypotension may develop.
- In some cases, heart rate may be inappropriately low for the degree of hypotension.

HEENT

Diplopia has been reported.

Dermatologic

Sweating and cyanosis may occur.

Cardiovascular

- With ingestion or inhalation exposure, hypotension, cold extremities, and various dysrhythmias and myocardial conduction disturbances (atrial fibrillation, junctional tachycardia, ventricular tachycardia, heart block, bundle branch block, and sinus arrest) have been observed.
- Ischemic changes also may occur in severe cases.
- Cardiac abnormalities have persisted for 3 weeks in some survivors.

Pulmonary

With inhalation exposure, patients may exhibit shortness of breath, chest tightness, cough, and tachypnea progressing to bilateral rales, pulmonary edema, and ARDS.

Gastrointestinal

Following ingestion, epigastric discomfort, profuse vomiting, watery diarrhea, and gastrointestinal bleeding are common.

Hepatic

- Elevated liver enzymes [aspartate aminotransferase (AST), alanine aminotransferase (ALT)] and jaundice are common in serious cases.
- Tender hepatomegaly has been reported.

Renal

- Glycosuria and ketonuria may develop.
- Nonoliguric renal failure and acute tubular necrosis have been observed.

Fluids and Electrolytes

- Hyperkalemia, hypomagnesemia, and hypermagnesemia are common in serious cases.
- Hypermagnesemia may be more pronounced at 12 to 24 hours postingestion compared with 6 to 12 hours postingestion.

Musculoskeletal

Skeletal muscle damage has been reported.

Neurologic

Effects range from anxiety, agitation, headache, and fatigue to ataxia, seizures, and coma.

Endocrine

Acute pancreatitis and hyperglycemia have been reported with zinc phosphide ingestion.

PROCEDURES AND LABORATORY TESTS

Essential Tests

No tests may be needed in asymptomatic patients after brief inhalation exposure.

Recommended Tests

- Serum electrolytes, glucose, BUN, and creatinine assess metabolic acidosis and hyperkalemia.
- Serum magnesium monitors occurrence of hypermagnesemia or hypomagnesemia.
- Pulse oximetry or arterial blood gases assess oxygenation in symptomatic patients.
- ALT, AST, and total bilirubin detect liver injury.
- ECG and creatine kinase monitoring detects myocardial injury.
- Serum amylase assesses pancreatitis.
- Urinalysis detects glycosuria, proteinuria, ketonuria.
- Complete blood count is used to detect various possible abnormalities.
- ECG, serum acetaminophen, and aspirin levels in suicidal ingestions are measured to detect occult ingestion.
- Chest radiography assesses the presence of infiltrates in symptomatic patients.
- Echocardiogram is used to check for global hypokinesia of the left ventricle and interventricular septum with decreased ejection fraction.

Not Recommended Tests

Phosphine blood levels are not helpful.

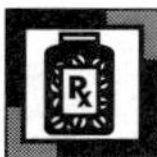

Treatment

- Treatment should focus on decontamination, airway management, and ensuring adequate oxygenation.
- Dose and time of exposure should be determined for all substances that could be involved.

DIRECTING PATIENT COURSE

The health-care provider should call the poison control center when:

- Shock, pulmonary symptoms, or other severe effects are present.
- Toxic effects are not consistent with phosphine toxicity.
- Coingestant, drug interaction, or underlying disease presents an unusual problem.

The patient should be referred to a health-care facility when:

- Attempted suicide or homicide is possible.
- Patient or caregiver seems unreliable.
- Toxic effects develop.
- Coingestant, drug interaction, or underlying disease presents an unusual problem.

Admission Considerations

Inpatient management is warranted for patients who:

- Exhibit ECG abnormalities, hypotension, or persistent pulmonary tract irritation or pulmonary dysfunction.
- Have more than a trivial inhalation exposure due to the delayed onset of pulmonary injury.

DECONTAMINATION

Out of Hospital

- Inhalation. Patient should be moved to fresh air; patent airway must be maintained.
- Ingestion. Emesis should not be induced.
- Eye exposure. Eyes should be irrigated for 15 to 20 minutes with room-temperature water.
- Skin exposure. Skin should be irrigated copiously with water.

In Hospital

- Inhalation. Airway, breathing, and circulation should be established as needed.
- Eye or skin exposure. Eyes and skin should be irrigated as needed.
- Ingestion

—Neither emesis nor lavage is recommended due to potential for increasing release of phosphine gas.
—One dose of activated charcoal (1–2 g/kg) should be administered without a cathartic if a substantial ingestion has occurred within the previous few hours.

ANTIDOTES

There is no specific antidote for phosphine poisoning.

ADJUNCTIVE TREATMENT

- Antacids and H_2-receptor blocking agents may be helpful for gastric irritation in cases of ingestion.
- In severe poisonings, adrenal function may be compromised; intravenous dosing of corticosteroid (e.g., hydrocortisone) should be considered, especially if hypotension is not responsive to dopamine infusion.

Hypotension

- Atropine can be used to correct hypotension related to bradycardia.
- The patient should be placed in the Trendelenburg position and 10 to 20 ml/kg 0.9% saline should be administered.
- Further fluid therapy can be guided by central pressure monitoring to avoid volume overload.
- Vasopressor such as dopamine may be added if needed.

Seizures

- Patent airway must be maintained.
- Benzodiazepine should be administered for initial control.
- If seizures persist or recur, another anticonvulsant such as phenobarbital can be added.

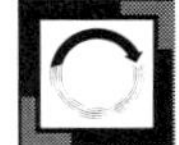

Follow-Up

PATIENT MONITORING

- Cardiac and respiratory function should be monitored continuously in symptomatic patients.
- Fluids, electrolytes, and acid-base status should also be followed closely.

EXPECTED COURSE AND PROGNOSIS

- Prognosis is favorable for the patient who survives the initial 24-hour period following ingestion.
- Fulminant toxicity may cause death within 12 to 24 hours.

DISCHARGE CRITERIA/INSTRUCTIONS

- From the emergency department. Asymptomatic patients with normal pulmonary function can be discharged following a 6-hour observation period and psychiatric evaluation, if needed.
- From the hospital. Patients can be discharged when pulmonary, cardiac, gastrointestinal, and renal effects resolve or stabilize.

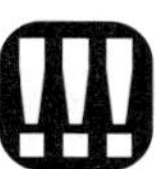

Pitfalls

DIAGNOSIS

Onset of pulmonary edema following inhalation exposure may be delayed up to 72 hours.

TREATMENT

- The addition of water to phosphide in the stomach during lavage may induce the release of more phosphine and is generally avoided.
- Shock and its sequelae are common following ingestion; renal failure may occur.

ICD-9-CM 987.9

Toxic effect of other gases, fumes, or vapors: unspecified gas, fume, or vapor.

See also: SECTION II, Hypotension and Seizures chapters.

RECOMMENDED READING

Gupta S, Ahlawat SK. Aluminum phosphide poisoning—a review. *Clin Toxicol* 1995;33:19–24.

Sarma PSA, Narula J. Acute pancreatitis due to zinc phosphide ingestion. *Postgrad Med J* 1996;846:237–238.

Singh S, Singh D, Wig N, Jit I, Sharma B. Aluminum phosphide ingestion—a clinico-pathologic study. *Clin Toxicol* 1996;34:703–706.

Author: Martha M. Foley

Reviewer: Richard C. Dart

Phosphorus

Basics

DESCRIPTION

Phosphorus is a nonmetallic element that is highly flammable.

FORMS AND USES

- "Red" phosphorus is used in safety matches and is nontoxic in single oral doses (see SECTION I, Nontoxic Ingestion chapter), although, rarely, repeated doses may result in systemic poisoning.
- "Black" phosphorus is the inert nontoxic form of elemental phosphorus.
- "Yellow" or "white" phosphorus is a translucent solid with a garliclike odor that is practically insoluble in water but soluble in most oils; spontaneous combustion occurs on exposure to air. It is highly toxic.

TOXIC DOSE

- An acute dose of about 1 mg/kg of yellow or white phosphorus may be fatal for an adult.
- A total dose of 3 mg was reported to be fatal for a 2-year-old.

EPIDEMIOLOGY

Poisoning is uncommon.

CAUSES

Child neglect or abuse should be considered if the patient is less than 1 year of age, suicide attempt if the patient is over 6 years of age.

PATHOPHYSIOLOGY

Phosphorus ions are taken into the kidneys and later into the liver and other organs, resulting in acute systemic phosphorus poisoning.

WORKPLACE STANDARDS

- OSHA. PEL TWA for yellow phosphorus is 0.1 mg/m^3. PEL TWA for phosphorus pentachloride is 1 mg/m^3.
- ACGIH. TLV TWA for yellow phosphorus is 0.02 ppm. TLV TWA for phosphorus pentachloride is 0.10 ppm.

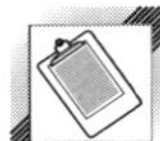

Diagnosis

SIGNS AND SYMPTOMS

Skin Exposure

Skin exposure may cause severely painful necrotic partial- and full-thickness yellowish burns from chemical and thermal effects.

Inhalation of Phosphorus Fumes

Vital Signs

Chronic inhalation may result in cachexia.

HEENT

Inhalation may have marked irritant effects on the eyes.

Pulmonary

Inhalation may cause upper airway irritation, dyspnea, and delayed noncardiogenic pulmonary edema; bronchitis may be seen in cases of chronic inhalation.

Gastrointestinal

Inhalation may cause nausea and vomiting.

Hepatic

Inhalation may cause acute hepatic damage and systemic phosphorus poisoning.

Hematologic

Chronic inhalation may produce anemia.

Musculoskeletal

Mandibular necrosis, such as "phossy" or "Lucifer's" jaw, may be seen with chronic inhalation.

Phosporus Ingestion

Toxicity is enhanced when it is dissolved in solvents (e.g., alcohol, oils). Phosphorus poisoning is classically divided into an initial gastrointestinal stage, followed by a relatively asymptomatic period, and terminating in acute liver failure with metabolic derangements.

Cardiovascular

Phosphorus ingestion may produce hypotension, tachycardia, and ECG with ST- and T-wave changes, QTc prolongation, low voltage QRS, and dysrhythmia.

Pulmonary

Ingestion may cause dyspnea, tachypnea, and pulmonary edema.

Gastrointestinal

Ingestion results in acute onset of nausea, vomiting, abdominal pain, diarrhea, and hematemesis.

Renal

Renal failure may develop within 24 hours.

Hepatic

Ingestion may, after delay of a day or more, produce liver injury and fulminant hepatic failure.

Hematologic

Ingestion may result in clotting abnormalities in severe cases.

Endocrine

- Early hypoglycemia has a grave prognosis.
- Normal or hypocalcemia, and hyper- or hypophosphatemia may occur.

Neurologic

Restlessness, irritability, lethargy, weakness, delirium, stupor, coma, or seizures may develop.

PROCEDURES AND LABORATORY TESTS

Essential Tests

- Serum electrolytes, BUN, creatinine, calcium, phosphorus, and urinalysis should be ordered to assess renal injury and electrolyte abnormalities.
- Serum liver function tests should be performed to assess liver injury.

Recommended Tests

- Complete blood count, international normalized ratio, and prothrombin time should be obtained to assess blood loss and coagulopathy.
- Arterial blood gas should be studied if respiratory symptoms are present.
- A chest radiograph should be obtained to assess pulmonary injury.

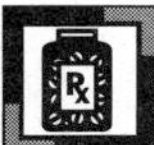

Treatment

- Supportive care with appropriate airway management is vital.
- The dose and time of exposure for all substances involved should be determined.

DIRECTING PATIENT COURSE

The health-care professional should call the poison control center when:

- Severe or persistent effects develop.
- Coingestant, drug interaction, or underlying disease presents an unusual problem.

The patient should be referred to a health-care facility when:

- Suicide or homicide attempt is possible.
- Toxic effects develop.
- Coingestant, drug interaction, or underlying disease presents an unusual problem.

Admission Considerations

Symptomatic patients should be admitted.

DECONTAMINATION

During decontamination, the patient and health-care provider should be protected from vomitus, gastric washings, and feces.

Skin or Eye Exposure

- The patient should be admitted to a burn unit.
- Exposed areas should be covered with wet dressings at all times.
- Exposed areas should be washed several times with a solution of 5% sodium bicarbonate–3% copper sulfate–1% hydroxy-ethyl-cellulose or 1% sodium lauryl sulphate, and rinsed thoroughly with saline between washings.
- Meticulous surgical debridement may be necessary.
- Exposed eyes should be continuously flushed with copious amounts of water; formal ophthalmologic examination should be performed.

Inhalation

- The patient should be moved to fresh air, and 100% oxygen with assisted ventilation should be administered as required.
- Careful observation for development of systemic effects or delayed pulmonary edema.

Ingestion

- The use of gastric lavage is controversial because of the corrosive effects of phosphorus poisoning.
- Gastric lavage with potassium permanganate (1:5,000 solution) is recommended to convert phosphorus to harmless oxidation products; however, there are no controlled clinical data regarding its efficacy.

ANTIDOTES

There is no specific antidote for phosphorus poisoning.

ADJUNCTIVE TREATMENT

Burns

Burned area should be thoroughly cleaned and debrided, followed by typical burn supportive care.

Hypotension

- The patient should receive normal saline 10 to 20 ml/kg and be placed in the Trendelenburg position.
- Further fluid therapy should be guided by central pressure monitoring.
- A vasopressor may be added.

—The dose of dopamine is 2 to 5 μg/kg/min titrated upward to effect; rates greater than 20 μg/kg/min are unlikely to provide further benefit.
—The dose of norepinephrine is 0.1 to 0.2 μg/kg/min, titrated upward to effect.
—High rates of infusion may cause tissue ischemia.

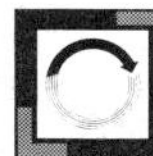

Follow-Up

PATIENT MONITORING

- Continuous respiratory and cardiac monitoring should be performed in symptomatic patients.
- In cases of inhalation, careful observation for development of systemic effects or delayed pulmonary edema is needed.

EXPECTED COURSE AND PROGNOSIS

Phosphorus poisoning is classically divided into an initial gastrointestinal stage, followed by a relatively asymptomatic period, and terminating in acute liver failure with metabolic derangements. The fatality rate after ingestion is approximately 50%.

DISCHARGE CRITERIA/INSTRUCTIONS

Patients may be discharged from the emergency department or hospital when toxic effects resolve or stabilize and after psychiatric evaluation, if needed.

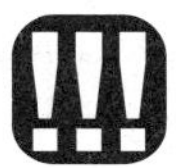

Pitfalls

DIAGNOSIS

Pulmonary injury may be delayed after inhalation.

ICD-9-CM 989

Toxic effect of other substances, chiefly nonmedicinal as to source.

See also: SECTION I, Nontoxic Ingestion chapter.

RECOMMENDED READING

Ben-Hur N. Phosphorus burns. *Prog Surg* 1978;16:180–181.

Blumenthal S. Lesser A. Acute phosphorus poisoning. *Am J Dis Child* 1938;55:1280–1287.

McCarnon MM, Gaddis GP. Acute yellow phosphorus poisoning from pesticide paste. *Clin Toxicol* 1981;18:693–711.

Author: Luke Yip

Reviewer: Richard C. Dart

Basics

DESCRIPTION

This chapter covers plants that have anticholinergic properties when ingested in sufficient amounts; for certain species, this amount can be quite small.

FORMS AND USES

- *Datura species* (jimsonweed, devil's apple, thorn apple, stinkweed, loco seeds, locoweed, Jamestown weed) contain hyoscyamine, scopolamine, and atropine.
- *Atropa belladonna* (belladonna, deadly nightshade) contains hyoscyamine, hyoscine, and atropine.
- *Hyoscyamus niger* (henbane, black henbane) contains hyoscyamine, hyoscine, and atropine.
- *Brugmansia* species (angel's trumpet) have anticholinergic properties similar to those of *Datura* species.
- *Lycium halimifolium* (matrimony vine) contains atropine, scopolamine, and hyoscyamine.
- *Cestrum nocturnum* and *C. diurnum* (night-blooming jessamine and day-blooming jessamine) contain solanine and various anticholinergic alkaloids.
- *Mandragora officinarum* contains hyoscyamine, scopolamine, and mandragorine.
- Several other plant species also cause anticholinergic effects.

TOXIC DOSE

Toxicity is difficult to estimate because concentration of toxin varies by species, with additional variation within each species. A few seeds or leaves of jimsonweed are usually sufficient to cause anticholinergic effects.

PATHOPHYSIOLOGY

- Plant parts contain tropane alkaloids (hyoscyamine, hyoscine, scopolamine, mandragorine, and atropine).
- These are anticholinergic compounds that competitively block muscarinic acetylcholine receptors.

EPIDEMIOLOGY

- Poisoning is common.
- Mild to moderate toxicity is common following accidental pediatric ingestion.
- Abuse commonly occurs by ingestion of plant material, ingestion of tea brewed from the plant, or inhalation of smoked plant material; toxicity also may follow ingestion of herbal preparations containing the plants.
- Death is rare and usually due to trauma sustained during delirium.

CAUSES

- Pediatric exposures are usually accidental.
- Exposures in teenagers and adults usually involve abuse or ingestion of herbal preparations.

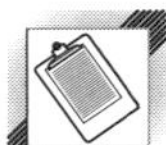

Diagnosis

DIFFERENTIAL DIAGNOSIS

- Toxic causes of anticholinergic effects include atropine, some mushrooms, and antihistamines. Due to pupillary dilation and tachycardia, sympathomimetic plants (e.g., ephedra) also may be confused with anticholinergic toxicity.
- Other drugs or conditions that produce hallucinations and delirium may be confused initially with anticholinergic syndrome (e.g., LSD, mescaline, peyote, phencyclidine).

SIGNS AND SYMPTOMS

- Anticholinergic compounds usually produce prompt onset of anticholinergic signs combined with delirium and hallucinations.
- Liquid preparations such as teas or herbal extracts often produce more acute onset and severe effects.
- Ingestion of plant parts may allow delay before toxicity develops.

VITAL SIGNS

Hyperthermia, tachycardia, and hypertension are common.

HEENT

- Dry mucous membranes, pupil dilation, and blurred vision are common.
- Isolated pupil dilation may occur following accidental contact secondary to rubbing eyes after handling an anticholinergic plant.

Dermatologic

Skin is commonly warm, dry, and flushed.

Cardiovascular

Tachycardia and hypertension are common.

Pulmonary

Smoke from burning of anticholinergic plants can cause respiratory irritation as well as systemic anticholinergic toxicity.

Gastrointestinal

Anticholinergic toxicity typically produces decreased gastrointestinal motility and bowel sounds; however, plants also may contain toxins that cause vomiting and diarrhea.

Renal

Acute renal injury may occur with rhabdomyolysis.

Fluids and Electrolytes

Dehydration is common secondary to increased insensible losses and decreased oral fluid intake caused by delirium.

Musculoskeletal

Agitation can produce rhabdomyolysis.

Neurologic

- Agitation, altered mental status, delirium, and hallucinations are common.
- Seizures occur infrequently.

PROCEDURES AND LABORATORY TESTS

Essential Tests

There are no essential tests for minimally symptomatic patients.

Recommended Tests

- Serum electrolytes, BUN, and creatinine are used to assess dehydration or kidney injury from rhabdomyolysis.
- Serum creatine kinase becomes elevated if rhabdomyolysis occurs.
- ECG should be monitored for patients with marked tachycardia; sinus tachycardia is common.
- Urinalysis should be performed to detect dehydration and myoglobin (positive dipstick for blood, but no red blood cells on microscopic analysis).

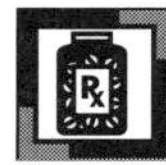

Treatment

- Treatment should focus on control of agitation and protecting the patient from self-harm.
- Dose and time of exposure should be determined for all substances involved.
- Physostigmine may be helpful in ruling out other causes of altered mental status.

DIRECTING PATIENT COURSE

The health-care provider should call the poison control center when:

- Seizure or other severe effects develop.
- Use of physostigmine is considered.
- Toxic effects are not consistent with anticholinergic toxicity.
- Coingestant, drug interaction, or underlying disease presents an unusual problem.

The patient should be referred to a health-care facility when:

- Attempted suicide or homicide is possible.
- Patient or caregiver seems unreliable.
- Undesired effects develop (hallucinations, blurred vision, seizure).
- Coingestant, drug interaction, or underlying disease presents an unusual problem.

Admission Considerations

Inpatient management is warranted if patient is in need of observation for agitation, delirium, or dysrhythmia, or if sedation is needed.

DECONTAMINATION

Out of Hospital

Emesis should be induced with ipecac within 1 hour of ingestion for alert pediatric or adult patients, especially if plant parts are involved.

In Hospital

- Emesis should be induced with ipecac within 1 hour of ingestion for alert patients who have ingested plant parts.
- Gastric lavage should be performed in pediatric (tube size 24–32 French) or adult (tube size 36–42 French) patients presenting within 1 hour of a large ingestion or if serious effects are present; lavage may be reasonable even several hours after ingestion due to gastrointestinal slowing.
- One dose of activated charcoal (1–2 g/kg) should be administered without a cathartic if a substantial ingestion has occurred; one repeat dose of activated charcoal may be helpful 4 to 6 hours following the first dose if a patient continues to exhibit signs of anticholinergic toxicity.
- Skin and mucous membranes should be washed copiously with water following mucous membrane or dermal exposure.

ANTIDOTES

Physostigmine is a specific antagonist to anticholinergic effects; however, it is used only to diagnose anticholinergic toxicity.

Indications

- Physostigmine is a diagnostic agent to distinguish altered mental status due to anticholinergic toxicity from other causes of agitation and hallucination.
- A positive response to a physostigmine test (clearing of delusion or hallucination) indicates an anticholinergic effect. Head CT and lumbar puncture may become unnecessary because the cause of altered mental status is known.

Contraindications

- A known allergy to a cholinergic agonist or to sulfites precludes the use of physostigmine.
- A tricyclic antidepressant overdose, or ECG findings suggestive of such an overdose (QRS widening, R-wave in ECG lead aVR), contraindicates use of physostigmine.
- Patients with a history of asthma, heart disease, diabetes, seizure disorder, or inflammation of the iris or ciliary body should not receive physostigmine.

Method of Administration

- Clinician should place the patient on a cardiac monitor and have atropine available at the bedside.
- Physostigmine should be given by slow intravenous push over 5 minutes.

—Adult dose is 0.5 to 2.0 mg.
—Pediatric dose is 0.02 mg/kg, up to 2.0 mg.
—Dose may be repeated once after 10 minutes if needed.

- Physostigmine effect typically wanes after 30 minutes.

Potential Adverse Effects

- Adverse effects are more common with larger doses and faster rates of administration.
- Muscarinic effects include vomiting, diarrhea, sweating, bronchorrhea, bradycardia, and hypotension; cardiac dysrhythmia may occur.
- Nicotinic effects (weakness, fasciculation) also may occur.
- Seizures occur rarely.

ADJUNCTIVE TREATMENT

Agitation or Hallucinosis

A benzodiazepine with which the provider has experience should be administered. Airway must be monitored closely.

Diazepam

- Adult dose is 5 to 10 mg intravenously.
- Pediatric dose is 0.2 to 0.5 mg/kg intravenously.
- Dose may be repeated at 10-minute intervals and titrated to effect.

Lorazepam

- Adult dose is 1 to 2 mg intravenously.
- Pediatric dose is 0.05 mg/kg intravenously.
- Dose may be repeated at 10-minute intervals and titrated to effect.

Seizure

- A patent airway must be assured.
- A benzodiazepine should be administered for initial control (see SECTION II, Seizures chapter, for further details).
- If seizures persist or recur, another anticonvulsant such as phenobarbital can be added.

Dysrhythmias or Conduction Abnormalities

Standard advanced cardiac life support guidelines should be followed.

Not Recommended Therapies

Physostigmine should not be used once the diagnosis is apparent.

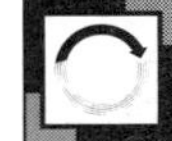

Follow-Up

PATIENT MONITORING

Vital signs, mental status, and volume status should be monitored until effects resolve.

EXPECTED COURSE AND PROGNOSIS

- Anticholinergic effects often persist for 24 to 48 hours and can last even longer following large exposure and if there is persistent gastrointestinal absorption.
- Hyperthermia and rhabdomyolysis can result from agitation that is improperly controlled (i.e., by the use of physical restraints alone).

DISCHARGE CRITERIA/INSTRUCTIONS

- From the emergency department. Asymptomatic patients may be discharged following decontamination and 4 to 6 hours of observation after the last dose of benzodiazepine; psychiatric evaluation should be obtained if needed.
- From the hospital. Patients may be discharged after resolution of toxic effects and psychiatric evaluation, if needed.

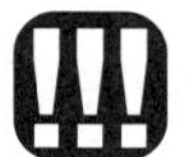

Pitfalls

DIAGNOSIS

- Minor partial improvement in mental status should not be attributed to physostigmine.

—The beneficial effect of physostigmine is usually obvious.
—Minor improvement may indicate that the patient has a component of anticholinergic toxicity, but life-threatening causes must be ruled out.

- Time should not be wasted attempting to identify the plant; instead, the patient should be treated symptomatically.

TREATMENT

- Physostigmine should not be used when the ECG suggests type 1a antidysrhythmic toxicity (widening of QRS or QTc, or R wave in lead aVR).
- It is important to maintain urinary output at 1 to 2 cc/kg/h; patients are usually dehydrated and may have rhabdomyolysis.

ICD-9-CM 971.1

Poisoning by drugs primarily affecting the autonomic nervous system: parasympatholytics (anticholinergics and antimuscarinics) and spasmolytics.

See also: SECTION II, Seizures; and SECTION III, Physostigmine chapter.

RECOMMENDED READING

Centers for Disease Control. Jimson weed poisoning: Texas, New York, and California, 1994. *MMWR* 1995;44:41–44.

Chan TYK. Anticholinergic poisoning due to Chinese herbal medicines. *Vet Hum Toxicol* 1995;37:156–157.

Author: Edwin K. Kuffner

Reviewer: Richard C. Dart

Plants—Cardiac Glycosides

Basics

DESCRIPTION

Cardiac glycoside is a term used to describe a group of naturally occurring plants that produce toxicity similar to digoxin.

FORMS AND USES

Plants that contain cardiac glycosides include:

- Common oleander (*Nerium oleander*).
- Yellow oleander (*Thevetia peruviana*).
- Lily-of-the-valley (*Convallaria majalis*).
- Types of foxglove (*Digitalis purpurea, Digitalis lantana*).
- Henbane (*Helleborus niger*).
- Sea onion (*Urginea maritima*) and squill (*Urginea indica*).
- Milkweed family, African arrow poisons, wintersweet, bushman's poison, frangipani, sea-mango, balloon cotton, redheaded cottonbush, king's crown, and rubber vine.
- Historically, plant glycosides were used as heart remedies.

TOXIC DOSE

- Toxicity varies widely depending on plant and preparation.
- An extract (e.g., tea made from plant) is generally the most toxic preparation.

PATHOPHYSIOLOGY

- The therapeutic mechanism is inhibition of the myocardial Na^+/K^+ exchange pump, increasing intracellular Na^+, decreasing Ca^{2+} excretion, and causing a net increase in intracellular Ca^{2+}, which augments myocardial contractility.
- Cardiac glycosides also increases vagal tone by decreasing baroreceptor sensitivity; the increased vagal tone results in decreased conduction velocity of the electrical impulse through the myocardium and atrioventricular (AV) node and increased AV node refractoriness.

EPIDEMIOLOGY

- Poisoning is rare.
- Toxic effects are typically mild.
- Death occurs following suicidal ingestion or consumption of brewed teas.

CAUSES

- Cardiac glycoside poisoning is usually an unintentional ingestion.
- Child neglect or abuse should be considered if the patient is less than 1 year of age; suicide if the patient is over 6 years of age.

DRUG AND DISEASE INTERACTIONS

- Any drug that inhibits myocardial conduction (β-receptor blocker, calcium channel blocker) may enhance cardiac glycoside toxicity.
- Underlying cardiac disease may predispose to dysrhythmia.
- Renal failure decreases digitalis elimination.
- Hypokalemia, hypercalcemia, hypomagnesemia, increased sympathetic nervous system activity, and hypothyroidism may exacerbate digitalis toxicity by different mechanisms.
- Nifedipine, spironolactone, triamterene, and amiloride decrease renal clearance of digoxin.
- Quinidine, quinine, verapamil, and amiodarone may increase digitalis levels.
- Warfarin can increase digoxin levels by displacement from protein binding sites.

PREGNANCY AND LACTATION

Digoxin. US FDA Pregnancy Category C. The drug exerts animal teratogenic or embryocidal effects, but there are no controlled studies in women, or no studies are available in either animals or women.

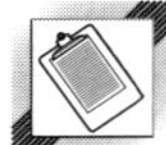

Diagnosis

DIFFERENTIAL DIAGNOSIS

- Other toxic agents that cause depression of cardiac conduction include β-receptor or calcium channel blockers and type 1 antidysrhythmics, among others.
- Nontoxic causes of cardiovascular depressant effects include myocardial ischemia and electrolyte abnormalities.

SIGNS AND SYMPTOMS

- Early signs of plant cardiac glycoside toxicity may be nonspecific, such as malaise, nausea and vomiting.
- As toxicity increases, cardiac conduction abnormalities emerge.

Vital Signs

Bradycardia, tachycardia, or hypotension may occur.

HEENT

Visual complaints, blurred vision, amblyopia, and colored halos may be present.

Cardiovascular

- Severe bradycardia, AV blocks, conduction delays, supraventricular and ventricular dysrhythmias, and congestive heart failure may occur.
- Cardiac arrest may develop suddenly.

Gastrointestinal

Nausea, vomiting, and abdominal pain may develop within a few hours and precede cardiac effects.

Fluids and Electrolytes

- Hyperkalemia is common with acute overdose.
- Hypokalemia is associated with chronic toxicity and use of diuretics.

Neurologic

Headache, lightheadedness, weakness, drowsiness, hallucinations, and confusion may develop in severe cases.

PROCEDURES AND LABORATORY TESTS

Essential Tests

- Serum digitalis level

—Some plant cardiac glycosides will cross-react with the standard digoxin assay, especially foxglove and oleander.
—The absolute level is not meaningful, but a positive result helps to confirm the diagnosis.
—The absence of detectable digoxin level does not rule out plant cardiac glycoside toxicity.

- ECG and continuous cardiac monitoring

—Prolonged PR interval and shortened QTc interval are common with cardiac glycoside toxicity.
—Atrial or junctional tachydysrhythmias, sinus bradycardia, and AV block are characteristic.
—Bidirectional ventricular tachycardia, atrial flutter with 2:1 block, and regularized atrial fibrillation are highly suggestive of cardiac glycoside toxicity.
—Peaked T waves, PR prolongation, and QRS prolongation may suggest hyperkalemia.

- Serum electrolytes, glucose, calcium, magnesium, BUN, and creatinine

—Hyperkalemia is an indication for digoxin-specific antibodies.
—Hypokalemia, hypercalcemia, or hypomagnesemia may predispose patients to dysrhythmias.
—Renal insufficiency impairs cardiac glycoside clearance.

Recommended Tests

- Liver function tests. Decreased hepatic function increases digitoxin levels.
- Serum acetaminophen and aspirin levels should be obtained in overdose setting to detect occult ingestion.
- Disorders that may alter laboratory results. Serum digoxin levels after administration of digoxin antibodies may be elevated because both free cardiac glycoside and bound glycoside may be measured by most laboratories.

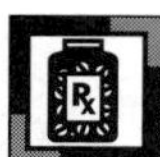

Treatment

• Therapy should focus on appropriate airway management and rapid assessment of need for digoxin immune Fab.
• Dose and time of exposure should be determined for all substances involved.

DIRECTING PATIENT COURSE

The health-care provider should call the poison control center when:

• Severe or persistent effects develop.
• Signs and symptoms are not consistent with cardiac glycoside poisoning.
• Coingestant, drug interaction, or underlying disease presents an unusual problem.

The patient should be referred to a health-care facility when:

• Toxic effects develop.
• Attempted suicide or homicide is possible.
• The patient or caregiver seems unreliable.
• Coingestant, drug interaction, or underlying disease presents an unusual problem.

Admission Considerations

Inpatient management in the intensive care unit is warranted for symptomatic patients and patients with ECG abnormalities.

DECONTAMINATION

Out of Hospital

Emesis should be induced with ipecac within 1 hour of ingestion for alert patients if health-care evaluation will be delayed.

In Hospital

• Ipecac-induced emesis should be considered because plant material is often not removed well by lavage, especially in children (due to small tube size).
• Gastric lavage should be performed in adult (tube size 36–42 French) patients presenting within 1 hour of a large ingestion or if serious effects are present.
• One dose of activated charcoal (1–2 g/kg) should be administered without a cathartic if a substantial ingestion has occurred within the previous few hours.

ANTIDOTES

Digoxin immune Fab is the antidote for cardiac glycoside poisoning.

Indications

• Any sign of cardiovascular instability should prompt administration of digoxin immune Fab.
• Rapid progression of toxicity, including gastrointestinal symptoms, is also an indication for digoxin immune Fab.
• Serum K^+ higher than 5.5 mEq/L indicates a poor prognosis and is an indication for Fab administration.

Dosage and Method of Administration

• If the patient is critically ill and cardiac glycoside toxicity is possible, 10 to 20 vials of Fab should be administered intravenously.
• In symptomatic but relatively stable patients, there are no data on empiric dosing; a typical initial empiric dose would be five vials intravenously, repeated if necessary.
• A digoxin level should not be used to calculate the dose because the toxin measured is from the plant, not from pure medication.
• See SECTION III, Digoxin Immune Fab for details of administration.

ADJUNCTIVE TREATMENT

• Atropine, isoproterenol, and cardiac pacing have been used for bradycardia or heart block if digoxin Fab is not available.
• Lidocaine and phenytoin have been used successfully for managing ventricular dysrhythmias.
• Phenytoin has been used for supraventricular tachydysrhythmias.
• Vasopressors may be helpful during initial stabilization or until digoxin Fab is available.
• Procainamide, quinidine, disopyramide and propranolol are not recommended because they may decrease conduction and worsen AV nodal block.
• Calcium is contraindicated because of the risk of cardiac tetany.

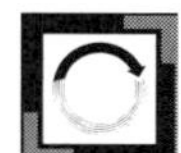

Follow-Up

PATIENT MONITORING

ECG should be obtained and continuous respiratory and hemodynamic monitoring should be instituted in all patients with cardiac glycoside toxicity.

EXPECTED COURSE AND PROGNOSIS

• Sequelae of hypotension or hypoxia may develop in some patients.
• Clinical improvement after administration of digoxin immune Fab is expected.

DISCHARGE CRITERIA/INSTRUCTIONS

• From the emergency department. Patients who are asymptomatic, have an undetectable digoxin level, and normal ECG and electrolytes may be discharged following gastrointestinal decontamination, 6 hours of observation, and psychiatric evaluation, if needed.
• From the hospital. Patients may be discharged following gastrointestinal decontamination, resolution of cardiac effects, and psychiatric evaluation, if needed.

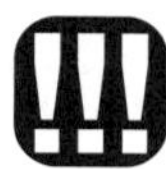

Pitfalls

DIAGNOSIS

• The symptoms of cardiac glycoside toxicity may be nonspecific, and a high index of suspicion is essential in arriving at the diagnosis.
• Patients may exhibit cardiac glycoside toxicity from plant ingestion despite undetectable serum digoxin levels.

TREATMENT

• Digoxin immune Fab should be administered even in the presence of cardiac arrest of short duration; survival rates of up to 50% for patients in cardiac arrest have been reported.
• Delay in treatment is dangerous because of rapid acute deterioration.
• Hospital pharmacies are often inadequately stocked with digoxin immune Fab.

ICD-9-CM 972

Poisoning by agents primarily affecting the cardiovascular system.

See also: SECTION II, Ventricular Dysrhythmias; SECTION III, Digoxin Immune Fab chapter.

RECOMMENDED READING

Lewin N. Digitalis. In: Goldfrank LR, Flomenbaum NE, Lewin NA, et al., eds. *Goldfrank's toxicologic emergencies,* 6th ed. Norwalk, CT: Appleton & Lange, 1998.

Author: Edwin K. Kuffner

Reviewer: Gerald F. O'Malley

Plants—Cyanogenic Glycosides

Basics

DESCRIPTION

Included in this chapter are plants that release cyanide during digestion or during preparation for eating.

FORMS AND USES

Plants containing cyanogenic glycosides include:

- Prunus species: apricot (laetrile is apricot pit kernel extract), cherry laurel, chokecherry, mountain mahogany, pin cherry, wild black cherry, plum, bitter almond, peach, pear seeds, apple seeds, crab apple seeds, and elderberry.
- *Manihot esculenta* (cassava), which is consumed as a staple carbohydrate source in many developing areas of the world.
- *Hydrangea* and *Linium* species.

TOXIC DOSE

- Ingestion of one or two seeds or pits is unlikely to produce toxicity.
- Ingestion of many seeds or pits (especially when chewed), or ingestion of tea, herbal preparations, or alternative medicines (e.g., laetrile) made with plants containing cyanogenic glycosides, can result in life-threatening cyanide toxicity.

PATHOPHYSIOLOGY

- Pits of the *Prunus* species contain varying amounts of amygdalin, which is not toxic unless the seed is disrupted and its contents metabolized by intestinal bacteria; thus, ingestion of whole seeds or pits is unlikely to cause toxicity.
- Enzymatic degradation of amygdalin produces benzaldehyde, glucose, and cyanide.
- Cassava contains the cyanogens linamarin and lotaustralin within the tuber; if the tuber is not properly processed prior to consumption, cyanide toxicity can result.

EPIDEMIOLOGY

- Poisoning is rare.
- Severe toxic effects are extremely rare, with death occurring usually in the settings of suicide attempt, ingestion of teas or herbal preparations, and use of alternative medicines.

CAUSES

- Poisoning from plants containing cyanide glycosides usually result from misuse of product caused by ignorance of potential toxicity.
- Child neglect should be considered if the patient is less than 1 year of age; suicide if the patient is over 6 years of age.

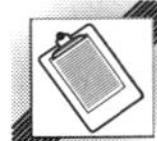

Diagnosis

DIFFERENTIAL DIAGNOSIS

- Other toxic agents that cause cyanide poisoning or symptoms resembling cyanide poisoning include inorganic cyanide (HCN, KCN), aliphatic nitriles (e.g., acetonitrile, acrylonitrile, etc.), carbon monoxide, hydrogen sulfide, iron, isoniazid, salicylates, and toxic alcohols.
- Nontoxic causes of dyspnea, confusion, and circulatory collapse include renal failure, diabetic or alcoholic ketoacidosis, and lactic acidosis, among others.

SIGNS AND SYMPTOMS

- Most accidental ingestions do not result in cyanide toxicity.
- Onset of symptoms of cyanide glycoside poisoning is usually delayed compared with that following exposure to inorganic cyanide.

Vital Signs

- Tachypnea and hyperpnea are commonly followed by respiratory depression and apnea in severe cases.
- Cardiorespiratory collapse is usually a preterminal event.

HEENT

- Arteriolarization (bright red appearance) of retinal vein on fundoscopic examination suggests cyanide toxicity.
- Glossitis often accompanies tropical ataxic neuropathy associated with chronic cassava consumption.
- Optic neuropathy or deafness may develop during chronic ingestion of cyanogenic plants.

Dermatologic

- Central cyanosis may be secondary to hypoventilation, and peripheral cyanosis may be secondary to hypoperfusion.
- Pallor, mottling, and decreased skin temperature are common with severe cyanide toxicity.
- Dermatitis often accompanies tropical ataxic neuropathy associated with chronic cassava consumption.

Cardiovascular

Cardiovascular collapse with bradycardia and hypotension is usually a preterminal event in cases of severe cyanide toxicity.

Pulmonary

- Chest pain and dyspnea are common in serious cases.
- Both cardiogenic and noncardiogenic pulmonary edema have been reported.

Gastrointestinal

Nausea, vomiting, and abdominal pain are common.

Fluids and Electrolytes

- Increased anion gap metabolic lactic acidosis is common.
- Severe and prolonged nausea, vomiting, and diarrhea can produce fluid and electrolyte abnormalities.

Neurologic

- Headache, lightheadedness, agitation, anxiety, confusion, lethargy, altered mental status, tremor, ataxia, coma, and seizures suggest cyanide toxicity.
- Chronic consumption of cassava has been associated with tropical ataxic neuropathy (a demyelinating disorder characterized by paresthesia, sensory ataxia, optic atrophy, and sensorineural hearing loss).
- Epidemic spastic paraparesis, characterized by lower extremity spastic paralysis, may occur in areas where cassava is a food staple.

PROCEDURES AND LABORATORY TESTS

Essential Tests

- Arterial blood gases should be obtained to evaluate for metabolic acidosis.
- Serum electrolytes, BUN, and creatinine levels may reveal an increased anion gap metabolic acidosis.

Recommended Tests

- Complete blood count should be performed, particularly to guide therapy if sodium nitrite therapy is needed; induction of methemoglobinemia can decrease oxygen-carrying capacity, especially in anemic patients.
- Serum lactate is increased in cyanide toxicity.
- Blood cyanide level may be helpful, but often is not available in time for clinical use.

—During acute intoxication, a level less than 0.2 μg/ml is generally not associated with symptoms; 0.5 to 1.0 μg/ml can produce tachycardia; 1.0 to 2.5 μg/ml can produce obtundation; 2.5 to 3.0 μg/ml can produce coma; and levels greater than 3.0 μg/ml can result in death.
—Results of blood cyanide level tests are unreliable in many laboratories.

- ECG should be performed on all patients who have signs or symptoms of cardiovascular instability.
- Serum acetaminophen and aspirin level in overdose setting to detect occult ingestion.
- A chest radiograph should be obtained for patients with signs of respiratory insufficiency.
- Head CT, lumbar puncture, and cultures may be needed to evaluate altered mental status.

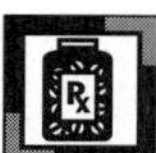

Treatment

• Therapy should focus on administration of 100% oxygen using a non-rebreather mask, aggressive supportive care, and determination of need for cyanide antidote kit.
• The dose and time of exposure should be determined for all substances involved.

DIRECTING PATIENT COURSE

The health-care provider should call the poison control center when:

• A history of cyanogenic plant ingestion is obtained or any toxic effect develops.
• Coingestant, drug interaction, or underlying disease presents an unusual problem.

The patient should be referred to a health-care facility when:

• Attempted suicide or homicide is possible.
• The patient or caregiver seems unreliable.
• Any toxic effects develop.
• Coingestant, drug interaction, or underlying disease presents an unusual problem.

Admission Considerations

Inpatient management is warranted for patients who have ingested potentially large amounts of plants containing cyanide glycosides (more than five pits or seeds) or who have signs of toxicity.

DECONTAMINATION

Out of Hospital

Emesis should be induced with ipecac within 1 hour of a large ingestion (greater than five chewed pits or seeds) in alert pediatric or adult patients if health-care evaluation will be delayed.

In Hospital

• Ipecac-induced emesis within 1 hour of a large ingestion (greater than five chewed pits or seeds) may be effective in retrieving plant material.
• Aspiration of gastric contents using a nasogastric tube may be helpful shortly after ingestion of a liquid preparation.
• Gastric lavage should be performed in pediatric (tube size 24–32 French) or adult (tube size 36–42 French) patients after a large ingestion, especially if toxic effects are present; the success rate for recovering plant material with gastric lavage, however, is usually low.
• One dose of activated charcoal (1–2 g/kg) should be administered without a cathartic if a substantial ingestion has occurred within the previous few hours.
• Dermal decontamination is performed by washing exposed skin with copious amounts of soap and water; exposed mucous membranes should be flushed with copious amounts of water.
• Whole-bowel irrigation is recommended following a large overdose of plant material.

ANTIDOTES

• Use of a complete cyanide antidote package is indicated for patients with known cyanide poisoning and serious clinical effects (hypotension, metabolic acidosis, altered mental status, etc.).

—For patients with known cyanide exposure but in whom clinical effects have not developed, treatment with the sodium thiosulfate component alone should be considered.

• The cyanide antidote package is not used for the treatment of chronic poisoning like tropical ataxic neuropathy or epidemic spastic paraparesis.

ADJUNCTIVE TREATMENT

• Tropical ataxic neuropathy treatment includes stopping cassava ingestion, placing patients on a balanced diet, and treating them with vitamin B_{12}.
• Hypotension

—Administration of 10 to 20 ml/kg 0.9% saline and Trendelenburg positioning may reduce hypotension.
—Further fluid therapy should be guided by central pressure monitoring to avoid volume overload.
—A vasopressor may be added if needed (see SECTION II, Hypotension chapter).

• Seizure

—Patent airway must be ensured.
—A benzodiazepine should be administered for initial control.
—If seizures persist or recur, another anticonvulsant such as phenobarbital should be added (see SECTION II, Seizures chapter).

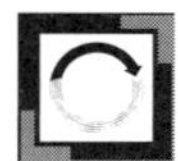

Follow-Up

PATIENT MONITORING

• Respiratory and cardiac function must be monitored continuously.
• Serum electrolyte, serum lactate, and arterial blood gas levels should be followed serially.

EXPECTED COURSE AND PROGNOSIS

• The onset of toxicity is longer in cardiac glycoside-containing plant toxicity than in toxicity from inorganic cyanide.
• Signs and symptoms of cyanide toxicity may develop within a few hours but may be delayed for 12 to 24 hours.
• Sequellae of hypoxia may persist.
• Toxic effects associated with spastic paraparesis and tropical ataxic neuropathy may be permanent.

DISCHARGE CRITERIA/INSTRUCTIONS

• From the emergency department. Patients who have accidentally ingested less than five seeds or pits need not be referred to the emergency department; if, however, they are seen in an emergency department, they should be given activated charcoal and may be discharged if they are asymptomatic.
• From the hospital. Patients may be discharged when toxic effects have resolved or stabilized for at least 24 hours.

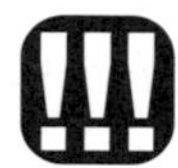

Pitfalls

DIAGNOSIS

It is important to admit an asymptomatic patient with a potentially large ingestion for at least 24 hours of observation.

TREATMENT

• Use of the cyanide antidote kit should be based on a patient's symptoms, not simply on the history of ingestion.
• Administering an adult dose of sodium nitrite to a pediatric patient can result in life-threatening methemoglobinemia.

ICD-9-CM 988.2

Toxic effect of noxious substances eaten as food: berries and other plants.

See also: SECTION II, Hypotension and Seizures chapters; and SECTION III, Cyanide Antidote Package chapter.

RECOMMENDED READING

Akinonwa A, Tunwashe OL. Fatal cyanide poisoning from Cassava-based meal. *Hum Exp Toxicol* 1992;11:47–49.

Author: Edwin K. Kuffner

Reviewer: Richard C. Dart

Plants—General

Basics

DESCRIPTION

This chapter covers all plants except those covered in other chapters (akee fruit; plants with anticholinergic properties; plants containing cardiac glycosides or cyanogenic glycosides; marijuana; mushrooms; pennyroyal) and plants that contain caffeine, capsaicin, colchicine/taxol, cyanogenic glycosides, ephedrine, ergot alkaloids, lysergic acid diethylamide (LSD), nicotine, pyrrolizidine alkaloids, quinine, or strychnine.

FORMS AND USES

Plants discussed in this chapter include:

- Betel nut, nutmeg, ergot alkaloids, morning glory, and peyote
- Rhubarb, sorrel, *Philodendron* species, and dumb-cane (*Dieffenbachia* species)
- Polygonaceae (*Rheum* and *Rumex* species), Chenopodiaceae (*Halogeton* species, *Glomeratus* species), *Spinaciae* (spinach), Oxalidaceae (*Oxalis cirnua*), Portulaceceae (*Portulaca* species), and Ficoidaceae (*Tetragonia* species).
- Mandrake, may apple, castor bean, jequirty bean, rosary pea, and daphne
- Elephants ear and skunk cabbage
- *Solanum* species (black nightshade, Jerusalem cherry, common potato, climbing nightshade)
- Buckeyes, horse chestnut, tonka bean, and tonco bean
- Globe thistle
- *Toxicodendron* species (nonclimbing poison ivy, poison ivy shrub or climbing vine, western poison oak, eastern poison oak, poison sumac), poinsettia, lime, parsley, celery, figs, and buttercups
- Holly, hyacinth, iris, daffodil, pyracantha, pokeweed, inkberry, crown of thorns, wisteria, *Aloe* species, and English ivy
- Mistletoe
- Water hemlock, western water hemlock, chinaberry, moonseed, and monkshood
- Nontoxic plants: *Episcia reptans,* African violet, aluminum plant, false aralia, coleus, gardenia, jade, wandering Jew, parlor palm, begonia, rubber plant, spider plant, zebra plant, baby's tears, bird's-nest fern, and Christmas cactus

Many plants share common names. If a plant is identified as nontoxic, the identification should be verified by an experienced individual.

PATHOPHYSIOLOGY

The toxic mechanisms of poisonous plants comprise a wide range of processes.

TOXIC DOSE

In general, it is difficult to produce toxicity from ingestion of most of these plants in their natural condition; concentration, solubilization, or large ingestion is needed for toxicity to develop.

EPIDEMIOLOGY

- Ingestion of a plant is common.
- Mild to moderate toxic effects are common.
- Severe toxic effects following exposure are extremely rare, with death occurring usually only in cases of misuse or suicide.

CAUSES

- Plant poisonings are usually accidents involving children.
- Adults have developed significant toxicity following the ingestion of teas or herbal preparations.

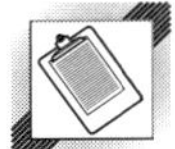

Diagnosis

DIFFERENTIAL DIAGNOSIS

- Plants causing nicotine toxicity include tree tobacco (*Nicotiana glauca*), Indian tobacco (*Lobelia inflata*), poison hemlock, spotted hemlock (*Conium maculatum*), golden chain tree (*Laburnum anagyroides*), and horsetail (*Equisetum*).
- Plants causing caffeine toxicity include coffee (*Coffea* species), chocolate, cola, cocoa (*Theobroma* species), and tea (*Camellia* species).
- Plants with hepatotoxic properties due to pyrrolizidine alkaloids include groundsel (*Senecio longilobus*), blue devil (*Echium* species), heliotrope (*Heliotropium europeaum*), and South African tuber (*Callilepsis laureola*).
- Akee fruit causes hypoglycemia.
- Hallucinogenic plants include ergots (*Claviceps purpurea*), nutmeg (*Myristica fragrans*), morning glory (*Ipomoea violacea*), and peyote (*Lophophora williamsii*).
- Autumn crocus (*Colchicum autumnale*) should be considered as a cause of renal toxicity.
- Bark of *cinchona* species should be considered as a cause of quinine toxicity.
- *Ephedra* species and mistletoe (*Phoradeudron flavesceus*) should be considered as a cause of sympathomimetic syndrome.
- *Strychnos nux-vomica* should be considered as a cause of seizures.
- Cardiac glycosides should be considered as a cause of bradycardia.
- Phytophotodermatitis may be caused by fig, lime, parsely, buttercup, and celery.

SIGNS AND SYMPTOMS

Physical signs may help identify the poison involved in a plant ingestion.

Vital Signs

- Tachycardia may result from significant gastrointestinal fluid losses due to toxic plant ingestion, as well as directly from ingestion of plants containing caffeine, nicotine, or coniine.
- Bradycardia may be caused by plants containing cardiac glycosides or muscarinic agonists.

HEENT

- Mucous membrane irritation is caused by plants containing calcium oxalate crystals; these may rarely cause airway compromise but should be considered in a child with persistent drooling, coughing, or respiratory distress.
- Salivation may result from mucous membrane irritation due to toxic plant exposure, as well as directly from nicotine.
- Lacrimation, conjunctivitis, rhinorrhea, and intense local burning pain are common with exposure to capsaicin.
- Mydriasis and dry mucous membranes occur with anticholinergic plant toxicity.
- Visual complaints and blindness may develop with quinine toxicity from *Cinchona* tree bark.
- Other visual complaints may result from cardiac glycoside plant toxicity.

Dermatologic

- Phytophotodermatitis (light-induced plant dermatitis) is caused by psoralens; lesions only occur on light-exposed areas.
- Contact dermatitis is caused by any of a number of plants, but particularly toxicodendron species.

Cardiovascular

Hypotension, tachycardia, and tachypnea may result from toxic effects of plants containing cyanide, caffeine, nicotine, or ephedrine.

Pulmonary

Cough, pulmonary inflammation, and edema result from inhalation of burning poison ivy, poison oak, or poison sumac smoke.

Gastrointestinal

- Vomiting or mild diarrhea is caused by many plants, especially those containing solanine, nicotine, caffeine, coniine, cicutoxin, or oxalate; nausea and vomiting also may be the first signs of cardiac glycoside toxicity.
- Decreased bowel sounds may be caused by anticholinergic plants.
- Severe diarrhea may indicate colchicine or toxalbumin (ricin and abrin) toxicity.

Hepatic

- Liver fibrosis may result from chronic pyrrolizidine alkaloid use.
- Hepatitis may be caused by water hemlock.

Renal

Renal toxicity may be caused by plants containing oxalates, or by colchicine, podophyllum, ricin, abrin, daphnin, and atractyloside.

Fluids and Electrolytes

- Hyperkalemia may indicate cardiac glycoside toxicity.
- Marked hypoglycemia may result from Akee fruit ingestion.

Musculoskeletal

Muscle contractions, tetany, and opisthotonos are caused by strychnine toxicity.

Neurologic

- Agitation, hallucinations, and seizures may be caused by anticholinergic plants.
- Seizures may be caused by water hemlock, poison hemlock, and plants containing nicotine, caffeine, or ephedrine.
- Headache, lightheadedness, altered mental status, metabolic acidosis, seizures, and coma indicate exposure to plants containing cyanogenic glycosides.
- Ascending motor paralysis may result from poison hemlock ingestion.

PROCEDURES AND LABORATORY TESTS

Essential Tests

No tests may be needed in asymptomatic patients.

Recommended Tests

- Serum electrolytes, BUN, and creatinine should be obtained for patients with protracted vomiting and diarrhea because of the risk of hypokalemia and dehydration and also to assess renal toxicity.
- Liver function tests should be obtained following the ingestion of plants that may cause hepatotoxicity.

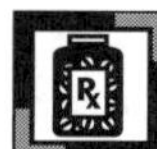

Treatment

- Treatment should focus on symptomatic and supportive care.
- The dose and time of exposure should be determined for all substances involved.

DIRECTING PATIENT COURSE

The health-care provider should call the poison control center when:

- Plant identification is needed.
- Toxic effects develop.
- Coingestant, drug interaction, or underlying disease presents an unusual problem.

The patient should be referred to a health-care facility when:

- Attempted suicide or homicide is possible.
- The patient or caregiver seems unreliable.
- Toxic effects develop.
- Coingestant, drug interaction, or underlying disease presents an unusual problem.

Admission Considerations

Inpatient management is warranted if renal injury or other serious effects develop or if persistent effects occur that preclude self-care at home.

DECONTAMINATION

Out of Hospital

Emesis should be induced with ipecac within 1 hour of ingestion for alert pediatric or adult patients if health-care evaluation will be delayed.

In Hospital

- Ipecac-induced emesis is recommended for pediatric patients and should be considered for adults because lavage is often ineffective in recovering plant material.
- Gastric lavage should be considered in adult (tube size 36–42 French) patients for large ingestion presenting within 1 hour of ingestion or if serious effects are present.
- One dose of activated charcoal (1–2 g/kg) should be administered without a cathartic if a substantial ingestion has occurred within the previous few hours.

ANTIDOTES

There are no specific antidotes for the plants covered in this chapter.

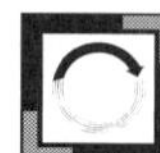

Follow-Up

DISCHARGE CRITERIA/INSTRUCTIONS

- From the emergency department. Asymptomatic or minimally symptomatic patients with normal examination may be discharged following decontamination, a 4- to 6-hour observation period, and psychiatric evaluation, if needed.
- From the hospital. Patients may be discharged after toxic effects have resolved or stabilized and a psychiatric evaluation, if needed, has been conducted.

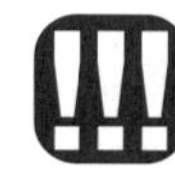

Pitfalls

DIAGNOSIS

- Plant ingestion rarely results in serious toxicity; if the toxin is concentrated (e.g., by making the plant into tea), however, serious toxicity may result.
- In most cases, the plant responsible for the toxic ingestion cannot be reliably identified; management should be supportive and based on a patient's symptoms.

TREATMENT

Most plants are not removed by lavage; a potentially serious ingestion is an indication for ipecac in the emergency department.

FOLLOW-UP

Hepatotoxic plants may not cause symptoms for several days.

ICD-9-CM 988.2

Poisoning effect of noxious substances eaten as food: berries and other plants.

See also: SECTION IV, Akee Fruit, Caffeine, Capsaicin, Colchicine, Ephedrine, Ergot Alkaloids, LSD and Other Psychedelic Compounds, Marijuana, Mushrooms, Nicotine, Pennyroyal, Plants—Anticholinergic, Plants—Cardiac Glycosides, Plants—Cyanogenic Glycosides, Pyrrolizidine Alkaloids, Quinine, Strychnine, and Water Hemlock chapters.

RECOMMENDED READING

Shih RD, Goldfrank LR. Plants. In: Goldfrank LR, Flomenbaum NE, Lewin NA, et al., eds. *Goldfrank's toxicologic emergencies.* 6th ed. Norwalk, CT: Appleton & Lange, 1998.

Author: Edwin K. Kuffner

Reviewer: Richard C. Dart

Podophyllum

Basics

DESCRIPTION

Podophyllum is a plant from the mayapple family, *Dysosma* or *Berberidaceae* species.

FORMS AND USES

- The dried roots and rhizomes have been used as herbal medications.
- Podophyllotoxin is the major active constituent of podophyllum resin.
- Pharmaceutical preparations of podophyllum or podophyllotoxin are topical resin solutions used as an alternative to cryotherapy for the topical treatment of external genital and perianal warts.
- Dermal application should be limited to less than 10 cm^2 of wart tissue and no more than 0.5 cc of solution/day.
- Podocon-25 (25%), Podofin (25%), Pod-Ben-25 (25%), and Podophyllum Resin Topical Solution USP (11.5%) can be applied once a week.
- Podofilox (0.5%) can be applied twice daily.
- Herbal products may contain podophyllum, but often the ingredient is not identified on the package.

TOXIC DOSE

- A single large topical application (5–10 ml) of 20% to 25% solution can cause serious toxicity in adults.
- The oral regimen used in some herbal products has produced severe toxicity.

PATHOPHYSIOLOGY

- Podophyllotoxin is a lipid-soluble compound that is readily absorbed dermally.
- Chemical effects are similar to colchicine and vinblastin:

—Antimitotic effect
—Inhibition of axoplasmic transport
—Inhibitory effects on protein, RNA, and DNA synthesis
—Blocking of oxidation enzymes in the tricarboxylic acid cycle

EPIDEMIOLOGY

- Podophyllum poisoning is rare.
- Toxic effects following dermal exposure are typically mild to moderate.
- However, death has occurred after oral or topical administration.

CAUSES

- Poisoning is usually via accidental overuse, such as excessive dermal application or accidental ingestion.
- Child abuse should be considered if the patient is less than 1 year of age; suicide attempt if the patient is over 6 years of age.

RISK FACTORS

The possibility of toxicity is increased if topical podophyllum resin is applied to friable, bleeding, or recently biopsied skin, or if the drug is inadvertently applied to normal skin and mucous membranes surrounding a condyloma.

PREGNANCY AND LACTATION

- Podofilox. US FDA Pregnancy Category C.

The drug exerts animal teratogenic or embryocidal effects, but there are no controlled studies in women, or no studies are available in either animals or women.

- Podophyllum, podophyllotoxin, and topical resin solution (Podocon-25, Podofin, Pod-Ben-25). US FDA Pregnancy Category X. Studies demonstrate fetal abnormalities or there is evidence of fetal risk based on human experience, or both, and the risk clearly outweighs any possible benefit.
- Podophyllum should not be used during pregnancy.

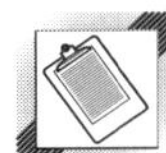

Diagnosis

DIFFERENTIAL DIAGNOSIS

- Toxic causes of rapid onset of nausea, vomiting, and hematemesis (especially if accompanied by acidosis and mental status changes) include colchicine, many antineoplastic agents, arsenic or other heavy metal, paraquat, ricin, or caustic agents.
- Other causes include severe infectious gastroenteritis, sepsis, meningitis, encephalitis, and organic brain syndromes.

SIGNS AND SYMPTOMS

- Toxicity generally begins 30 minutes to several hours after ingestion and 12 to 24 hours after dermal exposure.
- Early signs include vomiting, abdominal cramps and diarrhea, followed by confusion, altered mental status, and peripheral neuropathy.

Vital Signs

Tachycardia, hypotension, and tachypnea are common in severe overdose.

HEENT

Eye and mucosa exposures result in pain and irritation.

Dermatologic

Exposure is very irritating to skin and mucosa and may cause burns.

Cardiovascular

Tachycardia and hypotension are frequently reported following oral ingestion or topical exposure.

Pulmonary

Tachypnea and dyspnea occur frequently.

Gastrointestinal

Nausea, vomiting, abdominal pain, ileus, and severe diarrhea may occur after oral ingestion or dermal application.

Hepatic

Elevated alanine aminotransferase, aspartate aminotransferase, and lactate dehydrogenase may occur.

Renal

Oliguria, anuria, and complete renal failure have occurred rarely.

Hematologic

- Leukocytosis followed by leukopenia and thrombocytopenia may occur in severe cases.
- Thrombocytopenia generally reaches its nadir within 5 days and returns to normal within 20 days.

Neurologic

- Acute confusion, lethargy, stupor, coma, dizziness, fever, memory impairment, and convulsions have been reported following topical or oral exposure.
- Peripheral neuropathy, including stocking-and-glove paresthesia and sensory loss, areflexia, paralysis, and sensory ataxia, generally appears at 24 to 48 hours and peaks 4 to 7 days later.
- After topical use, neuropathy appears in the second week and progresses for 2 to 3 months.

Autonomic Nervous System

Autonomic dysfunction with sinus tachycardia, urinary retention, paralytic ileus, and orthostatic hypotension may persist for months.

Psychiatric

Visual and auditory hallucinations and paranoid delusions usually develop within 24 hours after ingestion and within 4 days after dermal application.

PROCEDURES AND LABORATORY TESTS

Essential Tests

- Complete blood count (CBC) to assess bone marrow effects
- Serum electrolytes, glucose, BUN, creatinine, and urinalysis to assess electrolyte abnormalities due to gastrointestinal losses and development of renal injury
- Liver function tests and amylase levels to assess organ injury

Recommended Tests

- ECG, serum acetaminophen, and aspirin levels in overdose setting to screen for occult ingestion
- Head CT, lumbar puncture, bacterial cultures, and other tests in patients with altered mental status of unknown etiology
- Electromyography and nerve conduction velocity in patients with peripheral neuropathy

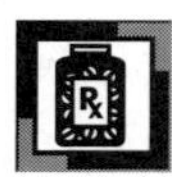

Treatment

- Treatment should focus on supportive care of severe gastroenteritis, altered mental status, and bone marrow suppression.
- Dose and time of exposure should be determined for all substances involved.

DIRECTING PATIENT COURSE

The health-care provider should call the poison control center when:

- A history of podophyllum ingestion is obtained.
- Toxic effects are not consistent with podophyllotoxin.
- Coingestant, drug interaction, or underlying disease presents an unusual problem.

The patient should be referred to a health-care facility when:

- Attempted suicide or homicide is possible.
- Patient or caregiver seems unreliable.
- Any excessive exposure has occurred.
- Coingestant, drug interaction, or underlying disease presents an unusual problem.

Admission Considerations

Inpatient management is required for patients with any toxic effects.

DECONTAMINATION

Out of Hospital

Emesis should be induced with ipecac within 1 hour of ingestion for alert pediatric or adult patients if vomiting has not occurred and health-care evaluation will be delayed.

In Hospital

- If vomiting has not occurred, ipecac-induced emesis should be administered within 1 hour of ingestion for the pediatric patient who is too small to have effective gastric lavage.
- If vomiting has not occurred, gastric lavage should be performed in pediatric (tube size 24–32 French) or adult (tube size 36–42 French) patients presenting within 1 hour of a large ingestion or if serious effects are present.
- One dose of activated charcoal (1–2 g/kg) should be administered without a cathartic if a substantial ingestion has occurred within the previous few hours.

ANTIDOTES

There is no specific antidote for podophyllotoxin.

ADJUNCTIVE TREATMENT

- Hypotension is treated with isotonic fluid infusion, Trendelenburg positioning, and a vasopressor if needed (dopamine is preferred, and norepinephrine is used for refractory hypotension).
- Although hemoperfusion is recommended by some, there is no conclusive information regarding its usefulness. Anecdotal experience reveals that either improvement or deterioration may occur following hemoperfusion.

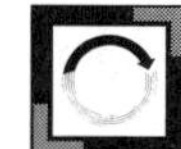

Follow-Up

PATIENT MONITORING

- Respiratory and cardiac function should be monitored continuously.
- CBC, electrolytes, renal and liver function tests, and amylase levels should be followed.

EXPECTED COURSE AND PROGNOSIS

- The peripheral neuropathy generally progresses to its peak within 1 week and tends to persist for months or years.
- Autonomic dysfunction may persist for months.
- Patients generally recover from leukocytopenia and thrombocytopenia within 1 month.
- Death, vegetative state, prolonged neuropathy, renal failure, and bone marrow suppression are all possible complications.

DISCHARGE CRITERIA/INSTRUCTIONS

- From the emergency department. Asymptomatic patients may be discharged after more than 24 hours has elapsed since exposure and following a psychiatric evaluation, if needed.
- From the hospital. Asymptomatic patients may be discharged when major effects are resolving, outpatient care has been arranged, and, if needed, a psychiatric evaluation has been completed.

PATIENT EDUCATION

Patients should be advised to wash therapeutically-applied podophyllin from the area after 1 to 4 hours.

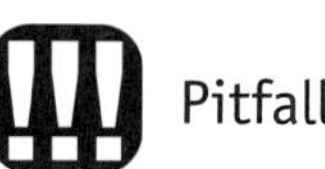

Pitfalls

DIAGNOSIS

- Early leukocytosis with fever, hypotension, and altered mental status may be mistaken for sepsis, meningitis, or encephalitis.
- Toxicity may be delayed following dermal application.

FOLLOW-UP

Prolonged follow-up of severe cases is usually needed.

ICD-9-CM 977

Poisoning by other and unspecified drugs and medicinal substances.

See also: SECTION II, Hypotension chapter.

RECOMMENDED READING

Chang LW, Yang CM, Chen CF, Deng JF. Experimental podophyllotoxin (Bajiaolian) poisoning: I. Effects on the liver, intestinal, kidney, pancreas and testis. *Biomed Environ Sci* 1992;5:283–292.

Chang LW, Yang CM, Chen CF, Deng JF. Experimental podophyllotoxin (Bajiaolian) poisoning: II. Effects on the nervous system. *Biomed Environ Sci* 1992;5:293–302.

Kao WF, Hung DZ, Tsai WJ, et al. Podophyllotoxin intoxication: toxic effects of Bajiaolian in herbal therapeutics. *Hum Exp Toxicol* 1992;11:480–487.

Yang CM, Deng JF, Chen CF, Chang LW. Experimental podophyllotoxin (Bajiaolian) poisoning: I. Biochemical bases for toxic effects. *Biomed Environ Sci* 1994;7:259–265.

Authors: Wei-Fong Kao and Jou-Fang Deng

Reviewer: Richard C. Dart

Polymer Fume Fever

Basics

DESCRIPTION

Polymer fume fever, also know as Teflon fever, is a flulike syndrome occurring after inhalation of fumes produced by decomposition of certain polymers, primarily polytetrafluoroethylene (PTFE) (Teflon).

TOXIC DOSE

The toxic dose is variable, depending on concentration and length of exposure.

PATHOPHYSIOLOGY

- The proposed mechanism of toxicity involves hydrolysis by the lung of carbonyl fluoride (a by-product of fluoropolymer combustion) to produce hydrofluoric acid, a pulmonary irritant.
- Other, small aerosolized particles that are liberated during polymer pyrolysis undoubtedly contribute to the pneumonitis, although an exact toxic species has not been identified.

EPIDEMIOLOGY

Toxic effects are common and underreported because of their self-limited nature.

CAUSES

Toxicity is generally caused by occupational accident or misadventure in the home (e.g., burning of Teflon coated item).

RISK FACTORS

- Occupational exposure to the by-products of combustion of fluoropolymers (e.g., Freon) is a hazard in the air conditioning repair industry.
- Disposal of products that contain fluorocarbons as part of the propellant is associated with a risk of exposure.
- Employment as a welder working on or near PTFE-coated wires or pipe fittings carries a risk of inhaling polymer fumes.

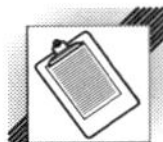

Diagnosis

DIFFERENTIAL DIAGNOSIS

- Chest discomfort and dyspnea with normal respiratory function and adequate oxygenation help to differentiate polymer fume fever from an infectious etiology or pulmonary embolism.
- History of occupational exposure to polymer fumes is the most important diagnostic factor.

SIGNS AND SYMPTOMS

Acute onset of flulike syndrome, including fatigue, chills, myalgia, and fever, is observed.

Vital Signs

- Other symptoms include fever of 39°C or higher, tachycardia secondary to fever, and tachypnea.
- Blood pressure, pulse oximetry results, and mental status are usually not affected.

HEENT

Mucosal irritation of eyes, mouth, and throat, and headache may occur.

Dermatologic

Diaphoresis may be seen.

Cardiovascular

Sinus tachycardia may coincide with fever and discomfort.

Pulmonary

Chest tightness or discomfort with dyspnea and nonproductive cough are common.

Gastrointestinal

Nausea, vomiting, and diffuse abdominal pain are common.

Musculoskeletal

Generalized arthralgia and myalgia may occur.

PROCEDURES AND LABORATORY TESTS

Essential Tests

Pulse oximetry or arterial blood gas analysis in patients with respiratory complaints.

Recommended Tests

- Urine fluoride levels may help to estimate chronic exposure.
- Carbon monoxide levels should be considered for all patients when concern about smoke inhalation exists.
- Pulmonary function tests and spirometry are variably affected by polymer fume fever.
- Chest radiography results are initially normal, but may develop diffuse infiltrates within hours in severe cases.

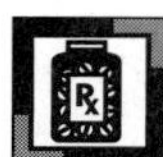

Treatment

- Treatment should focus on symptomatic and supportive care.
- The dose and time of exposure for all substances involved should be determined.

DIRECTING PATIENT COURSE

The health-care professional should call the poison control center when:

- Cause of respiratory symptoms is unclear.
- Severe or persistent effects develop.
- Coingestant, drug interaction, or underlying disease presents an unusual problem.

The patient should be referred to a health-care facility when:

- Suicide or homicide attempt is possible.
- Toxic effects develop.
- Coingestant, drug interaction, or underlying disease presents an unusual problem.

Admission Considerations

Patients with hypoxia or persistent complaints should be admitted.

DECONTAMINATION

Inhalation

The patient should be removed from the exposure and oxygen should be administered.

ANTIDOTES

There is no specific antidote for polymer fume fever.

ADJUNCTIVE TREATMENT

- Antipyretics should be administered to control fever.
- Hydration is warranted: either oral or, if the patient is too nauseated to drink, intravenous.
- Analgesics should be administered to control pain.
- Noncardiogenic pulmonary edema rarely develops, but should be treated in the usual manner.

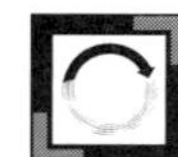

Follow-Up

EXPECTED COURSE AND PROGNOSIS

- Symptoms develop within 4 to 12 hours of exposure and disappear with only slight residual discomfort within 24 to 48 hours after removal from the source of the fumes.
- Recovery is typically complete, although a rare chemical pneumonitis and sometimes frank acute respiratory distress syndrome may complicate the exposure in susceptible individuals.

DISCHARGE CRITERIA/INSTRUCTIONS

Patients may be discharged from the emergency department or hospital when toxic effects resolve or stabilize during a 6-hour observation period.

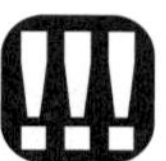

Pitfalls

FOLLOW-UP

It is important for health-care providers to educate patients as to the necessity of wearing pulmonary protective equipment.

ICD-9-CM 987

Toxic effect of other gases, fumes, or vapors.

See also: SECTION II, Pulmonary Edema chapter.

RECOMMENDED READING

Behrman A. Welders. In: Greenberg M, Phillips S, et al., eds. *Occupational, industrial and environmental toxicology.* St. Louis: Mosby, 1997:303–309.

Shusterman DJ. Polymer fume fever and other fluorocarbon pyrolysis related syndromes. *Occup Med* 1993;8:519.

Author: Gerald F. O'Malley

Reviewer: Luke Yip

Prednisone

Basics

DESCRIPTION

Prednisone (Prednicon-M, Sterapred) and prednisolone are steroids used for its antiinflammatory immunosuppressive activities.

FORMS AND USES

- It is used to treat allergic disease, dermatologic conditions, inflammatory bowel disease, bronchospasm, multiple sclerosis, myasthenia gravis, and pediatric bacterial meningitis and is used in various chemotherapeutic regimens.
- The dose of prednisone varies widely depending on the disorder but ranges from maintenance doses, which slightly exceed physiologic dosage (e.g., 5–15 mg/day in adults), to high dosages of 1 to 3 mg/kg/day.

TOXIC DOSE

- Ingestion of an acute massive dose is tolerated well.
- Chronic excessive dosing is needed to produce toxicity.

PATHOPHYSIOLOGY

- Prednisone has both antiinflammatory and immunosuppressant effects.
- It has mostly glucocorticoid properties, and minimal mineralocorticoid properties.

EPIDEMIOLOGY

Poisoning is uncommon.

CAUSES

- Toxicity is usually caused by chronic therapeutic ingestion.
- Child neglect or abuse should be considered if the patient is less than 1 year of age, suicide attempt if the patient is over 6 years of age.

DRUG AND DISEASE INTERACTIONS

- There is an increased risk of gastric ulcer when prednisone is used with aspirin or nonsteroidal antiinflammatory drugs.
- Severe muscle weakness may occur in patients with myasthenia gravis if given within 24 hours of pyridostigmine or other anticholinesterase.
- Potassium-depleting diuretics may enhance the potassium-wasting effect of prednisone.
- Cyclosporine and high-dose steroid therapy have produced several reports of seizures in both adult and pediatric patients.

PREGNANCY AND LACTATION

US FDA Pregnancy Category C. The drug exerts animal teratogenic or embryocidal effects, but there are no controlled studies in women, or no studies are available in animals or women.

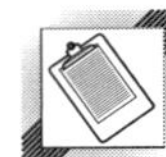

Diagnosis

SIGNS AND SYMPTOMS

Toxic effects occur during chronic administration.

HEENT

Posterior subcapsular cataracts and glaucoma may occur.

Gastrointestinal

Peptic ulcer may occur.

Fluids and Electrolytes

Hypokalemia and sodium retention, resulting in hypertension and edema, may occur during chronic use.

Musculoskeletal

Muscle wasting, weakness, pain, osteoporosis, vertebral compression fractures, and aseptic necrosis of femoral or humeral head have developed during chronic use.

Neurologic

Mental disturbances ranging from euphoria, depression, and anxiety to frank psychosis may follow acute large ingestion or chronic ingestion.

PROCEDURES AND LABORATORY TESTS

Essential Tests

No tests are usually needed in asymptomatic patients.

Recommended Tests

- Serum electrolytes, BUN, creatinine in symptomatic patients to assess hypokalemia and other potential causes of weakness.
- Radiography of appropriate areas if fractures are suspected
- Head CT, lumbar puncture, cultures, and other tests as needed in patients with altered mental status.
- ECG, serum acetaminophen and aspirin levels in overdose setting to detect occult ingestion.

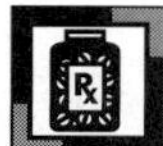

Treatment

Treatment consists mainly of reducing steroid dose and providing supportive care.

DIRECTING PATIENT COURSE

The health-care professional should call the poison control center when:

- Severe or persistent effects develop.
- Coingestant, drug interaction, or underlying disease presents an unusual problem.

The patient should be referred to a health-care facility when:

- Suicide or homicide attempt is possible.
- Toxic effects develop.
- Coingestant, drug interaction, or underlying disease presents an unusual problem.

Admission Considerations

Patients with severe fractures or gastrointestinal bleeding may require admission.

DECONTAMINATION

Out of Hospital

Induction of emesis is not needed due to low toxic potential after acute ingestion.

In Hospital

Lavage and activated charcoal may be appropriate if a coingestant is suspected. Please see appropriate chapter for suspected coingestant.

ANTIDOTE

There is no specific antidote.

ADJUNCTIVE TREATMENT

- Fractures, electrolyte abnormalities, and mental status change are all treated by reducing the steroid dose and providing symptomatic and supportive care.
- Unlike chronic ingestion, steroid tapering is not necessary after an acute overdose.

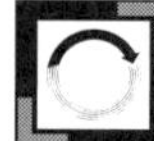

Follow-Up

PATIENT MONITORING

Intensive monitoring is not needed unless electrolyte or CNS abnormality is present.

EXPECTED COURSE AND PROGNOSIS

- Acute ingestion of prednisone, even in massive doses, is unlikely to cause clinical sequelae other than nausea and vomiting.
- Chronic effects are numerous, however, including increased susceptibility to infection.

DISCHARGE CRITERIA/INSTRUCTIONS

- From the emergency department. Asymptomatic patients may be discharged after decontamination and psychiatric evaluation, if needed.
- From the hospital. Patients may be discharged after toxic effects have stabilized or resolved.

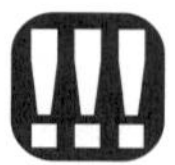

Pitfalls

DIAGNOSIS

Symptoms and signs of adrenocortical insufficiency, such as CNS depression and hypoglycemia, may occur with abrupt withdrawal of prednisone in a steroid-dependent patient.

ICD-9-CM 963.1

Poisoning by primarily systemic drugs: antineoplastic and immunosuppressive drugs.

RECOMMENDED READING

Kaufmann M, Kahaner K, Peselow RD, et al. Steroid psychosis: case report and brief overview. *J Clin Psychiatry* 1982;32:75–76.

Author: Robert E. Vander Leest

Reviewer: Richard C. Dart

Probenecid

Basics

DESCRIPTION

- Probenicid (Benemid) is a medication that prolongs the half-life of drugs (e.g., penicillins) in the blood.
- ColBENEMID contains both probenecid and colchicine.

FORMS AND USES

- When used for treatment of hyperuricemia and gout, the adult dosage of probenecid is 250 mg orally twice a day, which may be increased to up to 500 mg four times a day.
- When used to prolong the serum half-life of penicillin and cephalosporin antibiotics, as well as other drugs, the adult dosage is 500 mg orally four times a day.

TOXIC DOSE

- A toxic dose has not been well established.
- Severe toxicity has occurred after ingestion of 47 g.

PATHOPHYSIOLOGY

- Probenecid inhibits the secretion of organic acids (e.g., of uric acid and some drugs, such as penicillins) from the tubular cell into the renal tubule.
- This prolongs serum levels of the compounds normally excreted by this mechanism.
- Probenecid also blocks the resorption of uric acid from the renal tubule thereby increasing excretion of uric acid.

EPIDEMIOLOGY

Poisoning is uncommon.

CAUSES

- Toxicity is usually caused by deliberate overdose.
- Child neglect or abuse should be considered if the patient is less than 1 year of age, suicide attempt if the patient is over 6 years of age.

DRUG AND DISEASE INTERACTIONS

Hypoglycemic agents and several other drugs may prolong and increase the effect of probenecid.

PREGNANCY AND LACTATION

US FDA Pregnancy Category B. Animal studies indicate no fetal risk and there are no controlled human studies, or animal studies show an adverse fetal effect but well-controlled studies in women do not.

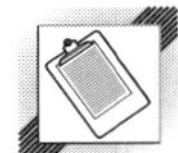

Diagnosis

SIGNS AND SYMPTOMS

Overdose is generally mild, but CNS depression can occur.

Vital Signs

Respiratory depression can occur.

Dermatologic

Rash is reported in 2% to 4% of patients.

Pulmonary

Respiratory depression and arrest can occur in large overdose.

Gastrointestinal

Nausea and vomiting are common in overdose and large therapeutic doses.

Renal

Nephrotic syndrome has been reported.

Hematologic

Bone marrow depression and blood dyscrasia have been reported.

Neurologic

- Somnolence progressing to coma occurs with large overdose.
- Tremors, hallucinations, and seizures also have been reported.

PROCEDURES AND LABORATORY TESTS

Essential Tests

No tests may be needed in asymptomatic patients.

Recommended Tests

- Pulse oximetry or arterial blood gases to evaluate oxygenation in symptomatic patients
- ECG, serum acetaminophen and aspirin levels in overdose setting to detect occult ingestion
- Serum electrolytes, BUN, creatinine, glucose, and other studies to evaluate other causes of altered mental status
- Head CT, lumbar puncture, cultures as appropriate to evaluate altered mental status.

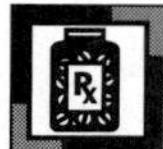

Treatment

- Symptomatic and supportive care is the mainstay of therapy.
- Dose and time of exposure should be determined for all substances involved.

DIRECTING PATIENT COURSE

The health-care professional should call the poison control center when:

- Severe or persistent effects develop.
- Coingestant, drug interaction, or underlying disease presents an unusual problem.

The patient should be referred to a health-care facility when:

- Suicide or homicide attempt is possible.
- Toxic effects develop.
- Coingestant, drug interaction, or underlying disease presents an unusual problem.

Admission Considerations

- Extended observation or hospital admission are rarely needed.
- Patients with seizure, altered mental status, or respiratory depression should be admitted.

DECONTAMINATION

Out of Hospital

Emesis is not recommended.

In Hospital

- Gastric lavage should be performed in pediatric (tube size 24–32 French) or adult (tube size 36–42 French) patients presenting within 1 hour of a large ingestion or if serious effects are present.
- One dose of activated charcoal (1–2 g/kg) should be administered without a cathartic if a substantial ingestion has occurred within the previous few hours.

ANTIDOTE

There is no specific antidote for probenecid poisoning.

ADJUNCTIVE TREATMENT

Seizures

A patent airway must be ensured, and a benzodiazepine should be administered for initial control; if seizures persist or recur, another anticonvulsant such as phenobarbital should be added.

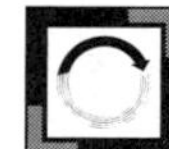

Follow-Up

PATIENT MONITORING

Respiratory and cardiac function should be monitored continuously in symptomatic patients.

DISCHARGE CRITERIA/INSTRUCTIONS

- From the emergency department. Asymptomatic patients may be discharged following decontamination, observation for 4 to 6 hours, and psychiatric evaluation, if needed.
- From the hospital. Patient may be discharged when CNS depression resolves, following psychiatric evaluation, if needed.

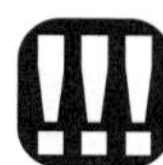

Pitfalls

FOLLOW-UP

- It is vital to realize that some formulations contain colchicine (see SECTION IV, Colchicine chapter).
- Health-care professionals should inform patients that probenecid may prolong the half-life of other drugs.

ICD-9-CM 974.7

Poisoning by water, mineral, and uric acid metabolism drugs: uric acid metabolism drugs.

See also: SECTION II, Seizures chapter; and SECTION IV, Colchicine chapter.

RECOMMENDED READING

Weiner IM, Mudge GH. Inhibitors of tubular transport of organic compounds. In: Goodman Gilman A, Goodman LS, Rall TW. *The pharmacological basis of therapeutics.* New York: McMillan, 1985:922–923.

Author: Kennon Heard

Reviewer: Richard C. Dart

Procainamide

Basics

DESCRIPTION

Procainamide (Pronestyl) is a medication used for the prevention and treatment of ventricular dysrhythmias.

FORMS AND USES

Oral Dosage

- Adult dose is 1 g, followed by 50 mg/kg in divided doses every 3 to 6 hours.
- Pediatric dosage is 15 to 50 mg/kg/day, given in divided doses every 3 to 6 hours.
- Sustained-release preparations (Procanbid) are available.

Intravenous Dosage

- Adult loading dose is 1 g infused at a rate of less than 50 mg/min to a maximum dose of 1 g.
- Adult maintenance dosage is 2 to 6 mg/min with cardiac monitoring.
- Pediatric loading dose is 10 to 15 mg/kg infused over 15 minutes.
- Pediatric maintenance dosage is 20 to 80 μg/kg/min.
- Infusion should be terminated if any of the following develop: hypotension, widening of QRS to more than 50% from baseline, or suppression of dysrhythmia.

TOXIC DOSE

- Toxicity may develop during rapid intravenous infusion of the therapeutic dose.
- Following ingestion, at least several grams are needed to produce toxicity.

PATHOPHYSIOLOGY

- The primary effect is to decrease myocardial impulse conduction velocity, manifested as widening of the QRS and PR intervals.
- Procainamide is metabolized in the liver to an active metabolite, *N*-acetylprocainamide (NAPA).
- Renal insufficiency can cause accumulation of NAPA.

EPIDEMIOLOGY

- Poisoning is uncommon.
- Adverse effects can occur in both therapeutic and overdose amounts.

CAUSES

- Poisoning usually results from an accidental incident.
- The possibility of child neglect or abuse should be considered if the patient is less than 1 year of age; suicide attempt in patients over 6 years of age.

RISK FACTORS

Preexisting liver or kidney dysfunction, heart block, severe heart disease, heart failure, and hypotension can all decrease metabolism.

DRUG AND DISEASE INTERACTIONS

- All other type 1 antidysrhythmics produce additive effects.
- Inhibitors of cytochrome P450 metabolism (e.g., cimetidine) increase procainamide levels.

PREGNANCY AND LACTATION

- US FDA Pregnancy Category C. The drug exerts animal teratogenic or embryocidal effects, but there are no controlled studies in women, or no studies are available in either animals or women.
- Procainamide is used in pregnancy to treat fetal arrhythmias.

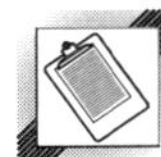

Diagnosis

DIFFERENTIAL DIAGNOSIS

- Toxic causes of CNS depression, seizure, and ECG conduction abnormality include type 1 antidysrhythmic agents, antihistamines, cocaine, β-receptor or calcium channel blockers, chloroquine, quinine, digoxin, phenothiazine, and cyclic antidepressants.
- Other causes of CNS depression and seizure are head trauma, elevated intracranial pressure, and severe electrolyte abnormality.

SIGNS AND SYMPTOMS

Primary manifestations are CNS depression, seizure, and ventricular dysrhythmia.

Vital Signs

Hypotension and decreased respirations may develop.

Dermatologic

Hypersensitivity reactions have occurred following a single dose.

Cardiovascular

- Intraventricular conduction delay, premature ventricular contractions, ventricular fibrillation, and torsade de pointes have been reported.
- Junctional and ventricular tachycardia may occur.

Pulmonary

Respiratory failure may develop.

Gastrointestinal

Anorexia, nausea, vomiting, and constipation are common.

Hepatic

Cholestatic jaundice and hepatitis occur rarely.

Neurologic

CNS depression, seizure, and obtundation may occur.

Immunologic

Systemic lupus erythematosus has occurred during chronic use.

Musculoskeletal

Skeletal muscle weakness associated with respiratory depression may occur.

PROCEDURES AND LABORATORY TESTS

Essential Tests

- ECG with continuous monitoring should be performed to assess QRS widening, QT prolongation, ST depression, or T-wave inversion; QT prolongation greater than 50% suggests toxicity.
- Serum electrolytes, BUN, creatinine, calcium, magnesium, and phosphorus should be determined to assess other causes of dysrhythmia.

Recommended Tests

- Arterial blood gases should be determined in patients with clinical effects or receiving bicarbonate therapy: pH should not exceed 7.55.
- Serum levels of procainamide and NAPA may be determined.

—Therapeutic level of procainamide ranges from 1.0 to 16.0 μg/ml.
—Normal values for the laboratory being used should be checked.
—A combined procainamide plus NAPA serum level in the range of 30 to 40 μg/ml indicates toxicity.

- Serum acetaminophen and aspirin levels should be measured in an overdose setting to detect occult ingestion.
- Complete blood count may be performed to detect thrombocytopenia.
- Liver function tests should be conducted to assess liver disease that may increase the procainamide level.

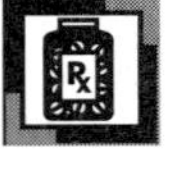

Treatment

- Treatment should focus on airway management and cardiac dysrhythmias.
- After decontamination, treatment should be supportive and symptomatic.
- Dose and time of exposure should be determined for substances involved.

DIRECTING PATIENT COURSE

The health-care provider should call the poison control center when:

- Altered mental status, cardiac dysrhythmia, or other severe effects are present.
- Toxic effects not consistent with the reported poisoning are present.
- Coingestant, drug interaction, or underlying disease presents unusual problems.

The patient should be referred to a health-care facility when:

- Attempted suicide or homicide is possible.
- Patient or caregiver seems unreliable.
- Patient has symptoms.
- Coingestant, drug interaction, or underlying disease presents unusual problems.

Admission Considerations

- Inpatient treatment in a cardiac-monitored setting is warranted when the patient develops CNS or cardiac toxicity.
- Admission should be considered for an asymptomatic patient with a history of ingestion exceeding 7 to 10 g, especially if a sustained-release preparation is involved.

DECONTAMINATION

Out of Hospital

Induction of emesis is not recommended.

In Hospital

- Gastric lavage should be performed in pediatric (tube size 24–32 French) or adult (tube size 36–42 French) patients presenting within 1 hour of a large ingestion or if serious effects are present.
- One dose of activated charcoal (1–2 g/kg) should be administered without a cathartic if a substantial ingestion has occurred within the previous few hours.
- Use of whole-bowel irrigation should be considered if a sustained-release preparation has been ingested.

ANTIDOTE

There is no specific antidote available.

ADJUNCTIVE TREATMENT

Hemodialysis increases clearance and may be of use in patients with refractory dysrhythmia or hypotension.

Bradycardia

- Standard agents, including atropine and isoproterenol, are usually ineffective.
- The early use of a pacemaker is recommended.

Ventricular Dysrhythmias

- An intravenous bolus of sodium bicarbonate, 1 to 2 mEq/kg, should be administered to narrow the QRS complex; however, the arterial pH should not exceed 7.55.
- Lidocaine

—Adult
 —Dose is 1.0 to 1.5 mg/kg by intravenous push.
 —Infusion is titrated from 1 to 4 mg/min to maintain suppression of ventricular dysrhythmia.
 —Dose is repeated in 0.5 to 0.75 mg/kg boluses, and maintenance infusion is increased every 5 to 10 minutes until ventricular tachycardia resolves or a total of 3 mg/kg has been given.
—Pediatric
 —Dose is 1 mg/kg given intravenously, intraosseously, or endotracheally.
 —The dose may be repeated in 10 to 15 minutes.
 —If a second dose is required, an infusion should be started at 20 to 50 μg/kg/min.
—The dose should be reduced in patients who have hepatic insufficiency, congestive heart failure, or cardiogenic shock or are over 70 years of age.

- Phenytoin or fosphenytoin may be useful for ventricular dysrhythmia refractory to the above therapies.

—Phenytoin loading dose
 —In adults and children, dose is 15 to 20 mg/kg intravenously.
 —Rate of infusion should not exceed 50 mg/min (adults) or 15 mg/kg/min (pediatric).
—Phenytoin maintenance dose for adults
 —Adult dose is 100 mg every 6 to 8 hours.
 —ECG and blood pressure should be monitored during infusion (for both loading and maintenance dose).
—Fosphenytoin loading dose is 15 to 20 mg of phenytoin equivalents/kg given at a rate of 100 to 150 mg phenytoin equivalents/min.

- Bretylium should be avoided because α-blocking effects may worsen hypotension.
- Other type 1a antidysrhythmic agents should be avoided because they may worsen dysrhythmias.
- Ventricular dysrhythmias may require cardioversion.

Torsade de Pointes

- Electrolyte abnormalities should be corrected, if present.
- Type 1a antidysrhythmic agents should be avoided because they also prolong the QT interval.
- Magnesium sulfate

—Adult
 —Dose is 1 to 2 g by intravenous push, and may be repeated in 10 to 15 minutes.
 —Intravenous infusion should begin at 2 to 20 mg/min, titrated to antidysrhythmic effect.
—Pediatric dose is 25 to 50 mg/kg administered intravenously over 5 minutes.

- Isoproterenol

—Adult initial dose is 2 to 4 μg/ml administered at 0.5 to 1.0 μg/min, titrated to effect.
—Pediatric dose is 0.1 μg/kg/min, titrated to effect.

- Electrical cardioversion or overdrive pacing at a rate of 130 to 150 beats/min may be required.

Hypotension

The primary treatment is correction of the dysrhythmia (see SECTION II, Hypotension chapter, for further details).

Seizures

Patent airway should be ensured (see SECTION II, Seizures chapter, for further information).

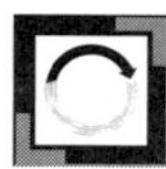

Follow-Up

PATIENT MONITORING

Cardiac rhythm, serum procainamide and NAPA levels, liver and kidney function, and electrolytes should be monitored for 24 hours or until dysrhythmia resolves.

EXPECTED COURSE AND PROGNOSIS

- Most toxic effects develop soon after overdose, peak in the first day, and then resolve.
- Cardiac and gastrointestinal side effects are seen in therapeutic doses.
- Sudden death from ventricular dysrhythmia may occur.

DISCHARGE CRITERIA/INSTRUCTIONS

- From the emergency department. Asymptomatic patients with normal ECG may be discharged after gastrointestinal decontamination, 6 hours of observation, and psychiatric evaluation, if needed.
- From the hospital. Patients may be discharged after toxic effects have resolved, ECG has been normal for 24 hours, and psychiatric evaluation has been performed, if needed.

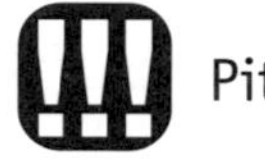

Pitfalls

DIAGNOSIS

- Signs of toxicity have occurred in patients taking therapeutic doses.
- Total procainamide levels should be determined.
- NAPA level may be toxic despite therapeutic procainamide level.

ICD-9-CM 972.0

Poisoning by agents primarily affecting the cardiovascular system: cardiac rhythm regulators.

See also: SECTION II, Bradycardia Toxidrome, Hypotension, Seizures, and Ventricular Dysrhythmias chapters; and SECTION III, Whole-Bowel Irrigation chapter.

RECOMMENDED READING

Procainamide. POISINDEX Editorial Staff. In: Rumack BH, Hess AJ, Gelman CR, eds. *POISINDEX system*. Englewood, CO: Micromedex, Inc. (edition expires May 31, 1998).

Author: David Nyman

Reviewer: Luke Yip

Propoxyphene

Basics

DESCRIPTION

Propoxyphene is a semisynthetic opioid analgesic medication.

FORMS AND USES

Propoxyphene is used to treat mild pain syndromes. It is generally considered less potent than codeine.

Propoxyphene Hydrochloride

- The adult dosage of propoxyphene hydrochloride is 65 mg orally every 4 hours.
- Formulations include Darvon (65 mg) and Darvon Compound (propoxyphene 65 mg, aspirin 389 mg, caffeine 32 mg).
- Wygesic (propoxyphene 65mg, acetaminophen 650 mg) is also available.

Propoxyphene Napsylate

- The adult dosage of propoxyphene napsylate is 100 mg orally every 4 hours.
- Formulations include Darvon-N (100 mg), Darvocet N 100 (propoxyphene napsylate 100 mg, acetaminophen 650 mg), and Darvocet N 50 (propoxyphene napsylate 50 mg, acetaminophen 325 mg).

TOXIC DOSE

- Toxic effects have been reported after ingestion of propoxyphene hydrochloride 10 mg/kg.
- Death may occur after ingestion of 20 mg/kg.

PATHOPHYSIOLOGY

- The analgesic effect of propoxyphene is mediated by activation of opioid receptors.
- Propoxyphene and its primary metabolite, norpropoxyphene, are cardiotoxic.
- This effect is thought to be mediated by inhibition of cardiac membrane sodium conduction, producing QRS interval widening and dysrhythmia in overdose.

EPIDEMIOLOGY

- Poisoning is uncommon.
- Toxic effects following exposure are typically moderate.
- Death occurs in patients with severe overdose associated with seizures and cardiac toxicity.

CAUSES

- Toxicity is caused usually by suicidal ingestion
- Child abuse should be considered if the patient is less than 1 year of age; suicide attempt if the patient is over 6 years of age.

DRUG AND DISEASE INTERACTIONS

- Respiratory and CNS depression may be exacerbated by concurrent use of ethanol or sedative-hypnotics, or any other agent causing CNS depression.
- *In utero* exposure may lead to neonatal withdrawal.
- Geriatric patients with underlying cardiac and renal disease may be predisposed to dysrhythmias.

PREGNANCY AND LACTATION

US FDA Pregnancy Category C. The drug exerts animal teratogenic or embryocidal effects, but there are no controlled studies in women, or no studies are available in either animals or women.

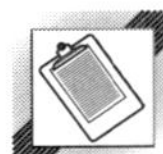

Diagnosis

DIFFERENTIAL DIAGNOSIS

- Toxic causes of respiratory and CNS depression include benzodiazepines, ethanol, barbiturates, numerous sedative-hypnotic drugs, tricyclic antidepressants and others.
- Nontoxic causes include hypoxia, severe electrolyte abnormality, hypoglycemia, intracranial bleed, meningitis, encephalitis, and postictal state, among others.

SIGNS AND SYMPTOMS

Propoxyphene overdose has a presentation similar to that of other opioids, with CNS, respiratory depression, and miosis, but is unique in that seizures and cardiac toxicity also may occur.

Vital Signs

- Bradypnea, bradycardia, and hypotension may occur.
- Hypothermia may occur in comatose individuals.

HEENT

Miosis is common.

Dermatologic

Injection may cause skin necrosis or abscess.

Cardiovascular

- QRS or QT interval prolongation may occur.
- Ventricular dysrhythmias and conduction defects including heart block may occur.

Pulmonary

- Respiratory depression, bradypnea, and hypoventilation may occur.
- Aspiration pneumonia may complicate respiratory depression or seizures.

Gastrointestinal

Nausea, vomiting, anorexia, abdominal pain, and constipation may occur.

Neurologic

Drowsiness, sedation, and coma, as well as confusion, hallucinations, and seizures, may occur in overdose.

Endocrine

Nephrogenic diabetes insipidus is a rare complication of propoxyphene use.

PROCEDURES AND LABORATORY TESTS

Essential Tests

No tests may be needed in asymptomatic patients.

Recommended Tests

- Serum electrolytes, glucose BUN, and creatinine levels are used to assess renal injury and altered mental status.
- Pulse oximetry or arterial blood gases are used for assessment of altered mental status.
- ECG assesses cardiac effects and potential toxicity of combination products; propoxyphene may cause cardiac conduction abnormalities similar to type 1a antidysrhythmics.
- Serum acetaminophen and aspirin levels should be evaluated to detect occult ingestion.
- Urinalysis and serum creatine kinase are used to evaluate comatose patients for rhabdomyolysis.

Not Recommended Tests

Many opiate immunoassays will not detect propoxyphene.

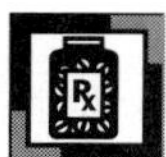

Treatment

- Treatment should focus on airway management and immediate treatment of seizures or cardiac toxicity.
- Dose and time of exposure for all substances involved must be determined.

DIRECTING PATIENT COURSE

The health-care provider should call the poison control center when:

- Seizure, ECG abnormality, or other serious effects are present.
- Toxic effects are not consistent with propoxyphene toxicity.
- Coingestant, drug interaction, or underlying disease presents an unusual problem.

The patient should be referred to a health-care facility when:

- Attempted suicide or homicide is possible.
- Patient or caregiver seems unreliable.
- Any toxic effects develop.
- Coingestant, drug interaction, or underlying disease presents an unusual problem.

Admission Considerations

Inpatient management is warranted for patients who develop cardiac conduction abnormality, seizure, or persistent CNS or respiratory depression.

DECONTAMINATION

Out of Hospital

Emesis should not be induced because CNS depression may develop rapidly.

In Hospital

- Gastric lavage should be performed in pediatric (tube size 24–32 French) or adult (tube size 36–42 French) patients presenting within 1 hour of a large ingestion or if serious effects are present.
- One dose of activated charcoal (1–2 g/kg) should be administered without a cathartic if a substantial ingestion has occurred within the previous few hours.
- Multiple-dose activated charcoal increases propoxyphene elimination but is not recommended due to potential for complications and lack of effect on duration of toxicity.

ANTIDOTES

Naloxone is used as an antidote.

- Indications: altered mental status of undetermined etiology (naloxone often does not effectively treat cardiac effects or respiratory depression).
- Absolute contraindications: none.
- Method of administration

—Adult or pediatric dose of 2.0 to 10.0 mg should be administered in 2.0-mg increments.
—Cumulative dose of 10.0 to 20.0 mg may be needed for propoxyphene.
—If only partial response is achieved, influence of another agent should be suspected.

- Potential adverse effects

—Naxolone may induce withdrawal syndrome.
—Reversal of opioid effects may unmask another underlying toxicity such as cocaine.

ADJUNCTIVE TREATMENT

Hypotension

- Hypotension related to bradycardia is corrected by atropine; an infusion of 10 to 20 ml/kg 0.9% saline also should be started and the patient placed in the Trendelenburg position.
- Further fluid therapy should be guided by central pressure monitoring to avoid volume overload.
- A vasopressor can be added, if needed.

Seizures

- Patency of airway must be ensured.
- A benzodiazepine should be administered for initial control.
- If seizures persist or recur, another anticonvulsant such as phenobarbital should be added.

Ventricular Dysrhythmia or Conduction Abnormality

- Seizures should be controlled rapidly and acidemia corrected.
- If QRS widening or dysrhythmia persists, sodium bicarbonate 1 to 2 mEq/kg intravenous bolus should be administered to increase the arterial pH to 7.45 to 7.55 and to narrow the complex width.
- An arterial pH of 7.55 should not be exceeded.
- Bretylium may be administered, 5 mg/kg over 1 minute; if unsuccessful, then a dose of 10 mg/kg over 1 minute should be administered and repeated as necessary for a total dose of 30 mg/kg.

Not Recommended Therapies

Procainamide, quinidine, and other type 1a antidysrhythmics should be avoided.

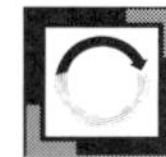

Follow-Up

PATIENT MONITORING

- Respiratory and cardiac parameters should be monitored continuously in all patients.
- Electroencephalographic (EEG) monitoring may be needed in patients with seizures that have been intubated and paralyzed.

EXPECTED COURSE AND PROGNOSIS

- Toxicity usually develops within hours and resolves over 24 hours.
- CNS depression following massive doses may require a longer recovery period.
- Possible complications include end-organ injury from hypotension or seizures.

DISCHARGE CRITERIA/INSTRUCTIONS

- From the emergency department

—Asymptomatic patients with a normal ECG may be discharged following decontamination, 6 hours of observation, and psychiatric evaluation, if needed.
—Patients receiving naloxone should be asymptomatic for 6 hours following naloxone administration before discharge.

- From the hospital. Patients may be discharged after resolution of toxic effects and psychiatric evaluation, if needed.

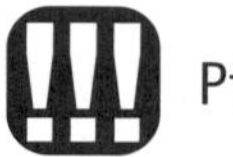

Pitfalls

DIAGNOSIS

Many products containing propoxyphene also contain acetaminophen or aspirin, and these coingestants may be overlooked.

TREATMENT

- Naloxone should not be used to treat cardiac conduction abnormalities.
- Large amounts of naloxone may be required to reverse the effects of propoxyphene intoxication causing hypotension or seizures.
- Due to short duration of action of naloxone, propoxyphene toxicity is likely to recur following naloxone administration.

ICD-9-CM 965.0

Poisoning by analgesics, antipyretics, and antirheumatics: opiates and related drugs.

See also: SECTION II, Hypotension, Seizures, and Ventricular Dysrhythmias chapters; SECTION III, Naloxone chapter; and SECTION IV, Acetaminophen and Salicylate chapters.

RECOMMENDED READING

POISINDEX Editorial Staff. Propoxyphene. In: Rumack BH, Sayre NK, Gelman CR, eds. *POISINDEX system.* Englewood, CO: Micromedex, Inc. (edition expires November 30, 1997).

Author: Lada Kokan

Reviewer: Katherine M. Hurlbut

Propylthiouracil

Basics

DESCRIPTION

Propylthiouracil (PTU) is an antithyroid agent used to treat hyperthyroidism, Graves' disease, and thyrotoxicosis.

FORMS AND USES

- PTU is available in 50-mg tablets.
- Pediatric dosage (>6 years of age) is 5 to 7 mg/kg/day divided every 6 to 8 hours.
- Adult dosage is 300 to 400 mg/day, up to 900 to 1,200 mg/day.
- Once an euthyroid state is achieved, the daily dose can usually be reduced and administered once daily.
- Clinical improvement usually begins within 24 to 36 hours of PTU initiation, and remissions usually require 1 to 2 years of therapy.
- Clinical improvement may be delayed until the stored supplies of thyroid hormone are used.

TOXIC DOSE

- The toxic dose after acute ingestion is unknown.
- A single ingestion of several grams has also proved nontoxic.
- Chronic administration of a therapeutic dose may rarely result in hepatitis.

PATHOPHYSIOLOGY

- PTU prevents the synthesis of thyroid hormone but does not block the release of previously synthesized and stored hormone.
- Toxicity is generally associated with chronic therapy.
- There are few reported cases of acute overdose.

EPIDEMIOLOGY

Poisoning is uncommon.

CAUSES

- Child neglect or abuse should be considered if the patient is less than 1 year of age, suicide attempt if the patient is over 6 years of age.

PREGNANCY AND LACTATION

- US FDA Pregnancy Category D. Evidence of human fetal risk exists, but benefits in certain situations (e.g., life-threatening situations or serious diseases) may make use of the drug acceptable despite its risks.
- Limited amounts of PTU are excreted in breast milk.
- Compared with methimazole, PTU is the preferred agent during breastfeeding because it has less of a tendency to cause neonatal hypothyroidism.
- Neonatal serum thyroxine and thyroid-stimulating hormone levels should be determined every 2 to 4 weeks during maternal therapy with PTU.

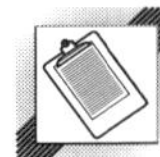

Diagnosis

SIGNS AND SYMPTOMS

Dermatologic

Rashes and alopecia have been reported with chronic therapy.

Cardiovascular

Vasculitides have been reported during chronic therapy.

Hematologic

Agranulocytosis, leukopenia, aplastic anemia, hemolytic anemia, and disseminated intravascular coagulation have been reported following chronic therapy but are rare.

Hepatic

Hepatotoxicity has been reported during chronic therapy and usually occurs within the first weeks to months of initiating treatment.

Musculoskeletal

Arthritis has been reported with chronic therapy.

Immunologic

Systemic lupus erythematosus occurs rarely during chronic therapy.

Endocrine

Hypothyroidism is a complication of chronic therapy.

PROCEDURES AND LABORATORY TESTS

Essential Tests

No tests are usually needed in asymptomatic patients.

Recommended Tests

- Serum liver enzymes should be monitored during chronic therapy to detect hepatitis.
- ECG, serum acetaminophen and aspirin levels should be checked in the overdose setting to detect occult ingestion.

Not Recommended Tests

PTU levels are usually not readily available or clinically useful.

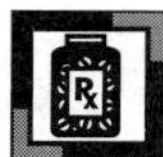

Treatment

- Treatment should focus on symptomatic and supportive care.
- The dose and time of exposure should be determined for all substances involved.

DIRECTING PATIENT COURSE

The health-care professional should call the poison control center when:

- Severe or persistent effects develop.
- Toxic effects are not consistent with PTU poisoning.
- Coingestant, drug interaction, or underlying disease presents an unusual problem.

The patient should be referred to a health-care facility when:

- Attempted suicide or homicide is possible.
- The patient or caregiver seems unreliable.
- Any toxic effects develop.
- Coingestant, drug interaction, or underlying disease presents an unusual problem.

Admission Considerations

Admission to the hospital is rarely needed.

DECONTAMINATION

Out of Hospital

Induced emesis is not recommended due to low toxic potential.

In Hospital

- Gastric lavage should be performed in pediatric (tube size 24–32 French) or adult (tube size 36–42 French) patients presenting within 1 hour of a large ingestion or if serious effects are present.
- One dose of activated charcoal (1–2 g/kg) should be administered without a cathartic if a substantial ingestion has occurred within the previous few hours.

ANTIDOTE

There is no specific antidote for PTU poisoning.

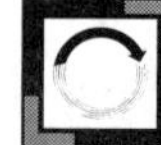

Follow-Up

PATIENT MONITORING

Patients on chronic therapy should have complete blood counts and liver function tests monitored regularly.

DISCHARGE CRITERIA/INSTRUCTIONS

- From the emergency department. Asymptomatic patients may be discharged following decontamination and psychiatric evaluation, if needed.
- From the hospital. Patients may be discharged when the toxic effects resolve.

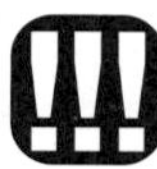

Pitfalls

FOLLOW-UP

- When treating thyrotoxicosis, the initial dose of PTU should be followed by administration of a dose of iodine in order to inhibit iodine utilization.
- Once a euthyroid state is maintained, administration of PTU should be withdrawn gradually and patients should be monitored closely for recurrence of hyperthyroidism.

ICD-9-CM 962.8

Poisoning by hormones and synthetic substitutes: antithyroid agents.

RECOMMENDED READINGS

POISINDEX Editorial staff. Propylthiouracil. In: Rumack BH, Toll LL, Gelman CR, eds. *POISINDEX system*. Englewood, CO: Micromedex, Inc. (edition expires August 31, 1997).

Author: Edwin K. Kuffner

Reviewer: Richard C. Dart

Psoralens

Basics

DESCRIPTION

Psoralens are used therapeutically in the treatment of psoriasis and vitiligo.

FORMS AND USES

- Methoxsalen (8-MOP, Oxsoralen) capsules: adult dose 10 to 70 mg orally 2 hours prior to ultraviolet (UV) light treatment.
- Trioxsalen (Trisoralen) capsules: adult dose 10 mg orally 2 to 4 hours prior to ultraviolet light treatment.
- Psoralens occur naturally in foods such as limes, figs, parsley, parsnips, mustard, carrots, and celery. Thus, patients may unintentionally expose themselves to additional sources of this substance.

TOXIC DOSE

Toxic doses have not been determined for these medications.

PATHOPHYSIOLOGY

- Psoralens are compounds that cause dermal photosensitivity.
- They are activated by UV light and bind to DNA, preventing cell replication.
- Psoralens are activated in the skin and produce little toxicity unless the person is exposed to UV light.
- Photosensitivity persists for up to 48 hours.

EPIDEMIOLOGY

Poisoning is uncommon.

CAUSES

- Poisoning is typically a therapeutic misadventure.
- Child neglect or abuse should be considered if the patient is less than 1 year of age, suicide attempt if the patient is over 6 years of age.

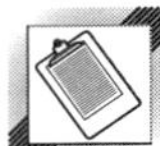

Diagnosis

DIFFERENTIAL DIAGNOSIS

- Toxic causes of skin injury include tetracyclines, antipsychotics, diuretics, oral hypoglycens, nonsteroidal antiinflammatory agents, antineoplastics, antihistamines, antidepressants, antihypertensives, many antibiotics, drug-induced Stevens-Johnson syndrome, and chemical burns.
- Nontoxic causes include Stevens-Johnson syndrome and environmental burns.

SIGNS AND SYMPTOMS

Dermatologic

- Increased sensitivity to UV light may result in skin burns.
- Redness and abnormal skin pigmentation can occur at therapeutic doses.
- Patients exposed to UV light in overdose may develop erythema, blisters, and bullae.

Gastrointestinal

Nausea and vomiting can occur in overdose and can occur with large therapeutic doses.

PROCEDURES AND LABORATORY TESTS

Essential Tests

No tests may be needed in asymptomatic patients.

Recommended Tests

- Serum electrolytes, BUN, creatinine, and glucose may be needed in severe cases.
- Serum acetaminophen and aspirin levels in an overdose setting are used to detect occult ingestion

Not Recommended Tests

Serum levels are not available.

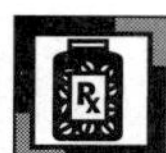

Treatment

- Supportive care and avoidance of UV light is the mainstay of therapy.
- Patients with extensive burns may require specialized burn care.
- Dose and time of exposure should be determined for all substances involved.

DIRECTING PATIENT COURSE

The health-care professional should call the poison control center when:

- Severe or persistent effects develop.
- Coingestant, drug interaction, or underlying disease presents an unusual problem.

The patient should be referred to a health-care facility when:

- Suicide or homicide attempt is possible.
- Toxic effects develop.
- Coingestant, drug interaction, or underlying disease presents an unusual problem.

Admission Considerations

Patients who may require specialized burn care (large area of involvement or possible third-degree burns) should be hospitalized.

DECONTAMINATION

- Gastric lavage is not recommended.
- One dose of activated charcoal (1–2 g/kg) should be administered without a cathartic if a substantial ingestion has occurred within the previous few hours.

ANTIDOTE

There is no specific antidote available for psoralen poisoning.

ADJUNCTIVE TREATMENT

Patient should be maintained in dark environment for 1 to 2 days to avoid UV light.

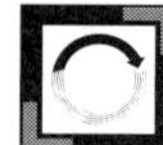

Follow-Up

EXPECTED COURSE AND PROGNOSIS

Skin burns heal gradually, depending on severity.

DISCHARGE CRITERIA/INSTRUCTIONS

- From the Emergency Department. Patient with known ingestion may be discharged after decontamination and psychiatric evaluation, if needed. However, patient should be kept in low UV light environment.
- From the Hospital. Patients may be discharged unless large area burns appear to be evolving.

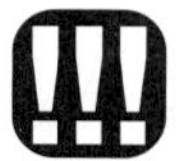

Pitfalls

DIAGNOSIS

Patients may develop skin reaction for several days following exposure.

ICD-9-CM 976

Poisoning by agents primarily affecting skin and mucous membrane: ophthalmological, otorhinolaryngological, and dental drugs.

RECOMMENDED READING

DRUGDEX Editorial Staff. Psoralens. In: Gelman CR, Rumack BH, Sayre NK, eds. *DRUGDEX system.* Englewood, CO: Micromedex, Inc. (edition expires November 30, 1997).

Author: Kennon Heard

Reviewer: Richard C. Dart

Pyrethrin/Pyrethrum

Basics

DESCRIPTION

- Pyrethrum refers to the crude extract made from the chrysanthemum plant.
- Refining of pyrethrum produces pyrethrin, an insecticide.
- Pyrethroids are totally synthetic insecticides similar to pyrethrin.

FORMS AND USES

- Synthetic products (pyrethroids) include Barthrin, Phenothrin, Resmethrin, Cypermethrin, Deltamethrin, Cyhalothrin, Fenvalerate, Cyfluthrinate, Cyfluthrin, Flucythrinate, Fenproponate, Fenproparthrin, Tralomethrin, and Tralocythrin.
- Naturally occurring products (pyrethrins) include Pyrethrin I, Pyrethrin II, Jasmolin I, Jasmolin II, Cinerin I, and Cinerin II.
- Pyrethrin and pyrethroid insecticides are characterized by their quick "knock down" insect toxicity.
- Pyrethrin and pyrethroid compounds are found in over 2,000 commercial compounds; many are marketed for home use, and the active ingredients may be in solution with hydrocarbon vehicles for spray use.

TOXIC DOSE

- Allergic reactions in susceptible individual may develop at any dose.
- Even large ingestions rarely produce toxicity.
- Oral toxic dose is estimated as 100 to 1,000 mg/kg.

PATHOPHYSIOLOGY

- Allergic reactions are the main toxic manifestations of pyrethrin exposure.
- Pyrethroids are less likely than pyrethrins to cause allergic reactions.
- Inhalation is the major route of exposure, and airway irritation is the primary toxic effect.
- Absorption is rapid and distribution is wide throughout all organ systems.
- Toxicity is usually limited because of rapid metabolism to nontoxic metabolites.
- Dermal or gastrointestinal absorption is possible, but toxicity rarely results.
- Carcinogenesis. Pyrethrins are categorized as IARC group 3: inadequate human evidence; inadequate animal evidence.

EPIDEMIOLOGY

- Exposure is common, but poisoning is rare.
- Toxic effects following exposure are typically mild.
- Children are considered more sensitive to pyrethrin exposure due to their inability to hydrolyze pyrethrin esters effectively.
- Death may occur after a massive ingestion.

CAUSES

- Poisoning usually occurs via inhalation exposures.
- Accidental ingestions also have been reported.
- Child abuse or neglect should be considered if the patient is less than 1 year of age; suicide attempt should be considered in patients over 6 years of age.

RISK FACTORS

- Occupations at risk for exposure are pesticide applicators, exterminators, and farmers.
- Individuals with ragweed allergy or history of severe environmental allergies are at increased risk for toxicity.

PREGNANCY AND LACTATION

- US FDA Pregnancy Category C. The drug exerts animal teratogenic or embryocidal effects, but there are no controlled studies in women, or no studies are available in either animals or women.
- No data exist on pregnancy complications other than the possibility of allergic reactions.

WORKPLACE STANDARDS

For pyrethrum:

- ACGIH. TLV TWA is 5 mg/m^3.
- OSHA. PEL TWA is 5 mg/m^3.
- NIOSH. REL is 5 mg/m^3; IDLH value is 5,000 mg/m^3.

Diagnosis

DIFFERENTIAL DIAGNOSIS

Toxic causes of acute respiratory irritation include acetylene, ammonia, carbon disulfide, chloramine, chlorine, chloroacetophenone (Mace), fluorine, hydrogen chloride, hydrogen fluoride, hydrogen sulfide, methyl bromide, methyl chloride, methyl iodide, and sulfur dioxide.

SIGNS AND SYMPTOMS

- Acute toxicity is usually attributable to irritant and sensitization properties.
- Respiratory system toxicity may develop because of mucous membrane and upper airway irritation.
- Contact and allergic dermatitis can occur.
- Massive ingestion (e.g., inadvertently preparing food in pyrethroid product) may cause headaches, fasciculation, and seizures.
- Chronic exposure may cause allergic dermatitis.
- Chronic dermal or inhalation exposure may lead to hypersensitivity reactions.
- Asthma or reactive airways disease syndrome is possible, as is hypersensitivity pneumonitis with chest pain, cough, dyspnea, and bronchospasm.

HEENT

- Following inhalation, a stuffy, runny nose and scratchy throat are common.
- Hypersensitivity reactions may occur, including wheezing, sneezing, shortness of breath, and bronchospasm.
- Eye exposures may result in mild to severe corneal damage, probably due to organic-solvent carrier.

Dermatologic

Contact dermatitis can occur with burning, intense pruritus and blistering, tingling, numbness, and erythema.

Pulmonary

- Inhalation may cause localized symptoms such as rhinitis, sneezing, throat irritation, laryngeal edema, and oral mucosal edema.
- Lower respiratory tract symptoms may include cough, shortness of breath, wheezing, and chest pain. Pulmonary edema is possible.
- Symptoms are enhanced in individuals sensitive to ragweed pollen (due to cross-sensitivity as ragweed) or having a strong allergic profile.

Gastrointestinal

Nausea, vomiting, cramping, diarrhea, and anorexia may occur.

Hematologic

Henoch-Schönlein purpura is a rare complication.

Neurologic

- CNS stimulation, numbness, tremors, incoordination, paralysis, seizures, and coma can occur following massive exposure.
- Stinging sensation of extremities in a stocking-and-glove distribution may occur.
- A large ingestion (200–500 cc) of concentrated formulations may cause coma and seizures within 20 minutes.

PROCEDURES AND LABORATORY TESTS

Essential Tests

No tests are usually needed for minimally symptomatic patients because most exposures involve limited local allergic reactions that can be diagnosed from the clinical examination.

Recommended Tests

- Peak flow measurements may be helpful to assess pulmonary function.
- In the rare case of severe toxicity, other tests, including complete blood count, serum electrolytes, BUN, creatinine, arterial blood gas, pulse oximetry, ECG, and chest radiograph, may be indicated.
- A chest radiograph is indicated for patients with severe respiratory exposures who have abnormal pulmonary examination results, tachypnea, or hypoxic or respiratory distress; it also may help evaluate the extent of injury and development of pulmonary edema.

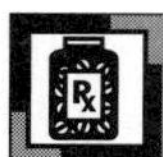

Treatment

- Treatment should focus on supportive respiratory care with provision of supplemental oxygen and airway management.
- Dose and time of exposure should be determined for all substances involved.

DIRECTING PATIENT COURSE

The health-care provider should call the poison control center when:

- Respiratory symptoms, altered mental status, or other severe effects are present.
- Toxic effects are not consistent with a simple upper respiratory irritant.
- Coingestant, drug interaction, or underlying disease presents an unusual problem.

The patient should be referred to a health-care facility when:

- Attempted suicide or homicide is possible.
- Patient or caregiver seems unreliable.
- Symptoms are present.
- Toxic effects are not consistent with a simple upper respiratory irritant.
- Coingestant, drug interaction, or underlying disease presents an unusual problem.

Admission Considerations

Inpatient management may be warranted for patients with persistent symptoms after exposure despite therapy.

DECONTAMINATION

Out of Hospital

- Emesis should not be induced routinely due to low toxicity of ingested pyrethrins.
- The patient should be removed from the source of exposure.

In Hospital

- Aspiration of gastric contents with a nasogastric tube may be used for the rare case of massive ingestion, especially if serious effects are present.
- One dose of activated charcoal (1–2 g/kg) should be administered if a substantial ingestion has occurred within the previous few hours.

ANTIDOTES

There is no specific antidote for pyrethrin or pyrethroid poisoning.

ADJUNCTIVE TREATMENT

Bronchospasm is treated as follows:

- Oxygen is administered, followed by albuterol, 0.15 mg/kg (maximum 10 mg) in saline with humidified oxygen via nebulizer every 20 to 30 minutes.

—The peak expiratory flow rate is often an objective indicator of the response to therapy.

—The response should be continually monitored.

- Methylprednisolone may be administered intravenously every 6 to 8 hours: adult dose, 1.0 to 1.5 mg/kg; pediatric dose, 1 to 2 mg/kg. This may be decreased to a single daily dose and tapered.
- Initiation of prednisone, 1 to 2 mg/kg orally for several days, may be considered for patients with severe bronchospasm or a history of asthma.

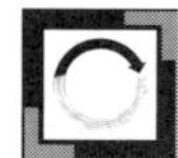

Follow-Up

PATIENT MONITORING

- Respiratory function should be monitored in symptomatic patients.
- Continuous cardiopulmonary monitoring should be performed in severe cases.

EXPECTED COURSE AND PROGNOSIS

- Respiratory effects develop soon after exposure, peak within an hour, and recover over hours to days with therapy.
- Dermal effects may take days to weeks for resolution.
- Long-term pulmonary or dermal allergic sensitization may be a complication.
- Chronic exposure may cause reactive airway disease.
- Occupational asthma from pyrethrin has been reported in exterminators and farmers.
- Sequelae of hypoxia or hypotension may occur in rare, life-threatening cases.

DISCHARGE CRITERIA/INSTRUCTIONS

From the emergency department or hospital. Asymptomatic patients may be discharged following decontamination, 4 to 6 hours of observation, and psychiatric evaluation, if needed.

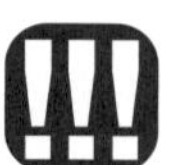

Pitfalls

DIAGNOSIS

- The possibility of coingestants should be considered, such as hydrocarbons and organophosphate or carbamate insecticides.
- It is important to observe the patient for 4 to 6 hours for the development of delayed pulmonary symptoms.

TREATMENT

It should not be assumed that pesticide exposure with respiratory symptoms is caused by an organophosphate or carbamate.

FOLLOW-UP

- It is important to arrange for a follow-up visit with an allergy/ immunology specialist for all patients with severe allergic symptoms.
- Delayed hypersensitivity to an acute exposure may develop, and patients should be instructed to avoid future exposures.

ICD-9-CM 989.4

Toxic effect of other substances, chiefly nonmedicinal as to source: other pesticides, not elsewhere classified.

RECOMMENDED READING

Dorman DC, Beasley VR. Neurotoxicology of pyrethrin and the pyrethroid insecticides. *Vet Hum Toxicol* 1991;33:238–243.

Paton DL, Walker JS. Pyrethrin poisoning from commercial-strength flea and tick spray. *Am J Emerg Med* 1988:6:232–235.

Ray DE. Pesticides derived from plants and other organisms. In: Hayes WJ, Laws ER, eds. *Handbook of pesticide toxicology.* San Diego: Academic, 1991:585–599.

Author: Alvin C. Bronstein

Reviewer: Gerald F. O'Malley

Pyrrolizidine Alkaloids

Basics

DESCRIPTION

- Pyrrolizidine alkaloids, also known as Senecio alkaloids, are found in more than 6,000 plant species worldwide.
- Human exposure is primarily limited to a few species: comfrey (*Symphytium*), groundsel, *Heliotroprium*, ragwort (*Senecio*), and coltsfoot (*Tussilago*).

FORMS AND USES

- There are no pharmaceutical-grade preparations.
- Herbs containing pyrrolizidine alkaloids are widely used in folk or "traditional" medicine for gastrointestinal complaints, infant colic, arthritis, sprains, bruises, and local wound care.
- Younger plants, roots, and seeds tend to have higher concentrations of alkaloid.
- Herbal teas concentrate toxins from the plant in hot water.
- The herbs are taken orally, topically, or as an enema.
- Honey from flowers has proven to be hepatotoxic.

TOXIC DOSES

- Toxic doses in nonfatal disease have ranged from 2 to 27 mg alkaloid/kg of body weight, and from 6 to 167 mg alkaloid/kg of body weight in fatal cases.
- Ingestion over several days or weeks is usually required to produce toxicity.

PATHOPHYSIOLOGY

- Pyrrolizidine alkaloids are metabolized by the liver to alkylating agents that cross-link DNA.
- Large acute (over several days) or chronic ingestion may cause centrilobular venoocclusive disease of the liver, followed by parenchymal necrosis and liver failure. In addition, chronic ingestion may produce venoocclusive disease of the lung (pulmonary hypertension).
- The substance is carcinogenic in all animal models; no long-term information in humans is available, but pyrrolizidine alkaloids are believed to be carcinogenic.

EPIDEMIOLOGY

- Poisoning is rare in developed countries.
- Toxicity is delayed weeks to months in chronic exposure, whereas acute ingestion manifests within days.
- Epidemics have followed contamination of grain stores in endemic areas.
- Death is common in patients who develop liver failure.

CAUSES

Toxicity usually occurs via accidental ingestion from contaminated food stores or from inadvertent poisoning from herbal remedies.

RISK FACTORS

- Young children are more susceptible to poisoning from pyrrolizidine alkaloids.
- Geriatric patients are at increased risk of toxicity due to decreased hepatic and renal function.

DRUG AND DISEASE INTERACTIONS

- Pyrrolizidine alkaloids act synergistically with aflatoxin and hepatitis B virus.
- Malnutrition may potentiate the action of pyrrolizidine alkaloids.

PREGNANCY AND LACTATION

- US FDA Pregnancy Category X. Studies have demonstrated fetal abnormalities or there is evidence of fetal risk based on human experience, or both, and the risk clearly outweighs any possible benefit.
- Transplacental toxicity with fatal infant disease has been reported.

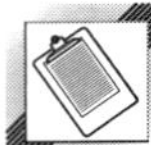

Diagnosis

DIFFERENTIAL DIAGNOSIS

- Toxicologic causes of acute hepatitis include acetaminophen, *Amanita* mushroom, yellow phosphorus, and carbon tetrachloride.
- Nontoxicologic causes of acute hepatitis include high-dose chemotherapy and bone marrow transplantation, Budd-Chiari syndrome, Reye's syndrome, infectious or alcoholic hepatitis, and others.
- Nontoxicologic causes of chronic hepatitis include hepatitis B, hepatitis C, autoimmune disease, and Wilson's disease.

SIGNS AND SYMPTOMS

- The liver is the principal target organ.
- After acute ingestion, onset of symptoms is typically remote by days from the ingestion, and the clinical picture is similar to that of Reye's syndrome.
- Onset is more insidious in chronic ingestion.

Vital Signs

- Tachypnea may occur.
- Fever is rare.

Dermatologic

Jaundice is a rare and inconstant finding.

Cardiovascular

- Right ventricular hypertrophy has been reported in animal models.
- Fibrosis of large venous vessels has occurred in humans.

Pulmonary

- Pulmonary hypertension and cor pulmonale may follow chronic ingestion.
- Alveolar edema and effusions have been reported.

Gastrointestinal

- In the acute form, gastroenteritis and abdominal pain develop unexpectedly over several days with rapidly developing ascites and hepatosplenomegaly.
- Chronic toxicity may result in hematemesis due to portal hypertension.
- Anorexia and weight loss are common to both acute and chronic forms.

Hepatic

- The hallmark of toxicity is centrilobular hepatic venoocclusive disease.
- The insidious development of ascites is associated with chronic ingestion.
- Chronic toxicity may cause signs of portal hypertension (prominent abdominal veins, ascites).

Renal

- Glomerulonephritis has been reported.
- Oliguria may occur in acute disease.

Fluids and Electrolytes

- Hypernatremia and hyperkalemia have both been described.
- Hypoglycemia may occur if liver failure develops.

Neurologic

Seizures, lassitude, and headache leading to encephalopathy from hepatic failure may develop.

Endocrine

Pancreatic lesions have been found.

PROCEDURES AND LABORATORY TESTS

Essential Tests

No tests may be needed in asymptomatic patients.

Recommended Tests

- Liver function tests and serum amylase in symptomatic patients are used to assess and monitor liver injury.
- Complete blood count, serum electrolytes, BUN, creatinine, glucose, and urinalysis are used to detect complications of liver injury.
- Abdominal CT or ultrasonography is used to evaluate other causes of hepatic injury.
- Liver biopsy is used to establish the diagnosis.
- Other tests. Testing of the plant or herbal preparation for alkaloid content has been used to confirm the source of toxicity.

Not Recommended Tests

Blood levels are not available.

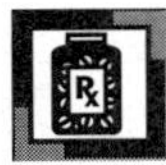

Treatment

- Treatment should focus on supportive measures for hepatic failure and removal of plant material.
- Dose, time of exposure, and method of preparation should be determined for all substances involved.
- Family members or friends who may have been exposed also may need to be examined.

DIRECTING PATIENT COURSE

The health-care provider should call the poison control center when:

- Hepatic failure or other severe effects are present.
- Toxic effects are not consistent with pyrrolizidine alkaloid poisoning.
- Coingestant, drug interaction, or underlying disease presents an unusual problem.

The patient should be referred to a health-care facility when:

- Patient or caregiver seems unreliable.
- Hepatic or pulmonary failure or other severe effects are present.
- Toxic effects are not consistent with pyrrolizidine alkaloid toxicity.
- Coingestant, drug interaction or underlying disease presents an unusual problem.

Admission Considerations

Inpatient management is warranted for patients with hepatic injury, respiratory distress, protracted vomiting, or hematemesis.

DECONTAMINATION

Most cases involve chronic ingestion, rendering gastrointestinal decontamination unnecessary.

Out of Hospital

Emesis should be induced with ipecac within 1 hour of ingestion for alert pediatric or adult patients if an acute, single ingestion has occurred.

In Hospital

- Ipecac-induced emesis is used within 1 hour of an acute, single ingestion in pediatric patients who are too small to have effective gastric lavage.
- Gastric lavage should be performed in pediatric (tube size 24–32 French) or adult (tube size 36–42 French) patients presenting within 1 hour of a large ingestion or if serious effects are present.
- One dose of activated charcoal (1–2 g/kg) should be administered without a cathartic if a substantial single ingestion has occurred within the previous few hours.

ANTIDOTES

There is no specific antidote for pyrrolizidine alkaloid poisoning.

ADJUNCTIVE TREATMENT

- Supportive therapy for hepatic failure will be needed in severe cases.
- A surgical portosystemic shunt may be required in severe cases.
- A patient with hepatic failure should be evaluated for liver transplantation.

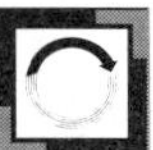

Follow-Up

PATIENT MONITORING

Patients with fulminant hepatic failure should have continuous respiratory and cardiac monitoring, frequent glucose levels, and daily levels of electrolyte and coagulation studies.

EXPECTED COURSE AND PROGNOSIS

- Course of illness is unpredictable; onset of symptoms varies between 19 days and 2 years.
- Progression to hepatic failure following a single ingestion is unusual, but has occurred.
- Mild illness tends to recover with minimal sequelae.
- Severe hepatotoxicity from chronic ingestion usually results in death.

DISCHARGE CRITERIA/INSTRUCTIONS

- From the emergency department

—Asymptomatic patients may be discharged with normal laboratory values and a reliable caregiver.
—Follow-up care should be arranged for evaluation of possible continuing or delayed liver injury.

- From the hospital

—Asymptomatic patients may be discharged with stable vital signs and stable or recovering liver function tests.
—Follow-up care should be arranged for evaluation of possible continuing liver injury.

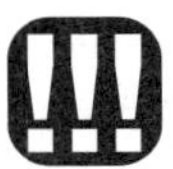

Pitfalls

DIAGNOSIS

- It is important to consider this cause of hepatotoxicity in patients taking herbal medication, with recent travel history to endemic areas or in outbreaks of hepatic failure.
- Use of herbal preparations in the recommended manner can result in toxic doses.

ICD-9-CM 988

Toxic effect of noxious substances eaten as food.

RECOMMENDED READING

Fox DW, Hart MC, Bergeson PS, et al. Pyrrolizidine (Senecio) intoxication mimicking Reye syndrome. *J Pediatr* 1978;93:980–982.

Ridker PM, Ohkuma S, McDermott NV, et al. Hepatic venocclusive disease associated with the consumption of pyrrolizidine-containing dietary supplements. *Gastroenterology* 1985;88:1050–1054.

Author: Michael Stackpool

Reviewer: Katherine M. Hurlbut

Quinine

Basics

DESCRIPTION

Quinine is an over-the-counter and prescription medication with a bitter taste that is derived from the bark of the cinchona tree.

FORMS AND USES

- Used to alleviate nighttime leg cramps: adult dose 260 mg orally at bedtime.
- Used rarely as an illicit abortifacient and to induce labor.
- Pharmaceutical preparations include:

—Quinine sulfate tablets or capsules
—Urea hydrochloride 5% for injection
—Quinine acid sulfate
—Quinine and aminophylline
—Quinine bisulfate

- Plants. Bark of the South American cinchona tree.
- Other. Quinine in tonic water at concentration of 50 mg/L.
- Used in the past as a type 1a antidysrhythmic agent and as an antimalarial agent.

TOXIC DOSE

Death in adults has followed the ingestion of 5 to 10 g, but symptoms may develop with 2 to 3 g.

PATHOPHYSIOLOGY

- Severe, intense flushing and pruritus is thought to be mediated by histamine release.
- Ocular toxicity is caused by a direct toxic effect on the retina.
- Cinchonism is a syndrome caused by "quinidine-like" drugs (derived from the cinchona tree), which is characterized by headache, fever, mydriasis, and tinnitus; transient or permanent blindness may develop.
- Type 1a antiarrhythmic, anticholinergic, and α-adrenergic effects may all contribute to cardiotoxicity.
- Antibodies to various blood elements have been found in individuals who developed the hemolytic uremic syndrome (HUS).

EPIDEMIOLOGY

- Poisoning is uncommon.
- Quinine has produced toxicity when used as an adulterant in street drugs.

CAUSES

- Toxic ingestion is usually intentional.
- Child neglect or abuse should be considered if the patient is less than 1 year of age; suicide attempt should be considered if the patient is over 6 years of age.

DRUG AND DISEASE INTERACTIONS

- Hepatic disease may increase toxicity by decreasing elimination.
- Glucose-6-phosphate dehydrogenase deficiency is a risk factor for quinine-induced hemolytic anemia.
- Preexisting cardiac conduction disturbances increase the risk of dysrhythmia.
- Pediatric patients have increased likelihood for seizures.
- Prochlorperazine may prolong the QTc interval seen on an ECG without increasing the quinine level.

PREGNANCY AND LACTATION

- US FDA Pregnancy Category D. Evidence of human fetal risk exists, but benefits in certain situations (e.g., life-threatening situations or serious diseases) may make use of the drug acceptable despite its risks.
- Intravenous administration leads to hyperinsulinemia and hypoglycemia during pregnancy.
- Quinine is a proven abortifacient and teratogen.
- Concentration in breast milk does not reach levels harmful to a nursing infant.

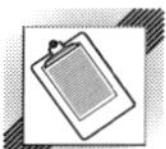

Diagnosis

DIFFERENTIAL DIAGNOSIS

Acute Visual Disturbance

- Toxic causes include digoxin, methanol, and methylmercury, among others.
- Nontoxic causes include amaurosis fugax, central retinal artery or vein occlusion, glaucoma, multiple sclerosis, and optic neuritis.

Tinnitus and Auditory Toxicity

- Toxic causes include furosemide, acetazolamide, aminoglycosides, salicylates, carbon monoxide, and heavy metals.
- Nontoxic causes include otitis media, mumps, penetrating trauma, barotrauma, and Ménière's disease.

SIGNS AND SYMPTOMS

- Severity of toxic effects is largely dose dependent.
- Cinchonism involves vomiting, decreased visual acuity, tinnitus, deafness, and headache following quinine ingestion.
- Severe toxicity may cause hypotension and syncope from ventricular dysrhythmias.

Vital Signs

- Tachycardia is typical, although bradycardia with heart block may occur.
- Blood pressure is usually normal or hypotensive.

HEENT

- Decreased visual acuity, which may suddenly progress to blindness, may develop.
- Tinnitus and reversible hearing loss may occur at therapeutic doses. High-pitched tones are affected first; by the time conversational hearing loss occurs, it may be permanent.

Dermatologic

- Photosensitivity reactions may occur with flushing and severe pruritus.
- Topical preparations may cause contact dermatitis.

Cardiovascular

Prolongation of PR, QRS, and QT intervals degenerating into ventricular tachycardia, torsade de pointes, and fibrillation may follow severe overdose.

Pulmonary

Respiratory depression and pulmonary edema may follow overdose.

Gastrointestinal

Vomiting, diarrhea, and abdominal pain are common.

Renal

- HUS may cause acute renal failure.
- Acute interstitial nephritis also has been reported.

Hematologic

Pancytopenia, coagulopathy, and disseminated intravascular coagulation have occurred, usually in association with HUS.

Neurologic

Ataxia, paresthesia, CNS depression, and seizures may occur.

Endocrine

Quinine can be associated with hyperinsulinemia, especially in pregnancy.

PROCEDURES AND LABORATORY TESTS

Essential Tests

ECG with continuous monitoring assesses QRS widening, QT prolongation, and ST- and T-wave abnormalities; QTc prolongation of more than 50% is associated with torsades de pointes.

Recommended Tests

- Complete blood count is used to follow platelets and hemoglobin if HUS is suspected.
- Serum electrolytes, glucose, BUN, creatinine, calcium, magnesium, and phosphorous assess other causes of dysrhythmia and renal dysfunction; hypoglycemia may develop.
- Serum acetaminophen and aspirin levels are measured in an overdose setting to detect occult ingestion.

• Pregnancy test is conducted owing to the risk of toxicity during pregnancy.
• Glucose-6-phosphate dehydrogenase quantitative assay is used if deficiency state is suspected.
• Head CT, lumbar puncture, bacterial cultures, and other tests are used to evaluate other causes of altered mental status.
• Visual acuity and ophthalmologic evaluation are used to assess visual abnormalities.
• Audiometry testing is used to assess hearing abnormality.

Not Recommended Tests

Blood levels of quinine are not clinically useful.

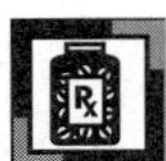

Treatment

• Therapy should focus on general supportive care, prompt treatment of dysrhythmias, and close monitoring of the airway.
• Dose and time of exposure should be determined for all substances involved.

DIRECTING PATIENT COURSE

The health-care provider should call the poison control center when:

• Life-threatening effects are present.
• Toxic effects are not consistent with quinine poisoning.
• Coingestant, drug interaction, or underlying disease presents an unusual problem.

The patient should be referred to a health-care facility when:

• Attempted suicide or homicide is possible.
• Patient or caregiver seems unreliable.
• Toxic effects have developed.
• Coingestant, drug interaction, or underlying disease presents an unusual problem.

Admission Considerations

Inpatient management is warranted if the patient exhibits neurologic, ocular, auditory, respiratory, hematologic, renal, or cardiac toxicity.

DECONTAMINATION

Out of Hospital

Emesis should not be induced; coma or seizure may develop abruptly.

In Hospital

• Gastric lavage should be performed in pediatric (tube size 24–32 French) or adult (tube size 36–42 French) patients presenting within 1 hour of a large ingestion or if serious effects are present.
• One dose of activated charcoal (1–2 g/kg) should be administered if a substantial ingestion has occurred within the previous few hours.

ANTIDOTES

There is no specific antidote for quinine toxicity.

ADJUNCTIVE TREATMENT

• The use of type 1a antiarrhythmic agents should be avoided.
• Multiple-dose activated charcoal enhances quinine elimination, but has not been shown to affect outcome.

Bradydysrhythmia

• Standard agents, including atropine and isoproterenol, are usually ineffective.
• Early use of a pacemaker is recommended.

Ventricular Dysrhythmias

• For stable patients, drug therapy should be initiated.
• For hypotensive patients, the Advanced Cardiac Life Support (ACLS) algorithm should be used: defibrillation followed by pharmacologic therapy. See also SECTION II, Ventricular Dysrhythmia chapter.

Torsade de Pointes

• For hypotensive patients, the ACLS algorithm should be used.
• For stable patients, electrolyte abnormalities should be corrected and magnesium sulfate administered.
• Quinidine, disopyramide, procainamide, amiodarone, and bretylium should be avoided; these drugs also prolong the QT interval.
• Isoproterenol is used to increase the heart rate.
• If rhythm is unresponsive, cardiac overdrive pacing may be required.

Hypotension

• Primary treatment is correction of dysrhythmia.
• Ten to 20 ml/kg 0.9% saline should be administered, along with a vasopressor if one is needed. Dopamine is preferred due to ready availability. Norepinephrine may be added in refactory cases.

Seizures

• Patent airway should be assured.
• A benzodiazepine should be used for initial control.
• If seizures persist, another anticonvulsant such as phenobarbital may be added.

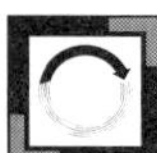

Follow-Up

PATIENT MONITORING

Cardiac and respiratory function should be monitored continuously in all patients with suspected quinine toxicity.

EXPECTED COURSE AND PROGNOSIS

• Blindness and deafness may be partial or complete, permanent or temporary.
• Recovery otherwise is likely to be complete with timely, supportive care.

DISCHARGE CRITERIA/INSTRUCTIONS

• From the emergency department. Asymptomatic patients can be discharged following decontamination, cardiac monitoring for 6 to 8 hours, and psychiatric evaluation, if needed.
• From the hospital. Patients can be discharged after toxic effects have resolved or stabilized and psychiatric evaluation is complete, if needed.

PATIENT EDUCATION

Patients with dermatologic toxicity due to quinine should be cautioned to avoid sunlight as well as ingestion of tonic water.

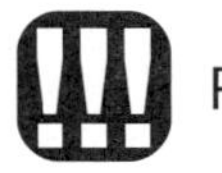

Pitfalls

DIAGNOSIS

Symptoms of cinchonism can be vague and overlooked.

ICD-9-CM 961.4

Poisoning by antiinfectives: antimalarials and drugs acting on other blood protozoa.

See also: SECTION II, Bradycardia, Hypotension, Seizures, and Ventricular Dysrhythmias chapters.

RECOMMENDED READING

Smilkstein MJ. Ophthalmologic principles. In: Goldfrank LR, et al., eds. *Goldfrank's toxicologic emergencies,* 6th ed. Norwalk, CT: Appleton & Lange, 1998.

Wolf LR, Otten EJ, Spadafora MP. Cinchonism: two case reports and review of acute quinine toxicity and treatment. *J Emerg Med* 1992;10:295–301.

Authors: Lada Kokan and Gerald F. O'Malley

Reviewer: Steven A. Seifert

Reserpine

Basics

DESCRIPTION

- Reserpine is an antihypertensive or a sedative medication.
- It also may be included with diuretic or other antihypertensive agents in combination products (e.g., reserpine and hydrochlorothiazide).

FORMS AND USES

- Formulations include Reserpine, Serpasil, and the plants, snake root, Rauwolfia alkaloids, and *Rauwolfia serpentina.*
- Combination products include Diupres, Hydropres, Ser-Ap-Es, Diutensen-R, Regroton, Demi-Regroton, Reserpine & Chlorothiazole, Salutensin, and Salutensin-Demi.
- As an antihypertensive, reserpine is prescribed at 0.5 mg/day orally, titrated to effect; the dose usually needs to be decreased after several days.
- Snake root tea is an herbal preparation used as a sedative.

TOXIC DOSE

The toxic dose has not been established, but coma for several days after a pediatric ingestion of 25 mg has been reported.

PATHOPHYSIOLOGY

- Reserpine depletes neurotransmitters from adrenergic neurons and serotonergic neurons.
- The decreased stores of catecholamine reduces sympathetic nervous system tone and thereby decreases blood pressure.
- In an overdose, depletion of catechols and serotonin results in hypotension and CNS depression.

EPIDEMIOLOGY

Poisoning is uncommon.

CAUSES

Child neglect or abuse should be considered if the patient is less than 1 year of age, suicide attempt if the patient is over 6 years of age.

PREGNANCY AND LACTATION

US FDA Pregnancy Category C. The drug exerts animal teratogenic or embryocidal effects, but there are no controlled studies in women, or no studies are available in animals or women.

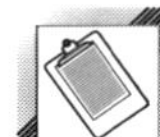

Diagnosis

DIFFERENTIAL DIAGNOSIS

Toxicologic causes of hypertension and hypotension associated with CNS depression include tricylic antidepressants, MAO inhibitors, and many others.

SIGNS AND SYMPTOMS

Hypotension and CNS depression predominate.

Vital Signs

- Initial tachycardia and hypertension can occur, followed by bradycardia and hypotension.
- Hypothermia has been reported.

HEENT

- Rhinorrhea has been reported.
- Nonreactive pupils may be observed.

Cardiovascular

Initial release of catecholamines may cause hypertension and tachycardia lasting up to 24 hours, followed by hypotension and hemodynamic collapse in severe cases.

Pulmonary

Respiratory depression may occur.

Gastrointestinal

Vomiting and diarrhea can occur with overdose.

Neurologic

- Somnolence progressing to coma occurs with overdose.
- Parkinson's disease has been reported during therapy.

Psychiatric

Reserpine can cause depression during therapeutic use.

PROCEDURES AND LABORATORY TESTS

Essential Tests

No tests may be needed in asymptomatic patients.

Recommended Tests

- Pulse oximetry or arterial blood gas analysis to evaluate oxygenation
- ECG to evaluate for heart block, to evaluate other causes of bradycardia
- Serum electrolytes, glucose, BUN, creatinine, and other studies as indicated to evaluate other causes of altered mental status
- Serum acetaminophen and aspirin levels in overdose setting to detect occult ingestion
- Serum catecholamines are increased for several days following ingestion, but levels are not clinically useful.

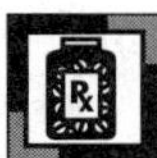

Treatment

- Supportive care is mainstay of therapy.
- Dose and time of exposure should be determined for all substances involved.

DIRECTING PATIENT COURSE

The health-care professional should call the poison control center when:

- Severe or persistent effects develop.
- Coingestant, drug interaction, or underlying disease presents an unusual problem.

The patient should be referred to a health-care facility when:

- Suicide or homicide attempt is possible.
- Toxic effects develop.
- Coingestant, drug interaction, or underlying disease presents an unusual problem.

Admission Considerations

Patients with symptoms or those with potentially toxic ingestion should be admitted.

DECONTAMINATION

Out of Hospital

Emesis should be induced with ipecac within 1 hour of ingestion for alert pediatric or adult patient if vomiting has not occurred and health-care evaluation will be delayed.

In Hospital

- Gastric lavage should be performed in pediatric (tube size 24–32 French) or adult (tube size 36–42 French) patients presenting within 1 hour of a large ingestion or if serious effects are present.
- One dose of activated charcoal (1–2 g/kg) should be administered without a cathartic if a substantial ingestion has occurred within the previous few hours.

ANTIDOTE

There is no specific antidote for reserpine poisoning.

ADJUNCTIVE TREATMENT

- Patients should be placed on a cardiac monitor, receive oxygen, and have intravenous access established.
- Symptomatic bradycardia should be treated with atropine and pacing.
- Hypotension is treated with infusion of 0.9% saline 10 to 20 ml/kg and Trendelenburg positioning. If blood pressure is unresponsive, dopamine may be infused at 2 to 5 μg/kg/min and titrated upward to 20 μg/kg/min to effect.
- Hypertension. If end-organ damage develops (rare), treatment is initiated with a titratable antihypertensive such as nitroprusside.

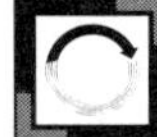

Follow-Up

PATIENT MONITORING

- Respiratory and cardiac function should be monitored continuously in symptomatic patients.
- Because the action of reserpine may be prolonged, patients with potentially significant ingestion should be monitored for 24 hours.

EXPECTED COURSE AND PROGNOSIS

- Toxic effects typically occur within 24 hours.
- Complete recovery is anticipated unless sequelae of hypoxia intercede.

DISCHARGE CRITERIA/INSTRUCTIONS

Patients with stable vital signs and normal mental status after 24-hour observation may be discharged from the hospital.

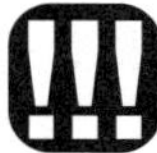

Pitfalls

TREATMENT

Hypertension may resolve and be followed by hypotension; thus, only short-acting antihypertensives should be used.

FOLLOW-UP

Reserpine should be avoided in patients with a history of depression.

ICD-9-CM 972.6

Poisoning by agents primarily affecting the cardiovascular system: other hypertensive agents.

See also: SECTION II, Bradycardia, Hypertension, and Hypotension chapters; Section III, Nitroprusside.

RECOMMENDED READING

Pfeifer HJ, Greenblatt DK, Koch-Wester J. Clinical toxicity of reserpine in hospitalized patients: a report from the Boston Collaborative Drug Survellaince Program. *Am J Med Sci* 1976;271:269–276.

Author: Kennon Heard

Reviewer: Richard C. Dart

Rifampin

Basics

DESCRIPTION

Rifampin is an oral antimicrobial used in the treatment of tuberculosis or *Neisseria meningitidis*.

FORMS AND USES

- Rifampin (Rifadin, Rimactane, and others): 150- and 300-mg capsules; for intravenous injection, available in a 600-mg ampule.
- Rifamate: rifampin (300 mg) with isoniazid (150 mg).
- Rifater: rifampin (120 mg) with isoniazid (50 mg) and pyrazinamide (300 mg).
- Rifampim used in combination therapy with other antimicrobials for tuberculosis

—Adult, 600 mg by mouth daily
—Pediatric, 10 to 20 mg/kg day (maximum dosage 600 mg/day)

- Prophylactic treatment of *N. meningitidis* (bacterial meningitis) exposures

—Adult, 600 mg by mouth twice a day for 2 days
—Pediatric
—Children under 1 month of age, 5 mg/kg twice a day for 2 days
—Children 1 month to 12 years of age, 10 mg/kg twice a day for 2 days (maximum dosage 600 mg/day)

TOXIC DOSE

Toxicity occurs with ingestion of more than 100 mg/kg/day by an adult or child.

PATHOPHYSIOLOGY

- The primary target organs are the gastrointestinal tract and liver.
- The most serious toxicity involves hepatic injury and jaundice, usually in patients with preexisting liver disease.
- The parent form of the drug is the toxic species; therefore, decreased hepatic function leads to accumulation of the parent compound and liver injury.
- Rifampin is widely distributed into most body tissues and fluids, discoloring tears, urine, and other secretions and excretory products with a red-orange tint.
- Rifampin is a potent inducer of the hepatic microenzyme system (CYP3A).

EPIDEMIOLOGY

- Poisoning is uncommon.
- Toxic effects following exposure are typically mild to moderate.
- Death is rare.

CAUSES

- Toxic ingestion is usually accidental.
- Child abuse or neglect must be considered if the patient is less than 1 year of age; a suicide attempt should be considered if the patient is over 6 years of age.

RISK FACTORS

Geriatric patients are at increased risk for liver injury.

DRUG AND DISEASE INTERACTIONS

- Coingestion with other hepatotoxic drugs increases risk.
- Fatalities are associated with preexisting liver disease, alcoholism, or lack of previous use of rifampin (no enzyme induction present as seen in chronic use).
- Chronic rifampin therapy may reduce the concentration of the following drugs metabolized by the cytochrome P450 system: oral anticoagulants, barbiturates, β-receptor blockers, clofibrate, oral contraceptives, corticosteroids, cyclosporine, dapsone, digitoxin, disopyramide, ethanol, fluconazole, halothane, oral hypoglycemics, ketoconazole, methadone, mexiletine, propranolol, protease inhibitors (e.g., indinavir), quinidine, sulfonylurea hypoglycemic agents, theophylline, oral verapamil, and zidovudine.

PREGNANCY AND LACTATION

- US FDA Pregnancy Category C. The drug exerts animal teratogenic or embryocidal effects but there are no studies in women, or no studies are available in either animals or women.
- Pregnant and lactating women should avoid rifampin due to teratogenic effects in high doses.

Diagnosis

DIFFERENTIAL DIAGNOSIS

- Toxic causes of vomiting possibly followed by hepatic injury include acetaminophen, chlorpromazine, phenylbutazone, tolbutamide, thiabendazole, chloral hydrate, pennyroyal oil, lead, and mercury.
- Other drugs may cause red- or orange-colored urine.

SIGNS AND SYMPTOMS

- Acute poisoning is characterized by nonspecific influenza-type symptoms (fever, chills, myalgia, malaise, gastrointestinal complaints), generalized pruritus, facial edema, gastrointestinal disturbances, and red to orange staining of skin (red-man syndrome) and body secretions.
- Chronic therapeutic use may cause hepatitis.
- Hypersensitivity reactions also may occur.

HEENT

- Facial edema, headache, and mouth, tongue, and throat soreness may occur.
- Red-orange coloration of sclera, tears, saliva, and sweat may occur and may permanently discolor contact lenses.

Dermatologic

- Red-orange skin coloration can be removed by washing.
- Pruritic rash, facial flushing, and urticaria can occur.

Gastrointestinal

- Nausea, vomiting, epigastric distress, abdominal cramps, and diarrhea can occur.
- Stool may become red-orange in acute overdose.

Hepatic

- During chronic therapeutic use, hepatitis occurs rarely, with jaundice and elevation of bilirubin, alanine aminotransferase (ALT), aspartate aminotransferase (AST), and alkaline phosphatase.
- Enzyme concentrations usually normalize over the next 48 hours.
- Hepatorenal syndrome occurs rarely during intermittent rifampin therapy.

Genitourinary

- Red-orange color of urine, hematuria, and proteinuria may occur.
- Acute renal failure is rare and usually occurs with chronic intermittent therapy.

Fluids and Electrolytes

Alterations in fluid and electrolyte balance may develop secondary to renal toxicity.

Hematologic

Thrombocytopenia, leukopenia, hemolytic anemia (hemolysis with hemoglobinuria), eosinophilia, and hemolysis are possible during therapy.

Neurologic

Fatigue, drowsiness, headache, dizziness, ataxia, confusion, inability to concentrate, generalized numbness, extremity pain, weakness, and (rarely) seizures may occur in an acute overdose.

PROCEDURES AND LABORATORY TESTS

Essential Tests

No tests may be needed in asymptomatic patients following acute overdose.

Recommended Tests

- Complete blood count (CBC), serum electrolytes, glucose, BUN, creatinine, AST, ALT, bilirubin, and urinalysis should be conducted in symptomatic patients to assess effects on liver, kidneys, or hematopoietic system.
- Prothrombin time/international normalized ratio and partial thromboplastin time should be tested to assess liver injury severity.
- ECG, serum acetaminophen, and aspirin levels should be determined in an overdose setting to detect occult ingestion.

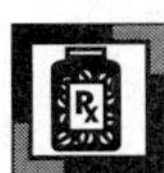

Treatment

- Treatment should focus on supportive care with appropriate airway management.
- Dose and time of exposure must be determined for all substances involved.

DIRECTING PATIENT COURSE

The health-care professional should call the poison control center when:

- Altered mental status, jaundice, hepatic failure, or other serious effects are present.
- Toxic effects are not consistent with rifampin toxicity.
- Coingestant, drug interaction, or underlying disease presents an unusual problem.

The patient should be referred to a health-care facility when:

- Any history of rifampin overdose ingestion is obtained.
- Patient or caregiver seems unreliable.
- Coingestant, drug interaction, or underlying disease presents an unusual problem.

Admission Considerations

Inpatient management is warranted if symptoms of hepatic damage or failure, or other serious concerns, are present.

DECONTAMINATION

Out of Hospital

Emesis should be induced with ipecac within 1 hour of ingestion for alert pediatric or adult patients if health-care evaluation will be delayed.

In Hospital

- Gastric lavage should be performed in pediatric (tube size 24–32 French) or adult (tube size 36–42 French) patients presenting within 1 hour of a large ingestion or if serious effects are present.
- One dose of activated charcoal (1–2 g/kg) should be administered if a substantial ingestion has occurred within the previous few hours.
- Because of extensive enterohepatic circulation, an additional dose of activated charcoal may be administered 2 to 4 hours later in symptomatic patients.

ANTIDOTES

There is no specific antidote for rifampin poisoning.

ADJUNCTIVE TREATMENT

- Standard symptomatic and supportive care should be provided based on the patient's complaints.
- In serious cases, replacement of coagulation factors with fresh frozen plasma may be needed.

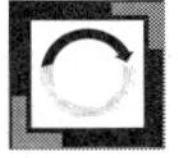

Follow-Up

PATIENT MONITORING

- In symptomatic patients with acute ingestion, cardiac and respiratory function should be monitored.
- CBC and liver enzymes should be monitored at least daily for 2 to 3 days in addition to cardiac and respiratory function.

EXPECTED COURSE AND PROGNOSIS

- Onset of effects after acute overdose occurs within hours.
- Following acute overdose, maximum liver enzyme elevations usually occur within 48 hours and resolve over the next week.
- Most patients recover over a period of 24 hours to 4 days, longer in cases with preexisting liver dysfunction or alcoholism.

DISCHARGE CRITERIA/INSTRUCTIONS

- From the emergency department. Asymptomatic patients with normal mental status may be discharged after a 6-hour observation period following gastrointestinal decontamination and psychiatric evaluation, if needed.
- From the hospital. Patients may be discharged after resolution of hepatic and neurologic effects and psychiatric evaluation, if needed.

PATIENT EDUCATION

Patients should be warned about body fluid discoloration and should be advised to remove contact lenses.

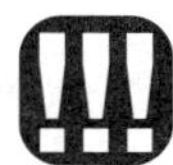

Pitfalls

DIAGNOSIS

- It is important to consider other causes of altered mental status and hepatic dysfunction.
- Impaired rifampin metabolism can occur with hepatic dysfunction (history of liver disease, alcoholics, patients on concomitant isoniazid therapy, the elderly).

TREATMENT

Intermittent rifampin therapy or high-dose rifampin therapy (≥1,200 mg) or restarting therapy after a rifampin-free interval may cause eosinophilia, hemolytic anemia, shock, thrombocytopenia, and acute tubular necrosis.

ICD-9-CM 960.6

Poisoning by antibiotics: antimycobacterial antibiotics.

See also: SECTION II, Urinary Color Change chapter.

RECOMMENDED READING

Mandell GL, Petri WA. Antimicrobial agents (continued): drugs used in the chemotherapy of tuberculosis, *Mycobacterium avium* complex disease, and leprosy. In: Hardman JG, Gilman AG, Limbird LE, eds. *Goodman and Gilman's pharmacological basis of therapeutics,* 9th ed. New York: McGraw-Hill, 1996:115–116.

Plomp TA, Battista HJ, Unterdorfer WC, et al. A case of fatal poisoning by rifampin. *Arch Toxicol* 1981;48:245–252.

Rifampin. In: Anderson PO, Knoben JE, eds. *1997-1998 Handbook of clinical drug data,* 8th ed. Stamford, CT: Appleton & Lange, 1997:69–72.

Author: Alvin C. Bronstein

Reviewer: Gerald F. O'Malley

Salicylates

Basics

DESCRIPTION

Salicylates include a variety of medications used for their analgesic and antiinflammatory effects.

FORMS AND USES

- The product packaging should be checked to determine whether a main ingredient is aspirin or acetaminophen and whether narcotics, decongestants, or barbiturates are present.
- Salicylates are available in a variety of forms for oral and topical use.
- Numerous brands contain aspirin alone, whereas others are combination products.
- Analgesic/antipyretic agents, such as aspirin [acetylsalicylic acid (ASA)], provide temporary relief of mild to moderate pain and reduce fever.
- Antiinflammatory agents (ASA, magnesium salicylate, salsalate, sulfasalazine) provide long-term maintenance in rheumatoid arthritis, systemic lupus erythematosus, ankylosing spondylitis, inflammatory bowel disease, and other diseases.
- Antiplatelet agents reduce deaths from myocardial infarction or unstable angina, and reduce transient ischemic attacks and stroke.
- Gastrointestinal agents (bismuth, subsalicylate, Pepto Bismol) are used to treat diarrhea and indigestion.
- Topical wart removers may contain 17% salicylate.
- Liniments and vaporizers contain high concentrations of methyl salicylate (up to 30%) in additives; oil of wintergreen is 100% methyl salicylate.
- The maximum recommended dosage for analgesic, antipyretic, and antiinflammatory indications is 4 g per day in divided doses (650 mg every 4 hours or 1 g every 6 hours), although some conditions are treated with larger amounts under a physician's supervision.

TOXIC DOSE

- An acute single ingestion of more than 150 mg/kg often causes toxicity, and the patient should be examined in a health-care facility.
- Chronic ingestion of more than 100 mg/kg/day may cause toxicity.
- One teaspoon (5 ml) of oil of wintergreen contains 1.4 g of salicylate and is a potentially lethal dose in a child who weighs less than 10 kg.

PATHOPHYSIOLOGY

- Aspirin (ASA) is hydrolyzed to salicylic acid (salicylate).
- Salicylate stimulates the medullary respiratory center, producing hyperventilation and respiratory alkalosis.
- Salicylate also uncouples oxidative phosphorylation at the cellular level, resulting in fever and decreased adenosine triphosphate production.
- Elevated lactic acid levels contribute to metabolic acidosis.
- Acidosis promotes the formation of the unionized form of salicylate, which readily penetrates the brain.
- Concentration of salicylate in the brain is directly correlated with lethality in animals.

EPIDEMIOLOGY

- Poisoning is common.
- Toxic effects following exposure are typically mild to moderate.
- Death occurs in patients who are inadequately treated or in whom the diagnosis is missed (usually the elderly with an underlying medical disease and chronic salicylate intoxication).

CAUSES

- Poisoning is usually caused by a suicidal ingestion.
- Chronic ingestion from therapeutic misadventure is also common.
- Child neglect should be considered if the patient is less than 1 year of age; suicide attempt in patients over 6 years of age.

RISK FACTORS

- Children between 4 and 12 years of age who ingest aspirin during a febrile illness may be at risk for Reye's syndrome.
- Elderly patients with underlying medical conditions have a 25% to 30% mortality rate from chronic salicylate when toxicity develops.

DRUG AND DISEASE INTERACTIONS

Acetazolamide increases salicylate toxicity by promoting CNS penetration.

PREGNANCY AND LACTATION

- US FDA Pregnancy Category C. The drug exerts animal teratogenic or embryocidal effects, but there are no controlled studies in women, or no studies are available in either animals or women.
- Therapeutic doses of aspirin during the first trimester of pregnancy and during breastfeeding are safe.
- Increased incidence of intracranial hemorrhage and premature closure of the ductus arteriosus in premature infants are associated with maternal ingestion of aspirin within 1 week of delivery.

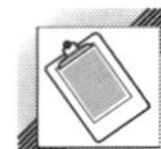

Diagnosis

DIFFERENTIAL DIAGNOSIS

- Toxicants causing increased anion gap metabolic acidosis include methanol, ethylene glycol, iron, metformin, lactic acidosis from any cause, and isoniazid (see SECTION II, Anion Gap Acidosis chapter).
- Nontoxic conditions causing metabolic acidosis include hypoxia or hypotension induced by any cause.

SIGNS AND SYMPTOMS

- Acute intoxication usually begins with nausea, vomiting, tinnitus, hearing loss, and respiratory alkalosis and may progress to severe toxicity over several hours.
- Chronic intoxication is insidious and often presents with altered mental status with a history consistent with volume depletion (anorexia, vomiting), perhaps in the setting of subacute pain such as toothache for several days.
- Either acute or chronic ingestion may result in dehydration, hypotension, hepatotoxicity, noncardiogenic pulmonary edema, lethargy, agitation, and seizures.

Vital Signs

Hyperventilation, tachycardia, fever, and hypotension may occur in moderate to severe overdose.

HEENT

- Tinnitus and transient hearing loss are common.
- Mucosal burns may occur from ingestion of topical wart removers (due to acid in product).

Cardiovascular

- Hypotension and shock are signs of severe poisoning.
- Malignant dysrhythmia may occur abruptly during severe toxicity.

Pulmonary

Tachypnea and hyperventilation are common; noncardiogenic pulmonary edema and respiratory failure occur in severe cases.

Gastrointestinal

- Nausea and vomiting are common.
- Aspirin bezoars may form after large ingestion or chronic ingestion of enteric-coated preparations, leading to prolonged absorption.
- Gastric stasis from pylorospasm, gastrointestinal bleeding, viscus perforation, and pancreatitis may occur.

Hepatic

Hepatic injury may occur in severe cases.

Renal

Proteinuria and acute renal insufficiency may develop.

Fluids and Electrolytes

- After acute ingestion, respiratory alkalosis develops initially, which may be followed by metabolic acidosis as the patient deteriorates.
- In small children, alkalosis may not occur and metabolic acidosis may be an early presenting sign.
- Dehydration and hypokalemia are common.
- Syndrome of inappropriate antidiuretic hormone may develop.
- Respiratory acidosis indicates severe toxicity or possibly coingestion of a CNS depressant.

Musculoskeletal

Rhabdomyolysis is a rare complication of severe poisoning.

Neurologic

In severe poisoning, lethargy, agitation, confusion, coma, seizures, cerebral edema, encephalopathy, asterixis, and focal neurologic findings may develop.

Endocrine

Hyperglycemia or hypoglycemia may occur.

Hematologic

Prolonged prothrombin time/partial thromboplastin time, disseminated intravascular coagulation, and inhibition of platelet aggregation are seen.

PROCEDURES AND LABORATORY TESTS

Essential Tests

Serial Serum Salicylate Levels

- Single acute ingestion

—Serum salicylate levels should be obtained every 2 hours for the first 4 to 8 hours to assess the rate of rise and absolute value of salicylate concentrations.
—Then levels should be obtained every 4 to 6 hours until sustained decline in levels is observed.
—Mild toxicity is associated with levels higher than 30 mg/dl.
—Hemodialysis is usually initiated for salicylate levels over 90 to 100 mg/dl, respiratory acidosis, or signs of end-organ damage (e.g., persistent hypotension, pulmonary edema, altered mental status, seizure).

- Chronic ingestion. A single level should be performed to screen for chronic intoxication. It is interpreted in the context of clinical signs. Interpretation of levels is as follows:

—Serious effects develop at salicylate levels lower than for acute ingestion.
—In the elderly, toxicity can occur at "therapeutic" levels, and seizures and death have occurred at a serum level of 35 mg/dl.
—Hemodialysis is often initiated for salicylate level greater than 50 mg/dl, respiratory acidosis, or signs of end-organ damage (e.g., pulmonary edema, altered mental status, or seizure).

- Diflunisal (Dolobid) may induce a false-positive salicylate level.

Serum Electrolytes, Glucose, BUN, and Creatinine

- Metabolic acidosis is common.
- Serial serum bicarbonate levels are used to assess acid-base status.
- Hyper- or hypoglycemia may develop.
- Elevated BUN and creatinine may develop.

Recommended Tests

- Arterial blood gases

—These are used to follow oxygenation and respiratory compensation for metabolic acidosis.
—Rising pCO_2 indicates respiratory failure and the need for endotracheal intubation as well as hemodialysis.

- ECG and serum acetaminophen level in an overdose setting are used to evaluate occult ingestion.
- Serum calcium is measured; hypocalcemia has been associated with aggressive bicarbonate therapy.
- Chest radiography in symptomatic patients can assess noncardiogenic pulmonary edema.
- Abdominal radiography may detect sustained-release or enteric-coated tablets.

Not Recommended Tests

Use of the Done nomogram is not recommended.

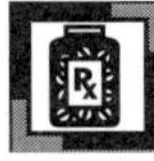

Treatment

- Treatment should focus on gastrointestinal decontamination, enhancement of renal excretion of salicylate, and deciding when hemodialysis is indicated.
- Treatment decisions should be based on signs of toxicity and the salicylate level.
- The salicylate level alone should not determine course of therapy.
- The dose and time of exposure must be determined for all substances involved.

DIRECTING PATIENT COURSE

The health-care provider should call the poison control center when:

- Altered mental status, seizure, respiratory acidosis, or hypoxia are present or dialysis is planned.
- Toxic effects are not consistent with salicylate poisoning.
- Coingestant, drug interaction, or underlying disease presents an unusual challenge.

The patient should be referred to a health-care facility when:

- Attempted suicide or homicide is possible.
- Patient or caregiver seems unreliable.
- Toxic effects are present.
- Coingestant, drug interaction, or underlying disease presents an unusual challenge.

Admission Considerations

Inpatient management is warranted for patients with a rising salicylate level or signs of end-organ damage (e.g., altered mental status, seizure, acidosis, or pulmonary edema).

DECONTAMINATION

Out of Hospital

Emesis should be induced with ipecac within 1 hour of ingestion for alert pediatric or adult patients if health-care evaluation will be delayed.

In Hospital

- Gastric lavage should be performed in pediatric (tube size 24–32 French) or adult (tube size 36–42 French) patients presenting within 1 hour of a large ingestion or if serious effects are present.
- Sustained-release formulations may be too large to be effectively removed by gastric lavage.
- One dose of activated charcoal (1–2 g/kg) is administered without a cathartic if a substantial ingestion has occurred; activated charcoal (0.5–1 g/kg) may be repeated every 4 to 6 hours for an additional one to two doses, provide bowel sounds are present.

ANTIDOTES

There is no specific antidote for salicylate poisoning.

ADJUNCTIVE TREATMENT

Endotracheal Intubation and Mechanical Ventilation

- Indications

—Altered mental status with inability to protect airway
—Rising pCO_2 level

- Method of administration

—Patient should be intubated in the standard manner.
—Ventilator setting should maintain the patient's previous minute volume, which is usually increased markedly.
—Settings should not be adjusted to produce pCO_2 of 40 mm Hg, which would probably produce relative respiratory acidosis and potentially worsen the patient's condition rapidly.

Hemodialysis

- Indications

—Clinical worsening, respiratory acidosis, particularly in conjunction with rising salicylate level despite gastrointestinal decontamination and urinary alkalinization
—Evidence of end-organ damage (persistent or recurrent hypotension, altered mental status, seizure, respiratory acidosis, noncardiogenic pulmonary edema, refractory metabolic acidosis)
—Oliguric renal failure
—Elderly patients with chronic salicylate ingestion and worsening clinical status
  —These patients have a high rate of mortality.
  —Early hemodialysis may be life saving.

- Method of administration

—Hemodialysis is terminated when clinical improvement, decline in the serum salicylate level approaching the therapeutic range, and correction of acid-base disturbances are achieved.

Whole-Bowel Irrigation

- Indications

—Large ingestion of enteric-coated or sustained-release tablet formulations
—Rising salicylate level despite gastrointestinal decontamination

- Contraindications

—Gastrointestinal ileus, perforation, bleeding, or obstruction

- Method of administration

—Adolescents and adults are administered a polyethylene glycol solution (Golytely, Colyte) at 2 L/h orally until rectal effluent is clear.
—The pediatric dose is 20 ml/kg/h orally until rectal effluent is clear.

- Adverse effects include vomiting, especially with rapid administration, and abdominal cramping.

Urinary Alkalinization

- Indications

—Symptomatic patients (tachypnea, tinnitus, recurrent vomiting) with history of salicylate ingestion should undergo empiric urinary alkalinization while awaiting initial salicylate level.
—Most patients with salicylate level of over 30 mg/dl should receive urinary alkalization while being further evaluated.
—All patients in whom hemodialysis is planned should receive urinary alkalization.

- Contraindications

—Encephalopathy, cerebral edema, renal failure, pulmonary edema, arterial pH higher than 7.55, serum sodium greater than 150 mEq/L

- Method of administration

—Adults are administered one to two ampules of sodium bicarbonate (44 or 50 mEq per ampule) by intravenous push. Three ampules of sodium bicarbonate are then mixed in 1 L of D5W and infused at 200 ml/h. The rate should be increased within clinically reasonable boundaries to produce urinary pH higher than 7.5. Urinary pH should be monitored hourly.
—Pediatric patients are administered sodium bicarbonate 1 to 2 mEq/kg by intravenous push. One to two ampules of sodium bicarbonate (44 or 50 mEq per ampule) are mixed in 1 L of D5W and infused at a rate within clinically reasonable boundaries starting at 1.5 to 2.0 times the maintenance rate and then adjusted to maintain the urinary pH above 7.5.
—When determining infusion rate, the influence on underlying medical conditions, such as congestive heart failure, myocardial ischemia, and renal insufficiency, should be considered.
—Urinary alkalinization continues until the patient has demonstrated clinical improvement with documented serial decline in serum salicylate levels toward the therapeutic range and correction of acid-base disturbances.
—Supplemental potassium is administered if serum level is less than 4.0 mEq/L.

- Adverse effects include pulmonary edema, metabolic alkalosis (rare), and hypernatremia (rare).

Hypotension

- The patient is treated with 10 to 20 ml/kg 0.9% saline intravenously and placed in the Trendelenburg position.
- Further fluid therapy is guided by central pressure monitoring to avoid volume overload.
- If hypotension is unresponsive, a vasopressor is administered.

Not Recommended Therapies

Acetazolamide should not be administered to alkalinize urine because it acidifies serum and increases salicylate penetration into the CNS.

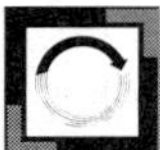

Follow-Up

PATIENT MONITORING

- Continuous respiratory and cardiac monitoring should be performed in symptomatic patients.
- Patients should be reassessed frequently for change in mental status and should have serial determinations of serum electrolyte and salicylate levels.
- Patients with rising salicylate levels, altered mental status, seizure, pulmonary edema, or respiratory acidosis should be monitored in an intensive care setting.

EXPECTED COURSE AND PROGNOSIS

- Acute intoxication typically begins within hours of ingestion and resolves within 24 to 48 hours depending on severity; a complete recovery is expected.
- Chronic intoxication may begin within days to weeks of salicylate ingestion and resolves over 48 to 72 hours once treatment is initiated.
- Permanent sequelae of hypoxia or cerebral edema may occur.

DISCHARGE CRITERIA/INSTRUCTIONS

- From the emergency department. Asymptomatic or minimally symptomatic patients may be discharged after gastrointestinal decontamination, observation for 4 to 6 hours, and a psychiatric evaluation, provided that serial serum salicylate levels decline significantlyand acid-base status is normal.
- From the hospital. Asymptomatic patients may be discharged after signs of toxicity resolve, serum electrolytes and renal function return to baseline, serial serum salicylate levels decline to 30 mg/dl, and a psychiatric evaluation is completed, if needed.

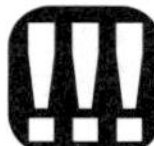

Pitfalls

DIAGNOSIS

- Use of the Done nomogram is not recommended.

—The specific conditions under which the nomogram was developed rarely mimic clinical conditions, so its use is not appropriate in many situations.
—Use of a 6-hour level often delays treatment of seriously ill patients.

- Use of salicylate concentration alone to guide therapy may lead to either overtreatment or undertreatment of seriously ill patients.

—Serum salicylate levels should be followed until at least two consecutive measurements demonstrate significant decline.
—Peak serum salicylate levels may be delayed from 10 to 60 hours with enteric-coated or sustained-release aspirin preparations.

- Methyl salicylate. Pure oil of wintergreen, a liquid formulation containing 100% methyl salicylate, is quickly absorbed in the gastrointestinal tract, resulting in rapid development of clinical salicylism.

TREATMENT

- Urinary alkalinization should be initiated empirically while awaiting initial serum salicylate levels if signs and symptoms consistent with salicylate toxicity are present.
- Ventilator settings of intubated and sedated patients should be adjusted (minute volume) to maintain pCO_2 at the patient's pCO_2 before intubation.

ICD-9-CM 965.1

Poisoning by analgesics, antipyretics, and antirheumatics: salicylates.

See also: SECTION II, Anion Gap Metabolic Acidosis and Hypotension chapters; and SECTION III, Sodium Bicarbonate chapter.

RECOMMENDED READING

Anderson RJ, Potts DE, Gabow PA. Unrecognized adult salicylate intoxication. *Ann Intern Med* 1976;85:745–748.

Gabow PA. How to avoid overlooking salicylate intoxication. *J Crit Illness* 1986;1:77–85.

Yip L, Jastremski MS, Dart RC. Salicylate intoxication. *J Intens Care Med* 1997;12:66–78.

Author: Luke Yip

Reviewer: Rivka S. Horowitz

Scombroid Fish Poisoning

Basics

DESCRIPTION

Scombroid fish poisoning is a syndrome of flushing, nausea, vomiting, and headache that occurs after eating fish.

FORMS AND USES

- Scombroid poisoning can be caused by eating raw or insufficiently cooked fish of the suborder Scombroidea; occasionally other fish species have been implicated.
- Toxic fish may have no abnormal taste or smell.
- Implicated fishes include skipjack, bonito, mackerel, Cero, albacore, tuna, mahi mahi or dolphinfish, bluefish, Bombay duck, kahawai, kingfish, pilchards, Pacific amberjack, salmon, trumpeter fish, sea perch, sprat, saury, striped marlin, and swordfish.
- Canned, dried, or smoked fish also may be the cause of this type of poisoning.

TOXIC DOSE

- U.S. Food and Drug Administration action level for histamine in tuna is 50 mg/100 g of meat.
- Most individuals will develop illness if the fish contains 100 mg of histamine per 100 g of flesh eaten.

PATHOPHYSIOLOGY

- Fishes implicated in scombroid fish poisoning contain large amounts of histidine, particularly in the dark meat.
- If improper refrigeration occurs, proliferation of normal marine microflora containing histidine decarboxylase will convert the histidine to histamine and saurine in quantities sufficient to cause poisoning, often without the appearance of putrefaction.

EPIDEMIOLOGY

- Poisoning is common; a small cluster of cases is not unusual.
- Toxic effects following exposure are typically mild to moderate, with death occurring rarely.
- All implicated fish species live in temperate or tropical waters.

CAUSES

Ingestion is unintentional as part of a meal.

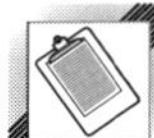

Diagnosis

DIFFERENTIAL DIAGNOSIS

- Scombroid fish poisoning may be confused with an allergic reaction, especially if there is only a single case and if the association with eating fish is not apparent.
- Ciguatera fish poisoning presents with gastroenteritis, paresthesias, hot/cold reversal, myalgia, and weakness.
- Domoic acid poisoning presents with gastroenteritis, myoclonus, seizures, and coma.
- Neurotoxic and paralytic shellfish poisoning present with gastroenteritis, paresthesias, ataxia, and respiratory paralysis.

SIGNS AND SYMPTOMS

Common effects include dermal flushing, throbbing headache, nausea, diarrhea, and vomiting, which may develop 5 minutes to 2 hours after ingestion.

Vital Signs

Tachycardia, hypotension, and shock may develop in the rare severe case.

HEENT

- Facial flushing or "feverish feeling" is common.
- Conjunctival injection and swelling of face, lips, and tongue may occur.
- Burning, hot, "sharp," or "peppery" sensation of the gingiva or throat may occur when eating the fish; oral blisters may develop.

Dermatologic

- Erythematous rash, pruritus, or burning sensation are common.
- Diaphoresis and urticaria occur less commonly.

Cardiovascular

- Palpitations are common.
- Tachycardia, hypotension, and shock are rare.

Pulmonary

- Chest tightness, dyspnea, bronchospasm, and mild respiratory distress may develop.
- Severe respiratory distress and respiratory collapse occur rarely.

Gastrointestinal

Nausea, vomiting, diarrhea, flatus, and abdominal cramps are common.

Neurologic

Headache is common; dizziness, weakness, apprehension, tingling, and anxiety also occur.

PROCEDURES AND LABORATORY TESTS

Essential Tests

No tests may be needed in minimally symptomatic patients.

Recommended

- Pulse oximetry and cardiac monitoring should be conducted to detect respiratory or cardiac toxicity in symptomatic patients.
- Serum electrolyte, BUN, and creatinine analyses are ordered to assess the effects of repeated vomiting or diarrhea.
- Laboratory confirmation of scombrotoxism is by quantitation of histamine in the flesh of implicated fish; illness is associated with 100 mg of histamine per 100 g of meat, but 20 mg of histamine per 100 g of flesh may cause illness in susceptible individuals.

Not Recommended Tests

Blood histamine level may be elevated, but it is not clinically useful.

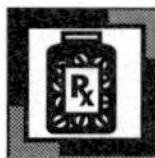

Treatment

• Treatment should focus on supportive care of respiratory and cardiovascular function.
• Dose and time of exposure should be determined for all substances involved.
• Most cases respond to antihistamines; bronchodilator and steroids may be necessary to treat bronchospasm.

DIRECTING PATIENT COURSE

The health-care provider should call the poison control center when:

• Pulmonary or cardiac toxicity develops.
• Toxic effects are not consistent with scombroid fish poisoning.
• Coingestant, drug interaction, or underlying disease presents an unusual problem.

The patient should be referred to a health-care facility when:

• Patient or caregiver seems unreliable.
• Severe vomiting or other toxic effects are present.
• Coingestant, drug interaction, or underlying disease presents an unusual problem.

Admission Considerations

Inpatient management is warranted if the patient exhibits severe persistent effects.

DECONTAMINATION

Out of Hospital

Induction of emesis is not recommended.

In Hospital

• Gastric lavage should be performed in pediatric (tube size 24–32 French) or adult (tube size 36–42 French) patients presenting within 1 hour of a large ingestion, if serious effects are present, and if vomiting has not already occurred.
• One dose of activated charcoal (1–2 g/kg) should be administered without a cathartic if a substantial ingestion has occurred within the previous few hours.

ANTIDOTES

There is no specific antidote for scombroid fish poisoning.

ADJUNCTIVE TREATMENT

• The histaminic effects usually respond to standard antihistamine agents; corticosteroids or epinephrine are rarely needed.
• Both H_1- and H_2-antihistamine receptor blockers should be administered:
  —H_1-antagonist (diphenhydramine)
  —Adult dosage is 50 mg intravenously over 2 minutes; dose should be repeated every 6 hours for 1 to 2 days.
  —Pediatric dosage is 1 mg/kg (up to 50 mg) intravenously over 2 minutes, not to exceed 5 mg/kg in 24 hours.
  —H_2 antagonists (cimetidine or ranitidine)
  —Adult dosage is cimetidine 300 mg intravenously or ranitidine 50 mg intravenously every 6 hours for a period of 1 to 2 days.
  —Pediatric dose is cimetidine 20 to 40 mg/kg intravenously per day divided every 6 hours up to 300 mg every 6 hours, or ranitidine 1 to 2 mg/kg intravenously per day divided every 6 to 8 hours.

• A corticosteroid may be useful in severe cases.

—Adult dose of methylprednisolone is 125 mg intravenously.
—Pediatric dose is 1 to 2 mg/kg (up to 60 mg/kg) intravenously.

• Epinephrine is rarely needed.

—Adult dose is 0.3 to 0.5 ml of 1/1,000 (1 mg/ml) subcutaneously.
—Pediatric dose is 0.01 ml/kg of 1/1,000 (1 mg/ml) subcutaneously, not to exceed 0.5 mg.

Seizure

• A patent airway must be ensured.
• A benzodiazepine is administered for initial control.
• If seizures persist or recur, another anticonvulsant such as phenobarbital or phenytoin may be added (see SECTION II, Seizures chapter).

Hypotension

• The patient should receive 10 to 20 ml/kg 0.9% saline intravenously and be placed in the Trendelenburg position.
• Further fluid therapy should be guided by central monitoring to avoid volume overload.
• If hypotension is unresponsive, a vasopressor should be administered (see SECTION II, Hypotension chapter).

Bronchospasm

• Administration of oxygen should be followed by albuterol 0.15 mg/kg (maximum of 10 mg) in saline with humidified oxygen via nebulizer every 20 to 30 minutes.

—If the peak expiratory flow rate is more than 90% of predicted flow rate after initial dose, additional doses may not be needed.
—Patient should be monitored continuously for response.

• Methylprednisolone may be administered intravenously every 6 to 8 hours in severe cases; this may be decreased to a single daily dose and tapered.

—Adult dose is 60 to 125 mg (1–1.5 mg/kg).
—Pediatric dose is 1 to 2 mg/kg.

• Initiation of prednisone, 2 mg/kg orally for several days, should be considered after discharge in patients treated with methylprednisolone.

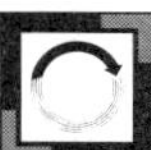

Follow-Up

PATIENT MONITORING

Respiratory and hemodynamic status should be monitored until patient is stable and improving.

EXPECTED COURSE AND PROGNOSIS

• Histamine reaction usually occurs within 60 minutes after eating the toxic fish but may be delayed 1 to 2 hours.
• Most cases are mild and self-limited, resolving in 3 to 36 hours.

DISCHARGE CRITERIA/INSTRUCTIONS

Patient may be discharged from emergency department or hospital when oral intake is tolerated and patient is asymptomatic for at least 6 hours.

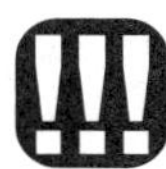

Pitfalls

DIAGNOSIS

Scombroid fish poisoning is often mistaken initially for an allergic reaction; thorough history taking is crucial to discover the true cause of illness.

ICD-9-CM 988.0

Toxic effect of noxious substances eaten as food: fish and shellfish.

See also: SECTION II, Hypotension and Seizures chapters.

RECOMMENDED READING

Morrow JF, Margolies GR, Rowland J et al. Evidence that histamine is the causative toxin of scombroid-fish poisoning. *N Engl J Med* 1991;324:716–720.

Taylor SL. Histamine food poisoning: toxicology and clinical aspects. *CRC Crit Rev Toxicol* 1987;17:91–128.

Author: Steven A. Seifert

Reviewer: Luke Yip

Scorpion Envenomation

Basics

DESCRIPTION

Scorpions are small invertebrates that look like small lobsters. They envenomate humans using a stinger at the end of their tail.

FORMS AND USES

- There are many species of scorpions in the United States; however, only the sting of the bark scorpion (*Centruroides exilicauda*) causes serious systemic symptoms.
- The bark scorpion is endemic to Arizona, the desert of southern California, western Texas, and southern Nevada.
- Other scorpion species in the United States may cause self-limited local pain.

TOXIC DOSE

A single sting causes mild to severe pain and has caused death in small children on rare occasions.

PATHOPHYSIOLOGY

- The primary toxin is a protein that increases sodium permeability of presynaptic neurons, resulting in continuous depolarization.
- This depolarization results in repetitive contraction of muscle fibers as well as sympathetic and parasympathetic stimulation.

EPIDEMIOLOGY

- Scorpion envenomation is relatively common in endemic areas.
- Toxic effects are typically mild in adults; most severe cases occur in children.
- Death is rare and is caused by respiratory failure.

CAUSES

- Most exposures involve inadvertent contact from a scorpion that has hidden in clothing, sleeping bags, bed sheets etc.
- Stings also may occur when scorpions are handled.

RISK FACTORS

- Children are more likely to develop severe systemic effects.
- Elderly patients may not tolerate the tachycardia and hypertension associated with severe envenomation.

PREGNANCY AND LACTATION

There is little information on scorpion envenomation in pregnancy; the patient should be treated as other patients.

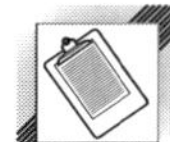

Diagnosis

DIFFERENTIAL DIAGNOSIS

- Toxic causes of acute localized pain include bite or sting from a wide variety of animals such as spiders, fire ants, bees, and wasps.
- Toxic causes of sympathetic and parasympathetic stimulation and movement disorders include cholinergic or sympathomimetic agents; in some cases, the patient also may appear to be hallucinating.
- Nontoxic causes of movement disorders, irritability, and seizures include meningitis, encephalitis, and intracranial bleeding.

SIGNS AND SYMPTOMS

- In adults, the sting usually causes localized pain that resolves over hours to days.
- In small children, pain may be followed by the characteristic effects of restlessness, roving eye movements, salivation, opisthotonos, and flailing extremities.

Vital Signs

- Tachycardia and hypertension are common.
- Mild hyperthermia is common in children.

HEENT

- Cranial nerve dysfunction leads to loss of pharyngeal muscle control, nystagmus, movements, double vision, and slurred speech.
- *Roving eye movements* refers to incessant, uncoordinated eye movements that occur in small children.
- Autonomic dysfunction leads to hypersalivation and mydriasis.
- Skeletal muscle dysfunction may result in tongue fasciculation.

Dermatologic

- Local skin findings are absent at the site of envenomation, although tapping on a bite site may cause sudden shooting pain.
- Diaphoresis is common.

Cardiovascular

Hypertension and tachycardia are common.

Pulmonary

- Increased secretions are common.
- Children may develop respiratory depression, stridor, wheezing, hypoxia, and, in severe cases, respiratory failure.

Gastrointestinal

- Nausea, vomiting, and increased salivation are common.
- Difficulty in swallowing may develop, particularly in children.

Musculoskeletal

- Muscle fasciculation is a sign of significant toxicity.
- Rhabdomyolysis has been reported, but is usually mild.

Neurologic

- The most common symptom in adults is pain and hyperesthesia at the sting site; the pain can migrate proximally and may be elicited by tapping on the sting site.
- In children, cranial nerve findings, especially abnormal eye movements and loss of pharyngeal muscle control, may occur.
- In children, jerking of the extremities and opisthotonos can occur and may be mistaken for seizures; however, the patient remains alert throughout the event.

PROCEDURES AND LABORATORY TESTS

Essential Tests

Pulse oximetry and serum electrolytes and glucose should be measured in patients with apparent altered mental status.

Recommended Tests

- Creatine kinase should be measured in patients with severe fasciculation or hyperactivity.
- EEG may be required if seizures are possible.

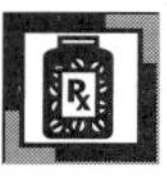

Treatment

- Treatment should focus on managing airway and controlling pain, anxiety, and movement disorders.
- The time of exposure should be determined.

DIRECTING PATIENT COURSE

The health-care provider should call the poison control center when:

- Severe systemic effects develop.
- Toxic effects are not consistent with scorpion envenomation.
- Underlying disease presents an unusual problem.

The patient should be referred to a health-care facility when:

- Patient is less than 2 years of age.
- Patient or caregiver seems unreliable.
- Respiratory distress, severe movement disorders, or other severe effects are present.
- Toxic effects are not consistent with scorpion envenomation.
- Underlying disease presents an unusual problem.

Admission Considerations

Inpatient management is warranted if:

- Adult patient has intractable pain despite administration of analgesics.
- Pediatric patient develops cranial nerve findings or fasciculation, in order to monitor airway patency.

DECONTAMINATION

Due to rapid absorption of a small volume of venom injected, decontamination is not recommended.

ANTIDOTES

Antivenom to bark scorpion venom is produced by Arizona State University; it has not been approved by the U.S. Food and Drug Administration and is available in Arizona only, but it has been shown to be effective.

Indications

Antivenom should be considered when severe systemic envenomation is unresponsive to sedation, especially if the airway is threatened by secretions.

Contraindications

A known allergy to goat-derived products contraindicates the use of antivenom.

Method of Administration

- Antivenom should be administered in a critical care setting, and the clinician should be prepared to manage the airway and treat anaphylaxis.
- Continuous respiratory and cardiac monitoring should be performed.
- A skin test should be performed by injecting 0.02 ml of antivenom intradermally and observing for wheal and flare reaction; a negative skin test result does not rule out the possibility of anaphylaxis.
- One to two vials of antivenom diluted in 50 to 100 ml of 0.9% saline should be administered intravenously over 20 to 30 minutes; if no clinical improvement is observed within 30 to 60 minutes, the dose can be repeated (up to a total of four vials).
- Consultation with a poison center or medical toxicologist is recommended.

Potential Adverse Effects

- Acute allergic reactions occur in up to 10% of patients; these may include rash and local swelling, and rarely wheezing or anaphylaxis.
- Serum sickness (fever, rash, myalgia) may develop in up to 60% of patients 5 to 14 days after administration (see SECTION III, Snake Antivenom chapter, for details of treatment).

ADJUNCTIVE TREATMENT

The selection of benzodiazepines administration versus antivenom is controversial. Currently, midazolam administration is recommended first. However the antivenom is appropriate in selected cases.

- Sedation with short-acting benzodiazepines has been used to control anxiety and hyperactivity associated with systemic envenomation.

—Midazolam infusion. Adult dosage is 5 mg/h, titrated to effect; the initial pediatric dosage is 100 μcg/kg/hr titrated upward to effect.
—Patient should be monitored for respiratory depression.

- Phenobarbital is not recommended.

—Sedation with long-acting agents may result in severe respiratory depression and prolonged ventilatory requirements.
—Shorter acting agents are preferred.

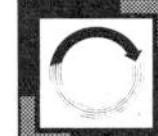

Follow-Up

PATIENT MONITORING

Patients developing systemic symptoms and those requiring sedation should be monitored for airway difficulties.

EXPECTED COURSE AND PROGNOSIS

- Adults typically develop pain and paresthesia only; these resolve over 24 hours.
- Venom effects may persist longer in patients who develop cranial nerve or skeletal muscle dysfunction.

—Systemic symptoms in children not receiving antivenom usually resolve within 12 hours but may persist for up to 36 hours.
—Systemic symptoms usually resolve within 1 hour in patients receiving antivenom, but pain may persist for over 24 hours.

DISCHARGE CRITERIA/INSTRUCTIONS

- From the emergency department

—A patient with pain that is managed by oral analgesics and with no systemic symptoms can be discharged.
—Patients treated with antivenom should be monitored for 4 to 6 hours.

- From the hospital. Patients may be discharged after resolution of systemic symptoms.

PATIENT EDUCATION

- Patients should be instructed to avoid areas of possible infestation, and to inspect and shake out clothes, shoes and sleeping bags prior to use.
- Patients who receive antivenom should be instructed about the symptoms to expect with serum sickness.

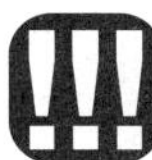

Pitfalls

DIAGNOSIS

- The failure to consider diagnosis of scorpion sting is common; the sting and the scorpion may not be noticed.
- In indigenous areas, scorpion sting should be considered in the infant with inconsolable crying or agitation.

TREATMENT

- Oversedation without airway protection may result in hypoxia and aspiration.
- Failure to prepare for treatment of antivenom-induced allergic reactions can lead to respiratory compromise

ICD-9-CM 989.5

Toxic effect of other substances, chiefly nonmedicinal as to source: venom.

See also: SECTION III, Snake Antivenon chapter.

RECOMMENDED READING

Gateau T, Bloom M, Clark R. Response to specific *Centruroides exilicauda* antivenom in 151 cases of scorpion stings. *J Toxicol Clin Toxicol* 1994;32:165–171.

Likes K, Banner W, Chavez M. *Centruroides exilicauda* envenomation in Arizona. *West J Med* 1984;141:634–637.

Rachesky IJ, Banner W, Dansky J, Tong T. Treatment for *Centruroides exilicauda* envenomation. *Am J Dis Child* 1984;138:1136–1138.

Author: Kennon Heard

Reviewer: Katherine M. Hurlbut

Sedative-Hypnotic Agents

Basics

DESCRIPTION

Sedative-hypnotic agents refers to nonbendiazepine drugs of various chemical structures whose predominant effect is CNS depression.

FORMS AND USES

These agents have sedative, hypnotic, anticonvulsant, and anxiolytic properties. Formulations include:

- Buspirone (Buspar) tablets
- Chloral hydrate (Aquachloral) suppositories, syrup, and tablets (triclofos sodium, Triclos, monosodium trichloroethyl phosphate)
- Chlormethiazole (Heminevrin, Distraneurine) caplets, syrup and tablets
- Glutethimide (Doriden) tablets
- Meprobamate (Miltown, Meprospan) tablets and elixir (Equanil, Equagesic, MB-TAB)
- Methaqualone (Quaalude) tablets and capsules
- Methyprylon (Noludar) tablets and capsules
- Ethchlorvynol
- Tramadol (Ultram)
- Zolpidem (Ambien)

Many of these drugs have been withdrawn from the U.S. market but are still available in other countries and from illicit sources. Some are used for treatment of and alcohol withdrawal syndromes.

Street Uses

- Glutethimide is used as a heroin potentiator or as an inexpensive heroin substitute; when combined with codeine, the mixes are called "loads."
- Methaqualone is used as an aphrodisiac and a "cocaine downer."

TOXIC DOSE

- Buspirone in doses of up to 300 mg causes minimal effects.
- Chloral hydrate causes toxicity in children at 1.5 g.
- One tablet of gluthethimide or meprobamate may produce sedation in a child.

PATHOPHYSIOLOGY

- All of these agents cause CNS and respiratory depression.
- The specific mechanism of action is often unclear (i.e., methaqualone, meprobamate); most are thought to enhance gamma-aminobutyric acid (GABA)-mediated activity in the CNS, thus increasing neuronal inhibition, similar to the effect of barbiturates.
- Chloral hydrate is metabolized to trichloroethanol, which produces its toxic effects.
- Buspirone may exert an effect on serotonin and dopamine-2 receptors in addition to enhancing norepinephrine metabolism in the locus ceruleus.
- The majority of these agents are hepatically metabolized; only meprobamate has significant renal elimination, and only glutethimide has enterohepatic circulation.

EPIDEMIOLOGY

- Poisoning is uncommon.
- Toxic effects are typically moderate.
- Death is rare and usually occurs in conjunction with other drug use (especially alcohol) and before reaching health care.

CAUSES

- Toxic ingestion is usually intentional.
- Child abuse or neglect must be considered if the patient is less than 1 year of age; suicide attempt if the patient is over 6 years of age.

RISK FACTORS

Liver disease may slow the metabolism of these compounds.

DRUG AND DISEASE INTERACTIONS

- Buspirone combined with a monoamine oxidase inhibitor may cause hypertension.
- Coingestion of any sedative-hypnotic agents with other CNS depressants increases toxicity.

PREGNANCY AND LACTATION

- Buspirone. US FDA Pregnancy Category B. Studies indicate no fetal risk, and there are no controlled human studies, or animal studies show an adverse fetal effect but well-controlled studies in pregnant women do not.
- Chloral hydrate, ethchlorvynol, and meprobamate. US FDA Pregnancy Category C. The drug exerts animal teratogenic or embryocidal effects, but there are no controlled studies in women, or no studies are available in either animals or women.
- Chloral hydrate, glutethimide, and meprobamate are excreted in breast milk and should not be taken during lactation.

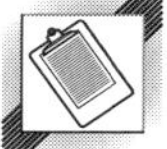

Diagnosis

DIFFERENTIAL DIAGNOSIS

- Toxic causes of generalized CNS depression are numerous: ethanol, antiseizure medications, and antidepressants, among others.
- Nontoxic causes include hypoxia, hypoglycemia, electrolyte abnormality, and intracranial infection or bleed, among others.

SIGNS AND SYMPTOMS

The predominant features are varying degrees of CNS depression, slurred speech, and impaired judgment and motor skills.

Vital Signs

Hypothermia, hypotension, and bradycardia may be present.

HEENT

- Occasional diplopia, blurred vision, nystagmus, or mydriasis may occur with any agent.
- Glutethimide may produce papilledema secondary to cerebral edema.
- Chlormethiazole may increase salivation.
- Ethchlorvynol has a pungent plastic or vinyl-like odor that may produce a mintlike aftertaste.
- Chloral hydrate has a pearlike odor.

Dermatologic

Chloral hydrate has irritant effects on skin and mucous membranes.

Cardiovascular

Chloral hydrate has negative inotropic effects, shortens the refractory period, increases automaticity, and may sensitize the myocardium to catecholamines, making the development of tachydysrhythmias more likely.

Pulmonary

- Respiratory depression is usually present.
- Pulmonary edema occurs in some cases (ethchlorvynol, methyprylon, meprobamate).
- Glutethimide produces thick, tenacious bronchial secretions.

Gastrointestinal

- Meprobamate, ethchlorvynol, and glutethimide may form concretions.
- Chloral hydrate has irritant effects in the gastrointestinal tract and can cause gastritis, esophagitis, and (rarely) gastrointestinal necrosis and esophageal stricture; it is also radiopaque.

Hepatic

Chloral hydrate can increase hepatic enzyme levels.

Renal

- Chloral hydrate can cause transient renal insufficiency.
- Myoglobinuria may develop with any sedative drug if prolonged coma occurs.

Hematologic

Glutethimide causes (rarely) leukopenia, thrombocytopenia, and aplastic anemia.

Fluids and Electrolytes

Lactic acidosis can occur in severe toxicity complicated by hypoxia and prolonged hypotension.

Neurologic

- Depression, lethargy, dysarthria, dystonia, headache, ataxia, prolonged or cyclic coma, amnesia, incoordination, hypertonicity, seizures, incontinence, myoclonus, tremor, hyperreflexia, vertigo, rare hyperexcited states, anxiety, and hallucinations, but rarely death, can occur due to CNS depression.

- Dysphoria may develop with buspirone.
- Muscular hypertonicity may occur with methaqualone.
- Glutethimide can produce an anticholinergic syndrome, along with loss of brainstem reflexes, hyporeflexia, and flaccid muscle tone; it also may cause cerebral edema.

Genitourinary

Buspirone can cause dysuria, enuresis, nocturia, and priapism with therapeutic use.

PROCEDURES AND LABORATORY TESTS

Essential Tests

No tests may be needed for minimally symptomatic patients.

Recommended Tests

- Serum electrolytes, glucose BUN, and creatinine are measured to assess the cause of CNS depression and seizures.
- ECG and pulse oximetry are used to assess cardiovascular effects.
- Serum acetaminophen, aspirin, and ethanol levels in an overdose setting are measured to detect occult ingestion.
- Urinalysis and serum creatine kinase are used to evaluate for rhabdomyolysis in comatose patients.
- Head CT, lumbar puncture, cultures, and other tests as needed are used to assess CNS depression.

Not Recommended Tests

Drug levels of any of these agents are not clinically useful.

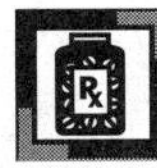

Treatment

Treatment should focus on

- Supportive care with appropriate airway management.
- Dose and time of exposure should be determined for all substances involved.

DIRECTING PATIENT COURSE

The health-care professional should call the poison control center when:

- CNS, respiratory, or myocardial depression or other serious effects are present.
- Toxic effects are not consistent with sedative-hypnotic poisoning.
- Coingestant, drug interaction, or underlying disease presents an unusual problem.

The patient should be referred to a health-care facility when:

- Attempted suicide or homicide is possible.
- Patient or caregiver seems unreliable.
- Any significant symptoms or history of coingestion with other CNS depressants are present.
- Drug interaction or underlying disease presents an unusual problem.

Admission Considerations

Inpatient management is warranted if the patient is persistently symptomatic or hemodynamically unstable, or has experienced a potentially large ingestion.

DECONTAMINATION

Out of Hospital

Ipecac is not recommended due to possibility of rapid patient deterioration.

In Hospital

- Gastric lavage should be performed in pediatric (tube size 24–32 French) or adult (tube size 36–42 French) patients presenting within 1 hour of a large ingestion or if serious effects are present.
- One dose of activated charcoal (1–2 g/kg) can be administered if a substantial ingestion has occurred within the previous few hours.
- Whole-bowel irrigation may be useful for treatment of meprobamate ingestion, but also may be helpful with other ingestions, due to slowed gastrointestinal motility.

ANTIDOTES

- There is no specific antidote for most sedative-hypnotic poisonings.
- In the case of chloral hydrate ingestion, there has been one anecdotal report of positive response to flumazenil (Romazicon) administration.

ADJUNCTIVE THERAPIES

- Hypotension

—Atropine should be used to correct hypotension related to bradycardia.
—Patient should also receive 10 to 20 ml/kg 0.9% saline intravenously and be placed in the Trendelenburg position.
—Further fluid therapy should be guided by central pressure monitoring to avoid volume overload.
—Vasopressor can be added if needed.

- Seizures

—Patent airway must be maintained.
—Benzodiazepine can be administered for initial control.
—If seizures persist or recur, another anticonvulsant such as phenobarbital may be added.

- Hemodialysis has been recommended in the treatment of chloral hydrate, meprobamate, and ethchlorvynol poisoning in the presence of hemodynamic instability that persists despite supportive care.
- β-blockers are considered the first line of drugs for the treatment of chloral hydrate–related cardiotoxicity.

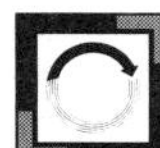

Follow-Up

PATIENT MONITORING

Respiratory and hemodynamic parameters should be monitored continuously.

EXPECTED COURSE AND PROGNOSIS

- Toxic effects may be delayed and prolonged due to decreased gastrointestinal motility and the long half-life of some agents; toxicity may persist for days after overdose.
- Recovery is usually complete unless complications of hypoxia, repeated seizures, or coma develop.
- Possible complications:

—Aspiration pneumonia and complications of prolonged coma may occur.
—Chloral hydrate may rarely cause renal failure, gastrointestinal bleed, esophageal stricture, and hepatitis.
—Ethchlorvynol may cause pulmonary edema due to direct capilloalveolar damage.

DISCHARGE CRITERIA/INSTRUCTIONS

- From the emergency department

—Asymptomatic patients may be discharged following 6 hours of observation and psychiatric evaluation, if needed.
—Prolonged observation may be needed for meprobamate poisoning due to its ability to form concretions and prolong drug absorption.

- From the hospital. Patient may be discharged following resolution or stabilization of toxic effects and after psychiatric evaluation, if needed.

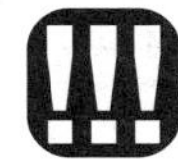

Pitfalls

DIAGNOSIS

Other sources of altered mental status such as intracranial injury or infection should be assessed.

ICD-9-CM 967

Poisoning by sedatives and hypnotics.

See also: SECTION II, Hypotension and Seizures chapters; SECTION III, Flumazenil chapter; and SECTION IV, Ethchlorvynol chapter.

RECOMMENDED READING

Ellenhorn MJ. Sedative-hypnotics. In: *Medical toxicology: diagnosis and treatment of human poisoning,* 2nd ed. Baltimore: Williams & Wilkins, 1996:684–703.

Author: Christopher Layton

Reviewer: Richard C. Dart

Selective Serotonin Reuptake Inhibitors

Basics

DESCRIPTION

Selective serotonin reuptake inhibitors (SSRIs) are antidepressant medications that do not share toxic mechanisms of the tricyclic antidepressants.

FORMS AND USES

- Fluoxetine (Prozac) is available as 10- and 20-mg tablets or as a 20 mg/5 ml solution and is prescribed at 5 to 80 mg/day.
- Fluvoxamine (Luvox) is available as 50- and 100-mg tablets and is prescribed at 100 to 300 mg/day.
- Paroxetine (Paxil) is available as 20- and 30-mg tablets and is prescribed at 10 to 50 mg/day.
- Sertraline (Zoloft) is available as 50- and 100-mg tablets and is prescribed at 50 to 200 mg/day.
- Psychiatric applications include depression, obsessive-compulsive disorder, and panic disorder.
- Other uses include appetite control, bulimia nervosa, diabetic neuropathy, headache, myoclonus, narcolepsy, obesity, and pain.

TOXIC DOSE

- A single ingestion of any of these agents by adults, even in gram quantities, generally leads to minimal toxicity.
- Very large pediatric ingestion has produced tachycardia, tremor, and coma.

PATHOPHYSIOLOGY

- SSRIs selectively block reuptake of serotonin (5-hydroxytryptamine) at presynaptic neuronal junctions.
- Therapeutic half-lives are 24 hours for sertraline, 12 to 18 hours for paroxetine, and 1 to 4 days for fluoxetine.
- Only fluoxetine has an active metabolite (norfluoxetine) with a prolonged half-life of 7 to 14 days.
- Effects can last from 1 to 6 weeks after discontinuation of the drug at therapeutic doses and longer in overdose.

EPIDEMIOLOGY

- Intentional overdose is common.
- Deaths are rare and usually due to coingestants.

CAUSES

- Poisoning is usually from suicidal ingestion.
- The possibility of child abuse or neglect should be considered in patients less than 1 year of age, suicide attempt in patients over 6 years of age.

RISK FACTORS

In geriatric patients, cardiac and liver dysfunction may lead to an elevated serum SSRI concentration.

DRUG AND DISEASE INTERACTIONS

- Serotonin syndrome may result from coingestion of SSRIs with monoamine oxidase inhibitors, stimulants (e.g., amphetamines), nonselective inhibitors of bioamine uptake, serotonin agonists, or other serotonin uptake inhibitors.
- Cimetidine inhibits the metabolism of paroxetine and may result in an increased serum paroxetine concentration.

PREGNANCY AND LACTATION

- Fluoxetine, paroxetine, and sertraline. US FDA Pregnancy Category B. Animal studies indicate no fetal risk and there are no controlled human studies, or animal studies show an adverse fetal effect but well-controlled studies in women do not.
- Fluvoxamine. US FDA Pregnancy Category C. The drug exerts animal teratogenic or embryocidal effects, but there are no controlled studies in women, or no studies are available in either animals or women.
- Withdrawal symptoms have occurred in the postpartum period in infants who were exposed to sertraline *in utero.*
- Pregnant patients should be monitored for premature labor or spontaneous abortion.

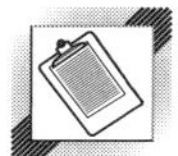

Diagnosis

DIFFERENTIAL DIAGNOSIS

- Toxic causes of altered mental status, tachycardia, and seizures include tricyclic antidepressants, theophylline, sympathomimetics, lithium, and others.
- Nontoxic causes include hyperthyroidism, electrolyte abnormalities, hyperpyrexia, hypoglycemia, encephalitis, severe dystonic reaction, drug withdrawal syndromes, and others.

SIGNS AND SYMPTOMS

- SSRI overdose is characterized by nonspecific effects.
- Drug interactions may result in serotonin syndrome, which is characterized by altered mental status, autonomic dysfunction, and neuromuscular abnormalities (included in a separate chapter).

Vital Signs

- Serotonin syndrome. Fluctuating blood pressure, tachycardia, tachypnea, and hyperthermia may occur.
- Acute overdose. Tachycardia or bradycardia may occur.

HEENT

Lacrimation, mydriasis, blurred vision, and, in severe cases, unreactive pupils may occur.

Dermatologic

Diaphoresis and flushing may occur.

Cardiovascular

- Sinus tachycardia or bradycardia is common.
- Premature ventricular contractions, QTc prolongation, junctional rhythms, and ventricular tachycardia may occur in very severe cases.

Gastrointestinal

Diarrhea, nausea, and vomiting are common.

Hepatic

Hepatic injury may occur in severe cases.

Renal

Rhabdomyolysis may occur in severe cases.

Neurologic

Akathesia, ataxia, hyperreflexia, myoclonus, restlessness, rigidity, shivering, trismus, coma, confusion, delirium, drowsiness, hallucinations (auditory and visual), mania, mutism, and seizures have occurred in severe cases.

Reproductive

Ejaculation failure and orgasmic inhibition may occur rarely.

PROCEDURES AND LABORATORY TESTS

Essential Tests

No tests may be needed in asymptomatic patients.

Recommended Tests

- Complete blood count, serum electrolytes, glucose, BUN, and creatinine should be determined in symptomatic patients to evaluate the causes of toxicity.
- Serum liver function tests should be performed in symptomatic patients to detect hepatic injury.
- ECG, serum acetaminophen and aspirin levels should be measured in an overdose setting to detect occult ingestion.

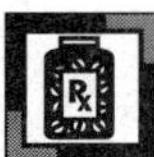

Treatment

• Treatment should focus on gastrointestinal decontamination and identification of coingestants.
• If serotonin syndrome is suspected, treatment should focus on protecting the airway, stabilizing blood pressure, and controlling fever.
• Dose and time of exposure should be determined for all substances involved.

DIRECTING PATIENT COURSE

The health-care provider should call the poison control center when:

• Coma, hyperthermia, or cardiovascular instability is present.
• Toxic effects are not consistent with SSRI toxicity.
• Coingestant, drug interaction, or underlying disease presents an unusual problem.

Patients should be referred to a health-care facility when:

• Attempted suicide or homicide is possible.
• Patient or caregiver seems unreliable.
• Toxic effects are present.
• Coingestant, drug interaction, or underlying disease presents an unusual problem.

Admission Considerations

Inpatient treatment is warranted when the patient has a change in mental status, fluctuating vital signs, fever, or seizures.

DECONTAMINATION

Out of Hospital

Emesis should be induced with ipecac within 1 hour of ingestion for alert pediatric or adult patients if health-care evaluation will be delayed.

In Hospital

• Emesis should be induced with ipecac within 1 hour of ingestion for the pediatric patient who is too small to have effective gastric lavage.
• Gastric lavage should be performed in pediatric (tube size 24–32 French) or adult (tube size 36–42 French) patients presenting within 1 hour of a large ingestion or if serious effects are present.
• One dose of activated charcoal (1–2 g/kg) should be administered without a cathartic if a substantial ingestion has occurred within the previous few hours.

ANTIDOTES

There is no specific antidote for SSRI poisoning.

ADJUNCTIVE TREATMENT

• Hemodialysis and multiple doses of activated charcoal are not effective for SSRI poisoning or serotonin syndrome.
• Seizures

—A patent airway should be ensured.
—A benzodiazepine should be administered for initial control.
—If seizures persist or recur, another anticonvulsant such as phenobarbital should be added.

• Serotonin syndrome is treated with temperature control, endotracheal intubation, muscle relaxation, and general supportive care.

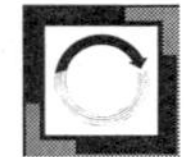

Follow-Up

PATIENT MONITORING

In patients with severe poisoning or serotonin syndrome, vital signs (especially temperature) as well as respiratory and cardiac function should be monitored continuously.

EXPECTED COURSE AND PROGNOSIS

• Acute SSRI toxicity typically resolves within 4 to 6 hours of ingestion.
• Patients with serotonin syndrome may be symptomatic for 24 to 48 hours.
• Fatalities have occurred from serotonin syndrome.
• Hyperpyrexia and status epilepticus may occur in serotonin syndrome.

DISCHARGE CRITERIA/INSTRUCTIONS

• From the emergency department. Asymptomatic patients may be discharged after 6 hours of observation following gastrointestinal decontamination and psychiatric evaluation, if needed.
• From the hospital

—Patients may be discharged after vital signs and mental status normalize.
—Psychiatric evaluation should be obtained for patients who have taken an intentional overdose.

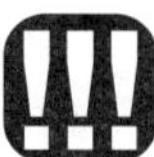

Pitfalls

DIAGNOSIS

• Toxicity resulting from SSRI drug interaction may not be identified.
• Careful drug history is needed to identify drug interactions.
• Long duration of action of SSRIs and fluoxetine metabolite can result in drug interactions up to 6 weeks after discontinuation of SSRI.

TREATMENT

Hyperthermia may cause serious injury if not adequately treated.

FOLLOW-UP

• Medications should be monitored carefully.
• Medications that interact adversely with SSRIs should be withheld for at least 6 weeks following discontinuation of the SSRI.

ICD-9-CM 969.0

Poisoning by psychotropic agents: antidepressants.

See also: SECTION II, Neuroleptic Malignant Syndrome and Serotonin Syndrome and Seizures chapters.

RECOMMENDED READING

Ellenhorn MJ, Schonwald S, Ordog G, et al. *Ellenhorn's medical toxicology: diagnosis and treatment of human poisoning,* 2nd ed. Baltimore: Williams & Wilkins, 1997:615–623,900–905.

Martin TG. Serotonin syndrome. *Ann Emerg Med* 1996;28:520–526.

Author: Timothy VanDuzer

Reviewer: Rivka S. Horowitz

Selenium

Basics

DESCRIPTION

Selenium (Se) is found as elemental selenium, inorganic selenium salts (sodium selenite), organic selenium, hydrogen selenide (gaseous form), selenium oxychloride (liquid, vesicant), selenium dioxide, and selenious acid.

FORMS AND USES

Industrial Uses

- Selenium is used to imbue a red pigment to glass and plastic.
- It is used in the electronics, copper, photography, and rubber industries, as well as in photocopy machines.
- It is a component of various substances, including gun bluing solution, sheep and cattle drench, and paint, varnish, and glue remover.

Food Sources of Selenium

- Grains grown in soil high in selenium, garlic, nuts, sunflower seeds, brown sugar, mushrooms, and egg noodles
- Seafood, especially swordfish, tuna, and oysters; liver; kidney; skimmed milk; egg yolk; beef; and chicken

Other

Selenium also is used as an antibacterial and antiseborrheic agent in shampoo.

TOXIC DOSE

Chronic ingestion of 30 to 60 mg/day has produced toxicity.

PATHOPHYSIOLOGY

- Selenium in toxic doses is thought to bind and interfere with sulfhydryl groups on enzymes needed for protein synthesis.
- Elemental selenium is minimally toxic.
- Selenium salts may produce toxicity by ingestion, inhalation, and percutaneous absorption.

EPIDEMIOLOGY

Poisoning is uncommon.

CAUSES

- Poisoning is usually accidental.
- The possibility of child neglect or abuse should be considered in patients less than 1 year of age; suicide attempt in patients over 6 years of age.

PREGNANCY AND LACTATION

- Selenium crosses the placenta and is transmitted in breast milk.
- Selenium is teratogenic in animals.

WORKPLACE STANDARDS

- ACGIH. TLV TWA is 0.2 mg/m^3.
- NIOSH. IDLH level is 1 mg/m^3.
- OSHA. PEL TWA is 0.2 mg/m^3.

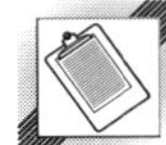

Diagnosis

DIFFERENTIAL DIAGNOSIS

Other causes of gastroenteritis include thallium toxicity, arsenic toxicity, and infectious gastroenteritis.

SIGNS AND SYMPTOMS

HEENT

Garlic or rotten horseradish breath, increased incidence of dental caries, chemosis, lacrimation, and "rose eye" (swelling and pink discoloration of the eyelids) may occur.

Dermatologic

- Dermatitis, alopecia, and brittle hair that breaks off at the scalp may occur.
- Selenious acid may cause chemical burn.

Cardiovascular

- Massive overdose causes hypotension, cardiomyopathy with ECG T-wave inversions, and elevated creatine kinase.
- Selenious acid may cause cardiomyopathy.

Pulmonary

- Inhalation of fumes or dust may cause respiratory mucosal irritation (sore throat, cough) that may last for 1 to 2 weeks after an acute exposure ("rose cold").
- High-dose exposure may cause pulmonary edema.

Gastrointestinal

- Gastrointestinal upset, abdominal pain, nausea, and vomiting may occur.
- Selenious acid may cause salivation and caustic gastrointestinal injury, hematemesis, and diarrhea.

Neurologic

- Dizziness, weakness, and peripheral painful paresthesia may occur.
- Hyperreflexia, convulsions, and motor disturbance can result.

Psychiatric

Languor, depression, and emotional instability can occur.

PROCEDURES AND LABORATORY TESTS

Essential Tests

No tests may be needed in asymptomatic patients.

Recommended Tests

- Complete blood count, arterial blood gas, serum electrolytes, BUN, creatinine, liver enzymes, and urinalysis should be obtained, especially after selenious acid ingestion.
- The selenium level in a 24-hour urine sample correlates well with dietary intake of selenium.
- Serum selenium levels also can be useful when renal dysfunction is present.
- Endoscopy may be needed for patients with caustic injury from ingestion of selenious acid.

Not Recommended Tests

Other body tissue levels (e.g., in hair or nails) are not useful.

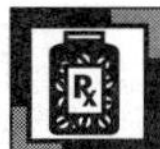

Treatment

- Therapy consists primarily of symptomatic and supportive care.
- Dose and time of exposure should be determined for all substances involved.

DIRECTING PATIENT COURSE

The health-care professional should call the poison control center when:

- Severe or persistent effects develop.
- Coingestant, drug interaction, or underlying disease presents an unusual problem.

The patient should be referred to a health-care facility when:

- Suicide or homicide attempt is possible.
- Toxic effects develop.
- Coingestant, drug interaction, or underlying disease presents an unusual problem.

Admission Considerations

Patients with serious end-organ injury (e.g., ECG changes, pulmonary edema) and patients with potential caustic injury from selenious acid should be admitted.

DECONTAMINATION

Out of Hospital

- The patient should be moved to fresh air following inhalation exposure.
- Skin exposures should be washed with copious amounts of water.

In Hospital

- Gastric emptying and activated charcoal are not recommended if caustic gastrointestinal injury has occurred.
- For acute ingestion, gastric lavage and activated charcoal are recommended.

—Gastric lavage should be performed in pediatric (tube size 24–32 French) or adult (tube size 36–42 French) patients presenting within 1 hour of a large ingestion or if serious effects are present.
—One dose of activated charcoal (1–2 g/kg) should be administered without a cathartic if a substantial ingestion has occurred within the previous few hours.

ANTIDOTE

There is no specific antidote for selenium poisoning.

ADJUNCTIVE TREATMENT

- Seizures, hypotension, bronchospasm, and pulmonary edema are treated in the usual manner.
- Not recommended treatments. Bromobenzene, British anti-Lewisite (BAL, dimercaprol), ethylenediaminetetraacetic acid (EDTA), and vitamin C have been tried and found to have inconsistent or harmful results.

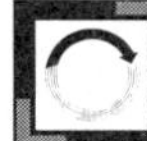

Follow-Up

PATIENT MONITORING

Future levels should be checked, especially if symptoms persist.

DISCHARGE CRITERIA/INSTRUCTIONS

Asymptomatic patients may be discharged from the emergency department or hospital following decontamination, 4 hours of observation, and psychiatric evaluation, if needed.

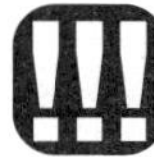

Pitfalls

DIAGNOSIS

- Selenium toxicity must be suspected in order to be diagnosed.
- Doses recommended in multivitamin bottles may exceed a dose causing chronic toxicity.

FOLLOW-UP

It is important to identify the source of selenium toxicity and remove it to avoid further poisonings.

ICD-9-CM 989

Toxic effect of other substances, chiefly nonmedicinal as to source.

See also: SECTION II, Seizures, Hypotension, and Pulmonary Edema chapters.

RECOMMENDED READING

Maejos MS, Romero CD. Urinary selenium concentrations. *Clin Chem* 1993;39:2040–2052.

Author: Gayle E. Long

Reviewer: Richard C. Dart

Sildenafil

Basics

DESCRIPTION

Sildenafil (Viagra) is an oral selective phosphodiesterase inhibitor that is used to treat erectile dysfunction.

FORMS AND USES

- Sildenafil is used to treat erectile dysfunction of either organic or psychogenic etiology.
- It is formulated as blue diamond-shaped tablets (25, 50, and 100 mg) for oral use.
- A dose of 25 to 100 mg is taken 0.5 to 4 hours before sexual activity once per day.

TOXIC DOSE

- Healthy volunteers tolerated single doses as large as 800 mg with a side effect profile similar to that seen at lower doses.
- Death or other serious effects following overdose have not been reported, although sudden death has occurred during therapeutic use and vigorous sexual activity.

PATHOPHYSIOLOGY

- Inflow of blood into the corpus cavernosum of the penis is increased by smooth muscle relaxation, a process that is enhanced by increased levels of cyclic guanosine monophosphate (cGMP).
- Phosphodiesterase type 5 (PDE5) is found in the penis and degrades cGMP.
- Through the inhibition of PDE5, sildenafil enhances the relaxation of vascular smooth muscle and allows an erection to occur.
- However, concurrent sexual stimulation is required to improve erectile dysfunction.
- Sildenafil inhibits other forms of PDE. Weak inhibition of PDE6 is thought to be the mechanism for the visual symptoms experienced by some patients who use sildenafil.

EPIDEMIOLOGY

- Sildenafil use has been described in an age group that ranges from 19 to 87 years.
- Toxic effects following exposure are typically minor; however, very large ingestions may cause hypotension, vasodilation, and tachycardia. This is particularly true when large doses of sildenafil are taken in the presence of organic nitrates.

CAUSES

- Poisoning is usually accidental.
- Child abuse or neglect should be considered if the patient is less than 1 year of age; suicide attempt in patients over 6 years of age.

DRUG AND DISEASE INTERACTIONS

- Sildenafil is eliminated via hepatic metabolism (predominantly CYP3A4) producing an active metabolite.
- Both the parent compound and the metabolite have similar elimination half-lives of approximately 4 hours.
- Healthy volunteers over the age of 65 had reduced clearance of sildenafil with plasma concentrations 40% higher than younger patients.
- Clearance of sildenafil is reduced in patients with hepatic insufficiency or significant renal impairment (creatinine clearance less than 30 ml/min).
- Concomitant use of cytochrome P450 inhibitors (especially those of the 3A4 isoforms) may reduce the clearance of sildenafil and increase serum concentrations. Examples include cimetidine, erythromycin, ketoconazole, itraconazole, and mibefradil.
- Because sildenafil has been shown to potentiate the hypotensive effects of nitrates, it is contraindicated in patients who use nitrates or other medications that could be nitric acid donors.

PREGNANCY AND LACTATION

- US FDA Pregnancy Category B. There is no evidence of teratogenicity, embryotoxicity, or fetotoxicity in animal models, but there are no controlled studies in pregnant women.
- The appearance of sildenafil in breast milk has not been studied. Sildenafil is not indicated in women or children.

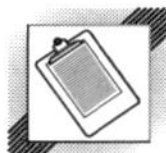

Diagnosis

DIFFERENTIAL DIAGNOSIS

- Other toxicants that cause flushing and headache include nitrates, niacin, calcium channel blockers such as nifedipine, α-adrenergic antagonists such as prazosin, and scombroid.
- Other toxicants that cause altered vision are digoxin, quinine, quinidine, chloroquine, hydroxychloroquine, and methanol.
- Nontoxic causes of flushing, headache, and altered vision include subarachnoid hemorrhage, pheochromocytoma, carcinoid, and anaphylaxis.

SIGNS AND SYMPTOMS

Adverse effects that have been noted in clinical trials include nausea, vomiting, headache, flushing, hypotension, dyspepsia, rhinitis, and abnormal vision (blue tinge to vision or sensitivity to light). Priapism has not been reported, but could occur, particularly in patients with sickle cell anemia, multiple myeloma, or leukemia.

Vital Signs

Tachycardia may be seen.

Cardiovascular

Hypotension, vasodilation, and tachycardia have been reported, and reduction of blood pressure of up to 10 mm Hg has been observed in healthy subjects.

Pulmonary

No effects have been reported.

Renal

No effects have been reported.

Fluids and Electrolytes

No effects have been reported.

Neurologic

Alterations in color vision, including a blue-green tinge, sensitivity to light, and decreased visual acuity have been noted in a small percentage of patients taking therapeutic doses. These effects appear to be dose related and resolve when the drug is discontinued.

Musculoskeletal

Brief myalgia has been described in individuals taking therapeutic doses.

PROCEDURES AND LABORATORY TESTS

Essential Tests

No tests may be needed in asymptomatic patients.

Recommended Tests

- An ECG with continuous cardiac monitoring is necessary.
- Serum electrolytes, glucose, BUN, and creatinine levels are measured to assess other causes of hypotension or dysrhythmia.
- Serum acetaminophen and aspirin levels in the overdose setting are used to detect occult ingestion.

Not Recommended Tests

Serum sildenafil levels are not clinically useful.

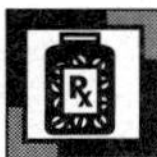

Treatment

- Treatment should focus on general supportive and symptomatic care.
- The dose and time of exposure must be determined for all substances involved.

DIRECTING PATIENT COURSE

The health-care provider should call the poison control center when:

- Hypotension, dysrhythmia, QRS widening, seizure, or coma are present.
- Toxic effects are not consistent with sildenafil poisoning.
- Coingestant, drug interaction, or underlying disease presents an unusual challenge.

The patient should be referred to a health-care facility when:

- Overdose effects are present (including persistent sinus tachycardia).
- Attempted suicide or homicide is possible.
- Patient or caregiver seems unreliable.
- Coingestant, drug interaction, or underlying disease presents an unusual challenge.

Admission Considerations

Inpatient management is warranted for all patients with altered mental status, hypotension, chest pain, or signs consistent with acute ischemic heart disease.

DECONTAMINATION

Out of Hospital

Emesis should not be induced because of low toxic potential.

In Hospital

- Gastric lavage should be performed in pediatric (tube size 24–32 French) or adult (tube size 36–42 French) patients. Following a massive ingestion, if serious effects are present or another toxic substance is likely to be present.
- If a substantial ingestion has occurred within the previous few hours, one dose of activated charcoal (1–2 g/kg) without cathartic should be administered.

ANTIDOTES

There is no specific antidote for sildenafil.

ADJUNCTIVE TREATMENT

Hypotension

- The patient should receive 10 to 20 ml/kg of 0.9% saline intravenously and be placed in the Trendelenburg position. Further fluid therapy is guided by central pressure monitoring in order to avoid fluid volume overload.
- If hypotension is unresponsive to the above treatment, a vasopressor should be administered.

—The dose of dopamine is 2 to 5 μg/kg/min intravenously, titrated upward to effect.
—Rates greater than 20 μg/kg/min are unlikely to provide further benefit.

- If hypotension is still unresponsive, norepinephrine is added at 0.1 to 0.2 μg/kg/min intravenously and titrated upward to effect.
- Caution must be exercised because too high a rate of infusion may cause tissue ischemia.

Not Recommended Therapies

Because sildenafil is highly bound to plasma proteins and is only minimally excreted in the urine, dialysis probably will not increase the rate of sildenafil clearance.

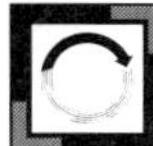

Follow-Up

PATIENT MONITORING

- In symptomatic patients, hemodynamic and rhythm monitoring should be performed continuously.
- In asymptomatic patients, 4 to 6 hours of observation with continuous blood pressure monitoring should be instituted in the emergency department.

EXPECTED COURSE AND PROGNOSIS

Most adverse effects are expected to be minor and temporary, resolving with the cessation of drug ingestion, unless sequelae of myocardial ischemia intercede.

DISCHARGE CRITERIA/INSTRUCTIONS

- From the emergency department. Asymptomatic patients may be discharged from the emergency department if their ECG is without ischemic changes and continuous cardiac monitoring does not show tachycardia or dysrhythmia for 4 to 6 hours.
- From hospital. Patients may be discharged from the hospital when clinical effects have resolved and vital signs are normal.

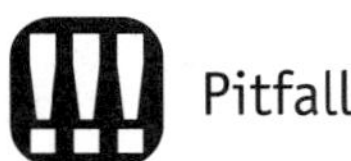

Pitfalls

DIAGNOSIS

Because of the nonspecific nature of the signs and symptoms of sildenafil toxicity, it is difficult to attribute these general complaints to sildenafil ingestion.

ICD-9-CM 975.1

Smooth muscle relaxants.

RECOMMENDED READING

Goldstein I, Lue TF, Padma-Nathan H, et al. Oral sildenafil in the treatment of erectile dysfunction. *N Engl J Med* 1998;338:1397–1404.

Morales A, Gingell C, Collins M, et al. Clinical safety of oral sildenafil citrate (Viagra) in the treatment of erectile dysfunction. *Impotence Res* 10:69–73.

Pfizer Laboratories. Viagra (sildenafil citrate), Product Information. Pfizer Laboratories, New York, 1998.

Authors: Jeffrey Rogers and Frank F.S. Daly

Reviewer: Richard C. Dart

Smoke Inhalation

Basics

DESCRIPTION

Smoke inhalation includes the inhalation of combustion products from synthetic or naturally occurring compounds.

FORMS AND USES

- The burning of wood, wood products, cotton, silk, natural fibers, and plants produces carbon dioxide (CO_2), carbon monoxide (CO), ammonia, aldehydes (e.g., acetaldehyde), and acrolein, as well as aliphatic and aromatic hydrocarbons.
- The burning of synthetic materials (plastics, flame retardants, upholstery, urethane foam cushions, etc.) produces cyanide (CN^-), hydrogen chloride, hydrogen bromide, halogenated hydrocarbons, isocyanates, nitrogen oxides, nitrates, nitrites, and benzene.
- Other common hazardous chemicals generated in fires include free radicals, hydrogen sulfide (H_2S), hydrogen fluoride, polyaromatic hydrocarbons, sulfur dioxide (SO_2), particulates, metals, chlorine, and oxyhydrocarbons.

PATHOPHYSIOLOGY

Asphyxiants

- Physical asphyxiants include CO_2, nitrogen, and others that reduce the concentration of oxygen in the air.
- Chemical asphyxiants include carbon monoxide, cyanide, hydrogen sulfide, nitrates, and nitrites (methemoglobin), which prevent the transport or use of oxygen absorbed by the lungs.

Pulmonary Irritants

Particulate matter includes dust, fumes, and smoke that may also contain such irritants as acrolein, acids, ammonia, nitrogen oxides, SO_2, phosgene, chlorine, and formaldehyde.

Thermal Injuries

- Upper and lower airway injury from inhalation of superheated ambient air or superheated steam may occur.
- Dermal burns may occur.

Lipid Peroxidation

Free radicals cause lipid peroxidation within the pulmonary surfactant system, altering the surface tension of the lungs and impairing respiratory function.

EPIDEMIOLOGY

- Smoke inhalation is common; toxic effects range from mild to severe.
- Most deaths from fires are caused by carbon monoxide or smoke inhalation, CO being the main toxic gas produced.

CAUSES

Usually exposure is accidental, but attempted suicide should be considered in patients over 6 years of age.

PREGNANCY AND LACTATION

Formation of carboxyhemoglobin is faster on the maternal side, but the half-life of carboxyhemoglobin is significantly longer in the fetus.

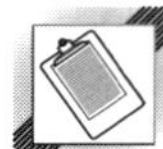

Diagnosis

SIGNS AND SYMPTOMS

- Dermal burns are obvious, but thermal injury to the upper and lower airways may be subtle initially.
- Chemical pneumonitis may be delayed.

Vital Signs

Tachycardia and tachypnea are common.

HEENT

- Hoarseness, dysphonia, stridor, and drooling may develop in serious cases.
- Eyes, mucous membranes, and respiratory tract may become irritated.
- Facial burns, singed nasal hairs, and carbonaceous sputum suggest serious smoke inhalation.

Cardiovascular

Myocardial ischemia or infarction from hypoxia may be seen.

Pulmonary

Cough, bronchospasm, rales, shortness of breath, rhonchi, and tracheobronchitis are common in serious exposures.

Neurologic

Headaches, altered mental status, dizziness, and coma may occur.

PROCEDURES AND LABORATORY TESTS

Essential Tests

- Arterial blood gases are used to assess oxygenation.
- Arterial or venous blood gases are studied to determine the presence of carboxyhemoglobin by cooximetry; a normal or low level does not exclude the diagnosis or necessarily reflect the severity of the poisoning, especially if oxygen was given to the patient or if there was a delay between exposure and blood sampling.
- ECG, serum electrolytes, BUN, creatinine, glucose, and lactate level are ordered to assess effects of hypoxia and other potential causes of CNS depression.

Recommended Tests

- Methemoglobin level should be ordered.
- Cyanide level will not be immediately available and should not affect initial treatment; it is used as a confirmatory test.
- Pulmonary function tests are used to assess bronchospasm.
- Serum acetaminophen and aspirin levels in an overdose setting are used to detect occult ingestion.
- A chest radiograph may initially be normal. Patchy pneumonitis or diffuse pulmonary edema may appear in the first 24 hours.
- A xenon lung scan may be useful in determining the extent of a parenchymal injury.
- Bronchoscopy may be needed to assess the extent of injuries to the upper and lower airways.

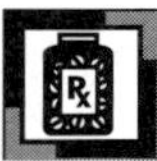

Treatment

- Initial treatment involves intensive supportive respiratory care and administration of 100% oxygen.
- Endotracheal intubation should be performed early.

DIRECTING PATIENT COURSE

The health-care provider should call the poison control center when:

- Carbon monoxide or cyanide poisoning or methemoglobinemia are suspected.
- Toxic effects are not consistent with smoke inhalation.
- A coingestant, drug interaction, or underlying disease presents an unusual problem.

The patient should be referred to a health-care facility when:

- Attempted suicide or homicide is possible.
- Any toxic effects develop.
- Patient or caregiver seems unreliable.
- A coingestant, drug interaction, or underlying disease presents an unusual problem.

Admission Considerations

Inpatient treatment is warranted for all patients who have sustained significant smoke inhalation (i.e., history of high or prolonged exposure).

DECONTAMINATION

Out of Hospital

The patient should be moved to fresh air and given supplemental oxygen.

In Hospital

- Oxygen (100%) should be administered.
- The patient's clothing should be removed and the skin should be washed copiously with water if skin contamination from the source is possible.

ANTIDOTES

Sodium Thiosulfate

• Indications. In order to treat unrecognized cyanide poisoning as early as possible, empiric treatment with the thiosulfate component of the cyanide antidote kit is recommended for unconscious victims from a fire.
• Contraindications. Treatment with the amyl nitrite and sodium nitrite components of the kit is not usually recommended (until levels of carboxyhemoglobin can be tested) because iatrogenic methemoglobinemia may further compromise the oxygen-carrying capacity of the victim.
• Method of administration. Adult dose is 50 ml of 25% solution (12.5 g) intravenously over several minutes; pediatric dose is 1.65 ml/kg of a 25% solution up to 50 ml (12.5 g) intravenously over several minutes.
• See SECTION III, Cyanide Antidote Package chapter for further detail.

Hyperbaric Oxygen

• Indications. Hyperbaric oxygen (HBO) is recommended for patients who are unconscious or symptomatic, have a markedly elevated carboxyhemoglobin level, or are pregnant with a carboxyhemoglobin level greater than 15%.
• Consulatation with a medical toxicologist is recommended in determining the need for HBO.
• Contraindications and adverse effects. See SECTION III, Hyperbaric Oxygen chapter.

ADJUNCTIVE TREATMENT

Seizures

• A patent airway should be ensured, and benzodiazepine should be administered for initial control.
• If seizures persist or recur, another anticonvulsant should be added, such as phenobarbital.

Hypotension

• The patient is given an isotonic fluid infusion and placed in the Trendelenburg position.
• A vasopressor is used if needed; dopamine is preferred, but norepinephrine is added for refractory hypotension.

Dysrhythmias or Conduction Abnormalities

• Lidocaine is used for ventricular tachycardia or multifocal preventricular contractions.

—Adult dose is 50 to 100 mg by intravenous bolus, followed by an infusion of 2 to 4 mg/min, titrated to the desired effect.
—Pediatric dose is 1 mg/kg bolus, followed by an infusion of 20 to 50 μg/kg/min, titrated to effect.
—One-half the bolus-dose may be repeated in 10 to 15 minutes.

• Bretylium dosage is 5 mg/kg over 1 minute; if the dose is unsuccessful, 10 mg/kg over 1 minute should be administered and repeated as necessary to a total dose of 30 mg/kg.

Bronchospasm

• Oxygen should be administered, followed by albuterol at 0.15 mg/kg (maximum of 10 mg) in saline with humidified oxygen via nebulizer every 20 to 30 minutes.
• If the peak expiratory flow rate is greater than 90% of predicted after the initial dose, additional doses may not be needed.
• The response should be monitored continually.
• Methylprednisolone dose is 60 to 125 mg (adults 1–1.5 mg/kg) given intravenously (pediatric 1–2 mg/kg), every 6 to 8 hours; this may be decreased to a single daily dose and tapered.
• Initiation of prednisone for outpatient treatment, 2 mg/kg orally for several days, should be considered.

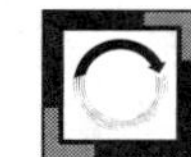

Follow-Up

PATIENT MONITORING

• Respiratory and cardiac function should be monitored continuously.
• Serial pulmonary function tests may be indicated.

EXPECTED COURSE AND PROGNOSIS

• Cough, dyspnea, cyanosis, and chest examination findings of wheezes, rales, and rhonchi in the hours following smoke inhalation are indicators of poor prognosis.
• Possible complications include long-term pulmonary complications or sequelae of hypoxia.

DISCHARGE CRITERIA/INSTRUCTIONS

• From the emergency department

—Discharge is warranted for asymptomatic patients without risk factors (i.e., for those who are not elderly, pregnant, or chronically ill) following decontamination and at least 6 hours of observation.
—Asymptomatic patients with high-risk exposures (i.e., facial or nasal burns, confined space exposure, elevated carboxyhemoglobin, or age over 40 years) should be admitted for observation for at least 24 hours.

• From the hospital. Discharge is warranted for patients following the resolution or stabilization of toxic effects.

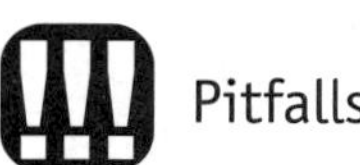

Pitfalls

DIAGNOSIS

• It is important to search for other injuries in addition to the obvious thermal injuries.
• Inhalation injuries are a dynamic process, and the initial presentation may seem trivial only to deteriorate over several hours.
• Absence of facial burns, singed nasal hairs, and carbonaceous sputum does not exclude airway injury.

TREATMENT

Updating the tetanus booster is important.

ICD-9-CM 987

Toxic effect of other gases, fumes, or vapors.

See also: SECTION II, Hypotension and Seizures chapters; and SECTION III, Cyanide Antidote Package and Hyperbaric Oxygen chapters.

RECOMMENDED READING

Ainslie G. Inhalation injuries produced by smoke and nitrogen dioxide. *Respir Med* 1993;87:169–174.

Kirk MA, Gerace R, Kulig K. Cyanide and methemoglobin kinetics in smoke inhalation victims treated with the cyanide antidote kit. *Ann Emerg Med* 1993;22:1413–1418.

Kulig K. Cyanide antidotes and fire toxicology. *N Engl J Med* 1991;325:1801–1802.

Tomaszewski CA, Thom SR. Use of hyperbaric oxygen in toxicology. *Emerg Med Clin North Am* 1994;12:437–459.

Author: Paul Bender

Reviewer: Luke Yip

Snakebite—Exotic

Basics

DESCRIPTION

Exotic snakes are those not indigenous to the United States.

FORMS AND USES

- Nonindigenous snakes are found in legitimate zoos throughout the United States.
- In addition, a large "underground zoo" exists, composed of snakes kept by collectors and snake fanciers.
- In recent years, bites have occurred from cobras, king cobras, green mambas, black mambas, saw scated vipers, and gaboon vipers.

TOXIC DOSE

One bite can be life threatening; however, 25% to 60% of venomous bites do not result in envenomation.

PATHOPHYSIOLOGY

- Snake venoms cause a wide range of effects, but most involve injury to one or all of the following: local bite site, the coagulation system, and the nervous and cardiovascular systems.
- During the act of biting, venom may be deposited on the skin, in subcutaneous tissue, or intramuscularly; the most common site is subcutaneous tissue.

EPIDEMIOLOGY

- Poisoning is rare.
- Toxic effects are typically mild to moderate, but may become life threatening.
- Death is unusual and occurs primarily in patients who present in shock or who do not pursue health care promptly.

CAUSES

Bites usually occur during the handling of snakes.

RISK FACTORS

- Snake keepers at legitimate zoos are often exposed to venomous exotic snakes.
- A history of a previous bite is more common in someone who routinely handles snakes.
- A bite on the hand nearly always indicates that the bite occurred during handling.

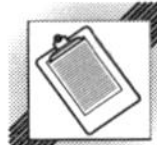

Diagnosis

DIFFERENTIAL DIAGNOSIS

- Puncture wounds also can be caused by inanimate objects (thorns, etc.) or bites from nonvenomous snakes.
- Swelling and ecchymosis can result from unrecognized trauma or coagulopathy.

SIGNS AND SYMPTOMS

Owing to the wide variety of snakes that may be involved, only those manifestations that should be considered in all cases are included.

- All bites should show evidence of skin wounds, although these may be scratches, small lacerations, or single puncture wounds in some cases.
- Toxic effects may begin within minutes, but in some cases toxicity does not develop for several hours.

Vital Signs

- Initial tachycardia and mild hypertension due to anxiety, pain, or venom effect are common.
- In severe cases the patient may become hypotensive.

HEENT

Venoms that cause muscular paralysis may cause ptosis, difficulty swallowing, and aspiration of oral secretions in severe cases.

Dermatologic

- Local effects should include bite marks.
- Swelling and ecchymosis may develop.

Cardiovascular

Shock may develop due to hypovolemia from soft-tissue swelling or hemorrhage, or due to myocardial depressant effects.

Pulmonary

Neurotoxic venoms may cause decreased depth of respiration and, rarely, pulmonary edema.

Gastrointestinal

- Nausea and vomiting are common with a wide range of snakes.
- Gastrointestinal hemorrhage may develop with venoms that cause coagulopathy.

Renal

- Hematuria may be the first sign of coagulopathy.
- Several venoms cause severe rhabdomyolysis, which can lead to acute renal failure.

Hematologic

- Many venoms cause coagulation abnormalities.
- Spontaneous hemorrhage may occur but is unusual.

Musculoskeletal

Compartment syndrome occurs infrequently.

Neurologic

Many venoms cause neuromuscular weakness and paralysis. The first sign often is blurred or double vision, followed by ptosis. Respiratory muscle weakness may result, leading to respiratory failure in severe cases.

PROCEDURES AND LABORATORY TESTS

The exact tests to be ordered depend on the snake that made the bite; however, the following laboratory tests are generally useful.

- Complete blood count and platelet count are made to assess blood loss and thrombocytopenia; peripheral smear may show evidence of red cell fragmentation.
- International normalized ratio (INR), prothrombin time, and partial thromboplastin time are often prolonged by venoms that consume coagulation factors; fibrinogen is often decreased.
- Serum electrolytes, BUN, creatinine, and creatine kinase can help assess volume status, renal function, and possible muscle injury.
- ECG may be needed in some cases to assess myocardial injury.
- Urinalysis may be performed to assess renal injury and blood loss.
- Intracompartmental pressure measurements may be needed if signs of compartment syndrome develop.

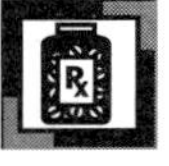

Treatment

- Treatment should focus on ensuring airway, appropriate intensive supportive care, and administration of antivenom, if needed.
- Time of bite and first aid measures that were performed should be determined.

DIRECTING PATIENT COURSE

The health-care provider should call the poison control center when:

- Patient presents with an exotic snakebite.
- Drug interaction or underlying disease presents an unusual problem.

The patient should be referred to a health-care facility when:

- History of exotic venomous snakebite is obtained.
- Patient or caregiver seems unreliable.
- Drug interaction or underlying disease presents an unusual problem.

Admission Considerations

Inpatient management in an intensive care setting is warranted for most patients who show signs of envenomation.

DECONTAMINATION

Out of Hospital

The only proven first aid measures are immobilization of the bitten limb and application of a firm bandage (crepe wrap) to limit movement of venom.

In Hospital

- Incision and suction, tourniquet application, ice, and electric shock therapy on any type of snake bite are strongly discouraged.
- Measures include immobilization of the bitten limb for all types of bites.
- Other first aid measures are not recommended in the hospital setting.

ANTIDOTES

- It is often possible to identify the snake because they are captive specimens; this information is needed to obtain the appropriate antivenom.
- An antivenom is produced for most venoms; due to their exotic nature, however, antivenoms are often not immediately available.
- A wide variety of antivenoms are available in the United States; however, they are stocked by zoos and aquariums for use if employees are bitten during the course of their duties.
- The antivenoms stocked by zoological parks can be provided for treatment of snakebite patients.
- All certified regional poison centers are provided a copy of the *Antivenom Index*, a catalog of antivenoms stocked by North American zoos and aquariums, as well as a list of professionals who are willing to provide medical assistance.
- The regional poison center should be contacted for this information.

ADJUNCTIVE TREATMENT

Coagulation Abnormalities

- In general, antivenom is the best treatment for coagulation defects.
- If it is not available, blood component therapy (e.g., fresh-frozen plasma or packed red blood cells) can be used to treat clinically significant bleeding.

Respiratory Failure

Endotracheal intubation should be performed at the first sign of impending respiratory failure from any type of poison.

Hypotension

- Patient should receive 10 to 20 ml/kg 0.9% saline and be placed in the Trendelenburg position.
- Large amounts may be needed if antivenom is not available.
- A vasopressor may be needed (see SECTION II, Hypotension chapter, for further details).

Tetanus

Prophylaxis should be provided if tetanus immunization status is not up to date.

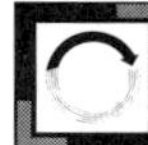

Follow-Up

PATIENT MONITORING

- Continuous respiratory and cardiac monitoring should be performed in symptomatic patients.
- Serial complete blood count, platelet count, prothrombin time or INR, and other coagulation tests may be needed in patients with coagulopathy.

EXPECTED COURSE AND PROGNOSIS

- Nearly all patients survive if adequate emergency and ICU care is provided.
- Permanent sequelae may occur, however, if severe local injury occurs or an adequate airway cannot be provided.

DISCHARGE CRITERIA/INSTRUCTIONS

- From the emergency department. Asymptomatic patients without presence of a coagulopathy may be discharged after observation for 8 hours.
- From the hospital. The patient may be discharged when local injury and coagulation effects or systemic effects have resolved.

PATIENT EDUCATION

All patients treated with antivenom should be warned that serum sickness may develop 1 to 2 weeks later (see SECTION II, Snake Antivenom chapter, for details of treatment for serum sickness).

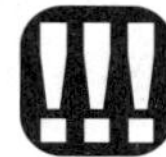

Pitfalls

DIAGNOSIS

For some bites, the signs of envenomation may be delayed several hours.

TREATMENT

The clinician must be prepared to treat anaphylaxis when antivenom from any source is administered.

FOLLOW-UP

Serum sickness from antivenom may develop after the patient has been discharged.

ICD-9-CM 989.5

Toxic effect of other substances, chiefly nonmedicinal as to source: venom.

See also: SECTION II, Hypotension chapter; and SECTION III, Snake Antivenom—Crotalid and Elapid Snakes chapter.

RECOMMENDED READING

Trestrail JH. The underground zoo: the problem of exotic venomous snakes in private possession in the United States. *Vet Hum Toxicol* 1982;24:144–149.

Author: Richard C. Dart

Reviewer: Katherine M. Hurlbut

Snakebite—North American Coral Snake

Basics

DESCRIPTION

Coral snakes are small, multicolored (black, red, yellow) venomous snakes.

FORMS AND USES

North American coral snakes include the following species and subspecies:

- Eastern coral snake (*Micrurus fulvius fulvius*)
- Texas coral snake (*Micrurus fulvius tenere*)
- Western coral snake (*Micruroides euryxanthus*)

Snake Identification

In North America only, coral snakes have colored bands that encircle their bodies in the following arrangements: if red and yellow bands are adjacent, the snake is venomous; if red and black bands are adjacent, the snake is nonvenomous.

TOXIC DOSE

One bite is potentially fatal; however, the coral snake usually has to hold on and chew to produce envenomation.

PATHOPHYSIOLOGY

- The venom produces an irreversible inhibition of neuromuscular transmission.
- Recovery takes weeks or months because receptors must regenerate.
- Unlike the pit vipers (e.g., rattlesnakes), coral snakes have fangs that are toothlike, fixed in erect position, and all of the same size.
- The bite deposits venom in subcutaneous tissues, but produces minimal local effects.

EPIDEMIOLOGY

- Coral snake bites are rare.
- Because prolonged contact is needed for envenomation to occur, nearly all coral snake bites occur during handling of snakes.
- Death may occur in patients who do not receive appropriate airway management.

CAUSES

Nearly all cases are associated with intentional handling of coral snakes.

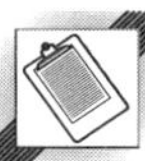

Diagnosis

DIFFERENTIAL DIAGNOSIS

- Fang marks may have the appearance of puncture wounds from inanimate objects (thorns, etc.) or the bite of a nonvenomous snake.
- Systemic effects may appear similar to any cause of bulbar palsy or progressive diffuse muscle paralysis.

SIGNS AND SYMPTOMS

- Venom effects may be delayed; however, if no effects occur over a period of 12 hours, it is likely a "dry bite."
- Reports of the snake holding on, being shaken or pulled to remove, or a history of drops of fluid coming through the puncture wound indicate bites with a high probability of envenomation.

Vital Signs

Tachycardia may develop, especially if hypotension is present.

HEENT

Difficult or slurred speech, or ptosis, may develop due to cranial nerve palsy.

Dermatologic

- The bite site will exhibit several puncture wounds, but these may be difficult to identify; the use of a magnifying glass is helpful.
- Injection of lidocaine or 0.9% saline beneath the suspected bite site may show exudation of fluid through unseen puncture wounds.
- Serious envenomation without fang marks has been reported.

Pulmonary

Dyspnea and respiratory insufficiency may develop.

Gastrointestinal

Nausea and vomiting may occur.

Musculoskeletal

Muscle tenderness may develop.

Neurologic

- Paresthesia, nausea, vomiting, lightheadedness, dizziness, and weakness are the most common effects; they may not appear immediately, but usually develop within hours.
- Fasciculation, diplopia, ptosis, or confusion may develop in serious envenomation cases.

PROCEDURES AND LABORATORY TESTS

Essential Tests

There are no diagnostic laboratory tests.

Recommended Tests

- Arterial blood gases may show evidence of hypoventilation.
- Serum electrolytes, glucose, BUN, creatinine, magnesium, calcium, and phosphate may be useful to evaluate causes of weakness.
- Serial evaluation of tidal volume or negative inspiratory force may be useful to monitor venom effects on ventilation.

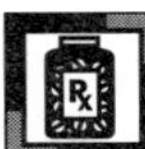

Treatment

- Supportive care with appropriate airway management is vital.
- Time of bite and first aid measures that were performed should be determined.
- The principle of management is to use antivenom to neutralize the venom before serious toxicity develops.

DIRECTING PATIENT COURSE

The health-care provider should call the poison control center when:

- A known coral snake bite has occurred, even if without apparent envenomation.
- Signs and symptoms are not consistent with coral snake envenomation.
- Underlying disease presents an unusual or difficult problem.

The patient should be referred to a health-care facility whenever a known coral snake bite has occurred.

Admission Considerations

Inpatient management is warranted if there is a high probability that a coral snake bite has occurred, or if any signs of envenomation develop.

DECONTAMINATION

Out of Hospital

- The bitten limb should be immobilized in functional position at or below heart level.
- Aspiration of the bite site may remove some venom, but should not involve incision of the bite marks; a venom extractor is marketed for this purpose.
- Intravenous access should be established, if possible, and the patient should be transported to the emergency department.

In Hospital

- The bitten limb should be immobilized and maintained at heart level or above.
- Decontamination is not useful by the time the patient reaches the hospital.
- If the hospital does not have antivenom, the limb should be immobilized until antivenom is obtained, or the patient should be transferred to a facility with antivenom available.

ANTIDOTES

• Coral snake antivenom (Antivenin, *Micrurus fulvius*) is commercially available and is the specific antidote for envenomation by this species of snake. The health-care worker should contact a regional poison center if antivenom is not available (see SECTION III, Antivenom chapter, for further details).
• Antivenin (Crotalidae) Polyvalent is not effective for coral snake bites.

Indications

• The determination of whether a bite has occurred is key to treatment; if bite marks are seen with the naked eye, through a magnifying glass, or by exudation of fluid through the puncture wounds, antivenom should be administered.
• Any confirmed bite (even if no effects are apparent) by the eastern or Texas coral snake should be treated.
• Bites by the western coral snake do not require antivenom treatment.

Contraindications

Severe allergy to horse serum or to coral snake antivenom is a relative contraindication.

Method of Administration

• Antivenom should be administered in a monitored critical care setting, and the clinician should be prepared to manage the airway and treat anaphylaxis.
• A skin test should be conducted once the decision to administer antivenom has been made.

—The skin test dose is 0.02 ml of test solution provided with the antivenom, injected intradermally, and observed for wheal and flare reaction.
—A negative skin test does not rule out hypersensitivity reaction to antivenom.

• Four to six vials of antivenom diluted in 250 ml of crystalloid should be administered intravenously over 1 hour.
• Antivenom should be administered as soon as possible after envenomation is confirmed.
• If symptoms develop or worsen, another four to five vials should be administered.

Potential Adverse Effects

• Localized phlebitis, rash, wheezing, or anaphylaxis may occur during infusion.
• Serum sickness may develop within 1 to 2 weeks of administration.

ADJUNCTIVE TREATMENT

• Electric shock therapy of the bite site is not recommended.
• The patient should be assessed repeatedly for development of complications of muscle weakness or respiratory insufficiency.
• Endotracheal intubation should be performed as soon as evidence of respiratory insufficiency develops (elevated pCO_2, declining negative inspiratory force).

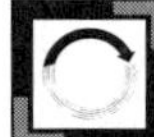

Follow-Up

PATIENT MONITORING

• Negative inspiratory force or tidal volume should be performed frequently for the first several hours to determine whether deterioration will occur.
• Respiratory function monitoring should continue until the patient recovers.
• Antivenom will likely stop progression of signs, but will not reverse effects that are present at time of administration.

EXPECTED COURSE AND PROGNOSIS

• If the bite did not penetrate the skin or no venom was injected, no effects will develop.
• If the patient is envenomated, but antivenom is administered early, venom effects should stabilize and then resolve over a period of weeks.
• Severe effects (muscle weakness, respiratory insufficiency) may take weeks to resolve despite the use of antivenom.

DISCHARGE CRITERIA/INSTRUCTIONS

• From the emergency department. Patient may be discharged after several hours of observation if it appears that the bite did not penetrate the skin, no venom was injected, and no toxic effects are developing.
• From the hospital. Patient may be discharged if symptoms and signs of envenomation do not develop or have resolved following treatment with antivenom.

PATIENT EDUCATION

Venomous snakes should not be handled.

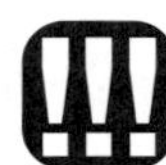

Pitfalls

DIAGNOSIS

Serious envenomation without apparent fang marks has been reported.

TREATMENT

Delay in the administration of antivenom allows irreversible venom effects to develop.

FOLLOW-UP

Serum sickness may occur 3 to 14 days following antivenom infusion (see SECTION III, Snake Antivenom chapter, for details of treatment).

ICD-9-CM 989.5

Toxic effect of: venom.

See also: SECTION III, Snake Antivenom—Crotalid and Elapid Snakes chapter.

RECOMMENDED READING

Kitchens CS, Van Mierop LHS. Envenomation by the eastern coral snake (*Micrurus fulvius fulvius*). *JAMA* 1987;258:1615–1618.

Author: Richard C. Dart

Reviewer: Rivka S. Horowitz

Snakebite—North American Crotalids

Basics

Nearly all venomous snakebites in North America are caused by snakes from the family Crotalidae (pit vipers).

DESCRIPTION

Crotalidae includes the following genera:

- *Agkistrodon*: Copperhead, cottonmouth, and water moccasin snakes
- *Crotalus*: Rattlesnakes
- *Sistrurus*: Massasauga and pigmy rattlesnakes

PATHOPHYSIOLOGY

- Crotalid snake venom contains dozens of components ranging from individual ions (e.g., zinc) to peptides and large-molecular-weight molecules.
- Crotalid snake bite produces three types of effects: local wound injury (pain, swelling, ecchymosis), coagulopathy (low platelet count, low fibrinogen, increased prothrombin time/international normalized ratio), and systemic effects (hypotension).
- The venom is usually injected subcutaneously; however, intramuscular (uncommon) and intravenous (rare) injection may occur.

EPIDEMIOLOGY

- The approximate 8,000 snake bites each year in North America cause about five deaths.
- The elderly and young children are at the highest risk of death.

CAUSES

- Bite on the hand is usually due to handling of the snake.
- Bite on the foot is usually accidental.

PREGNANCY AND LACTATION

Moderate to severe envenomation may cause vaginal bleeding and miscarriage.

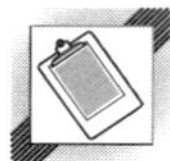

Diagnosis

DIFFERENTIAL DIAGNOSIS

- Bite by a venomous snake in which venom is not injected (dry bite)
- Bite by a nonvenomous snake
- Puncture wounds from inanimate objects (e.g., thorns)
- Swelling or ecchymosis due to unrecognized trauma or coagulopathy

SIGNS AND SYMPTOMS

Venom effects may appear immediately or develop over several hours. If no effects occur within 8 to 12 hours, a dry bite is likely. If life-threatening effects develop, they typically occur within a few hours.

Vital Signs

Heart rate and blood pressure are often increased soon after the bite occurs and may be followed by hypotension with continued tachycardia.

HEENT

Cranial nerve paralysis manifested as ptosis has been reported occasionally, usually after the bite of the Mojave rattlesnake.

Dermatologic

- The bite will show one, two, or more puncture wounds. Scratches or small lacerations also may produce envenomation.
- Faint ecchymosis may develop around the site of the bite.
- Localized pain and edema usually start early and progress proximally; however, they may be delayed for hours. Rapid progression indicates more serious envenomation.

Cardiovascular

Hypotension may occur early, although rarely. Generally, it develops after several hours due to volume depletion caused by loss of volume into the edematous limb.

Pulmonary

Noncardiogenic and cardiogenic pulmonary edema rarely develop.

Gastrointestinal

Nausea and vomiting are common. Gastrointestinal hemorrhage rarely occurs.

Renal

- Volume depletion is common and may become severe.
- Acute renal failure may occur if hypotension is prolonged or rhabdomyolysis develops.

Hematologic

Anemia, thrombocytopenia, and hypofibrinogenemia are common.

Musculoskeletal

- Fasciculation has been reported after bites by some species.
- Compartment syndrome is rare. Severe pain, distal paresthesia, pallor, and pulselessness are indicators.

Neurologic

Altered mental status may occur in cases of severe envenomation.

PROCEDURES AND LABORATORY TESTS

Essential Tests

- Complete blood count. Blood counts will decrease over the first few days; hemoconcentration may occur to third-spacing of fluid into edematous area; and the platelet count, used to monitor the effectiveness of antivenom therapy, is often decreased and may fall below $20,000/mm^3$.
- Serum electrolytes, BUN, and creatinine measurements are used to assess volume status and renal injury.
- Prothrombin time (PT) and international normalized ratio (INR) are often increased, sometimes dramatically. Measurement is used to monitor the effectiveness of antivenom therapy.
- Urinalysis

—Red cells indicate hemorrhage.
—Positive hemoglobin without cells may indicate myoglobinuria.

Recommended Tests

- Fibrinogen level is often decreased and may reach zero. Measurement is used to monitor the effectiveness of antivenom therapy.
- Fibrin split product concentration is often increased.
- The leading edge of swelling should be marked with an indelible marker every 15 to 30 minutes because progression of swelling is one indicator for use of antivenom.
- Creatine kinase concentration is measured to monitor venom-related muscle injury.
- Imaging. Chest x-ray is needed only if pulmonary symptoms develop.
- Intracompartmental pressure monitoring is necessary for all patients with suspected compartment syndrome.

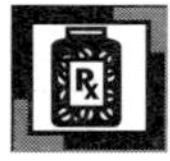

Treatment

- The principle of therapy is to neutralize the venom using antivenom.
- Supportive care of local injury, coagulopathy, and systemic toxicity is performed until antivenom can be administered.
- Time of bite and any first-aid measures already performed must be determined.

DIRECTING PATIENT COURSE

The health-care provider should call the poison control center when:

- Shock or other life-threatening effects are present.
- Signs and symptoms are not consistent with pit viper envenomation.
- Underlying disease presents an unusual diagnostic or therapeutic challenge.

The patient should be referred to a health-care facility any time that a history of a venomous snake bite is obtained.

DECONTAMINATION

Out of Hospital

- Supportive care of local injury, coagulopathy, and systemic effects, with appropriate airway management, is vital.

—The affected limb should be immobilized in a functional position at heart level or below until antivenom can be administered.
—Aspiration of the bite site using an extractor may remove some venom. This should not involve the incision of the bite marks.

- An intravenous line should be inserted, if possible, and the patient transported to an emergency department.

In Hospital

- First aid is probably not useful after the patient has reached the emergency department. The patient should be placed in a monitored bed, and venom effects should be assessed; if progressing, an antivenom agent should be administered.
- After an intravenous line has been started, the affected limb should be elevated above heart level.

ANTIDOTES

- The principle of management is to neutralize the injected venom using an antivenom agent. Antivenom should be administered if the effects of the venom are worsening.
- Crotalidae Polyvalent immune Fab (ovine) (see SECTION III, Snake Antivenom chapter)

—Indications include evidence of local wound worsening (e.g., progression of swelling), coagulopathy, or systemic signs or symptoms.
—Contraindications include a history of allergy to the product (relative contraindication).
—Dose. Initially 4 to 6 vials are administered, repeated up to two times to achieve control, and then two vials are administered every 6 hours for three additional doses. Further doses may be needed at physician discretion.
—Administration. The dose is diluted in 250 ml of crystalloid and infused intravenously over 1 hour
—Adverse effects. Acute adverse effects occur during infusion in 20% of patients. Anaphylaxis has not been reported to occur.

- Antivenin (Crotalidae) Polyvalent (Wyeth-Ayerst) (see SECTION III, Snake Antivenom—Crotalid and Elapid Snakes chapter, for details).

—Indications include evidence of local wound worsening (e.g., progression of swelling), coagulopathy, or systemic signs and symptoms.
—Contraindications include a history of allergy to the product (a relative contraindication).
—Dose. Smaller doses than those listed may be appropriate if the bite is made by a copperhead snake.
    —No antivenom is administered if the envenomation is minimal.
    —Ten vials should be administered if the envenomation is moderate or if the envenomation syndrome is worsening.
    —Ten to thirty, or more, vials should be administered in the presence of life-threatening envenomation or if the syndrome is worsening rapidly. At least 20 vials should be given initially if the patient demonstrates cardiovascular instability.

—Administration
    —Epinephrine and equipment for endotracheal intubation should be immediately available. A skin test should be conducted by injecting 0.02 cc of the skin test material intradermally. A positive response is a wheal and flare reaction within 15 to 30 minutes.
    —Ten milliliters of normal saline should be added to each vial of antivenom. It is mixed by rolling the vial between the hands. The mixture is diluted by injecting it into a normal saline intravenous bag (5–10 vials in 250 ml normal saline). The vials should not be shaken. The volume of saline should be reduced in pediatric patients (total volume should equal 20 ml/kg).
    —Initially, the antivenom should be administered intravenously at a slow rate (10 to 25 cc/h), then titrated upward (250 cc/hr) if no reaction occurs. The initial dose should be completed during the first hour, if possible.

—Adverse effects
    —Acute allergy or anaphylaxis occurs in 25% of patients.
    —Serum sickness occurs in 75% of patients.

ADJUNCTIVE TREATMENT

- Adequate analgesia (e.g., meperidine or morphine) should be provided as needed.
- Hypotension is treated in the usual manner (see SECTION II, Hypotension chapter).
- A tetanus immunization should be administered, if needed.

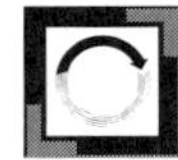

Follow-Up

PATIENT MONITORING

- Continuous respiratory and cardiac monitoring should be performed in symptomatic patients.
- The patient should be assessed repeatedly for development of elevated compartment pressure, evidence of bleeding, and progression of tissue injury.

EXPECTED COURSE AND PROGNOSIS

- The effects of venom usually peak during the first day and then abate over several days. Edema may recur repeatedly for weeks to months.
- The patient should be monitored for bleeding. Coagulation abnormality may return within the first week.
- Approximately 40% of patients bitten on the hand and 15% of patients bitten on the lower extremity have long-term complaints.

DISCHARGE CRITERIA/INSTRUCTIONS

- From the emergency department. The patient can be discharged if swelling, coagulation abnormality, and systemic signs fail to develop for 8 to 12 hours.
- From the hospital. The patient can be discharged when all venom effects have clearly begun to resolve and when antivenom therapy is complete (usually within 36 hours after admission).

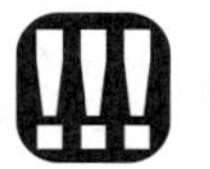

Pitfalls

DIAGNOSIS

Venom effects may take hours to develop; therefore, patients should be observed for 8 to 12 hours.

TREATMENT

- Delay in antivenom administration may allow irreversible venom effects to develop.
- The patient should not be left unattended during antivenom infusion.
- Fasciotomy has been used to treat compartment syndrome; however, research suggests that it is ineffective. The procedure should not be considered unless true compartment syndrome exists.
- Additional antivenom and mannitol should be administered instead.
- Electric shock treatment and tourniquets should not be used.

FOLLOW-UP

- Serum sickness may develop; it usually becomes evident 1 to 2 weeks after treatment.
- Venom effects may recur 3 to 7 days after the antivenom agent has been excreted.

ICD-9-CM 989.5

Toxic effect of other substances, chiefly nonmedicinal as to source: venom.

See also: SECTION II, Hypotension chapter; SECTION III, Snake Antivenom—Crotalid and Elapid Snakes chapter.

RECOMMENDED READING

Gomez H, Dart RC. Clinical toxicology of snake bite in North America. In: Meier J, White J, eds. *Clinical toxicology of animal venoms and poisons.* Boca Raton, FL: CRC Press, 1995:619–644.

Author: Richard C. Dart

Reviewer: Katherine M. Hurlbut

Sodium Fluoride

Basics

DESCRIPTION

Sodium fluoride and stannous fluoride are used in toothpaste to prevent dental caries.

FORMS AND USES

- The maximum allowable amount of fluoride in a tube of toothpaste is 260 mg.
- Fluoride is also available in dental fluoride products (e.g., sodium fluoride chewable tablets).
- Fluoride in various forms is present in rodenticides, insecticides, and veterinary products
- Hydrogen fluoride and ammonium fluoride are covered in a separate chapter.

TOXIC DOSE

The estimated toxic dose is 5 to 10 mg/kg of fluoride ions (in a small child, the equivalent of an entire tube of toothpaste).

PATHOPHYSIOLOGY

- Free fluoride ions interfere with oxidative phosphorylation, leading to anaerobic metabolism and lactic acidosis.
- Free fluoride ions will precipitate calcium, leading to severe hypocalcemia.

EPIDEMIOLOGY

- Poisoning is uncommon.
- Toxic effects are typically mild unless large amounts or a concentrated form is ingested.

PREGNANCY AND LACTATION

- No information is available concerning overdose.
- Appropriate fluoride supplementation is considered safe during pregnancy.

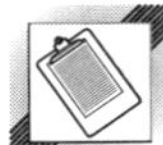

Diagnosis

SIGNS AND SYMPTOMS

Cardiac dysrhythmias caused by hypocalcemia are the primary concern.

HEENT

Some concentrated forms may cause mucosal erosion.

Cardiovascular

Dysrhythmia and hypotension consistent with hyperkalemia or hypocalcemia may be seen, and ventricular dysrhythmias may develop suddenly.

Respiratory

Tachypnea is common.

Gastrointestinal

- Epigastric pain, nausea, vomiting, dysphagia, hematemesis, and diarrhea may be noted, but typically do not occur immediately.
- High-concentration products may cause mucosal burns.

Fluids and Electrolytes

Hypocalcemia, hyperkalemia, and hypomagnesemia may occur.

Neurologic

Generalized muscle spasms and weakness, tetany, and hyperreflexia secondary to hypocalcemia can occur.

PROCEDURES AND LABORATORY TESTS

Essential Tests

No tests may be needed in asymptomatic patients with small ingestion.

Recommended Tests

- Serum electrolytes (including calcium, and magnesium) should be monitored frequently in all symptomatic patients.
- Complete blood count should be ordered in symptomatic patients following ingestion for hemorrhagic gastritis.
- Serial ECG and continuous cardiac rhythm monitoring may provide early evidence of hyperkalemia or hypocalcemia; ECG effects may include QT prolongation, ST changes, T-wave inversion, and ventricular tachycardia for fibrillation.
- Pulse oximetry or arterial blood gases are measured to monitor for respiratory depression or development of pneumonitis.
- Endoscopy may be needed following ingestion of caustic products (see SECTION IV, Hydrogen Fluoride chapter).

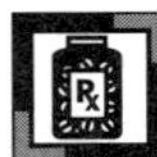

Treatment

- Therapy should focus on serial evaluation for signs of hypocalcemia, maintenance of airway, and administration of calcium.
- Dose and time of exposure should be determined for all substances involved.

DIRECTING PATIENT COURSE

The health-care professional should call the poison control center when:

- Severe or persistent effects develop.
- Coingestant, drug interaction, or underlying disease presents an unusual problem.

The patient should be referred to a health-care facility when:

- Suicide or homicide attempt is possible.
- Toxic effects develop.
- Coingestant, drug interaction, or underlying disease presents an unusual problem.

Admission Considerations

All symptomatic patients should be admitted to an intensive care unit.

DECONTAMINATION

Out of Hospital

- Ipecac is not recommended.
- In alert patients, 8 ounces of milk, 30 cc of milk of magnesia, or two to four calcium carbonate tablets (e.g., Tums) are administered to form insoluble complexes with fluoride and decrease absorption.

In Hospital

- Lavage is not recommended.
- In alert patients, 8 ounces of milk, 30 cc of milk of magnesia, or two to four calcium carbonate tablets (e.g., Tums) should be administered orally.
- Activated charcoal does not bind fluoride.

ANTIDOTES

Calcium Chloride

- 10% solution is indicated if signs of hypocalcemia develop.
- An infusion of 5 to 10 cc should be administered intravenously over 10 minutes; the dose may be repeated based on the response of the QTc interval.
- See SECTION III, Calcium chapter.

Magnesium Sulfate

- Magnesium sulfate is a second line agent for treatment of hypocalcemia.
- An infusion of 2 to 4 g should be administered intravenously over 10 minutes; the dose may be repeated hourly, as needed.
- See SECTION IV, Magnesium chapter.

ADJUNCTIVE TREATMENT

- Patients with digital burns may benefit from local application of calcium gluconate gel.
- See SECTION IV, Hydrogen Fluoride chapter, for details of therapy.

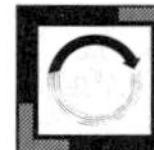

Follow-Up

PATIENT MONITORING

Asymptomatic patients should undergo cardiac monitoring with serial ECGs and calcium, potassium, and magnesium measurements for at least 4 to 6 hours.

EXPECTED COURSE AND PROGNOSIS

Most patients make a full recovery if treatment is available before hypocalcemia develops.

DISCHARGE CRITERIA/INSTRUCTIONS

- From the emergency department. Children with self-limited effects after ingesting less than 10 mg/kg fluoride (more than 10 g toothpaste/kg) may be discharged.
- From the hospital. Patient may be discharged when toxic effects have resolved and serum calcium has been normal for 24 hours.

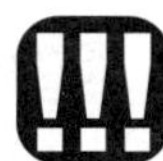

Pitfalls

FOLLOW-UP

Patients who sustain gastric mucosal damage should be advised of the possible development of strictures and scarring.

ICD-9-CM 989

Toxic effect of other substances, chiefly nonmedicinal as to source.

See also: SECTION III, Calcium and Magnesium chapters; SECTION IV, Hydrogen Fluoride.

RECOMMENDED READING

Augenstein WL, Spoerke DG, Kulig KW, et al. Fluoride ingestion in children: a review of 87 cases. *Pediatr* 1991;88:907–912.

Author: Julie Seaman

Reviewer: Kennon Heard

Sotalol

Basics

DESCRIPTION

Sotalol (Betapace) is a class III antidysrhythmic medication.

FORMS AND USES

- Sotalol (Betapace, Sotacor) is used to treat high-risk ventricular dysrhythmia.
- Adult oral dosage is 120 to 480 mg/day.
- Adult intravenous dosage is 20 to 60 mg over 2 to 3 minutes.
- Pediatric oral dosage is 2 to 4 mg/kg/day in two divided doses.

TOXIC DOSE

A therapeutic dose has been associated with torsade de pointes, particularly in patients with predisposing conditions.

PATHOPHYSIOLOGY

- A noncardioselective β-blocker, sotalol lacks significant intrinsic sympathomimetic activity and membrane-stabilizing properties.
- Sotalol lengthens the action potential duration, resulting in class III antidysrhythmic activity.
- The combined effects of bradycardia and lengthened action potential may produce torsade de pointes.

EPIDEMIOLOGY

- Poisoning is rare.
- Toxic effects following exposure are typically moderate.
- Death occurs in patients who have ingested a large quantity, who have underlying electrolyte disorders, or who have cardiovascular disease.

CAUSES

- Poisoning usually occurs as a suicidal ingestion in an adult.
- Child abuse or neglect should be considered if the patient is less than 1 year of age; suicide attempt in patients over 6 years of age.

RISK FACTORS

Patients with underlying heart disease, electrolyte abnormality (hyperkalemia, hypomagnesemia, hypocalcemia), renal insufficiency, or congenital QT prolongation are at increased risk of torsade de pointes.

DRUG AND DISEASE INTERACTIONS

Drugs that prolong QT interval (tricyclic antidepressants, type 1a antidysrhythmic agents) increase the risk of dysrhythmia.

PREGNANCY AND LACTATION

- US FDA Pregnancy Category B. Animal studies indicate no fetal risk and there are no controlled human studies, or animal studies show an adverse fetal effect but well-controlled studies in pregnant women do not.
- Sotalol is concentrated in breast milk, but there are no reports of infant toxicity.

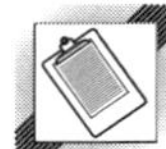

Diagnosis

DIFFERENTIAL DIAGNOSIS

- Toxic agents that produce prolongation of QT interval include quinidine, disopyramide, procainamide, ibutilide, pentamidine, propoxyphene, thioridazine, and cyclic antidepressants.
- Other conditions that prolong QT interval include congenital QT prolongation, hyperkalemia, and ventricular dysrhythmia secondary to ischemia or other etiology.

SIGNS AND SYMPTOMS

An overdose may cause bradycardia, hypotension, syncope, ventricular dysrhythmia, or asystole.

Vital Signs

Mild bradycardia and hypotension are common and may become severe after a large ingestion.

Cardiovascular

Severe hypotension generally only develops with serious ventricular dysrhythmias (QT prolongation, torsade de pointes, premature ventricular contractions, ventricular tachycardia, or ventricular fibrillation).

Pulmonary

Respiratory depression may develop in severe cases.

Neurologic

Syncope, seizures, and altered mental status may occur in patients with ventricular dysrhythmia.

PROCEDURES AND LABORATORY TESTS

Essential Tests

- Serum electrolytes, BUN, and creatinine are ordered to evaluate other causes of dysrhythmia.
- ECG with continuous cardiac monitoring is used to detect QT prolongation and ventricular dysrhythmia.

Recommended Tests

- Serum magnesium and calcium levels are assayed in patients with dysrhythmia to assess other causes.
- Serum acetaminophen and aspirin levels in overdose setting are tested to detect occult ingestion.

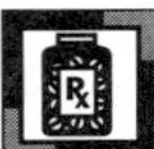

Treatment

- Treatment should focus on cardiac monitoring, supportive care, and treatment of ventricular dysrhythmia.
- The dose and time of exposure must be determined for all substances involved.

DIRECTING PATIENT COURSE

The health-care provider should call the poison control center when:

- Ventricular dysrhythmia, hypotension or other serious effects are present.
- Toxic effects are not consistent with sotalol ingestion.
- Coingestant, drug interaction, or underlying disease presents an unusual challenge.

The patient should be referred to a health-care facility when:

- Attempted suicide or homicide is possible.
- Patient or caregiver seems unreliable.
- Any symptoms develop.
- Coingestant, drug interaction, or underlying disease presents an unusual challenge.

Admission Considerations

Inpatient management is warranted for patients with prolonged QTc, dysrhythmia, hypotension, or a CNS complaint such as syncope.

DECONTAMINATION

Out of Hospital

Emesis should not be induced; coma or seizure may develop abruptly.

In Hospital

- Gastric lavage should be performed in pediatric (tube size 24–32 French) or adult patients (tube size 36–42 French) presenting within 1 hour of a large ingestion or if serious effects are present.
- One dose of activated charcoal (1–2 g/kg) should be administered without a cathartic if a substantial ingestion has occurred within the previous few hours.

ANTIDOTES

There is no specific antidote available.

ADJUNCTIVE TREATMENT

An arterial line or Swan-Ganz catheterization may be needed to manage persistent hypotension and dysrhythmias.

Torsade de Pointes

- Electrolyte abnormalities should be corrected, if present.
- If the patient is hemodynamically unstable, electrical cardioversion should be performed immediately.

- The clinician should avoid quinidine, disopyramide, procainamide, amiodarone, or bretylium, or any other agents that prolong QT interval.
- Magnesium sulfate is the primary treatment.

—Adult dose is 1 to 2 g, given as an intravenous push and repeated if needed in 10 to 15 minutes; intravenous infusion also should be initiated at a rate of 2 to 10 mg/min, titrated to antidysrhythmic effect.
—Pediatric dosage is 25 to 50 mg/kg intravenously over 5 minutes followed by continuous infusion.

- If magnesium is not effective, isoproterenol (2 to 4 μg/ml) is administered at an initial rate of 0.5 to 1.0 μg/min, titrated to effect; pediatric dose is 0.1 μg/kg/min, titrated to effect.

Bradycardia

- If bradycardia is associated with hypotension, atropine is administered.

—Adult dose is 0.5 to 1 mg intravenously, repeated in 5 minutes if necessary to a maximum of 2 mg.
—Pediatric dose is 0.02 mg/kg intravenously, repeated every 5 minutes as needed; the maximum dose is 1 mg for children, 2 mg for adolescents.

- If the patient is unresponsive to atropine, isoproterenol may be added; adult infusion is 5.0 μg/min, titrated to effect; pediatric infusion is 0.1 μg/kg/min, titrated to effect.
- The unresponsive patient should undergo cardiac pacing.

Hypotension

- In patients with hypotension and no evidence of volume overload, intravenous 0.9% saline is administered at 10 to 20 ml/kg; volume overload must be avoided because many agents that cause bradycardia are also myocardial depressants.
- Dopamine may be administered for persistent hypotension at 2 to 5 μg/kg/min by intravenous infusion, titrated to effect; doses above 20 mg/kg/min are unlikely to have further effect.
- If the patient is unresponsive to dopamine, norepinephrine is added, 0.1 to 0.2 μg/kg/min in a continuous infusion, and titrated to effect.

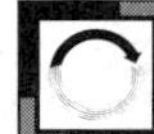

Follow-Up

PATIENT MONITORING

Electrolytes as well as cardiac rhythm and respiratory function should be monitored throughout the patient's hospitalization.

EXPECTED COURSE AND PROGNOSIS

- Survival and full recovery are expected if the patient receives appropriate aggressive care before anoxic injury intercedes.
- Permanent neurologic injury from sustained hypotension, seizures, or hypoxia may result.

PATIENT EDUCATION

Patients with renal insufficiency should avoid sotalol.

DISCHARGE CRITERIA/INSTRUCTIONS

- From the emergency department. If electrolytes are normal and no dysrhythmia or QTc prolongation develops for 6 hours after ingestion, the patient may be discharged after gastrointestinal decontamination and psychiatric evaluation, if needed.
- From the hospital. Patient may be discharged approximately 24 hours after QTc and dysrhythmia normalize and after a psychiatric evaluation, if needed.

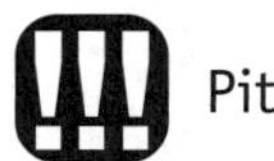

Pitfalls

DIAGNOSIS

Toxicity can occur at therapeutic doses in a patient who has an electrolyte disorder or who uses drugs that prolong the QT interval.

TREATMENT

High doses of magnesium may be required to control torsade de pointes.

ICD-9-CM 972

Poisoning by agents primarily affecting the cardiovascular system.

See also: SECTION II, Hypotension and Ventricular Dysrhythmia chapters; and SECTION III, Atropine and Magnesium Sulfate chapters.

RECOMMENDED READING

Neuvonen PJ, Elonen E, Vuorenmaa T, et al. Prolonged Q-T interval and severe tachyarrhythmias, common features of sotalol intoxication. *Eur J Clin Pharmacol* 1981;20:85–89.

Author: Katherine M. Hurlbut

Reviewer: Richard C. Dart

Basics

DESCRIPTION

Stingrays are aquatic, bottom-dwelling animals with a whiplike tail.

FORMS AND USES

- The stingrays (round, southern, blunt-nosed, eagle, and other rays) have one to four spines on the dorsal surface of the elongated tail; when the ray is provoked, its tail whips upward, thrusting the spine or spines into the victim.
- Other common names for stingrays include "demons of the deep," devilfish, guitarfish, skates, electric rays, eagle rays, and mantas.

TOXIC DOSE

Depending on size and species, one strike can cause severe mechanical trauma or envenomation.

PATHOPHYSIOLOGY

- The lash of a stingray tail often causes severe lacerations as well as envenomation.
- Pieces of the tail may contaminate the wound.
- The venom is a complex heat-labile protein that induces proteolytic local effects as well as systemic toxicity, most notably in the cardiovascular, respiratory, and nervous systems.

EPIDEMIOLOGY

- Envenomation is common along the Pacific coast and the Gulf of Mexico, as well as along the southeastern U.S. coast.
- Poisoning is most common during the summer and autumn months coinciding with seaside vacations.
- Death is rare, most often a complication of thoracic or abdominal penetration.

CAUSES

Stingrays are nonaggressive bottom feeders that strike as a defensive mechanism, most commonly after the submerged ray is stepped on in shallow water.

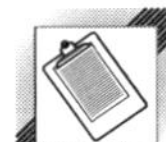

Diagnosis

DIFFERENTIAL DIAGNOSIS

- Toxic causes of puncture wounds and pain include envenomation by scorpionfish, weeverfish, and fire coral.
- Nontoxic causes include trauma from stepping on or being struck by rocks or other underwater debris, or bites by nonvenomous marine organisms.

SIGNS AND SYMPTOMS

- Immediate pain occurs at the site of envenomation, which peaks 2 to 4 hours later and may begin to subside over the next 6 to 12 hours.
- Systemic effects are uncommon; they may begin soon after envenomation and usually resolve within 24 hours.
- Barbs and spines that remain embedded in the victim may continue to secrete venom for days.

Vital Signs

Tachycardia (more common) or bradycardia with hypo- or hypertension may occur.

Dermatologic

- The wound initially may develop a dusky or cyanotic rim, advancing to an erythematous discoloration with hemorrhage, usually within the first 2 hours.
- Local dermal, fat, and muscle necrosis occurs rapidly.
- Secondary bacterial infection is common.

Cardiovascular

- Tachycardia is common.
- Bradycardia secondary to direct myocardial depression and atrioventricular blockade may occur.
- Dysrhythmias due to direct myocardial toxicity have been reported.

Pulmonary

Respiratory difficulty due to systemic effects occurs rarely.

Gastrointestinal

Nausea, vomiting, and diarrhea may develop.

Musculoskeletal

- Extensive local tissue damage may develop.
- Osteomyelitis may occur with bone penetration.

Neurologic

Headache, vertigo, syncope, weakness, axillary or inguinal pain, fasciculation, paresthesia, paralysis, and seizures may occur.

PROCEDURES AND LABORATORY TESTS

Essential Tests

No tests may be needed for mildly painful envenomation.

Recommended Tests

- Complete blood count, serum electrolytes, BUN, creatinine, coagulation studies, blood and wound cultures, and other tests are used in symptomatic patients as clinically indicated.
- ECG and cardiac monitoring are used in cases of severe envenomation to monitor dysrhythmias.
- A radiograph of the injured part helps to evaluate the presence of foreign bodies or bone injury.
- Ultrasonography of the area of envenomation helps to locate and extract embedded barbs and spines.

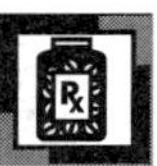

Treatment

- Treatment should focus on immersion in hot water and meticulous decontamination and local wound care.
- Extent of envenomation and trauma and time of exposure should be determined, including all other substances that could be involved.

DIRECTING PATIENT COURSE

The health-care provider should call the poison control center when:

- Persistent pain or major trauma are present.
- Toxic effects are not consistent with stingray envenomation.
- Drug interaction or underlying disease presents an unusual problem.

The patient should be referred to a health-care facility when:

- Patient or caregiver seems unreliable.
- Any toxic effects develop.
- Drug interaction or underlying disease presents an unusual problem.

Admission Considerations

Inpatient management is warranted if the patient exhibits persistent systemic effects, serious trauma, or pain requiring parenteral analgesics.

DECONTAMINATION

Out of Hospital

- Wound should be irrigated immediately with the coldest water available to remove venom, provide some slight anesthesia, and cause vasoconstriction of blood vessels in the immediate area.
- If sterile water is not available, tap or ocean water may be used.
- There is no indication for the addition of ammonia, magnesium sulfate, potassium permanganate, or formalin to the irrigation bath.
- Visible spines or integumentary sheath should be removed carefully in order to alleviate the ongoing envenomation.
- Affected part should be submerged in hot water (if available) to tolerance (upper limit 45°C or 113°F) for 30 to 90 minutes.
- Ice or cryotherapy is contraindicated.

In Hospital

- If the correct prehospital decontamination has not occurred, it should be instituted immediately.
- Wound exploration should be performed, and any spine or integumentary sheath remaining embedded in the wound should be extracted.

ANTIDOTES

There is no specific antidote for stingray envenomation.

ADJUNCTIVE TREATMENT

Tetanus immunization should be updated if necessary.

Pain

- Affected area should be immersed in hot saline or water without causing burns (upper limit 45°C or 113°F) until pain is relieved; hot water should be replaced every 15 minutes.
- Wound can be infiltrated with local anesthetic without epinephrine; regional block or systemic (intravenous) analgesia should be considered for persistent pain.

Wound Care

- After meticulous cleaning and copious irrigation, the wound should be left open or primary closure delayed.
- Infection is treated in the standard manner with reexploration and use of antimicrobials; third-generation cephalosporin and ciprofloxacin are reasonable choices.

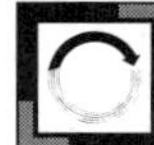

Follow-Up

PATIENT MONITORING

- In severe cases, respiratory and cardiac function should be monitored continuously.
- Follow-up for wound evaluation should be provided.

EXPECTED COURSE AND PROGNOSIS

- Toxic effects develop quickly and typically peak in the first few hours.
- Systemic effects occur, but are uncommon and usually resolve over 24 hours.
- Most patients suffer several weeks of discomfort at the wound site, but recover completely.
- Some residual scarring of the site is common.

DISCHARGE CRITERIA/INSTRUCTIONS

- From the emergency department

—Patients with only local trauma and pain that can be managed by oral pain medication may be discharged.
—Follow-up wound care should be arranged.

- From the hospital

—Patient can be discharged when systemic effects resolve and pain can be managed with oral pain medication.
—Follow-up wound care should be arranged.

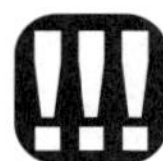

Pitfalls

DIAGNOSIS

- Focusing too much on the local tissue damage may allow cardiovascular and neurologic toxic effects to develop unnoticed.
- The possibility of envenomation by alternative organisms, such as the scorpionfish, should be considered.

TREATMENT

- It is important to meticulously clean the wound and search for embedded foreign objects.
- Administration of narcotic pain relievers instead of immersion of affected part into hot water is inappropriate.
- It is important to consider updating the tetanus immunization.

ICD-9-CM 989.5

Toxic effect of other substances, chiefly nonmedicinal as to source: venom.

See also: SECTION IV, Fish Stings chapter.

RECOMMENDED READING

Auerbach PS. Marine envenomation. In: Auerbach PS, ed. *Wilderness medicine: management of wilderness and environmental emergencies.* St. Louis: Mosby, 1995.

Author: Martha M. Foley

Reviewers: Gerald F. O'Malley and Luke Yip

Strychnine

Basics

DESCRIPTION

Strychnine tablets were formerly used as human and veterinary analeptics, analgesics, cathartics, stimulants, aphrodisiacs, and tonics.

FORMS AND USES

Strychnine is available in bulk forms from chemical supply companies.

Pharmaceutical Preparations

- Eastons tablets. Formula A contains iron phosphate 200 mg, quinine sulfate 50 mg, strychnine hydrochloride 1 mg; formula F contains half the strength of formula A.
- Strychiomel tablets. Each contains 1.5 mg strychnine, 10 mg thioridazine, and 2.5 mg yohimbine.
- Strychnine (0.1 mg/kg orally) has been studied in the treatment of sleep apnea and in the treatment of nonketotic hyperglycinemia and glycine encephalopathy.
- Strychnine-containing pills are no longer marketed, but may be found in old medicine cabinets.

Plants

- *Strychnos nux-vomica*. Dried seeds of the tree are used by herbalists and indigenous healers. Death has been reported in the United States as recently as 1996. Seeds are disk shaped, 2 to 3 cm in diameter, and 2 to 4 mm thick, and grey-green in color but become darker with drying.
- *Strychnos ignatii*. The beans contain strychnine.
- *Strychnos tiente* (Upas tree). Resins from this tree were used in Malaysia to make poison darts.

Commercial Products

- The primary use of strychnine today is in rodenticides.
- Preparations available to the public contain 0.3% to 0.5% strychnine; 5% preparations are available to licensed exterminators.
- Common trade names include El Roy Mouse Bait, Mologen Mouse Lure, Mice Doom Pellets, Hot Spring Buttons, Sparrow Cracks, Pied Piper Kwik Kill, Sweeney's Poison Wheat, Mole-nots, Mouse Maiz, Mo-go, Rad Seed, Pigeon-9, Kilmice, Gopher Bait/Mix/Tabs, Gopher Getter, Orco Gopher Bait, Gopher Death, Gopher Go, and Senco Poison Oats.
- Strychnine also is used in poison for pigeons, rabbits, and other animals considered pests.

Other Sources

- In adulterated street drugs, strychnine has been used to "cut" heroin, cocaine, and amphetamines.
- For laboratory and research uses, strychnine can be obtained in bulk form from chemical supply companies.
- Strychnine also has been used in criminal homicide and executions.

TOXIC DOSE

- The lethal oral dose of pure strychnine for children is 5 to 10 mg; for adults, 100 to 150 mg is toxic.
- Chronic exposure to lower doses does not appear to cause toxicity.

PATHOPHYSIOLOGY

- Toxic effects are due to blockade of glycine-mediated inhibition in the spinal cord.
- Strychnine competes with glycine for inhibitory postsynaptic receptors in the spinal cord, resulting in disinhibition of motor neurons and producing muscular activity that appears to be a seizure.

EPIDEMIOLOGY

Poisoning is uncommon and extremely rare in the United States due to restrictions on the sale of strychnine-containing products.

Causes

- Three types of exposure predominate:

—Accidental ingestion of "tonics" or rodenticides by children
—Suicide attempts
—Exposure to adulterated illicit drugs, especially powdered cocaine

- Child neglect or abuse should be considered if the patient is less than 1 year of age; attempted suicide in patients over 6 years of age.

PREGNANCY AND LACTATION

Data are not available for humans, but strychnine has caused spontaneous abortion in animal models.

WORKPLACE STANDARDS

- OSHA. PEL TWA is 0.15 mg/m^3.
- NIOSH. IDLH level is 3 mg/m^3.

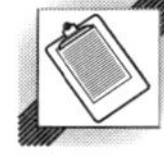

Diagnosis

DIFFERENTIAL DIAGNOSIS

- Convulsive activity in an awake patient without a postictal phase is the hallmark of strychnine poisoning.
- Differential diagnosis includes any cause of seizures, particularly repeated seizurelike activity.

SIGNS AND SYMPTOMS

- The onset of symptoms may occur within 30 minutes of ingestion, faster after inhalation.
- Prodromal symptoms include apprehension, heightened awareness, myoclonus, and muscle twitching, which may proceed to generalized convulsions.
- Sensory stimuli (touching and sounds) seem to trigger convulsive activity.

Vital Signs

Tachycardia, tachypnea, hypertension, and hyperthermia may occur.

HEENT

Blurred vision, nystagmus, mydriasis, and proptosis may develop.

Cardiovascular

- Strychnine has no direct toxic effect.
- Hypertension and tachycardia may accompany neuromuscular hyperactivity.
- Nonspecific ST- or T-wave abnormalities have been reported on the ECG.

Pulmonary

- Spasm or paralysis of the respiratory muscles may lead to respiratory failure, the primary cause of death.
- Adult respiratory distress syndrome and pulmonary embolism have been reported.

Gastrointestinal

Nausea and vomiting occur and pose a risk of aspiration.

Hepatic

- Elevated lactic dehydrogenase, alanine aminotransferase, and aspartate aminotransferase levels have been reported.
- Multiple organ failure with hepatic necrosis may complicate hyperthermia.

Renal

Acute renal failure due to rhabdomyolysis may follow repeated seizures.

Hematologic

Leukocytosis is common after seizures.

Fluids and Electrolytes

- Lactic acidosis, hyperkalemia, hypocalcemia, and hypophosphatemia may result from acute renal failure.
- Lactic acidosis usually resolves once seizures are controlled.

Musculoskeletal

- Muscle spasms and tightness are common and painful.
- Trismus, risus sardonicus (sardonic smile), and opisthotonos are characteristic.

• The most powerful muscle acting on the joint tends to control the type of posturing seen: flexion of upper extremities or extension of lower extremities.
• Edema and compartment syndrome have been reported.

Neurologic

• In contrast to epileptiform seizures, patients develop tonic-tetanic activity as opposed to tonic-clonic activity.
• Patients usually remain alert during and after the seizures unless anoxic encephalopathy ensues; there is no postictal state.
• Auditory, tactile, and visual stimuli can provoke violent, painful muscle spasms and seizures lasting 30 seconds to 2 minutes.
• Muscle relaxation for 5 to 10 minutes between seizures is typical.

PROCEDURES AND LABORATORY TESTS

Essential Tests

• Serum electrolytes, glucose, creatinine, BUN, creatinine kinase, and urinalysis to assess acidosis and other causes of seizures and muscle injury
• Arterial blood gas analysis to assess acidosis and oxygenation

Recommended Tests

• Serum calcium, magnesium, phosphorus, and liver function test to assess causes of seizure and liver injury
• ECG, serum acetaminophen, aspirin levels, and urine toxicology screen in an overdose setting to detect occult ingestion

Not Recommended Tests

Blood tests for strychnine correlate poorly with toxic effects and are not used clinically.

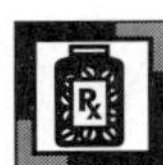

Treatment

• Treatment should focus on control of seizures and general supportive care.
• Endotracheal intubation and airway management should be performed early.
• The dose and time of exposure should be determined for all substances involved.

DIRECTING PATIENT CARE

The health-care provider should call the poison control center when:

• A history of strychnine ingestion is obtained or any toxic effects develop.
• A coingestant, drug interaction, or underlying disease presents an unusual problem.

The patient should be referred to a health-care facility when:

• Suicide or homicide attempt is possible.
• Ingestion of a strychnine-containing product is possible, or any toxic effects develop.
• A coingestant, drug interaction, or underlying disease presents an unusual problem.

Admission Considerations

Inpatient treatment is warranted for patients with persistent minor effects or those that develop seizures, acidosis, hypoxia, bradycardia, hypotension, hypercarbia, or rhabdomyolysis.

DECONTAMINATION

Out of Hospital

Emesis should not be induced because seizures may develop abruptly.

In Hospital

• Gastric lavage should be performed in pediatric (tube size 24–32 French) or adult (tube size 36–42 French) patients presenting within 1 hour of a large ingestion or if serious effects are present.
• One dose of activated charcoal (1–2 g/kg) should be administered without a cathartic if a substantial amount has been ingested within the previous few hours.
• Activated charcoal is highly effective in absorbing strychnine; preliminary data suggest a potential benefit from multiple-dose activated charcoal.

ANTIDOTES

There are no specific antidotes for strychnine toxicity.

ADJUNCTIVE TREATMENT

• For initial control of seizures, a benzodiazepine should be administered, repeating the dose every 10 minutes as needed and monitoring the patient's airway closely.

—Diazepam. Adult dose, 5 to 10 mg initially; pediatric dose, 0.2 to 0.5 mg/kg.
—Lorazepam. Adult dose, 2 to 4 mg intravenous push over 2 to 5 minutes; pediatric dose, 0.1 mg/kg intravenous push over 2 to 5 minutes, not to exceed 4 mg/dose.

• If seizures persist or recur, another anticonvulsant, such as phenobarbital or phenytoin, may be added.
• General anesthesia and neuromuscular paralysis may be needed to terminate seizure activity.
• Hemodialysis does not increase elimination effectively but may be useful if renal failure develops.
• Not recommended therapies. Acid diuresis is no longer recommended and may worsen renal failure.

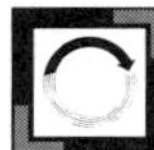

Follow-Up

PATIENT MONITORING

Respiratory function and cardiac rhythm should be monitored continuously.

EXPECTED COURSE AND PROGNOSIS

• Aggressive initial management is the key to a good prognosis. Strychnine exposure is rapidly fatal in the untreated patient.
• Prognosis is good for patients who survive beyond 5 hours with airway and seizure control.
• Seizure activity usually resolves by 24 hours.
• Possible complications include aspiration; sequelae of hypoxia, ischemia, or repeated seizures; and renal injury from rhabdomyolysis.

DISCHARGE CRITERIA/INSTRUCTIONS

• From the emergency department. Asymptomatic patients may be discharged following decontamination, 4 to 6 hours of observation and a psychiatric evaluation, if needed.
• From the hospital. Patients should be discharged when toxic effects have resolved or stabilized and following psychiatric evaluation, if needed.

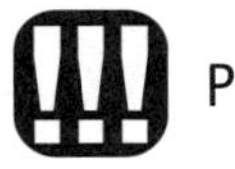

Pitfalls

DIAGNOSIS

The key to diagnosis is recognition of tonic-tetanic seizures in an alert patient without a postictal state.

TREATMENT

• Gastric lavage or other procedures may precipitate seizures and aspiration if endotracheal intubation is not performed first.
• Failure to control seizures rapidly may lead to a significantly worse prognosis.

ICD-9-CM 989.1

Toxic effect of other substances, chiefly nonmedicinal as to use: strychnine and salts.

See also: SECTION II, Seizures chapter.

RECOMMENDED READING

Smith BA. Strychnine poisoning. *J Emerg Med* 1990;8:321–325.

Bryson P. Strychnine. In: *Comprehensive review in toxicology for emergency clinicians,* 3rd ed. Washington, DC: Taylor & Francis, 1996:790–792.

Author: Michael Anderson

Reviewer: Richard C. Dart

Succinamide Anticonvulsants

Basics

DESCRIPTION

Succinamide anticonvulsants are used to control petit mal seizures.

FORMS AND USES

- Ethosuximide (Zarontin). Dose is titrated up to 1,500 mg/day in adults.
- Methsuximide (Celontin). Dose is titrated up to 1,200 mg/day in adults.
- Phensuximide (Milontin). Dose is titrated up to 3,000 mg/day in adults.

TOXIC DOSE

Toxic doses have not been well established in humans.

PATHOPHYSIOLOGY

Succinamide anticonvulsants suppress the paradoxical brain activity responsible for the lapse of consciousness caused by absence seizures.

DRUG INTERACTIONS

- Phenytoin levels may be increased with concurrent administration of succinamide.
- Other antiseizure medications also may exhibit altered metabolism.

PREGNANCY AND LACTATION

- Ethosuximide and methsuximide. US FDA Pregnancy Category C. Studies have shown that the drug exerts animal teratogenic or embryocidal effects, but there are no controlled studies in women, or no studies are available in either animals or women.
- Phensuximide. US FDA Pregnancy Category D. Evidence of human fetal risk exists, but benefits in certain situations may make use of the drug acceptable despite its risks.

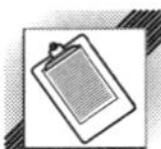

Diagnosis

Toxic causes of depressed mental status include alcohol, anticonvulsants, narcotics, and sedative-hypnotics, among others.

SIGNS AND SYMPTOMS

Primary effects are neurologic and may be prolonged due to the long half-lives of active metabolites.

Gastrointestinal

Nausea and vomiting are common.

Neurologic

- Irritability, euphoria, lightheadedness, headache, ataxia, parkinsonian-like symptoms, and photophobia have been reported on therapeutic doses.
- Acute overdose may cause CNS depression and coma.
- Coma may resolve only to recur several hours later.

Hematologic

- Side effects on therapeutic dose include leukopenia, monocytosis, eosinophilia, granulocytopenia, agranulocytosis, thrombocytopenia, and aplastic anemia.
- Blood dyscrasias are more common with ethosuximide.

PROCEDURES AND LABORATORY TESTS

Essential Tests

No tests may be needed in asymptomatic patients.

Recommended Tests

- Complete blood count, serum electrolytes, glucose, BUN, creatinine and liver function tests, and other antiseizure medication levels should be measured.
- Plasma levels should be obtained.
- Methsuximide. It is the metabolite that should be determined in overdose. Therapeutic levels are 20 to 40 μg/ml of *N*-demethylsuximide. Coma is associated with *N*-demethylsuximide levels above 150 μg/ml.
- Phensuximide. Therapeutic range is 10 to 20 μg/ml.

Ethosuximide. Therapeutic levels range from 40 to 100 μg/ml. Levels greater than 150 μg/ml are usually associated with toxicity.

- ECG, serum acetaminophen and aspirin in overdose setting to detect occult ingestion.
- Head CT, lumbar puncture, cultures, urine toxicology, and other tests as needed to assess CNS depression.

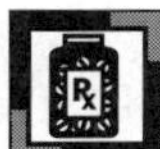

Treatment

- Treatment should focus on airway management and treatment of coma.
- The dose and time of exposure should be determined for all substances involved.

DIRECTING PATIENT COURSE

The health-care professional should call the poison control center when:

- Severe or persistent effects develop.
- Coingestant, drug interaction, or underlying disease presents an unusual problem.

The patient should be referred to a health-care facility when:

- Suicide or homicide attempt is possible.
- Toxic effects develop.
- Coingestant, drug interaction, or underlying disease presents an unusual problem.

Admission Considerations

Patients with depressed mental status after a 6-hour observation period should be admitted.

DECONTAMINATION

- Gastric lavage should be performed for substantial ingestion presenting within 1 hour of ingestion or if serious effects are present.
- Activated charcoal (1–2 g/kg) should be administered if ingestion has occurred within the past few hours.
- Enhanced elimination

—Ethosuximide and methsuximide. Hemodialysis may be useful in enhancing elimination and should be considered with patients with persistent severe respiratory depression.

ANTIDOTE

There is no specific antidote for succinamide poisoning.

ADJUNCTIVE TREATMENT

Hemodialysis increases ethosuximide elimination and may be useful in serious poisoning.

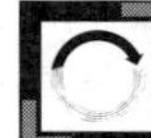

Follow-Up

PATIENT MONITORING

- Respiratory and cardiac monitoring should be performed continuously in symptomatic patients.
- Patients with methsuximide overdose should be observed for at least 24 hours following clinical improvement.

EXPECTED COURSE AND PROGNOSIS

- Recovery is expected with supportive and symptomatic care.
- Clinical course with methsuximide may exhibit improvement, followed by relapse to coma within 24 hours, secondary to accumulation of active metabolite.

DISCHARGE CRITERIA/INSTRUCTIONS

Asymptomatic patients may be discharged after decontamination, 6 hours of observation and, if needed, a psychiatric evaluation.

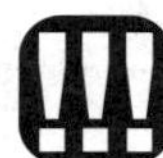

Pitfalls

FOLLOW-UP

Relapse with recurrence of coma may occur with methsuximide overdose.

ICD-9-CM 966.2

Poisoning by anticonvulsants and antiparkinsonism drugs: succinimides.

RECOMMENDED READING

Baehler RW, Wark J, Smith W, et al. Charcoal hemoperfusion in the therapy for methsuximide and phenytoin overdose. *Arch Intern Med* 1980;140:1466–1468.

Karch SB. Methsuximide overdose: delayed onset of profound coma. *JAMA* 1973;223:1463–1465.

Author: Steven A. Seifert

Reviewer: Kennon Heard

Sucralfate

Basics

DESCRIPTION

Sucralfate is a sucrose-aluminum preparation that is used for a variety of peptic pathologic conditions; toxicity is rare.

FORMS AND USES

- Sucralfate (Carafate) is used for therapy of acute duodenal ulcers and for maintenance therapy after healing.
- It is also used in a variety of gastrointestinal peptic conditions, including treatment of gastroesophageal reflux disease.

—Adult dosage for ulcer therapy is 1 g by mouth four times a day.
—Pediatric dosage has not been established.

TOXIC DOSE

No toxic dose has been established.

PATHOPHYSIOLOGY

Sucralfate is a poorly absorbed sucrose-aluminum preparation that binds to the gastrointestinal mucosa, thereby offering protection from local acid injury.

EPIDEMIOLOGY

Poisoning is uncommon.

CAUSES

Child neglect or abuse should be considered if the patient is less than 1 year of age, suicide attempt if the patient is over 6 years of age.

DRUG AND DISEASE INTERACTIONS

Patients on dialysis who are treated with sucralfate may develop aluminum toxicity.

PREGNANCY AND LACTATION

US FDA Pregnancy Category B. Animal studies indicate no fetal risk and there are no controlled human studies, or animal studies show an adverse fetal effect but well-controlled studies in women do not.

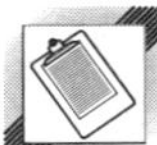

Diagnosis

DIFFERENTIAL DIAGNOSIS

Aluminum toxicity may appear similar to lithium toxicity, alcohol intoxication, and phenytoin, carbamezepine, and phenobarbital toxicity.

SIGNS AND SYMPTOMS

Dermatologic

Rashes and urticaria may develop.

Gastrointestinal

- Constipation is most common.
- Patient may also develop diarrhea, indigestion, or mechanical obstruction of gastrointestinal tract (sucralfate bezoar or "sucralith").

Fluids and Electrolytes

In patients on dialysis, aluminum toxicity may occur.

Musculoskeletal

In patients on dialysis, aluminum toxicity may occur, including osteodystrophy, bone pain, and bone microfractures.

Neurologic

In patients on dialysis, aluminum toxicity may occur, including dysarthria, acute encephalopathy, myoclonic jerks, and seizures.

PROCEDURES AND LABORATORY TESTS

Essential Tests

No tests are usually needed on asymptomatic patients.

Recommended Tests

- Aluminum level

—The aluminum level should be measured in dialysis patients demonstrating signs of aluminum toxicity.
—Aluminum levels may be obtained on blood, water, and dialysate, most commonly by atomic absorption.
—Normal serum levels are less than 15 μg/L.

- Barium swallow may help diagnose sucralfate bezoars.
- ECG, serum acetaminophen and aspirin in overdose setting to detect occult ingestion.

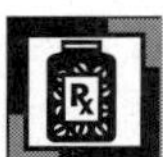

Treatment

- Treatment should focus on supportive care with appropriate airway management.
- Dose and time of ingestion should be determined for all substances involved.

DIRECTING PATIENT COURSE

The health-care professional should call the poison control center when:

- Severe or persistent effects develop.
- Coingestant, drug interaction, or underlying disease presents an unusual problem.

The patient should be referred to a health-care facility when:

- Suicide or homicide attempt is possible.
- Toxic effects develop.
- Coingestant, drug interaction, or underlying disease presents an unusual problem.

Admission Considerations

Dialysis patients exhibiting signs of aluminum require intensive care monitoring.

DECONTAMINATION

Out of Hospital

Induction of emesis is not recommended due to low toxic potential.

In Hospital

Gastric lavage and activated charcoal administration are not needed due to the benign nature of overdose.

ANTIDOTES

Dialysis patients may require deferoxamine chelation therapy for aluminum toxicity, related encephalopathy, and bone demineralization.

ADJUNCTIVE TREATMENT

Oral calcium carbonate may be substituted for aluminum- or magnesium-containing phosphate binders to prevent or treat aluminum toxicity.

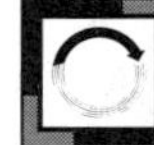

Follow-Up

PATIENT MONITORING

Aluminum levels must be followed for end-stage renal patients on dialysis who are using sucralfate.

EXPECTED COURSE AND PROGNOSIS

Sucralfate ingestions are typically benign in patients with normal renal function.

DISCHARGE CRITERIA/INSTRUCTIONS

Discharge asymptomatic patients from the emergency department or hospital following decontamination and psychiatric evaluation, if needed.

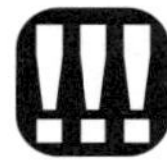

Pitfalls

DIAGNOSIS

Failure to consider aluminum toxicity as an etiology of dementia in patients with renal failure

TREATMENT

Use in end-stage renal failure patients may lead to aluminum toxicity, especially if these patients are taking other aluminum-containing medicines.

ICD-9-CM 976.3

Poisoning by agents primarily affecting skin and mucous membrane, ophthalmological, otorhinolaryngological, and dental drugs: emollients, demulcents, and protectants.

See also: SECTION III, Deferoxamine chapter.

RECOMMENDED READING

McCarthy DM. Sucralfate. *N Engl J Med* 1991;325:1017–1025.

Author: Kathleen Graham

Reviewer: Gerald F. O'Malley

Sulfur Dioxide

Basics

DESCRIPTION

Sulfur dioxide is a colorless, highly irritating, nonflammable gas.

FORMS AND USES

- Sulfur dioxide is a common pollutant from combustion of fossil fuels; the most common sources are automobiles and smelters and industries that burn soft coal and other fossil fuels.
- It is used in metal ore refining, chemical manufacturing, treatment of wood pulp to make paper, and extraction of lubricating oils.
- It is used as a preservative, disinfectant, reducing agent, bleaching agent, fumigant, fungicide, insecticide, and a food additive or preservative.

TOXIC DOSE

- Many patients can detect a sharp odor or taste of sulfur at an air concentration range of 3 to 5 ppm.
- Tissue irritation begins at approximately 8 to 12 ppm, and severe irritation may occur at levels up to and exceeding 50 ppm.

PATHOPHYSIOLOGY

- Sulfur dioxide combines with water to form sulfurous acid, which is caustic, and this may be further oxidized to sulfuric acid.
- Due to its moderate water solubility, it is typically absorbed in the nose and upper airways when inhaled.
- However, if the minute ventilation of the patient is large, or if large exposure occurs, sufficient gas may reach the lower airways to produce pneumonitis and pulmonary edema in severe cases.

EPIDEMIOLOGY

Poisoning is uncommon.

CAUSES

Toxicity above simple mucous membrane irritation is usually from occupational exposure.

WORKPLACE STANDARDS

- ACGIH. TLV TWA is 2 ppm; STEL is 5 ppm.
- OSHA. PEL TWA is 5 ppm.
- NIOSH. IDLH level is 100 ppm.

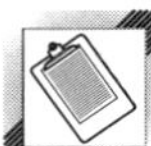

Diagnosis

DIFFERENTIAL DIAGNOSIS

Toxic causes of mucous membrane irritation include inhalation of chlorine, ammonia, isocyanates, ozone, chloramine, and many others.

SIGNS AND SYMPTOMS

The majority of exposures result in only irritation of the upper respiratory tract and mucous membranes.

HEENT

Mucous membrane irritation, cough, and rhinorrhea are common.

Dermatologic

Liquid sulfur dioxide may cause frostbite.

Pulmonary

- Cough, chest pain, and bronchospasm are common.
- Pulmonary edema may develop in severe cases and may be delayed in onset.

PROCEDURES AND LABORATORY TESTS

Essential Tests

No tests may be needed in mildly symptomatic patients with a history of brief exposure.

Recommended Tests

- Arterial blood gases, pulse oximetry, and chest radiography are warranted in symptomatic patients.
- Complete blood count, serum electrolytes, BUN, and creatinine are useful in symptomatic patients to assess injury.
- Sulfhemoglobin levels may be useful to confirm exposure, but are performed only by referral laboratories.

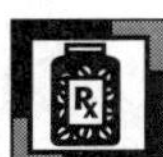

Treatment

- Treatment should focus on airway management and supportive care.
- Endotracheal intubation may be needed for severe exposure.
- Dose and time of exposure should be determined for all substances involved.

DIRECTING PATIENT COURSE

The health-care professional should call the poison control center when:

- Severe or persistent effects develop.
- Underlying disease presents an unusual problem.

The patient should be referred to a health-care facility when:

- Toxic effects develop.
- Underlying disease presents an unusual problem.

Admission Considerations

Inpatient management is warranted for patients with a history of significant exposure, who should be admitted for observation.

DECONTAMINATION

- The patient should be removed from the source and administered 100% oxygen.
- The eyes or skin, if exposed, should be irrigated.

ANTIDOTES

There is no specific antidote for sulfur dioxide poisoning.

ADJUNCTIVE TREATMENT

- Bronchospasm is treated in the same manner as asthma; the role of corticosteroids is controversial, and some investigators recommend early use.
- Pulmonary edema is treated as the noncardiogenic type (see SECTION II, Pulmonary Edema chapter).
- Burn or frostbite, caused by direct contact with liquid, is treated in the usual manner with conservative local wound care.
- Ocular injury is treated in the standard manner for caustic eye exposure.

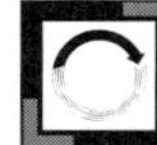

Follow-Up

PATIENT MONITORING

- Continuous respiratory and cardiac monitoring should be performed during the acute episode.
- Most individuals with mild to moderate exposure will not require follow-up.
- Individuals who are exposed to larger amounts, or who are susceptible because of underlying asthma may require monitoring of expiratory flow rates and volumes, as well as a follow-up evaluation.

EXPECTED COURSE AND PROGNOSIS

- Development of injury may be delayed more than 24 hours.
- Certain individuals may develop asthma following pulmonary acid exposure.

DISCHARGE CRITERIA/INSTRUCTIONS

- From the emergency department. Asymptomatic or minimally symptomatic patients may be discharged after a 4- to 6-hour observation period (unless large exposure is suspected).
- From the hospital. Patient may be discharged after appropriate observation (usually at least 24 hours) for potentially serious inhalation.

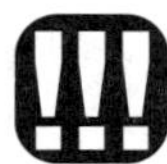

Pitfalls

DIAGNOSIS

Development of pulmonary edema may be delayed more than 24 hours after exposure.

ICD-9-CM 987.3

Toxic effect of other gases, fumes, or vapors: sulfur dioxide.

See also: SECTION II, Pulmonary Edema chapter.

RECOMMENDED READING

Charan MB, Myers CG, Lakshminarayan S, et al. Pulmonary injuries associated with acute sulfur dioxide inhalation. *Am Rev Respir Dis* 1979;119:555–560.

Balmes JR, Fine JM, Shepherd D. Symptomatic bronchoconstriction after short term inhalation of sulfur dioxide. *Am Rev Respir Dis* 1997;136:1117–1121.

Author: Scott D. Phillips

Reviewer: Richard C. Dart

Sumatriptan

Basics

DESCRIPTION

Sumatriptan (Imitrex) is an ergot alkaloid derivative used in the treatment of migraine headache.

FORMS AND USES

The typical dose is 6 mg subcutaneously, 25 to 100 mg orally.

TOXIC DOSE

- Sumatriptan is minimally toxic in acute overdose; a dose of 200 mg has been ingested without toxic effect.
- However, therapeutic doses have caused coronary vasospasm in susceptible individuals.

PATHOPHYSIOLOGY

- Sumatriptan should not be administered intravenously because of its potential to cause coronary vasospasm.
- Acute myocardial infarction, ventricular dysrhythmias, and coronary vasospasm have occurred with therapeutic doses of subcutaneous sumatriptan.

EPIDEMIOLOGY

Poisoning is uncommon.

CAUSES

- Toxic effects are usually caused by an adverse drug event during therapeutic use.
- Child neglect or abuse should be considered if the patient is less than 1 year of age, suicide attempt if the patient is over 6 years of age.

DRUG AND DISEASE INTERACTIONS

- Subcutaneous sumatriptan should not be administered to individuals with signs or symptoms of ischemic heart disease, history of myocardial infarction, documented silent ischemia, or Prinzmetal's angina.
- Sumatriptan should not be administered to patients who have recently received dihydroergotamine.

PREGNANCY AND LACTATION

US FDA Pregnancy Category C. The drug exerts animal teratogenic or embryocidal effects, but there are no controlled studies in women, or no studies are available in animals or women.

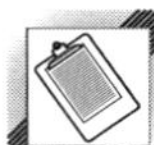

Diagnosis

SIGNS AND SYMPTOMS

Vital Signs

Acute onset of hypertension may occur.

Dermatologic

Injection site reaction commonly occurs.

Cardiovascular

Coronary artery spasm may cause nausea, vomiting, diaphoresis, chest pain, dysrhythmia, or other manifestations of myocardial ischemia.

Gastrointestinal

Nausea, vomiting, and abnormal taste have occurred.

Neurologic

- Tingling and dizziness are common.
- Hemiparesis has occurred in association with sumatriptan use.
- Drowsiness, sensation of warmth, and fatigue occur.

PROCEDURES AND LABORATORY TESTS

Essential Tests

No tests may be needed in asymptomatic patients.

Recommended Tests

- ECG, serum creatine kinase, and other tests as appropriate in symptomatic patients for management of myocardial ischemia
- Other tests as needed to evaluate other adverse effects
- Serum acetaminophen and aspirin in overdose setting to detect occult ingestion.

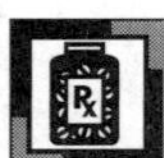

Treatment

- Therapy should focus on supportive care and detection of cardiac ischemia.
- Standard treatment of myocardial ischemia is initiated while supportive care continues.

DIRECTING PATIENT COURSE

The health-care professional should call the poison control center when:

- Severe or persistent effects develop.
- Coingestant, drug interaction, or underlying disease presents an unusual problem.

The patient should be referred to a health-care facility when:

- Suicide or homicide attempt is possible.
- Toxic effects develop.
- Coingestant, drug interaction, or underlying disease presents an unusual problem.

Admission Considerations

All symptomatic patients should be admitted to an intensive-care setting.

DECONTAMINATION

Out of Hospital

Decontamination is not recommended because is usually associated with therapeutic dose.

In Hospital

- Gastric lavage is not recommended.
- One dose of activated charcoal (1–2 g/kg) should be administered without a cathartic if a substantial ingestion has occurred within the previous few hours.

ANTIDOTES

There is no specific antidote for sumatriptan toxicity.

ADJUNCTIVE TREATMENT

Myocardial ischemia and dysrhythmias are treated in the same manner as atherosclerotic heart disease.

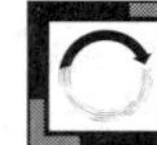

Follow-Up

PATIENT MONITORING

ECG, cardiac monitoring, and laboratory tests are performed for myocardial ischemia in symptomatic patients.

EXPECTED COURSE AND PROGNOSIS

Full recovery over several hours is expected unless sequelae of myocardial or cerebral ischemia intercedes.

DISCHARGE CRITERIA/INSTRUCTIONS

Asymptomatic patients may be discharged from the emergency department or hospital following decontamination, a 6-hour observation period, and psychiatric evaluation, if needed.

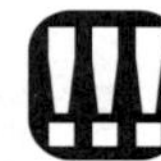

Pitfalls

DIAGNOSIS

Patient's history of headache often have other potentially lethal drugs available for coingestion.

ICD-9-CM 972

Poisoning by agents primarily affecting the cardiovascular system.

Recommended Reading

Brown EG, Endersby CA, Smith RN, et al. The safety and tolerability of sumatriptan. *Eur Neurol* 1991;311:339–344.

Author: Luke Yip

Reviewer: Katherine M. Hurlbut

Basics

DESCRIPTION

Tacrine is a centrally acting, reversible, cholinesterase inhibitor.

FORMS AND USES

- Tacrine (Cognex) is used in the treatment of Alzheimer's disease.
- It also has been used occasionally as a long-acting inhibitor of acetylcholinesterase in anticholinergic overdose.

TOXIC DOSE

The estimated lethal dose in an adult is 30 mg/kg.

PATHOPHYSIOLOGY

- Tacrine is a reversible cholinesterase inhibitor that is active mainly within the CNS.
- This results in increased brain acetylcholine levels, which improves cognitive function.
- Tacrine has minimal peripheral effect.
- The most likely toxic effects would be those of cholinergic excess.

EPIDEMIOLOGY

- There are few reports of overdose in humans.
- Poisoning is expected to be mild, treatable, and unlikely to be fatal unless a coingestant is involved.

CAUSES

Child neglect or abuse should be considered if the patient is less than 1 year of age, suicide attempt if the patient is over 6 years of age.

PREGNANCY AND LACTATION

US FDA Pregnancy Category C. The drug exerts animal teratogenic or embryocidal effects, but there are no controlled studies in women, or no studies are available in animals or women.

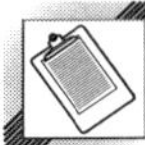

Diagnosis

DIFFERENTIAL DIAGNOSIS

Toxicologic causes of acute vomiting, diarrhea, diaphoresis, and miosis are organophosphate or carbamate insecticides, nerve agents used in war, and edrophonium, among others.

SIGNS AND SYMPTOMS

Vital Signs

Bradycardia may occur.

HEENT

Miosis may occur.

Dermatologic

Diaphoresis may occur.

Cardiovascular

Bradycardia, heart block, and asystole may occur with large overdose.

Pulmonary

Bronchospasm and pulmonary edema can occur with overdose.

Gastrointestinal

Severe vomiting and diarrhea may occur with overdose.

Hepatic

- Hepatotoxicity occurs in 50% of patients within 1 to 3 months of starting therapeutic dose.
- It is usually reversible upon discontinuation, but permanent hepatic damage and hepatic failure have been reported.

Fluids and Electrolytes

Vomiting and diarrhea may lead to fluid loss, alkalosis, and hypokalemia.

Neurologic

- Seizures may occur with overdose.
- Worsening of parkinsonian symptoms was reported in an animal model and one human report.

PROCEDURES AND LABORATORY TESTS

Essential Tests

No tests may be needed in asymptomatic patients.

Recommended Tests

- Pulse oximetry or arterial blood gases are used to evaluate oxygenation.
- ECG is performed to evaluate for conduction abnormalities.
- Serum electrolytes, glucose, BUN, and creatinine levels are measured if fluid loss has been significant or altered mental status develops.
- Liver function tests are ordered in acute overdose or in symptomatic patients on chronic therapy.
- Decreased cholinesterase activity in plasma and serum indicates toxicity.
- Serum acetaminophen and aspirin levels in an overdose setting are measured to detect occult ingestion.
- Head CT, lumbar puncture, cultures, toxicology screening as appropriate in patients with altered mental status.

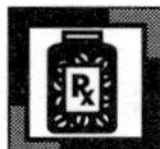

Treatment

- Treatment focuses on supportive care and symptomatic therapy with atropine.
- Severe cases may need endotracheal intubation.
- Dose and time of exposure should be determined for all substances involved.

DIRECTING PATIENT COURSE

The health-care professional should call the poison control center when:

- Severe or persistent effects develop.
- Coingestant, drug interaction, or underlying disease presents an unusual problem.

The patient should be referred to a health-care facility when:

- Suicide or homicide attempt is possible.
- Toxic effects develop.
- Coingestant, drug interaction, or underlying disease presents an unusual problem.

Admission Considerations

Patients with persistent cholinergic symptoms or complications such as hypotension or seizure should be admitted.

DECONTAMINATION

Out of Hospital

Induction of emesis is not recommended.

In Hospital

- Gastric lavage should be performed in pediatric (tube size 24–32 French) or adult (tube size 36–42 French) patients presenting within 1 hour of a large ingestion or if serious effects are present.
- One dose of activated charcoal (1–2 g/kg) should be administered without a cathartic if a substantial ingestion has occurred within the previous few hours.

ANTIDOTES

- Atropine is the antidote for cholinergic poisoning induced by tacrine.
- The primary goal is to reduce pulmonary secretions.
- The adult dose of atropine is 1 to 2 mg and the pediatric dose is 0.05 mg/kg, given intravenously every 5 to 10 minutes and titrated until symptoms resolve (see SECTION III, Atropine chapter).

ADJUNCTIVE TREATMENT

- Seizures are treated initially with benzodiazepines in the usual manner (see SECTION II, Seizures chapter).
- Bronchospasm is treated with atropine as described above and nebulized albuterol or other bronchodilator.

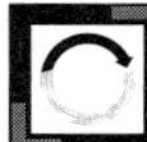

Follow-Up

PATIENT MONITORING

- Patients should be placed on a cardiac monitor and have intravenous access established.
- Liver enzymes should be tested serially to determine the course of injury.

EXPECTED COURSE AND PROGNOSIS

- Toxic effects are expected to develop within hours.
- Complete recovery is expected unless sequelae of prolonged hypotension or seizures develop.

DISCHARGE CRITERIA/INSTRUCTIONS

- From the emergency department. Asymptomatic patients may be discharged after gastrointestinal decontamination, observation for 6 hours, and psychiatric evaluation, if needed.
- From the hospital. Patients may be discharged when symptoms are resolving, liver enzymes improving, and following psychiatric evaluation, if needed.

ICD-9-CM 971

Poisoning by drugs primarily affecting the autonomic nervous system.

See also: SECTION II, Hypotension and Seizures chapters; and SECTION III, Atropine chapter.

RECOMMENDED READING

Ellenhorn MJ. Unclassified drugs: Tacrine. In: *Ellenhorn's medical toxicology,* 2nd ed. Baltimore: Williams & Wilkins, 1997:963–965.

Author: Kennon Heard

Reviewer: Richard C. Dart

Tamoxifen

Basics

DESCRIPTION

Tamoxifen (Tamofen, Nolvadex) is an antiestrogen hormone.

FORMS AND USES

The usual dose is 20 to 40 mg daily; however, doses as high as 200 mg per day have been used in the treatment of breast cancer.

TOXIC DOSE

Toxic dose has not been established.

PATHOPHYSIOLOGY

- Tamoxifen is a competitive inhibitor of estradiol binding to estrogen receptors and is considered the treatment of choice for both pre- and postmenopausal women with estrogen receptor–positive tumors of the breast.
- The most specific and dangerous complication of therapy with tamoxifen is hypercalcemia, a direct consequence of the successful treatment of neoplastic metastases to bone.
- Gynecologic malignancies appear related to tamoxifen therapy.

EPIDEMIOLOGY

Poisoning is uncommon.

CAUSES

Child neglect or abuse should be considered if the patient is less than 1 year of age, suicide attempt if the patient is over 6 years of age.

PREGNANCY AND LACTATION

US FDA Pregnancy Category D. Evidence of human fetal risk exists, but benefits in certain situations (e.g., life-threatening situations or serious diseases) may make use of the drug acceptable despite its risks.

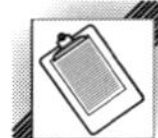

Diagnosis

DIFFERENTIAL DIAGNOSIS

Toxic causes of hypercalcemia include vitamin D, vitamin A analogs, calcium administration, estrogen administration, aluminum hydroxide, hydrochlorothiazide, and furosemide.

SIGNS AND SYMPTOMS

- Acute exposure causes gastrointestinal symptoms.
- Chronic changes such as malignancy or hepatic injury may take days, weeks, or longer to appear.

HEENT

- Retinal degeneration has been seen with high-dose therapy.
- Additional ophthalmologic complications during therapeutic use include macular edema and keratopathy.

Cardiovascular

- QT interval prolongation may develop following massive overdose.
- Myocardial infarction has occurred secondary to thromboemboli.
- Dysrhythmias have not been reported.

Pulmonary

Pulmonary embolism is a rare complication of therapy.

Gastrointestinal

Nausea and vomiting are common.

Hepatic

Liver enzyme elevations may develop during therapy.

Hematologic

- Thrombosis with pulmonary embolism may occur.
- Thrombocytopenia has been reported following overdose.

Neurologic

- Acute exposure may cause tremor
- Hyperreflexia, unsteady gait, and dizziness often develop at doses above 400 mg.

PROCEDURES AND LABORATORY TESTS

Essential Tests

No tests may be needed in asymptomatic patients.

Recommended Tests

- Complete blood count (CBC), serum electrolytes, glucose, calcium, BUN, creatinine, liver transaminases in symptomatic patients or following overdose.
- ECG to monitor for QT prolongation and to identify possible ischemia or infarction.
- Pulse oximetry or arterial blood gases in patients with respiratory complaints.
- Evaluation for pulmonary embolism in patients with appropriate signs.

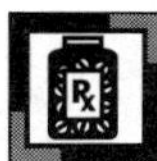

Treatment

- Treatment should focus on supportive care with appropriate airway management.
- Dose and time of exposure should be determined for all substances involved.

DIRECTING PATIENT COURSE

The health-care professional should call the poison control center when:

- Severe or persistent effects develop.
- Coingestant, drug interaction, or underlying disease presents an unusual problem.

The patient should be referred to a health-care facility when:

- Suicide or homicide attempt is possible.
- Toxic effects develop.
- Coingestant, drug interaction, or underlying disease presents an unusual problem.

Admission Considerations

Patients with hypercalcemia or evidence of thrombosis or dysrhythmia should be admitted to a monitored bed.

DECONTAMINATION

- Gastric lavage should be performed in pediatric (tube size 24–32 French) or adult (tube size 36–42 French) patients presenting within 1 hour of a large ingestion or if serious effects are present.
- One dose of activated charcoal (1–2 g/kg) should be administered without a cathartic if a substantial ingestion has occurred within the previous few hours.

ANTIDOTES

There is no specific antidote for tamoxifen poisoning.

ADJUNCTIVE TREATMENT

- Hypercalcemia is treated initially with fluid resuscitation.
- Seizures. A benzodiazepine is administered for initial control; if seizures persist or recur, another anticonvulsant such as phenobarbital is added. The airway should be monitored closely.
- Cardiac dysrhythmias. Treatment is discussed in SECTION II, Ventricular Dysrhythmias chapter.

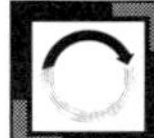

Follow-Up

PATIENT MONITORING

- ECG and cardiac rhythm monitoring are indicated.
- Liver enzymes, calcium, and CBC should be repeated in 24 hours.

EXPECTED COURSE AND PROGNOSIS

Complete recovery is anticipated unless sequelae of hypercalcemia or hypoxia intercede.

DISCHARGE CRITERIA/INSTRUCTIONS

Patients may be discharged from the emergency department of hospital when serum calcium is normal and complications have resolved and following psychiatric evaluation, if needed.

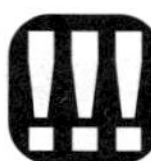

Pitfalls

DIAGNOSIS

Due to nonspecific symptoms and the use of multiple medications, the diagnosis of tamoxifen toxicity in an obtunded patient may be overlooked.

FOLLOW-UP

- Follow-up over several weeks is needed after acute overdose to detect the development of hepatic injury or thrombocytopenia.
- Patients that are chronically supertherapeutic need close follow-up to monitor for ophthalmologic complications and thromboembolic disease.

ICD-9-CM 963.1

Poisoning by primarily systemic agents: antineoplastic and immunosuppressive drugs.

See also: SECTION II, Seizure and Ventricular Dysrhythmia chapters.

RECOMMENDED READING

Jordan VC. Tamoxifen: toxicities and drug resistance during the treatment and prevention of breast cancer. *Annu Rev Pharmacol Toxicol* 1995:35:195–212.

Author: Lada Kokan

Reviewer: Kennon Heard

Basics

DESCRIPTION

• A teratogen is an agent or condition that may cause a permanent alteration in form or function in the offspring when present during prenatal growth. The term does not include agents that cause fetal death or affect the rate of growth. Chemical, drug, infectious, or physical agents, or nutritional deficiencies can all be teratogens.
• Anomaly and malformation refer to a structural abnormality.
• A birth defect or a congenital defect is a morphologic, enzymatic, genetic, or chromosomal abnormality.
• A syndrome is a collection of abnormalities that, if some or all of the abnormalities are present in an individual, constitute a syndrome. A syndrome is generally associated with a specific agent.

PATHOPHYSIOLOGY

Mechanisms of teratogenesis may include:

• Disruption of chromosomal structure or replication.
• Alteration of the hormonal environment of the fetus.
• Depletion of essential nutrients or oxygen.
• Deposition of compounds into developing tissues.

EPIDEMIOLOGY

• Approximately 3% of newborns have an identified congenital defect.
• Additional abnormalities identified in older children result in a 6% overall incidence of congenital defects.
• Premature and stillborn infants and spontaneously aborted embryos and fetuses have a higher rate of congenital defects.

PREGNANCY AND LACTATION

US FDA Pregnancy Categories

• Category A. Controlled studies in women fail to demonstrate a risk to the fetus in the first trimester, and the possibility of fetal harm appears remote.
• Category B. Animal studies do not indicate a risk to the fetus and there are no controlled human studies, or animal studies do show an adverse effect on the fetus but well-controlled studies in pregnant women have failed to demonstrate a risk to the fetus.
• Category C. Studies have shown that the drug exerts animal teratogenic or embryocidal effects, but there are no controlled studies in women, or no studies are available in either animals or women.
• Category D. Positive evidence of human fetal risk exists, but benefits in certain situations (e.g., life-threatening situations or serious diseases for which safer drugs cannot be used or are ineffective) may make use of the drug acceptable despite its risks.
• Category X. Studies in animals or humans have demonstrated fetal abnormalities or there is evidence of fetal risk based on human experience, or both, and the risk clearly outweighs any possible benefit.

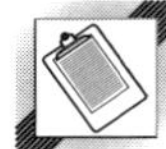

Diagnosis

DIFFERENTIAL DIAGNOSIS

Known Teratogens

• Androgenic hormones (testosterone, methyltestosterone, norlutin, pranone, lutocylol, danazol, and normethandrone).

—Masculinization of the female fetus may occur if exposure occurs during the first 90 days of gestation.
—Clitoral hypertrophy and labial fusion also have been described.

• Anticoagulants [warfarin (Coumadin)].

—One of six pregnancies exposed to coumadin results in abortion or stillbirth; one out of six results in deformity.
—Coumadin derivatives taken in the first 100 days of gestation are associated with fetal nasal hypoplasia, small birth size, and Conradi's syndrome, which is calcific stippling of the secondary skeletal epiphyses.
—Blindness, hydrocephalus, mental retardation, and other abnormalities have been described in offspring exposed after 100 days of gestation.

• Antineoplastic agents (azauridine, bleomycin, busulfan, chlorambucil, cisplastin, cyclophosphamide, cytarabine, danorubicin, 5-fluorouracil, hydroxyurea, mechlorethamine, melphalam, and methotrexate).

—A multitude of abnormalities involving almost every organ system and a total incidence of 10% to 50% for congenital abnormalities has been reported.
—Folate supplementation for mothers receiving antifolates such as methotrexate has been recommended.

• Carbamazepine

—The risk of neural tube defects is increased to 1%.
—Maternal folate supplementation is recommended.

• Carbon monoxide. A variety of neurologic abnormalities have been reported: cerebral atrophy, mental retardation, microcephaly, seizures, cerebral palsy, and increased risk of fetal loss.
• Diethylstilbestrol (DES)

—Clear cell carcinoma of the vagina or cervix is associated with a high incidence of maternal use of DES before the 18th week of gestation.
—Oligomenorrhea, a reduced number of pregnancies, and an increased rate of spontaneous abortions, preterm pregnancies, and perinatal mortality, were found in exposed daughters.
—Genital abnormalities and spermatozoal changes were found in sons.

• Ethanol

—Fetal alcohol syndrome is associated with chronic maternal alcohol use during pregnancy. Growth retardation, neurologic abnormalities (including mental retardation), and craniofacial abnormalities (microcephaly, maxillary hypoplasia, cleft palate, and micrognathia) constitute the syndrome.
—Chronic maternal ethanol use is associated with a perinatal mortality of 17% and a 44% incidence of mental deficiency in offspring.

• Iodine and antithyroid medications (methimazole and propylthiouracil)

—Thyroid hypertrophy and hypothyroidism may occur in the offspring of mothers taking these medications, particularly if exposed during the third trimester.
—Neonatal hypothyroidism results in cretinism if untreated.

• Isoretinoin (cis-retinoin, etretinate, accutane)

—Craniofacial abnormalities, cardiac defects, hydrocephalus, and microcephaly may occur.
—The risk of fetal abnormalities with isoretinoin exposure is 38%, with neurologic defects predominating (80%).

• Lead. Lower scores in developmental tests have been found in children of mothers with high blood lead levels. An increased risk of developmental delays is possible with a maternal blood lead level greater than 10 μg/dl.
• Lithium. There is an increased risk of Ebstein's cardiac abnormality.
• Mercury. The risks of cerebral palsy, mental retardation, ocular malformations, microcephaly, and dental malocclusion are increased; the greatest risk is if exposure occurs during the 6th to 8th months of gestation.
• Methimazole (Tepazole). Scalp defects were associated with methimazole use in pregnancy in several reports.
• D-penicillamine is associated with the hyperelastosis of the skin.
• Phenytoin

—Fetal hydantoin syndrome includes craniofacial defects (including a low nasal bridge, hypertelorism, and abnormal ears), phalangeal hypoplasia, skeletal abnormalities, mental retardation, microcephaly, growth deficiency, neuroblastoma, and cardiac abnormalities.
—An 11% risk of developing the typical syndrome and a 31% risk of a partial syndrome development have been reported in children following maternal phenytoin use.

• Polychlorobiphenyls (PCBs)

—The development of a "cola-colored baby" has been associated with maternal exposure to polychlorobiphenyls in an incident involving PCB-contaminated rice oil.
—Other abnormalities included intrauterine

growth retardation, ocular abnormalities, and teeth present at birth.

- Thalidomide. Use of thalidomide during days 21 to 40 of gestation has resulted in a 20% risk of limb phocomelia or other abnormalities, including facial, gastrointestinal, cardiac, and renal abnormalities.
- Tetracycline (doxycycline). Dental discoloration in the fetus may occur after maternal use.

—Exposure after more than 120 days of gestation discolors primary teeth in 50% of cases.
—Exposure after 250 days may discolor permanent teeth.
—Before 120 days there is no known risk.

- Trimethadione (paramethadione) is associated with a syndrome which includes mental retardation, V-shaped eyebrows, epicanthus, low-set ears with folded helices, intrauterine growth retardation, palatal defects, cardiac abnormalities, and irregular teeth.
- Valproate increases the risk of neural tube defects to 1.2%; other abnormalities also may be associated with valproate use (microcephaly and cardiac defects) but have not been proven.

Possible Teratogens

- Aminoglycosides (gentamicin, kanamycin, streptomycin, and tobramycin). Neonatal auditory dysfunction has occurred following maternal treatment.
- Angiotensin-converting enzyme (ACE) inhibitors (captopril, enalapril, lisinopril, and ramipril). Renal defects, intrauterine growth retardation, hypocalvarium, pulmonary hypoplasia, and newborn hypotension may be associated with ACE inhibitor use during the second or third trimesters.
- Barbiturates (including amobarbital, butabarbital, methohexital, pentobarbital, phenobarbital, primidone, secobarbital, and thiopental). A variety of defects have been associated with barbiturate use during pregnancy; however, there is a lack of consistency between studies.
- Benzodiazepines (diazepam)

—Exposure to diazepam during the first trimester in animals has been associated with increased fetal death and thoracic vertebral anomalies.
—No consistent risk of abnormalities was found in human studies.

- Bromides. Skeletal and gastrointestinal abnormalities; exposure near term has been associated with hypotonia and central nervous system depression that resolved.
- Chenodiol. Animal studies have found fetal hepatotoxicity and necrosis of adrenal glands and kidneys.
- Cigarettes

—Maternal cigarette smoking may cause growth retardation, abruptio placentae, placenta previa, and placental changes that suggest decreased placental blood flow.
—Increased perinatal mortality and sudden infant death syndrome have been associated with maternal smoking.

- Cocaine

—Use during pregnancy has been associated with premature delivery, spontaneous abortion, abruptio placentae, and growth retardation.
—Malformations of the genitourinary and cardiac systems, face and limbs, as well as neurobehavioral and neurophysiologic effects in newborns, also have been reported.

- Colchicine

—Maternal use for gout has not been shown to result in a consistent human teratogenicity; however, teratogenicity occurs in animals.
—Azoospermia after paternal use may occur.

- Corticosteroids (cortisone, dexamethasone, hydrocortisone, methylprednisolone, prednisolone, prednisone, and triamcinolone). Despite a number of congenital anomalies associated with maternal corticosteroid use, there is no conclusive evidence of a relationship between corticosteroid use and congenital anomalies.
- Diuretics (chlorothiazide, hydrochlorothiazide, furosemide, and triamterene)

—At high doses, loop diuretics have been associated with some abnormalities in animals; however, the risks of defects in humans have not been demonstrated.
—Thiazide diuretics may be associated with an increased risk of congenital defects if used during the first trimester but not later in pregnancy.

- Ergots (dihydroergotamine, ergonovine, ergotamine, and methylergonovine). Limited use does not appear to be teratogenic.
- Estrogenic hormones (estradiol, ethinyl estradiol, and mestranol). An increase in congenital anomalies has not been consistently found.
- Marijuana may be associated with growth retardation.
- Mifepristone (RU 486). Human data are lacking; teratogenicity has been shown in some animal species but not others.
- Minoxidil. Exposure is associated with neonatal hypertrichosis.
- Oral contraceptives. There is no conclusive evidence of congenital anomalies.
- Phencyclidine. Irritability, hypertonicity, poor feeding and sucking, nystagmus, poor head control, respiratory distress, and facial abnormalities have been described.
- Progesterone hormones (ethynodiol, levonorgestrel, norethindrone, and norgestrel). An increase in congenital anomalies has not been consistently found. A 0.3% risk of masculinization of female fetuses has been found.
- Rifampin. There is a possible risk of hypoprothrombinemia and bleeding with maternal rifampin use.
- Quinine. No increased teratogenic effect with therapeutic use for malarial prophylaxis has been proved.
- Ribavarin. Although experience is limited, animal studies show teratogenicity in all species tested.
- Solvents are associated with congenital bowel atresia.
- Sulfonylureas (including acetohexamide, chlorpropamide, glipizide, glyburide, and tolbutamide). Persistent hypoglycemia is seen in neonates born to mothers taking an oral hypoglycemic near term.
- Tricyclic antidepressants (amitriptyline, doxepin, imipramine, desipramine, and nortriptyline). Limb reduction anomalies as well as a number of other individual anomalies have been reported following amitriptyline use; however, the bulk of the data indicates that tricyclic antidepressants are relatively safe during pregnancy.
- Vaccines. Maternal measles infection may result in an increased abortion rate and congenital malformations. Use of the vaccine during pregnancy is not recommended because maternal polio infection may result in congenital anomalies.

PROCEDURES AND LABORATORY TESTS

A pregnancy test is recommended in all female patients of potential childbearing age (10–45 years) exposed to a teratogen.

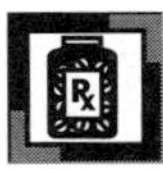

Treatment

- The general principle is that good maternal care is likely to result in a good fetal outcome.
- If a pregnant patient is exposed to a teratogen, she should be referred to an obstetrician who can initiate monitoring.

ICD-9-CM 760.0-779.9

Drug reaction and poisoning affecting a newborn.

RECOMMENDED READING

Briggs GG, Freeman RK, Yaffe SJ. *Drugs in pregnancy and lactation.* Baltimore: Williams & Wilkins, 1990.

Koren G, ed. *Maternal-fetal toxicology: a clinician's guide.* New York: Marcel Dekker, 1990.

Author: Lada Kokan

Reviewer: Kennon Heard

Terfenadine

Basics

DESCRIPTION

Terfenadine (Seldane) is a nonsedating antihistamine (H_1) medication.

FORMS AND USES

- Typical adult dose is 60 mg orally.
- Terfenadine was removed from the United States market in 1997.

TOXIC DOSE

The parent form (terfenadine) is the toxic species; metabolites are less toxic.

PATHOPHYSIOLOGY

Torsade de pointes have been reported when terfenadine was used concomitantly with drugs that interfere with hepatic cytochrome P450 enzyme.

EPIDEMIOLOGY

Torsade de pointes have been reported to occur when terfenadine was taken in an intentional overdose, taken in dosage higher than the recommended dosage, in patients with cirrhosis or a history of alcohol abuse, and during use with a contraindicated medication.

CAUSES

- Toxicity is usually caused by drug interaction.
- Child neglect or abuse should be considered if the patient is less than 1 year of age, suicide attempt if the patient is over 6 years of age.

DRUG AND DISEASE INTERACTIONS

Drug interactions occur with ketoconazole, itraconazole, metronidazole, fluconazole, miconazole, and macrolide antibiotics (e.g., erythromycin), all of which increase terfenadine levels by interfering with terfenadine metabolism.

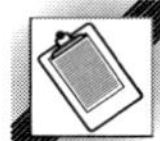

Diagnosis

A meticulous patient history including concomitant medications is important because a drug interaction is the most likely cause of toxicity.

DIFFERENTIAL DIAGNOSIS

Terfenadine-induced toxicity should be considered in the differential diagnosis of syncope, seizures, ventricular tachydysrhythmia, or prolonged QTc on ECG.

SIGNS AND SYMPTOMS

Cardiovascular

Syncope, seizures, ventricular tachydysrhythmia, prolonged QTc on ECG, and torsade de pointes may occur.

Neurologic

Lightheadedness and syncope may occur secondary to cardiac effects.

PROCEDURES AND LABORATORY TESTS

Essential Tests

- Serum electrolytes, complete blood count, BUN, and creatinine to assess causes of syncope
- ECG and cardiac monitoring to detect cardiac effects
- Serum acetaminophen and aspirin levels in overdose setting to detect occult ingestion.

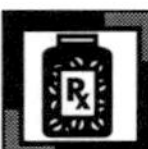

Treatment

Treatment should focus on supportive cardiac care and treatment of ventricular tachydysrhythmias.

DIRECTING PATIENT COURSE

The health-care professional should call the poison control center when:

- Severe or persistent effects develop.
- Coingestant, drug interaction, or underlying disease presents an unusual problem.

The patient should be referred to a health-care facility when:

- Suicide or homicide attempt is possible.
- Toxic effects develop.
- Coingestant, drug interaction, or underlying disease presents an unusual problem.

Admission Considerations

Patients with syncope or prolonged QTc on the ECG should be admitted to an intensive care setting, with continuous cardiac monitoring until at least 24 hours after the patient has been asymptomatic and the QTc has returned to baseline.

DECONTAMINATION

Out of Hospital

Ipecac-induced emesis should be avoided.

In Hospital

One dose of activated charcoal (1–2 g/kg) should be administered without a cathartic if a substantial ingestion has occurred within the previous few hours.

ANTIDOTES

There is no specific antidote for terfenadine poisoning.

ADJUNCTIVE TREATMENT

- Intravenous magnesium sulfate has been successful in the management of torsade de pointes.
- Isoproterenol, cardioversion, and temporary cardiac pacing may also be necessary.

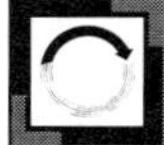

Follow-Up

PATIENT MONITORING

Patients should be placed on a cardiac monitor and an ECG obtained.

EXPECTED COURSE AND PROGNOSIS

Complete recovery is anticipated unless sequelae of hypotension intercede.

DISCHARGE CRITERIA/INSTRUCTIONS

Asymptomatic patients with normal ECG results may be discharged following decontamination, 6 hour observation period, and psychiatric evaluation, if needed.

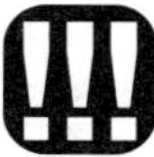

Pitfalls

- Physicians should avoid combining terfenadine with drugs that interfere with terfenadine metabolism [ketoconazole, itraconazole, metronidazole, fluconazole, miconazole, macrolide antibiotics (e.g., erythromycin)], cause torsade de pointes, or prolong QTc (e.g., quinidine, procainamide, disopyramide, sotalol, haloperidol, thioridazine, probucol, pentamidine).
- Terfenadine should be avoided in patients with congenital long QT syndrome.

ICD-9-CM 963.0

Poisoning primarily by systemic agents: antiallergic and antiemetic drugs.

See also: SECTION II, Ventricular dysrhythmia chapter.

RECOMMENDED READING

Safety of terfenadine and astemizole. *Med Lett Drugs Ther* 1992;34:9–10.

Author: Steven A. Seifert

Reviewer: Richard C. Dart

Testosterone and Methyltestosterone

Basics

DESCRIPTION

Testosterone is a naturally occurring hormone that may be abused by body builders.

FORMS AND USES

- Steroids are commonly abused by teenagers and athletes attempting to improve physical attributes and performance.
- Veterinary steroids, with a number of different names, are also commonly abused.
- Abusers will frequently "stack" multiple steroids and "cycle" drug-free periods between periods of use.

TOXIC DOSE

Toxic dose varies greatly by specific agent and by individual, and typically requires repeated administration.

PATHOPHYSIOLOGY

Toxicity is caused by CNS effects leading to aggression as well as cardiac disease caused by promotion of atherogenesis.

EPIDEMIOLOGY

Poisoning is common.

CAUSES

Toxicity is primarily the result of chronic abuse and unlikely in acute overdose.

PREGNANCY AND LACTATION

US FDA Pregnancy Category X. Studies in animals or humans have demonstrated fetal abnormalities or there is evidence of fetal risk based on human experience, or both, and the risk clearly outweighs any possible benefit.

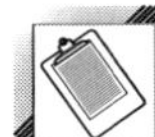

Diagnosis

DIFFERENTIAL DIAGNOSIS

Diagnosis of testosterone toxicity is based on history of use and a clinical scenario suggestive of androgenic effects.

SIGNS AND SYMPTOMS

Dermatologic

Increased skin oils resulting in furunculosis, folliculitis, and acne may occur.

Cardiovascular

Thrombosis and myocardial infarction have been reported.

Gastrointestinal

Nausea and vomiting occur.

Hepatic

Cholestasis and hepatomas may develop.

Musculoskeletal

Growth arrest in children is secondary to early epiphyseal fusion.

Neurologic

Thrombosis may result in cerebrovascular accident.

Genitourinary

Hypogonadism and aspermia may occur.

Endocrine

- Serum testing will show increased levels of low-density lipoprotein and growth hormone, with decreased levels of high-density lipoprotein, luteinizing hormone, and follicle-stimulating hormone.
- Men experience gynecomastia and impaired spermatogenesis.
- Women report androgenic effects such as alopecia, hirsutism, low-pitched voice, clitoromegaly, amenorrhea, aggressiveness, and diminished breast size.

Psychiatric

- Mania and euphoria are not uncommon.
- Psychotic behavior has been described.
- Depressive withdrawal symptoms may occur after discontinuation of steroid use.

PROCEDURES AND LABORATORY TESTS

Essential Tests

No tests are usually needed in asymptomatic patients, particularly after acute ingestion.

Recommended Tests

- Serum testosterone and epitestosterone levels may be obtained; a ratio greater than 6 to 1, respectively, indicates supplemental testosterone use.
- Liver function tests and cholesterol levels may be useful.
- Cardiac and neurologic evaluation should be instituted in patients with potential myocardial or cerebrovascular ischemia.
- Semen analysis may demonstrate gonadal effect.
- Urine testing can detect exogenous steroid use.

Not Recommended Tests

Isolated steroid levels are generally not useful.

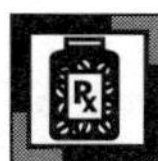

Treatment

Appropriate supportive care should be initiated first, although toxicity from acute ingestion is unlikely.

DIRECTING PATIENT COURSE

The health-care professional should call the poison control center when:

- Severe or persistent effects develop.
- Coingestant, drug interaction, or underlying disease presents an unusual problem.

The patient should be referred to a health-care facility when:

- Suicide or homicide attempt is possible.
- Toxic effects develop.
- Coingestant, drug interaction, or underlying disease presents an unusual problem.

Admission Considerations

Admission to a detoxification facility may be necessary for acute withdrawal. Admission for complications (e.g., myocardial ischemia) is used as appropriate.

DECONTAMINATION

Out of Hospital

Induction of emesis is not recommended due to low toxic potential.

In Hospital

- Gastric lavage (in the setting of oral overdose) should be performed in pediatric (tube size 24–32 French) or adult (tube size 36–42 French) patients presenting within 1 hour of a massive ingestion or if serious effects are present.
- One dose of activated charcoal (1–2 g/kg) should be administered without a cathartic if a substantial ingestion has occurred within the previous few hours.

ANTIDOTES

There is no antidote for testosterone or methyltestosterone.

ADJUNCTIVE TREATMENT

Psychiatric evaluation should be initiated for patients who ingest an overdose amount or manifest behavioral symptoms.

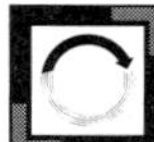

Follow-Up

PATIENT MONITORING

Monitoring is not typically needed for acute ingestion, but may be needed for chronic effects (e.g., infarction or behavioral effects).

EXPECTED COURSE AND PROGNOSIS

Minimal effects with complete recovery is expected after acute ingestion.

DISCHARGE CRITERIA/INSTRUCTIONS

- From the emergency department. Asymptomatic patients may be discharged after decontamination and psychiatric evaluation, if needed.
- From the hospital. Patients may be discharged following resolution of complications.

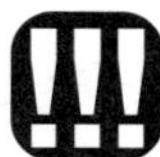

Pitfalls

FOLLOW-UP

- Human immunodeficiency virus testing should be recommended to those abusing injectable steroids.
- Drug abuse counseling is necessary in all identified steroid abusers; inappropriate use should be considered a serious addiction.

ICD-9-CM 962

Poisoning by hormones and synthetic substitutes.

RECOMMENDED READING

Brower KJ. Clinical assessment and treatment of anabolic steroid users. *Psychiatr Ann* 1992;22:31–33.

Pope HG, Katz DL. Psychiatric and medical effects of anabolic-androgenic steroid use. *Arch Gen Psychiatry* 1994;51:375–382.

Author: John P. Marshall

Reviewer: Richard C. Dart

Tetrodotoxin

Basics

DESCRIPTION

Tetrodotoxin is a nonprotein toxin found in several different animal species.

FORMS AND USES

• Animals containing tetrodotoxin include members of the puffer fish order Tetraodontinae (100 species of puffer fish, blowfish, balloonfish, and porcupine fish), newts (*Taricha granulosa*), salamanders (*Tarichatorosa* species), and the blue-ringed octopus (*Hapalochlaena maculosa*).
• The most toxic portions are the liver, viscera, gonads, and skin.

TOXIC DOSE

The toxicity of a particular specimen varies with species, area, and season.

PATHOPHYSIOLOGY

• Tetrodotoxin selectively blocks sodium movement through voltage-gated sodium channels and sodium-potassium pumps.

—Tetrodotoxin produces respiratory depression by its direct effects on the respiratory center in the medulla and by axonal blockade of the nerves innervating the respiratory muscles.
—It also affects the chemoreceptor trigger zone to cause emesis or hyperemesis.

• The toxin is heat stable and water soluble.
• Tolerance does not develop upon repeated exposure to tetrodotoxin.

EPIDEMIOLOGY

• Poisoning is increasingly common due to culinary adventuring.
• Toxic effects following exposure may be severe.
• Death may occur in untreated cases.

CAUSES

• Poisoning is usually accidental, involving improperly prepared puffer fish.
• Many people (especially Japanese) consider the puffer fish a delicacy.
• In Japan, puffer fish dishes (fugu) are prepared by licensed chefs.

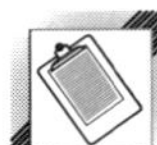

Diagnosis

Diagnosis is based on a history of ingestion and presentation with vomiting, progressive depression of mental status, and respiratory insufficiency.

DIFFERENTIAL DIAGNOSIS

• Toxic causes of nausea and vomiting include other causes of food poisoning (scombroid fish, staphylococcus, *Bacillus cereus*, and many others) and caustic ingestion.
• Nontoxic causes include gastritis, infectious gastroenteritis, bowel obstruction, and increased intracranial pressure.

SIGNS AND SYMPTOMS

• Many cases are mild and are associated with anxiety reaction to the possibility of poisoning.
• Symptoms typically begin within 30 minutes of ingestion; speed of onset is directly related to the quantity of toxin consumed.
• The syndrome may include headache, vomiting, paresthesia, fasciculation, dysphagia, diaphoresis, weakness, and ascending paralysis.
• Death results from respiratory paralysis or cardiovascular collapse.

Vital Signs

• Hypothermia may occur.
• Hypotension, bradycardia, and respiratory arrest may occur up to 24 hours postingestion.

HEENT

Headache, hypersalivation, and peculiar taste sensations are common.

Dermatologic

• Diaphoresis is common.
• Blistering and exfoliative dermatitis have been reported during recovery.

Cardiovascular

Hypotension and cardiac dysrhythmia may develop in serious cases.

Pulmonary

Dyspnea, cyanosis, and acute respiratory failure may occur.

Gastrointestinal

• Nausea, vomiting, and abdominal pain are common.
• Hyperemesis and diarrhea may occur.

Neurologic

• Paresthesia of the lips, tongue, mouth, face, fingers, and toes begins 10 to 45 minutes after ingestion.
• Dysarthria, dysphagia, weakness, and ataxia are common.
• Cranial nerve palsies, fasciculation, pupillary alterations, seizures, loss of deep tendon and spinal reflexes, and progressive ascending paralysis may develop in severe poisoning.

PROCEDURES AND LABORATORY TESTS

Essential Tests

No tests may be needed for asymptomatic patients.

Recommended Tests

• Serum electrolytes, glucose, BUN, creatinine. Acid-base imbalances and dehydration may occur from hyperemesis.
• ECG. Cardiac dysrhythmia may develop, especially if the patient is hypoxic; sinus bradycardia, tachycardia, asystole, and atrioventricular node conduction abnormalities have been reported.
• Arterial blood gases or pulse oximetry. Hypercapnia or hypoxia indicates pulmonary involvement.
• Pulmonary function testing. Depression of forced expiratory volume or negative inspiratory force may indicate pulmonary involvement.

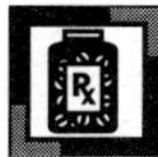

Treatment

• Treatment should focus on supportive care with airway protection.
• Endotracheal intubation should be performed early if respiratory function begins to deteriorate.

DIRECTING PATIENT COURSE

The health-care provider should call the poison control center when:

• Hypotension, cardiac dysrhythmia, respiratory failure, ascending paralysis, or other severe effects are present.
• Signs and symptoms are not consistent with tetrodotoxin poisoning.
• Underlying disease presents an unusual challenge.

The patient should be referred to a health-care facility when:

• Attempted suicide or homicide is possible.
• Patient or caregiver seems unreliable.
• Symptoms develop.
• Underlying disease presents an unusual challenge.

Admission Considerations

Inpatient treatment is warranted when the patient has respiratory, cardiac, or CNS effects, or if mild symptoms or signs of intoxication (e.g., paresthesia) persist more than 4 hours.

DECONTAMINATION

Out of Hospital

Induction of emesis with ipecac is not recommended.

In Hospital

• Ipecac-induced emesis is not recommended.
• Gastric lavage should be performed in pediatric (tube size 24–32 French) or adult (tube size 36–42 French) patients presenting within 1 hour of a large ingestion or if serious effects are present.
• One dose of activated charcoal (1–2 g/kg) should be administered without a cathartic if ingestion has occurred within the previous few hours.

ANTIDOTES

There is no specific antidote available.

ADJUNCTIVE TREATMENT

Hypotension

• The patient should be treated with 10 to 20 ml/kg 0.9% saline intravenously and placed in the Trendelenburg position.
• Further fluid therapy should be guided by central pressure monitoring to avoid volume overload.
• If hypotension does not respond to treatment, a vasopressor is administered.

—Dopamine
 —The dosage for adults or children is 2 to 5 μg/kg/min, titrated to effect.
 —Rates greater than 20 μg/kg/min are unlikely to provide further benefit.

—Norepinephrine may be added if blood pressure is unresponsive.
 —The dosage is 0.1 to 0.2 μg/kg/min, titrated to effect.
 —High rates of infusion may cause tissue ischemia.

Seizures

Seizures may occur and are treated initially with endotracheal intubation and benzodiazepine administration (see SECTION II, Seizures chapter).

Naloxone

• Tetrodotoxin and opioids have similar molecular configurations.
• The use of naloxone has theoretical benefit but has not been tested clinically.

Not Recommended Therapies

Antihistamines, corticosteroids, edrophonium, pyridostigmine, and neostigmine have all been advocated, but are not recommended due to lack of evidence of benefit.

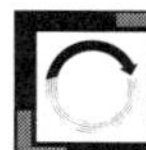

Follow-Up

EXPECTED COURSE AND PROGNOSIS

• Most patients develop minor symptoms and may be discharged after observation.
• Patients who receive treatment before hypoxia occurs recover after a prolonged episode of supportive care.
• Sequelae of hypoxia may occur in patients who do not receive timely medical therapy.

DISCHARGE CRITERIA/INSTRUCTIONS

• From the emergency department. Patients who do not develop toxic effects for 6 hours may be discharged after gastrointestinal decontamination.
• From the hospital. Patients may be discharged after recovery of adequate respiratory function.

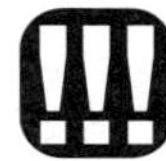

Pitfalls

TREATMENT

Endotracheal intubation is the key to successful therapy in serious cases; it should be performed early in deteriorating patients to prevent aspiration.

ICD-9-CM 989.5

Toxic effect of other substances, chiefly nonmedicinal as to source: venom.

See also: SECTION II, Hypotension and Seizures chapters; and SECTION IV, Food Poisoning—Shellfish chapter.

RECOMMENDED READING

Sims JK, Ostmas DC. Puffer fish poisoning: emergency diagnosis and management of mild human tetrodotoxication. *Ann Emerg Med* 1986;15:1094–1098.

Weisman RS. Marine animals. In: Goldfrank LR, et al., eds. *Goldfrank's toxicologic emergencies,* 6th ed. East Norwalk, CT: Appleton & Lange, 1998.

Author: Netti Riggs

Reviewer: Richard C. Dart

Thallium

Basics

DESCRIPTION

Thallium is a heavy metal.

FORMS AND USES

- Thallium salts (e.g., sulfate or carbonate) are used as pesticides and rodenticides.
- They are no longer available in the United States, but are available in some countries.

TOXIC DOSE

The fatal dose in an adult is approximately 1 g of absorbed thallium.

PATHOPHYSIOLOGY

- Absorption of thallium from dermal, inhalational, and gastrointestinal routes is rapid and almost total.
- Thallium salts are highly toxic.
- Solubility of most thallium salts, except for thallium fluoride, increases with decreasing pH.

EPIDEMIOLOGY

Poisoning is uncommon.

CAUSES

- Toxic ingestion is usually suicidal.
- Child neglect or abuse should be considered if the patient is less than 1 year of age, suicide attempt if the patient is over 6 years of age.

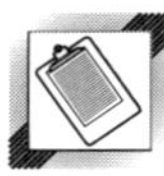

Diagnosis

DIFFERENTIAL DIAGNOSIS

Other toxic causes of painful peripheral neuropathy include chronic arsenic poisoning and selenium poisoning.

SIGNS AND SYMPTOMS

Transient nausea and vomiting are initially seen, followed by alopecia, Mee's lines, and a painful peripheral sensory neuropathy over the next 1 to 2 weeks.

HEENT

Optic neuritis, decreased visual acuity, and impaired color vision can occur.

Dermatologic

Severe acne, Mee's lines, and alopecia may occur.

Cardiovascular

Systemic hypertension, cardiac dysrhythmias, ventricular tachycardia, and bradycardia can occur.

Pulmonary

- Respiratory muscle weakness may occur.
- Respiratory failure or acute respiratory distress syndrome may occur in severe cases.

Gastrointestinal

Symptoms may include salivation, stomatitis, nausea, vomiting (may have green color), diarrhea, hemorrhage, anorexia, severe paroxysmal abdominal pain, and a bloating sensation.

Renal

- Urine may have a green color.
- Proteinuria, hematuria, and renal failure may develop.

Musculoskeletal

Myalgia, muscle weakness/atrophy, ataxia, and choreiform movements can occur.

Neurologic

- Early peripheral and CNS disturbances (e.g., insomnia, paresthesias, myalgias, peripheral burning sensation, headache, cranial nerve palsies, seizures, delirium, coma, painful peripheral neuropathy, and severe pain) may occur.
- Patients with protracted cases may develop dementia, depression, and psychosis.

PROCEDURES AND LABORATORY TESTS

Essential Tests

In asymptomatic patients, thallium concentration in a 24-hour urine collection is needed to document exposure.

Recommended Tests

- Serum electrolytes, BUN, creatinine, glucose, and calcium levels.
- Urinalysis, spot urine, and 24-hour urine collection for thallium are used.
- ECG is used in symptomatic patients to detect dysrhythmias and prolongation of QTc.
- Because thallium is radiopaque, abdominal radiographs may help to guide decontamination.
- Head CT, lumbar puncture, cultures as appropriate for altered mental status.

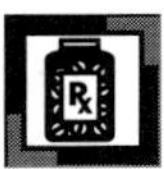

Treatment

- Treatment should focus on supportive care and advanced cardiac life support.
- Dose and time of ingestion should be determined for all substances involved.

DIRECTING PATIENT COURSE

The health-care professional should call the poison control center when:

- Severe or persistent effects develop.
- Coingestant, drug interaction, or underlying disease presents an unusual problem.

The patient should be referred to a health-care facility when:

- Suicide or homicide attempt is possible.
- Toxic effects develop.
- Coingestant, drug interaction, or underlying disease presents an unusual problem.

Admission Considerations

Symptomatic patients should be admitted for evaluation.

DECONTAMINATION

Out of Hospital

- Exposed skin areas should be washed thoroughly.
- Ipecac is unlikely to be needed due to spontaneous vomiting.

In Hospital

- Following acute skin exposure, the patient's clothing should be removed and skin washed copiously with water.
- Emesis or gastric lavage is recommended for recent substantial ingestion, followed by an initial dose of activated charcoal (1–2 g/kg) orally.

ANTIDOTES

There is no specific antidote for thallium poisoning.

ADJUNCTIVE TREATMENT

- Endotracheal intubation and ventilatory support for respiratory failure should be provided.
- Shock related to gastrointestinal hemorrhage may require volume and blood replacement.
- Prussian blue increases thallium excretion and has been used successfully in Europe, but is not commercially available in the United States.
- Potassium chloride loading has been suggested to enhance thallium elimination and may be considered.
- Consultation with a toxicologist or poison center is recommended.
- Hemodialysis has been reported to be useful in the treatment of thallium poisoning.

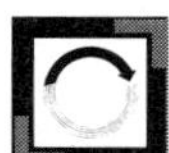

Follow-Up

PATIENT MONITORING

Cardiac, renal, and hepatic function should be monitored as well as 24-hour urine thallium collection.

EXPECTED COURSE AND PROGNOSIS

- Symptoms may be delayed 12 to 24 hours in acute poisoning and peak 1 to 2 weeks after exposure.
- Neurologic damage resolves slowly and may be permanent.
- Paresthesias have occurred as early as 12 to 13 hours after massive ingestion.

DISCHARGE CRITERIA AND INSTRUCTIONS

- From the emergency department. Asymptomatic patients may be discharged after 6 hour observation period, decontamination, a psychiatric evaluation, if needed.
- From the hospital. The patient may be discharged when signs and symptoms are stable.

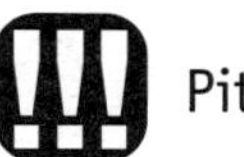

Pitfalls

DIAGNOSIS

History is often key to differentiation from other causes of peripheral neuropathy, but is often difficult to obtain or unreliable.

ICD-9-CM 989.4

Toxic effect of other substances, chiefly nonmedicinal as to source: other pesticides, not elsewhere classified.

See also: SECTION II, Hypotension chapter.

RECOMMENDED READING

Moore D, House I, Dixon A. Thallium poisoning. *BMJ* 1993;306:1527–1529.

Author: Gregory M. Bogdan

Reviewer: Luke Yip

Theophylline

Basics

DESCRIPTION

Theophylline is a methylxanthine derivative medication used in the treatment of asthma and chronic obstructive pulmonary disease.

FORMS AND USES

Pharmaceutical preparations include Accurbron, Aerolate tablets and liquid, Aminophylline, Aquaphyllin, Asmalix, Bronkodyl, Constant-T, Diolor, Duraphyl, Dyphylline, Elixicon, Elixomin, Elixophyllin capsules, solution, and liquid, Lanophyllin, Lufyllin, Marax tablets and syrup (which also contains ephedrine and hydroxyzine), Mudrane (which also contains ephedrine and phenobarbital), Primatene (which also contains ephedrine), Quadrinal (which also contains ephedrine and phenobarbital), Quibron, Quibron 300 (which also contains guaifenesin), Quibron SR (sustained release), Respbid (sustained release), Slo-bid (sustained release), Slo-phyllin (sustained release), Sustaire, Theo-24 (sustained release), Theobid, Theochron, Theoclear, Theoclear LA (sustained release), Theodur (sustained release), Theo-X (sustained release), Theolair liquid and tablets, Theolair SR (sustained release), Theolate, Theophylline, Theospan, Theovent, Uni-Dur (sustained release), and Uniphyl (sustained release).

- Theophylline is used for bronchospasm, asthma, neonatal apnea, and maintenance therapy of chronic obstructive pulmonary disease.
- The adult oral loading dose is 5 mg/kg, and the oral maintenance dose is 300 to 600 mg/day divided every 6 to 8 hours.
- The pediatric oral loading dose is 5 mg/kg; the oral maintenance dosage is 12 to 20 mg/kg/day divided every 4 to 6 hours, up to a maximum of 600 mg/day.

TOXIC DOSE

- Individual patient tolerance to theophylline varies widely.
- An acute ingestion of several times the daily dose will cause nonlethal toxic effects.
- Ingestion of just one or two extra doses per day for several days can be lethal.

PATHOPHYSIOLOGY

- Theophylline antagonizes the activity of adenosine and increases the intracellular concentration of cyclic adenosine monophosphate (cAMP) by increasing cAMP production and decreasing its degradation.
- In an overdose setting, theophylline is associated with elevated levels of epinephrine and norepinephrine; these effects result in smooth muscle relaxation, vasodilation, and cardiac and CNS stimulation.

EPIDEMIOLOGY

- Poisoning is uncommon.
- Toxic effects following exposure are typically mild to moderate after acute overdose and moderate to severe after chronic overdose.
- Death is more likely after chronic overdose and in infants or the elderly.

CAUSES

- Excessive therapeutic dosing is the most common cause of toxicity; serum theophylline levels should be monitored closely when increasing maintenance dose.
- Decreased metabolism leading to increased serum levels may result from drug interactions, alcoholic liver disease, and congestive heart failure.
- Chronic overdose is usually accidental, iatrogenic, or the result of drug interactions.
- Acute overdose is usually a nonaccidental incident in adults and accidental in children.
- Child abuse should be considered if the patient is less than 1 year of age; suicide attempt if the patient is more than 6 years of age.

RISK FACTORS

- Patients over 60 or under 3 years of age are at greatest risk for severe complications (dysrhythmia, seizure) after chronic overdose.
- Hepatic dysfunction may predispose a patient to theophylline intoxication.

DRUG AND DISEASE INTERACTIONS

Many drugs reduce the rate of theophylline metabolism and may cause toxicity: allopurinol, cimetidine, ciprofloxacin, clarithromycin, disulfiram, enoxacin, erythromycin, ethanol, estrogen, idrocilamide, interferon A, methotrexate, mexiletine, norfloxacin, ofloxacin, pefloxacin, pentoxifylline, pipenidic acid, propafenone, propranolol, tacrine, thiabendazole, ticlopidine, troleandomycin, and verapamil.

PREGNANCY AND LACTATION

US FDA Pregnancy Category C. The drug exerts animal teratogenic or embryocidal effects, but there are no controlled studies in women, or no studies are available in either animals or women.

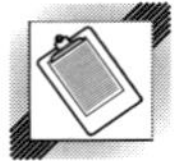

Diagnosis

DIFFERENTIAL DIAGNOSIS

- Other toxic causes of tachycardia and agitation include sympathomimetic drugs (caffeine, cocaine, amphetamines, ephedrine, and phenylpropanolamine, among others), lithium, monoamine oxidase inhibitors, or serotonin syndrome.
- Other causes include nondrug causes of sympathomimetic excess (withdrawal from alcohol or sedative-hypnotic agents, pheochromocytoma, psychiatric disease, hyperthyroidism).

SIGNS AND SYMPTOMS

Acute Overdose

- Nausea, vomiting, agitation, tremors, abdominal pain, mild metabolic acidosis, hypokalemia, hyperglycemia, and tachycardia are all common.
- Severe effects such as dysrhythmia and seizure are usually associated with serum theophylline levels greater than 100 μg/ml.

Chronic Overdose

- Gastrointestinal effects do not characterize the clinical presentation as with acute overdose.
- Agitation, tremor, and severe effects such as dysrhythmias and seizures may occur at moderately elevated serum levels (35–40 μg/ml), most often in patients over 60 or less than 3 years of age.

Vital Signs

- Tachycardia, tachypnea, and hypertension are common as toxicity begins.
- Hypotension develops if cardiovascular effects are severe.

Cardiovascular

- Sinus tachycardia is common.
- Other dysrhythmias include supraventricular tachycardia, multifocal atrial tachycardia, atrial fibrillation, and premature ventricular contractions.
- Ventricular tachycardia and ventricular fibrillation may occur, most often with chronic overdose or in acute overdose with levels exceeding 100 μg/ml.

Gastrointestinal

- Nausea, vomiting, and abdominal pain are common and often persistent with acute overdose.
- Bezoar may form with sustained-release formulations.

Hematologic

Leukocytosis is common.

Fluids and Electrolytes

- Hypokalemia is common with acute overdose.
- Hypomagnesemia and hypophosphatemia also may occur.
- Mild metabolic acidosis is common with acute overdose.
- Severe metabolic acidosis may occur with hypotension or seizures.

Musculoskeletal

- Rhabdomyolysis may occur with prolonged seizures.
- Compartment syndrome occurs rarely, usually after prolonged seizures.

Neurologic

- Tremor, agitation, and nervousness are common.
- Seizures may occur, most often with chronic overdose or in acute overdose with levels exceeding 100 μg/ml.

Genitourinary

Acute renal failure may occur in the rare patient who develops rhabdomyolysis.

Endocrine

Hyperglycemia is common with acute overdose.

PROCEDURES AND LABORATORY TESTS

Essential Tests

Serial serum theophylline levels should be repeated every 2 hours until levels decrease and patient is clinically improved; therapeutic level is 10 to 20 μg/ml for both adults and children.

- Acute ingestion

—The level should be repeated to ensure it is not increasing.
—An increasing serum theophylline level implies continued absorption (inadequate decontamination, sustained-release formulation, bezoar formation) and increased risk for severe toxicity.

- Chronic ingestion

—At a given theophylline level, chronic patients are at greater risk for toxicity than patients with acute ingestion.
—Severe dysrhythmia or seizures may occur at theophylline levels of 35 to 40 μg/ml.

ECG

- Sinus tachycardia is common.
- Various atrial or ventricular dysrhythmias may develop and are more common with chronic toxicity than with acute exposure.

Serum Electrolytes

Mild metabolic acidosis and hypokalemia are consistent with acute overdose.

Recommended Tests

- Arterial blood gases

—Mild, compensated metabolic acidosis is consistent with acute toxicity.
—Severe metabolic acidosis or acidemia should prompt search for another cause (unless hypotension or seizure have complicated course).

- BUN and creatinine. Renal insufficiency may develop following severe poisoning.
- Serum creatine kinase is measured in patients with prolonged seizure to detect rhabdomyolysis due to seizures or compartment syndrome.
- Serum acetaminophen and aspirin levels are measured in an overdose setting to detect occult overdose.
- Abdominal radiography may show sustained-release tablets.
- Endoscopy or upper gastrointestinal series should be considered to rule out bezoar formation in patients with persistently increasing levels despite gastrointestinal decontamination and administration of activated charcoal.
- Intracompartmental pressure should be determined if compartment syndrome is suspected clinically.

Treatment

- Treatment focuses on prevention of gastrointestinal absorption, support of hemodynamic function, and enhancement of theophylline elimination.
- Aggressive use of antiemetics may be needed for protracted vomiting.
- Dose and time of exposure should be determined for all substances involved.

DIRECTING PATIENT COURSE

The health-care provider should call the poison control center when:

- Hemodialysis is being considered.
- Seizure, hypotension, or serious dysrhythmia are present.
- Signs and symptoms are not consistent with theophylline poisoning.
- Coingestant, drug interaction, or underlying disease presents an unusual challenge.

A patient should be referred to a health-care facility when:

- The provider suspects chronic toxicity.
- A person not chronically taking theophylline may have ingested more than 10 mg/kg.
- Attempted suicide or homicide is possible.
- Patient or caregiver seems unreliable.
- Symptoms develop.
- Coingestant, drug interaction, or underlying disease presents an unusual challenge.

Admission Considerations

ICU management is needed for:

- Chronic intoxication and serum theophylline levels above 25 to 30 μg/ml or persistent signs and symptoms of intoxication.
- Acute intoxication with persistent signs or symptoms (intractable vomiting, tachycardia, dysrhythmia, seizures, agitation) or increasing levels.
- Acute ingestion of a sustained-release product.

Theophylline

DECONTAMINATION

Out of Hospital

Ipecac is not recommended because of the risk of seizures.

In Hospital

- Ipecac is not recommended.
- Gastric lavage should be performed in pediatric (tube size 24–32 French) or adult (tube size 36–42 French) patients presenting within 1 hour of a large ingestion or if serious effects are present.
- One dose of activated charcoal (1–2 g/kg) should be administered without a cathartic if a substantial ingestion has occurred within the previous few hours.
- Whole-bowel irrigation with polyethylene glycol solution (Golytely, Colyte) has been recommended in patients who have ingested sustained-release preparations or in patients with increasing levels despite standard decontamination.

—Studies of efficacy are lacking.
—Usual dose is 1 to 2 L/h in adults until rectal effluent is clear.

ANTIDOTES

There is no specific antidote for theophylline poisoning.

ADJUNCTIVE TREATMENT

- Seizures should be controlled with benzodiazepines and phenobarbital.
- Hypotension should be treated with isotonic intravenous fluids and vasopressors if needed; α-adrenergic drugs (phenylephrine, norepinephrine) are theoretically preferred because theophylline causes excessive β-adrenergic receptor stimulation.
- Hypokalemia is common and electrolytes should be replaced as needed.
- Persistent vomiting

—Suggested antiemetic adult regimens include the intravenous administration of metoclopramide 0.5 to 1.0 mg/kg plus diphenhydramine 25 to 50 mg combined with prochlorperazine 10 mg or droperidol 2.5 mg.
—Ondansetron, 8 mg intravenously infused over 15 minutes, is an alternative.

- Tachydysrhythmias are often resistant to therapy because the initiating stimulus (theophylline) cannot be removed quickly. Therefore, hemodialysis is the procedure of choice. However, if the heart rate compromises the blood pressure before dialysis can be performed, esmolol administration is a temporizing measure.

—Intravenous bolus of 500 μg/kg is infused over 1 minute followed by an infusion of 50 μg/kg/min for 4 minutes.
—If response is inadequate, the loading dose is repeated and infused at 100 μg/kg/min for 4 minutes.
—This titration is repeated as needed until the heart rate is controlled or toxicity (hypotension) develops.
—β-receptor blockers may precipitate bronchospasm in susceptible patients; esmolol should be discontinued immediately if bronchospasm occurs.
—Unopposed α-receptor stimulation is a theoretical concern during β-blockade; if blood pressure increases dangerously during infusion, α-receptor stimulation may be the cause.

- Multiple-dose activated charcoal increases theophylline clearance but has not been shown to alter outcome.

—A typical treatment regimen is 25 to 50 g (0.5–1.0 g/kg) of activated charcoal orally every 2 to 4 hours.
—A cathartic can be administered with the first dose.
—The treatment is recommended for:
  —Mild to moderate effects after acute overdose and serum theophylline levels below 80 to 100 μg/ml
  —Patients with chronic overdose with mild to moderate effects and levels less than 40 to 60 μg/ml and age between 3 and 60 years

—The treatment should be discontinued if ileus or obstruction develop, if the patient is not passing charcoal stools, or when level falls below 30 μg/ml.

- Hemodialysis substantially increases clearance.

—It is indicated for acute ingestion when:
  —Clinically significant dysrhythmias, seizures, or hypotension occur.
  —Theophylline level is greater than 80 to 100 μg/ml, especially if increasing.
  —Patients have taken an acute overdose and have a level greater than 60 μg/ml that is rising despite multiple-dose activated charcoal.

—It is indicated for treatment of chronic intoxication when:
  —Theophylline level is greater than 40 to 60 μg/ml and age is greater than 60 years or less than 3 years.
  —Significant underlying disease is present (especially cardiovascular, alcoholic liver disease, severe congestive heart failure) that might predispose to complications or reduce theophylline clearance.
  —Serum theophylline level is not rapidly falling with multiple-dose activated charcoal.

- Hemoperfusion also substantially increases theophylline clearance, but it is not widely available and frequently produces thrombocytopenia; its indications are similar to those for hemodialysis.

Not Recommended Therapies

Long-acting β-blocking agents are not recommended.

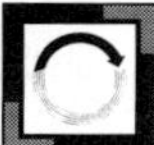

Follow-Up

PATIENT MONITORING

- Serial serum theophylline levels should be monitored every 2 to 4 hours until levels are falling and patient improves clinically.
- An ECG should be obtained and continuous cardiac monitoring instituted.
- Serum electrolytes should be monitored daily, more often during acute illness as indicated.

EXPECTED COURSE AND PROGNOSIS

- Acute intoxication

—Patients generally do well with adequate gastrointestinal decontamination and multiple-dose activated charcoal.
—Effects usually peak in the first 12 hours and then abate.
—Toxicity may be delayed or prolonged after ingestion of sustained-release products.

- Chronic intoxication

—There is a greater risk of complications and death than with acute intoxication, particularly for patients over 60 or under 3 years of age and those with significant underlying disease.
—Aggressive management with early hemodialysis may improve the outcome in these patients.

- Possible complications include neurologic impairment from intractable seizures, dysrhythmia, or hypotension.
- Obstruction, ileus, and constipation from multiple-dose activated charcoal may be life threatening.
- Myocardial ischemia may result from increased oxygen demand.

DISCHARGE CRITERIA/INSTRUCTIONS

From the Emergency Department

Patients may be discharged when:

- Serum levels fall below 25 μg/ml.
- Signs of toxicity are improved.
- Psychiatric evaluation, if needed, has been completed.

All medications should be reviewed before discharge to avoid recurrent drug interactions.

From the Hospital

Patients may be discharged when:

- Serum levels fall below 25 μg/ml.
- Signs of toxicity are improved.
- Patient is passing activated charcoal.
- Psychiatric evaluation, if needed, has been completed.

All medications should be reviewed before discharge to avoid recurrent drug interactions.

PATIENT EDUCATION

Patients should be educated about potential drug interactions and the dangers of increasing dose without monitoring serum levels.

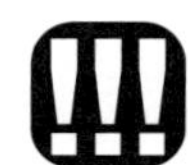

Pitfalls

DIAGNOSIS

- Signs and symptoms may be mild in patients with chronic overdose until severe effects develop suddenly (seizures, dysrhythmias).
- Sustained-release preparations may cause a delayed increase in serum levels (6–8 hours or more after acute ingestion).
- Over-the-counter preparations (e.g., Primatene) may contain theophylline.
- Abdominal radiography without apparent opaque pills cannot exclude the presence of theophylline in the gastrointestinal tract.

TREATMENT

- The health-care provider should avoid prescribing drugs that interfere with theophylline metabolism.
- Hemodialysis should be considered in any patient who has chronic intoxication and a level greater than 40 to 60 μg/ml and who is less than 3 or greater than 60 years of age or has significant underlying medical (particularly cardiac) conditions, because severe toxicity may develop abruptly and is associated with a poorer outcome.

ICD-9-CM 975.7

Poisoning by agents primarily acting on the smooth and skeletal muscles and respiratory system.

See also: SECTION II, Hypotension, Tachycardia and Seizures chapters; and SECTION III, Aminophylline and Activated Charcoal chapters.

RECOMMENDED READING

Shannon M. Predictors of major toxicity after theophylline overdose. *Ann Intern Med* 1993;119:1161–1167.

Shannon M, Lovejoy FH. The influence of age vs peak serum concentration on life-threatening events after chronic theophylline intoxication. *Arch Intern Med* 1990;150:2045–2048.

Shannon M, Lovejoy FH. Effect of acute vs chronic intoxication on clinical features of theophylline poisoning in children. *J Pediatr* 1992;121:125–130.

Author: Katherine M. Hurlbut

Reviewer: Richard C. Dart

Thioridazine

Basics

DESCRIPTION

Preparations include thioridazine (Mellaril) and mesoridazine (metabolite of thioridazine).

FORMS AND USES

- Used in the treatment of psychiatric disorders.
- The adult dosage is 150 to 300 mg/day, up to 800 mg/day orally; the pediatric dosage is 0.5 to 3 mg/kg/day orally.

TOXIC DOSE

Ingestion of a few grams by an adult can be lethal.

PATHOPHYSIOLOGY

- Thioridazine and mesoridazine have anticholinergic, α-adrenergic-blocking, sodium channel-blocking, and extrapyramidal effects.
- They block dopamine D_2 receptors and disrupt neurotransmission in the nigrostrial, mesolimbic, and mesocortical dopaminergic pathways, hypothalamic dopamine neurons, and peripheral dopaminergic areas.

EPIDEMIOLOGY

- Poisoning is uncommon.
- Toxic effects following exposure are typically mild.
- Death may occur in patients who have ingested large quantities and have intractable dysrhythmias.
- Elderly patients may be more at risk than younger patients for hypotension and dysrhythmias.

CAUSES

- Ingestion is usually suicidal.
- Child neglect should be considered if the patient is younger than 1 year of age; attempted suicide if the patient is over 6 years of age.

DRUG AND DISEASE INTERACTIONS

- Liver disease may result in drug accumulation from therapeutic doses.
- Patients with electrolyte abnormalities (hypomagnesemia, hypocalcemia), prolonged QT syndrome, or other underlying cardiac disorder are at a greater risk for dysrhythmia.

PREGNANCY AND LACTATION

US FDA Pregnancy Category C. The drug exerts animal teratogenic or embryocidal effects, but there are no controlled studies in women, or no studies are available in either animals or women.

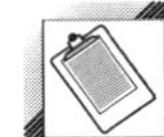

Diagnosis

DIFFERENTIAL DIAGNOSIS

- Toxic causes of ventricular dysrhythmias include type 1 antidysrhythmics, other phenothiazines, tricyclic antidepressants, antihistamines, cocaine, β-receptor or calcium channel blocker, quinine, digoxin, phenothiazine, nticholinergics, amiodarone, sotalol, and procainamide.
- Nontoxic causes include CNS bleed, mass or infection, congenital prolonged QT syndrome, hypomagnesemia, hypocalcemia, hypokalemia, and dysrhythmias secondary to ischemia.

SIGNS AND SYMPTOMS

- CNS depression is common.
- Seizures and cardiac dysrhythmias may develop in a large overdose.

Vital Signs

Fever and hypotension may occur.

HEENT

- Mydriasis is common.
- Pigmentary retinopathy may occur with chronic use, particularly with doses higher than 800 mg/day.

Cardiovascular

- QT prolongation, hypotension, ventricular dysrhythmia, torsade de pointes, and conduction blocks may occur after an overdose.
- The onset of dysrhythmias may be delayed up to 10 hours.

Pulmonary

Pulmonary edema has been reported after an overdose.

Gastrointestinal

Constipation and ileus are common.

Hepatic

Cholestatic jaundice or mixed cholestatic and hepatocellular jaundice may occur after an overdose or with therapeutic use.

Renal

Urinary retention may occur.

Hematologic

Leukopenia and agranulocytosis are rare adverse effects of therapeutic use.

Musculoskeletal

Rhabdomyolysis may occur in poisoning complicated by seizures.

Neurologic

- Agitation, CNS depression, coma, seizures, extrapyramidal symptoms, and tardive dyskinesia (acute overdose or chronic use) occur.
- Neuroleptic malignant syndrome (NMS) is a rare complication.

PROCEDURES AND LABORATORY TESTS

Essential Tests

ECG and continuous monitoring to detect prolongation of QTc, conduction block, or ventricular dysrhythmia.

Recommended Tests

- Serum acetaminophen and aspirin levels in an overdose setting can detect occult ingestion.
- Serum electrolytes, including calcium and magnesium, in patients with ECG abnormalities can assess their contributions to dysrhythmia.
- Other tests (lumbar puncture, toxicology screen) as needed can rule out other causes of altered mental status.
- Head CT as needed is used to evaluate other causes of coma and seizures.

Not Recommended Tests

Serum levels of thioridazine/mesoridazine are not clinically useful after overdose.

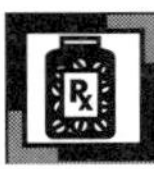

Treatment

- Treatment should focus on airway management, blood pressure support, and treatment of dysrhythmia.
- The dose and time of exposure should be determined for all the substances involved.

DIRECTING PATIENT COURSE

The health-care provider should call the poison control center when:

- Coma, QT prolongation, ventricular dysrhythmias, seizure, hyperthermia, or other severe effects are present.
- Toxic effects are not consistent with thioridazine/mesoridazine poisoning.
- Coingestant, drug interaction, or underlying disease presents an unusual problem.

The patient should be referred to a health-care facility when:

- Attempted suicide or homicide is possible.
- Patient or caregiver seems unreliable.
- Any toxic effects are present.
- Coingestant, drug interaction, or underlying disease presents an unusual problem.

Admission Considerations

Inpatient treatment is warranted for patients with CNS depression, hypotension, seizure, hyperthermia, prolonged QTc, and dysrhythmias, and for those who have ingested a sustained-release product.

DECONTAMINATION

Out of Hospital

Emesis should not be induced because a coma or seizures may develop abruptly.

In Hospital

- Gastric lavage should be performed in pediatric (tube size 24–32 French) or adult (tube size 36–42 French) patients presenting within 1 hour of a large ingestion or if serious effects are present.
- One dose of activated charcoal (1–2 g/kg) should be administered without a cathartic if a substantial ingestion has occurred within the previous few hours.

ANTIDOTES

There are no antidotes for thioridazine/mesoridazine poisoning.

ADJUNCTIVE TREATMENT

Seizures

A benzodiazepine should be administered for initial control, monitoring the airway closely.

- Diazepam. Adult dose is 5 to 10 mg initially, repeated every 10 minutes if needed; pediatric dose is 0.2 to 0.5 mg/kg every 10 minutes as needed.
- Lorazepam. Adult dose is 2 to 4 mg intravenous push over 2 to 5 minutes, repeated every 10 minutes as needed; pediatric dose is 0.1 mg/kg intravenous push over 2 to 5 minutes, not to exceed 4 mg/dose; may be repeated every 10 minutes as needed.
- If seizures persist or recur, another anticonvulsant (e.g., phenobarbital or phenytoin) can be added.

Hypotension

- The patient should be given 10 to 20 ml/kg 0.9% NaCl and placed in the Trendelenburg position; further fluid therapy should be guided by central pressure monitoring to avoid a volume overload.
- If the hypotension is unresponsive, a vasopressor should be administered.

—Dopamine. Adult dosage is 2 to 5 μg/kg/min, titrated to effect (rates above 20 μg/kg/min are unlikely to provide further benefit).
—Norepinephrine. Adult dosage is 0.1 to 0.2 μg/kg/min, titrated to effect.
—A high rate of infusion may cause tissue ischemia.

Dysrhythmia or Conduction Abnormality

- It is important to control seizures and correct acidemia.
- If QRS widening or dysrhythmias persist, $NaHCO_3$ should be administered in a 1 to 2 mEq/kg intravenous bolus and repeat as needed to maintain an arterial pH of 7.45 to 7.55.
- Lidocaine may be used for ventricular tachycardia or multifocal premature ventricular contractions.

—Adult dose is 50 to 100 mg intravenous bolus followed by an infusion of 2 to 4 mg/min, titrated to effect.
—Pediatric dose is 1 mg/kg bolus followed by an infusion of 20 to 50 μg/kg/min, titrated to effect.
—The bolus dose may be repeated in 10 to 15 minutes.

- Cardiac pacing may be required for an atrioventricular block.
- Ventricular dysrhythmias also may be treated with magnesium, overdrive pacing, or cardioversion (see SECTION II, Ventricular Dysrhythmias chapter).

Other Disorders

- For extrapyramidal symptoms, diphenhydramine is administered at 0.5 to 1.0 mg/kg/dose intravenously over 1 to 2 minutes, or benztropine at 1 to 2 mg intravenously. Maintenance for 1 to 2 days of diphenhydramine or benztropine for continuing symptoms is recommended.
- For NMS, the primary treatment is aggressive supportive care.

Not Recommended Therapies

Forced diuresis, hemodialysis, and hemoperfusion are not helpful.

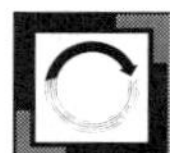

Follow-Up

PATIENT MONITORING

- Continuous respiratory and cardiac monitoring and serial ECG should be performed.
- Fluid and electrolytes, liver and renal function, and clinical indicators of toxicity should be followed.

EXPECTED COURSE AND PROGNOSIS

- Most patients recover with supportive care.
- Rarely, patients sustain hypoxic brain injury from prolonged dysrhythmias.

DISCHARGE CRITERIA/INSTRUCTIONS

- From the emergency department. Patients may be discharged after gastrointestinal decontamination if they are asymptomatic after ingestion of a non-sustained-release product, with normal ECG and vital signs after 6 to 8 hours of observation, and after psychiatric evaluation, if needed.
- From the hospital. Patients may be discharged when their mental status has returned to baseline, their hypotension has resolved, and their ECG has been normal for 24 hours.

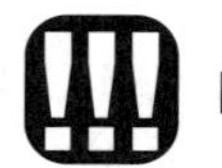

Pitfalls

DIAGNOSIS

Extended-release products may require extended observation and treatment.

TREATMENT

Incomplete decontamination may result in prolonged symptoms or delayed deterioration.

FOLLOW-UP

Inadequate observation time may result in missing late complications of extrapyramidal symptoms or NMS.

ICD-9-CM 969.1

Poisoning by phenothiazine-based tranquilizers.

See also: SECTION II, Hypotension, Ventricular Dysrhythmias, Neuroleptic Malignant Syndrome and Serotonin Syndrome, and Seizures chapters.

RECOMMENDED READING

Blaye IL, Donatini B, Hall M, et al. Acute overdosage with thioridazine: a review of the available clinical literature. *Vet Hum Toxicol* 1993;35:147–150.

Burda CD. Electrocardiographic abnormalities induced by thioridazine (Mellaril). *Am Heart J* 1968;76:153–156.

Author: Katherine M. Hurlbut

Reviewer: Richard C. Dart

Thyroid Products

Basics

DESCRIPTION

- Thyroid products are medications used to replace thyroid hormone.
- Substances include thyroxine (T_4) (Levothyroxine, Levothroid, Synthroid), Liothyronine (T_3) (Cytomel), desiccated thyroid (Thyroid USP), T_3/T_4 combination (Euthroid, Thyrolar), thyroglobulin (Proloid), and Liotrix (Thyrolar, Euthroid).

FORMS AND USES

The typical adult starting dosage for the treatment of hypothyroidism is:

- Thyroxin, 50 μg/day
- Desiccated thyroid, 30 mg/day
- Liothyronine, 25 μg/day
- Liotrix, 1 tablet/day
- Thyroglobulin, 32 to 130 mg/day
- Levothyroxin, 0.05 to 0.2 mg/day

TOXIC DOSE

- One-time ingestion of several milligrams of levothyroxine or 350 mg of desiccated thyroid may cause symptoms in adults.
- Children have developed symptoms after 1.5 mg of levothyroxine or 600 mg of desiccated thyroid.
- Repeated ingestion over several days is usually required to produce serious toxicity.

PATHOPHYSIOLOGY

- Thyroid hormone interacts with growth hormone, accelerates cellular oxidation, increases energy expenditure, and leads to increased heat production and oxygen consumption.
- Thyroid hormone potentiates the effects of catecholamines.
- T_4 and T_3 are both metabolically active; T_3 is three to five times more active than T_4.
- Multiple mechanisms function to maintain a relatively euthyroid status despite the presence of elevated serum thyroid hormone levels; this may prevent acute toxicity from developing after thyroid hormone overdose.

EPIDEMIOLOGY

- Poisoning is rare.
- Toxic effects following exposure are typically mild, with death occurring only with long-term chronic ingestion.

CAUSES

- Poisoning is usually the result of accidental ingestion.
- Child neglect or abuse should be considered if the patient is less than 1 year of age; suicide attempt should be considered if the patient is more than 6 years of age.

RISK FACTORS

Elderly patients are more susceptible to toxicity, especially if underlying cardiovascular disease is present.

DRUG AND DISEASE INTERACTIONS

- Cholestyramine binds thyroid hormone in the intestine and reduces thyroid hormone absorption.
- Phenytoin may decrease serum T_4 levels.
- All forms increase the effect of oral anticoagulants.
- Pregnancy causes decreased T_4 elimination because of increased thyroid-binding globulin production; thus, thyroid gland activity is increased.

PREGNANCY AND LACTATION

- US FDA Pregnancy Category A. Controlled studies in women fail to demonstrate a risk to the fetus in the first trimester, and the possibility of fetal harm appears remote.
- Mild hyperthyroidism has little effect on the course of pregnancy; severe and uncontrolled thyrotoxicosis is complicated by an increased frequency of abortion, premature labor, and toxemia of pregnancy.
- Infants may be born with a transient, neonatal hyperthyroidism (weight loss, hyperkinesis, tachycardia, and diarrhea), which regresses within 3 to 4 weeks of birth.

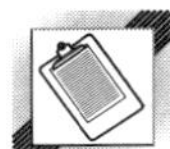

Diagnosis

DIFFERENTIAL DIAGNOSIS

- Toxic causes of tachycardia, tachypnea, and nervousness include numerous compounds: anticholinergics, caffeine or theophylline, disulfiram reaction, inorganic mercury, monoamine oxidase inhibitors, neuroleptic malignant syndrome, salicylate, serotonin syndrome, and sympathomimetic drugs, among others.
- Nontoxic causes include endogenous thyrotoxicosis, hypoglycemia, and adrenergic storm from any cause.

SIGNS AND SYMPTOMS

Primary symptoms are anxiousness, tachycardia, and tremor.

Vital Signs

Hypertension, tachycardia, tachypnea, and fever can occur.

HEENT

Mydriasis may occur.

Dermatologic

Diaphoresis and flushed, moist skin may be observed.

Cardiovascular

Tachycardia, palpitations, dysrhythmia (usually supraventricular tachycardia), hypertension or hypotension, angina, congestive heart failure, and, rarely, cardiovascular collapse may occur.

Gastrointestinal

Vomiting, diarrhea, abdominal pain, and increased appetite may occur.

Fluids and Electrolytes

Dehydration may develop.

Musculoskeletal

Weakness is common, and rhabdomyolysis may develop in severe cases.

Neurologic

Anxiety, intolerance to heat or cold, restlessness, insomnia, apprehension, headache, confusion, agitation, tremor, psychosis, seizures, and coma may be observed.

PROCEDURES AND LABORATORY TESTS

Essential Tests

No tests may be needed in minimally symptomatic patients.

Recommended Tests

- Elevated T_4 and T_3 levels help confirm ingestion of thyroid preparations, if rapidly available.
- Markedly elevated T_4 level may be helpful in identifying those patients requiring close follow-up over the next 1 to 2 weeks.
- Thyroglobulin level is suppressed during exogenous thyrotoxicosis.
- Serum electrolytes, BUN, creatinine, and glucose levels evaluate other causes of fever, tachycardia, and altered mental status.
- Liver function tests, coagulation studies, and serum creatine kinase may be elevated in patients with hyperthermia or severe agitation.
- ECG and serum acetaminophen and aspirin levels in an overdose setting are used to detect occult ingestion.
- Head CT, lumbar puncture, and toxicology studies are used as needed to evaluate other causes of altered mental status.

Not Recommended Tests

T_4 and T_3 levels are of minimal value in determining prognosis or treatment if not available within 48 hours.

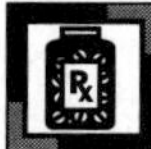

Treatment

- Treatment should focus on gastric decontamination, evaluation of coingestions, and follow-up of initially asymptomatic patients.
- In symptomatic patients, discontinuation of exposure and general supportive care are usually appropriate therapy due to the self-limited and benign course.
- Dose and time of exposure should be determined for all substances involved.

DIRECTING PATIENT COURSE

The health-care provider should call the poison control center when:

- Marked tachycardia, hypotension, or other severe effects are present.
- Toxic effects are not consistent with thyroid hormone poisoning.
- Coingestant, drug interaction, or underlying disease presents an unusual problem.

The patient should be referred to a health-care facility when:

- Attempted suicide or homicide is possible.
- Patient or caregiver seems unreliable.
- Toxic effects are present.
- Coingestant, drug interaction, or underlying disease presents an unusual problem.

Admission Considerations

Inpatient management is warranted for patients with:

- Moderate to severe toxicity.
- Underlying cardiopulmonary disease.
- Advanced age, with an ingestion of more than 100 μg/kg T_4 or 30 μg/kg T_3.
- Serum T_4 concentration greater than 50 μg/dl or T_3 level higher than 350 ng/ml.
- Evidence of massive ingestion.

DECONTAMINATION

Out of Hospital

Emesis should be induced with ipecac within 1 hour of an acute ingestion for alert pediatric or adult patients if health-care evaluation will be delayed.

In Hospital

- Ipecac is not recommended in adults.
- Ipecac-induced emesis may be administered within 1 hour of acute ingestion for the pediatric patient who is too small to have effective gastric lavage.
- Gastric lavage should be performed in pediatric (tube size 24–32 French) or adult (tube size 36–42 French) patients presenting within 1 hour of a large ingestion or if serious effects are present.
- One dose of activated charcoal (1–2 g/kg) should be administered without a cathartic if a substantial ingestion has occurred within the previous few hours.

ANTIDOTES

There is no specific antidote for thyroid hormone toxicity.

ADJUNCTIVE TREATMENT

- Cholestyramine increases elimination of thyroid hormones. The adult dose is 4 g orally four times a day to symptomatic patients until toxic effects resolve. The dose for children 6 to 12 years of age is 80 mg/kg three times a day.
- Hyperthermia is treated using standard measures; dantrolene has been used with success in thyrotoxicosis.
- Propranolol is used to treat tachycardia, systolic hypertension, and tremulousness.

—Adult dose is 10 to 40 mg orally every 4 to 6 hours or 1 mg intravenously every 5 minutes until response or total of 5 mg has been administered.
—Pediatric oral dose is 0.5 to 1.0 mg/kg every 6 hours; the intravenous dose is 0.01 to 0.1 mg/kg over 10 minutes up to a total dose of 1 mg.
—Esmolol has been used for severe cases to achieve more rapid control.

- Sodium ipodate (Oragrafin) may be indicated. It inhibits peripheral conversion of T_4 to T_3 by shunting the conversion of T_4 to rT_3; onset of action is 6 hours with a duration of action of 36 to 48 hours. Oral dose is 1 g/kg, and it may be repeated for recurrence of symptoms.
- Propylthiouracil (PTU) inhibits T_4 to T_3 conversion.

—Adult dose is 333 mg every 8 hours for 5 to 7 days.
—Pediatric dose is 2 to 3 mg/kg every 8 hours.

- Plasmapheresis increases T_4 elimination 30 fold.
- Hemoperfusion increases T_4 elimination 5 fold.

Not Recommended Therapies

Prophylactic treatment with propranolol, propylthiouracil, corticosteroids, or extracorporeal detoxification may be instituted in the early asymptomatic phase.

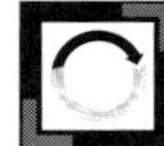

Follow-Up

PATIENT MONITORING

- Patients with signs of thyroid storm should have continuous respiratory and cardiac monitoring.
- Asymptomatic patients do not require cardiac monitoring (unless a coingestion is suspected), but may require serial clinical evaluation for symptoms over the following 1 to 2 weeks.

EXPECTED COURSE AND PROGNOSIS

- Patients may not develop symptoms for several days after a single acute ingestion.
- If severe toxicity develops, resolution with supportive care usually requires several days.
- Thyroid toxicity may cause sequelae of thyroid storm such as end-organ damage from hyperthyroidism.

DISCHARGE CRITERIA/INSTRUCTIONS

- From the emergency department

—Asymptomatic patients may be discharged following gastrointestinal decontamination and psychiatric evaluation, if needed.
—Clinical monitoring for signs of hyperthyroidism must be arranged for 7 to 10 days.

- From the hospital. Patients may be discharged when symptoms have resolved and the serum T_3 has dropped below 350 to 400 ng/ml.

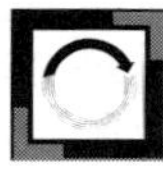

Follow-Up

PATIENT MONITORING

Patients should be followed closely for symptoms of toxicity and treated aggressively if symptoms develop.

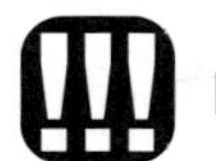

Pitfalls

DIAGNOSIS

- Clinical effects of T_4 ingestion often do not occur until approximately 4 days after ingestion.
- If the thyroid preparation is pure T_3 or a mixture of T_4 and T_3, clinical symptoms may occur within 24 hours after ingestion; mixtures of T_4 and T_3 have both immediate and delayed clinical effects.
- In contrast to a single acute ingestion, the chronic ingestion of supratherapeutic doses of T_4 can cause serious injury, which is usually evident at presentation.

ICD-9-CM 962.7

Poisoning by hormones and synthetic substitutes: thyroid and thyroid derivatives.

RECOMMENDED READING

Lewander WJ, Lacouture PG, Silva JE, et al. Acute thyroxine ingestion in pediatric patients. *Pediatr* 1989;84:262–265.

Mohamed Shakir KM, Ladenson PW. Thyroid. In: Haddad LM, Shannon MW, Winchester JF, eds. *Clinical management of poisoning and drug overdose,* 3rd ed. Philadelphia: WB Saunders, 1998:1133–1142.

Author: Luke Yip

Reviewer: Richard C. Dart

Tick Paralysis

Basics

DESCRIPTION

Tick paralysis involves progressive weakness leading to generalized paralysis.

- Ticks in the United States that cause tick paralysis include:

—Pacific Northwest. *Dermacentor andersoni* (wood tick).
—Southeast. *D. variabilis* (dog tick), *Amblyomma americanum* (lone star tick), *A. maculatum* (Gulf Coast tick), and *Ixodes scapularis* (black-legged deer tick).

- Outside the United States, ticks causing paralysis may be found in:

—Crete. *Hyalomma truncata* and *I. ricinus*.
—Australia. *I. cornatus, I. holocyclus*, and *I. hirsti*.
—South Africa. *Rhinicephalus simus* and *R. evertsi*.

PATHOPHYSIOLOGY

- Adult female ticks bite painlessly to feed on blood.
- A neurotoxin is secreted from an attached and engorging pregnant female tick's salivary glands.
- The mechanism of neurotoxin effect is unclear; the toxin may interfere with the release of acetylcholine at the neuromuscular junction and slow motor conduction.

TOXIC DOSE

One tick is sufficient to produce toxicity; however, it must remain attached and feed for several days before symptoms develop.

EPIDEMIOLOGY

- Poisoning is rare.
- Toxic effects following exposure are typically mild to moderate, with death occurring rarely.
- Most cases in the United States occur in the Northwest and Southeast during the spring and summer months.

CAUSES

Poisoning usually occurs via an accidental environmental encounter.

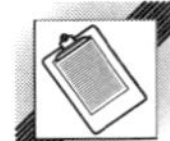

Diagnosis

DIFFERENTIAL DIAGNOSIS

- Toxic causes of progressive weakness and paralysis include diphtheria, tetanus, botulism, arsenic, thallium, and selenium, among others.
- Nontoxic causes include periodic paralysis, Guillain-Barré syndrome, transverse myelitis, myasthenia gravis, and Eaton-Lambert syndrome, among others.

SIGNS AND SYMPTOMS

- Ticks typically attach in relatively concealed areas of the body, including the scalp, axilla, ear, groin, or popliteal areas.
- Tick paralysis usually presents as an ascending flaccid paralysis that develops several days following tick attachment. Sensory function is typically preserved.

Vital Signs

Fever (tick-induced fever) is a separate condition that has rarely been associated with motor dysfunction.

HEENT

- Ticks are commonly found in the scalp concealed by hair.
- Diplopia and dysarthria may be early signs of bulbar weakness.
- Nystagmus has been reported.
- Bulbar paralysis and upper airway obstruction or aspiration can result in death if not recognized.

Dermatologic

- Local reaction to a tick bite often produces a pruritic papule.
- Bacterial superinfection is common, with excoriation due to pruritus.

Pulmonary

- Dyspnea may be an early sign of respiratory muscle weakness.
- Respiratory paralysis can result in death if it is not recognized.

Gastrointestinal

- Dysphagia may be an early sign of bulbar involvement.
- Nausea, vomiting, and diarrhea can be associated with tick-induced fever.

Neurologic

- Muscle weakness usually starts in the distal muscles of the lower extremities and ascends over 24 to 48 hours to involve the proximal lower extremities, the trunk, the upper extremities, and the head.
- Muscle weakness originating in proximal muscles has occurred rarely.
- Decreased deep tendon reflexes usually develop after the onset of muscle weakness and may progress to areflexia over 24 to 48 hours.
- Sensation usually remains intact, although paresthesia has been reported.
- Ataxia may be an early sign of muscle weakness.

PROCEDURES AND LABORATORY TESTS

Essential Tests

No tests may be needed in a minimally symptomatic patient on whom the tick has been discovered and removed.

Recommended Tests

- Serum electrolytes, glucose, BUN, creatinine, magnesium, calcium, and phosphate levels are used to evaluate metabolic causes of weakness, such as hypokalemia.
- Arterial blood gases, pulse oximetry, and serial vital capacity measurements are used to assess respiratory function and the need for intubation.
- Lumbar puncture is used to detect elevated cerebrospinal fluid protein without cells, which is common with Guillain-Barré or lymphocytosis (e.g., viral-induced transverse myelitis).
- Heavy metal screening is used to evaluate patients with suspected exposure.
- A chest radiograph may be useful in ruling out Eaton-Lambert syndrome, which is often associated with underlying neoplasms.
- Motor nerve conduction studies will usually show normal to slightly slowed conduction velocities with normal distal latencies.
- Sensory nerve conduction is usually normal.
- Electromyographic studies will usually show that compound muscle action potentials are abnormally low.

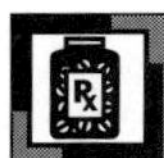

Treatment

- Treatment should focus on removing the tick and supporting respiratory function.
- Supportive care with appropriate airway management is vital, with specific treatment initiated while supportive care continues.

DIRECTING PATIENT COURSE

The health-care provider should call the poison control center when:

- Diplopia, dysphagia, muscle weakness, or other severe effects are present.
- Symptoms and signs are not consistent with tick paralysis.
- Underlying disease presents an unusual problem.

The patient should be referred to a health-care facility when:

- Patient or caregiver seems unreliable.
- Any toxic effects are noted.
- Underlying disease presents an unusual problem.

Admission Considerations

Inpatient management is warranted for patients with neurologic effects.

DECONTAMINATION

- The area is washed with soap and water.
- The tick is then removed.

—Using a magnifying glass, the tick is grasped as close to the skin surface as possible with fine forceps, blunt forceps, or gloved fingers.
—A gentle steady traction is applied, being careful not to squeeze, crush, or puncture the body of the tick.
—Grasping the tick by the side of the mouth may facilitate removal.
—Application of oil or solvent is rarely helpful and may make grasping the tick more difficult.
—Retained mouth parts must be removed and sometimes require excision under local anesthesia.

- The area must be reexamined with a magnification system to make sure the entire tick has been fully removed.
- The area is rewashed with soap and water.

ANTIDOTES

There is no specific antidote for tick paralysis.

ADJUNCTIVE TREATMENT

- Incomplete removal of a tick can produce a pruritic nodule (granuloma) that may require surgical excision.
- Endotracheal intubation and mechanical ventilation may be needed in severe cases.

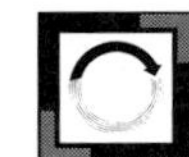

Follow-Up

PATIENT MONITORING

- Airway patency and respiratory function must be monitored continuously.
- Pulmonary function tests, specifically the negative inspiratory force, is a useful serial indicator of respiratory muscle strength.

EXPECTED COURSE AND PROGNOSIS

- Gradual improvement of motor function should begin within a few hours of tick removal.
- Complete recovery usually occurs within 48 hours but may take up to a week. One case reported weakness lasting months.
- Respiratory compromise can lead to hypoxic injury.

DISCHARGE CRITERIA/INSTRUCTIONS

Asymptomatic patients may be discharged from the emergency department or hospital after tick removal has been accomplished.

PATIENT EDUCATION

- Patients should wear long sleeves and long pants when travelling outdoors in tick-endemic areas.
- Chemical tick repellents are recommended.

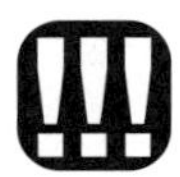

Pitfalls

DIAGNOSIS

- More than one tick may be involved and must be removed.
- Ticks also may be vectors for infectious diseases, including Rocky Mountain spotted fever, Q fever, tularemia, relapsing fever, borreliosis, babesiosis, Colorado tick fever, Boutoneneuse fever, ehrlichiosis, encephalitis, and Lyme disease.

TREATMENT

- The health-care professional must ensure that tetanus immunization status is up to date.
- Using a hot instrument is not recommended due to the risk of inflicting thermal injury.

FOLLOW-UP

The patient should not be discharged immediately after tick removal because muscle weakness may continue to progress after the removal of the tick due to further absorption of venom, failure to identify other ticks, or absorption of venom from retained mouth parts.

ICD-9-CM 989.5

Toxic effect of other substances, chiefly nonmedicinal as to source: venom.

RECOMMENDED READING

Doan-Wiggins L. Tick-borne diseases. *Emerg Med Clin North Am* 1991;9:303–324.

Author: Edwin K. Kuffner

Reviewer: Richard C. Dart

Ticlopidine

Basics

DESCRIPTION

Ticlopidine hydrochloride (Ticlid) is an oral antithrombotic medication that inhibits platelet function.

FORMS AND USES

- It is used for prevention of stroke, myocardial infarction, or complications from sickle cell disease (250 mg orally twice a day).
- It is also used to maintain vascular graft patency.

TOXIC DOSE

Ingestion of 10 g in an adult may result in life-threatening hemodynamic instability and coagulopathy.

PATHOPHYSIOLOGY

- Ticlopidine prolongs bleeding time by irreversibly inhibiting aggregation for the life of the platelet.
- Minimal effects can be demonstrated within 6 hours, and peak platelet inhibitory effects occur in 3 to 5 days.

EPIDEMIOLOGY

Poisoning is uncommon.

CAUSES

- Severe poisoning is usually the result of suicidal ingestion.
- Child neglect or abuse should be considered if the patient is less than 1 year of age, suicide attempt if the patient is over 6 years of age.

DRUG AND DISEASE INTERACTIONS

- The safety of combining ticlopidine with other anticoagulants, such as aspirin or coumadin, is controversial, and the practice is generally not recommended.
- Serum levels of phenytoin and theophylline are often increased by ticlopidine.

PREGNANCY AND LACTATION

FDA Pregnancy Category B. Animal studies indicate no fetal risk and there are no controlled human studies, or animal studies show an adverse fetal effect but well-controlled studies in women do not.

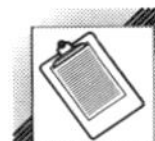

Diagnosis

DIFFERENTIAL DIAGNOSIS

Toxic causes of coagulopathy include brodifacoum, warfarin, or other anticoagulants.

SIGNS AND SYMPTOMS

Cardiovascular

Large overdose may cause agitation, hypotension, and tachycardia.

Gastrointestinal

- Nausea, vomiting, and diarrhea are common.
- Cholestatic jaundice has occurred during therapy.

Hematologic

- In overdose, spontaneous bleeding may develop.
- Reversible neutropenia may develop during therapy using ticlopidine.
- Thrombocytopenic thrombotic purpura has been reported during therapy using ticlopidine.

Fluids and Electrolytes

Metabolic acidosis results from large overdose.

Neurologic

Agitation, CNS depression, and seizures may develop.

PROCEDURES AND LABORATORY TESTS

Essential Tests

No tests may be needed in asymptomatic patients.

Recommended Tests

- Serum elecrolytes, glucose, BUN, and creatinine in symptomatic patients to assess acidosis and renal function.
- Arterial blood gas in symptomatic patients to assess acid-base status.
- Coagulation studies and serum liver enzymes are used to assess toxicity.
- ECG, serum acetaminophen and aspirin levels in overdose setting to detect occult ingestion.

Not Recommended Tests

Drug levels in the serum are not typically available and do not correlate well with clinical effects.

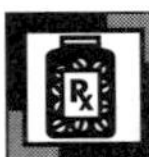

Treatment

- Treatment should focus on control of seizures, correction of electrolyte abnormalities, and replacement of coagulation factors in patients with bleeding.
- Dose and time of exposure should be determined for all substances involved.

DIRECTING PATIENT COURSE

The health-care professional should call the poison control center when:

- Severe or persistent effects develop.
- Coingestant, drug interaction, or underlying disease presents an unusual problem.

The patient should be referred to a health-care facility when:

- Suicide or homicide attempt is possible.
- Toxic effects develop.
- Coingestant, drug interaction, or underlying disease presents an unusual problem.

Admission Considerations

Patients who develop major toxicity (seizures, metabolic acidosis, coagulopathy, spontaneous hemorrhage) should be admitted.

DECONTAMINATION

Out of Hospital

Emesis should be induced with ipecac within 1 hour of ingestion for alert pediatric or adult patient if health-care evaluation will be delayed.

In Hospital

- Gastric lavage should be performed in pediatric (tube size 24–32 French) or adult (tube size 36–42 French) patients presenting within 1 hour of a large ingestion or if serious effects are present.
- One dose of activated charcoal (1–2 g/kg) should be administered without a cathartic if a substantial ingestion has occurred within the previous few hours.

ANTIDOTES

There is no specific antidote for ticlopidine poisoning.

ADJUNCTIVE TREATMENT

- Seizures should be controlled using a benzodiazepine, followed by phenobarbitol in resistant cases.
- Blood components should be replaced as needed.

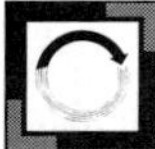

Follow-Up

PATIENT MONITORING

- Blood count should be monitored, including differential at baseline and every 2 weeks during the first 3 months of therapy to monitor for neutropenia and thrombocytopenia.
- Liver function tests should be considered in any patient in whom liver dysfunction is suspected.
- Complete recovery is anticipated unless sequelae of acidosis or hemorrhage develop.

DISCHARGE CRITERIA/INSTRUCTIONS

- From the emergency department. Asymptomatic patients may be discharged after a 6-hour observation period, decontamination, and psychiatric evaluation, if needed.
- From the hospital. Patient may be discharged when toxic effects resolve.

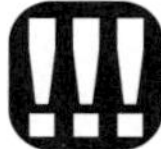

Pitfalls

FOLLOW-UP

- The patient's laboratory values should be monitored closely during the first 3 months of therapy, when most adverse reactions are noted.
- It is vital to recognize interactions between ticlopidine and other anticoagulants.

ICD-9-CM 964.2

Poisoning by agents primarily affecting blood constituents: anticoagulants.

See also: SECTION II, Seizures chapter.

RECOMMENDED READING

Farver DK, Hansen LA. Delayed neutropenia with ticlopidine. *Ann Pharmacother* 1994;28:1344–1346.

Horowitz RS, et al. Cardiopulmonary instability, mental status changes and hemorrhage associated with overdose of ticlopidine. *Vet Hum Toxicol* 1993;35:344.

Author: Robert E. Vander Leest

Reviewer: Richard C. Dart

Tin

Basics

DESCRIPTION

Tin is available in a variety of consumer and industrial products.

FORMS AND USES

- *Organotin* refers to tin with an organic group (triphenyltin, trialkyltin, trimethyltin).
- Tin is a metal primarily encountered in paint, toothpaste additive, and utensils, as well as in industrial substances, such as solders, fungicides, catalysts, stabilizers, electroplating, alloys (e.g., bronzes), and ceramics.
- The role of tin as a cause of metal fume fever is covered in SECTION II, Metal Fume Fever chapter.

TOXIC DOSE

- Metallic tin or its inorganic salts typically require large doses over prolonged periods to produce toxicity.
- Organic tins are more toxic, but precise doses are unknown.

PATHOPHYSIOLOGY

- Inorganic noncaustic tin compounds are not toxic when ingested.
- Pulmonary symptoms may result from inhalation exposure.
- Potassium, sodium, chloride, or sulfate salts of tin may cause gastrointestinal caustic injury.
- Organic tin compounds are the most caustic, and some, such as triphenyltin, can be dermally absorbed.
- Triphenyltin may result in toxicity following oral, dermal, or inhalation exposure.
- Tetralkyltin is converted to trialkyltin.

EPIDEMIOLOGY

- Exposure is common, but toxicity is uncommon.
- Massive exposure is required to cause death.

PREGNANCY AND LACTATION

Genotoxicity has been found in numerous animal studies.

WORKPLACE STANDARDS

- ACGIH. TLV TWA is 2 mg/m^3.
- OSHA. PEL TWA is 2 mg/m^3.
- NIOSH. IDLH level is 100 mg/m^3 for metal and inorganic compounds; 25 mg/m^3 for organic compounds.

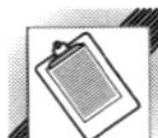

Diagnosis

SIGNS AND SYMPTOMS

HEENT

- Headaches and visual disturbances may occur.
- Tin chloride salt reacts with water to create fumes that may result in mucous membrane irritation.
- Acute inhalation, dermal exposure, or ingestion of organotins such as trimethyltin may cause hearing loss.

Pulmonary

- Organotin inhalation may include dyspnea, cough, wheeze, and occupational asthma.
- Delayed pulmonary edema may occur in severe cases.
- Pneumoconiosis, with no lung function test abnormalities and no known long-term associated mortality, has been described following chronic tin oxide inhalation.

Gastrointestinal

- Symptoms following ingestion of caustic tin salts may include nausea, vomiting, diarrhea, and abdominal pain.
- Dialkyl tin is most caustic and may cause hematemesis.

Neurologic

- Organotins primarily affect the CNS, and encephalopathy and cerebral edema may occur with acute or chronic exposure.
- Acute inhalation, dermal exposure, or ingestion of organotins such as trimethyltin may cause delirium, cerebellar dysfunction, unresponsiveness, nystagmus, seizures, sensory neuropathy, confabulation, and visual disturbances.
- Polyneuropathy may follow, and recovery may take months to years.

PROCEDURES AND LABORATORY TESTS

Essential Tests

No tests may be needed following ingestion of noncaustic inorganic tin compounds.

Recommended Tests

- Complete blood count, serum electrolytes, BUN, and creatinine should be monitored in patients with gastrointestinal symptoms or bleeding.
- ECG, serum acetaminophen, and aspirin levels should be screened in an overdose setting to detect occult ingestion.
- Urinary tin concentration. Normal urine level of 16.6 μg/L or total excretion of 23.4 μg/day has been reported.
- Patients with pulmonary symptoms should have chest radiograph and an assessment of oxygenation.
- Tin levels are available from referral laboratories for confirmation of exposure.

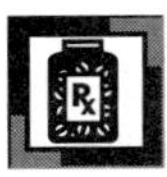

Treatment

- Treatment should focus on general supportive care and on close monitoring of airway.
- Dose and time of exposure should be determined for all substances involved.

DIRECTING PATIENT COURSE

The health-care professional should call the poison control center when:

- Severe or persistent effects develop.
- Coingestant, drug interaction, or underlying disease presents an unusual problem.

The patient should be referred to a health-care facility when:

- Suicide or homicide attempt is possible.
- Toxic effects develop.
- Coingestant, drug interaction, or underlying disease presents an unusual problem.

Admission Considerations

Patients with any evidence of caustic injury should be admitted for complete evaluation and intensive supportive care.

DECONTAMINATION

Out of Hospital

- Induction of emesis is not recommended.
- Gastric dilution with up to 250 ml water or milk is used for an adult following ingestion of caustic tin salts.
- Dilution should be avoided in the event of tin chloride ingestion because of its reactivity with water.
- For an inhalation exposure, the patient should be moved to fresh air and administered oxygen.
- Immediate irrigation should be performed following ocular or dermal exposure.

In Hospital

- Emesis is not recommended due to the caustic nature of many tin compounds.
- Activated charcoal and lavage may help decrease absorption following organotin ingestion; however, a charcoal should be avoided if gastrointestinal endoscopy is planned.

ANTIDOTES

There is no specific antidote for tin poisoning.

ADJUNCTIVE TREATMENT

- Bronchospasm or respiratory tract irritation are treated with humidified oxygen and bronchodilators as needed.
- Pulmonary edema is treated as the noncardiogenic type (see SECTION II, Pulmonary Edema chapter, for details).
- Hypotension is treated as the hypovolemic type with intravenous infusion of 10 to 20 ml/kg of 0.9% saline. If blood pressure is unresponsive, vasopressors may be needed (see SECTION II, Hypotension chapter).

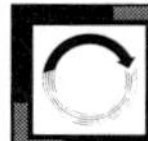

Follow-Up

PATIENT MONITORING

Symptomatic patients should receive continuous respiratory and cardiac monitoring.

EXPECTED COURSE AND PROGNOSIS

- Caustic gastrointestinal effects develop soon after ingestion, peak within hours, and may persist for days in serious cases.
- Sequelae of stricture or motility dysfunction may persist.
- Inhalation injury typically begins immediately, but may take 24 hours to become severe and resolves over days.

DISCHARGE CRITERIA/INSTRUCTIONS

- From emergency department. Asymptomatic patients may be discharged following decontamination (if appropriate), observation for 4 to 6 hours, and psychiatric evaluation, if needed.
- From hospital. Patients with improving symptoms may be discharged following endoscopy (if needed).

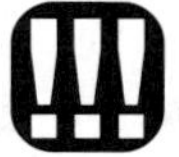

Pitfalls

TREATMENT

The health-care provider should expect and prepare for delayed symptoms, including pulmonary edema and neurotoxicity following organotin exposure.

ICD-9-CM 985.9

Toxic effect of other metals: unspecified metal.

See also: SECTION II, Hypotension and Pulmonary Edema chapters; SECTION IV, Metal Fume Fever chapter.

RECOMMENDED READING

Kreyburg S, Torvilc A, Bjorneboe A, et al. Trimethyl tin poisoning: report of a case with postmortem examination. *Clin Neuropathol* 1992;11:256–259.

Wax PM, Dockstader L. Tributyl tin use in interior paints: a continuing health hazard. *J Toxicol Clin Toxicol* 1995;33:239–241.

Author: Lada Kokan

Reviewer: Richard C. Dart

Tolazoline

Basics

DESCRIPTION

Tolazoline is an imidazoline derivative that is structurally related to phentolamine.

FORMS AND USES

- Substances include tolazoline hydrochloride, benzazoline hydrochloride, Priscol, Priscoline, and Vaso-Dilatan.
- Tolazoline is used in the treatment of pulmonary hypertension.

—Pediatric dosage, 1 to 2 mg/kg intravenously over 10 minutes followed by an infusion of 1 to 2 mg/kg/h
—Adult dosage, 1 to 2 mg/kg intravenously every 12 hours (has been used to treat cor pulmonale)

- It is also used in the treatment of peripheral vascular disease at a dosage of 25 to 50 mg orally four times daily.
- Tolazoline has been suggested as a treatment for clonidine overdose; however, no good data are available on this use.

TOXIC DOSE

Insufficient data are available to evaluate.

PATHOPHYSIOLOGY

Tolazoline causes peripheral vasodilation by competitively antagonizing α-adrenergic receptors.

EPIDEMIOLOGY

Poisoning is uncommon.

DRUG AND DISEASE INTERACTIONS

- Ingestion of tolazoline with alcohol may precipitate a disulfiram-like reaction.
- Hyperchloremic metabolic acidosis, acute renal failure, and duodenal perforation have been in infants given tolazoline.

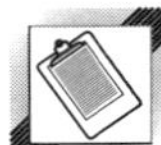

Diagnosis

SIGNS AND SYMPTOMS

Predominant effects are those of α-adrenergic blockade.

Vital Signs

Orthostatic hypotension, tachycardia, hypertension and shock may occur.

Dermatologic

Increased pilomotor activity, peripheral vasodilation, skin flushing, and sweating may occur.

Cardiovascular

- Tachycardia, hypotension, and cardiac dysrhythmias may occur.
- Intraarterial injection may be followed by a burning sensation in the limb.

Gastrointestinal

- Patient may experience nausea, vomiting, diarrhea, and epigastric pain.
- Tolazoline stimulates gastric acid secretion and may exacerbate ulcers.
- Gastrointestinal hemorrhage occurs rarely.

Renal

Oliguria and hematuria may occur.

Hematologic

Thrombocytopenia and other blood dyscrasias have been reported.

PROCEDURES AND LABORATORY TESTS

Essential Tests

No tests may be needed in asymptomatic patients.

Recommended Tests

- Patients with hypotension should have an ECG and cardiac monitor to evaluate ischemia.
- CBC, serum electrolytes, BUN, creatinine, and other tests may be useful to determine cause of hypotension.

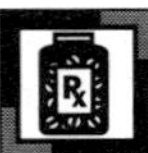

Treatment

- Therapy should focus on discontinuing drug and providing supportive care.
- Dose and time of exposure should be determined for all substances involved.

DIRECTING PATIENT COURSE

The health-care professional should call the poison control center when:

- Severe or persistent effects develop.
- Coingestant, drug interaction, or underlying disease presents an unusual problem.

The patient should be referred to a health-care facility when:

- Toxic effects develop.
- Coingestant, drug interaction, or underlying disease presents an unusual problem.

Admission Considerations

Extended observation or hospital admission are typically needed for patients with persistent hypotension.

DECONTAMINATION

Gastrointestinal decontamination is not usually needed because of the intravenous route of administration.

ANTIDOTES

There is no specific antidote available for tolazoline.

ADJUNCTIVE TREATMENT

Hypotension may be refractory to initial therapy because of the direct α-receptor blockade.

- Patient should receive 10 to 20 ml/kg 0.9% saline and be placed in the Trendelenburg position.
- Further fluid therapy should be guided by central monitoring or right heart catheterization to avoid volume overload.
- Beta adrenergic agents may be ineffective.
- Clinically significant hypotension may be treated using an alpha adrenergic agent such as phenylephrine (1%).

—A slow intravenous push injection of 100 to 500 μg, repeated if necessary in 15 minutes.
—This may be followed by a continuous infusion of 10 mg in 500 ml of D_5W at a rate up to 180 μg/minute and then titrated to response (often the rate can be decreased).

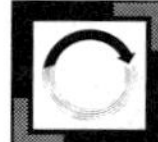

Follow-Up

PATIENT MONITORING

The patient's cardiac rhythm and vital signs should be monitored continuously.

EXPECTED COURSE AND PROGNOSIS

Most patients recover uneventfully over a few hours.

DISCHARGE CRITERIA/INSTRUCTIONS

Asymptomatic patients may be discharged from the emergency department or hospital following observation for 6 hours and psychiatric evaluation, if needed.

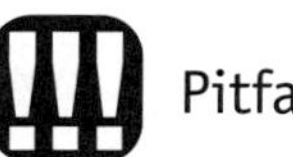

Pitfalls

TREATMENT

Hypotension may be refractory to dopamine therapy; rapid progression to phenylephrine therapy may be indicated.

ICD-9-CM 971.3

Poisoning by drugs primarily affecting the autonomic nervous system: sympatholytics (antiadrenergics).

See also: SECTION II, Hypotension chapter.

RECOMMENDED READING

Butt W, Auldist A, McDougall P, et al. Duodenal ulceration: a complication of tolazoline therapy. *Aust Paediatr J* 1986;22:221–223.

Author: Luke Yip

Reviewer: Richard C. Dart

Toluene

Basics

DESCRIPTION

Toluene (methylbenzene, methyl benzol, phenyl methane, toluol) is a common aromatic hydrocarbon solvent.

FORMS AND USES

- Toluene is a component of paints, varnishes, paint removers, dyes, lacquers, inks, glues, cleaners, transmission fluid, and degreasers.
- The primary sources of toluene exposure are in the production and use of gasoline and the intentional abuse of inhaled products containing toluene.

TOXIC DOSE

- Adult ingestion of 2 ounces has resulted in death.
- Inhalation causes acute intoxication, but permanent effects develop only with chronic abuse.
- Pulmonary aspiration of a few milliliters can produce aspiration pneumonitis.

PATHOPHYSIOLOGY

- Inhalation is the major route of exposure, although toluene is very well absorbed following ingestion and upon dermal contact.
- Toluene causes direct cellular toxicity to the lung and gastrointestinal tract, but toxic metabolites cause injury in the CNS and in the renal, cardiac, hepatic, and hematopoietic systems.
- Toluene abuse is performed by sniffing directly from the bottle or "huffing" from a rag or plastic bag saturated with toluene.

EPIDEMIOLOGY

- Exposure is common and underreported.
- Toxic effects following exposure are typically related to the dose (concentration × time).
- Death is rare and generally secondary to cardiac dysrhythmia or respiratory depression.
- Adolescents are more likely to be abusers of inhaled toluene than are older or younger people.

CAUSES

- Exposure occurs primarily by occupational inhalation and intentionally during abuse (sniffing or huffing).
- Child abuse or neglect should be considered in patients younger than 6 years of age, intentional misuse in patients over 6 years of age.

RISK FACTORS

Certain occupations are especially hazardous: aviation fuel blenders, gasoline blenders, benzene production, laboratory workers, coke oven workers, lacquer workers, painters, perfume makers, petrochemical workers, rubber cement manufacturers, saccharin manufacturers, printers, and rotogravure printers.

PREGNANCY AND LACTATION

- Maternal toluene abuse is teratogenic.
- There is an increased incidence of spontaneous abortions and preterm deliveries.

WORKPLACE STANDARDS

- ACGIH. TLV TWA is 50 ppm; STEL is 150 ppm.
- OSHA. PEL TWA is 200 ppm; PEL STEL is 300 ppm.
- NIOSH. IDLH is 500 ppm.

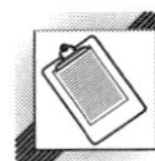

Diagnosis

DIFFERENTIAL DIAGNOSIS

- Toxic causes of altered mental status include opioids, sedative-hypnotics, ethanol, gamma-hydroxybutyrate, rohypnol, clonidine, methanol, anticonvulsants, and ethylene glycol, among others.
- Nontoxic causes of altered mental status include intracranial trauma or infection, hypoglycemia or other metabolic disturbances, and electrolyte abnormalities.

SIGNS AND SYMPTOMS

- Acute exposure can involve CNS excitation, euphoria, and nervousness, followed by somnolence, confusion, vertigo, ataxia, seizures, and coma with prolonged or high-dose exposure.
- Chronic exposure can involve muscle weakness, hyporeflexia, myalgias, ataxia, electrolyte abnormalities, predominantly hypokalemia, and serious cognitive and memory deficits.

Vital Signs

Fever and tachycardia are common.

HEENT

- Splash contact may cause blepharospasm, corneal abrasion, chemical conjunctivitis, and lacrimation.
- Optic atrophy with decreased vision, abnormal color vision, nystagmus, and ototoxicity/sensorineural hearing loss are rare complications of chronic inhalational exposure.

Dermatologic

Prolonged skin exposure can cause dermatitis and rarely burns.

Cardiovascular

- Sudden death after acute inhalation is believed to be related to ventricular dysrhythmia, caused by sudden surges in sympathetic outflow with catecholamine release, sensitization of the myocardium to catecholamines, hypoxia induced by simple asphyxiant effects and electrolyte abnormalities.
- Dilated cardiomyopathy and myocardial infarction occur in chronic abusers.

Pulmonary

- Aspiration can cause a chemical pneumonitis.
- Pneumothorax and pneumomediastinum may occur after forceful sniffing or huffing.
- Reactive airway disease may occur in chronic abusers.

Gastrointestinal

Vomiting, abdominal cramps, and diarrhea are common following ingestion.

Hepatic

Increased aminotransferase levels (alanine aminotransferase, aspartate aminotransferase) may occur.

Renal

- Reversible distal renal tubular acidosis (RTA) is common, and hyperchloremic nonanion gap metabolic acidosis, low serum bicarbonate, and marked hypokalemia may occur.
- Some patients may have features of both distal and proximal RTA.
- Renal insufficiency and glomerulopathy occur rarely and are usually reversible.

Musculoskeletal

- Rhabdomyolysis with elevated creatine kinase levels is common, but rarely severe.
- Muscle weakness is common due to hypokalemia.

Neurologic

- Initial CNS excitation may involve euphoria, nervousness, tremor, insomnia, nystagmus, headache, nausea, and vomiting.
- Subsequent CNS depression may involve somnolence, confusion, vertigo, ataxia, seizures, and coma.
- Peripheral neuropathy, cognitive deficits, memory impairment, psychiatric disorders, encephalopathy, and emotional lability may develop during chronic exposure.

PROCEDURES AND LABORATORY TESTS

Essential Tests

No tests may be needed in minimally symptomatic patients.

Recommended Tests

- Serum electrolytes, glucose, BUN, creatinine, and urinalysis are advised to detect hypokalemia, acidosis, or renal injury.
- An ECG and continuous monitoring are recommended. Hypokalemia may cause PR prolongation, low-voltage QRS complexes, ST depression, T-wave flattening, U waves, or QT prolongation.
- Complete blood count, liver function tests, creatine kinase, serum lactate, and arterial blood gases may be indicated to assess acidosis and liver or muscle injury.

• Serum acetaminophen and salicylate levels are recommended in an overdose setting to evaluate occult ingestion.
• Chronic abuse may cause changes on CT or MRI, such as abnormal gray-white differentiation, cerebral and cerebellar atrophy, low-density lesions in the basal ganglia, and hyperdensities in the brainstem and cerebellum.

Not Recommended Tests

Levels of toluene and its metabolites are not clinically useful, but may be used for medical monitoring of the workplace.

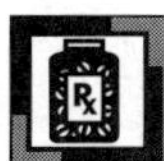

Treatment

• Treatment should focus on airway management and hemodynamic support.
• The dose and time of exposure should be determined for all substances involved.

DIRECTING PATIENT COURSE

The health-care provider should call the poison control center when:

• Severe metabolic acidosis, electrolyte abnormality, or other serious effects are present.
• Toxic effects are not consistent with toluene poisoning.
• A coingestant, drug interaction or underlying disease presents an unusual problem.

The patient should be referred to a health-care facility when:

• Attempted suicide or homicide is possible.
• Patient or caregiver seems unreliable.
• Toxic effects are present.
• Coingestant, drug interaction or underlying disease presents an unusual problem.

Admission Considerations

Inpatient care is warranted for patients with persistent mental status depression, cardiac toxicity, severe metabolic abnormality, renal failure, or rhabdomyolysis.

DECONTAMINATION

Out of Hospital

• Inhalation. Patients should be removed from exposure and administered supplemental oxygen.
• Ingestion. Emesis should not be induced due to the rapid onset of CNS depression.

In Hospital

• Gastric aspiration should be performed in adult or pediatric patients presenting within 1 hour of a large ingestion or if serious effects are present. A standard nasogastric tube may be used because toluene is liquid.
• One dose of activated charcoal (1–2 g/kg) should be administered without a cathartic if a substantial ingestion has occurred within the previous hour.

ANTIDOTES

There are no specific antidotes for toluene toxicity.

ADJUNCTIVE TREATMENT

• Potassium deficits may be very large and may require replacement (after ensuring that renal failure is not present). Potassium chloride 10 mEq/h should be administered until the deficit has been corrected.
• Serum bicarbonate level may be extremely low, but there is no consensus on whether hypobicarbonatemia should be treated.
• With or without treatment, it will require several days for the bicarbonate and potassium levels to normalize after discontinuation of toluene abuse.

In cases of severe pulmonary aspiration with hypoxemia, treatment with bypass methods of oxygenation (extracorporeal membrane oxygenation) has been successful.

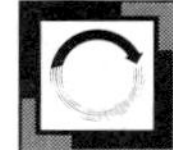

Follow-Up

PATIENT MONITORING

Respiratory function, cardiac rhythm, and electrolytes should be monitored in symptomatic patients.

EXPECTED COURSE AND PROGNOSIS

• Acute effects from inhalation peaks rapidly.
• Chronic inhalation causes CNS injury that is only partially reversible.
• Acid-base and electrolyte abnormalities may be dramatic, but they respond over several days to supportive care and repletion of deficits.
• Possible complications include permanent CNS damage and optic atrophy; sudden death has occurred from dysrhythmia.

DISCHARGE CRITERIA/INSTRUCTIONS

From the Emergency Department

• Acute exposure. Asymptomatic patients may be discharged if they have a normal (i.e., baseline for patient) neurologic examination result, no cardiac effects after a 6-hour observation period, and psychiatric evaluation, if needed.
• Chronic exposure. Stable patients may be discharged if they do not have severe electrolyte abnormalities and after psychiatric evaluation, if needed.

From the Hospital

• Patients may be discharged after resolution or stabilization of CNS, cardiac, musculoskeletal, and electrolyte effects.
• A psychiatric evaluation should be obtained, if needed.

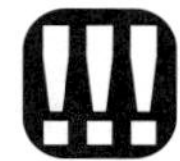

Pitfalls

DIAGNOSIS

• It is important to consider alternative diagnoses for alteration and depression in mental status.
• The patient must be checked for hypokalemia and renal failure.

TREATMENT

• Hypokalemia should be treated promptly.
• Fetal monitoring should be performed in pregnant patients who have been exposed to toluene.

ICD-9-CM 989.8

Toxic effect of other substances, chiefly nonmedicinal as to source: other substances, chiefly nonmedicinal as to source; or

987.1

Toxic effect of other gases, fumes or vapors: other hydrocarbon gas.

RECOMMENDED READING

Arnold GL, Kirby RS, Langendoerfer S, Wilkins-Haug L. Toluene embryopathy: clinical delineation and developmental follow-up. *Pediatr* 1994;93:216–220.

Wilkins-Haug L, Gabow PA. Toluene abuse during pregnancy: obstetric complications and perinatal outcomes. *Obstet Gynecol* 1991;77:504–509.

Author: Gerald F. O'Malley

Reviewer: Luke Yip

Basics

DESCRIPTION

Tramadol is a synthetic, opioid agonist analgesic medication.

FORMS AND USES

- Tramadol (Ultram) is an analgesic similar to opioid analgesics, but has fewer effects at opioid receptors.
- Typical adult dose is 50 to 100 mg orally, subcutaneously, intramuscularly, rectally, or intravenously.

TOXIC DOSE

- Toxic dose is poorly defined.
- Ingestion of several grams is needed for fatality in an adult.

PATHOPHYSIOLOGY

Tramadol blocks norepinephrine and serotonin reuptake, which may result in respiratory depression and hypotension.

EPIDEMIOLOGY

Poisoning is uncommon.

CAUSES

Child neglect or abuse should be considered if the patient is less than 1 year of age, suicide attempt if the patient is over 6 years of age.

DRUG AND DISEASE INTERACTIONS

Drugs that have a depressant activity on the CNS have an additive effect when combined with tramadol.

PREGNANCY AND LACTATION

- US FDA Pregnancy Category C. The drug exerts animal teratogenic or embryocidal effects, but there are no controlled studies in women, or no studies are available in animals or women.
- Tramadol is excreted in breast milk at a concentration of 0.1% that of the maternal dose.

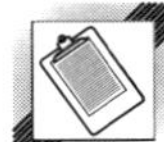

Diagnosis

DIFFERENTIAL DIAGNOSIS

- Toxic causes of CNS depression include opioids, benzodiazepines, barbiturates, ethanol, baclofen, and gamma-hydroxybutyrate.
- Nontoxic causes include trauma, infection, and metabolic derangements (hypoglycemia, hypoxia, electrolyte disturbances).

SIGNS AND SYMPTOMS

Vital Signs

Tachycardia and hypertension occur rarely.

HEENT

Miosis is common following acute overdose.

Cardiovascular

Hypotension and myocardial ischemia may occur with large overdose.

Pulmonary

- Respiratory depression is common.
- Pulmonary edema occurs rarely.

Gastrointestinal

Nausea and vomiting are common.

Renal

Urinary retention is common in overdose.

Musculoskeletal

Hypertonia and rhabdomyolysis may occur.

Neurologic

- CNS depression is common following overdose.
- Seizures may occur rarely.

PROCEDURES AND LABORATORY TESTS

Essential Tests

No tests may be needed for minimally symptomatic patients.

Recommended Tests

- Serum electrolytes, glucose, BUN, creatinine, creatine kinase, blood glucose, and pulse oximetry should be obtained in patients with altered mental status.
- ECG, serum acetaminophen and aspirin levels in overdose setting to detect occult ingestion.
- Head CT, lumbar puncture, toxicology screening and other tests as indicated should be performed for patients with CNS depression.

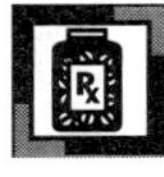

Treatment

- General approach to tramadol toxicity is the same as for opioid agents.
- Supportive care with appropriate airway management is vital.
- Dose and time of exposure should be determined for all substances involved.

DIRECTING PATIENT COURSE

The health-care professional should call the poison control center when:

- Severe or persistent effects develop.
- Coingestant, drug interaction, or underlying disease presents an unusual problem.

The patient should be referred to a health-care facility when:

- Suicide or homicide attempt is possible.
- Toxic effects develop.
- Coingestant, drug interaction, or underlying disease presents an unusual problem.

Admission Considerations

Inpatient management is warranted if the patient exhibits CNS depression, hypotension, or respiratory depression.

DECONTAMINATION

Out of Hospital

Induction of emesis is not recommended.

In Hospital

- Gastric lavage should be performed in pediatric (tube size 24–32 French) or adult (tube size 36–42 French) patients presenting within 1 hour of a large ingestion or if serious effects are present.
- One dose of activated charcoal (1– 2 g/kg) should be administered without a cathartic if a substantial ingestion has occurred within the previous few hours.

ANTIDOTES

Naloxone is the specific antidote for tramadol poisoning.

- The dose is 2 mg intravenously
- If no improvement is noted, the dose should be doubled to 4 mg intravenously.
- If there is still no improvement, more naloxone is unlikely to be effective.

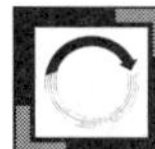

Follow-Up

PATIENT MONITORING

- Respiratory and cardiac function should be monitored continuously.
- Arterial blood gases and pulse oximetry should be monitored in patients with respiratory depression.
- Patients should be observed for 6 hours after treatment to monitor for symptoms.

EXPECTED COURSE AND PROGNOSIS

If adequate supportive care is provided, most patients survive tramadol overdose without serious sequelae.

DISCHARGE CRITERIA/INSTRUCTIONS

- From the emergency department. After 6 hours of observation, asymptomatic patients may be discharged from the emergency department following decontamination and appropriate psychiatric referral.
- From the hospital. Patients may be discharged when toxic effects resolve and after 6 hours without naloxone therapy.

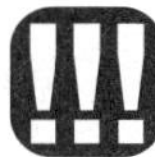

Pitfalls

DIAGNOSIS

Failure to evaluate for other serious causes of CNS depression may lead to misdiagnosis.

ICD-9-CM 965

Poisoning by analgesics, antipyretics, and antirheumatics.

See also: SECTION III, Naloxone and Nalmephene chapter.

RECOMMENDED READING

Lee SR, McTavish D, Sorkin EM. Tramadol: a preliminary review of its pharmacodynamic and pharmacokinetic properties and therapeutic potential in acute and chronic pain status. *Drugs* 1993;46:313–347.

Author: Richard C. Dart

Reviewer: Gerald F. O'Malley

Trazodone and Nefazodone

Basics

DESCRIPTION

Trazodone and nefazodone are atypical antidepressant medications.

FORMS AND USES

- Trazodone (Desyrel). Adult dose is 150 to 600 mg/day orally in divided doses for depression; the recommended starting dosage is 150 mg/day, with an increase of 50 mg/day every 3 to 4 days. It is not recommended for children.
- Nefazodone (Serzone). Adult dosage is 200 to 600 mg/day orally in divided doses for depression; the recommended starting dosage is 200 mg/day, with an increase of 100 to 200 mg/day at intervals of no less than 1 week. It is not recommended for children.
- Elderly or debilitated patients should be started at 100 mg/day with a more cautious increase in dose.

TOXIC DOSE

- An oral trazodone overdose of 2 to 3 g may cause respiratory depression in an adult.
- There is little information available about nefazodone, but it is expected to be similar to trazodone.

PATHOPHYSIOLOGY

- Therapeutic effects are produced by the inhibition of serotonin reuptake and the blockade of 5-hydroxytryptamine 2 (5-HT_2) of serotonin receptors.
- Their actions also include α_1-receptor blockade and weak α_2-receptor blockade.
- The cardiac conduction effects are qualitatively similar to but quantitatively much less severe than those of the tricyclic antidepressants.
- Anticholinergic activity is minimal.
- No evidence of carcinogenesis has been reported.

EPIDEMIOLOGY

- Poisoning is common.
- Toxic effects following exposure are typically mild to moderate, with death occurring in cases involving coingestants or massive overdose.

CAUSES

- Ingestion is usually intentional.
- Child neglect or abuse should be considered if the patient is less than 1 year of age, attempted suicide in patients over 6 years of age.

DRUG AND DISEASE INTERACTIONS

- Additive effects occur with other CNS depressants (ethanol, benzodiazepines, barbiturates, narcotics, etc.).
- Serotonin syndrome may develop when the drug is taken with monoamine oxidase inhibitors or other serotonin reuptake inhibitors.
- Increased or decreased prothrombin times may be induced when taken with warfarin.
- Increase in serum levels of astemizole, alprazolam, triazolam, and other drugs metabolized by cytochrome P450 may be observed.

PREGNANCY AND LACTATION

- Experience with trazodone and nefazedone overdose in pregnancy is limited.
- US FDA Pregnancy Category C. The drug exerts animal teratogenic or embryocidal effects, but there are no controlled studies available in women, or no studies in either animals or women.

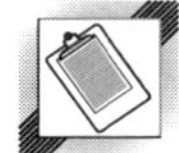

Diagnosis

DIFFERENTIAL DIAGNOSIS

- Toxic causes of CNS depression include other serotonin reuptake inhibitors, tricyclic antidepressants, ethanol, benzodiazepines, barbiturates, and narcotics, among others.
- Nontoxic causes include electrolyte disorders (e.g., hyper- or hyponatremia and hypoglycemia), any cause of hypoxia, infection, and intracranial events (e.g., bleed and stroke).

SIGNS AND SYMPTOMS

Primary effects of clinical concern are CNS depression, lethargy, ataxia, and myoclonus; coma may occur following a large ingestion.

Vital Signs

Temperature may be elevated as part of serotonin syndrome, hypertension (rare) or hypotension (common), bradycardia (common), or respiratory depression.

HEENT

Tinnitus, blurred vision, and dry mouth occur rarely.

Cardiovascular

- Bradycardia is common; transient first-degree atrioventricular block sometimes occurs.
- Prolonged QTc and torsade de pointes develop rarely.

Pulmonary

Respiratory depression is seen in severe cases.

Gastrointestinal

Nausea and vomiting occur.

Hepatic

Liver enzyme elevations occur rarely during therapy.

Hematologic

Leukopenia has developed during therapy.

Fluids and Electrolytes

- Hyponatremia may occur with an overdose.
- Peripheral edema is common during therapy.

Musculoskeletal

Muscle weakness and rhabdomyolysis appear with serotonin syndrome.

Neurologic

- Dizziness, CNS depression, ataxia, seizures, and serotonin syndrome occur.
- Mania may occur at therapeutic doses. Coma may be prolonged.

Urologic

Priapism has been reported following an overdose.

PROCEDURES AND LABORATORY TESTS

Essential Tests

No tests may be needed in asymptomatic patients.

Recommended Tests

- Serum electrolytes, glucose, BUN, creatinine, glucose to evaluate other causes of altered mental status
- ECG, serum acetaminophen and aspirin levels in an overdose setting to evaluate for occult ingestion
- Head CT, lumbar puncture, bacterial cultures, and toxicology studies as needed to evaluate other causes of altered mental status

Not Recommended Tests

Quantitative serum levels are not clinically useful.

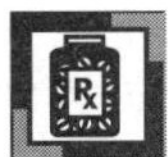

Treatment

- Treatment should focus on decontamination and supportive care with appropriate airway management.
- The dose and time of exposure should be determined for all substances involved.

DIRECTING PATIENT COURSE

The health-care provider should call the poison control center when:

- Altered mental status, dysrhythmia, or other severe effects are present.
- Toxic effects are not consistent with trazodone or nefazodone poisoning.
- Coingestant, drug interaction, or underlying disease presents an unusual problem.

The patient should be referred to a health-care facility when:

- Attempted suicide or homicide is possible.
- Patient or caregiver seems unreliable.
- Any toxic effects are present.
- Coingestant, drug interaction or underlying disease presents an unusual problem.

Admission Considerations

Inpatient treatment is warranted for patients who demonstrate persistent CNS abnormalities or hypotension, dysrhythmia, or ECG abnormalities.

DECONTAMINATION

Out of Hospital

Induction of emesis is not recommended.

In Hospital

- Gastric lavage should be performed in pediatric (tube size 24–32 French) or adult (tube size 36–42 French) patients presenting within 1 hour of a large ingestion or if serious effects are present.
- One dose of activated charcoal (1–2 g/kg) should be administered without a cathartic if a substantial ingestion has occurred within the previous few hours.

ANTIDOTES

There are no specific antidotes for trazodone or nefazodone poisoning.

ADJUNCTIVE TREATMENT

- Intravenous magnesium, isoproterenol, and overdrive pacing may be required for torsade de pointes.
- Hypotension should be treated with isotonic fluid infusion (10–20 ml/kg), Trendelenburg positioning, and a vasopressor (e.g., dopamine) if needed. Norepinephrine is recommended for refractory hypotension.
- For seizures, after assuring the patient's airway, a benzodiazepine should be administered for initial control; if seizures persist or recur, another anticonvulsant such as phenobarbital should be added.
- Serotonin syndrome is treated with temperature control, muscle relaxation, endotracheal intubation, and general supportive care.
- Intracavernosal injection of norepinephrine or surgical intervention for priapism may be necessary; immediate consultation with a urologist is recommended.

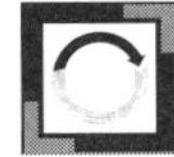

Follow-Up

PATIENT MONITORING

- Continuous respiratory, cardiac, and blood pressure monitoring should be instituted.
- The patient should be monitored for CNS depression.

EXPECTED COURSE AND PROGNOSIS

- Most patients who overdose on trazodone or nefazodone exclusively will recover fully.
- Patients with CNS depression may require 24 to 48 hours to recover.
- Aspiration from emesis may occur during periods of CNS depression.
- Seizures, cardiac arrhythmias, and the serotonin syndrome may all result in potentially fatal outcomes.

DISCHARGE CRITERIA/INSTRUCTIONS

- From the emergency department. Asymptomatic patients may be discharged after 6 hours of observation following gastrointestinal decontamination and psychiatric evaluation, if needed.
- From the hospital. Patients may be discharged following recovery, gastrointestinal decontamination, resolution of CNS depression, and psychiatric evaluation if needed.

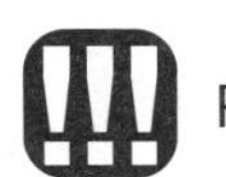

Pitfalls

TREATMENT

- Inadequate early airway management and ventilatory support may result in aspiration or hypoxia.
- Quinidine, procainamide, disopyramide, isoproterenol, amiodarone, and other drugs known to prolong the QTc are generally contraindicated.
- If priapism is not addressed immediately, impotence may result.

ICD-9-CM 969

Poisoning by psychotropic agents.

See also: SECTION II, Hypotension, Neuroleptic Malignant Syndrome and Serotonin Syndrome, Seizures and Ventricular Dysrhythmia chapters.

RECOMMENDED READING

Fishbain DA. Priapism associated with trazodone therapy [Letter]. *J Urol* 1989;142:831.

Henry JA, Ali CJ, Caldwell R, et al. Acute trazodone poisoning: clinical signs and plasma concentrations. *Psychopathology* 1984;17(suppl 2):77–81.

Lesar T, Kingston R, Dahms R, et al. Trazodone overdose. *Ann Emerg Med* 1983;12:221–223.

Author: Steven A. Seifert

Reviewer: Richard C. Dart

Trimethobenzamide

Basics

DESCRIPTION

Trimethobenzamide (Tigan) is an antiemetic medication.

FORMS AND USES

The usual dosage is 250 mg orally three times a day or 200 mg intramuscularly or by rectum every 6 to 8 hours.

TOXIC DOSE

Toxic dose is poorly characterized; very large doses would have to be ingested to induce toxicity.

PATHOPHYSIOLOGY

- Trimethobenzamide is a nonphenothiazine antiemetic that directly depresses the chemoreceptor trigger zone.
- Toxic effects arise primarily from anticholinergic action; however, in some cases, α-receptor blockade is apparent (e.g., miosis).

EPIDEMIOLOGY

Poisoning is uncommon and toxic effects are typically mild.

CAUSES

- Poisoning is usually suicidal.
- Child abuse or neglect should be considered in patients less than 1 year of age; suicide attempt in patients over 6 years of age.

PREGNANCY AND LACTATION

US FDA Pregnancy Category C. The drug exerts animal teratogenic or embryocidal effects, but there are no controlled studies in women, or no studies are available in animals or women.

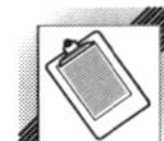

Diagnosis

DIFFERENTIAL DIAGNOSIS

Toxic causes of anticholinergic effects include atropine, scopolamine, or antihistamines.

SIGNS AND SYMPTOMS

Acute overdose primarily produces anticholinergic symptoms.

Vital Signs

Tachycardia, hyperthermia, and either hypertension or hypotension can occur.

HEENT

- Dry mouth and dysphagia have been reported.
- Mydriasis is most common, but miosis also may occur.

Cardiovascular

- Hypotension can occur due to vasodilation.
- Quinidine-like effects may result in myocardial depression and ventricular dysrhythmia in massive overdose.

Pulmonary

Respiratory depression can occur due to muscle weakness.

Gastrointestinal

Vomiting can occur with overdose.

Hepatic

Hepatitis has been reported.

Musculoskeletal

- Dystonic reactions may occur.
- In large overdoses muscle paralysis may occur.

Neurologic

- Somnolence progressing to coma occurs with overdose.
- Tremors, hallucinations, and seizures also have been reported.

PROCEDURES AND LABORATORY TESTS

Essential Tests

No tests may be needed in asymptomatic patients.

Recommended Tests

- Serum electrolytes, BUN, creatinine, glucose, and other studies may be needed to evaluate other causes of altered mental status.
- Pulse oximetry or arterial blood gases are performed to evaluate oxygenation in symptomatic patients.
- ECG is used to evaluate for widened QRS complex interval.
- Serum acetaminophen and aspirin levels are obtained in an overdose setting to detect occult ingestion.

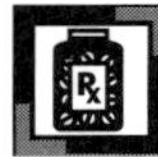

Treatment

- Supportive care is the mainstay of therapy.
- Dose and time of exposure should be determined for all substances involved.

DIRECTING PATIENT COURSE

The health-care professional should call the poison control center when:

- Severe or persistent effects develop.
- Coingestant, drug interaction, or underlying disease presents an unusual problem.

The patient should be referred to a health-care facility when:

- Suicide or homicide attempt is possible.
- Toxic effects develop.
- Coingestant, drug interaction, or underlying disease presents an unusual problem.

Admission Considerations

Extended observation or hospital admission is rarely needed, but would be appropriate for CNS depression or cardiovascular effects.

DECONTAMINATION

Out of Hospital

Induction of emesis is not recommended.

In Hospital

- Gastric lavage should be performed in pediatric (tube size 24–32 French) or adult (tube size 36–42 French) patients presenting within 1 hour of a large ingestion or if serious effects are present.
- One dose of activated charcoal (1–2 g/kg) should be administered without a cathartic if a substantial ingestion has occurred within the previous few hours.

ANTIDOTES

There is no specific antidote available for trimethobenzamide poisoning.

ADJUNCTIVE TREATMENT

Seizures

- Patent airway must be maintained.
- A benzodiazepine should be administered for initial control.
- If seizures persist or recur, another anticonvulsant such as phenobarbital can be added.

Dystonic Reactions

- These should be treated with diphenhydramine 25 to 50 mg intravenously, intramuscularly, or orally, every 6 hours.
- Patients should have oral treatment continued for 3 to 5 days to prevent recurrence.

Hypotension

- Atropine can be used to correct hypotension related to bradycardia.
- Patient should receive 10 to 20 ml/kg 0.9% saline intravenously and be placed in the Trendelenburg position.
- Further fluid therapy should be guided by central pressure monitoring to avoid volume overload.
- Vasopressor may be added if needed.

—Dopamine. 2 to 5 μg/kg/min should be infused intravenously and titrated upward to effect.
—Rates above 20 μg/kg/min is unlikely to offer additional benefit.
—If pressure is unresponsive, norepinephrine (0.1–0.2 μg/kg/min) may be added and titrated upward to effect.
—High infusion rates may cause tissue ischemia.

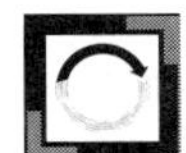

Follow-Up

PATIENT MONITORING

Patients with symptoms should be placed on a cardiac monitor, given oxygen, and have intravenous access established.

EXPECTED COURSE AND PROGNOSIS

Anticholinergic effects peak within hours, but may require 24 hours or more for resolution.

DISCHARGE CRITERIA/INSTRUCTIONS

- From emergency department. Asymptomatic patients with normal vital signs can be discharged after decontamination, 4 to 6 hours of observation, and psychiatric evaluation, if needed.
- From hospital. Patients may be discharged when capable of caring for themselves and following psychiatric evaluation, if needed.

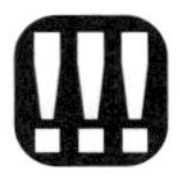

Pitfalls

TREATMENT

Failure to treat dystonic reactions for 3 to 5 days may allow recurrence.

ICD-9-CM 973

Poisoning by agents primarily affecting the gastrointestinal system.

See also: SECTION II, Hypotension and Seizures chapters.

RECOMMENDED READING

POISINDEX editorial staff. Trimethobenzamide. In: Rumack BH, Sayre NK, Gelman CR, eds. *POISINDEX system.* Englewood, CO: Micromedex, Inc. (edition expires May 31, 1998).

Author: Kennon Heard

Reviewer: Richard C. Dart

Valproic Acid

Basics

DESCRIPTION

Valproic acid is used to treat seizure disorders, bipolar affective disorder, and migraine headache.

FORMS AND USES

Pharmaceutical preparations of valproic acid include sodium valproate (Depakene) and divalproex sodium (Depakote).

- For seizures, the adult starting dosage is 15 mg/kg/day orally in one to three divided doses, increasing to a maximum of 60 mg/kg/day over several weeks.
- For migraine, the adult dosage is 250 to 1,000 mg/day orally.
- For mania, the starting dosage for adults is 750 mg/day, titrated up to a maximum dose of 60 mg/kg/day divided into three doses per day.

TOXIC DOSE

- Toxic effects may begin at doses near therapeutic levels in drug-naive individuals.
- Coma has occurred in children ingesting more than 200 mg/kg, and death has been reported in a 20-month-old who ingested 750 mg/kg.

PATHOPHYSIOLOGY

Both therapeutic and toxic mechanisms are poorly characterized; valproic acid may increase brain concentrations of gamma-aminobutyric acid.

EPIDEMIOLOGY

- Poisoning is uncommon.
- The toxic effects that follow exposure are typically mild, with death occurring after a massive overdose or due to a coingestant.

CAUSES

- Usually ingestion is intentional.
- Child neglect should be considered if the patient is less than 1 year of age; attempted suicide in patients over 6 years of age.

RISK FACTORS

Patients with underlying cardiovascular disease may be predisposed to more severe cardiovascular effects.

DRUG AND DISEASE INTERACTIONS

- Coingestion with other sedative, hypnotic, or anticonvulsant drugs will increase CNS depressant effects.
- Therapeutic administration with cimetidine, ranitidine, aspirin, and isoniazid may increase valproate levels.
- Coadministration with other anticonvulsants may increase concentration of the valproate metabolite and cause liver injury.

PREGNANCY AND LACTATION

- US FDA Pregnancy Category D. Evidence of human fetal risk exists, but benefits in certain situations (e.g., life-threatening situations or serious diseases) may make use of the drug acceptable despite its risks.
- Valproic acid is a known human teratogen and has been associated with an increased risk of spina bifida (1%–2%) and minor craniofacial abnormalities.

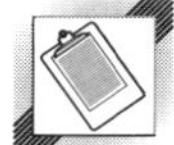

Diagnosis

DIFFERENTIAL DIAGNOSIS

- Toxic causes of CNS depression include barbiturates, other anticonvulsants, ethanol, and sedative-hypnotics, among many others.
- Other causes include metabolic or electrolyte derangements, CNS mass or bleed, and infection.

SIGNS AND SYMPTOMS

- Mild CNS depression is common, progressing in serious cases to coma, respiratory depression, and hypotension.
- Fever occurs rarely.

HEENT

Pinpoint pupils have been reported but are uncommon.

Cardiovascular

- Cardiac arrest may occur with a severe overdose, usually secondary to respiratory failure.
- Profound hypotension may occur with a severe overdose.

Pulmonary

Respiratory failure may occur with a severe overdose.

Gastrointestinal

Pancreatitis has been noted after a severe overdose and may also occur during chronic therapeutic use.

Hepatic

- Hepatitis may develop during chronic therapeutic use and may occasionally be fatal.
- Hepatitis occurs primarily in children during their first 6 months of therapy with multiple anticonvulsants.
- Mild elevations in hepatic enzymes occur rarely after acute overdose.

Renal

Acute renal failure occurs rarely, probably due to hypotension.

Hematologic

- Bone marrow depression (anemia, thrombocytopenia, and leukopenia) occurs rarely after an overdose.
- Leukopenia may develop during chronic therapeutic use.

Fluids and Electrolytes

Hypernatremia and hypocalcemia are rare effects after an acute overdose.

Neurologic

- CNS depression is common after an overdose and ranges from lethargy to coma.
- Hypertonia and seizures have been reported after an overdose.
- Parkinsonism and cerebellar atrophy have been reported with chronic use.

Acid-Base

Metabolic acidosis occurs rarely, probably due to hypotension.

PROCEDURES AND LABORATORY TESTS

Essential Tests

Valproic acid level:

- The therapeutic level is 50 to 100 μg/ml.
- Acute toxicity may develop above 100 μg/ml.

Recommended Tests

- Serum electrolytes, glucose, BUN, creatinine to assess altered mental status or presence of metabolic acidosis
- Pulse oximetry and arterial blood gases in symptomatic patients to assess hypoxia and metabolic acidosis
- Serum levels of other anticonvulsants to assess CNS depression
- Complete blood count, platelet count, and serum amylase to assess bone marrow depression and pancreatitis after a severe overdose
- ECG, serum acetaminophen, and aspirin levels in an overdose setting to detect occult overdose
- Other tests (serum ethanol, urine toxicology screen, lumbar puncture, and bacterial cultures) as needed to rule out other causes of CNS depression
- Chest radiograph in patients with hypoxia, coma, respiratory depression or suspected aspiration
- Head CT as needed to rule out other causes of CNS depression

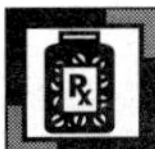

Treatment

- Treatment should focus on airway management and support of hemodynamic function.
- The dose and time of exposure should be determined for all substances that could be involved.

DIRECTING PATIENT COURSE

The health-care provider should call the poison control center when:

- Coma, respiratory depression, hypotension, or other severe effects are present.
- Toxic effects are not consistent with valproic acid poisoning.
- Coingestant, drug interaction, or underlying disease presents an unusual problem.

A patient should be referred to a health-care facility when:

- Attempted suicide or homicide is possible.
- Patient or caregiver seems unreliable.
- Toxic effects are present.
- Coingestant, drug interaction, or underlying disease presents an unusual problem.

Admission Considerations

ICU treatment is warranted in patients with altered mental status or hemodynamic instability.

DECONTAMINATION

Out of Hospital

Emesis should not be induced because CNS depression may develop.

In Hospital

- Gastric lavage should be performed in pediatric (tube size 24–32 French) or adult (tube size 36–42 French) patients presenting within 1 hour of a large ingestion or if serious effects are present.
- A dose of activated charcoal (1–2 g/kg) should be administered without a cathartic if a substantial ingestion has occurred within the previous few hours.
- Hemodialysis

—Valproic acid is highly protein bound, but the percentage of unbound drug increases substantially at toxic levels.
—Hemodialysis has been used in case reports, but hemodialysis clearance rates have not been reported.
—Routine use of hemodialysis is not recommended, but it may be of use in patients with severe intoxication and hemodynamic instability.

- Hemoperfusion. Routine use of hemoperfusion is not recommended, but it may be of use in patients with severe intoxication with hemodynamic instability.
- Multiple-dose activated charcoal

—Case reports suggest that its use shortens elimination half-life, but no controlled studies have been undertaken.
—Routine use is not recommended, but one or two additional doses of activated charcoal without a cathartic should be used if valproate levels are increasing.

- Whole-bowel irrigation is recommended in patients with increasing serum levels despite gastric decontamination, particularly after ingestion of enteric-coated or divalproex containing products.

ANTIDOTES

There are no specific antidotes for valproic acid toxicity.

ADJUNCTIVE TREATMENT

Naloxone is reported to reverse CNS depression in some cases of valproic acid overdose, but results have been inconsistent. The usual initial adult dose is 2 mg by intravenous push.

Hypotension

- Use atropine first if hypotension is related to bradycardia.
- The patient should be given 10 to 20 ml/kg 0.9% saline and placed in the Trendelenburg position.
- Further fluid therapy should be guided by central pressure monitoring to avoid volume overload.
- A vasopressor may be added if needed.

Seizures

After assuring airway patency, a benzodiazepine should be administered for initial control. If seizures persist or recur, another anticonvulsant can be added, such as phenobarbital.

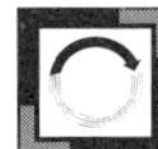

Follow-Up

PATIENT MONITORING

- Respiratory and cardiac parameters in symptomatic patients should be monitored continuously.
- Sequelae of prolonged hypotension or hypoxia occur rarely.

EXPECTED COURSE AND PROGNOSIS

Most patients recover within 24 to 48 hours; however, patients with severe hypotension and CNS depression may require 4 to 5 days or longer to recover.

DISCHARGE CRITERIA/INSTRUCTIONS

- From the emergency department

—Asymptomatic patients with decreasing serum levels after decontamination and 6 to 8 hours of observation should be discharged.
—Psychiatric evaluation should be completed, if appropriate.

- From the hospital

—Patient may be discharged when hypotension and respiratory depression have resolved, CNS depression has improved, and serum levels are decreasing.
—Psychiatric evaluation should be completed, if appropriate.

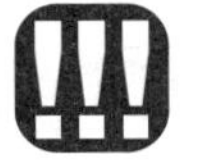

Pitfalls

DIAGNOSIS

Peak serum levels and the onset of symptoms may be delayed 8 hours or longer after ingestion of divalproex sodium.

ICD-9-CM 968

Poisoning by other central nervous system depressants and anesthetics.

See also: SECTION II, Hypotension and Seizures chapters; and SECTION III, Whole-Bowel Irrigation chapter.

RECOMMENDED READING

Dupois RE, Lichtman SN, Pollack GM. Acute valproic acid overdose: clinical course and pharmacokinetic disposition of valproic acid and metabolites. *Drug Safety* 1990;5:65–71.

Osborn H. Anticonvulsants. In: *Goldfrank's toxicologic emergencies,* 6th ed. Norwalk, CT: Appleton & Lange, 1998.

Author: Katherine M. Hurlbut

Reviewer: Richard C. Dart

Vinyl Chloride

Basics

DESCRIPTION

Vinyl chloride monomer (vinyl chloride, chloroethylene, chloroethene) is a highly flammable, colorless gas with a sweet odor. It is usually handled and transported as a liquid under its own vapor pressure and is used to manufacture protective clothing, medical equipment, car parts, adhesives, and methylchloroform. It is involved in the production of polyvinyl chloride.

FORMS AND USES

Vinyl chloride is ubiquitous in industry in many forms and as the component of many other chemicals.

TOXIC DOSE

Inhalation of a 10,000-ppm concentration may cause symptoms; inhalation of a concentration over 120,000 ppm may cause death.

PATHOPHYSIOLOGY

- The vinyl chloride monomer is thought to be the cause of interstitial pulmonary disease.
- The polymer is essentially nontoxic.

EPIDEMIOLOGY

Poisoning is uncommon.

CAUSES

- Exposure is typically occupational in origin.
- Chronic occupational exposure has been associated with acroosteolysis and hepatic angiosarcoma with latencies of 1–2 years and 20 years, respectively.

WORKPLACE STANDARDS

- ACGIH. TLV TWA is 5 ppm; no STEL.
- OSHA. PEL TWA is 1 ppm; ceiling is 5 ppm.
- NIOSH. IDLH not determined.

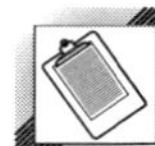

Diagnosis

DIFFERENTIAL DIAGNOSIS

- Toxic causes of interstitial pulmonary disease include asbestosis, silicosis, and paraquat poisoning.
- Nontoxic causes include connective tissue disease and infectious pneumonitis.

SIGNS AND SYMPTOMS

The primary acute health risk is respiratory depression.

HEENT

Vinyl chloride spray can cause frostbite.

Dermatologic

- Chronic exposure may cause acroosteolysis.
- Primary triad of Raynaud's phenomenon, osteolysis in the terminal phalanges of the fingers, and scleroderma-like lesions (thickening of the skin or raised nodules) on the hands and forearm may be present.

Cardiovascular

Ventricular dysrhythmias have occurred after large exposure.

Pulmonary

- Pulmonary effects include dyspnea, asthma, and pneumoconiosis.
- Chronic interstitial disease, independent from pneumoconiosis, also may occur.

Hepatic

Chronic exposure may cause hepatic injury, enlargement, and increased incidence of hepatic angiosarcoma.

Neurologic

Headache, ataxia, euphoria, visual disturbances, paresthesia, and CNS depression leading to death from respiratory failure are possible.

Reproductive

Loss of libido and decreased sperm count are possible during chronic exposure.

PROCEDURES AND LABORATORY TESTS

Essential Tests

No tests may be needed for asymptomatic patients with acute exposure.

Recommended Tests

- Complete blood count, serum electrolytes, glucose, BUN, creatinine, and liver enzymes should be obtained for symptomatic patients.
- Arterial blood gases or pulse oximetry should be determined if respiratory symptoms develop.
- Hand radiographs are used to assess acroosteolysis in patients with chronic exposure.

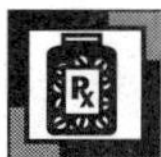

Treatment

Following acute exposure, treatment should focus on airway management and general supportive care.

DIRECTING PATIENT COURSE

The health-care professional should call the poison control center when:

- Severe or persistent effects develop.
- Underlying disease presents an unusual problem.

The patient should be referred to a health-care facility when:

- Toxic effects develop.
- Underlying disease presents an unusual problem.

Admission Considerations

Any patient with tachypnea, chest pain, or hypoxia should be admitted.

DECONTAMINATION

- For dermal exposure, the affected area should be washed thoroughly with soap and water.
- For inhalational exposure, remove the patient from source of exposure and administer oxygen.

ANTIDOTES

There are no specific antidotes for vinyl chloride poisoning.

ADJUNCTIVE TREATMENT

- Frostbite should be treated in the standard fashion.
- Acute inhalational syndrome involves symptomatic treatment of respiratory tract irritation, pneumonitis and depression.
- Chronic exposure

—Provide general supportive care and symptomatic treatment of Raynaud's phenomenon and scleroderma-like skin lesions.

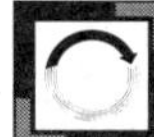

Follow-Up

PATIENT MONITORING

- Proper authorities should be notified, source of exposure identified, and exposure terminated.
- Other exposed individuals should be evaluated.

EXPECTED COURSE AND PROGNOSIS

Outcome is dependent on concentration of solution and length of time and exposure.

DISCHARGE CRITERIA/INSTRUCTIONS

Asymptomatic patients may be discharged from the emergency department or hospital after a 6-hour observation period and following decontamination.

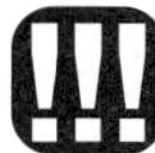

Pitfalls

DIAGNOSIS

- As is the case with all occupation-related illnesses, other individuals may be exposed and become symptomatic.
- Acroosteolysis and hepatic angiosarcoma are rare diseases and should be considered sentinal cases.

ICD-9-CM 987

Toxic effect of other gases, fumes, or vapors.

RECOMMENDED READING

Cordasco EM, Demeter SZ, Uerkay J, et al. Pulmonary manifestations of vinyl and polyvinyl chloride (interstitial lung disease). *Chest* 1980;78:828–834.

Danziger H. Accidental poisoning by vinyl chloride. *Can Med Assoc J* 1960;82:828–830.

Author: Luke Yip

Reviewer: Gerald F. O'Malley

Vitamin A and Retinoids

Basics

DESCRIPTION

Vitamin A is a commonly available dietary supplement.

FORMS AND USES

- Substances include vitamin A and various retinoids (Aquasol A, Materna, Megadose, ACES, Lazer, Vi-Daylin), etretinate (Tegason), acitretin (Tigason), isotretinoin (Accutane), and tretinoin (Renova, Retin A, Vesanoid).
- Isotretinoin (Accutane) is used to treat nodulocystic acne unresponsive to conventional therapy.
- Etretinate (Tegason) and acitretin (Tigason) are used to treat severe psoriasis unresponsive to standard therapies and other disorders of dyskeratinization.
- Tretinoin (Renova, Retin A, Vesanoid) is used to treat acne vulgaris, fine wrinkles, mottled hyperpigmentation, tactile facial skin roughness, and acute promyelocytic leukemia.

TOXIC DOSE

- Acute ingestion of 300,000 U of vitamin A is toxic to children.
- Adult toxicity may be produced by an acute ingestion of 4 million U (pregnant women should not exceed 8,000 U/day).
- Chronic ingestion above 25,000 U/day may produce toxicity.
- Toxicity has not been reported from beta carotene ingestion.
- Retinoic acid syndrome may occur in the treatment of leukemia at 45 mg/m^2.

PATHOPHYSIOLOGY

Carotene is converted to vitamin A in the body.

EPIDEMIOLOGY

Poisoning is uncommon.

CAUSES

Child neglect or abuse should be considered if the patient is less than 1 year of age, suicide attempt if the patient is over 6 years of age.

PREGNANCY AND LACTATION

- Beta carotene. US FDA Category C. The drug exerts animal teratogenic or embryocidal effects, but there are no controlled studies in women, or no studies are available in animals or women.
- Etretinate. US FDA Category X. Studies in animals or humans have demonstrated fetal abnormalities or there is evidence of fetal risk based on human experience, or both, and the risk clearly outweighs any possible benefit.
- Tretinoin. US FDA Category B. Animal studies indicate no fetal risk and there are no controlled human studies, or animal studies show an adverse fetal effect but well-controlled studies in women do not.
- Vitamin A (do not exceed 8,000 U/day). US FDA Category A. Controlled studies in women fail to demonstrate a risk to the fetus in the first trimester, and the possibility of fetal harm appears remote.
- Excretion in breast milk is small until massive doses are ingested by the mother.

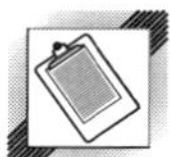

Diagnosis

SIGNS AND SYMPTOMS

- Target organs for vitamin A are the CNS and liver.
- Tretinoin produces toxic effects similar to those seen with vitamin A, except for retinoic acid syndrome, which is characterized by fever, dyspnea, infiltrates, and pleural or pericardial effusions developing during therapy of leukemia.
- In retinoic acid syndrome, the patient also may have liver or renal injury culminating in death.

HEENT

Double vision and papilledema may occur.

Dermatologic

Dryness, seborrhea, pruritus, and generalized desquamation may be present.

Hepatic

Patient may exhibit increased transaminase levels, jaundice, and hepatic fibrosis.

Hematologic

Coagulopathy may occur in patients with liver injury.

Fluids and Electrolytes

Hypercalcemia is possible.

Neurologic

- Anorexia, vomiting, headache, irritability, CNS depression, and pseudotumor cerebri may occur.
- Seizures occur rarely.

PROCEDURES AND LABORATORY TESTS

Essential Tests

No tests are usually needed in asymptomatic patients who have ingested less than 300,000 U of vitamin A.

Recommended Tests

- Complete blood count, serum electrolytes, BUN, creatinine, calcium, liver function tests, prothrombin time, international normalized ratio, and bone radiography
- Bone radiography to show osteopenia and periosteal new bone growth in children
- Chest radiography in patient with pulmonary symptoms
- Vitamin A level to help establish diagnosis (does not affect management)

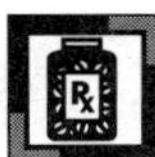

Treatment

- Supportive care and termination of exposure are the mainstay of therapy.
- Dose and time of exposure should be determined for all substances involved.

DIRECTING PATIENT COURSE

The health-care professional should call the poison control center when:

- Toxic amount may have been ingested.
- Severe or persistent effects develop.
- Coingestant, drug interaction, or underlying disease presents an unusual problem.

The patient should be referred to a health-care facility when:

- Suicide or homicide attempt is possible.
- Toxic effects develop.
- Coingestant, drug interaction, or underlying disease presents an unusual problem.

Admission Considerations

Inpatient management is warranted if CNS depression, hypotension, or cardiac dysrhythmias develop.

DECONTAMINATION

Out of Hospital

Emesis should be induced with ipecac within 1 hour of ingestion for alert pediatric or adult patients if health-care evaluation will be delayed.

In Hospital

- Gastric lavage should be performed in pediatric (tube size 24–32 French) or adult (tube size 36–42 French) patients presenting within 1 hour of a large ingestion or if serious effects are present.
- One dose of activated charcoal (1–2 g/kg) should be administered without a cathartic if a substantial ingestion has occurred within the previous few hours.

ANTIDOTES

There is no specific antidote for vitamin A or tretinoin poisoning.

ADJUNCTIVE TREATMENT

Naloxone has been recommended but is often ineffective for CNS depression caused by vitamin A.

- The initial dose is 2 mg intravenously.
- If no improvement is noted, the dose is doubled to 4 mg intravenously.
- If no improvement is noted, more naloxone is unlikely to be effective.

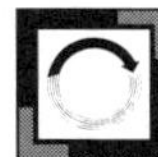

Follow-Up

EXPECTED COURSE AND PROGNOSIS

Effect may not begin to resolve for several days due to lipophilic nature of compounds.

DISCHARGE CRITERIA/INSTRUCTIONS

Patients may be discharged from the emergency department or hospital when toxic effects resolve or stabilize and after psychiatric evaluation, if needed.

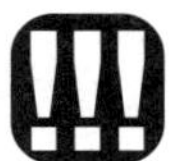

Pitfalls

DIAGNOSIS

Unusual dietary sources should be investigated. Polar bear liver may contain lethal levels of vitamin A.

ICD-9-CM 963.5

Poisoning by primarily systemic agents: vitamins, not elsewhere classified.

See also: SECTION III, Naloxone chapter.

Author: Chris Fleming

Reviewer: Richard C. Dart

Water Hemlock

Basics

DESCRIPTION

Water hemlock (*Cicuta maculata, C. douglasii*) is a poisonous plant of the carrot family.

FORMS AND USES

- Water hemlock grows in swampy areas (e.g., irrigation ditches) near bodies of water.
- Other names for water hemlock are beaver poison, *carotte à moreau,* cowbane, false parsley, false parsnip, poison parsnip, snake root, snake weed, spotted cowbane, spotted parsley, wild carrot, and wild parsnip.

TOXIC DOSE

One small bite is sufficient to produce serious toxicity in an adult or child.

PATHOPHYSIOLOGY

- Cicutoxin, the primary toxin in water hemlock, is found in all portions of the plant and is most concentrated in the roots.
- Although its mechanism of action is unclear, cicutoxin is thought to cause overstimulation of central cholinergic pathways.

EPIDEMIOLOGY

- Poisoning is rare.
- Toxic effects following exposure are typically severe, with death occurring in 30% to 70% of ingestions.

CAUSES

- Poisoning is usually the result of the accidental ingestion of water hemlock misidentified as an edible root (e.g., wild carrot, Jerusalem artichoke).
- Child neglect or abuse should be considered if the patient is less than 1 year of age.

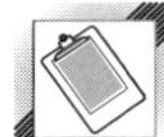

Diagnosis

DIFFERENTIAL DIAGNOSIS

- Other plants known to cause seizures include poison hemlock (*Conium maculatum*), tobacco (nicotine), and false morel mushroom.
- Other causes may include organophosphate pesticides and isonicotinic acid hydrazide.

SIGNS AND SYMPTOMS

Severe gastroenteritis develops within 30 to 60 minutes and is quickly followed by diaphoresis, dizziness, weakness, seizures, and coma.

Vital Signs

Tachycardia, bradycardia, and hypertension may occur during seizures. Status epilepticus may cause cardiopulmonary arrest.

HEENT

Mydriasis, blurred vision, and salivation may occur.

Dermatologic

Pallor or flushing, as well as diaphoresis, may be seen.

Cardiovascular

Tachycardia and hypertension may be seen early; cardiac arrest and hypotension may occur in severe cases.

Pulmonary

Respiratory arrest or pulmonary edema may result from prolonged seizure activity.

Gastrointestinal

Nausea, vomiting, diarrhea, and abdominal cramping are common.

Hepatic

Liver function test elevation has been reported.

Renal

Acute tubular necrosis may develop from dehydration, hypotension, or rhabdomyolysis.

Hematologic

Coagulopathy may develop.

Fluids and Electrolytes

Metabolic acidosis may ensue as a result of seizure activity and suggests severe intoxication.

Musculoskeletal

Rhabdomyolysis may develop due to seizure activity.

Neurologic

Altered mental status may occur, ranging from lethargy and confusion to coma and status epilepticus.

PROCEDURES AND LABORATORY TESTS

Essential Tests

Laboratory testing may not be needed in asymptomatic patients.

Recommended Tests

- Serum electrolytes, glucose, BUN, and creatinine should be measured to detect metabolic acidosis (which suggests severe intoxication).
- Arterial blood gas is used to assess oxygenation and acid-base status in symptomatic patients.
- Liver function, coagulation studies, and serum creatine kinase may be elevated in patients with protracted seizures.
- Unless water hemlock is confirmed as the toxin responsible, an altered mental status workup, including head CT and lumbar puncture, should be pursued to rule out other causes of seizures.
- A chest radiograph may be helpful to rule out aspiration.

Not Recommended Tests

Testing for cicutoxin in blood or urine is not clinically helpful.

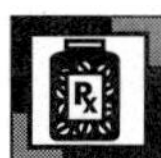

Treatment

- Treatment should focus on maintaining an adequate airway, on oxygenation, and on the immediate treatment of seizures.
- The dose and time of exposure should be determined for all substances involved.

DIRECTING PATIENT COURSE

The health-care provider should call the poison control center when:

- Seizures or other severe effects are present.
- Toxic effects are not consistent with water hemlock poisoning.
- Coingestant or underlying disease presents an unusual problem.

The patient should be referred to a health-care facility when:

- Attempted suicide or homicide is possible.
- Patient or caregiver seems unreliable.
- Toxic effects develop.
- Coingestant or underlying disease presents an unusual problem.

Admission Considerations

Inpatient treatment is warranted when patients develop refractory vomiting, seizures, or altered mental status.

DECONTAMINATION

Out of Hospital

Emesis should not be induced due to the potential for seizures.

In Hospital

- Gastric lavage should be performed in pediatric (tube size 24–32 French) or adult (tube size 36–42 French) patients presenting within 1 hour of a large ingestion or if serious effects are present.
- One dose of activated charcoal (1–2 g/kg) should be administered without a cathartic if a substantial ingestion has occurred within the previous few hours.

ANTIDOTES

There is no specific antidote for water hemlock poisoning.

ADJUNCTIVE TREATMENT

Seizure

- Because water hemlock-induced seizures can be protracted and refractory to treatment, aggressive seizure control with one or more anticonvulsants is recommended.
- Rapid sequence induction and endotracheal intubation are often needed.
- Adequate airway and oxygenation must be ensured.

—Benzodiazepine should be administered for initial control.
—Diazepam. Adult dose is 5 to 10 mg initially, repeated every 10 minutes if needed; pediatric dose is 0.2 to 0.5 mg/kg, repeated every 10 minutes if needed.
—Lorazepam. Adult dose is 2 to 4 mg intravenous push over 2 to 5 minutes, repeated every 10 minutes if needed; pediatric dose is 0.1 mg/kg intravenous push over 2 to 5 minutes, not to exceed 4 mg/dose. The dose can be repeated every 10 minutes if necessary.

- The need for intubation should be closely monitored.
- If seizures persist or recur, another anticonvulsant should be added, such as phenobarbital.
- Other options for repeated seizures despite therapy include neuromuscular blockade with EEG monitoring and general anesthesia.

Hypotension

Hypotension should be treated with isotonic fluid infusion (10–20 cc/kg), Trendelenburg positioning, and a vasopressor if needed (preferably dopamine); norepinephrine is used for refractory hypotension.

Rhabdomyolysis

Seizures should be terminated as quickly as possible, and adequate hydration and urine output (1–2 ml/kg/h) should be ensured.

Not Recommended Therapies

The use of anticholinergic agents has not been shown to be beneficial in animal models of water hemlock poisoning.

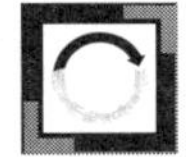

Follow-Up

PATIENT MONITORING

Electrolytes and hemodynamic and pulmonary functions should be monitored continuously during acute illness.

EXPECTED COURSE AND PROGNOSIS

- If patients are successfully supported through their seizures, recovery is common.
- Possible complications include cerebral injury, secondary to protracted seizures and/or hypoxia, acute renal failure from rhabdomyolysis, and aspiration pneumonia.

DISCHARGE CRITERIA/INSTRUCTIONS

- From the emergency department

—Asymptomatic patients with normal mental status may be discharged following decontamination and observation for 4 to 6 hours.
—All patients with seizures should be admitted.

- From the hospital. The patient may be discharged after seizures have resolved, mental status has returned to baseline, and laboratory values normalize.

PATIENT EDUCATION

Because most water hemlock poisonings are the result of the ingestion of a misidentified plant, education could be an effective preventive measure.

Pitfalls

DIAGNOSIS

- The patient's history of wild plant ingestion is essential in making a diagnosis.
- Nontoxicologic etiologies for seizures or altered mental status should be ruled out as well.

TREATMENT

- Early airway management is essential.
- Seizures may be difficult to control and often require more than one anticonvulsive agent or neuromuscular blockade.

ICD-9-CM 988.2

Toxic effect of noxious substances eaten as food: berries and other plants.

See also: SECTION II, Hypotension and Seizures chapters.

RECOMMENDED READING

Landers D, Seppi K, Blauer W. Seizures and death on white river float trip. *West J Med* 1985;142:637–640.

Starreveld E, Hope CE. Cicutoxin poisoning (water hemlock). *Neurology* 1975;25:730–734.

Author: Edward W. Cetaruk

Reviewer: Luke Yip

Zinc

Basics

DESCRIPTION

Zinc is an element used as both a medication and in occupational settings.

FORMS AND USES

- Substances include metallic zinc, zinc gluconate, zinc chloride, and zinc sulfate.
- Zinc is an essential dietary supplement, and zinc gluconate has been used as a symptomatic treatment for colds.
- See SECTION II, Metal Fume Fever chapter, for respiratory effects of zinc alloys; see SECTION IV, Phosphine chapter, for zinc phosphide.

TOXIC DOSE

- Ingestion of 10 to 30 g of zinc sulfate has resulted in death.
- Massive ingestion of zinc gluconate has caused little toxicity.

PATHOPHYSIOLOGY

- The toxicity of zinc salts (zinc chloride, sulfate) is expressed primarily in gastrointestinal corrosiveness and pulmonary irritation.
- Zinc phosphide may release phosphine gas when mixed with gastric contents.
- Zinc supplements appear to interfere with copper absorption.

EPIDEMIOLOGY

- Poisoning is uncommon.
- Toxic effects are mild unless a zinc salt is involved.

CAUSES

Most ingestions are suicidal.

WORKPLACE STANDARDS

For zinc chloride:

- ACGIH. TLV TWA is 1 mg/m^3 (fume); STEL is 2 mg/m^3.
- OSHA. PEL TWA is 1 mg/m^3
- NIOSH. IDLH level is 50 mg/m^3.

Data for other zinc compounds are not available.

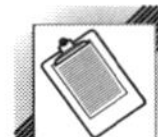

Diagnosis

DIFFERENTIAL DIAGNOSIS

Toxic causes of acute gastroenteritis includes arsenic, mercuric chloride, caustic agents, and many others.

SIGNS AND SYMPTOMS

- The severity of the symptoms is related to the form of zinc salt involved and the route of exposure.
- In general, zinc chloride is the most corrosive, followed by phosphide, and sulfate.
- Inhalation causes pulmonary irritation and may result in severe pulmonary edema; ingestion causes corrosive gastrointestinal effects.

Vital Signs

Tachypnea can occur with pulmonary irritation.

HEENT

Eye, nasal, and oral irritation can occur.

Dermatologic

Skin irritation is common with dermal exposure to zinc salts.

Pulmonary

Inhalation of zinc salts causes pulmonary irritation and may progress to edema in severe cases.

Gastrointestinal

- Nausea and vomiting are common in overdose and can occur with large therapeutic doses.
- Serious corrosive injury can occur, particularly with chloride or sulfate salts.

Renal

Renal failure and nephritis have been reported after ingestion of caustic zinc salts.

Hematologic

Anemia due to copper deficiency has been reported with chronic ingestion.

Neurologic

CNS depression can occur with zinc ingestion.

PROCEDURES AND LABORATORY TESTS

Essential Tests

No tests may be needed for asymptomatic patients following ingestion of zinc gluconate.

Recommended Tests

- Complete blood count (CBC), serum electrolytes, BUN, and creatinine should be monitored in patients with significant gastrointestinal fluid loss or bleeding.
- Patients with pulmonary symptoms should have chest radiographs and assessment of oxygenation.
- ECG, serum acetaminophen and aspirin levels should be screened in an overdose setting to detect occult ingestion.
- Patients on chronic high-dose zinc therapy should have a CBC to evaluate for possible anemia.
- Metallic zinc and zinc salts are usually seen on radiographs.
- Gastrointestinal endoscopy for caustic effects may be needed for patients with gastrointestinal toxicity.
- Zinc levels are of little use clinically.

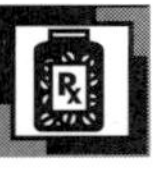

Treatment

- Supportive care is the mainstay of therapy.
- Dose and time of exposure should be determined for all substances involved.

DIRECTING PATIENT COURSE

The health-care professional should call the poison control center when:

- Severe or persistent effects develop.
- Coingestant, drug interaction, or underlying disease presents an unusual problem.

The patient should be referred to a health-care facility when:

- Suicide or homicide attempt is possible.
- Toxic effects develop.
- Coingestant, drug interaction, or underlying disease presents an unusual problem.

Admission Considerations

Patients with vomiting or evidence of end organ injury following any type of zinc ingestion should be admitted for evaluation.

DECONTAMINATION

Out of Hospital

Patients ingesting zinc chloride should be given 100 to 200 cc of water to dilute the products.

In Hospital

- Zinc sulfate ingestion should be treated with lavage and whole-bowel irrigation if ingestion was recent and there is no evidence of acute caustic injury.
- Zinc gluconate ingestion should be treated via lavage only after a massive ingestion.
- Gastric lavage should be performed in pediatric (tube size 24 to 32 French) or adult (tube size 36 to 42 French) patients for large ingestion presenting within 1 hour of ingestion or if serious effects are present.

ANTIDOTES

There is no specific antidote available for zinc poisoning.

ADJUNCTIVE TREATMENT

- Bronchospasm or respiratory tract irritation are treated with humidified oxygen and bronchodilators as needed.
- Patients with copper deficiency should receive copper supplementation and should discontinue zinc supplements.
- Calcium EDTA has been used to treat patients with significant CNS depression after zinc chloride ingestion, but is of questionable value.
- Steroid therapy is of unproven benefit in caustic burns of this type, but have been recommended for specific types of alkaline corrosive burns.

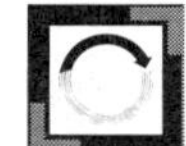

Follow-Up

PATIENT MONITORING

- Cardiac and respiratory function should be monitored continuously in symptomatic patients.
- Patients should be placed on a cardiac monitor, on oxygen, and have intravenous access established.

EXPECTED COURSE AND PROGNOSIS

- Zinc gluconate produces few effects, and complete recovery is expected.
- Zinc chloride may result in caustic injury and may leave sequelae of strictures and esophageal dysfunction.

DISCHARGE CRITERIA/INSTRUCTIONS

- From emergency department. Patients with adequate decontamination, minimal symptoms, and normal mental status and vital signs for 4 hours of observation may be discharged following psychiatric evaluation, if needed.
- From hospital. Patient may be discharged following evaluation and stabilization of caustic injury.

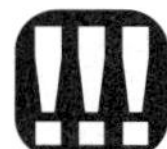

Pitfalls

DIAGNOSIS

- Failure to realize ingestion of zinc salts can result in significant gastrointestinal burns.
- Patients with vomiting, drooling, stridor, or refusal to take oral fluids should undergo endoscopy.

FOLLOW-UP

Failure to admit patients with inhalation exposure who remain symptomatic in the emergency department can result in deterioration.

ICD-9-CM 97

Poisoning by other and unspecified drugs and medicinal substances.

See also: SECTION II, Metal Fume Fever chapter; and SECTION IV, Caustics—Acidic and Phosphine chapters.

RECOMMENDED READING

POISINDEX editorial staff. Zinc compounds. In: Rumack BH, Sayre NK, Gelman CR, eds. *POISINDEX system.* Englewood, CO: Micromedex, Inc. (edition expires November 30, 1997).

Author: Kennon Heard

Reviewer: Richard C. Dart

Zolpidem

Basics

DESCRIPTION

Zolpidem is a short-acting hypnotic agent used as a sleep aid.

FORMS AND USES

- Preparations include zolpidem (Ambien).
- Typical dose is 10 mg orally.

TOXIC DOSE

Toxic dose is poorly defined; ingestion of several times the daily dose has caused only mild CNS depression.

PATHOPHYSIOLOGY

- Zolpidem is a short-acting hypnotic agent that acts at specific CNS benzodiazepine receptors.
- Two deaths have been reported; one patient ingested a combination of zolpidem, carisoprodol, and meprobamate, and the other patient ingested a phenothiazine sedative used in veterinary practice.

EPIDEMIOLOGY

Poisoning is uncommon.

CAUSES

- Poisoning usually arises from suicidal ingestion.
- Child neglect or abuse should be considered if the patient is less than 1 year of age, suicide attempt if the patient is over 6 years of age.

PREGNANCY AND LACTATION

US FDA Pregnancy Category C. The drug exerts animal teratogenic or embryocidal effects, but there are no controlled studies in women, or no studies are available in animals or women.

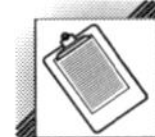

Diagnosis

SIGNS AND SYMPTOMS

Vital Signs

- Hypotension has been reported, but usually in mixed ingestions.
- Tachycardia occurs occasionally.

HEENT

Mydriasis occurs but is uncommon.

Cardiovascular

Tachycardia, bradycardia, and hypotension occur rarely.

Pulmonary

Depression of respiration is uncommon in isolated ingestion but is frequently seen in mixed ingestions.

Gastrointestinal

Nausea and vomiting have been reported.

Fluids and Electrolytes

Mild hypokalemia and transient elevation of creatinine have been reported.

Neurologic

- Drowsiness is the most common effect.
- Confusion, amnesia, dizziness, ataxia, headache, and coma without respiratory depression also may occur.

PROCEDURES AND LABORATORY TESTS

Essential Tests

No tests may be needed in asymptomatic patients.

Recommended Tests

- Serum electrolytes, BUN, creatinine, glucose, and pulse oximetry should be obtained in patients with altered mental status.
- ECG, serum acetaminophen, and aspirin levels should be performed to detect occult ingestion.
- Zolpidem may be detected as a benzodiazepine on routine screening.
- Head CT, lumbar puncture, cultures, and other tests as indicated to evaluate other causes of CNS depression may be needed.

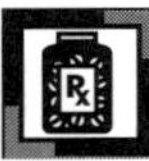

Treatment

- Management should be focused on maintenance of airway and determination of cause for CNS depression.
- Dose and time of exposure should be determined for all substances involved.

DIRECTING PATIENT COURSE

The health-care professional should call the poison control center when:

- Severe or persistent effects develop.
- Coingestant, drug interaction, or underlying disease presents an unusual problem.

The patient should be referred to a health-care facility when:

- Suicide or homicide attempt is possible.
- Toxic effects develop.
- Coingestant, drug interaction, or underlying disease presents an unusual problem.

Admission Considerations

Inpatient management is warranted if the patient has persistent CNS depression following a 6-hour observation period.

DECONTAMINATION

• Gastric lavage should be performed in pediatric (tube size 24–32 French) or adult (tube size 36–42 French) patients presenting within 1 hour of a large ingestion or if serious effects are present.
• One dose of activated charcoal (1–2 g/kg) should be administered without a cathartic if a substantial ingestion has occurred within the previous few hours.

ANTIDOTES

Flumazenil is often effective in the reversal of CNS depression.

• Adult dose is 0.1 to 0.2 mg intravenous push every 1 to 2 minutes until clinical effect occurs or a total of 1 to 2 mg is given; if resedation occurs, 1 mg may be given every 20 minutes to a maximum of 3 mg/h.
• Pediatric dose is 10 μg/kg intravenous push, titrated to effect; resedation may occur.

ADJUNCTIVE TREATMENT

Endotracheal intubation should be performed if airway becomes compromised.

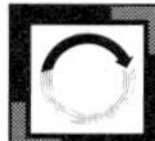

Follow-Up

PATIENT MONITORING

• Respiratory and cardiac function should be monitored continuously.
• Patients should be observed for 6 hours after treatment to monitor for symptoms.

EXPECTED COURSE AND PROGNOSIS

• Toxicity usually occurs quickly, peaks within hours, and resolves over 24 hours.
• Complete recovery occurs unless sequelae of hypoxia intercede.

DISCHARGE CRITERIA/INSTRUCTIONS

Patients with normal mental status and vital signs may be discharged from the emergency department or hospital following decontamination, a 6-hour observation period, and psychiatric evaluation, if needed.

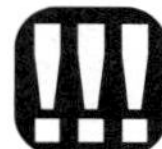

Pitfalls

DIAGNOSIS

Failure to evaluate for other serious causes of altered mental status can lead to misdiagnosis.

ICD-9-CM 967

Poisoning by sedatives and hypnotics.

See also: SECTION III, Flumazenil chapter.

RECOMMENDED READING

Garnier R, Gueralte EE, Muzard D, et al. Acute zolpidem poisoning: analysis of 344 cases. *J Toxicol Clin Toxicol* 1993;32:391–404.

Author: Kennon Heard

Reviewer: Richard C. Dart

Index

Page numbers in boldface indicate major discussion; page numbers in italics denote figures; those followed by "t" denote tables.

Index

Index

Index

Index

Index

Index

Index

Index

Index

Index

Index

Index

Index

Index

Index

Index